nj gerstner 9/95

MANUAL OF CLIN
IN ADULT AMBUL
WITH ANNOTATED

MANUAL OF CLINICAL PROBLEMS IN ADULT AMBULATORY CARE
WITH ANNOTATED KEY REFERENCES

SECOND EDITION

EDITED BY

LAURIE DORNBRAND, M.D.
Clinical Assistant Professor, Department of Medicine, Stanford University School of Medicine, Stanford; Director, Geriatrics Clinic, Geriatric Research Education and Clinical Center (GRECC), Palo Alto Veterans Administration Medical Center, Palo Alto, California

AXALLA J. HOOLE, M.D.
Professor of Medicine and Social Medicine, Division of General Medicine and Clinical Epidemiology, University of North Carolina at Chapel Hill School of Medicine; Attending Physician, Department of Medicine, University of North Carolina Hospitals, Chapel Hill

C. GLENN PICKARD, JR., M.D.
Professor of Medicine and Social Medicine, Division of General Medicine and Clinical Epidemiology, University of North Carolina at Chapel Hill School of Medicine; Attending Physician, Department of Medicine, University of North Carolina Hospitals, Chapel Hill

Little, Brown and Company
Boston/Toronto/London

Copyright © 1992 by Laurie Dornbrand, Axalla J. Hoole, and
C. Glenn Pickard, Jr.

Second Edition

Third Printing

Previous edition copyright © 1985 by Laurie Dornbrand, Axalla J. Hoole,
Robert H. Fletcher, and C. Glenn Pickard, Jr.

All rights reserved. No part of this book may be reproduced in any form
or by any electronic or mechanical means, including information storage
and retrieval systems, without permission in writing from the publisher,
except by a reviewer who may quote brief passages in a review.

Library of Congress Cataloging-in-Publication Data

Manual of clinical problems in adult ambulatory care / edited by
Laurie Dornbrand, Axalla J. Hoole, C. Glenn Pickard, Jr.—2nd ed.
    p.   cm.
  Includes bibliographical references and index.
  ISBN 0-316-19019-5
  1. Family medicine—Handbooks, manuals, etc. 2. Ambulatory
medical care—Handbooks, manuals, etc. I. Dornbrand, Laurie.
II. Hoole, Axalla J., 1938–   III. Pickard, C. Glenn (Carl
Glenn), 1936–
  [DNLM: 1. Ambulatory Care. 2. Internal Medicine.
WB 115 M2935]
RC55.M264 1992
616—dc20
DNLM/DLC
for Library of Congress   91-45998
                                                                                     CIP

Printed in the United States of America

SEM

CONTENTS

Contributing Authors	xiii
Preface	xxi
Acknowledgments	xxiii

I. CONSTITUTIONAL SYMPTOMS

1.	**Dizziness**	1
	James P. Browder	
2.	**Fatigue**	5
	Mack Lipkin and Robert A. McNutt	
3.	**Obesity**	8
	Robert B. Baron	
4.	**Weight Loss**	15
	William D. Heizer	

II. EYE PROBLEMS

5.	**Ocular Foreign Bodies**	21
	Hunter R. Stokes	
6.	**Corneal Abrasion**	24
	Hunter R. Stokes	
7.	**Conjunctivitis**	26
	Hunter R. Stokes	
8.	**Eyelid Disorders**	31
	Hunter R. Stokes	
9.	**Cataracts**	32
	Hunter R. Stokes	
10.	**Glaucoma**	36
	Jan A. Kylstra	
11.	**Visual Impairment**	41
	Hunter R. Stokes	

III. EAR PROBLEMS

12.	**Deafness and Tinnitus**	45
	James P. Browder	
13.	**Otitis Externa**	50
	Marion Danis	
14.	**Otitis Media**	53
	Desmond K. Runyan	
15.	**Earwax**	56
	Terry L. Fry	

IV. UPPER RESPIRATORY PROBLEMS

16.	**Colds and Influenza** Timothy W. Lane	59
17.	**Sinusitis** Suzanne W. Fletcher and Amelia F. Drake	66
18.	**Sore Throat** Robert M. Centor and Frederick A. Meier	70
19.	**Hoarseness** James P. Browder and Duncan S. Postma	75
20.	**Rhinitis** W. Paul Biggers	79

V. LOWER RESPIRATORY PROBLEMS

21.	**Asthma** James F. Donohue	87
22.	**Chronic Obstructive Pulmonary Disease** James F. Donohue	95
23.	**Acute Lower Respiratory Tract Infection** C. Glenn Pickard, Jr.	103
24.	**Solitary Pulmonary Nodule** Raymond F. Bianchi	107

VI. CARDIOVASCULAR PROBLEMS

25.	**Hypertension: Who Needs Treatment?** C. Stewart Rogers	110
26.	**Evaluation and Treatment of Hypertension** C. Stewart Rogers	114
27.	**Angina Pectoris** Mark A. Hlatky and Daniel B. Mark	126
28.	**Congestive Heart Failure** Laurence O. Watkins	133
29.	**Rehabilitation After Myocardial Infarction** Thomas E. Kottke and Mark A. Hlatky	139
30.	**Paroxysmal Supraventricular Tachycardia** Ross J. Simpson, Jr.	142
31.	**Premature Ventricuiar Contractions** Ross J. Simpson, Jr.	147
32.	**Atrial Fibrillation** Ross J. Simpson, Jr.	151
33.	**Pacemakers** Andreas T. Wielgosz	155

34.	**Heart Murmurs**	157
	Park W. Willis IV	
35.	**Mitral Valve Prolapse**	162
	Henry J. Kahn	
36.	**Prosthetic Valves**	166
	Andreas T. Wielgosz	
37.	**Endocarditis Prophylaxis**	168
	Park W. Willis IV	

VII. PERIPHERAL VASCULAR PROBLEMS

38.	**Chronic Venous Disorders**	173
	Robert S. Grossman	
39.	**Arterial Disease of the Extremities**	177
	John S. Kizer	
40.	**Thrombophlebitis**	182
	Thomas McAfee and Christopher Bogert	

VIII. GASTROINTESTINAL PROBLEMS

41.	**Dysphagia**	187
	Eugene M. Bozymski and John W. Garrett	
42.	**Esophagitis**	191
	Brentley D. Jeffries and Sidney E. Levinson	
43.	**Functional Dyspepsia**	197
	Douglas A. Drossman	
44.	**Peptic Ulcer Disease**	200
	Eugene M. Bozymski and John W. Garrett	
45.	**Irritable Bowel Syndrome**	206
	Douglas A. Drossman	
46.	**Diverticular Disease of the Colon**	209
	Douglas A. Drossman	
47.	**Acute Diarrhea**	212
	C. Glenn Pickard, Jr.	
48.	**Chronic Diarrhea**	218
	R. Balfour Sartor	
49.	**Constipation**	221
	R. Balfour Sartor	
50.	**Anorectal Disorders**	225
	C. Glenn Pickard, Jr.	
51.	**Hematochezia and Occult Gastrointestinal Bleeding**	230
	Robert A. McNutt and Sidney E. Levinson	
52.	**Gallstones**	233
	Michael D. Apstein	

IX. URINARY PROBLEMS

53. Urinary Tract Infections in Women — 241
Axalla J. Hoole

54. Urinary Tract Infections in Men — 245
Axalla J. Hoole

55. Benign Prostatic Hyperplasia — 249
J. Pack Hindsley, Jr., and James L. Fry, Jr.

56. Chronic Renal Failure — 252
William D. Mattern

57. Renal Stones — 258
Romulo E. Colindres and C. Richard Morris

58. Hematuria — 265
John E. Anderson

59. Proteinuria — 270
Katherine A. Huffman

60. Urinary Incontinence in the Elderly — 274
Mark E. Williams

61. Urinary Catheterization — 278
Todd A. Linsenmeyer

X. MUSCULOSKELETAL PROBLEMS

62. Osteoarthritis — 283
L. Celeste Robb-Nicholson and Matthew H. Liang

63. Rheumatoid Arthritis — 287
Suzanne V. Sauter

64. Nonsteroidal Anti-inflammatory Drugs — 296
Bernard Lo

65. Gout — 304
Kenneth E. Sack

66. Osteoporosis — 307
Philip D. Sloane and Steven R. Cummings

67. Neck Pain — 312
Peter Curtis

68. Shoulder Pain — 315
Peter Curtis

69. Low Back Pain — 320
Nortin M. Hadler and Timothy S. Carey

70. Knee Pain — 326
Axalla J. Hoole and Laurence E. Dahners

71. Tendinitis and Bursitis — 332
Kenneth E. Sack

72. Nonarticular Musculoskeletal Pain — 335
Kenneth E. Sack

73. Nocturnal Leg Cramps — 337
Laurie Dornbrand

XI. REPRODUCTIVE SYSTEM PROBLEMS

74. Vaginitis — 341
Jack D. McCue and Laurie Dornbrand

75. Birth Control — 346
Axalla J. Hoole

76. Abnormal Uterine Bleeding — 357
Deborah J. Dotters

77. Dysmenorrhea — 360
Nancy Milliken

78. Premenstrual Syndrome — 362
Linn Parsons and Laurie Dornbrand

79. Pelvic Inflammatory Disease — 365
John S. Kizer

80. Breast Lumps, Breast Pain, and Nipple Discharge — 369
William H. Goodson III

81. Menopause — 373
Thomas C. Keyserling and Robert H. Fletcher

82. Female Sexual Dysfunction — 380
Cheryl F. McCartney

83. Male Sexual Dysfunction: Erectile Failure — 384
Todd A. Linsenmeyer and Laurie Dornbrand

XII. ENDOCRINE AND METABOLIC PROBLEMS

84. Diagnosis of Diabetes Mellitus — 391
John T. Gwynne and Jorge J. Gonzalez

85. Management of Type I Diabetes — 394
John T. Gwynne and Jorge J. Gonzalez

86. Management of Type II Diabetes — 401
John T. Gwynne

87. Management of Complications of Diabetes — 406
John T. Gwynne

88. Hypoglycemia — 409
Rebecca A. Silliman

89. Evaluation of Thyroid Function — 412
Robert D. Utiger

90. Hyperthyroidism — 416
Robert D. Utiger

91. Hypothyroidism — 422
Robert D. Utiger

92. Thyroid Nodules — 425
Robert D. Utiger

93. Goiter — 428
Robert D. Utiger

94. Hypercalcemia — 431
Robert H. Fletcher

95. Asymptomatic Hyperuricemia	435
Kenneth E. Sack	
96. Corticosteroid Therapy and Withdrawal	437
David R. Clemmons	

XIII. BLOOD PROBLEMS

97. Anemia	443
Peter C. Ungaro	
98. Abnormal Bleeding	449
Katherine A. High and Robert H. Fletcher	
99. Polycythemia	453
James A. Bryan II	

XIV. NERVOUS SYSTEM PROBLEMS

100. Headache	457
Robert W. Eckel and J. Douglas Mann	
101. Seizures: Evaluation	469
John A. Messenheimer	
102. Treatment of Seizures	474
John A. Messenheimer	
103. Transient Ischemic Attacks and Carotid Bruits	481
John S. Kizer	
104. Parkinsonism	488
Axalla J. Hoole and Colin D. Hall	
105. Bell's Palsy	493
Robert S. Dittus	
106. Dementia in the Elderly	495
Alan K. Halperin and Mary K. Goldstein	

XV. PSYCHIATRIC PROBLEMS

107. Anxiety	501
John J. Haggerty, Jr.	
108. Depression	506
John J. Haggerty, Jr.	
109. Insomnia	513
Jeffery J. Fahs	
110. Problem Patients	519
Douglas A. Drossman	
111. Grief	522
Eric W. Jensen	
112. Alcoholism	526
JudyAnn Bigby	

XVI. INFECTIOUS DISEASES

113. Sexually Transmitted Diseases — 533
Eliseo J. Pérez-Stable

114. Management of HIV-Infected Patients — 549
Mitchell H. Katz

115. Herpes Zoster — 560
Terrie Mendelson

116. Infectious Mononucleosis — 563
Jack D. McCue

117. Intestinal Parasites — 567
Richard A. Davidson and Terrie Mendelson

118. Tuberculosis — 572
Eliseo J. Pérez-Stable

119. Viral Hepatitis — 579
Terrie Mendelson and Bernard Lo

XVII. ALLERGIC CONDITIONS

120. Urticaria — 587
Rebecca A. Silliman

121. "Bee" Stings — 590
Rebecca A. Silliman

XVIII. HEALTH MAINTENANCE

122. Preventive Care — 593
Russell Harris

123. Athletic Physicals — 603
Desmond K. Runyan and Sally S. Harris

124. Immunizations — 608
Eliseo J. Pérez-Stable

125. Cardiac Risk Factor Modification — 616
Mark A. Hlatky and Stephen B. Hulley

126. High Blood Cholesterol: Screening and Interventions — 619
Robert B. Baron

127. Exercise — 626
David S. Siscovick

128. Medical Advice for Travelers — 630
Robert B. Baron

129. Occupational Diseases and Disability Determination — 637
Gary Pasternak and Timothy S. Carey

130. Cigarette Smoking Cessation — 640
Elizabeth E. Campbell

131. Breast Cancer Screening — 646
Suzanne W. Fletcher

132.	**Prostate Cancer Screening** James L. Fry, Jr.	650

XIX. MISCELLANEOUS

133.	**Syncope** M. Andrew Greganti	653
134.	**Edema** William F. Finn	658
135.	**Lymphadenopathy** Robert H. Fletcher and David J. Weber	662
136.	**Hypothermia and Cold Injury** Alan K. Halperin	667
137.	**Heat Injury** Alan K. Halperin	671
138.	**Minor Soft Tissue Injuries and Infections** Sally J. Trued	674
139.	**Hiccups** Raymond F. Bianchi	681
140.	**Chronic Idiopathic Pain** Douglas A. Drossman	682
141.	**Medications in Pregnancy and Lactation** Ronald J. Ruggiero	688
142.	**Mouth Lesions** E. Jefferson Burkes, Jr.	696

XX. DIETS

143.	**Low-Salt Diets** C. Stewart Rogers	701
144.	**High-Fiber Diets** R. Balfour Sartor	704
145.	**Cholesterol-Lowering Diets** Robert B. Baron	706

INDEX   713

CONTRIBUTING AUTHORS

John E. Anderson, M.D.
Assistant Professor of Medicine, Johns Hopkins University School of Medicine; Attending Physician, Renal Division, Francis Scott Key Medical Center, Baltimore

Michael D. Apstein, M.D.
Assistant Professor of Medicine, Harvard Medical School; Chief, Gastroenterology Section, Brockton/West Roxbury Veterans Administration Medical Center, Boston

Robert B. Baron, M.D., M.S.
Associate Professor of Clinical Medicine and Director, Primary Care Internal Medicine Residency Program, University of California, San Francisco, School of Medicine, San Francisco

Raymond F. Bianchi, M.D.
Clinical Associate Professor of Medicine, University of North Carolina at Chapel Hill School of Medicine, Chapel Hill; Senior Attending Physician, Department of Medicine, Carolinas Medical Center, Charlotte, North Carolina

JudyAnn Bigby, M.D.
Associate Physician, Brigham and Women's Hospital, Boston

W. Paul Biggers, M.D.
Professor of Surgery, Division of Otolaryngology, University of North Carolina at Chapel Hill School of Medicine; Attending Physician, Department of Surgery, University of North Carolina Hospitals, Chapel Hill

Christopher Bogert, M.D.
Emergency Physician, Department of Medicine, City Hospital, Martinsburg, West Virginia

Eugene M. Bozymski, M.D.
Professor of Medicine, University of North Carolina at Chapel Hill School of Medicine; Co-Chief, Division of Digestive Diseases and Nutrition, University of North Carolina Hospitals, Chapel Hill

James P. Browder, M.D., Ph.D.
Department of Otolaryngology, Kaiser-Permanente, Raleigh, North Carolina

James A. Bryan II, M.D., M.P.H.
Professor of Medicine and Social Medicine, Division of General Medicine and Clinical Epidemiology, University of North Carolina at Chapel Hill School of Medicine; Attending Physician, The North Carolina Memorial Hospital, Chapel Hill

E. Jefferson Burkes, Jr., D.D.S., M.S.
Professor of Oral Pathology, University of North Carolina at Chapel Hill School of Medicine, Chapel Hill

Elizabeth E. Campbell, M.D.
Assistant Professor of Medicine, University of North Carolina at Chapel Hill School of Medicine, Chapel Hill; Assistant Professor of Medicine, Wake Area Health Education Center, Raleigh, North Carolina

Timothy S. Carey, M.D., M.P.H.
Associate Professor of Medicine and Chief, Division of General Medicine and Clinical Epidemiology, University of North Carolina at Chapel Hill School of Medicine; Associate Attending Physician, University of North Carolina Hospitals, Chapel Hill

Robert M. Centor, M.D.
Chair, Division of General Internal Medicine, Virginia Commonwealth University, Medical College of Virginia School of Medicine, Richmond

David R. Clemmons, M.D.
Professor of Medicine, Division of Endocrinology and Metabolism, University of North Carolina at Chapel Hill School of Medicine; Attending Physician, Department of Medicine, University of North Carolina Hospitals, Chapel Hill

Romulo E. Colindres, M.D.
Professor of Medicine and Associate Chair, Department of Medicine, University of North Carolina at Chapel Hill School of Medicine; Attending Physician, University of North Carolina Hospitals, Chapel Hill

Steven R. Cummings, M.D.
Associate Professor of Medicine and Epidemiology, University of California, San Francisco, School of Medicine; Attending Physician, Moffitt-Long Hospital, San Francisco

Peter Curtis, M.R.C.P., F.R.C.C.P.
Professor of Family Medicine, University of North Carolina at Chapel Hill School of Medicine; Attending Physician, Department of Family Medicine, University of North Carolina Hospitals, Chapel Hill

Laurence E. Dahners, M.D.
Associate Professor of Surgery, Division of Orthopaedics, University of North Carolina at Chapel Hill School of Medicine; Associate Attending Physician, Department of Surgery, University of North Carolina Hospitals, Chapel Hill

Marion Danis, M.D.
Associate Professor of Medicine, Division of General Medicine and Clinical Epidemiology, University of North Carolina at Chapel Hill School of Medicine; Associate Attending Physician, University of North Carolina Hospitals, Chapel Hill

Richard A. Davidson, M.D., M.P.H.
Associate Professor of Medicine, University of Florida College of Medicine; Staff Physician, Shands Teaching Hospital and Clinics, Inc., Gainesville, Florida

Robert S. Dittus, M.D.
Associate Professor of Medicine, Indiana University School of Medicine; Attending Physician, Indiana University Hospitals, William N. Wishard Memorial Hospital, and Richard L. Roudebush Department of Veterans Affairs Medical Center, Indianapolis

James F. Donohue, M.D.
Professor of Medicine, Division of Pulmonary Medicine, University of North Carolina at Chapel Hill School of Medicine; Attending Physician, Department of Medicine, University of North Carolina Hospitals, Chapel Hill

Laurie Dornbrand, M.D.
Clinical Assistant Professor, Department of Medicine, Stanford University School of Medicine, Stanford; Director, Geriatrics Clinic, Geriatric Research Education and Clinical Center (GRECC), Palo Alto Veterans Administration Medical Center, Palo Alto, California

Deborah J. Dotters, M.D.
Assistant Professor of Obstetrics and Gynecology, University of North Carolina at Chapel Hill School of Medicine; Assistant Attending Physician, Department of Obstetrics and Gynecology, University of North Carolina Hospitals, Chapel Hill

Amelia F. Drake, M.D.
Assistant Professor of Surgery, Division of Otolaryngology, University of North Carolina at Chapel Hill School of Medicine; Assistant Attending Physician, Department of Surgery, University of North Carolina Hospitals, Chapel Hill

Douglas A. Drossman, M.D.
Professor of Medicine and Psychiatry, University of North Carolina at Chapel Hill School of Medicine; Attending Physician, Department of Medicine, University of North Carolina Hospitals, Chapel Hill

Robert W. Eckel, M.D.
Clinical Assistant Professor, Georgetown University School of Medicine, Washington, D.C.; Neurologist, Kaiser-Permanente, Kensington Center, Kensington, Maryland

Jeffery J. Fahs, M.D.
Clinical Assistant Professor of Psychiatry, University of North Carolina at Chapel Hill School of Medicine, Chapel Hill; Director, Psychiatric Services, Murdoch Center, Butner, North Carolina

William F. Finn, M.D.
Professor of Medicine, Division of Nephrology, University of North Carolina at Chapel Hill School of Medicine; Attending Physician, Department of Medicine, University of North Carolina Hospitals, Chapel Hill

Robert H. Fletcher, M.D.
Co-Editor, *Annals of Internal Medicine*, American College of Physicians, Philadelphia

Suzanne W. Fletcher, M.D., M.Sc.
Adjunct Professor of Medicine, University of Pennsylvania and Thomas Jefferson University; Editor, *Annals of Internal Medicine*, American College of Physicians, Philadelphia

James L. Fry, Jr., M.D.
Attending Physician, Department of Urology, Georgetown Memorial Hospital, Georgetown, South Carolina

Terry L. Fry, M.D.
Attending Physician, Department of Otolaryngology, Georgetown Memorial Hospital, Georgetown, South Carolina

John W. Garrett, M.D.
Clinical Assistant Professor of Medicine, Division of Digestive Diseases and Nutrition, University of North Carolina at Chapel Hill School of Medicine, Chapel Hill; Clinical Assistant Attending Physician, Asheville Area Health Education Center, Asheville; Asheville Gastroenterology Associates, Asheville, North Carolina

Mary K. Goldstein, M.D.
Fellow in Health Sciences, Department of Medicine, Stanford University School of Medicine, Stanford; Director, Graduate Medical Education, Geriatric Research Education and Clinical Center (GRECC), Palo Alto Veterans Administration Medical Center, Palo Alto, California

Jorge J. Gonzalez, M.D.
Associate Professor of Medicine, Division of Endocrinology, University of North Carolina at Chapel Hill School of Medicine, Chapel Hill; Associate Attending Physician, Wilmington Area Health Education Center, Wilmington, North Carolina

William H. Goodson III, M.D.
Professor of Surgery, University of California, San Francisco, School of Medicine; Attending Physician, The Medical Center at the University of California, San Francisco, San Francisco

M. Andrew Greganti, M.D.
Professor and Associate Chair for Clinical Affairs, Department of Medicine, Division of General Medicine and Clinical Epidemiology, University of North Carolina at Chapel Hill School of Medicine; Attending Physician, Department of Medicine, University of North Carolina Hospitals, Chapel Hill

Robert S. Grossman, M.D.
Vice Chair, Department of Medicine, Pennsylvania State University College of Medicine, Hershey; Chair, Department of Medicine, Harrisburg Hospital, Harrisburg, Pennsylvania

John T. Gwynne, M.D.
Professor of Medicine, Division of Endocrinology, University of North Carolina at Chapel Hill School of Medicine; Attending Physician, Department of Medicine, University of North Carolina Hospitals, Chapel Hill

Nortin M. Hadler, M.D., F.A.C.P.
Professor of Medicine and Microbiology/Immunology, Division of Rheumatology and Immunology, University of North Carolina at Chapel Hill School of Medicine; Attending Physician, Department of Medicine, University of North Carolina Hospitals, Chapel Hill

John J. Haggerty, Jr., M.D.
Associate Professor of Psychiatry, University of North Carolina at Chapel Hill School of Medicine; Associate Attending Psychiatrist and Director, 4-S Inpatient Unit, Department of Psychiatry, University of North Carolina Hospitals, Chapel Hill

Colin D. Hall, M.B.Ch.B.
Vice Chair and Professor, Department of Neurology, and Professor of Medicine, University of North Carolina at Chapel Hill School of Medicine; Attending Physician, Department of Neurology, University of North Carolina Hospitals, Chapel Hill

Alan K. Halperin, M.D.
Associate Professor and Co-Chief of General Medicine, University of New Mexico School of Medicine; Associate Chief of Staff, Ambulatory Care, Veterans Administration Medical Center, Albuquerque, New Mexico

Russell Harris, M.D., M.P.H.
Assistant Professor of Medicine and Epidemiology, Division of General Medicine and Clinical Epidemiology, University of North Carolina at Chapel Hill School of Medicine; Assistant Attending Physician, University of North Carolina Hospitals, Chapel Hill

Sally S. Harris, M.D., M.P.H.
Clinical Assistant Professor of Pediatrics, Stanford University School of Medicine, and Team Physician, Stanford University, Stanford; Sports Medicine Specialist, Palo Alto Medical Clinic, Palo Alto, California

William D. Heizer, M.D.
Professor of Medicine, Division of Digestive Diseases and Nutrition, University of North Carolina at Chapel Hill School of Medicine; Attending Physician, University of North Carolina Hospitals, Chapel Hill

Katherine A. High, M.D.
Assistant Professor of Medicine and Pathology, University of North Carolina at Chapel Hill School of Medicine; Attending Physician and Director, Clinical Coagulation Laboratory, University of North Carolina Hospitals, Chapel Hill

J. Pack Hindsley, Jr., M.D.
Clinical Assistant Professor, East Carolina University School of Medicine, Greenville; Attending Physician, Beaufort County Hospital, Washington, North Carolina

Mark A. Hlatky, M.D.
Associate Professor of Health Research and Policy and Medicine, Stanford University School of Medicine; Attending Cardiologist, Stanford University Hospital, Stanford, California

Axalla J. Hoole, M.D.
Professor of Medicine and Social Medicine, Division of General Medicine and Clinical Epidemiology, University of North Carolina at Chapel Hill School of Medicine; Attending Physician, Department of Medicine, University of North Carolina Hospitals, Chapel Hill

Katherine A. Huffman, M.D.
Clinical Associate Professor of Medicine, Division of Nephrology, University of North Carolina at Chapel Hill School of Medicine; Clinical Associate Attending Physician, Department of Medicine, University of North Carolina Hospitals, Chapel Hill

Stephen B. Hulley, M.D., M.P.H.
Professor and Chief, Division of Clinical Epidemiology, Department of Epidemiology and Biostatistics, University of California, San Francisco, School of Medicine, San Francisco

Brentley D. Jeffries, M.D.
Clinical Instructor of Medicine, Division of Digestive Diseases and Nutrition, University of North Carolina at Chapel Hill School of Medicine, Chapel Hill; Clinical Instructor and Attending Physician, Asheville Area Health Education Center, Asheville; Asheville Gastroenterology Associates, Asheville, North Carolina

Eric W. Jensen, M.D.
Associate Professor of Psychiatry and Medicine, University of North Carolina at Chapel Hill School of Medicine, Chapel Hill

Henry J. Kahn, M.D.
Associate Clinical Professor of Medicine, Division of General Internal Medicine, University of California, San Francisco, School of Medicine; Attending Physician, Moffitt-Long Hospital, San Francisco

Mitchell H. Katz, M.D.
Chief of Research Branch, AIDS Office, Department of Public Health, San Francisco

Thomas C. Keyserling, M.D., M.P.H.
Research Assistant Professor of Medicine, Division of General Medicine and Clinical Epidemiology, University of North Carolina at Chapel Hill School of Medicine; Attending Physician, Department of Medicine, University of North Carolina Hospitals, Chapel Hill

John S. Kizer, M.D.
Professor of Medicine and Pharmacology, Division of General Medicine and Clinical Epidemiology, University of North Carolina at Chapel Hill School of Medicine; Associate Director and Research Scientist, Brain and Development Research Center, University of North Carolina Hospitals, Chapel Hill

Thomas E. Kottke, M.D.
Associate Professor of Medicine and Consultant, Division of Cardiovascular Diseases, Mayo Foundation, Rochester, Minnesota

Jan A. Kylstra, M.D.
Assistant Professor of Ophthalmology, University of North Carolina at Chapel Hill School of Medicine; Assistant Attending Physician, Department of Ophthalmology, University of North Carolina Hospitals, Chapel Hill

Timothy W. Lane, M.D.
Associate Professor of Medicine, University of North Carolina at Chapel Hill School of Medicine, Chapel Hill; Director, Internal Medicine Training Program, Moses H. Cone Memorial Hospital, Greensboro, North Carolina

Sidney E. Levinson, M.D.
Clinical Associate Professor of Medicine, Division of Digestive Diseases and Nutrition, University of North Carolina at Chapel Hill School of Medicine; Clinical Associate Attending Physician, University of North Carolina Hospitals, Chapel Hill

Matthew H. Liang, M.D., M.P.H.
Associate Professor of Medicine, Harvard Medical School; Attending Physician, Departments of Medicine and Rheumatology/Immunology, Brigham and Women's Hospital, Boston

Todd A. Linsenmeyer, M.D.
Clinical Assistant Professor of Surgery (Urology) and Assistant Professor of Physical Medicine and Rehabilitation, University of Medicine and Dentistry of New Jersey-New Jersey Medical School, Newark; Director of Urology, Kessler Institute for Rehabilitation Medicine, West Orange, New Jersey

Mack Lipkin, M.D.[*]
Visiting Professor of Clinical Medicine, University of North Carolina at Chapel Hill School of Medicine, Chapel Hill; President, Zlinkoff Foundation, New York

Bernard Lo, M.D.
Associate Professor of Medicine and Co-Director, Robert Wood Johnson Clinical Scholars Program, University of California, San Francisco, School of Medicine; Attending Physician, Moffitt-Long Hospital, San Francisco

---

[*] Deceased.

J. Douglas Mann, M.D.
Associate Professor of Neurology, University of North Carolina at Chapel Hill School of Medicine; Associate Attending Physician, Department of Neurology, University of North Carolina Hospitals, Chapel Hill

Daniel B. Mark, M.D., M.P.H.
Assistant Professor of Medicine, Duke University School of Medicine; Co-Director, Cardiac Care Unit, Duke University Medical Center, Durham, North Carolina

William D. Mattern, M.D.
Associate Dean for Academic Affairs and Professor of Medicine, Division of Nephrology, University of North Carolina at Chapel Hill School of Medicine; Attending Physician, Department of Medicine, University of North Carolina Hospitals, Chapel Hill

Thomas McAfee, M.D.
Assistant Clinical Professor, University of California, San Francisco, School of Medicine; Attending Physician, Division of General Internal Medicine, Moffitt-Long Hospital, San Francisco

Cheryl F. McCartney, M.D.
Associate Dean for Student Affairs and Associate Professor of Psychiatry, University of North Carolina at Chapel Hill School of Medicine; Associate Attending Psychiatrist, Department of Psychiatry, University of North Carolina Hospitals, Chapel Hill

Jack D. McCue, M.D.
Professor of Medicine, Tufts University School of Medicine, Boston; Vice Chair, Department of Medicine, Baystate Medical Center, Springfield, Massachusetts

Robert A. McNutt, M.D.
Assistant Professor of Medicine, Division of General Medicine and Clinical Epidemiology, University of North Carolina at Chapel Hill School of Medicine; Assistant Attending Physician, Department of Medicine, University of North Carolina Hospitals, Chapel Hill

Frederick A. Meier, M.D., C.M.
Associate Professor of Pathology and Medicine, Virginia Commonwealth University, Medical College of Virginia School of Medicine; Director, Clinical Laboratories, Medical College of Virginia Hospitals, Richmond

Terrie Mendelson, M.D.
Assistant Clinical Professor of Medicine, Division of General Internal Medicine, University of California, San Francisco, School of Medicine; Attending Physician, Moffitt-Long Hospital, San Francisco

John A. Messenheimer, M.D.
Associate Professor of Neurology and Medicine, University of North Carolina at Chapel Hill School of Medicine; Associate Attending Physician, Department of Neurology, University of North Carolina Hospitals, Chapel Hill

Nancy Milliken, M.D.
Assistant Professor of Obstetrics, Gynecology, and Reproduction Sciences, University of California, San Francisco, School of Medicine, San Francisco

C. Richard Morris, M.D.
Associate Professor of Pediatrics, University of North Carolina at Chapel Hill School of Medicine; Associate Attending Physician, Department of Pediatrics, University of North Carolina Hospitals, Chapel Hill

Linn Parsons, M.D.
Assistant Professor of Obstetrics and Gynecology, Bowman Gray School of Medicine of Wake Forest University; Attending Physician, Department of Gynecology, North Carolina Baptist Hospital, Winston-Salem, North Carolina

Gary Pasternak, M.D., M.P.H.
Associate Chief of Occupational Medicine and Employee Health Services, Department of Medicine, Santa Clara Valley Medical Center, San Jose, California

Eliseo J. Pérez-Stable, M.D.
Associate Professor of Medicine, University of California, San Francisco, School of Medicine; Attending Physician, Division of General Internal Medicine, Moffitt-Long Hospital, San Francisco

C. Glenn Pickard, Jr., M.D.
Professor of Medicine and Social Medicine, Division of General Medicine and Clinical Epidemiology, University of North Carolina at Chapel Hill School of Medicine; Attending Physician, Department of Medicine, University of North Carolina Hospitals, Chapel Hill

Duncan S. Postma, M.D.
Clinical Associate Professor of Surgery, Division of Otolaryngology (Head and Neck Surgery), University of North Carolina at Chapel Hill School of Medicine, Chapel Hill; Associate Attending Physician, Tallahassee Regional Memorial Medical Center, Tallahassee, Florida

L. Celeste Robb-Nicholson, M.D., M.P.H.
Instructor in Medicine, Harvard Medical School; Associate Physician, Massachusetts General Hospital, Boston

C. Stewart Rogers, M.D.
Associate Professor of Medicine, University of North Carolina at Chapel Hill School of Medicine, Chapel Hill; Associate Attending Physician, Internal Medicine Training Program, Moses H. Cone Memorial Hospital, Greensboro, North Carolina

Ronald J. Ruggiero, Pharm.D.
Associate Clinical Professor, University of California, San Francisco, School of Pharmacy; Pharmacist Specialist, Pharmaceutical Services, The Medical Center at the University of California, San Francisco

Desmond K. Runyan, M.D., D.P.H.
Associate Professor of Social Medicine and Pediatrics, University of North Carolina at Chapel Hill School of Medicine; Associate Attending Physician, Department of Pediatrics, University of North Carolina Hospitals, Chapel Hill

Kenneth E. Sack, M.D.
Director of Clinical Program in Rheumatology and Clinical Professor of Medicine, University of California, San Francisco, School of Medicine; Attending Physician, Moffitt-Long Hospital, San Francisco

R. Balfour Sartor, M.D.
Associate Professor of Medicine, Division of Digestive Diseases and Nutrition, University of North Carolina at Chapel Hill School of Medicine; Associate Attending Physician, Department of Medicine, University of North Carolina Hospitals, Chapel Hill

Suzanne V. Sauter, M.D.
Clinical Associate Professor of Medicine, Division of Rheumatology, University of North Carolina at Chapel Hill School of Medicine; Director, Rehabilitation, and Clinical Associate Attending Physician, Department of Medicine, University of North Carolina Hospitals, Chapel Hill

Rebecca A. Silliman, M.D., Ph.D.
Associate Professor of Medicine, Tufts University School of Medicine; Attending Physician, Department of Medicine, New England Medical Center Hospitals, Boston

Ross J. Simpson, Jr., M.D.
Associate Professor of Medicine, Division of Cardiology, University of North Carolina at Chapel Hill School of Medicine; Director, Coronary Care Unit, and Associate Attending Physician, Department of Medicine, University of North Carolina Hospitals, Chapel Hill

David S. Siscovick, M.D., M.P.H.
Associate Professor of Medicine and Epidemiology, University of Washington School of Medicine; Attending Physician, Department of Medicine, Harborview Medical Center, Seattle

Philip D. Sloane, M.D., M.P.H.
Associate Professor of Family Medicine, University of North Carolina at Chapel Hill School of Medicine; Associate Attending Physician, Department of Family Medicine, University of North Carolina Hospitals, Chapel Hill

Hunter R. Stokes, M.D., F.A.C.S.
Clinical Professor of Ophthalmology, University of South Carolina School of Medicine, Columbia; Department of Ophthalmology, McLeod Regional Medical Center, Florence, South Carolina

Sally J. Trued, M.D., M.P.H., F.A.C.E.P.
Assistant Professor of Clinical Medicine and Community and Family Medicine, Dartmouth Medical School, Hanover; Attending Physician, Dartmouth-Hitchcock Medical Center, Lebanon, New Hampshire

Peter C. Ungaro, M.D.
Professor of Medicine, University of North Carolina at Chapel Hill School of Medicine, Chapel Hill; Senior Attending Physician, Department of Medicine, New Hanover Memorial Hospital, Wilmington, North Carolina

Robert D. Utiger, M.D.
Clinical Professor of Medicine, Harvard Medical School; Attending Physician, Brigham and Women's Hospital, Boston

Laurence O. Watkins, M.D., M.P.H., F.A.C.C.
Attending Physician, Department of Medicine, Broward General Medical Center, Fort Lauderdale, Florida

David J. Weber, M.D., M.P.H.
Associate Professor of Medicine, Pediatrics, and Epidemiology, University of North Carolina at Chapel Hill School of Medicine; Medical Director, Hospital Epidemiology, and Associate Attending Physician, Department of Medicine, University of North Carolina Hospitals, Chapel Hill

Andreas T. Wielgosz, M.D., Ph.D.
Associate Professor of Medicine, Community Medicine, and Epidemiology, University of Ottawa Faculty of Medicine; Head, Division of Cardiology, Ottawa General Hospital, Ottawa, Ontario

Mark E. Williams, M.D.
Associate Professor of Medicine, Division of General Medicine and Clinical Epidemiology, University of North Carolina at Chapel Hill School of Medicine; Director, Program on Aging, and Associate Attending Physician, Department of Medicine, University of North Carolina Hospitals, Chapel Hill

Park W. Willis IV, M.D.
Associate Professor of Medicine and Pediatrics, Division of Cardiology, University of North Carolina at Chapel Hill School of Medicine; Director, Cardiac Graphics Laboratory, and Associate Attending Physician, Department of Medicine, University of North Carolina Hospitals, Chapel Hill

PREFACE

Clinicians often perceive a gap between the information supplied in traditional medical texts and the day-to-day concerns of patient care. In *Manual of Clinical Problems in Adult Ambulatory Care,* Second Edition, we have endeavored to bridge this gap and meet the needs of general care clinicians at all levels.

The topics reviewed in the Manual were selected because of their frequency in ambulatory medical practice. Throughout we have used both diagnosis-oriented and problem-oriented approaches, depending on the level of resolution with which medical conditions typically present. Chapters therefore cover specific diagnostic entities, such as asthma and parkinsonism, and problems, such as proteinuria and shoulder pain. We have added chapters on Atrial Fibrillation, Chronic Diarrhea, Chronic Idiopathic Pain, Cholesterol-Lowering Diets, Hematuria, Herpes Zoster, Management of HIV-Infected Patients, Minor Soft Tissue Injuries and Infection, and Tuberculosis. We have also added separate chapters on important topics in clinical pharmacy including Nonsteroidal Anti-inflammatory Drugs and Medications in Pregnancy and Lactation. The section on Health Care Maintenance has been reorganized with increased emphasis on preventive care and screening: Preventive Care replaces Periodic Medical Examination, Medical Advice for Travelers is now a separate chapter, and the Immunizations chapter has been completely rewritten.

While we have attempted to make this text comprehensive, it is not meant to be all-inclusive. Discussion is directed toward questions that must be answered by clinicians in order to provide effective patient care. Each chapter is accompanied by an annotated bibliography of articles that are particularly influential, well done, or provocative. When answers to clinical problems were not available from published research, we explained that customary practice was not documented in the literature.

In *Manual of Clinical Problems in Adult Ambulatory Care,* we have endeavored to present information in a way that will be immediately useful in both office and clinical settings. We hope readers will find we have accomplished this goal and that the Manual will prove a practical, scholarly companion in the complex task of adult ambulatory care.

L.D.
A.J.H.
C.G.P., Jr.

ACKNOWLEDGMENTS

We are grateful to the contributing authors for their scholarship and for the graciousness with which they adapted their individual styles to conform to our editorial needs. Many helped with chapters in addition to the ones they were writing. Special thanks to Tim Carey for his helpful reviews of many chapters and to Bernard Lo for valuable comments on much of the book and major editorial contributions to several chapters. We are grateful to Martin C. Carey for his critical review of the chapter on gallstones, and for the assistance of Kirk Adams, Eddie Atwood, Chris Brymer, Peter Davol, Elena Gates, Leslie Goldberg, Peter Greenberg, Ellen Hughes, John Parker, Barbara Stumpf, Ed Wang, Phil Wasserstein, and Toni Zeiss, who gave helpful comments on various chapters.

All manuscripts were edited in the offices of the Division of General Medicine and Clinical Epidemiology at the University of North Carolina at Chapel Hill, and at the Geriatric Research Education and Clinical Center at the Palo Alto Veterans Administration Medical Center. We are deeply indebted to Sherri Sturdivant Woodcock at Chapel Hill; she provided heroic secretarial support, superb organizational skills, and unfailing cheerfulness, without which our complicated cross-country editorial process would have faltered. Thanks also to Yolanda Keyes in Palo Alto for splendid technical support in preparation of the final manuscript and for general mothering.

Finally, we would like to thank our editor at Little, Brown, Kristin Odmark, for extraordinary support and patience in enduring our lengthy delays in completing this project, and Paula Noonan in the production department, for remaining upbeat even when a substantial portion of the copyedited manuscript was destroyed in the Oakland hills fire.

Notice

The indications and dosages of all drugs in this book have been recommended in the medical literature and conform to the practices of the general medical community. The medications described do not necessarily have specific approval by the Food and Drug Administration for use in the diseases and dosages for which they are recommended. The package insert for each drug should be consulted for use and dosage as approved by the FDA. Because standards for usage change, it is advisable to keep abreast of revised recommendations, particularly those concerning new drugs.

I. CONSTITUTIONAL SYMPTOMS

1. DIZZINESS
James P. Browder

Patients who complain of "dizziness" present a major diagnostic problem. Most will prove to have benign, self-limited disease. In many cases the complaint is attributed to simple situational tension and anxiety; however, this "diagnosis" is made only by ruling out other illnesses, which occasionally are quite serious and in some cases life-threatening.

Surveys of patients with dizziness, derived from emergency rooms, referral centers, and primary care centers, find that up to one-third of cases are attributable to vestibular problems; another large group (up to 20%), to hyperventilation; and the remainder, divided among a number of neurologic, psychiatric, and cardiovascular problems. Those patients who present to an emergency room are more likely to have dizziness associated with a serious problem (heart failure, gastrointestinal bleeding, or neurologic catastrophe) than are those who present to a primary care or referral center. Dizziness is a much more frequent complaint in the elderly, but the reported prevalence varies widely. In most series patients complaining of syncope and presyncope were included under the general category of dizziness, but these symptoms are associated with a particular subset of problems that are discussed separately in Chapter 133.

Patients with a complaint of dizziness initially may be divided, largely on the basis of history, into four categories: (1) patients who have acute readily definable problems for which dizziness is only one complaint, (2) patients with syncope and presyncope, (3) patients who have clear-cut vertigo, and (4) patients who have an ill-defined complaint of dizziness.

Evaluation

The evaluation of patients with dizziness and vertigo is based primarily on the patient's description of symptoms and the physical examination. Few laboratory tests are indicated. In patients with recurrent dizziness, a diagnosis may only be obtained after a medical evaluation over several visits.

The physical examination of the patient with vertigo or dizziness should always include an aural, a neurologic, and a cardiac examination as well as an examination directed toward evaluating the problems identified by history. Testing for orthostatic hypotension and symptom reproduction with hyperventilation is also useful.

A detailed neurologic examination is not necessary unless focal symptoms or signs suggest an intracranial lesion. A "mini" or "screening" examination should include the following, with abnormal findings directing a more thorough and specific evaluation:

1. Cranial nerve evaluation with specific attention to nystagmus, a pathologic finding if present in mid gaze or moderate lateral gaze. A few beats of transient end-point (stretch receptor) nystagmus are present in everyone and have little clinical significance. Horizontally beating nystagmus strongly suggests unilateral vestibular pathology, whereas vertical nystagmus suggests a lesion in the brain stem. Failure to demonstrate nystagmus in a patient who is complaining of acute, severe vertigo is most unusual and should cast doubt on the complaint.
2. Tests of cerebellar function and the Romberg test.
3. Specific vestibular testing. The Dix-Hallpike maneuver should be done on all patients complaining of positional vertigo whose symptoms are evoked by a change in position and who are symptomless at rest. The test maneuver consists of the forcible and rapid change from a sitting position to a lying position with the head turned and neck extended. It should be performed with great caution, if at all, in elderly subjects or those suspected of significant atherosclerotic disease of the carotid or vertebral systems. The test should be done at least twice, once with the head turned to the left and again with the head turned to the right. The classic findings described below are pathognomonic of paroxysmal positional vertigo and obviate any further testing:
    a. Subjective vertigo, usually moderate to severe
    b. Rotatory nystagmus, that is, nystagmus in which the globe torques around a central axis in either a clockwise or a counterclockwise direction

c. A latent period of several seconds after completion of the maneuver before the onset of nystagmus
d. Fatigue in the response on repetition of the testing (if the subject can be induced to repeat the maneuver)

After these evaluations the majority of patients fall into the category of the ill-defined complaint of dizziness. Only this problem and vertigo are discussed in this chapter.

Vertigo

Vertigo is the sensation of spatial disorientation resulting from a mismatch of stimuli from the vestibular, visual, and somatosensory systems. It can be caused by local or systemic problems that affect the vestibular system or can be of primary vestibular origin.

Patients with vertigo have a sensation of moving, usually spinning, when no apparent cause of movement is present. Often the patient spontaneously reports that the room spins. A key question to distinguish vertigo from ill-defined dizziness is: "Does it feel like the room is spinning around you or does it feel like you are spinning around on the inside?" Patients who describe the sensation as "spinning on the inside" are much less likely to have vertigo. Nausea and vomiting often accompany vertigo and represent stimulation of the vegetative nervous system by the vestibular nuclei. Vertigo is typically episodic; it occurs in discrete attacks, is sudden in onset, and lasts no longer than a few hours, although a residual "queasy" feeling may persist for several days. Patients who complain of constant, unremitting dizziness rarely have vertigo. Vertigo is almost always made worse by changes in head position and most patients with vertigo prefer to lie very still. Vertigo can be intense; although patients may not have the words to adequately describe the problem, it is clear to them that something serious has happened.

Secondary Causes of Vertigo

Problems that may involve the vestibular system, thereby causing vertigo, include disease of the external and middle ear, lesions of the central nervous system, systemic illnesses, and drug effects or toxicity. Eye problems may give the feeling of disorientation, but not the physical finding of nystagmus.

EAR PROBLEMS. External and middle ear problems occasionally are associated with vertigo, although vertigo is usually neither the most prominent nor the presenting symptom. Otitis externa, "swimmer's ear," can sometimes produce vertigo, presumably by changing the blood flow and thus the temperature in the affected ear. Direct involvement of the vestibular system by infection occurs only in malignant otitis externa, which occurs in diabetics and immunocompromised patients.

Acute and chronic otitis media are also occasionally associated with vertigo, but uncomplicated perforations of the tympanic membrane do not cause vertigo. Cholesteatoma (foul-smelling drainage with or without squamous debris) and vertigo suggest erosion of the bone over the horizontal canal and the need for prompt surgical decompression. If mastoiditis is present (mastoid tenderness and/or cellulitis), vertigo may signal impending bacterial labyrinthitis and constitutes a surgical emergency.

CENTRAL NERVOUS SYSTEM PROBLEMS. Vertebrobasilar ischemia and lesions of the brain stem may lead to vertigo. Vertigo is not a finding of hemispheric disease. Although vertigo is frequently found in patients with vertebrobasilar disease, it may be associated with other findings such as diplopia, dysphagia, or dysarthria to suggest vertebrobasilar involvement. Symptoms and signs of facial and somatic paresthesias, Horner's syndrome, and cerebellar ataxia accompanying vertigo also strongly point to compromise of the basilar arterial system. Vertigo resulting from central causes usually is milder and persistent with less fluctuation in symptoms, and is accompanied by less easily detectable nystagmus. Nausea is rarely a prominent feature.

Vertigo also arises from ischemia of the vestibular nuclei and/or the labyrinth itself or can be a manifestation of cranial nerve involvement in polyarteritis nodosa with polyneuropathy. By definition, there must be other accompanying symptoms or signs involving both spinal and cranial nerves, usually asymmetrically. Vertigo is a symptom in 20% of patients with multiple sclerosis, but must always be associated with other neurologic symptoms for the diagnosis to be made.

DRUGS. Although many drugs cause nonvertiginous sensations or are accompanied by orthostatic symptoms, a few drugs, such as the anticonvulsants Dilantin, phenobarbital, and primidone, cause vertigo at toxic levels. Alcohol, tobacco, and caffeine may also cause dizziness, but usually these substances do not cause true vertigo.

Primary Vestibular Problems

The most frequently encountered vestibular problems discussed here are positional vertigo, Meniere's disease, and labyrinthitis. Vertigo may also be associated with injuries from barotrauma on both ascent and descent during scuba diving and from pressure changes in airplanes.

POSITIONAL VERTIGO. Although most vertigo is aggravated by changes in head position, positional vertigo is elicited *only* by such changes and does not occur when the patient is still. Two types of positional vertigo can be readily described.

Benign positional vertigo characteristically occurs at night when the patient is recumbent, is of very brief duration and mild intensity, and is usually provoked by turning *on to one side but not the other*. The physical findings are entirely normal, and if the classic story is given, no other assessment is indicated. Treatment is reassurance that the symptoms will disappear over several weeks, although brief but widely spaced recurrences are not uncommon. Meclizine can be used at bedtime if desired; for severe dizziness, diazepam may be needed.

Paroxysmal positional vertigo often occurs after trauma and involves mild-to-moderate symptoms provoked by *vertically* oriented head movements. It has been attributed to the temporary displacement of one of the otoliths onto the gelatinous capsule of the posterior semicircular canal. Symptoms persist until the otolith is resorbed. A classic response to the Dix-Hallpike maneuver is pathognomonic for paroxysmal positional vertigo. Vestibular suppression with meclizine and avoidance of the precipitating movement (usually extending the neck while looking up) allows symptomatic resolution within a few weeks. Some advocate vestibular habituation by provocative head movements that elicit the vertigo, theorizing that by this means the central nervous system will more quickly compensate for the disordered vestibular input.

MENIERE'S DISEASE. *Meniere's disease* is the most important lesion primarily involving the vestibular system. The diagnosis is suspected only if the classic triad of symptoms described by Meniere is present: episodic vertigo, fluctuating hearing loss (typically low frequency), and roaring tinnitus; fullness or stuffiness in the ears, particularly during acute episodes, is also frequently present. A reasonable search for systemic metabolic disease or regional infection should be undertaken, since as many as 50% of those with Meniere's disease will have significant intercurrent illness. The primary goal of treatment is the control of the potentially disabling vertigo. Treatment is initially a salt-restriction diet and diuretics. Surgery on the endolymphatic system is reserved for those who cannot be managed medically.

LABYRINTHITIS. *Vestibular neuritis (acute labyrinthitis)* is the term usually given to an acute attack of severe, incapacitating vertigo that may recur, although not with the ferocity of the initial attack. Results of a physical examination and audiologic assessment are entirely normal, ruling out Meniere's disease, but caloric testing shows a unilateral vestibular defect ("unilateral weakness") that is usually permanent. Viral labyrinthitis is the name given to a similar condition that differs only by its close temporal association with viral illness. These names presume more about the disease than is actually known, and a name such as vestibular apoplexy may be more accurate though probably less popular. The condition is self-limited and resolves when the central nervous system, primarily the cerebellum, adjusts to the asymmetric vestibular input. Audiometric assessment is essential to rule out cochlear involvement, which would suggest another diagnosis. Electronystagmography (ENG) is not essential. Of greater importance is continued follow-up to make sure that the clinical course corresponds to the diagnosis and to reassure the patient that the condition is not degenerative. Treatment consists of symptomatic relief, with either meclizine if symptoms are mild or benzodiazepine for more severe symptoms, and reassurance that the illness is self-limited.

Unsteadiness or Light-headedness

Patients who cannot be described as having vertigo or in whom the description is in doubt are better described as having "unsteadiness" or "light-headedness." They often readily agree that this is a more accurate description of the complaint. The cause of discomfort is a heterogeneous group of problems that range from gastrointestinal bleeding or aortic stenosis to mild, self-limited drug reactions or a state of tension or anxiety. In almost all patients (> 85% in some series), the underlying problem can be determined by the initial history and physical examination. Among the most common causes of unsteadiness are drugs (particularly antihypertensive and psychotropic drugs, as well as many over-the-counter preparations such as antihistamines), any of the causes of syncope when the syndrome is not fully expressed (e.g., postural hypotension and arrhythmias), and psychiatric conditions (e.g., depression, chronic anxiety, and anxiety attacks, particularly with hyperventilation). Other less common conditions causing unsteadiness are anemia and cardiovascular disease. Although hypertension has been frequently associated with dizziness, its causal relationship is unclear.

Older patients frequently complain of dizziness. Although there is demonstrable aging of the vestibular system (in one series 46% of elderly patients who complained of dizziness had a lesion of the vestibular system), age-related changes by themselves are not thought to be sufficient to cause dizziness. The deteriorating vestibular system may be unable to compensate for visual and neurologic dysfunction, and older patients may present with dizziness or a gait disturbance from a combination of these problems. Failing eyesight is frequently seen in isolation or in combination with other processes in elderly patients complaining of dizziness.

Acute stress as well as chronic affective disorders often present as "dizziness" or "light-headedness," because these terms provide the most acceptable language for the patient to describe the condition. Assigning this etiology to a patient, however, depends on ruling out somatic pathology.

Treatment of unsteadiness depends on the underlying cause. Patients who seem to have unsteadiness because of anxiety or tension present a dilemma; reassurance is occasionally therapeutic, but most often will not suffice. Many of these patients demand that medicines be given; using tranquilizers or the sedating antihistamines in treating vertigo is a matter of clinical judgment.

Referral

In those instances of vertigo in which one of the above-mentioned syndromes is not clearly defined, the patient should be referred to an otolaryngologist for further evaluation. If a neurologic problem is identified or suspected as the key condition, a neurologic consultation would be appropriate.

Sloane P, Baloh RW. Persistent dizziness in the geriatric patient. J Am Geriatr Soc 1989; 37:1031–8.
An evaluation of patients over 70 years old who complained of dizziness for over a year.

Herr RD, Zun L. A directed approach to the dizzy patient. Ann Emerg Med 1989; 18:664–72.
A review of patients with dizziness who presented to an emergency room.

Sloane PD, Baloh RW, Honrubia V. The vestibular system in the elderly: clinical implications. Am J Otolaryngol 1989; 10:422–9.
An excellent discussion of this topic.

Lehrer JF, Poole DC. Diagnosis and management of vertigo. Compr Ther 1987; 13(9):31–40.
A thorough but readable review of the diagnosis and management of the symptom of vertigo, providing "a clear path for the physician who is consulted by a patient with vertigo."

Baloh RW, Honrubia V, Jacobson K. Benign positional vertigo: clinical and oculographic features in 240 cases. Neurology 1987; 37:371–8.
A large and carefully described study.

McGee ML. Electronystagmography in peripheral lesions. Ear Hear 1986; 7:167–75.
A review of labyrinthine (peripheral vestibular) pathology and the classic ENG findings associated with labyrinthine injury, with a discussion of the most common clinical disorders affecting the peripheral vestibular system and their ENG manifestations.

Madlon-Kay D. Evaluation and outcome of the dizzy patient. J Fam Pract 1985; 21:109–13.
A study derived from patients' complaints of dizziness who reported to an emergency room.

Miyamoto RT. Meniere's disease. Indiana Med 1986; 79:961–5.
Review of the etiology, clinical manifestations, functional tests, differential diagnosis, and medical and surgical treatment of Meniere's disease.

Drachman D, Hart CW. An approach to the dizzy patient. Neurology 1972; 22:323–34.
An early systematic effort to find the cause of dizziness.

2. FATIGUE
Mack Lipkin and Robert A. McNutt

The complaint of fatigue is a challenge to clinicians because possible causes range from the trivial to the lethal. Fatigue is a common complaint and often the first symptom of physical or mental illness, unhealthy life-styles, unhappy experiences, or any combination of these. It may be presented in varied language: "I can't get out of bed in the morning," "I have no pep," "I'm tired all the time," or "I just don't feel good."

Fatigue can be both an effect of many disorders and itself a cause of further morbidity. For example, hepatitis and infectious mononucleosis are accompanied by both lassitude and depression, which in turn can lead to problems in work, social life, and nutrition, resulting in more depression and fatigue. This interweaving of cause and effect, along with imprecise language, has made it difficult to find reliable data on the frequency of various causes of fatigue in ambulatory practice. Primarily physical causes are seen in 3 to 50% of patients. Viral infections, cardiopulmonary, and endocrine (diabetes and hypothyroidism) disorders lead the list. Drugs are common causes, especially psychotropic, antihypertensive, and cardiovascular medications. Primarily psychosocial causes are diagnosed in 10 to 50% of patients, with life-style problems, anxiety, and depression being the most common. Physical and psychosocial disorders often occur together.

The natural history of fatigued patients is as varied as the causes. One prospective study, however, found that more than 50% of fatigued patients remained so after 1 year. In addition, 21% of previously nonfatigued patients became fatigued.

A meticulous history, physical examination, and focused laboratory review can identify the cause of fatigue in about 85% of patients. A sensitive social and family history is often revealing. Many patients are often anxious about possible causes, especially cancer, and a thorough examination may be needed to reassure both patient and physician. Clinical experience suggests that several findings make primarily physical causes less likely, but do not rule them out. These include: (1) fatigue present longer than 4 months without associated symptoms and signs; (2) fatigue that is worse in the morning, especially if it disappears with activity; (3) a fluctuating course; (4) a stressful social history; (5) a life-style conducive to tiredness; and (6) a history of psychological disturbance.

Life-style Problems
Fatigue associated with unhealthy life-styles and habits is probably the most common type seen in ambulatory practice. What we know about this cause of fatigue is based mainly on clinical observations; there have been few rigorous studies of the relationship between life-style and symptoms. Inquiry to elicit such problems should explore the following areas.

Occupational History
A detailed description of the patient's work may uncover such factors as problems with associates and supervisors, limited future prospects, monotony, or chronic dissatisfaction, all of which may contribute to chronic fatigue or even exhaustion. "Overwork" is a common complaint and often misleading; most people enjoy hard work if it is satisfying. Those who are unhappy in their jobs or who work compulsively are more likely to complain to physicians. The elderly usually decrease their work effort gradually as their energy and endurance fade; those who insist on maintaining their former patterns may complain of fatigue.

Domestic Environment
Evaluation of the domestic environment should include compatibility with spouse or other companions, degree of mutual support, financial problems, sexual satisfaction, and troubles with children or other relatives.

Exercise Patterns
Inadequate exercise over a long period of time may lead to decreased vigor and ready fatigability. Patients with depression, anxiety, and tension often report temporary relief with exercise, whereas those whose fatigue stems from disease often feel worse after exercise.

Eating Habits
People who do not eat properly often feel tired. This includes both those who grossly overeat and those who substitute coffee and carbohydrates for meals.

Rest and Recreation
Imbalance in work, play, and rest, patterns of recreation, and the range of hobbies and interests can result in fatigue.

Drug Use
The excessive use of substances with stimulant or depressive effects, including alcohol, caffeine, and tobacco as well as amphetamines, sedative-hypnotics, and minor tranquilizers, may also result in cyclical patterns of activity and fatigue.

Treatment
When problems in any of the above-mentioned areas are elicited, simply pointing them out to the patient may be a useful first step in dealing with the associated physical symptoms. Changes in diet, exercise, and recreation patterns may be suggested. Some problems at work and home may be amenable to counseling from the primary physician; others require more specialized intervention.

Depression

Depressive reactions are seen in many forms and degrees of severity. The term *depression* is applied, often quite vaguely, to a miscellany of clinical conditions ranging from an endogenous disorder to a situational reaction, normal or excessive, to unfortunate life events.

Regardless of the type of depression, it is commonly accompanied by morning fatigue, whether or not the patient slept well. Although many depressed patients blame poor sleep for their fatigue, the two are probably not cause-and-effect but associated manifestations of the underlying mechanism. The patient who describes feeling abysmally tired in the morning, but less fatigued a few hours later, is almost always a depressed person. In contrast, people with chronic disease seldom show such diurnal rhythm and, unlike depressed patients, generally feel somewhat better after resting.

The suspicion of depression should lead to a search for further evidence, such as a history of previous depression, dysphoric mood, sleep disturbance, loss of an important person, disappointment, or failure. Obsessive-compulsive patients are prone to recurring depressions. The elderly, especially the physically ill, are notoriously subject to depressions, and the presentation is often deceptive, masked by physical complaints.

Once again, obtaining the patient's history of drug use is essential. Depression may be a side effect of a number of commonly prescribed drugs, including reserpine, alpha-methyldopa, propranolol, benzodiazepines, chlorpromazine, and birth control pills. Improper use of prescribed sedatives, tranquilizers, or amphetamines can result in cycles in which symptoms are temporarily relieved, followed by a feeling of letdown, which causes more drug use and results in more fatigue and/or depression.

In any case, the diagnosis of depression should always be made on positive evidence, not solely on an inability to find an "organic" cause. Positive evidence, properly elicited, often offers clues to appropriate management. Further information on evaluation and treatment of depression is contained in Chapter 108.

The Chronic Fatigue Syndrome

The chronic fatigue syndrome ("chronic mono," chronic Epstein-Barr virus, or chronic fatigue and immune dysfunction syndrome) is a name given to the constellation of debilitating fatigue and associated nonspecific symptoms and signs. The term *chronic fatigue syndrome* is preferred because other terms imply cause, and the cause is not established. In addition, terms such as *immune dysfunction* can cause undue concern for patients. Patients with this syndrome can usually pinpoint the onset of symptoms, and are typically female, young, and high achievers. The latter demographic groups are, however, more likely to consult with physicians.

In an attempt to define chronic fatigue syndrome, a consensus committee has outlined 2 major and 14 minor diagnostic criteria. A case of the chronic fatigue syndrome must fulfill major criteria 1 and 2, and the following minor criteria: 6 or more of the 11 symptom criteria and 2 or more of the 3 physical criteria; or 8 or more of the 11 symptom criteria. The major criteria are: (1) the new onset of debilitating fatigue, reducing daily activity below 50%, of at least 6 months' duration; and (2) the absence of a clinical condition that may produce similar symptoms. The minor criteria must also have persisted or recurred over a 6-month period. These include: (1) *symptoms* of fever, sore throat, painful lymph nodes, muscle weakness or discomfort, prolonged fatigue following exercise, headaches, migratory arthralgia, difficulty thinking or concentrating, and sleep disturbance; and (2) *physical signs* of low-grade fever, nonexudative pharyngitis, or palpable or tender lymph nodes in the anterior or posterior cervical areas. The list of clinical conditions to be considered before making the diagnosis of chronic fatigue syndrome reads like an index to a general textbook of medicine.

The cause of chronic fatigue syndrome was originally attributed to reactivation of latent Epstein-Barr virus, but recent data have discredited this theory. Stronger associations have been found to other viruses such as measles and herpes simplex types 1 and 2. Testing for the Epstein-Barr virus should, therefore, not be done in patients with chronic fatigue syndrome. The cause of this syndrome is likely to be multifactorial. Causative hypotheses now include viruses, stress, depression, and immune deficiency. While no specific therapies exist, patients can be reassured that most improve over time.

Time will show whether the chronic fatigue syndrome is simply a trendy label for a miscellany of symptoms, or an entity with a specific etiology, course, and treatment. Patients so labeled may suffer both from their symptoms and from the false security of a diagnosis. Physicians ought not to assume fatigue is due to such an entity and look no further. It is helpful to remember that many patients in ambulatory medical clinics have symptoms that do not fit properly in any standard category. Once appropriate diagnostic maneuvers have been performed, the challenge is to assist the patient to maximize function and cope with the remaining symptoms. A number of organizations offer support to patients with chronic fatigue syndrome. These include:

Chronic Fatigue and Immune Deficiency Syndrome (CFIDS)
c/o Community Health Services
1401 E. 7th Street
Charlotte, NC
($15 membership, with monthly newsletter)

Chronic Fatigue Syndrome Society
P.O. Box 230108
Portland, OR 97223
($20 membership, with newsletter)

National Chronic Fatigue Syndrome Association
919 Scott Avenue
Kansas City, KS 66105
($10 membership, with newsletter)

Lipkin M. The care of patients: perspectives and practices. New Haven: Yale University Press, 1987.
Useful background material.

Solberg LI. Lassitude. JAMA 1984; 251:3272–6.
Helpful review with many references. Takes an algorithmic approach to patients presenting with fatigue.

Morrison JD. Fatigue as a presenting complaint in family practice. J Fam Pract 1980; 10:795–800.
Review of 176 patients with a diagnosis of fatigue, taken from a medical record data base. Helpful epidemiologic data.

Sugarman JR. Evaluation of fatigue in a family practice. J Fam Pract 1984; 19:643–7.
Retrospective chart review of patients with a diagnosis of fatigue, after failure to make a specific diagnosis on the first medical encounter.

Katerndahl DA. Fatigue of uncertain etiology. Fam Med Rev 1983; 1:26–38.
More useful epidemiologic data.

Valdini AF. A one-year follow up of fatigued patients. J Fam Pract 1988; 26:33–8.
Prospective study of patients identified by the Rand Index of Vitality, rather than by patient complaint.

Barsky AJ. Hidden reasons some patients visit doctors. Ann Intern Med 1981; 94:492–8.
Sensible discussion of psychological problems in ambulatory practice.

Holms GP. The chronic fatigue syndrome: a working case definition. Ann Intern Med 1988; 108:387–9.
Discussion of the chronic fatigue syndrome, with useful references.

Dale J, Straus SE. Psychiatric diagnoses in patients who have chronic fatigue syndrome. J Clin Psychiatry 1989; 50:53–6.
Reviews 28 patients with chronic fatigue syndrome for the prevalence of psychiatric disease.

Wessely S, David A. Management of chronic (post-viral) fatigue syndrome. J R Coll Gen Pract 1989; 39:26–9.
Discussion of a strategy of rehabilitation based on an understanding of the interplay between physical and psychological factors.

Gold D, et al. Chronic fatigue: a prospective clinical and virologic study. JAMA 1990; 264:48–53.
No evidence of ongoing Epstein-Barr virus infection was demonstrated in a population of patients with chronic fatigue.

3. OBESITY
Robert B. Baron

Obesity is one of the most common disorders encountered in clinical practice and has major public health implications. Using current definitions, approximately 25% of Americans are obese. If all Americans were to achieve a normal body weight, it has been estimated that there would be a 3-year increase in life expectancy, 25% less coronary heart disease (CHD), and 35% less congestive heart failure and stroke.

Table 3-1. Weight ranges for men and women*

Height	Age group			
	19–24	25–44	45–65	> 65
5-0	97–123	102–133	112–143	123–148
5-1	100–127	106–137	116–148	127–153
5-2	104–131	109–141	119–152	130–157
5-3	107–135	113–146	124–156	135–163
5-4	110–139	116–150	127–162	139–168
5-5	114–143	120–156	132–167	144–178
5-6	117–147	123–159	135–172	147–178
5-7	121–152	127–165	140–178	152–185
5-8	124–157	131–170	144–183	157–189
5-9	128–161	135–175	144–188	161–196
5-10	131–166	138–180	152–193	166–202
5-11	135–171	142–185	157–198	171–207
6-0	139–175	146–190	161–204	175–213
6-1	143–181	151–196	166–211	181–219
6-2	147–187	154–201	170–216	185–226

*Proposed recommendations from the National Academy of Sciences. Heights are measured without shoes, and weights without clothing.

Unfortunately, obesity is also one of the most difficult and frustrating disorders to manage successfully. Considerable effort is expended by primary care providers and patients, with little benefit. Using standard treatments, only 20% of patients lose 20 pounds at 2-year follow-up, while only 5% of patients lose 40 pounds. The challenge is, therefore, to identify those patients with obesity who are most likely to benefit medically from treatment and most likely to succeed at losing and maintaining weight loss. Those patients unable to successfully lose weight should not be blamed or berated for their failure, but should be provided additional information about the medical need for weight loss, and provided ongoing support and care for their obesity-related medical problems. Treatment failures should be used to identify those factors that contributed to failure, in an attempt to improve success in future attempts.

Definitions
Obesity is an excess of body fat. In practical terms, obesity is most often defined as excess body weight for height. The two most commonly used terms are the relative weight (RW) and the body mass index (BMI). The RW is the actual weight divided by the "desirable weight," the midpoint value recommended by the National Academy of Sciences (Table 3-1); it is often expressed as a percent. The BMI, or Quetelet index, is the actual body weight divided by the height squared (kg/m^2). This index more closely corresponds to measurements of body fat and better differentiates "overweight" due to an increase in muscle mass from obesity.

A recent National Institutes of Health Consensus Conference defined obesity as an RW of greater than 120%, or a BMI greater than 27.5 kg/mg^2. Morbid obesity is commonly defined as an RW greater than 200%, or a BMI greater than 40 kg/m^2.

Health Consequences of Obesity
The relationship between body weight and mortality is curvilinear, similar to other cardiovascular risk factors. Most studies have demonstrated a J-shaped or U-shaped relationship, suggesting that the thinnest portion of the population also has an excess mortality. This is thought to be due to the higher rate of cigarette smoking in the thinnest group.

The relationship of body weight to mortality is further modified by two other factors, age and location of body fat. The body weights associated with the lowest mortality increase with age. Newer age-specific weight tables such as those published by Metropolitan

Life Insurance Company in 1983 and those proposed by the National Academy of Sciences recommend weights approximately 10 to 20 pounds (depending on height) more than those listed in older weight tables. More important is the observation that the location of the excess body fat is a major determinant of the degree of excess mortality due to obesity. Excess body fat around the waist and flank is associated with a markedly greater health risk than a similar amount of excess fat in the thighs and buttocks. The greater the amount of abdominal obesity, the greater the health risk at any given body weight. Further subdivision of the abdominal fat may also be important. Preliminary evidence suggests that excess fat located around the viscera may be more dangerous than a similar quantity of subcutaneous fat.

The increase in total mortality related to obesity results predominantly from CHD. Obesity is an independent risk factor for CHD, and is associated with a two- to threefold greater prevalence of other major risk factors for CHD including hypertension, hypercholesterolemia, and diabetes mellitus. Obesity is also associated with a variety of other medical disorders including degenerative joint disease of both weight-bearing and non–weight-bearing joints, certain cancers (colon, rectum, and prostate in men, and uterus, biliary tract, breast, and ovary in women), cerebrovascular disease, diseases of the digestive tract (gallstones, reflux esophagitis), and thromboembolic disorders. Obese patients also have a greater incidence of surgical and obstetric complications and are more prone to accidents. Although obesity is not associated with an increased risk of major psychiatric disorders, obese patients are at increased risk of psychological disorders and social discrimination.

Evaluation of Obese Patients

The diagnostic evaluation of an obese patient should focus on relevant historical information, the degree of obesity, medical consequences, potential secondary causes of obesity, and motivation for treatment.

History should identify significant obstacles to treatment and/or behaviors that can be changed specifically to achieve weight loss. A strong family history of obesity and onset of obesity during childhood may identify individuals with obesity particularly resistant to treatment. Recent weight gain is often a clue to affective disorders, or less commonly, an endocrinopathy. Determining eating and exercise behaviors is particularly important for identifying those behaviors amenable to change. Alcohol intake, for example, is often a significant source of unneeded calories and an impediment to behavior change. Information about prior attempts at weight loss is also important to identify treatments that are less likely to succeed. The use of laxatives, diuretics, hormones, over-the-counter medications, and nutritional supplements should also be addressed to identify potential side effects. The use of such substances may also be a clue to an underlying eating disorder such as bulimia.

Degree of obesity is assessed by dividing the patient's current weight by the "desirable weight" to obtain the RW as described above. The degree of abdominal obesity should be assessed by measurement of the waist-hip ratio (W/H). A normal ratio is 1.0 in men and 0.8 in women. Screening for the medical consequences of obesity is performed by physical examination and simple laboratory tests. Blood pressure and fasting blood sugar and lipid levels (total cholesterol, low-density-lipoprotein cholesterol, high-density-lipoprotein cholesterol, and triglycerides) are particularly important.

Secondary causes of obesity are rare and account for less than 1% of all cases. Endocrine causes such as hypothyroidism and Cushing's syndrome are the most important and can usually be excluded by physical examination. Patients with recent unexplained weight gain or ambiguous physical findings can be further evaluated with a serum thyroid-stimulating hormone (TSH) and dexamethasone suppression test as needed. Other secondary causes are extremely rare and most often present during childhood. Medications that cause weight gain include phenothiazines, tricyclic antidepressants, cyproheptadine, and corticosteroids.

Motivation for treatment should be formally assessed prior to beginning any treatment regimen. Patients' attitudes toward their body weight and their desire to change it should be discussed. Motivation can be further assessed by asking the patient to complete specific pretreatment tasks. Most useful is the completion of a 3-day diet diary.

Treatment

Although many problems encountered in medical practice can be treated by weight loss alone, only motivated patients should be aggressively begun on weight loss programs. Weight loss treatments vary considerably in terms of risk, cost, and efficacy, and treatment plans should be individualized. For most patients with mild or moderate obesity, a multifactorial approach including diet, exercise, behavior modification, and social support can be prescribed. Close patient-provider contact and long-term follow-up are key ingredients for success.

Diet Therapy

Standard dietary treatment of obesity should utilize the same nutritional principles as diet recommendations for healthy people, emphasizing a high-carbohydrate, low-fat, high-fiber diet. Total fat intake should be limited to 30% or less of total calories; protein, to 15%; and carbohydrate, to 55% or greater. Since typical US diets currently contain approximately 37% of total calories as fat, the replacement of foods high in fat with foods higher in carbohydrates and dietary fiber is quite useful.

Total calorie intake should be designed to create a daily calorie deficit of 500 to 1000 calories per day. Since 1 pound of fat equals approximately 3500 calories, these deficits will result in a 1- to 2-pound weight loss per week. Total calorie intake can be estimated by multiplying the patient's "desirable weight" (obtained from weight tables) by 30 calories per kilogram, and then subtracting the desired calorie deficit. For example, a 40-year-old 5-ft, 10-in. man who weighs 200 pounds has a desirable weight of 159 pounds (73 kg). His estimated energy requirement is approximately 2190 kcal. To lose 2 pounds per week, he should be prescribed 1190 kcal per day.

Referral to a clinical dietician is often useful to teach quantitative aspects of diet therapy. Patients can be taught to count calories, use dietary exchanges, or use computer software for diet analysis. More qualitative aspects of diet can easily be taught by primary care providers, by emphasizing those aspects of the diet that are high in calories but provide little additional nutritional benefit, such as dietary fat, sucrose, and alcohol. With the patient's diet record in hand, the primary care provider can help the patient identify these dietary factors and suggest low-calorie, high-fiber alternatives.

No dietary manipulation of macronutrients or other nutritional components can change the basic thermodynamic concepts described above. Virtually all popular diets, however, are based on attempts to circumvent thermodynamics. It is impossible for the clinician to keep up with each new popular diet. Categorizing the most common diets, however, can allow generalizations that provide a basic understanding of their approaches. Major categories of standard diets include low-carbohydrate diets, vegetarian diets, single-food diets, high-carbohydrate diets, and very-low-calorie diets. (VLCDs). These are summarized at the end of this chapter.

Exercise

Few patients can lose a significant amount of weight and maintain the weight loss without a concurrent aerobic exercise program. Aerobic exercise offers a number of significant advantages to patients attempting to lose weight. Most important is the prevention of the decrease in metabolic rate commonly seen with dieting. Additional advantages include the preservation of lean body mass, increased calorie expenditure both during and after exercise, cardiovascular training effect, decreased appetite (per calorie expended), and a general sense of well-being. Aerobic exercise also lowers blood sugar levels in diabetics, improves lipid levels in patients with high blood cholesterol, lowers blood pressure in hypertensives, and decreases overall cardiovascular-related mortality.

Young patients with mild-to-moderate obesity can be started directly on a regular aerobic exercise program. Patients are commonly instructed to select two exercises and to perform one of them four to five times per week for 20 to 25 minutes per day. Patients are taught to take their pulse and to generate a sustained tachycardia at 70 to 80% of their maximum predicted heart rate. Men over 40 and women over 50 years old, patients with symptomatic CHD, and patients with multiple CHD risk factors should undergo an exercise treadmill test prior to prescribing exercise.

Behavior Modification and Social Support
Sustained weight loss requires long-term changes in eating behavior. Patients must learn specific skills to facilitate decreased calorie intake and increased energy expenditure. Although formal behavior modification programs are available in most communities, most patients can be taught basic behavioral strategies in the office.

The single most useful behavioral skill is planning and record-keeping. Patients can be taught to plan both menus and exercise programs in advance. They are then instructed to record actual dietary and exercise behaviors. While the act of record-keeping itself will aid in behavioral change, the availability of records will also help the health care provider assess progress and make specific suggestions for additional problem-solving. Specific reward systems such as refundable financial contracts have been shown to be effective for many patients.

Social support is an additional essential component for any successful weight loss program. Most successful programs use peer group support. Involvement of family members is also important. A comprehensive review of published results of weight loss programs strongly suggests that close provider-patient contact is a better predictor of success than the particular weight loss intervention.

Management of Severe Obesity

Very-Low-Calorie Diets
A major new development in the dietary treatment of severe obesity is the development of safe and effective VLCDs. Also known as protein-sparing modified fasts, these diets restrict calorie intake to 300 to 500 kcal per day. Patients ingest only preformulated, usually liquid, food that provides adequate protein, vitamins, and minerals. Additional intake is limited to 2 to 3 qt of calorie-free beverages per day. The major advantage of these diets is the complete removal of patients from the food environment, facilitating greater dietary compliance. In addition, the greater calorie deficit results in more rapid weight loss, usually 3 to 4 pounds per week, encouraging the patient to continue. Patients on VLCDs have marked improvements in obesity-related metabolic parameters such as blood sugar and blood lipid levels, and blood pressure. Most diabetic, hypertensive, and hypercholesterolemic patients can have medications markedly reduced or discontinued soon after initiation of the diet.

VLCDs have been only slowly accepted by the medical community due to the tragic history of the Last Chance Diet and other "liquid protein supplements" (60 deaths), and to the marketing disaster of the Cambridge diet program (sold by lay salespeople without medical supervision). Currently marketed VLCDs (Optifast, Medibase, Health Management Resources [HMR], Medifast) can be obtained only through trained physicians. Patients are examined weekly and closely monitored with frequent laboratory tests. Programs usually restrict enrollment to patients who are more than 40% overweight. Common side effects include orthostatic hypotension, fatigue, cold intolerance, and transient hair loss (up to 10% of patients). Other less common complications include electrolyte disorders, gout, cholecystitis, and cardiac arrhythmias. No increase in mortality has been reported.

As with standard-diet therapy of obesity, VLCDs require compliance during the diet and long-term nutritional and behavioral changes to maintain weight loss. Even well-planned programs that combine VLCDs with behavior modification, exercise, and social support report variable long-term results. Eighteen-month follow-up for over 4000 such patients showed a 25% early dropout rate. Of those remaining in the program, 68% lost considerable weight but did not reach their goal. Of this group only 5 to 10% maintained weight loss after 18 months. Of the 32% of patients who attained their goal weight, 30% of women and 50% of men maintained their weight loss at 18 months.

Surgery
Although indications for surgical therapy remain controversial, over 100,000 obese patients have had such operations. Gastric operations are now the procedures of choice. Most popular are the vertical-banded (Mason) gastroplasty, in which a smaller stomach pouch is created, and gastric bypass procedures. Although both procedures result in significant weight loss, randomized trials comparing the two tend to favor gastric bypass procedures. In experienced centers, perioperative mortality averages less than 1%. Complications such

as wound dehiscence, peritonitis, nausea and vomiting, vitamin deficiencies, and hair loss occur in 25 to 50% of patients.

Jejunoileal bypass, the first major surgical procedure popularized for the treatment of obesity, has been abandoned by most surgeons. Although weight loss was effectively produced and maintained (average of 100 pounds in 5 years), diarrhea and fluid and electrolyte disorders occurred chronically in over half of the patients and one-third of patients developed progressive liver disease. Two newer bypass operations under investigation are a biliointestinal operation and a biliopancreatic operation. Jaw wiring is another commonly used, but not recommended, surgical treatment. On average, the initial weight loss is similar to that after gastric procedures but the data on weight maintenance are quite variable. Suction lipectomy, or liposuction, is a surgical procedure permitting the removal of fat from specific areas of the body. Usually performed by plastic surgeons, 5 pounds of fat can be removed with each procedure in an attempt to reshape thighs and waists resistant to more traditional weight loss and exercise treatments. No advantageous metabolic changes are induced by the procedure.

Other Treatments

Medications for obesity are widely available over the counter and with prescription. The most commonly used medications include the nonamphetamine appetite suppressants, fenfluramine, phentermine, and mazindol; the antihistamine phenylpropanolamine; and the antidepressant fluoxetine. Fenfluramine and fluoxetine are most frequently prescribed. Although some studies demonstrate short-term effectiveness as compared with placebo, many others show no effect. Only one study has shown long-term benefit when compared to either placebo or behavioral treatments. Most authorities either avoid medications completely or limit their use to patients beginning long-term treatment programs who need assistance with initial weight loss.

Despite numerous studies demonstrating the lack of efficacy of human chorionic gonadotropin hormone for the treatment of obesity, this injectable substance is still widely used. A recent random survey of weight loss programs in Los Angeles County showed 19 of 40 still using human chorionic gonadotropin. Thyroid hormone is also often used to treat obesity, but weight loss is produced only if patients become chemically hyperthyroid.

In controlled studies, a weight loss "device," the Garren-Edwards gastric bubble, failed to consistently demonstrate any benefit compared to diet alone; it was withdrawn from the market in 1988.

Review of Popular Diets

Low carbohydrate diets are the most resilient popular diet concept. Examples include the Atkins diet, the Stillman diet, and the Scarsdale diet. These diets are based on the correct observation that at equal-calorie intakes, low-carbohydrate diets result in more rapid weight loss than do high-carbohydrate diets. Unfortunately, the greater weight loss observed during low-carbohydrate feeding is entirely due to changes in water balance. During carbohydrate restriction, ketonuria increases and results in greater sodium excretion and water loss. The resumption of carbohydrate feeding reverses this process and results in sodium and water retention. No other changes in body composition or degree of weight loss are observed. Low-carbohydrate diets are by definition high in fat and/or protein and are thus unsuitable for long-term weight loss. These diets are also commonly deficient in calcium and dietary fiber.

Vegetarian diets are typically low-fat, high-carbohydrate, high-fiber diets and thus consistent with dietary goals. Vegetarian diets, however, can be either nutritionally adequate or inadequate depending on the food selected. Diets that restrict all animal products (vegan) require particular attention to protein intake and vitamin B_{12}. Diets that include dairy products (lactovegetarian) or dairy and eggs (lacto-ovovegetarian) are easier to plan.

Single-food diets are based on the concept that it is not only what you eat but when you eat it that is important. The Beverly Hills diet, for example, suggests that by ingesting foods one at a time, digestion is made more efficient, resulting in fewer calories getting "stuck" and less weight gain. This diet, which relies primarily on fresh fruit, is inadequate in protein, niacin, calcium, and iron. As expected, it commonly results in diarrhea.

High-carbohydrate diets are commonly balanced, hypocaloric diets. Most are high in fiber. Although dietary fiber has no unique weight loss quality, these diets are consistent with US dietary goals and can be encouraged. Most large commercial diet programs such as Weight Watchers and TOPS use high-carbohydrate diets and can be recommended to patients.

Atkinson RL, et al. A comprehensive approach to outpatient obesity management. J Am Diet Assoc 1984; 84:439.
An example of a well-thought-out program.

Bray GA, Gray DS. Obesity: part I—pathogenesis; part II—treatment. West J Med 1988; 149:429–41, 555–71.
A superb two-part review covering all major aspects of the subject.

Byerley L, et al. Popular diets: how they rate. 2nd ed. Santa Monica, Cal: California Dietetic Association, 1987.
A useful compendium of popular diets.

Council on Scientific Affairs. Treatment of obesity in adults. JAMA 1988; 260:2547–51.
The American Medical Association perspective.

Fujioka S, et al. Contribution of intra-abdominal fat accumulation to the impairment of glucose and lipid metabolism in human obesity. Metabolism 1987; 36:54–9.
Visceral fat is associated with a greater risk of metabolic abnormalities than is subcutaneous fat, as detected by CT scan.

Kirshner MA, et al. An eight-year experience with a very-low calorie formula diet for control of major obesity. Int J Obesity 1988; 12:69–80.
Long-term follow-up of the Optifast experience. Those patients who achieve weight goal do significantly better.

Larsson B, et al. Abdominal adipose tissue distribution, obesity, and risk of cardiovascular disease and death: 13 year follow up of participants in the study of men born in 1913. Br Med J 1984; 288:1401.

Lapidus L, et al. Distribution of adipose tissue and risk of cardiovascular disease and death: a 12 year follow up of participants in the population study of women in Gothenburg, Sweden. Br Med J 1984; 289:1257.
The W/H ratio is a very strong predictor of obesity-related morbidity and mortality in both men and women.

NIH Consensus Development Panel on the Health Implications of Obesity. Health implications of obesity. Ann Intern Med 1985; 103:1073.
A RW of 120% is defined as obesity.

Stunkard AJ. Conservative treatments for obesity. Am J Clin Nutr 1987; 45:1142–54.
An excellent review.

Stunkard AJ, et al. The body mass index of twins who have been reared apart. N Engl J Med 1990; 322:1483–7.
A recent study suggesting a very strong genetic component to obesity.

Wadden TA, Van Itallie TB, Blackburn GL. Responsible and irresponsible use of very-low-calorie-diets in the treatment of obesity. JAMA 1990; 263:83–5.
Emphasizes the need for careful patient selection and medical monitoring by specially trained physicians.

Weinsier AL. Recommended therapeutic guidelines for professional weight control programs. Am J Clin Nutr 1984; 40:865.
Excellent guidelines for initiating and evaluating programs.

4. WEIGHT LOSS
William D. Heizer

Body weight normally fluctuates as much as 1.5% from day to day as a result of short-term imbalances in the intake and output of water and food. Over long periods of time, however, the weight of most healthy adults remains remarkably constant. Investigation of unexplained losses of more than 5% of the usual body weight should be considered, although this does not necessarily indicate a serious physical problem.

Documentation of Weight Loss

The surest evidence of weight loss is comparison of the current weight with previously recorded values. Single values should be interpreted with caution; a recent survey of all 97 scales used for weighing adults in a university medical center showed that 10% were in error by more than 1%; home scales may be even less accurate. These findings underscore the importance of establishing a baseline by obtaining and recording accurate weights at every patient encounter, regardless of the reason for the visit.

In the absence of documentation, a history of weight loss may be corroborated if the patient recalls the amount of measured weight at one or more times in the previous years (although large persons tend to underestimate and small persons to overestimate their weights); if there has been a recent change in clothing size, especially the belt size; or if friends or relatives think the patient has lost weight. Pathologic weight loss should also be considered in an obese patient who is having unusual success on a weight reduction program.

Occasionally, the loss of body tissue is accompanied by a nearly equal gain in extracellular fluid; in such instances, the loss of soft tissue mass may be most noticeable in the face and limbs. When patients with edema or ascites are weighed, some estimate of the quantity of extracellular fluid present should be recorded so that both prior and subsequent weights can be interpreted correctly.

Causes and Mechanisms of Weight Loss

The list of conditions that cause weight loss is long, and the prevalence of various causes of weight loss has not been investigated extensively. In a study of patients at a Veterans Administration medical center who had involuntarily lost 5% or more of their usual body weight in 6 months, a specific cause for the weight loss was found in 74% and no cause was found in 26%, despite extensive diagnostic evaluation and prolonged follow-up. Cancer and gastrointestinal diseases were the most common causes, found in 19% and 14% of the patients, respectively. Depression, congestive heart failure, alcoholism, and chronic obstructive pulmonary disease each accounted for the weight loss in 5 to 10% of the patients. A variety of other disorders, including diabetes, thyrotoxicosis, infection, sarcoidosis, rheumatoid arthritis, drug-induced gastrointestinal symptoms, and neurologic diseases, each accounted for the weight loss in less than 5% of the total group of patients. A 2-year study of admissions to a general hospital medical service in Israel yielded very similar results. Unintentional weight loss of at least 5% of the usual body weight was a presenting or prominent symptom in 2.8% of all admissions; no cause for weight loss was found in 23%. Cancer, usually involving the gastrointestinal tract, was present in 36%, while 17% had various other gastrointestinal disorders and 10% had psychiatric disorders as the apparent cause for weight loss. A similar study done today might yield substantially different results, including some patients with human immunodeficiency virus (HIV) infection as the underlying cause of weight loss.

The three basic mechanisms of weight loss include decreased intake, increased rate of calorie utilization, and excessive calorie loss. Whatever the underlying cause, decreased food intake is almost always the most important mechanism, even when the other mechanisms contribute.

Decreased intake may result from physical and financial factors that limit food intake, unpleasant symptoms associated with eating, dietary idiosyncracies, and psychiatric conditions such as depression and anorexia nervosa.

Increased metabolic rate (energy expenditure) can contribute to weight loss in many disease states. Hyperthyroidism, by increasing energy expenditure and activity, can cause profound weight loss, even in patients with normal or increased calorie intake. Inflammation, burns, bone fractures, and sometimes cancer can also increase resting energy expenditure. Weight loss from these causes is usually modest, because the resulting increase in energy utilization rarely exceeds twice the normal resting energy expenditure. The increase in energy expenditure due to fever is 10 to 13% for each 1°C (33.8°F) increment above normal.

Increased physical activity rarely causes significant weight loss because of the relatively small amount of energy expended in even strenuous activities, compared to the large number of calories in body fat. A 70-kg person running 6 miles will use 500 calories, but an expenditure of 3500 calories is required to consume a pound of fat. Therefore, with an increase in activity equivalent to running 6 miles every day, a 70-kg person would lose only about 1 pound per week.

A loss of calories due to malabsorption, especially from pancreatic insufficiency, and uncontrolled diabetes mellitus can cause weight loss, with normal or even supranormal food intake.

Psychological Causes of Weight Loss

The major psychological causes for weight loss include depression, drug abuse, and anorexia.

Depression is probably the leading psychological cause for weight loss seen in the outpatient setting and can be recognized by appetite and sleep disturbance, anhedonia (low energy, poor motivation, decreased libido), feelings of sadness, agitation or psychomotor retardation, and poor concentration or memory (see Chap. 108). A diagnosis of depression or other psychosocial problems does not, of course, rule out the simultaneous presence of a physical cause for weight loss, because both may be present independently or they may be related (e.g., depression appearing as an early manifestation of malignancy).

Drug abuse may result in decreased food ingestion due to altered moods, preoccupation with obtaining drugs, and unwillingness or inability to spend money for food.

Anorexia nervosa most often occurs in adolescent women who lose weight as a result of decreased intake, frequently accompanied by self-induced vomiting, laxative abuse, or excessive physical activity. The disorder often first appears shortly after separation from previous social support (e.g., leaving home, death of parent). The diagnosis should be considered in any young female who is losing weight. Diagnostic criteria outlined in the *Diagnostic and Statistical Manual of Mental Disorders* (DSM-IIIR) include intense fear of becoming obese, which is not diminished by progressive weight loss; disturbance of body image (i.e., claiming to feel fat even when very thin); refusal to maintain a body weight over a minimal normal weight for age and height; and absence of physical illnesses that would account for the weight loss. Failure to recognize the syndrome is likely to precipitate an inappropriately extensive medical evaluation. On the other hand, few cases are so clearly evident initially that all diagnostic testing can be avoided. Patients with inflammatory bowel disease and brain tumors have been mistakenly diagnosed as having anorexia nervosa.

Determining the Cause of Weight Loss

In the majority of instances in which a physical cause for weight loss can be found, the cause will be obvious after the history, physical examination, and a minimal laboratory investigation are completed. For example, of 91 male veterans evaluated for involuntary weight loss, the cause was clinically evident on the initial evaluation in 55 of the 59 patients with identified physical causes. The likelihood of physical cause was increased in the presence of nausea or vomiting; recent change in cough; and a variety of physical findings such as cachexia, abdominal mass, adenopathy, or thyromegaly. Physical causes were less likely in patients who did not smoke heavily (< 20 pack-years) or who maintained their usual activity level.

History

In attempting to determine how changes in food intake or physical activity may be contributing to weight loss, it is helpful to ask a patient to describe a typical day: time of arising, meals, snacks, activities, time of going to bed, and amount of sleep. Eliciting the circumstances contributing to decreased food intake may suggest a specific cause, such as:

1. The thought, sight, and/or odor of food is not appealing (malignancy, many drugs, depression).
2. The sensation of taste is abnormal or the patient complains of a bad taste in the mouth (hepatitis, drugs, sinusitis, vitamin B deficiencies, zinc deficiency, psychological disorders).
3. Mechanical problems, pain, or dyspnea limits chewing or swallowing (neurologic, dental, oral, esophageal, or pulmonary abnormalities).
4. Unpleasant symptoms curtail food intake, such as abdominal pain (gastritis, peptic ulcer, gallbladder disease, intestinal ischemia, partial intestinal obstruction, inflammatory bowel disease, abdominal malignancy), diarrhea (infectious enteritis, inflammatory bowel disease, occasionally lactase deficiency, rarely irritable bowel syndrome), or nausea and vomiting.
5. The patient experiences lethargy or weakness (neurologic and muscular disease, alcohol or drug abuse).
6. The patient has idiosyncratic food preferences or overzealous adherence to diets, sometimes prescribed or self-initiated for gastrointestinal symptoms or for real or presumed allergies to various foods.
7. Adequate food is unavailable due to infirmity or poverty.
8. There is an exaggerated fear of obesity and/or inappropriate pursuit of thinness (anorexia nervosa).

Physical Examination
The physical examination should assess nutritional status as well as identify underlying causes of weight loss. In addition to general findings, such as wasting, fever, tachycardia, and apathetic appearance, specific attention should be paid to evidence of glossitis or other mouth lesions; poor dentition; goiter; adenopathy; masses in the abdomen, rectum, or pelvis; organomegaly; and peripheral neuropathy.

Laboratory Evaluation
Laboratory evaluation should be guided by the results of the history and physical examination. An initial battery of tests might include three stool specimens for occult blood; complete blood cell count with differential; urinalysis and chemistry profile for glucose, creatinine, and albumin; and other liver tests. Thyroid function tests should be performed for all elderly patients with weight loss because of the high incidence of thyroid dysfunction in this age group, and should be considered for other patients in whom the history strongly suggests that food intake has not decreased. Additional studies to be considered include chest x-ray, sigmoidoscopy, and upper gastrointestinal series with small bowel followthrough. Colonoscopy and mammograms should be done if there is a clinical suspicion of breast or colon cancer of if there is a history of these cancers in first-degree relatives.

Laboratory studies for malabsorption should be considered when food intake is normal and there is no evidence of causes of increased metabolic rate from diabetes, thyroid disease, or tumor. However, many causes of malabsorption, for example, celiac sprue, often cause anorexia. Screening tests for malabsorption should include a Sudan stain of the stool for fat and tests for serum carotene and folic acid. These tests are only valid when the patient has been eating an adequate diet for several weeks. The definitive test for malabsorption is a quantitative determination of fat absorption by means of a 72-hour stool collection or possibly a breath test for fat absorption where available.

If the cause of the patient's weight loss is not apparent on history and physical examination, and results of the tests mentioned are normal, the best management might then be watchful waiting, with further investigation primarily dictated by continuing weight loss or development of new symptoms. Follow-up visits should also be used to reevaluate any possible psychological causes for weight loss.

Treatment
Management of the patient with weight loss is directed toward diagnosing and treating the underlying medical problem. In the ambulatory care setting, weight loss is often more

important as an indication of the presence and severity of underlying disease than as a medical problem requiring treatment.

At some point, weight loss itself may become a significant medical problem, but deciding when that point has been reached is not easy. Many studies show that life expectancy is greatest for individuals with weights 5 to 20% below the US average, excluding cigarette smokers and people with preexisting disease. Furthermore, a modest degree of weight loss is probably a beneficial adaptive response in some illnesses, including chronic obstructive pulmonary disease, congestive heart failure, and possibly some cancers.

Although data are sketchy, it is likely that at a loss of 10 to 20% of normal body weight, medically significant manifestations of malnutrition begin to appear. These include weakness, decreased stamina, depressed immune function, increased tendency for breakdown of the skin, increased susceptibility to infection, and emotional changes of apathy and irritability. An individual of average weight would be expected to lose approximately 15% of body weight in 3 weeks of total starvation, 3 months of one-half normal food intake, and 3 weeks of one-half the normal nutrient intake if severely traumatized.

There are no measures of nutritional status suitable for clinical use that are specific and sensitive. In addition to weight loss, measurements that may provide some quantitative assessment of the degree of protein-calorie malnutrition include skinfold thickness, serum albumin and transferrin concentrations, total lymphocyte count, and delayed hypersensitivity by skin testing.

It is preferable to prevent rather than treat serious nutritional deficiency, and prevention should begin early. Most important is to discover and eliminate the cause of the weight loss. In addition, attention should be directed toward increasing oral intake. This may include:

1. More frequent feeding of foods with high-calorie density
2. Use of community resources such as senior center lunch programs and Meals on Wheels
3. Arranging for properly fitting dentures
4. Avoiding restrictive diets of unproved benefit
5. Avoiding drugs that suppress appetite or hinder gastrointestinal function whenever possible (This usually means eliminating all drugs that are not required.)
6. Avoiding accidental or unnecessary restriction or intake in association with diagnostic procedures
7. Using commercial dietary supplements

A number of nutritionally complete liquid diets are commercially available for use as supplements or meal replacement. Many are lactose-free. They require little or no preparation, but few patients find them as palatable as ordinary food. Most of the formulas have a calorie density of 1 cal per milliliter. A few with greater calorie densities may be especially useful for patients with early satiety.

Marton KI, Sox HC Jr, Krupp JR. Involuntary weight loss: diagnostic and prognostic significance. Ann Intern Med 1981; 95:568–74.
A prospective study of the causes of weight loss in patients evaluated at a Veteran's Administration medical center.

Rabinovitz MKR, et al. Unintentional weight loss. A retrospective analysis of 154 cases. Arch Intern Med 1986; 146:186–7.
A retrospective analysis of the incidence and causes of weight loss in patients admitted to an internal medicine service in Tel Aviv, Israel.

Forbes GB. Body composition: influence of nutrition, disease, growth, and aging. In: Shils ME, Young VR, eds. Modern nutrition in health and disease. Philadelphia: Lea & Febiger, 1988: 533–56.
A general discussion of normal body weight, body composition, and the relationship between changes in body composition and changes in calorie balance.

Grant JP, Custer PB, Thurlow J. Current techniques of nutritional assessment. Surg Clin North Am 1981; 61:437–63.
Good summary of clinically available methods of nutritional assessment, including history, physical examination, body composition analysis, anthropometric measurements, and biochemical measurements.

Floch MH. Weight loss and nutritional assessment. In: Floch MH, ed. Nutrition and diet therapy in gastrointestinal disease. New York: Plenum, 1981:101.
Categorizes diseases that often cause weight loss and reviews methods for assessing nutritional status.

Balaa MA, Drossman DA. Anorexia nervosa and bulimia: the eating disorders. Dis Mon 1985; 31(6):1–52.
Review of the psychosocial, endocrine, medical, and nutritional features of anorexia and bulimia, with current management of the conditions.

Halmi KA. Anorexia nervosa and bulimia. Annu Rev Med 1987; 38:373–80.
An update on the research and treatment of anorexia nervosa and bulimia.

Garfinkel PE, et al. Differential diagnosis of emotional disorders that cause weight loss. Can Med Assoc J 1983; 129:939–45.
A practical discussion and illustrated cases of weight loss resulting from anorexia, conversion disorder, schizophrenia, and depression. Discusses differential diagnosis and treatment of each condition and emphasizes the importance of properly diagnosing the various emotional disorders that cause weight loss.

Shil ME, Bloch AS, Chernoff R. Liquid formulas for oral and tube feeding. Order from Nutrition Support Kitchen, Box 279, Memorial Sloan-Kettering Cancer Center, 1275 York Avenue, New York, NY 10021.
Tables listing the composition of a large number of commercially available liquid diets and supplements. An excellent starting point but incomplete because of the number of new products being marketed.

Hill GL, Beddoe AH. Dimensions of the human body and its compartments. In: Kinney JM, et al., eds. Nutrition and metabolism in patient care. Philadelphia: Saunders, 1988:89.
A comprehensive review of the measurement, determinants, and components of body weight loss and its functional effects, and the changes in body weight in health and disease.

DeWys WD. Nutritional abnormalities in cancer. Weight loss in cancer patients: prognostic and pathophysiologic considerations. In: Kluthe R, Lohr GW, eds. Nutrition and metabolism in cancer. New York: Thieme-Stratton, 1981:8.
Frequency, magnitude, and prognostic implication of weight loss among more than 3000 cancer patients, by type of cancer.

Robbins LJ. Evaluation of weight loss in the elderly. Geriatrics 1989; 44:31–7.
Discusses the distinction between physiologic weight loss with advancing age and pathologic weight loss in the elderly. Concludes that up to 50% of elderly patients claiming weight loss will not have that complaint corroborated by medical records or family members. The benign "d's" of weight loss in the elderly: dentition, dysgeusia, dysphagia, diarrhea, disease (chronic), depression, dementia, dysfunction (social), and drugs.

II. EYE PROBLEMS

5. OCULAR FOREIGN BODIES
Hunter R. Stokes

Foreign bodies in and around the eye are usually quite painful and can cause significant permanent loss of vision if not properly managed. They may be embedded in the skin of the lid, sometimes penetrating the lid onto or into the conjunctiva, or embedded in the cornea, either superficially or deeply.

Lid and Periocular Foreign Bodies
Lid and periocular orbital foreign bodies are usually from shattered particles in a work-related accident (nails, wood) or from explosions (gunshot, fireworks). Retained foreign bodies from projectiles (shotguns, BB guns) may be in the soft tissue of the lid, in the orbit, or within the eyeball. The immediate danger is related to the depth of penetration and the resultant damage to the eyeball. It is important to know the exact location of the foreign body, but routine x-ray studies are usually of little value.

Penetrating lid injuries by large foreign bodies (nails, sticks) are very painful. Immediate removal is indicated but is best done by an ophthalmologist, because the distal end of the foreign body may have penetrated the globe. For transport of patients with retained foreign bodies, the primary consideration is protection from further damage by preventing any movement (e.g., rubbing) of the foreign body, especially if a portion of the object protrudes from the eye or eyelids. A simple paper cup, either flat-bottomed or pointed, can be taped over the eye. This allows the foreign body to remain in place and puts no pressure on the eye.

Conjunctival Foreign Bodies
Foreign bodies in the cul-de-sacs and under the upper lid can occur without any noticeable trauma, coming on a gust of wind or from an automobile air-conditioner duct. Common foreign bodies causing trauma include work-related particles (from drilling, sanding) and sand or dirt. Typical complaints are the obvious foreign body sensation ("trash in my eye") or the foreign body seems to "move around in the eye." Actually, the foreign body is almost always lodged in the substance of the conjunctiva under the upper lid and is not moving. But with each blink, a different area of the cornea is irritated, giving the impression that the foreign body is moving.

Evaluation
If the foreign body is in the inferior cul-de-sac, it can be seen by having the patient look up while the lower lid is pulled down. Foreign bodies in the superior cul-de-sac can sometimes be seen with elevation of the upper lid while the patient looks down. However, most of these foreign bodies will be lodged in the conjunctiva on the undersurface of the upper lid and can only be seen by eversion of the lid. The presence of such a foreign body is suggested by abrasions of the superior aspect of the cornea in a multiple linear pattern (vertical) usually confined to one quadrant, which can be seen by fluorescein stain.

Eversion of the upper lid is essential in locating foreign bodies under the upper lid. The proper method is to (1) have the patient look down with both eyes open and (2) grasp the lashes of the upper lid and lift up while depressing the midportion of the upper lid laterally with a blunt instrument. As long as the patient continues to look down, the upper lid will remain relaxed and everted so that a careful examination can be performed. As soon as the patient looks up or attempts to squeeze the eye shut, the lid will return to its usual position.

The best "instrument" for everting the lid is a double-tipped cotton swab, with one end moistened with a local anesthetic such as proparacaine (Ophthetic or Ophthaine) or tetracaine (Pontocaine). The dry end is used as a fulcrum to evert the lid and the damp end is available to sweep across the conjunctival undersurface of the lid to remove any foreign body that may be found. The small sulcus just under the lid margin must be carefully examined; small foreign bodies lodged in this indentation can be easily overlooked.

If a foreign body seems likely but is not found with lid eversion, it either is still there but has not been found, or else has been washed out and the eye is still painful. Fluorescein instillation may then reveal a "spot" of dye, indicating a relatively transparent foreign body (sand, insect wing, fiberglass particle) that can usually be wiped away with the cotton swab.

If no foreign body has been found with inspection of fluorescein staining, it is a good idea to sweep the moist cotton swab completely across the conjunctival surface underneath the upper lid, to wipe away a missed foreign body. If still no foreign body is seen, it may have become dislodged by tears and is no longer in the eye. This is a diagnosis of exclusion.

Patients complaining of a foreign body sensation days after exposure to glass fragments (e.g., a broken light bulb or windshield) must be re-examined. If no foreign body is seen, a thin sliver of glass may have been embedded in the conjunctiva and is intermittently presenting itself at the surface to create a scratchy sensation. These patients should be referred to an ophthalmologist for a slit-lamp examination.

Treatment
Visual acuity should be measured prior to initiation of efforts to remove any foreign body. This may have prognostic and later medicolegal importance.

Conjunctival foreign bodies that are on the surface of the conjunctiva or that have superficially penetrated the conjunctiva of the eyeball (bulbar conjunctiva) can usually be wiped off with the cotton swab as described already or lifted off with a toothless forceps after the eye is anesthetized. If there is any difficulty in removing the foreign body, if it appears to be deeply embedded, or if there is severe pain when the foreign body is touched, then attempts at removal should be discontinued and the patient immediately referred to an ophthalmologist.

Sometimes an underlying laceration of the conjunctiva is discovered after a foreign body is removed. Exploration of the wound is important, as it may reveal an additional subconjunctival foreign body or laceration of sclera, which may need specialized treatment. Such patients should be referred to an ophthalmologist.

Corneal Foreign Bodies

While conjunctival foreign bodies may be wind-borne or entrapped as a part of a conjunctival laceration, corneal foreign bodies most often arrive at the corneal surface with significant force. They therefore vary from conjunctival foreign bodies in two respects: First, they tend to be more deeply embedded, making them less likely to wash out by tears; and second, they usually consist of clipped or broken particles, most often metallic particles.

Treatment
As with conjunctival foreign bodies, visual acuity should be measured before removal is attempted. The prognosis is good for most corneal foreign bodies because treatment is usually instituted in time to avoid damage to vision and complications. Removal of corneal foreign bodies cannot be attempted without anesthetizing the cornea with a topical anesthetic. Irrigation of the cornea with sterile saline, directing the flow toward the foreign body, will dislodge many foreign objects. If this fails, wiping with a damp cotton swab is indicated, but because corneal foreign bodies are easily embedded, removal with a cotton swab may not be possible. In these cases, a spud or 25-gauge needle can be used if the patient's head can be held still and the physician has excellent near vision. An excellent light source and some form of magnification (examiner loupe) are necessary. The cornea is only 1 mm thick, and the slightest unpredicted movement of the head can cause more damage by the spud or the needle than by the foreign body. If spud or needle effort is not immediately successful, removal efforts should be discontinued and referral made for removal under a slit lamp. Also, if removal of the foreign body is immediately followed by a shallowing of the anterior chamber or an obvious leakage of fluid, perforation of the cornea must be suspected and the patient immediately referred to an ophthalmologist.

Many corneal foreign bodies are metallic, but the use of a magnet for removal is not recommended. Many metallic bodies are nonmagnetic or weakly magnetic, and even if magnetic, may be only partially removed by the magnet.

Iron foreign bodies (quite common from drilling or hammering steel) cause rust in the underlying corneal tissue within only 2 to 4 hours. A metallic foreign body present for 8 hours may have a complete rust ring around or beneath it, which remains after the foreign body is removed. Patients with a rust ring should be referred to an ophthalmologist for removal with a hand drill under slit-lamp magnification.

If a metallic corneal foreign body has been embedded for 2 to 4 days before medical attention is sought, the necrosis of tissue underlying the rust ring may permit removal of the foreign body and the entire ring rather easily. While this makes removal of the foreign body easier, there is a greater risk of infection leading to corneal ulceration and subsequent scar formation. These patients should also be referred to an ophthalmologist.

After a foreign body has been removed from the cornea, the management is similar to that for a corneal abrasion: prevention of infection, avoidance of steroids, pain control, and careful monitoring of the healing process.

Antibiotic coverage is essential because few, if any, foreign bodies are sterile when they are embedded in the cornea. If there is any hint of infection, such as haze in the surrounding cornea or marked injection of adjacent conjunctiva, when the foreign body is removed, ophthalmology consultation is indicated. Otherwise, a solution such as any specific or broad-spectrum ophthalmic antibiotic solution—examples include Neosporin, gentamicin (Garamycin), sulfacetamide (Sulamyd), or tobramycin—should be instilled and a pressure bandage applied for 24 hours. The latter encourages rapid healing of the corneal wound, but should not be applied in the presence of infection. All patients who have had a corneal foreign body removed must be seen 24 hours later to ensure that no infection is present and to monitor healing. The development of any haze in the base of the defect where the foreign body was removed suggests early corneal ulceration, and requires referral to an ophthalmologist. After 24 hours, antibiotics should be used four times a day, until the epithelium is healed. Healing should be monitored with fluorescein staining; if staining is still present after 72 hours, referral to an ophthalmologist is indicated.

The pain following removal of a corneal foreign body may last for several days, and is caused by ciliary spasm, a reflex reaction to stimulation of exposed corneal nerve endings. This spasm may be relieved by paralyzing the ciliary body muscle with administration of a cycloplegic. For abrasions greater than 3 mm long, a long-acting cycloplegic, such as scopolamine (0.25% Isopto Hyoscine) should be instilled along with the antibiotic solution. Topical anesthetics interfere with healing of corneal defects, and should never be dispensed or prescribed.

Topical steroids should be avoided in the management of corneal defects after the foreign body is removed. Steroids inhibit wound-healing, encourage fungal infections (a real consideration when the foreign body is vegetable matter, such as wood or pine needles), and in susceptible patients, may increase intraocular pressure to levels high enough to cause damage to the optic nerve.

Many primary care physicians who initially see patients with corneal foreign bodies choose to remove only superficial foreign bodies and refer all others to an ophthalmologist. Also, they elect to refer all patients for follow-up care after the foreign body is removed. All foreign bodies located in the central region of the cornea should at least be referred for follow-up slit-lamp examination. Even a faint scar, if located centrally, in or near the visual axis, can lead to a permanent reduction in vision.

Havener WH. Synopsis of ophthalmology. 2nd ed. St. Louis: Mosby, 1963.
Contains an excellent discussion of situations related to foreign bodies and also an excellent photographic demonstration of eversion of the lids.

Gardiner PA. Accident and first aid—ABC of ophthalmology series. Br Med J 1978; 2:1347–50.
This series covers a variety of ocular problems; the one on injuries is complementary to this discussion of corneal foreign bodies.

Chiapella AP, Rosenthal AR. One year in an eye casualty clinic. Br J Ophthalmol 1985; 69:865–70.

Edwards RS. Ophthalmic emergencies in a district general hospital casualty department. Br J Ophthalmol 1987; 71:938–42.
Surveys that put things into perspective. These two articles record the frequency and origin of eye injuries. Foreign bodies lead the list in both studies.

6. Corneal Abrasion
Hunter R. Stokes

Corneal abrasions are common and quite painful. Any superficial contact with the anterior surface of the eyeball, as well as extensive exposure of the cornea to ultraviolet light (sunlamp, welder's arc), may remove a portion of the epithelial surface of the cornea. Uncomplicated corneal abrasions almost always heal without scarring or visual impairment. Most corneal abrasions, especially smaller ones, can be managed by primary care or emergency room physicians.

Diagnosis
Corneal abrasion should be suspected when pain or the sensation of a foreign body follows trauma to the eye. Oblique illumination of the cornea with a penlight usually discloses an irregular area of the normally smooth, glistening corneal surface. Direct or slightly tangential illumination may reveal a shadow on the surface of the iris that moves in the opposite direction of the movement of the light. Fluorescein instillation into the inferior cul-de-sac facilitates diagnosis; any area of abrasion will be outlined by absorbed dye and will be more visible. Cobalt blue filter (a small filter that can be attached to the tip of a penlight) will further illuminate the fluorescein. Fluorescein strips should be used instead of solution because the latter is an excellent culture medium for *Pseudomonas*. The strips should be dampened with water or sterile saline, or lightly touched to the moist conjunctival surface of the lower lid if the eye is tearing.

Differential Diagnosis
The most important problem that may be confused with an abrasion is herpes simplex keratitis. Immediate ophthalmology referral is indicated if this condition is identified or suspected, because herpetic corneal lesions always leave a scar, and delayed management can lead to significant permanent loss of vision. Herpes keratitis is most frequently seen in the winter, with the seasonal increase in viral infections, and in the early weeks of hot summer weather. Suggestive diagnostic findings include (1) a history of herpes keratitis, (2) a coexisting fever blister, (3) recent upper respiratory tract infection, (4) an absent or vague history of corneal trauma, (5) a dendritic (branching) corneal stain pattern, and (6) reduced corneal sensitivity (the latter is impossible to test if a topical anesthetic has been instilled or used to dampen the fluorescein strip).

The persistence of pain and a linear stain in a patient with no history of ocular trauma and no foreign body under the upper lid dictates referral to an ophthalmologist, because the dendritic pattern of herpes keratitis may be very difficult to appreciate without a slit lamp. If the history and symptoms suggest a corneal abrasion, even when none is seen using fluorescein, it is appropriate to treat the eye for an abrasion for 24 hours. If symptoms persist after 24 hours, referral to an ophthalmologist is necessary.

Specific antiviral therapy is instituted immediately by the ophthalmologist if herpes simplex keratitis is strongly suspected. If herpes keratitis is not strongly suspected, only an antibiotic is used in the first 24 hours.

Treatment
The first step in the management of corneal abrasion is to make certain that there is no retained foreign body either on or in the cornea or under the upper lid. It may be necessary to instill a topical anesthetic in order to examine the eye adequately, especially when dealing with ultraviolet burns. However, topical anesthetic should *never* be prescribed or dispensed for use by the patient. The anesthetized cornea may be exposed to further trauma as the natural blink reflex is diminished, and the anesthetic precludes adequate healing by delaying re-epithelialization. Patients may also use the leftover portion of the anesthetic for the next "scratched eye," which may instead be a corneal ulcer, a penetrating foreign body, or some other serious, potentially blinding eye problem.

A very small, uncomplicated corneal abrasion often heals spontaneously within 12 to 24 hours. However, if an abrasion is large enough to be visible to the naked eye of the examiner, it should be treated with antibiotic drops and a pressure patch.

Antibiotic or sulfonamide solution, not ointment, should be instilled before a patch is placed. There is some evidence that ointment may lead to delayed healing and a higher incidence of recurrent erosion because ointment particles may be trapped under the healing epithelium.

A pressure patch is placed over the injured eye unless the other eye does not have good vision. Bilateral abrasions (as with ultraviolet burns) may require bilateral patches or patching of the more seriously injured eye. Healing is improved by applying the patch with pressure sufficient to keep the eyelids from rubbing over the abrasion. This is accomplished by applying tape strips, usually three to five parallel strips of 1-in. tape, with the superior ends pointing toward the central part of the forehead and the inferior ends toward the lateral part of the cheek on the injured side. Patients should not attempt to reapply pressure patches that fall off because in doing so they may cause further irritation.

Patching the eye will help to reduce the pain of a corneal abrasion, but additional analgesia may be needed, particularly if the abrasion is large. Instillation of moderately long-acting cycloplegic drops such as scopolamine (0.25% Isopto Hyoscine) prior to patching will reduce ciliary spasm (a major cause of pain) and dilate the pupil for approximately 72 hours. An oral analgesic such as codeine may sometimes also be needed.

After 24 hours the patch should be removed and the eye re-examined to monitor the healing process and look for signs of infection. Antibiotic should be continued four times a day for 24 to 48 hours, even if re-epithelialization has occurred. A haze noted around an abrasion suggests infection, which can develop into a superficial ulcer and results in slower healing and a permanent scar. The finding of a haze therefore dictates immediate ophthalmologic referral. An abrasion that does not heal in 48 to 72 hours should also prompt a referral. A transparent embedded foreign body or a missed foreign body under the upper lid may be present, and slit-lamp examination is indicated.

Topical steroids and topical medications containing steroids should never be used to treat corneal abrasions. Not only can the steroid enhance the growth of herpes lesions of the cornea, but it also encourages the growth of fungal lesions that can cause an elevation of intraocular pressure. Most importantly, topical steroids inhibit corneal wound-healing.

Complications

In up to 10% of corneal abrasions, recurrent epithelial erosions result from failure of the epithelium to adhere to the underlying basement membrane. The classic picture of recurrent erosion is the spontaneous onset of severe pain in an injured eye, occurring weeks or months after apparent healing. This often occurs during the night or on awakening. Many cases of recurrent erosion occur in patients who have an underlying problem of the superficial aspect of the cornea known as anterior membrane dystrophy. Dystrophy must be suspected in all patients with recurrent erosion after abrasion and may also cause recurrent erosions in patients without a history of corneal abrasion. Ophthalmology referral is necessary for diagnosis. The treatment may be simple (lubricant drops during the day and ointment at bedtime), but the erosion may be a long-term problem.

Referral

Many primary care and emergency room physicians treat corneal abrasions initially and refer the patient to an ophthalmologist for follow-up the next day. Patients with large or deep abrasions, suspected herpes lesions, and abrasion with haze (possible ulcer) should be referred to an ophthalmologist at the time of injury. Continued pain or stain after 48 hours, failure to heal after 48 to 72 hours, or presentation that suggests a recurrent erosion also requires immediate referral to an ophthalmologist.

Adreine J, et al. Symposium on ocular pharmacology and therapeutics. St. Louis: Mosby, 1970.
An old, but classic reference. The discussion focuses on the treatment of the conjunctiva, but is also appropriate for the cornea.

Eiferman RA. Recurrent corneal epithelial erosions. Perspect Ophthalmol 1981; 4:3–7.
An excellent discussion, with photographs.

Baum JL, Silbert AM. Aspects of corneal wound healing in health and disease. Trans Ophthalm Soc UK 1978; 98:348—51.

This is an excellent description of the potential for recurrent erosion when ointment is used, as opposed to solutions. The process of wound-healing by the sliding of epithelial cells and adhesion of epithelium to the basement membrane is demonstrated.

Stern GA, et al. Effect of topical antibiotic solutions on corneal epithelial wound healing. Arch J Ophthalmol 1983; 101:644–7.
An excellent discussion of the relative toxicity of the more commonly used topical antibiotic solutions.

Dua HS, et al. Clinical patterns of corneal epithelial wound healing. Am J Ophthalmol 1987; 104:481–9.
An excellent review of exactly how the corneal epithelium heals, which should help primary care physicians understand the physiology of this unique form of healing by the migration of epithelial sheets.

Woods TO. Recurrent erosion. Trans Am Ophthalmol Soc 1984; 82:850.
An excellent discussion of recurrent erosion.

The treatment of recurrent corneal erosion. JAMA 1987; 257:1898–9.
Contains several letters to the editor which describe standard and newer treatments of recurrent erosion.

7. CONJUNCTIVITIS
Hunter R. Stokes

The conjunctiva is a thin, transparent tissue that covers the inner surface of the lids (palpebral conjunctiva) and the anterior surface of the sclera (bulbar conjunctiva). Inflammation and/or infection of the conjunctiva is the most common eye disease in the western hemisphere.

The common causes of conjunctivitis include bacteria, chlamydia, viruses, and allergies. Other, less common types—fungal, chemical, and idiopathic—are important but uncommon and rarely need to be considered by the primary care practitioner. Trachoma, a form of chlamydial conjunctivitis that is rare in the United States, is the most common infectious disease in the world.

Differential Diagnosis
The red eye is the most common eye problem that leads a patient to seek medical attention. Conjunctivitis must be distinguished from other conditions that can present as a red eye, such as trauma to the cornea (discussed in detail in Chaps. 5 and 6), acute iritis, acute glaucoma (discussed in Chap. 10), and subconjunctival hemorrhage. Key features in differential diagnosis are summarized in Table 7-1.

Acute conjunctivitis is characterized by marked drainage tending to be mucoid or purulent and injection of the palpebral conjunctiva. It is often associated with swelling of the lids. Conjunctival redness is diffuse; in contrast to the other causes of the red eye, pain is minimal. There may, however, be a scratchy foreign body sensation. Vision, pupil size and reactivity, and intraocular pressure all are normal.

Corneal trauma typically presents with significant pain and a foreign body sensation. Redness may be localized or diffuse. Visual acuity depends on the area of cornea involved; blurred vision results when the central part of the cornea is affected. Pupil size may be normal or, if marked ciliary spasm is present, reduced. Clouding of the cornea suggests a corneal ulcer and mandates immediate ophthalmology referral. Fluorescein stain of the cornea is used to elucidate the type and extent of corneal involvement. Keratitis (inflammation of the cornea, often caused by exposure to a sunlamp, arc-welding, overuse of contact lenses, or cross-country snow skiing) shows a diffuse stain, whereas abrasions, foreign bodies, or ulcers show a stain pattern isolated to a segment of the cornea.

Acute iritis presents with photophobia, a constricted, poorly reactive pupil, and a "ciliary flush," or injection of the bulbar conjunctiva around the limbus (the junction of the conjunc-

Table 7-1. Differential diagnosis of the red eye

	Conjunctivitis	Corneal: abrasion, ulcer, foreign body, keratitis	Acute iritis	Acute glaucoma
SYMPTOMS				
Pain	Minimal	Moderate to severe	Moderate to severe	Severe (often with associated nausea and vomiting)
Foreign body sensation	Mild	Moderate to severe	None	None
Vision	Usually normal	Blurred (depends on area of cornea involved)	Blurred, with photophobia	Severely reduced—often less than 20/200
SIGNS				
Drainage	Watery to purulent	Often watery	None	None
Conjunctiva	Marked injection—more away from limbus; palpebral more than bulbar	Mild-to-moderate bulbar injection	Moderate injection, usually bulbar near limbus	Moderate-to-marked injection, usually bulbar near limbus
Cornea	Clear	Abnormal—depends on cause*; use fluorescein stain	Clear	Diffusely cloudy
Pupil size	Normal	Normal or slightly small	Small	Mid-dilated
Pupil reaction to light	Normal	Normal	Normal	Usually nonreactive
Intraocular pressure	Normal	Normal	Normal	Normal
INCIDENCE	Very common	Common	Infrequent	Rare
OTHER INFORMATION	May see associated blepharitis	History important for foreign body, abrasion; history of contact lens wear, arc-welding for keratitis		Anterior chamber is shallow

*See discussion.

tiva and cornea). Pain is moderate, often described as a deep aching sensation, and vision is blurred. The presentation may be confused with acute glaucoma but in iritis, the vision is better, the intraocular pressure is normal, and the anterior chamber is of normal depth. Immediate ophthalmology consultation is indicated to evaluate and manage potential complications; timely institution of pupillary dilatation may prevent scarring, which may impair pupillary movement and cause secondary glaucoma.

Acute glaucoma results from a sudden obstruction to aqueous outflow of the anterior chamber, with an extreme rise in intraocular pressure and a marked reduction of vision. It usually occurs in patients with shallow anterior chambers who are anatomically predisposed. Pain is severe and often accompanied by nausea and vomiting. The bulbar conjunctiva is usually injected near the limbus. The intraocular pressure in acute glaucoma can be estimated by palpating the eyeball through closed eyelids. The globe will be impressively firm or even rock-hard. Depth of the anterior chamber can be estimated using penlight illumination of the anterior chamber. Light directed across the eye from the temporal side should illuminate the entire iris surface. With a shallow anterior chamber, the iris is bowed forward, and the nasal portion of the iris will not be illuminated. This procedure is not possible if the pressure is high enough to cause significant corneal clouding. Urgent ophthalmology consultation is mandatory; delay may result in permanent loss of vision in the affected eye.

Subconjunctival hemorrhage is a dramatic but usually benign condition that results from bleeding in the small, fragile vessels of the conjunctiva. It is sharply circumscribed in appearance and appears acutely. It may be caused by minor trauma, or occur spontaneously, usually from increases in venous pressure due to coughing, sneezing, or straining. There is no associated pain, and both vision and pupillary responses are normal. Rarely a systemic disease like blood dyscrasia or severe hypertension causes the hemorrhage. In most cases, patients may be reassured that the hemorrhage will clear spontaneously, over 1 to 2 weeks.

Approach to Diagnosis

Once other conditions have been ruled out, the cause of conjunctivitis can usually be determined from the history and physical examination. In general, bacterial conjunctivitis is associated with mucopurulent discharge, smooth, inflamed conjunctiva with red dots (papillae), and no preauricular lymphadenopathy. Viral conjunctivitis is associated with a watery discharge and follicles (hypertrophied translucent lymph tissue surrounded by blood vessels); enlarged preauricular lymph nodes may be present. Allergic conjunctivitis is associated with chemosis and mucoid discharge. In studies comparing laboratory analysis with clinical diagnosis of bacterial, viral, and allergic conjunctivitis, correlations range from poor to 75%. Most authorities agree, however, that in primary care practices, smears and cultures are impractical and are not indicated unless management proves difficult or an unusual or virulent organism, such as *Neisseria gonorrhoeae,* is suspected.

Bacterial Conjunctivitis

Bacterial conjunctivitis, the most common type of conjunctivitis, is most often caused by *Staphylococcus aureus, Pneumococcus,* and *Hemophilus influenzae.* It has a rather sudden onset, beginning usually in one eye, to be followed in the other eye in 2 to 5 days. There is severe irritation with a foreign body sensation and a purulent exudate. The reaction is more prominent in the palpebral conjunctiva than in the bulbar conjunctiva, with mild injection of the conjunctival vessels. Usually there is edema of the lid. In the chronic bacterial conjunctivitis caused by *S. aureus* colonization of the lid margins and eyelash follicles, there may be an associated blepharitis. This is often described as granulated eyelids because of swelling of the lid margins and crusting of the lashes. A stye (external hordeolum) may also occur. These conditions are discussed further in Chapter 8.

Conjunctival secretions in bacterial conjunctivitis are infectious for 24 to 48 hours after therapy begins. Family members must take care when applying medication to the eyes of infected patients.

Treatment

Acute bacterial conjunctivitis is self-limited and usually clears in 2 weeks without treatment. With treatment, dramatic clearing occurs in 48 to 72 hours. A variety of topical antibiotics (sulfonamides, chloramphenicol, neomycin, polymyxin, bacitracin, gentamicin, tobramycin, erythromycin) are equally effective and may be used as solutions or ointments. Neomycin is frequently associated with allergic reactions. In such cases, the purulence and exudate of infection clear, but are shortly replaced by severe itching and burning of the eyes, red swollen lids, and a dry, almost scaly appearance to the skin of the lid. The drug should be stopped and cold compresses applied.

Referral
Patients with recurrent or chronic conjunctivitis should be referred to an ophthalmologist. In chronic bacterial conjunctivitis, a combination of steroid and sulfonamide (e.g., Blephamide, Vasocidin), or steroid and antibiotic (e.g., Maxitrol, NeoDecadron) has been demonstrated to be more effective than either alone. However, a steroid-containing compound should be prescribed only by an ophthalmologist. See Chapter 6 for a discussion of the dangers of ophthalmic steroids.

Viral Conjunctivitis
Many viruses can cause conjunctivitis, and many milder cases are not brought to medical attention. Two syndromes caused by adenoviruses are responsible for most outbreaks: adenopharyngeal conjunctivitis and epidemic keratoconjunctivitis. Herpes simplex conjunctivitis may result in corneal ulceration and scarring.

Adenopharyngeal conjunctivitis (APC) is associated with fever of 100°F to 104°F (37.7–40.0°C) and a severe pharyngitis; large preauricular nodes are usually present. There is a bilateral follicular conjunctivitis with marked redness and watery discharge. Multiple, small subepithelial corneal infiltrates may occur and reduce vision. Swimming pool conjunctivitis is commonly caused by the APC virus and occasionally by the EKC virus, neither of which is eliminated by proper chlorination.

Epidemic keratoconjunctivitis (EKC) usually begins in one eye with marked conjunctival injection, follicles, and tearing. A huge preauricular node is not unusual. About half of patients develop a keratitis, with marked chemosis. Corneal involvement is associated with pain and blurred vision, which may persist for months after the infection clears. The infectivity of EKC is dramatic, and it is often the explanation for a summer outbreak of severe pink eye. The virus is shed for about 14 days, during which time patients must take precautions to avoid spreading the disease to others. Precautions must be taken with hands, ophthalmic solutions, and bathroom linen. Hand towels used by those with EKC must be washed in hot water to reduce the chance of spread. Physicians must be careful because hand-to-eye as well as tonometer contamination has been implicated in epidemics.

Herpes simplex conjunctivitis is associated with a fever blister on the lip or upper face, typical vesicular lesions on the skin of the eyelids, and/or dendritic corneal herpes lesions. The conjunctivitis is typically unilateral with follicles. If herpes is suspected, the patient should be referred to an ophthalmologist for detection and treatment of corneal ulcerations.

Treatment
There is no specific therapy for viral conjunctivitis. However, a topical antibiotic is usually prescribed for 10 to 14 days to prevent secondary bacterial infection. Topical lubricants (e.g., methylcellulose) may relieve eye redness and discomfort. Symptomatic treatment is indicated for the fever and sore throat of APC. Referral to an ophthalmologist is indicated for management of EKC with painful corneal involvement.

The possibility of herpetic infection should discourage primary care practitioners from prescribing steroid medication for any conjunctival infections. Even though herpetic infection is not always associated with a typical corneal ulcer, topical steroid preparations can dramatically enhance proliferation of herpes simplex, resulting in permanent vision loss from a corneal scar.

Allergic Conjunctivitis
There are several forms of allergic conjunctivitis, characterized by itching, the presence of eosinophils in the eye, discharge or conjunctival scrapings, and a history of exposure to an allergen.

Allergic Reactions to Topical Medications
A contact inflammation, which may involve lids as well as the conjunctiva, may occur with use of many medications including Neosporin, idoxuridine, and atropine. Often the condition for which the patient was treated will resolve in 3 to 5 days, but a week later the redness is worse because of an allergy to the medication, and the lids may be dry and scaly. A vicious cycle may develop, with additional medication resulting in worsening of the allergic response. Discontinuing all topical medications is diagnostic as well as therapeutic in such cases. Symptomatic relief may be achieved with cool compresses and an ocular lubricant.

Hay Fever Conjunctivitis
Hay fever conjunctivitis is an acute seasonal or environmental condition that is mild but sometimes frightening in appearance. The patient notes a sudden onset of itching, tearing, and "fullness" of one or both eyes, and finds redness of the conjunctiva with associated marked chemosis. With marked edema, the eye seems to "sink" into the conjunctiva, and the conjunctiva may protrude beyond the lid margins when the eyelids are closed. There is almost always a history of an immediate past confrontation with a known allergen (e.g., pollen, grass). Treatment includes cold compresses, vasoconstrictors for 24 to 48 hours (Albalon-A Liquifilm or Vasocon-A Ophthalmic Solution), and systemic antihistamines for 24 hours. The condition clears as rapidly as it appears.

Vernal Conjunctivitis
Vernal keratoconjunctivitis occurs annually in the spring or early summer, usually in warm climates, and typically affects adolescents, more often males than females. It is bilateral, and causes severe itching, with watery discharge and severe papillary conjunctivitis. The papillae are so large that they are described as "cobblestone," and are most frequently noted on the upper palpebral conjunctiva. Each huge papilla has a flat surface and a tuft of capillaries that are readily visible. Lesions may also be prominent at the limbus, where the papillae form a gelatinous mound.

This condition is recurrent for 5 to 10 years, after which it often spontaneously disappears. Symptomatic patients are, however, quite uncomfortable. Cold compresses help. Topical steroids usually relieve the symptoms, but the chronicity of the condition often leads to prolonged use of steroids and its associated dangers. Patients with vernal conjunctivitis should be referred to an ophthalmologist. Although the diagnosis is easy, conjunctival and corneal scarring may occur, and expertise in the management of corticosteroid therapy is important.

Recently topical cromolyn sodium (Opticrom) has been found useful in treating vernal keratoconjunctivitis and is much safer than steroids.

Wilson LA, et al. Treatment of external eye infections: a double-masked trial of tobramycin and gentamycin. J Ocular Ther Surg 1982; 1:364–7.
Discusses the relative values of two antibiotics, with an excellent clinical description of many cases of bacterial conjunctivitis.

Eiferman RA. A primer of conjunctivitis. Prim Care 1979; 6(3):561–86.
An overview of the treatment of conjunctivitis.

Stenson S, et al. Studies in acute conjunctivitis. Arch Ophthalmol 1982; 100:1275–7.
An analysis of 700 cases of conjunctivitis comparing laboratory and clinical findings.

Leibowitz H, et al. Human conjunctivitis. Arch Ophthalmol 1976; 94:1747–9, 1752–6.
A two-part report. The first found poor correlation between laboratory and clinical findings. The second examined treatment and found steroid antibiotic preparations were better than antibiotics alone and both were better than placebos in relieving symptoms.

Vaughn D, Asbury T, Tabbara K. General ophthalmology. 12th ed. Norwalk, Conn: Appleton and Lange, 1989.
An excellent general ophthalmology text, revised every 2 years and used as the standard in many medical schools. References and discussions throughout the book refer to the red eye, beginning with a differential diagnosis chart inside the front cover.

8. EYELID DISORDERS
Hunter R. Stokes

Blepharitis

Blepharitis is inflammation of the lid margins where the lash follicles are located, occurring with or without active infection. It is the most common affection of the eyelids and is usually a chronic condition with acute exacerbations.

Chronic blepharitis ("granulated eyelids") presents with moderate swelling of the lids along the lash line, with scaling of the skin. Management is directed toward keeping the lid margins clean. The lid margins should be vigorously scrubbed with a warm cloth twice a day and the lashes scrubbed with undiluted baby shampoo applied to cotton-tip applicators. The lower lids (almost always the ones involved) are pulled down so that the scrubbing of the lash margins is against the inferior orbital rim. After the lashes are cleansed, the warm cloth is again used to wipe away the shampoo as well as any material in the lashes that is produced by the scrubbing. In severe cases, this process may be preceded by 1 to 2 minutes of warm compresses, to aid in loosening secretions. Chronic blepharitis is often associated with seborrhea and/or dandruff and if either of these conditions is present, then the skin or scalp problem also requires vigorous treatment.

Acute infectious flare-ups should be managed with applications of topical antibiotics four times a day (e.g., bacitracin, erythromycin, or tobramycin [Tobrex] ointment or drops) as well as the above cleansing schedule. Frequent flare-ups may be prevented by nightly applications of an antibiotic ointment. Sulfacetamide (Sulamyd, Bleph-10) may be used as an alternative to the previously mentioned preparations, but it contains sulfur, a potential allergen, as the active ingredient. Neosporin should generally be avoided for long-term use because of the rather frequent incidence of neomycin allergy. Steroid-containing preparations, such as Blephamide, Vasocidin, and NeoDecadron, should *not* be prescribed except by an ophthalmologist after an appropriate examination; while their immediate effects may be dramatic, long-term or inappropriate use of steroids in the eye can have dangerous complications.

Chalazion and Hordeolum

Almost all localized swollen masses of the eyelids are either chalazia or hordeola. The two are often confused and to some extent are managed similarly. However, the history, anatomic position of the swelling, and degree of inflammation are usually sufficiently different to distinguish between them and allow specific therapy.

Chalazion is a chronic, granulomatous inflammation of a meibomian gland, a sebaceous gland in the tarsal plate of the eyelid. Chalazia occur in patients of any age, and are always located deep within the lid tissue adjacent to the inner (conjunctival) surface. On physical examination, a small, nontender nodule ("English pea") is palpable within the lid, and there is a corresponding area of redness and elevation on the everted lid.

Small, chronic chalazia do not require treatment. If they are large enough to cause an obvious cosmetic swelling or to create pressure on the eyeball (which can actually blur vision by creating astigmatism), surgical excision by an ophthalmologist is indicated.

Infected chalazia can present with painful swelling. This complication is managed with warm compresses, applied for 15 minutes four times a day, as well as topical sulfonamides or other antibiotics, applied four times a day as either ophthalmic solution or ointment. Systemic antibiotics are almost never necessary.

Since a chalazion is an inflammatory lesion, steroid injection has been used as primary treatment for a recurrence. However, surgical excision remains the most effective management. Recurrence of a chalazion is rare, but recurrence in the same section of the lid requires biopsy to rule out malignancy.

Hordeolum (stye) is essentially a localized, superficial abscess of one of the sweat or sebaceous glands of the eyelids, usually caused by *Staphylococcus aureus*. It presents as a red, swollen, and quite tender mass, which most commonly points to the skin surface of the lid (external hordeolum). Less often an internal hordeolum occurs; it is usually larger than an external one and points toward the inner conjunctival surface. Styes are more common in children and teenagers.

Treatment for a hordeolum is similar to that for an infected chalazion: warm compresses for 15 minutes four times a day, followed by topical antibiotics, in either ophthalmic solution or ointment. If improvement does not occur in 24 to 48 hours, incision and drainage at the area of pointing, either internal or external, may occasionally be necessary. The procedure can be done by a nonspecialist. Systemic antibiotics are not necessary for simple, localized hordeola.

A large hordeolum (usually internal) can sometimes progress to localized cellulitis that involves the entire lid and potentially threatens cavernous sinus thrombosis. With the first hint of cellulitis, systemic antibiotics to treat *S. aureus* should be added to the local therapy.

Recurrent hordeola occasionally occur. They are usually in one eye and are caused by a chronic staphylococcal infection of the lid. Systemic antibiotics may help; usually referral to an ophthalmologist is indicated for recurrent lid infection.

Entropion and Ectropion

Entropion, a turning in of the lid, usually involves the lower lid, and is most often seen in patients over 50 years old. In the United States, entropion usually occurs in elderly individuals, due to weakening of the layers and support attachments of the lower lid. Entropion from scarring of the conjunctival surface of the lid can also involve the upper lid; it usually results from trachoma, which is rare in the United States.

In entropion, the turning in of the lash margin causes the lashes to rub against the cornea. This condition, trichiasis, is quite symptomatic and surgical repair of the entropion may be required.

Ectropion, the outward turning of the lash margins of the lid, always involves the lower lid and leads to chronic irritation and tearing. It may result from aging, with relaxation of the orbicularis muscle, or from scarring of layers or skin of the lower lid. With either type, outward turning of the lash margin exposes the conjunctival surface, which may then become progressively thickened and keratinized. Management is difficult and often requires surgery.

Abramson IA Jr. Color atlas of anterior segment eye disease. New York: McGraw-Hill, 1964.
Includes excellent photographs of blepharitis, chalazia, and hordeola.

McCulley JP, Moore MB, Batoba AY. Mucous fishing syndrome. Ophthalmology 1985; 92:1262–5.
Has a catchy title and describes an interesting chronic condition (usually dry eyes), that leads to excess mucus production. Patients are so concerned with this bothersome but minor problem that they traumatize the conjunctiva, which leads to more mucus. This condition should be considered in all cases of blepharitis.

9. Cataracts
Hunter R. Stokes

A cataract is a clouding of the lens, which normally is transparent, colorless, and biconvex. Cataracts are the most common cause of severe visual impairment in the United States, as well as the most common cause of correctable severe visual disability. More than 90% of all cataracts result from the normal aging process of the human lens. They occur more often in diabetics and are also associated with hypoparathyroidism, myotonic dystrophy, and atopic dermatitis. Less commonly, cataracts are congenital, the result of traumatic injury to the lens or lens capsule, or associated with the use of certain drugs, such as systemic corticosteroids and topical echothiaphate iodide (used for glaucoma treatment).

Cataracts are present to some degree in at least 70% of patients over 70 years old. They are usually bilateral; however, the degree of opacification and rate of progression may differ from one eye to the other. Cataracts are often classified according to the location of the most significant opacities. In *nuclear* cataracts, the central portion or nucleus of the lens becomes denser or sclerotic; yellow, brown, or gray discoloration may be present. In *cortical* cataracts, the opacities are localized to the more peripheral portions of the lens, and may have the appearance of radiating spokes in slit-lamp examination. Both nuclear and cortical cataracts are common in elderly patients, and the two types may coexist. Of *subcapsular* cataracts, posterior subcapsular cataracts, in which there is opacity and irregularity of the posterior surface of the lens, are the most rapidly progressive type. They are more commonly seen in younger patients and patients who are on corticosteroids. Cataracts are also often classified by stage of development. In immature cataracts, opacities are separated by areas of clear lens, whereas total lens opacification is present in a mature cataract. In a hypermature cataract, liquefaction of the lens cortex has occurred, with loss of fluid through the lens capsule; the latter may cause an inflammatory reaction within the eye and associated glaucoma.

Clinical Findings

The type and extent of visual impairment resulting from a cataract reflect the location and density of the lens opacities. Patients with cataracts characteristically note a gradually progressive reduction in vision, which they may describe as a "clouding" or "fogging." Patients with cortical cataracts may not experience significant visual impairment until late in the development of the opacities. Some patients with nuclear cataracts may actually report an improvement in near vision, even discarding glasses for some visual functions ("second sight"). This occurs because sclerotic changes in the lens nucleus alter its shape as well as its transparency. The change in shape can result in relative myopia, which changes the refractive error and may allow some farsighted patients to perform close work without glasses for the first time in many years. The perception of color may be affected, usually with advanced nuclear sclerotic cataracts in which the lens has become pigmented; blues tend to be filtered out and the color that objects appear is shifted to the yellow and red end of the spectrum. Patients with central opacities (e.g., nuclear and posterior subcapsular cataracts) may find their vision is worse in bright light; because of pupillary constriction, light enters through the area of greatest opacification, and is both blocked and diffused. These patients may complain of glare and often find that their vision is better in low light, when the pupil is dilated.

Evaluation

Cataracts are detected by directing a penlight into the pupil or, more easily, by looking through the ophthalmoscope. Opacities of the lens can best be seen with the ophthalmoscope set at approximately +10 and with the examiner approximately 12 in. from the patient's face. They appear as dark areas against the background of the red-orange pupillary light reflex. The examination can be facilitated by dilating the pupil with phenylephrine hydrochloride (10% Neo-Synephrine [ophthalmic] solution), which is not cycloplegic and does not affect close vision. The risk of causing acute angle-closure glaucoma with pupillary dilation is small. The location, degree of opacification, and maturity of a cataract should then be further elucidated with a slit-lamp biomicroscope.

When a patient is found to have a cataract, referral to an ophthalmologist is indicated. This does not mean that the patient will immediately have cataract surgery. In addition to characterizing the type and severity of the cataract, a thorough ophthalmologic examination must be performed to detect possible coexisting eye conditions (glaucoma, retinal disorders, retinal holes and/or detachment). An assessment of visual acuity, including a refraction, should also be performed. Often a change in the patient's glasses, indicated by a careful refraction, will improve the visual acuity so that the patient may continue to function visually without surgery. Occasionally, dilating drops may also improve vision and preclude immediate surgery. In addition to an objective assessment of the patient's visual acuity, a history should be obtained of the patient's visual impairment in activities such as driving, reading, and pursuit of work or hobbies.

Because most cataract operations are performed on elderly patients, other eye problems, including macular degeneration, retinal vascular occlusive disorders, retinopathy of diabetes, hypertension, and arteriosclerosis, may reduce the final visual acuity. When the opacification of the cataract precludes good visualization of the fundus, specialized tests can usually predict postoperative visual outcomes to some extent. Such assessment is important so that patients can have realistic expectations for the outcome of surgery. Elderly patients and their families may be disappointed when the patient cannot "read the phone book" or renew a driver's license after surgery; this level of vision may not have been achievable because of other ocular problems, which are best identified prior to surgery.

After the initial visit, semiannual or annual examinations by the ophthalmologist are continued until surgery is ultimately indicated.

Treatment

The only specific treatment for a cataract is surgical removal of the lens (cataract extraction). This procedure is indicated when the level of visual impairment reduces the ability of the patient to perform daily activities and/or significantly alters the patient's life-style. Cataract surgery is usually quite successful. Over 90% of patients will achieve correctable vision of 20/40 or better; however, some patients will receive less benefit, even without surgical complications. An appropriate preoperative examination will identify most patients in the latter group prior to surgery and reduce disappointment from unrealistic expectations.

Over 95% of cataract operations are now done on an outpatient basis, either in a hospital or in an ambulatory surgery center. A preoperative examination, preferably performed by the patient's primary physician, is done to ensure that medical conditions are stable. Infections of any kind, but particularly those involving the skin, should be resolved prior to surgery to avoid possible contamination of the eye. Most ophthalmologists also prescribe a regimen of preoperative cleansing of the lids, with both pre- and intraoperative administration of topical antibiotics. The surgical procedure itself usually takes about 1 hour or less, and is usually done under local anesthesia. Patients are able to ambulate immediately after the procedure. Outpatient surgery is safe even if the patient is quite elderly ($\geq$ 80 years old) or a diabetic, or has other significant medical conditions. Anesthesia personnel are usually present in the operating room to monitor the patient's vital signs, to give appropriate preoperative intravenous medications to prevent pain from the local anesthesia block performed by the surgeon, and to manage medical problems that may arise during surgery. Indications for inpatient surgery are unstable medical conditions that require additional monitoring in the pre- or postoperative period.

Surgical Techniques

More than 95% of cataract extractions are now done by one of the extracapsular techniques, in which the lens nucleus is removed through an incision in the anterior lens capsule, and the back membrane of the lens (posterior capsule) is polished and left intact. This permits more "stability" of remaining internal components of the eye and also serves as the "hammock" into which most intraocular lenses are implanted. In younger patients, the lens nucleus is soft and may be fragmented ultrasonically and the lens components then aspirated (phacoemulsification). This procedure may not be suitable for elderly patients, in whom the nucleus is very firm and may not easily emulsify.

Intracapsular surgery, in which the entire lens, including the capsule, is removed from the eye was the most common method of cataract extraction until the mid-1980s. It is usually performed with a cryoextractor; the lens is removed after being frozen to the extractor tip. Use of the intracapsular technique has declined because extracapsular surgery offers a smaller incision, reduced incidence of complications, and more support for the implanted lens.

Operative and postoperative pain is minimal with all techniques unless complications occur.

Complications

The most serious postoperative complication is infection, which usually occurs in the first week. Although fulminant endophthalmitis (infection inside the eye, most often caused by *Staphylococcus* or *Streptococcus* species) is rare, with an estimated incidence of about 0.1%, and loss of vision in 0.02%, it can destroy the potential for vision in 24 hours. Other conditions that require medical and/or surgical intervention include glaucoma (especially in the first 1–4 days), hemorrhage, suture breakage, intraocular lens displacement, inflammation (iritis), and a variety of retinal problems. While the complication rate after cataract extraction exceeds 30% if one includes all the minor complications and inconveniences that may require an additional visit to the ophthalmic surgeon's office, most of these are not vision-threatening. They must all, however, be promptly evaluated. The incidence of major complications is closer to 5%. The final vision is significantly improved in 95% of patients after cataract surgery.

Clouding of the posterior capsule may occur 6 months to several years after extracapsular surgery and is more a consequence of the surgery than a complication. This opacification occurs in up to 50% of patients, and unless corrected may reduce vision just as the cataract did. It may safely be treated using the neodymium YAG laser, which by a microexplosion, causes tissue disruption and optical breakdown of the opaque posterior capsule. This is the primary use of the laser in cataract surgery; contrary to popular mythology, *cataracts cannot be removed by laser.*

Surgical Referrals
Effective 1989, cataract extraction is one of the procedures for which every state requires prior approval by the state professional review organization (PRO). Advertisements of "free cataract surgery" (not permitted by Medicare), laser cataract surgery, or cataract surgery without suture are misleading, and patients attracted by these clinics should receive a second opinion. Likewise, a diagnosis of cataracts that must be operated on immediately should signal to the primary care physician that a second opinion is needed. Medicare will pay for the second opinion.

Postoperative Care
Patients are usually seen by the operating surgeon within 24 hours after surgery and again in 2 to 4 days. Thereafter, periodic examinations are provided until the final refraction and prescribing of lenses, usually 2 to 3 months after surgery. Temporary restrictions of activity in the early postoperative period are imposed primarily to prevent inadvertent trauma to the eye and elevations in the intraocular pressure. These include avoidance of strenuous physical activity and bending, and the use of eyeshields or glasses at all times. Any change in the appearance or "feeling" of the eye in the postoperative period should result in an immediate examination by an ophthalmologist. After the first postoperative week, the eye is usually patched only at night and reasonable activities are permitted, including driving an automobile if the other eye has adequate vision to permit safe driving. Topical medications, usually an antibiotic and a steroid, are ordinarily used for 3 to 4 weeks. Sutures used in cataract extraction are extremely small (usually 10-0 nylon) and may not need removal. If removal is necessary, it is done at 6 to 8 weeks postoperatively. The healing process is sufficiently complete at about 3 months for a final refraction to be obtained and a permanent lens prescribed, either eyeglasses or contact lenses.

Optical Correction After Cataract Extraction
Surgical aphakia (absence of the lens) results in improved light transmission, but vision is blurred unless it is corrected by an artificial lens. This lens may be in the form of an intraocular lens, a contact lens, or spectacles.

Intraocular lenses are now implanted in more than 95% of all eyes operated on for a cataract in the United States; while all patients are not candidates for implants, newer surgical techniques and improvements in lens design make this the preferred method of correction of aphakia. An intraocular lens can be implanted years after previous cataract extraction has been performed. This is called a secondary implant.

Contact lenses provide a satisfactory visual result for aphakic patients. However, many elderly patients are unable to handle contact lenses because of arthritis, tremor, or anxiety. Others have insufficient tearing.

Any type of contact lens may be used after cataract surgery. Hard contact lenses are less expensive, and more durable, and may be used for a wider range of visual problems than can soft lenses. Also, their tinting makes them easier to find, and their relative inflexibility makes them easier to handle. Some soft contact lenses are inserted daily, while others may be inserted by a vision care specialist and left in place for weeks. Not all eyes can be fitted with an extended-wear contact lens, and if fitted, the patient should have the lens removed at least bimonthly to be examined, in order to reduce the chance for damage to the eye. Soft lenses are more likely to be lost. The average postoperative cataract patient may require up to three soft lenses in the first year (Medicare only pays for the first one). A new type of contact lens, the gas-permeable lens, has the vision and durability traits of a hard lens, and its comfort is almost as good as the soft lens.

Aphakic spectacles are the least desirable alternative. Although they require a shorter surgical time than do intraocular lenses and less effort from the patient than do contact lenses, they provide a substantially less satisfactory visual result. They magnify (by about 33%), distort images, and severely limit peripheral vision. Because of the magnification, aphakic spectacles cannot be used comfortably by patients who have had only one eye operated on for cataract; if the other eye still has useful vision, the difference in image size is intolerable. For these patients, the option is either to wear a contact lens or to have an intraocular lens implanted.

Liesgang TJ. Cataracts and cataract operations (two parts). Mayo Clin Proc 1984; 59:556–67, 622–32.
A thorough and well-referenced review, with helpful diagrams of types of cataracts, surgical techniques, and optical corrections.

Straatsma BR, et al. Aging-related cataract: laboratory investigation and clinical management. Ann Intern Med 1985; 192:82–92.
Report from a UCLA conference, covering pathology and biochemical aspects of cataract as well as medical and surgical management, with color photographs of cataract patterns.

Capino D, Leibowitz HM. The elderly patient with cataract. Hosp Pract March 30, 1987; 22(3A):19–37.
A concise review, with photographs of cataracts and diagrams of procedures.

Wong WW. Indications for cataract surgery: psycholinguistic considerations. Arch Ophthalmol 1978; 96:526–8.
An excellent philosophical discussion on when cataract surgery should be performed, concluding that successful cataract extraction should permit the patient to function better visually postoperatively. A related editorial is on p. 247.

Obstbaum SA. Cataracts and intraocular lens surgery: the pursuit of excellence. In: Deutsch E, ed. Year book of ophthalmology. Chicago: Year Book, 1989: Chapter 6.
Discusses recent issues and advances in cataract surgery and highlights many of the recent additions to the literature on the subject.

Applegate WB, et al. Impact of cataract surgery with lens implantation on vision and physical function in elderly patients. JAMA 1987; 257:1064–5.
Documents improved vision and improved objective function in areas ranging from mental status to timed manual performance.

10. GLAUCOMA
Jan A. Kylstra

Glaucoma is a group of diseases, rather than a single entity, characterized by elevated intraocular pressure, progressive changes in the optic disk, and progressive visual field loss. It is one of the three leading causes of blindness in the United States and the leading cause of blindness in nonwhite Americans. An estimated 2 million people have glaucoma, half of whom are under treatment; 80,000 people are blind from glaucoma.

Physiology of Intraocular Pressure
The eye is not a rigid sphere, but is in fact more like a balloon. Its relatively stable shape is due to the intraocular pressure, which keeps the eye "inflated." Intraocular pressure is determined by the rate of production of aqueous humor by the ciliary body and the resistance to aqueous outflow, primarily through the trabecular meshwork and canal of Schlemm. Increased production of aqueous humor or increased outflow resistance will

elevate the intraocular pressure. Conversely, decreased aqueous production or decreased outflow resistance will lower the intraocular pressure.

Significant individual variation exists in the susceptibility of optic nerves to elevated intraocular pressure. Many individuals with elevated intraocular pressures (> 2 standard deviations above the mean) will never develop optic nerve damage. In contrast, some patients without elevated pressures develop progressive, "glaucomatous" cupping of the optic disk and visual field loss. It is not even known why high intraocular pressures cause optic nerve damage, although mounting evidence suggests that pressure-induced collapse of the structural support of the optic nerve head destroys axons by mechanical compression. Despite these considerations, it is generally correct to state that glaucoma is caused by increased intraocular pressure.

Classification

The primary glaucomas are best classified according to the clinical appearance of the anterior chamber angle. The "angle" is the intersection of the cornea, iris, and ciliary body, where the major outflow channel for aqueous humor is found.

In primary open-angle glaucoma, the increased resistance to aqueous outflow results from a microscopic abnormality of the outflow tract itself; angle structures appear normal when viewed through a gonioscope. The latter is an ophthalmologic instrument that allows visualization of the trabecular meshwork and surrounding structures by means of a special contact lens. In primary angle-closure glaucoma, increased outflow resistance is caused by physical blockage of the outflow tract by the base of the iris. This occurs only in eyes with narrow angles, in which the iris is bowed forward and the angle structures are obscured by the base of the iris or by scar tissue.

Risk Factors

Primary open-angle glaucoma is the most common type of glaucoma, comprising up to 89% of all cases. The prevalence of this disease increases with age. Few cases can be found in patients below the age of 40, whereas some studies estimate that 14% of persons over the age of 80 have the disease. Numerous studies suggest that glaucoma occurs at an earlier age and is more severe in black Americans than in white Americans. The risk of developing the disease if a first-degree relative is affected is between 4 and 16%. In addition to increasing age, black race, and family history, other apparent but less-well-established risk factors are diabetes and nearsightedness.

Primary angle-closure glaucoma is a relatively rare disease. Risk factors for the development of angle-closure glaucoma include increasing age, farsightedness, a positive family history, a history of angle-closure glaucoma in the contralateral eye, and pupillary dilation. The common denominator between all these risk factors is that they are all associated with "narrowing" of the angle.

Evaluation

Clincial Features

Primary open-angle glaucoma is a chronic disease that progresses over many years. It is usually bilateral but often asymmetric, and is asymptomatic until severe visual field loss or loss of central vision occurs. An eye with primary open-angle glaucoma outwardly looks normal. Severe loss of visual field and visual acuity due to open-angle glaucoma is irreversible, but some studies suggest that early field changes are reversible by reducing intraocular pressure.

Primary angle-closure glaucoma usually presents as an acute, symptomatic disease that can progress to severe visual loss in hours to days. The patient complains of severe eye pain, headache, nausea, or abdominal discomfort and presents with a red, painful eye, decreased vision, mid-dilated and unreactive pupil, and a hazy cornea. Many cases of angle-closure glaucoma are initially misdiagnosed as gastroenteritis or migraine. Primary angle-closure glaucoma can also present as a subacute attack characterized by mild ocular discomfort and the appearance of colored halos around streetlights, due to corneal edema.

Diagnosis

The diagnosis of open-angle glaucoma is based on finding an elevated intraocular pressure, glaucomatous changes in the optic disk, and visual field changes in the presence of an open angle. Angle-closure glaucoma is diagnosed by demonstrating elevated intraocular pressure in the presence of a closed angle.

Intraocular pressure may be measured with several different instruments, including Shiotz or applanation tonometers. As with systemic hypertension, there is no sharp delineation between normal and abnormal ocular tension. Pressures below 22 mm Hg are generally considered normal, as long as the optic nerves appear normal. Pressures in the 22- to 30-mm Hg range are regarded with suspicion, and those greater than 31 mm Hg are probably abnormal. When such elevated pressures are found, nerves and visual fields must be examined closely for abnormalities consistent with glaucoma.

The optic disk changes found in all forms of chronic glaucoma result from the death of axons. As more axons are lost, the "cup," or depression in the center of the optic nerve head, gets larger. This enlargement usually occurs in a focal pattern but can be generalized. The major changes to look for are the following: (1) asymmetric cups; (2) focal thinning of the neural rim (the nerve tissue lying between the edge of the cup and the edge of the disk itself), usually seen at the superotemporal or inferotemporal disk margin; and (3) a superficial hemorrhage overlying the edge of the disk.

The visual field defects of glaucoma usually start with small blind spots near the point of fixation. These small blind spots or scotomas gradually enlarge to involve the peripheral visual field and, finally, the central vision.

Treatment

While a clinically important elevation of intraocular pressure is due to an increased resistance to aqueous outflow rather than an overproduction of aqueous humor, glaucoma treatment is aimed at both reducing aqueous humor production and decreasing outflow resistance.

Open-angle glaucoma is treated medically unless the disease progresses despite maximal tolerated therapy. Currently, laser treatment and intraocular surgery are reserved for medical failures.

Angle-closure glaucoma is a surgical disease. Following medical treatment of the acute attack and to reverse corneal edema, a laser is used to make a hole in the peripheral iris. This almost always results in a cure. The contralateral eye is usually treated with the laser prophylactically since there is a 50% risk of having an attack in the initially uninvolved eye within 5 years.

Drug Therapy

Medications used to treat chronic glaucoma of all types generally fall into four classes: beta-blockers, cholinergics, adrenergics, and carbonic anhydrase inhibitors. The first three of these are administered topically, usually in the form of drops, whereas the carbonic anhydrase inhibitors are taken orally. Treatment is usually begun with a beta-blocker, often used twice daily. The cholinergic drugs such as pilocarpine (formerly the first-line drug of choice) require more frequent administration and induce miosis and ciliary muscle contraction which some patients find troublesome; cholinergic drugs are now usually used as a second-line drug when intraocular pressure is not adequately controlled by a beta-blocker or in patients who cannot tolerate beta-blockers. The adrenergic drugs are likewise usually used as adjunctive therapy. The carbonic anhydrase inhibitors cause side effects that limit their use in about 50% of patients, so they are usually reserved for severe, poorly responsive, chronic glaucoma or for acute elevations in pressure. While the choice and adjustment of medications are usually made by an ophthalmologist, primary care clinicians must be aware of the potential systemic side effects of these drugs. Medications given as eyedrops can be absorbed through the blood vessels of the conjunctiva and nasal mucosa in sufficient quantities to produce significant systemic effects; while they occur less frequently than reactions to the orally administered carbonic anhydrase inhibitors, reactions can be serious.

BETA-ADRENERGIC BLOCKERS. Timolol, the most commonly prescribed antiglaucoma medication, is the most commonly used of the beta-blockers. Alternative agents include betaxolol, which like timolol is used twice daily, and levobunolol, used once daily. These medications are thought to act by decreasing aqueous production. Timolol drops have been associated with fatal bronchospasm. Besides worsening of asthma or emphysema, other complications associated with beta-blockers include decompensation of congestive heart failure, cardiac conduction disturbances, and depression.

CHOLINERGIC AGENTS. Pilocarpine, the most commonly used cholinergic agent, acts by decreasing the resistance to aqueous outflow; its pressure-lowering effect is independent of the pupillary constriction it invariably induces. Although pilocarpine has a low incidence of systemic side effects, it has been associated with nausea, vomiting, diarrhea, sweating, tremor, hypotension, sinus bradycardia, and atrioventricular block. A related drug, echothiophate iodide (Phospholine Iodide), which is a cholinesterase inhibitor, can inhibit the breakdown of succinylcholine and produce markedly prolonged postoperative paralysis.

ADRENERGIC AGENTS. Epinephrine and its prodrug, dipivefrin, are the commonly used adrenergic agents. They act by decreasing outflow resistance and also by decreasing aqueous production. They may cause tachypnea, and in sufficient doses, tachycardia, hypertension, tremor, restlessness, and headache.

CARBONIC ANHYDRASE INHIBITORS. Acetazolamide (Diamox) and the newer carbonic anhydrase inhibitor methazolamide (Neptazane) reduce aqueous production. Both produce paresthesias of the hands and face in a majority of patients. They often produce a syndrome of malaise, anorexia, and severe weight loss, and can cause hypokalemia, especially when taken in conjunction with potassium-depleting diuretics. They are also associated with the development of kidney stones.

Screening for Open-Angle Glaucoma

There are currently no established guidelines for screening patients for open-angle glaucoma. None of the three components of diagnosis (elevated intraocular pressures, glaucomatous disk changes, and visual field defects) offers a simple and reliable screening test.

Although tonometry is easily performed and provides objective measurement of intraocular pressure, its sensitivity and specificity are less than 50%. Several large population studies have shown that half of all patients with known glaucoma were classified as "normal" on the basis of a single measurement of intraocular pressure, probably because intraocular pressure varies during the day and a glaucomatous eye does not always have elevated pressures. Patients with "low-tension" glaucoma have optic nerves so susceptible to pressure-induced damage that they experience progressive disk cupping and visual field loss, with pressures in the high-normal range. Furthermore, many patients with elevated intraocular pressure on random screening will have normal pressure on repeat testing. Of those patients with elevated intraocular pressure on multiple examinations, only 5% actually have glaucoma and those who do not have only a 0.5% to 1.0% chance of developing glaucoma each year.

Evaluation of the optic disk for evidence of glaucomatous cupping is a subjective test with significant interobserver variability. While this may be a useful screening test for glaucoma when carried out by experienced examiners, it is not reliable when performed by nonexpert clinicians.

Visual field testing is quite sensitive but impractical for screening, as it requires skilled technicians or very expensive computerized visual field machines to produce accurate results.

It is clearly desirable to make the diagnosis of open-angle glaucoma before it results in irreversible loss of vision, but a useful screening test for the primary care setting is not currently available. Until a better approach is worked out, it is appropriate to refer high-risk patients to an ophthalmologist for screening with a complete eye examination. High-risk patients include whites over the age of 50, blacks over the age of 40, or anyone with a family history of glaucoma in a first-degree relative.

Ocular Side Effects of Systemic Medications

In addition to the systemic side effects of glaucoma medications as discussed above, primary care clinicians must also understand the effects that systemic medications may have on glaucoma.

The only systemic medications that frequently elevate the intraocular pressure in patients with open-angle glaucoma are the corticosteroids. A high percentage of these patients demonstrate elevations of intraocular pressure in response to both systemic and topical corticosteroids. This response is usually reversible. A smaller percentage of patients without a history of glaucoma also demonstrate steroid-induced elevations of intraocular pressure. It is therefore wise to refer any patient on chronic topical or systemic steroid treatment for ophthalmic evaluation.

Many physicians worry about harming glaucoma patients by giving them systemic medications with weak adrenergic or anticholinergic side effects, such as cold medications, antidepressants, and antidiarrheals. These medications, however, are dangerous only insofar as they weakly dilate the pupil and thereby predispose to angle-closure glaucoma. They have no significant effect on the intraocular pressure in patients with open-angle glaucoma. Patients with diagnosed angle-closure glaucoma have, in all likelihood, already been treated with a laser iridotomy in both eyes and can therefore be dilated with impunity. These medications are therefore *not* contraindicated in the patient with diagnosed glaucoma.

Johnson DH, Brubaker RF. Glaucoma: an overview. Mayo Clin Proc 1986; 61:59–67.
Reviews clinical findings, diagnostic tests, and available medical, surgical, and laser treatment options.

American Academy of Ophthalmology, Quality of Care Committee Glaucoma Panel. Preferred practice pattern: primary open angle glaucoma. San Francisco: American Academy Ophthalmology, 1989.
A consensus view of the American Academy of Ophthalmology on how best to diagnose and manage patients with open-angle glaucoma, with excellent and readable discussions on definition, diagnosis, rationale for treatment, and screening. It may be obtained without charge by writing to The American Academy of Ophthalmology, P.O. Box 7424, San Francisco, CA 94120-7424.

Shields MB. Textbook of glaucoma. 2nd ed. Baltimore: Williams & Wilkins, 1987.
An eminently readable, comprehensive, and well-referenced textbook that is a favorite of ophthalmology residents and suitable for the nonophthalmic physician as well. The sections on angle-closure glaucoma and glaucoma medications are particularly useful.

Anderson DR. Glaucoma: the damage caused by pressure. XLVI Edward Jackson Memorial Lecture. Am J Ophthalmol 1989; 108:485–95.
A thoughtful discussion, emphasizing that the damage produced, rather than the pressure, is the important feature of the disease.

Margolis KL, Rich EC. Open-angle glaucoma. Prim Care 1989; 16:197–209.
Includes both diagrams and photographs illustrating the process of cupping, and a review of screening methods, from a primary care perspective.

Capino DG, Leibowitz HM. Glaucoma: screening, diagnosis, and therapy. Hosp Pract May 30, 1990; 25(5A):73–91.
Reviews physiology, diagnosis, and treatment, with diagrams of aqueous humor flow and funduscopic photographs of cupping.

Everitt DE, Avorn J. Systemic effects of medications used to treat glaucoma. Ann Intern Med 1990; 112:120–5.
A helpful discussion and literature review on the systemic effects of glaucoma medications.

Leske MC. The epidemiology of open angle glaucoma: a review. Am J Epidemiol 1983; 118:166–91.
An excellent, comprehensive review of the epidemiology of primary open-angle glaucoma, discussing definitions, incidence, prevalence, risk factors, and public health impact.

Mason RP, et al. National survey of the prevalence and risk factors of glaucoma in St. Lucia, West Indies. Ophthalmology 1989; 96:1363–8.
One of the only population-based epidemiology studies of glaucoma in a black population; it demonstrates a prevalence rate of 8.8% for individuals 30 years or older, significantly higher than the rate of 1.9% in the predominantly white, over 50, population of Framingham, Mass.

11. VISUAL IMPAIRMENT
Hunter R. Stokes

The measurement of visual acuity is the most important and revealing test of ocular function. It is appropriate for primary care physicians to check distance acuity in their offices. Careful measurements of the visual acuity should be recorded for all patients with ocular and facial trauma. Besides establishing visual acuity at the time of the accident, this data will prove to be extremely valuable in assessing progression of the injury and in determining treatment.

Patients whose visual acuity must be measured for the purpose of jobs, legal blindness and disability determinations, military induction, and medicolegal cases should be referred to an ophthalmologist. Often these requests for vision examination require documentation of distance and near vision with and without correction, visual field measurement, and sometimes a refraction. While legal blindness is usually described as vision of 20/200 or less, other factors, such as the field of vision and the degree of ocular motility (including the presence or absence of diplopia), are often a part of the formula necessary to make the final determination.

The most common causes of visual impairment include hereditary defects in people under the age of 20, diabetic retinopathy in those 21 to 60 years old, and macular degeneration in those over 60. Cataracts are a common cause of visual impairment, and are present to some degree in most patients over 70, but most cataracts are operated on when significant impairment occurs. (See Chap. 9.)

Evaluation

Vision Testing

DISTANCE VISION. The major component of the office visual acuity examination is testing of distance vision. A hallway is sufficient for testing if the proper distance (20 ft) and lighting are available. In addition to the usual Snellen chart, charts should be available for children and the illiterate (E chart). The examiner should measure vision in patients with acuity less than 20/200 by recording finger counting (CF) at various distances (e.g., CF 1 ft, CF 6 in.), hand movements (HM), light perception (LP), or total blindness (no light perception [NLP]). Improvement of vision by a pinhole is objective evidence of myopia in preteens and teenagers.

NEAR VISION. The measurement of near vision is not as important as the measurement of distance acuity and need not be measured by primary care physicians. Children and young adults usually have good near vision, and refractive errors (especially myopia) affect distance vision more than near vision. After the age of 40, all patients begin to develop presbyopia and cannot see "up close" as well as before.

COLOR VISION. Six percent of males have some degree of color blindness or at least a red and green deficiency. Rarely is color blindness associated with other ocular problems. The only limitations for color-deficient people are certain color-related jobs (interior design, clothing sales, and airplane piloting) and appointments to the military academies. Poor color vision is not considered a disability.

Intraocular Pressure Measurements

Two percent of Americans over the age of 40 have chronic open-angle glaucoma, a disease that leads to elevated intraocular pressures and blindness if it is not diagnosed and treated. Primary care physicians can measure intraocular pressure with a Schiotz tonometer; this is not accurate as a screening test, however, and patients at increased risk for glaucoma should be referred for ophthalmologic examination (See Chap. 10).

Refraction

A refraction measures the optical error of the eyes and determines the corrective lenses that are necessary for the best vision. A refraction is indicated whenever the vision drops, both in patients who wear glasses and in those who do not. It is not uncommon for young people who are nearsighted (myopic) to require a change in glasses every year from age 9 or 10 to age 15 or 16. Optometrists as well as ophthalmologists are trained to perform refractions, and patients whose eyes are otherwise healthy can appropriately be refracted by optometrists. A refraction in isolation, however, represents only a portion of a comprehensive ophthalmologic examination; in some circumstances, examination of the entire visual system is needed to evaluate the eyes for any ocular manifestations of systemic disease. Children from birth to age 6 and adults over 50 have the highest incidence of disease and generally should see an ophthalmologist.

Methods to Correct Refractive Errors

Spectacles

Refractive errors are most commonly corrected by glasses. Modern frames are sufficiently attractive and durable so that most patients including children are more or less willing to wear them. Lenses may be glass or plastic; the plastic lenses, which are now more scratch-resistant and can be tinted, have become much more popular.

Most patients over 40 require correction for near vision ("presbyopia"); this can be accomplished with either full or half glasses or with bifocals. Bifocals have distance correction in the top and near correction in the bottom (bifocal segment). Graduated or invisible bifocals eliminate the image jump that bothers some patients. The absence of a line in the lenses also allows patients in their early 40s to camouflage the need of bifocals. The disadvantages of the graduated bifocals are the additional costs and the slightly smaller field of vision available for near vision.

Contact Lenses

The original hard contact lenses were relatively inexpensive and quite durable. But because they were not permeable to oxygen, they were uncomfortable to many wearers and could be worn only for a very limited time. Recently, available rigid gas-permeable lenses have most of the optical properties of the older hard lenses and much of the comfort features of the soft lenses.

Soft contact lenses are made of a hydrophilic plastic material that is oxygen-permeable. They are quite comfortable and can be worn longer than hard lenses. The most gas-permeable of these soft lenses are marketed as extended-wear lenses and previously were advertised as "30-day wear" lenses. In 1989, a study demonstrated a much higher incidence of corneal ulcer when extended-wear lenses were worn for more than 7 days, so removal of the lenses at least once a week is encouraged. Disposable soft contact lenses are advertised to be worn for 7 days and then discarded. They were developed to reduce the risk of corneal ulcers, to reduce the damage of soft lenses by deposit buildup, and to make the care of contact lenses easier by eliminating the need for various solutions in contact lens maintenance. This system is more expensive as many lenses are needed each year. There are dangers: Corneal ulcers have been reported and there is always a temptation to wear the lenses for longer than 1 week, increasing the risk of complications.

Special Problems

Diabetes Mellitus

Patients with diabetes mellitus are at increased risk for ocular problems. Transient myopia with reduction in distance visual acuity is induced by hyperglycemia. Cataracts occur earlier than in nondiabetics and with twice the incidence; moreover, the complication rate with cataract surgery is four to five times greater. Chronic simple glaucoma occurs three times more often, and other forms of glaucoma occur more frequently and with greater severity. The retinopathy of diabetes mellitus is the fastest rising cause of severe visual impairment and occurs as a function of the duration of the disease.

All diabetics noted to have neovascularities and microaneurysms should be referred immediately to an ophthalmologist for a complete evaluation. Because primary care physicians can easily miss eye findings, early referral for a complete ophthalmologic examination is appropriate. At a minimum, all insulin-dependent diabetics should be referred to an ophthalmologist after they have had the disease for 10 years, and thereafter should be seen at least annually. The ophthalmologic examination sometimes includes an intravenous fluorescein angiogram to study the dynamics of the retinal circulation. This examination should identify those patients who may benefit from laser treatment. During the past decade, lasers have reduced the number of diabetics who eventually become blind from proliferative retinopathy.

Floaters

Patients who complain of a "skim over the eyes" are often having visual disturbances from an uncorrected or undercorrected refractive error. However, the presence of floaters is a common complaint among patients over the age of 35 and is often associated with detachment of the vitreous base; this is not a serious problem and is infrequently associated with detachment of the retina or an intraocular hemorrhage. This differentiation can only be made by an ophthalmologist. All patients who suddenly develop new or additional floaters need ophthalmologic evaluation. This is particularly important in patients who have a higher likelihood of retinal problems associated with the floaters, including very nearsighted patients, diabetics (especially insulin-dependent, long-standing diabetics, and those with significant retinopathy), and those with a previous history of retinal disorders.

Acute Vision Loss

The primary care physician may be the first consulted when acute vision loss occurs. In most cases, evaluation by an ophthalmologist is indicated. If the patient has known medical problems such as diabetes mellitus, hypertension, cardiac arrhythmias, or carotid insufficiency, the ophthalmologist can best evaluate the fundus findings while the primary care physician manages or arranges management of the medical condition.

Sudden loss of vision with pain has many causes, including glaucoma, iritis, corneal ulcer, and temporal arteritis. Temporal arteritis usually occurs in patients over 60 years old; although retinopathy and temporal pain are usually noted, it may present as sudden, painless blindness with a normal fundus. Rapid identification and treatment of this condition are essential, because up to 50% of patients may go blind in the other eye in 1 to 2 weeks without systemic steroid treatment. Optic neuritis causes sudden vision loss, with or without pain, and in young adults is often the first sign of multiple sclerosis. The disk is usually swollen and this must be differentiated from papilledema. The ophthalmologist can evaluate the fundus, obtain visual fields, and then refer the patient to a neurologist if indicated.

Retinal detachment often presents as a sudden painless loss of vision. Ocular tumors (e.g., malignant melanomas in adults) may present as sudden vision loss if the tumor suddenly extends into the visual axis or involves the macular region.

Amaurosis fugax, "fleeting blindness," is sudden painless, unilateral blindness, with the vision returning to normal in minutes. Frequently, the problem is embolic disease from an atheromatous lesion of the ipsilateral internal carotid artery. If the embolus lodges in the central retinal artery just behind the disk, all blood flow to the retina is blocked; the clinical picture includes "box-carring" of both arteries and veins on funduscopic examination, and a "cherry red spot" in the macula due to edema throughout the retina, with the macula region being spared. If the embolus passes into the eye and is lodged in the main central retinal artery on the disk, then it may be visible. Often, the embolus fragments and sticks at bifurcations of more peripheral arterioles, and is visible as "Hollenhorst plaques"—glistening orange-yellow flakes. The risk of blockage and vision loss is much less if the embolus travels toward the retinal periphery. It is essential that these patients be evaluated for neck bruits and have ophthalmodynamometry performed by the ophthalmologist, to measure the pressures in the retinal arteries. Doppler studies, pneumoplethysmography, and arteriography may also be required to define the lesions.

Unless there is a typical associated finding, that is, hemiplegia with sudden vision loss or severe headache, projectile vomiting, and sudden vision loss, patients with acute vision loss should first be seen by the ophthalmologist, although definitive care by another specialist (neurologist, neurosurgeon, vascular surgeon) may also be needed.

Low Vision

As the population in the United States continues to age and as medical care allows patients with many diseases to have a significantly extended life expectancy, many people, especially older citizens, ultimately have a significant loss of vision in one or both eyes. There are approximately 500,000 legally blind people in the United States; about 50,000 become legally blind annually.

Each state has one or more agencies which assist visually handicapped people. Services include large-print books, books on tape, special glasses, projection screens, special radios, mobility training, and "seeing-eye dogs." Also in each state there are programs to assist the visually handicapped who are still in school. Although any ophthalmologist or optometrist can provide information on these programs, "low-vision specialists" are particularly skilled in training patients to maximize any remaining vision.

When a patient presents with a chronic problem of low vision, the primary physician should perform a comprehensive, ophthalmologic examination to identify problems that may be treated, and see that referral is made for low-vision services.

Fonda G. Management of the patient with subnormal vision. 2nd ed. St Louis: Mosby, 1970:3–5.
Excellent reference on the causes of poor vision as defined by age groups.

Faye EE. Clinical low vision. 2nd ed. Boston: Little, Brown, 1984.
The essential reference on low vision, written by the medical director of the Lighthouse for the Blind in New York City.

Grey RHB, et al. Ophthalmic survey of a diabetic clinic: I—ocular findings, II—requirements for treatment of retinopathy. Br J Ophthalmol 1986; 70:797–803, 804–7.
Two excellent articles providing general guidance to primary care physicians on the diagnosis and treatment of ocular findings in diabetes mellitus.

Vaughn D, Asbury T, Tabbara K. General ophthalmology. 12th ed. Norwalk, Conn: Appleton and Lange, 1989.
An excellent general text, updated every 3 years, with discussions on many of the issues included in this chapter.

Contact lenses: what to consider. Consumer Rep 1989; 54:411–5.
A review that is helpful to both laymen and professionals.

Mertz PD, et al. Corneal infiltrates associated with disposable extended wear soft contact lenses: a report of nine cases. CLAO J 1990; 16:269–72.
Describes complications with the lenses previously presumed to be the safest, with a good discussion of the complications related to various types of contact lenses.

III. EAR PROBLEMS

12. DEAFNESS AND TINNITUS
James P. Browder

Hearing loss is a complaint at the extremes of life; most adults spend their middle years relatively unperturbed by disorders of hearing. In primary care practices acute deafness is rarely a presenting complaint; much more frequently chronic deafness is discovered during the evaluation for other complaints. In fact, losses acquired during the perinatal period can go undetected for years if they are relatively mild or unilateral. Rarely does acute or chronic presentation signal a life-threatening condition, such as an acoustic tumor; however, neither should be treated as trivial.

Evaluation

History
The major questions to be answered when confronted with deafness are: Is the condition treatable? Is it a manifestation of a serious underlying disease? Is the deafness interfering with daily activities? The history should consider whether the hearing loss is acute or chronic; whether only one or both ears are affected; whether the hearing loss is stable, progressive, or episodic since onset; and whether pain, otorrhea, or vertigo is present. Exposure to ototoxic drugs, such as aspirin and caffeine as well as antibiotics (aminoglycosides, streptomycin, vancomycin, erythromycin, or chloramphenicol), diuretics (ethacrynic acid, furosemide), salicylates, quinine, or antineoplastic drugs (cisplatin, vinca alkaloids, nitrogen mustard), should be considered. A history of congenital or progressive hearing loss in younger members of the family or significant deafness in older ones should be elicited, as should work exposure to high levels of noise.

Physical Examination
Abnormalities may be found in the external ear or the canal, but the presence of a normal tympanic membrane and external auditory canal does not eliminate significant middle and/or inner ear pathology.

Pneumatic otoscopy is useful to indicate membrane compliance, but only if movement of the membrane can be demonstrated. Lack of movement may indicate a stiff membrane or middle ear fluid, or only a poor fit of the instrument in the ear canal. Confirmation of a nonmoving membrane is best accomplished, if necessary, with tympanometry.

Assessment of the Eighth Cranial Nerve Function
The whispered voice is the best clinical test of hearing and should be done with the patient using a finger to occlude the opposite ear to prevent crossover. A person with normal hearing should be able to respond appropriately to simple questions directed at the test ear, spoken at a level that can be barely heard by the examiner. Ticking watches, snapping fingers, and other similar sounds are too narrow and poorly controlled auditory stimuli.

Tuning forks are of limited clinical value. The 256- and 512-Hz (but *not* the 128-Hz) forks can be used to discriminate between mild and moderately severe conductive losses when comparing ipsilateral bone and air conduction (Rinne test). Tuning forks are most useful in following patients with known unilateral conductive loss and are less helpful in evaluating new hearing loss or in losses that are bilateral or complex (mixed conductive and sensorineural).

Causes of Deafness
Deafness can be categorized as conductive deafness or sensorineural deafness, each occurring in particular age groups and with typical findings. In the young, hearing loss is most often conductive in origin and acute in onset; in the elderly, hearing loss is most often chronic sensorineural deafness and frequently accompanied by tinnitus.

Conductive Hearing Loss
Conductive hearing loss is the most common cause of hearing loss and is usually secondary to a middle ear effusion resulting from a eustachian tube malfunction. This may follow

an upper respiratory tract infection, allergy, or less commonly, nasopharyngeal tumor, cleft palate, or trauma. Other causes are otosclerosis, fixation of the ossicles, or cholesteatoma.

Sensorineural Hearing Loss

Sensorineural hearing loss (SNHL) is most commonly seen in older people as a consequence of aging. Uncommon causes include Meniere's disease, ototoxic drug exposure, acoustic tumors, congenital deafness, childhood viral illness (e.g., mumps), and trauma.

Presentation of Deafness

Acute Deafness

The causes of acute deafness may be found anywhere from the external ear to the central nervous system. Wax in the external ear canal decreases hearing, but only if it completely occludes the canal or impedes the movement of the tympanic membrane. Acute deafness that results from problems of the middle ear is usually associated with trauma to the head or to barotrauma incurred during rapid descent in the air or under water or with physical straining. Infections of the middle ear (otitis media) can present as acute deafness especially in children; in adults infection is usually an exacerbation of a chronic middle ear problem. Fever, elevated white bood cell count, periauricular inflammation, diabetes, and vertigo are all signs of infection that may indicate mastoiditis or spread to the meninges. Any of these associated findings may indicate the need for parenteral antibiotics and ear-nose-throat (ENT) consultation. Serous otitis media that leads to deafness is most often associated with an upper respiratory tract infection or acute allergic reaction. Serous otitis media in an adult that is insidious in onset and fails to respond to therapy suggests a lesion in the nasopharynx.

Acute hearing loss is usually accompanied by a straightforward history and a diagnostic physical examination. However, acute unilateral hearing loss unassociated with trauma or other obvious causes can occur. If there is no history of antecedent trauma or straining, otoscopic findings are normal, and audiometry reveals moderate-to-severe sensorineural deafness, the cause is presumed to be vascular or viral and confined to the inner ear. Vertigo, tinnitus, and/or pain usually indicate a poorer prognosis for recovery of hearing. Some observers have reported the associated finding of subtle, multiple cranial nerve defects, indicating a polyneuropathy, probably viral.

Functional Hearing Loss

Occasionally an acute hearing loss develops during adolescence or in association with an affective disorder, but in the absence of other organic symptoms. This form of deafness is thought to be of functional origin. Comparison between pure tone reception and speech reception thresholds may be used to distinguish functional from organic causes of deafness.

Subacute/Chronic Deafness

Subacute/chronic deafness occasionally may be caused by a lesion of the external canal such as long-term buildup of wax, or of the surrounding bones such as a carcinoma or osteoma. More frequently, the problems reside in the middle or inner ear. The hallmark of chronic deafness from the middle ear is a conductive hearing loss demonstrable by testing with a tuning fork or audiometry. Causes of chronic deafness found in the middle ear may be classified according to the appearance of the canal and tympanic membrane. Patients with both a normal canal and membrane usually have chronic deafness from otosclerosis or an ossicular discontinuity. Otosclerosis is the end result of osteitis of unknown cause that involves the oval window and produces ankylosis of the stapes footplate. Ossicular discontinuity is a disruption of the ossicular chain, most often caused by trauma, chronic infection, or occasionally otosclerosis. Tympanometry may help to differentiate between these two problems.

A normal canal with an abnormal membrane usually suggests a chronic otitis media due to chronic effusion of the middle ear. This presents as a painless hearing loss accompanied by a feeling of fullness in the ear. From the relatively reversible secretory phase, it can progress to chronic purulent otitis media, and less commonly to adhesive otitis media. The early phase of secretory otitis media represents a chronic effusion usually indicative of eustachian tube malfunction from causes that include infection, allergy, or other problems such as cleft palate or neoplasia. In secretory otitis media the tympanic membrane is dull, amber or dark-colored, and often retracted. Conductive hearing loss presents with an immobile membrane seen on pneumatic otoscopy or a characteristic tympanogram pattern found on audiometry. Diagnosis and treatment of the secretory phase are crucial if permanent middle ear damage is to be avoided; patients who do not respond symptomatically or with improved hearing may be referred to an ENT specialist. Adhesive otitis media, an uncommon late sequela of untreated secretory otitis media, represents the fibrous organization of a chronic effusion that remained sterile. The membrane is typically opaque, off-white, minimally retracted, and immobile. Adhesive disease is associated with a complete hearing loss (45–55 dB), as opposed to secretory otitis media, which usually is associated with conductive hearing loss of 30 dB or less.

Problems in the inner ear occur primarily in older patients. Sensorineural deafness most commonly is a manifestation of chronic hair cell loss thought to be caused by repeated exposure to noise and/or impaired blood supply to the cochlea.

Specific Hearing Loss Syndromes

Presbycusis often associated with tinnitus occurs as a slowly progressive sensorineural hearing loss in persons over 65 years old. There is recruitment (abnormal hypersensitivity to noise) and a decrease in speech discrimination (poor understanding of speech even when spoken loudly enough). Often patients who do not think their hearing is impaired are brought in by their families. Demonstration of these characteristics by audiometry and acoustic reflex testing is sufficient to make the diagnosis.

Noise-induced hearing loss can occur from exposure in the workplace (e.g., textile mills) or during recreational activities (e.g., firearms, rock concerts). Early in the disease there is an isolated pure tone loss at 4000 Hz in one or both ears; pure tone loss progresses to other frequencies with repeated exposures. Patients with abnormal findings on screening audiometry should be referred to an ENT specialist.

Acoustic neuroma, if large, may be associated with definite, often multiple, cranial nerve deficits, but small tumors may present with subtle changes in hearing or a recent onset of tinnitus. Because early detection carries a significantly higher success rate with much less morbidity, anyone who has significant tinnitus lasting longer than a month, unilateral unexplained hearing loss, or any persistent unilateral hearing complaint without clear cause deserves audiometric assessment that includes acoustic reflex testing and, if needed, auditory brainstem reflex (ABR) testing.

Meniere's disease is associated with the triad of fluctuating sensorineural hearing loss, episodic vertigo, and roaring tinnitus which is diagnostic of this condition; vertigo is usually the most prominent and troublesome symptom. For a more complete discussion of the evaluation and management of the patient with Meniere's disease, see Chapter 1.

Referral

Referral to an otolaryngologist is appropriate for anyone with acute deafness for whom there is not an apparent diagnosis or for those with an apparent treatable acute or chronic cause but continued deafness after appropriate treatment. Referral to an *audiologist* is usually appropriate for patients with chronic deficits in whom a hearing device is being considered. These patients usually require other tests, listed below, to determine the level of injury or whether a hearing aid is appropriate.

Speech reception threshold (SRT) is the level at which 50% of speech is intelligible. Significant discrepancy between speech and pure tone reception (a measure of sensitivity) suggests poor compliance or malingering, particularly if speech thresholds are much higher than pure tones.

Speech discrimination (SD) scores are an assessment of speech comprehension rather than threshold. SD levels less than 85 to 90% are considered abnormal. Levels below 50% severely compromise comprehension, making amplification merely the delivery of noise and not useful to the patient.

Tympanometry provides an indirect, objective measurement of the tympanic membrane and/or ossicular stiffness, and is recorded as a pressure-versus-compliance curve. A tympanogram is indicated when audiometry shows a conductive loss but a diagnosis is not apparent on clinical examination. Specific patterns may discriminate between otosclerosis, middle ear effusion, or eustachian tube dysfunction.

Auditory Aids

Hearing Aids

Hearing aids are the most widely used form of auditory rehabilitation. Whether or not someone can benefit from a hearing aid, particularly in the presence of other disabilities or advanced age, is a judgment based on several factors. First, the patient must have sufficient speech discrimination to understand what is amplified. A patient who is able to comprehend less than half of what is said, even though the sound is amplified, will find a hearing aid more a source of frustration than a benefit. Second, the patient must also have a sufficiently wide dynamic range. With SNHL, the threshold of discomfort from loud sounds is often lowered. Hearing aids may thus be limited in their ability to produce sounds loud enough to be heard but not so loud that they cause pain. An assessment of the limitations and capabilities of the wearer to adapt to the device over time is necessary. Vendors who are willing to sell an aid without such an assessment and without a prepurchase trial period should be avoided. Good practice requires that the patient be allowed to rent the device for a moderate fee for a trial at home and at work for at least 1 month, and that appropriate servicing and a limited warranty be available. Which of the many types of hearing aids is best suited for any given individual is a judgment best made jointly by a professionally trained and certified audiologist and the prospective wearer.

Other Devices

A variety of inexpensive auditory amplifiers are also available and should be considered for those who could benefit from amplification but who lack the manual dexterity to use a standard aid or whose need for amplification is limited. Such devices include: telephone receiver amplifier, radio and television earphones, and stereophonic headphones. Electronic retail outlets market a device much like a "Walkman" that is inexpensive and simple to use.

Cochlear Implants

Cochlear implantation of a device to stimulate the eighth cranial nerve directly can provide sound awareness for those with complete deafness, whether acquired before or after learning to speak. The device must be implanted surgically and requires an intensive period of postimplantation therapy to be successfully used.

Tinnitus

All cases of atypical tinnitus in which the cause is not immediately apparent should be referred to an otolaryngologist for audiometric evaluation and a thorough head and neck examination.

"Garden Variety" Tinnitus

A high-pitched ringing sound localized to one ear and of varying degrees of intensity and duration is an exceedingly common occurrence in the general population. It may be associated with ototoxic drug exposure, especially aspirin. Occasionally, tinnitus of this nature can be so disturbing that a physician is consulted. Unfortunately, no effective treatment exists except for discontinuing any ototoxic drugs. Because the symptom is most disturbing at night, a soft, monotonous noise, such as a fan or radio, may help mask the tinnitus. Some patients with mild SNHL and tinnitus may benefit from a hearing aid that is used not so much to amplify what is heard as to provide a source of external background noise to mask the tinnitus. In every case where a patient's primary complaint is tinnitus, an audiogram should be obtained, since tinnitus may signal the onset of progressive deafness or acoustic tumor.

Roaring Tinnitus

Roaring tinnitus, especially if linked with hearing loss and/or vertigo, suggests Meniere's syndrome.

Pulsatile Tinnitus

Pulsatile tinnitus may accompany a middle ear effusion or may represent a transmitted sound from a cardiac murmur or cervical bruit. It may also be an early sign of increased intracranial pressure. If the tinnitus can be shown to be in synchrony with the heartbeat, careful auscultation of the heart, cervical vessels, eyes, and the mastoid and parietal areas of the skull may reveal a bruit signaling a cardiovascular anomaly, an aneurysm or fistula, or an arteriovenous malformation. A CT scan of the head is mandatory for patients with persistent pulsatile tinnitus without clear cause.

Fluttering Tinnitus
Fluttering tinnitus may be caused by intermittent spasm of the tensor tympani muscle or even the presence of an insect in the external auditory canal. Tympanometry is helpful in documenting the former condition. Tensor tympani spasm is normally associated with an acute eye irritation, by a reflex phenomenon, or it may be a manifestation of acute anxiety.

Clicking Tinnitus
Clicking tinnitus is the hallmark of palatal myoclonus. This is a disorder of uncertain etiology that responds to mild sedation. The diagnosis is confirmed by observing a rapid, rhythmic twitching of the ipsilateral palate while the tinnitus is present.

Crunching Tinnitus
Crunching tinnitus in association with chewing may represent temporomandibular joint arthritis or a foreign body, such as a hair in the external auditory canal that rubs against the tympanic membrane.

Glassock ME, ed. Sensorineural deafness. Otolaryngol Clin North Am 1978; 11(1).
Over 25 articles by an international panel covering in depth such topics as noise-induced hearing loss, sudden hearing loss, cochlear otospongiosis (otosclerosis), hearing aids, and cochlear implants.

Page JM, ed. Audiology. Otolaryngol Clin North Am 1978; 11(3).
A complete discussion in a number of articles of contemporary audiometric evaluation including testing for central auditory dysfunction, brain stem–evoked response audiometry, impedance testing (tympanometry), and evaluation for hearing aids.

Arenberg IK, Meniere's disease. Otolaryngol Clin North Am 1980; 13(4).
A thorough presentation of both the known and the problematic concerning the pathophysiology, diagnosis/staging, and treatment of Meniere's disease.

Ryback LP. Drug ototoxicity. Annu Rev Pharmacol Toxicol 1986; 7:29–55.
A review of the therapeutic agents most likely to cause hearing loss in humans. Includes a review of the anatomy and physiology of the auditory periphery and a discussion of the morphologic changes, pharmacokinetic studies, physiologic effects, and possible mechanisms of ototoxicity for each class of drug reviewed.

Coles RRA, Hallam RS. Tinnitus and its management. Br Med Bull 1987; 43:983–98.
A discussion of the types of tinnitus, its measurement, and management, with particular emphasis on psychological therapy and tinnitus masking.

Levine SB, Snow JB Jr. Pulsatile tinnitus. Laryngoscope 1987; 97:401–6.
A thorough review with case reports of a rare but usually treatable condition that may herald significant intra- and extracranial disease.

Marion MS, Cevette MJ. Tinnitus. Mayo Clinic Proceedings 1991; 66(6):614–20.
A concise review of types of tinnitus.

13. OTITIS EXTERNA
Marion Danis

Otitis externa is an inflammation of the skin of the auricle and external auditory canal. It is most commonly caused by bacterial infection; fungal and herpetic infections occur considerably less frequently. Diffuse infectious otitis is five times more common in swimmers than in nonswimmers and occurs with greater frequency in hot, humid climates because of the macerating effect of water on the epithelium of the external auditory canal. Other causes of otitis externa include allergic reactions such as contact or eczematoid dermatoses, generalized skin conditions such as psoriasis or seborrhea, and trauma or irritation from foreign bodies such as cotton swabs, matchsticks, hairpins, or earplugs.

Clinical Presentation
Ear pain is the presenting complaint in approximately 85% of patients with otitis externa, and varies in severity from slight discomfort that is difficult to distinguish from itching, to excruciating aching or throbbing. The severity of pain is due to the direct attachment of the skin of the external ear to the periosteum and perichondrium, so that edema of the dermis compresses nerve fibers against the cartilage or bone. Any movement of the auricle, such as chewing, can be painful. Itching is present in two-thirds of patients and often precedes the pain. If the condition becomes chronic, itching is often the chief complaint. Conductive hearing loss may occur from occlusion of the lumen of the external auditory canal by edema, secretions, cerumen, or other debris.

Physical findings classically include erythema and edema of the skin of the auditory canal, a greenish-tinged discharge, and pain on manipulating the auricle. Regional lymph node enlargement and tenderness may be present. Involvement of both ears occurs almost 20% of the time.

Differential Diagnosis

Otitis Media

When the lumen of the external auditory canal is obliterated by pus and debris, it becomes difficult to differentiate otitis externa from otitis media, particularly if the latter is chronic otitis media with perforation and drainage. Table 13-1 presents some clinical features that are useful in making the distinction. Cultures may be warranted in rare instances where differentiation of otitis externa from otitis media is unusually difficult; the different spectrum of organisms seen in the two conditions may help to distinguish between them. Organisms seen in diffuse otitis externa, listed in order of decreasing prevalence, are *Pseudomonas* species, *Staphylococcus aureus*, *Proteus*, *Escherichia coli*, anaerobes, and a few less common organisms. The organisms that cause otitis media are those usually seen in respiratory tract infections, such as pneumococci, *Hemophilus influenzae*, and group A beta streptococcus.

Localized Otitis Externa

A staphylococcal folliculitis may, in its early stages, present as a diffuse red swelling of the ear canal. Exquisite tenderness on manipulation of the auricle may suggest the presence of a furuncle; occasionally the accompanying swelling is so severe that the canal is obliterated and visualization of the furuncle is difficult. Spontaneous rupture of the furuncle is followed by marked relief of pain; purulent drainage may also be seen.

Other Infectious Causes

Fungal infections of the external ear are not common and usually occur in extremely moist, hot climates or when the external ear has been a site of chronic bacterial infection. Itching is often a more prominent symptom than pain. Typically responsible are the saprophytes, opportunists that colonize the skin (e.g., *Aspergillus*, *Actinomyces*), and superficial pathogenic fungi (e.g., *Candida*, *Trichophyton* species). If a patient has had a protracted case of otitis externa, then a fungal infection might be suspected. The diagnosis may be supported by observation of fungal hyphae on a 10% potassium hydroxide slide preparation of scrapings and confirmed by culture on Sabouraud medium.

Table 13-1. Clinical features of acute diffuse otitis externa and acute otitis media

Feature	Otitis externa	Otitis media
Pain	Aggravated by moving jaw, manipulating auricle	Aggravated by swallowing, belching
Tenderness	Prominent	Absent
Systemic symptoms	Usually absent	Fever, rhinitis, sore throat
Regional lymphadenopathy	Often present	Usually absent
Swelling of ear canal	Prominent	Absent
Discharge	Not profuse; may be malodorous	Occurs with tympanic perforation
Tympanic membrane	Normal or inflamed, but intact; no middle ear fluid	May be perforated; fluid in middle ear

Mycobacterial infections of the ear are extremely rare and need only be considered when chronic granulomatous and ulcerative lesions occur in the ear canal. *Myocoplasma* infections involving the ear can cause bullous lesions on the tympanic membrane, as can viral infections. Herpes simplex and herpes zoster can affect the external ear and present with typical vesicles.

Noninfectious Inflammatory Reactions
Contact dermatitis of the external ear can result from exposure to irritating substances or a reaction to allergens such as poison ivy, cosmetics, and nickel and rubber compounds. Patients with inflammation of the external ear should be asked about any exposure to hair sprays, shampoos, soaps, dyes, earrings, or local medication (particularly those containing neomycin) and use of foreign objects in the ear such as hairpins, matches, earplugs, and headphones.

Seborrhea, psoriasis, and eczematoid dermatoses may involve the external ear; the presence of characteristic lesions elsewhere on the skin, particularly the scalp, assists the diagnosis.

The ear is a favorite site of itching and scratching, and neurodermatitis should be considered once other conditions are ruled out. In early cases, erythema, edema, vesiculations, and crusting may occur, leading to dry, thickened, lichenified skin; these findings are difficult to distinguish morphologically from those due to other causes.

Other Causes of Ear Pain
Pain in the ear due to impacted cerumen or a foreign body should be excluded. When the external ear canal and tympanic membrane appear normal, pain due to parotitis, periauricular adenitis, mastoiditis, dental caries, temporomandibular joint dysfunction, and pharyngitis should be considered.

Treatment
Diffuse otitis externa should be treated with a topical antimicrobial agent until symptoms and signs are resolved. If the ear canal is not occluded, an otic solution can be applied three times a day, using the following technique: The patient should lie down with the affected ear upward, and the auricle should be pulled up and back to straighten the canal while the solution is instilled. This position should be maintained for 1 or 2 minutes. Although combined antibiotic and steroid preparations (e.g., Cortisporin Otic) are often used, controlled trials have shown equivalent results using preparations of 2% acetic acid solution. These are available commercially as either an aqueous acetic acid solution (Otic Domeboro) or propylene glycol solution of acetic acid (Vosol, Orlex). A 1:1 mixture of clear white vinegar (5% acetic acid) and rubbing alcohol is less expensive and probably as effective. External otitis caused by fungal infection also usually responds to the above-

mentioned acetic acid solutions. Persistent otomycosis will respond to tolnaftate drops (Tinactin) unless it is a reflection of a systemic fungal infection.

Topical antibiotic mixtures are indicated when the tympanic membrane is perforated, because the entry of acetic acid and alcohol into the middle ear can cause stinging and burning. Cortisporin suspension, because of its higher pH, may be less irritating than the solution. Corticosteroid-containing otic preparations are also useful for coexisting dermatoses.

If the canal is at all occluded, a wick should be inserted in the external canal. Cotton, gauze, or compressed hydroxycellulose, available commercially as Otowick, may be used. The latter is a stiff, expandable wick that can be inserted into the inflamed canal more easily and with less pain. The wick should be kept moist with the solution, thus ensuring continuous application to the inflamed tissue and preventing the drops from simply rolling out of the canal.

Cleaning the ear canal is often very difficult and is not necessary unless accumulated secretions or debris prevent contact with the otic solution. Very gentle suctioning, if available, or irrigation with an acetic acid solution (e.g., 1:1 dilution of clear white vinegar with saline solution, water, or rubbing alcohol) are appropriate techniques.

Oral analgesic medication should be prescribed for the first 24 to 48 hours. Topical analgesics are ineffective. Severe itching that is not relieved by application of otic solution may respond to an oral antihistamine.

Localized otitis externa should be treated like any other localized staphylococcal skin infection, with warm compresses and observation. Most furuncles resolve spontaneously, but incision and drainage are sometimes necessary. Inflammation of the surrounding tissue, fever, and lymphadenopathy are indications for oral antibiotics. A penicillinase-resistant drug such as dicloxacillin is usually used.

Mycoplasma infections of the ear need not be treated with erythromycin since it is difficult to distinguish *Mycoplasma* infections from viral infections and because there is little evidence that antibiotics alter the course of nonrespiratory symptoms of *Mycoplasma* infections. The bullae may be lanced to relieve pain.

Prevention of otitis externa can be accomplished in individuals who have repeated attacks, by administering one of the acetic acid solutions described above or aluminum acetate (Burow's solution) daily, and particularly after swimming. Bathing caps and earplugs do not prevent infection.

Malignant Otitis Externa

The most serious complication of otitis externa is a spreading *Pseudomonas* infection, which occurs primarily in elderly diabetic patients, and has a reported 20% mortality rate. Characteristic features include severe, unrelenting ear pain, persistent discharge, and a markedly elevated erythrocyte sedimentation rate. Cranial neuropathies may develop. Any elderly, diabetic, or immunocompromised patient with otitis externa should be observed carefully for this complication. Some authorities recommend beginning such patients on an oral antibiotic, selected on the basis of antipseudomonal coverage or on the basis of culture and sensitivity of the aural discharge, if the patient has not responded to topical management within 2 weeks. If the condition is suspected, prompt intervention is imperative; infectious disease and ENT consultations are appropriate. Antipseudomonal antibiotics are administered for 4 to 8 weeks and surgical débridement is sometimes necessary.

Senturia BH, Marcus MD, Lucente FE. Disease of the external ear. 2nd ed. New York: Grune & Stratton, 1980.
  A complete reference on diseases of the external ear, which includes an excellent discussion of various causes of external otitis.

Marcy SM. Infections of the external ear. Pediatr Infect Dis J 1985; 4:192–201.
  A well-referenced review of the microbiology, pathogenesis, clinical findings, treatment, and prevention of external ear infections.

Cassini N, et al. Diffuse otitis externa: clinical and microbiologic findings in the course of a multicenter study on a new otic solution. Ann Otol Rhinol Laryngol 1977; 86;Suppl 39:1–16.

Reviews the literature on the epidemiology, pathogenesis, and bacteriology of diffuse otitis externa, and provides results of a trial comparing two antibiotic and corticosteroid formulations. Both formulations had a clinical efficacy rate of 97%.

Taylor JS. Otitis externa: treatment using a new expandable wick. Eye Ear Nose Throat Mon 1974; 53:458–9.
A stiff, expandable Weck cell ear wick (Weck cell sponge) is used to deliver medication to the edematous auditory canal, and much less pain is incurred in its use.

Lambert IF. A comparison of the treatment of otitis externa with "Otosporin" and aluminum acetate: a report from a services practice in Cyprus. J R Coll Gen Pract 1981; 31:291–4.
A useful article that characterizes the presentation of otitis externa in a general practice and compares the results of treatment with either aluminum acetate or an antibiotic and steroid combination (Otosporin). This randomized trial shows no difference in outcome with the two treatments.

Maher A, et al. Otomycosis: an experimental evaluation of six antimycotic agents. J Laryngol Otol 1982; 96:205–13.
Clotrimazole and tolnaftate inhibited the greatest number of fungal isolates from infected ears, at the lowest minimal inhibitory concentrations.

Rubin J, Yu VL. Malignant external otitis: insights into pathogenesis, clinical manifestations, diagnosis and therapy. Am J Med 1988; 85:391–7.
Reviews the literature on this potentially devastating condition. Remarks that the erythrocyte sedimentation rate may be valuable in making the diagnosis and monitoring treatment.

Corey JP, Levandowski RA, Ranwalker AP. Prognostic implications of therapy for necrotizing external otitis. Am J Otol 1985; 6:353–7.
The value of antipseudomonal antibiotics with or without surgery is demonstrated.

14. OTITIS MEDIA
Desmond K. Runyan

Although less common in adults than in children, acute otitis media remains a painful problem that may be followed by complications, including mastoiditis, bacterial meningitis, and other central nervous system infections. The clinical diagnosis is sometimes difficult to make, even for experienced physicians, and despite years of research, many aspects of the treatment remain controversial.

The offending infectious agent in otitis media is almost always bacterial. An antecedent viral infection may predispose the patient to the disease, and the highest attack rates occur in the winter months during viral epidemics. However, primary viral infection of the middle ear appears to be uncommon. *Pneumococcus* is the most frequent bacterial pathogen in both adults and children and is found in 24 to 44% of middle ear cultures during acute otitis. *Hemophilus influenzae*, the second most common bacteria isolated, is the presumed pathogen for about one-fifth of all middle ear infections. Conventional wisdom held that *H. influenzae* had a declining role with advancing age and was rarely recovered in patients over age 8. However, there are now a number of reports of *H. influenzae* disease in older children and adults. In series of adolescents and adults, *H. influenzae* was present in 17 to 33% of cultures from the middle ear. Less than 10% of *H. influenzae* isolates are type B, which is more often associated with resistance to ampicillin and central nervous system infection; the remainder are usually nontypeable. Other known pathogens of the middle ear include group A streptococcus, *Branhamella catarrhalis*, *Staphylococcus aureus*, *Escherichia coli*, and *Pseudomonas*.

Diagnosis

The clinical presentation of acute otitis media is usually quite specific in adults: ear pain, otorrhea, hearing loss, and/or vertigo. Fever is common but not universal. Conjunctivitis, rhinitis, and pharyngitis occur if there is a concomitant upper respiratory tract infection, often with adenopathy of the posterior auricular and posterior cervical nodes.

Differential Diagnosis

Otorrhea may make it difficult to differentiate otitis media with perforation from otitis externa. The former typically has a history of antecedent viral infection and of intense pain, followed by acute relief at the time of perforation. Otitis externa often follows exposure to water, and is accompanied by tenderness on movement of the outer ear (see Chap. 13). In the absence of complete occlusion of the external canal, hearing in otitis externa should be normal whereas it usually is impaired in otitis media. Other entities in the differential diagnosis of earache include mumps, dental abscess, ear canal furuncle, ear canal foreign body, trauma, and tonsillitis.

Clinical Diagnosis

The diagnosis of acute otitis media is made on clinical grounds alone. A sealed otoscope with the capability of pneumatic otoscopy is the most appropriate instrument to use in making the diagnosis. The standard operating head otoscope can be used to facilitate the removal of cerumen in order to visualize the tympanic membrane. The ear canal can often be cleansed well enough to visualize the tympanic membrane when the diagnosis is otitis media, but the canal may be too tender and swollen to clean if the patient has otitis externa. Techniques for cleaning the ear include swabbing the canal with cotton twisted onto a probe or wooden stick, using a cerumen spoon or loop, and irrigating with half-strength white vinegar or Burow's solution. If the ear canal cannot be cleaned adequately for visualization of the tympanic membrane and other surfaces, treatment may be begun, based on the history, with or without an audiogram.

The tympanic membrane should be observed for contour, color, translucence, and mobility. The classic description of otitis media is a red, opaque, bulging tympanic membrane that has "lost" its bony landmarks. Distortion of the luster or "light reflex" of the anterior-inferior portion of the tympanic membrane has been suggested as a useful indicator of the presence or absence of otitis media, but this sign is frequently inaccurate. In contrast, the mobility of the tympanic membrane during pneumatic otoscopy has been shown to be moderately sensitive and quite specific for otitis media. The normal tympanic membrane should move briskly as small amounts of air are introduced into the sealed otoscope head. Pus accumulated behind the drum impedes normal membrane motility.

Impedance tympanometry is a sensitive and reliable method of detecting middle ear effusion. The tympanometer measures the resonance of the ear canal for a fixed sound as the air pressure is systematically varied; it is now being widely used in clinical practice to confirm the presence of fluid in the middle ear.

Bacteriologic Diagnosis

Definitive bacteriologic diagnosis is usually not necessary for treatment of otitis media. Rarely, it may be necessary to perform a tap of the middle ear, using a 20-gauge spinal needle and a tuberculin syringe, to identify the specific infecting organism. Culture of the middle ear is most helpful for immunosuppressed patients with otitis or when otitis develops during antibiotic therapy. Nasopharyngeal cultures do not accurately reflect middle ear flora and so have no clinical utility in routine practice or for either of the above-mentioned situations.

Treatment

Currently, it is standard practice to prescribe an antibiotic for acute otitis media. Although existing data suggest that the acute clinical course of otitis is affected minimally by the addition of antibiotics, antimicrobial therapy may play an important role in reducing the incidence of suppurative complications. The usual clinical course of otitis media is nearly complete resolution of pain and fever in less than 48 hours. In one study, the duration of pain and fever among patients with otitis did not differ markedly for patients treated with antibiotics than for those treated with antihistamines only. On the other hand, it is clear that there has been a marked decline in the incidence of complications, such as perforation, coincident with the routine use of antimicrobials.

Antibiotics

Amoxicillin (250–500 mg tid) is the usual first choice, as it will cover all of the usual organisms responsible for otitis media, including most *H. influenzae*, and is inexpensive. Penicillin (200–500 mg qid) with the addition of sulfonamide (4 g to start, then 1 g qid) is an alternative. Erythromycin (250–500 mg qid) may be substituted for the penicillin in penicillin-sensitive patients.

Trimethoprim-sulfamethoxazole (1–2 tablets bid) is frequently prescribed because it has good *H. influenzae* coverage, but failure to eliminate pneumococcal isolates is not uncommon. The usual course of therapy is 10 days. Cefaclor (250–500 mg tid), the most commonly used cephalosporin, is expensive and recent reports suggest that the recurrence rate of infection is higher with cefaclor than with other regimens. Cefuroxime axetil covers the range of pathogens but is much more expensive than amoxicillin.

Adjunctive Therapies

ANTIHISTAMINES AND ORAL DECONGESTANTS. These medications have been advocated as adjuncts to the medical management of acute otitis. Animal studies in the 1960s and 1970s supported their theoretic utility. However, there are now a large number of clinical trials that demonstrate that these medications are of no use. In a few studies, the addition of these drugs appeared to delay the clearance of middle ear fluid. They have no place in the routine management of uncomplicated otitis media. Decongestants delivered by nasal spray have not been shown to be useful, but the number of studies is small.

ANALGESICS. For pain relief, topical analgesics for the ear (e.g., Auralgan) appear to be minimally effective. The epithelium of the tympanic membrane inhibits adequate absorption unless the membrane is very distended by middle ear infection. Oral analgesics, including aspirin and acetaminophen, are effective for mild-to-moderate pain. Narcotic preparations may be necessary for a few patients during the first 24 to 48 hours.

Complications

Complications of otitis media include central nervous system infection, mastoiditis, and cholesteatoma. The relationship between acute otitis media and serous otitis is less clear. Middle ear effusion frequently persists after acute infection, but serous otitis is also identified as a cause of conductive hearing loss in the absence of a history of acute infection. Mastoiditis is thought to accompany almost all cases of otitis, and routine antibiotic therapy of the otitis is adequate to treat the mastoid infection. Untreated mastoid infection can become a surgical emergency if osteitis and thrombosis of the proximate venous sinuses develop. The chronically infected middle ear may develop a cholesteatoma, which is a mass of desquamated epithelial cells with or without cholesterol crystals. This mass can lead to eventual destruction of middle ear structures and result in a conductive hearing loss.

Serous Otitis

Serous otitis is diagnosed when a middle ear is not acutely inflamed but appears to contain fluid, seen as decreased translucence, a horizontal fluid level (when the patient is upright), bubbles behind the eardrum, and often retraction of the eardrum. Synonyms include "glue ear" and "secretory otitis." The causes and natural history of serous otitis are unclear, but subacute infection, allergy, barotrauma, eustachian tube dysfunction, and persistent fluid following acute otitis are all believed to play a role. It has recently been established that effusion may persist for as long as 10 weeks after an acute infection. Some investigators have found a variety of bacterial pathogens in middle ear fluid despite the lack of clinical evidence of acute inflammation. The long-term consequences of serous otitis are not known; the relationship to permanent hearing loss remains controversial.

Treatment of serous otitis remains problematic. Antihistamines and decongestants have been advocated as logical and appropriate; however, recent clinical trials have demonstrated a lack of effectiveness. The discovery of bacteria in some "serous" middle ear fluid at tympanostomy tube placement has prompted most experts to recommend antimicrobial treatment. Other options include surgical drainage with or without tympanostomy tube placement, and mechanical efforts at middle ear inflation (i.e., gum-chewing or holding one's nose while inflating the nasopharynx). Because of a lack of data regarding treatment, a conservative medical approach, including antibiotic treatment, mechanical efforts, and watchful waiting, is most prudent for the first 2 to 4 weeks. Because of the remote possibility of a nasopharyngeal cancer, consultation with an otolaryngologist should follow if the middle ear effusion persists in an otherwise healthy adult.

Paradise J. Otitis media in infants and children. Pediatrics 1980; 65:917–43.
Probably the most extensive and authoritative review of otitis media ever published. This article should be the basis of any further reading on otitis.

Giebink GS. The microbiology of otitis media. Pediatr Infect Dis J 1989; 8:Suppl 1:S18–20.
A current review of the microbiologic spectrum encountered in middle ear disease.

Henderson F, et al. A longitudinal study of respiratory viruses and bacteria in the etiology of acute otitis with effusion. N Engl J Med 1982; 306:1377–83.
A longitudinal study of the incidence and microbiology of otitis in a known population of children. The best work of its kind to date.

Schwartz R. Bacteriology of otitis media: a review. Otolaryngol Head Neck Surg 1981; 89:444–50.
A review of clinical techniques for ear cultures, and a discussion of the microbiologic findings of more than 2800 ear cultures.

Cantekin E, et al. Lack of efficacy of a decongestant-antihistamine combination for otitis media with effusion in children: results of a double blind randomized trial. N Engl J Med 1983; 308:297–301.
A study that is conclusive in its dismissal of antihistamine adjunctive therapy.

Greunfast K. A review of the efficacy of systemically administered decongestants in the prevention and treatment of otitis media. Otolaryngol Head Neck Surg 1981; 89:432–9.
A summary of the pharmacology of these drugs and the clinical and animal studies supporting their use.

Gates GA, Avery CA, Prihoda TJ. Effectiveness of adeniodectomy and tympanostomy tubes in the treatment of chronic otitis media with effusion. N Engl J Med 1987; 317:1444–51.
A randomized study strongly supporting the use of surgical interventions in chronic middle ear disease.

Perlman PE, Ginn DR. Respiratory infections in ambulatory adults. Choosing the best treatment. Postgrad Med 1990; 87:175–84.
A current review.

15. EARWAX
Terry L. Fry

Earwax (cerumen) is created by the secretions of the sebaceous glands located in the skin that line the outer, cartilaginous half of the ear canal. The quantity and consistency of the wax vary with the individual. Environmental factors may also contribute; swimming or showering can result in water being absorbed by otherwise dry cerumen, causing expansion and displacement of wax into deeper portions of the ear canal.

Significant quantities of cerumen may be present, with no noticeable hearing impairment as long as there is even a tiny area of patency through which sound waves can travel. There may be no other symptoms if cerumen is soft and does not traumatize the external canal with excursions of the temporomandibular joint or touch the tympanic membrane. Ear pain may result if firm cerumen touches the tympanic membrane, or traumatizes the external canal, and is associated with otitis externa. Disequilibrium may occur if the impaction is against the tympanic membrane.

Cerumen exerts a protective, antibacterial effect by helping to maintain an acid pH in the ear canal. However, when excessive or impacted secretions result in a hearing deficit or the symptoms described above, or when they obscure the tympanic membrane during an otoscopic examination, removal of the cerumen becomes necessary.

Cerumen Removal

Cotton swabs may be used by clinicians to remove cerumen from widely patent, nontortuous, non–hair-bearing ear canals. When used by patients, swabs may serve only to impact the wax more deeply within the medial, bony half of the ear canal, which normally should not contain cerumen. For this reason, patients should be discouraged from using cotton swabs. Several safe and simple methods, used singly or in combination, are effective in removing cerumen. These include instrumentation, irrigation, suction, and chemical softeners.

Instrumentation

Firm cerumen may be removed with a smooth cerumen spoon or wire loop. Preferably this should be performed under direct vision, through an operator-held otoscope. The examiner's hand should be stabilized against the patient's head to avoid inadvertent trauma with patient movement. The cerumen is most readily removed if the instrument is placed in an area where the cerumen is separated from the ear canal or in an area of central patency; always keep in mind the distance to the patient's tympanic membrane. This can often be determined by first examining the opposite nonimpacted ear.

Irrigation

Irrigation should be done with a liquid warmed to body temperature, to avoid caloric stimulation that can result in vertigo. A solution of 1.5% acetic acid is preferable to tap water because the low pH retards the overgrowth of *Pseudomonas* in the wet ear canal. Such an irrigating solution may be readily approximated by diluting 1 part commercially available white vinegar (5% acetic acid) with 2 parts water. Adding to this solution an equal volume of hydrogen peroxide or 1:750 benzalkonium chloride (Zephiran Chloride) supplies a detergent effect, which aids in separating the wax from the ear canal.

Irrigation should be done under gentle pressure, with the tip of an ear bulb syringe held carefully at the entrance of the ear canal while the pinna is retracted superiorly and posteriorly (in the adult) or posteriorly (in the child); forceful irrigation can traumatize the tympanic membrane and ossicular chain. The fluid should be directed toward the superior aspect of the ear canal or wherever there is a separation between the impaction and the ear canal or toward a central patency. A direct blast against cerumen mass will only cause it to become more deeply impacted. In experienced hands, the Water Pik is also an effective irrigating device when used as described above. However, if it is used improperly, the turbulence it creates may cause trauma.

Irrigation is relatively contraindicated in any individual with a known perforation of the tympanic membrane because it may cause middle ear infection. However, this complication is very unusual when diluted vinegar is used as an irrigant, even when an ear with an unrecognized perforation is inadvertently irrigated. Patients with perforations may find that the lower pH of the irrigant causes discomfort once it gains access to the middle ear, which is an excellent clue to discontinue irrigation.

Suction

Soft, semifluid cerumen can often be removed most efficaciously under direct vision with a blunt-tipped 14-gauge needle attached to a wall- or portable-suction device, with the suction pressure equivalent to approximately 10 cm H_2O. By compressing the connecting tubing, suction can be terminated immediately if necessary. Excessive suction can cause caloric stimulation and result in vertigo. Suction irrigation or other instrumentation should be reserved for a specialist if the patient has had previous radical mastoid surgery or has tympanostomy tubes.

Chemical Softeners
Some cerumen impactions may resist all of the above-described techniques but may respond to softening agents instilled in the ear canal over a 7- to 14-day period. When used alone, these agents will not usually be effective on dense, hard, inspissated cerumen and must be followed by suction, wire loop, or irrigation for final removal. Softening agents are also the method of choice when a thin layer of cerumen persists against the tympanic membrane. The most commonly used softening agents are Debrox, Cerumenex, acetic acid (1.5%) in combination with water, peroxide, or an emulsifying agent such as benzalkonium chloride. Stool softeners are sometimes suggested for this purpose but are not indicated for softening the cerumen because they may cause a severe inflammatory reaction in the ear canal.

Debrox Drops (carbamide peroxide 6.5% in anhydrous glycerol) act as a peroxide by releasing oxygen and thereby débriding and cleansing the ear canal. These drops offer a safe and effective means for softening minimal-to-moderate amounts of cerumen; 3 to 5 drops are instilled in the affected ear(s) twice a day. Results are seen in several days.

Cerumenex Drops (10% triethanolamine polypeptide oleate condensate in propylene glycol with chlorbutanol 0.5%) emulsify cerumen while maintaining an acid pH. Action is usually complete in 15 to 30 minutes. Cerumenex is appropriate for office rather than outpatient use. At least 1% of patients using these drops develop a hypersensitivity reaction, with a local dermatitis ranging from mild erythema to a severe eczematoid reaction involving any areas originally in contact with the drops. Even in those patients not hypersensitive to Cerumenex, local reaction may occur if the drops are accidentally applied to the periaural area.

Hydrogen peroxide is a safe and effective agent for loosening the attachment of cerumen to the underlying ear canal. An alternative is sterile benzalkonium chloride (Zephiran). Mixing either of these solutions in a 1:1 ratio with diluted white vinegar maintains an acid pH that retards development of an infection resulting from solution remaining in the ear canal after cleaning is finished. Applications once or twice a day are usually effective in 4 to 14 days. There is some evidence that these aqueous preparations are more effective than the commercial organic solvents.

Chronic Care
Many patients ask, "If I can't use cotton swabs or stick anything in my ears, how can I keep them clean?" In response to this question, the clinician should explain the protective role of cerumen, stressing that its presence does not indicate that the ear is "dirty." Patients with increased cerumen production can use diluted white vinegar warmed to body temperature as an irrigant one to two times per week for an effective, safe, and economic means of cerumen removal. Irrigation may be done with a bulb syringe. To avoid impactions, patients with narrow or tortuous ear canals may require periodic scheduled visits for cerumen removal. Even with regular irrigations, the use of cotton swabs may cause impactions of cerumen.

Caruso VG, Meyerhoff WC. Trauma and infection of the external ear. In: Paparella M, Shumrick D, eds. Otolaryngology. 2nd ed. Philadelphia: Saunders, 1980:1345–6.
  A good discussion of cerumen and its function in the ear canal.

Senturia BH, Marcus MD, Lucente FE. Diseases of the external ear. New York: Grune & Stratton, 1981:26–30.
  Discusses role of bacteria in the pathogenesis of otitis externa, supporting the use of solutions with acid pH.

Robinson AC, Hawke M. The efficacy of ceruminolytics: everything old is new again. J Otolaryngol 1989; 18:263–7.
  In in vitro tests of a variety of ceruminolytics, preparations with an aqueous base were most effective, the best being a 10% solution of sodium bicarbonate!

IV. UPPER RESPIRATORY PROBLEMS

16. COLDS AND INFLUENZA
Timothy W. Lane

The term *flu* is commonly used interchangeably to describe both the mildly symptomatic common cold and the more dramatic febrile illnesses associated with acute influenza. Morbidity is typically minor, but colds and other respiratory tract infections cause about one-third of all school and work absenteeism. And the estimated annual expenditure on nonprescription cold medications is over $3 billion.

The viral etiologies of upper respiratory infections (URIs) are numerous and may cause overlapping clinical syndromes. Distinguishing one cause from another in clinical practice is usually not important because of the lack of any specific treatment. Influenza, however, accounts for far greater morbidity and mortality and its identification is much more important because of the availability of treatment and prevention strategies.

The Common Cold

The common cold is a popular generic term for the benign clinical syndrome marked by sneezing, increased nasal secretions, and mild malaise that can be caused by one of several viruses. It is estimated that rhinoviruses account for 30 to 50% of colds, and coronaviruses, parainfluenza, adenoviruses, enteroviruses, and respiratory syncytial viruses cause about 20 to 25%. Milder forms of influenza and bacterial infections of the upper airway such as those caused by *Chlamydia pneumoniae* or *Mycoplasma pneumoniae* and group A streptococcal pharyngitis can mimic the cold syndrome and cause 10 to 15% of cases. Sporadic cases of mumps, rubella, rubeola, and cytomegalovirus infection may occasionally present as colds. However, 35% or more of colds have no identifiable cause, perhaps because diagnostic methods are not sufficiently sensitive.

The viruses responsible for colds primarily infect ciliated epithelial cells of the nasal mucosa, and secondarily, other epithelial cells in the upper respiratory tract. A mild cellular inflammatory response occurs, resulting in increased local production of mucus and immunoglobulin, which along with shedding epithelial cells constitute the nasal discharge. Viral shedding peaks with severity of illness and may continue for 2 to 3 weeks afterward at lower titers. Local bacterial adherence to epithelial cells increases during colds and may be responsible for subsequent development of bacterial sinusitis and otitis media.

Epidemiology

Colds predominantly occur from September through March in temperate climates and during the rainy season in the tropics. This periodicity may result from exposure at school and at home. Despite popular belief, wet weather and chilling do not enhance the experimental induction of rhinoviral infections, nor have a variety of other environmental conditions been shown to be related to the development of colds.

Children average six to eight colds per season and adults, two to four. These rates appear to be higher for children in day care and for adults who work with young children.

The exact method of transmission of cold viruses is not entirely clear. Aerosol transmission appears to be most important. Several studies have demonstrated that the hands are contaminated with virally infected secretions 60% of the time, and that these secretions can be spread directly to the hands of susceptible individuals, who in turn inadvertently inoculate their nasal and conjunctival mucous membranes. The reduction of rhinovirus transmission by virucidal hand-cleansing agents supports direct person-to-person contact. Secretions contaminating commonly handled objects do not appear to be an efficient vehicle for transmission. The incubation period for most colds is 48 to 72 hours, but may be as long as 7 days.

Clinical Manifestations

The usual symptoms of the common cold are nonspecific and do not allow the distinction of one viral cause from another. Nasal "stuffiness" and mucus discharge are typically the first and most prominent symptoms, accompanied by sneezing and followed a day or so later by a mildly sore throat, often described as "scratchy," mild burning and tearing of the eyes, low-grade malaise and achiness, and at most a modest elevation in temperature (i.e., ≤ 101°F or ≤ 38.5°C). A dry nonproductive cough is present by the second or third day of symptoms in 40 to 60% of patients. Less common symptoms (in 15–30%) are hoarseness, headache, and chills. Symptoms peak by the third to fifth day and then begin to abate. Cough and hoarseness may continue for another week or so. Cigarette smokers are more likely to have prolonged cough and to develop purulent bacterial bronchitis, and probably sinusitis as well.

Physical findings are usually limited to nasal mucosal edema, erythema, and copious nasal secretions. The pharynx may be mildly erythematous and without exudate, but is more often normal in appearance. Occasionally, palpable and slightly tender cervical lymph nodes are present.

Complications of colds include acute sinusitis and otitis media, which occur in an estimated 1 to 2% of patients. The cold viruses including rhinoviruses can occasionally involve the lower tracheobronchial tree and may cause pneumonitis. Alterations in mucociliary transport and increased secretions in the sinuses and eustachian tubes may predispose to these sequelae. The viruses commonly associated with colds might predispose to bacterial pneumonia, but except for influenza viruses A and B, sound epidemiologic evidence for this association is lacking.

Diagnosis

The typical manifestations of the common cold are so consistent that self-diagnosis is the rule and a specific etiologic diagnosis is not necessary for supportive treatment. Patients typically consult physicians for reassurance and/or work or school excuses. Acute debilitating symptoms and a fever of 101°F (38.3°C) or higher should lead to consideration of other causes, such as acute sinusitis, tracheobronchitis, pneumonia, or influenza or adenovirus infection. Purulent nasal discharge or sputum production suggests a complication, such as sinusitis or lower respiratory tract infection; otitis media can usually be excluded by otoscopic examination. It may be difficult to differentiate purulent bacterial sinusitis from viral infection of the sinuses, especially if the sinuses are not draining; the use of transillumination and sinus films is discussed further in Chapter 17. Fever and vasomotor rhinitis may also be confused with the common cold, but their differences in chronic patterns should be evident from the history. Bacterial superinfection of chronic allergic rhinitis and sinusitis is suggested by a history of chronic nasal discharge, especially in association with exposure to allergens, and itchy conjunctivitis.

Mycoplasma pneumoniae and *Chlamydia pneumoniae* infection can present as a cold syndrome. These species often cause laryngitis and protracted nonproductive cough of 2 or more weeks' duration. Although the infection may progress to pneumonia, there are no clinical trials to show a benefit of treating URIs caused by these organisms.

Treatment

Since no specific antiviral therapy is currently available for the common cold viruses (although several are under investigation), relief of symptoms is the therapeutic goal. Over 800 nonprescription cold remedies are currently available, many containing the same or similar agents. The most popular over-the-counter preparations are combination products, generally containing an antihistamine, a sympathomimetic decongestant, an analgesic (often aspirin or acetaminophen), and ethanol if it is a liquid preparation. None of the combination remedies has been rigorously examined, and studies of single agents or combinations of two have been small, often with inconsistent results. No study has yet demonstrated that symptomatic therapy reduces complications.

Nasal Symptoms

Nasal sympotns include sneezing, "stuffiness" or relative obstruction secondary to nasal mucosal edema, and nasal discharge. Topical sympathomimetic decongestants such as sprays or drops of 0.25 to 0.5% phenylephrine or 1% ephedrine effectively reduce nasal congestion and discharge when used at 4-hour intervals. Xylometazoline (Otrivin) and oxymetazoline (Afrin), longer-acting sympathomimetics, need to be used only two to three times per day. Patients should be cautioned that use of any of these decongestants beyond 5 to 7 days or too frequent daily applications can lead to rebound congestion; topical agents should therefore be used only when warranted by severity of symptoms.

High-dose oral pseudoephedrine, 60 mg four times a day, also reduces nasal discharge. The oral adrenergic decongestant phenylpropanolamine has similar benefits at 25 mg to 50 mg four times a day, but can induce marked hypertension in those with moderate-to-severe hypertension and those taking monoamine oxidase inhibitors.

Antihistamines with anticholinergic properties such as chlorpheniramine and brompheniramine at 4 to 8 mg, taken orally four times a day, have been shown to be marginally helpful in decreasing nasal congestion and sneezing; the nonsedating antihistamine terfenadine (Seldane) has no anticholinergic activity, and has not improved nasal symptoms in a controlled trial. In general, the widespread reliance on the antihistamines exceeds their very modest and inconsistently demonstrated efficacy.

Petroleum-base jellies (e.g., Vaseline) may lessen the irritation and fissures that occur about the nostrils from frequent blowing. Inhaled moist air from sources ranging from hot chicken soup to a variety of vaporizers has been shown to reduce the weight of nasal mucus and improve the overall subjective resolution of symptoms.

Cough

Codeine, 30 mg three to four times a day, or dextromethorphan, 30 mg three to four times a day, are equally effective cough suppressants. Comparative trials suggest more nausea and drowsiness with dextromethorphan, but it is available in over-the-counter formulations. Despite the fact that most coughs with colds probably are induced by postnasal drip, antihistamines and decongestants have not been shown to consistently reduce cough.

Expectorants such as terpin hydrate or guaifenesin (also known as glyceryl guaiacolate) are useful as placebos, but have been shown to have no additional efficacy in removing secretions.

Sore Throat

Although no therapy is entirely satisfactory for sore throat, the generally mild throat discomfort associated with the common cold can be temporarily alleviated by gargles with warm water and table salt (1 teaspoon/qt), soothing throat lozenges (some over-the-counter preparations contain benzocaine or other local anesthetics), or gargles with diphenhydramine (Benadryl) elixir. The latter has a topical anesthetic effect, but use should be limited to 2 teaspoons (25 mg) every 4 to 6 hours to avoid sedation or other antihistamine side effects from swallowed medication.

Muscle Aches, Fever, and Chills

The common over-the-counter analgesics, aspirin or acetaminophen, have long been recommended for colds. The antipyretic effects are less important since fevers are usually mild. Controlled evaluations of aspirin revealed a decrease in musculoskeletal complaints in treatment groups, but most have not shown statistical differences from placebo. Ibuprofen has been examined in a comparative trial and is no more effective than aspirin.

Prevention

The prevention of transmission of colds has focused on frequent hand-washing, careful disposal of tissues, and limiting contact with others. Few of these strategies have been clinically examined, but this commonsense hygiene may help to reduce spread. Washing the hands with a virucidal cleanser has decreased transmission in an experimental setting, but impregnating nasal tissues with virucidal organic acids has not been of benefit. Vitamin C emerged as a preventive fad two decades ago, but the weight of evidence of well-designed studies is against any prophylactic or therapeutic benefit. Significant (80%) reduction in household transmission of natural and experimentally induced rhinovirus colds has been achieved with nasal application of interferon alfa-2, with tolerable nasal drying in 10%. Interferon used in a much higher dose for active treatment causes severe nasal discomfort and bleeding and is a classic example of the cure being worse than the disease. Low-dose interferon for prophylaxis of rhinovirus colds in the household setting might be a feasible clinical strategy when it is available and if it is reasonably priced.

Influenza

Influenza viruses occur worldwide, causing frequent outbreaks during the wintertime in temperate areas and throughout the year in the tropics. As with other respiratory tract viruses, this seasonal periodicity may reflect exposure in schools and homes. Influenza viruses A and B cause recurrent epidemics of respiratory infections. Despite the availability of vaccines for influenza viruses A and B, waves of epidemic disease continue worldwide because of constant minor genetic mutations. These lead to "drift" in the critical viral surface antigens, hemagglutinin and neuraminidase, that are responsible for virulence and infectivity. Antigenic drifts occur more commonly for influenza A and explain its dominant role in epidemic disease. Major antigenic changes or shifts often result in a pandemic because of the immunologic susceptibility of large segments of the global population to a new strain. Despite yearly formulations of vaccines, these unpredictable antigenic changes may result in vaccines that are immunologically unprotective.

Epidemiology

Influenza is transmitted by both large- and small-particle aerosols generated by coughing and sneezing. It may also be spread by contact contamination but its explosive onset favors aerosol transmission as the main vector. Influenzas A and B almost always appear between October and March in temperate areas and the outbreaks, caused primarily by A, wane over 6 to 8 weeks as the majority of susceptible patients are exposed. Rarely a sporadic case of influenza will be documented at other times during the year.

Attack rates of influenza vary from year to year, but in epidemics 20 to 30% of a population may develop clinical disease, with attack rates as high as 50% where a major antigenic shift has occurred. Children have the highest attack rates of influenza illness in outbreaks, with the elderly least likely to become infected. However, the relative risk to the elderly of serious complications from influenza is much greater, as reflected in a 5- to 10-fold increase in rates of hospitalization and a fivefold increase in mortality, when compared to children and young adults. Furthermore, it has been shown during outbreaks that over 80% of the deaths attributed to influenza occur in those older than 65.

Seasonal influenza activity is monitored in the United States by the Centers for Disease Control (CDC), by observing the mortality ascribed to "pneumonia and influenza" in selected cities and by obtaining viral cultures from patients with appropriate symptoms in sentinel primary care settings. Reports of influenza activity are usually a month behind. This information lag has impeded wider use of antivirals and the annual application of vaccine.

Clinical Presentation

The classic symptomatic presentation of both influenzas A and B is prostration, chills, nasal stuffiness, sore throat, prominent headache, myalgias, and a dry to minimally productive cough. Nausea, vomiting, and dizziness are less common (20–40%). Accompanying clinical findings include high fever up to 104°F (40°C), nonexudative pharyngitis, nasal congestion, and muscle tenderness. Less common signs include cervical adenopathy (20%) and conjunctival injection. These acute signs and symptoms usually resolve rather quickly over 4 to 5 days. Acute recovery appears to depend on both humoral immunity and the production of interferon. Healthy hosts, however, often experience fatigue, malaise, and a lingering nonproductive cough for 2 to 3 more weeks. Necrosis of infected respiratory epithelial cells and subsequent repair are presumed to cause some of these persistent manifestations.

The usual incubation period of influenza is 2 to 3 days, with a range of 1 to 7 days. Viral shedding in respiratory secretions begins within 1 day before the onset of symptoms, peaks with severity, and declines over 4 to 5 days. Patients hospitalized with known or suspected acute influenza require respiratory isolation during this time of viral shedding to prevent nosocomial transmission.

The most frequent complications of influenza are related to the respiratory tract. Bacterial tracheobronchitis occurs in up to 30% of adults and sinusitis occurs in 5 to 10%. These sequelae probably result from the destruction of mucociliary cells as well as decreased granulocyte phagocytic ability and increased adherence of potential bacterial pathogens to virally infected epithelial cells. Smoking enhances the risk of these complications.

Chest radiographic "screening" in influenza outbreaks has shown a 5% prevalence of pneumonic infiltrates. Primary symptomatic influenza pneumonia occurs in about 1% of adults with influenza and can occasionally be fatal even in the young adult. Bacterial pneumonia causes greater morbidity, but less mortality than bilateral primary viral pneumonia. In both, clinical onset is about 1 week after the onset of classic symptoms, and both are heralded by recrudescence of fever and clinical relapse with pulmonary symptoms. (Cough with purulent sputum is a clue to bacterial infection.) The most common putative causes of bacterial pneumonia are *Pneumococcus,* nontypeable *Hemophilus influenzae,* and staphylococci. Susceptibility to pneumonia is greater in the elderly (> 65 years old) and those with chronic renal, metabolic (including diabetes), hematologic, immunodeficiency, or cardiopulmonary disorders.

Rare central nervous system complications include meningoencephalitis, transverse myelitis, Reye's syndrome, and Guillain-Barré syndrome. Other infrequent manifestations are myositis, myoglobinuric renal failure, myocarditis, pericarditis, glomerulonephritis, and parotitis.

Diagnosis

The chance that a patient presenting with typical symptoms has influenza is related directly to the prevalence of influenza. The clinical diagnosis of influenza during an outbreak approaches 85% sensitivity and is generally sufficient for clinical management. Cases of "flu" in nonepidemic circumstances are most often not caused by influenza, but by respiratory syncytial virus, parainfluenza, and adenoviruses, which may mimic the symptoms and signs of influenza.

Findings on routine laboratory testing are nonspecific. Usually the only abnormality in a healthy person is a slight-to-moderately elevated peripheral WBC (12–15,000/μl). Confirmation of a clinical diagnosis is not currently practical since isolation of influenza virus from nasal and throat swab specimens requires 3 to 5 days. Serologic specimens collected 3 to 4 weeks apart can be examined for a fourfold or greater rise in either complement-fixing or hemagglutination-inhibition antibodies. Delays and expense limit the usefulness of these methods in the clinic. Direct and rapid means of viral diagnosis are under development.

Treatment

Most healthy children and adults less than 65 years old are unlikely to develop complications of influenza and require only supportive therapy. Symptomatic treatment of nasal congestion, cough, sore throat, muscle aches, and fever is similar to that for colds, as discussed above. In children and young adults in their early 20s aspirin used to treat influenza enhances the development of Reye's syndrome; acetaminophen should be substituted if symptomatic relief is needed.

Amantadine (Symmetrel) and a new antiviral agent, rimantadine (Flumadine), have activity against influenza A, but not B. Several randomized, prospective, and placebo-controlled trials have demonstrated that amantadine reduces the duration of fever by 50% and reduces the duration of other systemic manifestations of influenza A by 1 to 2 days. Similar benefits have been shown for rimantadine. Chemotherapy is effective in all ages only when it is begun within 48 hours of symptomatic onset of influenza A.

The dose of amantadine currently recommended by the Food and Drug Administration (FDA) for therapy is 200 mg by mouth daily (in one or two divided doses) for 5 days. Five to 10% of patients taking amantadine at this dose experience dizziness, nausea, and difficulty with mental concentration. These effects are quickly reversible when the drug is stopped. Amantadine's clearance depends on renal function and the dose should be reduced to 100 mg daily in those 65 or older and/or for those with creatinine clearances estimated to be less than 50 ml per minute. Several studies of amantadine, 100 mg daily, in all ages showed the same benefit as 200 mg daily, but with less toxicity. Many experts now recommend this 100-mg daily dose. Rimantadine, which undergoes hepatic clearance, has less adverse effects at a dose of 200 mg/day, when compared to amantadine at 200 mg/day, but further comparative trials using amantadine at 100 mg daily are needed to establish a clear preference. Amantadine and rimantadine are contraindicated in pregnancy. Influenza A strains resistant to both amantadine and rimantadine appear to be responsible for failure of postexposure prophylaxis when the index patient is also treated.

No other active agent is routinely available for influenza B, but recent experimental trials of aerosolized or oral ribavirin have suggested a treatment and prophylaxis benefit for influenzas A and B.

The greatest impediment to proper use of amantadine or rimantadine is difficulty in making a secure diagnosis. Nonetheless in outbreaks, these agents should be prescribed, particularly for those at high risk of complications, for example, the elderly and those with chronic cardiac or pulmonary diseases such as chronic obstructive pulmonary disease (COPD) and asthma. The use of either agent in severe and advanced influenza A infections has not been studied.

Prevention

Well-designed prospective studies have shown amantadine and rimantadine to be equally effective in all ages in preventing 50 to 80% of infections with influenza A. Efficacy of prophylactic treatment has been established if it is given over the usual 6-week period of influenza A activity. The results of controlled trials of amantadine and rimantadine prophylaxis of household members after exposure to an index case are conflicting. A recent large, prospective study of household prophylaxis with rimantadine showed no benefit because of the emergence of drug-resistant isolates from both the index case and secondary cases. Further study is needed to clarify this issue.

When there is epidemiologic evidence of influenza A, however, early use of chemoprophylaxis should be considered especially for the elderly, chronically ill, nursing home residents, and health care workers responsible for direct patient care. Because influenza vaccine is not completely protective, supplemental chemoprophylaxis may be used for those at the highest risk of complications even if they have been vaccinated. The dose approved for prophylaxis is 200 mg daily of amantadine or rimantadine, but recent clinical trials have demonstrated that 100 mg of amantadine daily is equally effective prophylactically and should lessen adverse effects. Chemoprophylaxis must be administered over the usual 6- to 8-week period of an outbreak to be of benefit. A practical option for the unvaccinated is to administer chemoprophylaxis and influenza vaccine simultaneously. Immunogenicity is not compromised, and chemoprophylaxis can be discontinued safely after 2 weeks when over 80% of subjects will have developed protective antibodies. When applied topically, interferon is effective in the prevention of experimentally induced influenza, but local drying and cracking of mucous membranes limit its usefulness.

Influenza vaccine has been shown to be 70 to 90% effective in reducing clinical infection in young healthy adults when there is a good antigenic match with naturally circulating strains. In case-control studies, vaccine efficacy in persons 65 years or older has been estimated to range from 30 to 70%. More importantly, a 30 to 40% reduction in morbidity, hospitalization, and mortality has been consistently demonstrated in these studies of vaccinated residents of nursing homes and other chronic care settings. See Chapter 124 about the use and indications for influenza vaccine.

Gwaltney JM. The common cold. In: Mandell GL, Douglas RG Jr, and Bennett JE, eds. Principles and practices of infectious diseases. New York: Wiley, 1989:489–93.

Lowenstein SR, Parrino TA. Management of the common cold. Adv Intern Med 1987; 32:207–34.
Two comprehensive reviews that sort out the major issues.

A symposium on antihistamines in rhinovirus colds. Pediatr Infect Dis J 1988; 7:215–42.
In separate trials of antihistamines, terfenadine (Seldane) was ineffective in a large study ($n > 200$ patients) and chlorpheniramine was of modest benefit ($n = 40$ patients). Consensus of experts in cold research concludes that antihistamines offer little in symptomatic management.

Howard JC, et al. Effectiveness of antihistamines in the symptomatic management of the common cold. JAMA 1979; 242:2414–7.
A purportedly positive study supporting use of chlorpheniramine versus placebo in 271 randomized patients. Patients and physicians rated symptoms subjectively but were blinded to treatment categories. A few nasal symptoms rated by patients were statistically better for the treatment group, but none of the physician ratings were.

Gaffey MJ, et al. Ipratropium bromide treatment of experimental rhinovirus infection. Antimicrob Agents Chemother 1988; 32:1644–7.
Ipratropium (Atrovent), an anticholinergic currently used to treat asthma and COPD, had some benefit in reducing nasal symptoms when used intranasally, 80 g three times a day for 5 days. It may be an adjunct to topical sympathomimetics, but an expensive and not-yet-approved one.

Sperber S, Hayden F. Chemotherapy of rhinovirus colds. Antimicrob Agents Chemother 1988; 32:409–19.
An excellent review of what has been tried and what is in trial, including experimental antivirals.

Cold remedies: which ones work best? Consumer Rep 1989; 54:8–12.
A good overview of nonprescription products, for both physician and patients. Aimed at the educated consumer, and especially appropriate for this topic, it is written in the usual adversarial and critical style.

Tyrell D, et al. Local hyperthermia benefits natural and experimental common colds. Br Med J 1989; 298:1280–3.

Macknin ME, et al. Effect of inhaling heated vapor on symptoms of the common cold. JAMA 1990; 264:989–91.
Two randomized and blinded trials of 40 to 43°C (104.0–109.4°F) moist air three times a day versus 20 to 30°C (68–86°F) "control" air. The first, conducted in more than 180 subjects, demonstrated significant reduction in overall symptoms, duration of illness (mean of 3.0 versus 4.7 days), and weight of nasal secretions in group treated with 43°C moist air. The second study did not confirm any benefits to therapy. Frequency of application differed in the trials and more clinical investigation is needed.

Hayden FG, et al. Prevention of natural colds by contact prophylaxis with nasal alpha$_2$ interferon. N Engl J Med 1986; 314:71–5.
Nearly 80% reduction in rhinovirus colds and 40% prophylactic efficacy overall. Adverse nasal drying was tolerable, unlike in previous therapeutic trials with high-dose interferon. May be practical in certain situations in the future if cost is tolerable.

Marlin SW, et al. A soluble form of intercellular adhesion molecule-1 inhibits rhinovirus infection. Nature 1990; 344:70–2.
A glimpse of the future? The predominant human receptor adhesion molecule-1 for rhinoviruses has been cloned, and this preliminary work demonstrates that recombinant receptor can prevent infection by blocking viral-binding sites. Raises possibilities for therapy and even vaccine by inducing receptor-blocking antibodies.

Douglas RG Jr, Betts RF. Influenza virus. In: Mandell GL, Douglas RG Jr, Bennett, JE, eds. Principals and practice of infectious diseases. New York: Wiley, 1989:1306–25.
Up-to-date and thorough clinical review of the topic by experienced clinical investigators, with an extensive bibliography.

Glezen WP, et al. Acute respiratory disease associated with influenza epidemics in Houston, 1981–83. J Infect Dis 1987; 144:1119–26.
Studies of the "microepidemiology" of influenza in Houston via a citywide surveillance system, identifying its considerable and often hidden annual morbidity and mortality.

Morbidity and Mortality Weekly Report (MMWR).
Publishes updates on influenza activity worldwide and annual recommendations for influenza vaccine formulation and use of antiviral drugs. Perusal of the MMWR will keep one informed of influenza activity during the winter season.

Douglas RG Jr. Prophylaxis and treatment of influenza. N Engl J Med 1990; 322:443–50.
An in-depth review of the evidence for the efficacy of vaccine prevention, chemotherapy, and chemoprophylaxis with either amantadine or rimantadine. Comparative trials of rimantadine versus amantadine favor rimantadine because of reduced adverse effects, but "high"-dose (200-mg/day) amantadine was used. Next study should be a comparative trial using 100 mg of amantadine daily.

Hayden FG, et al. Emergence and apparent transmission of rimantadine-resistant influenza A virus in families. N Engl J Med 1989; 321:1696–702.

In a placebo-controlled trial among 57 families whose members received rimantadine prophylaxis after identification of a household index, rimantadine failed because rimantadine-resistant strains were transmitted from the treated index patients. Amantadine resistance has also been described. Assuming that treating patients with established influenza induces resistance suggests that the index cases should not be treated if at all possible when attempting household prophylaxis.

Sears S, Clements ML. Protective efficacy of low dose amantadine in adults when challenged with mild-type influenza A. Antimicrob Agents Chemother 1987; 31:1470–3.

Well-designed study supporting efficacy of "low-dose," 100 mg orally daily, amantadine.

Patriarca PA, et al. Prevention and control of type A influenza infections in nursing homes. Ann Intern Med 1987; 107:732–40.

Analysis of the cost-effectiveness of the possible preventive strategies of vaccination and antiviral prophylaxis, reviewing the evidence for vaccine efficacy in the elderly. Strongly justifies the cost of vaccine.

17. SINUSITIS
Suzanne W. Fletcher and Amelia F. Drake

Sinusitis is inflammation of the mucosal lining of the paranasal sinuses. Irritation and edema in the area of the ostia, the apertures through which the sinuses drain, lead to obstruction, stasis, and subsequent infection. Factors that may induce such a response include allergens and environmental irritants such as nicotine or other air pollutants. Polyps or tumors of the nasal or paranasal cavities can also obstruct sinus drainage. Sinusitis is a common diagnosis in ambulatory care, accounting for about 1% of office visits in the United States. Approximately 25% of people develop sinusitis some time during their lives.

Sinusitis is subdivided by duration into acute sinusitis, with symptoms lasting up to 3 weeks; subacute sinusitis, with symptoms lasting from 3 weeks to 3 months; and chronic sinusitis, with symptoms occurring over 3 months. Figure 17-1 shows three of the four pairs of sinuses. The maxillary sinuses are thought to be most frequently involved in adults with acute sinusitis, and because these sinuses are also most accessible, the majority of studies have been carried out on them. Most of what is known about "sinusitis" is really about maxillary sinusitis. Frontal sinusitis is the next most frequently occurring form in adults, while ethmoid sinusitis is most common in children. Isolated sphenoid sinusitis is rare.

Diagnosis

Symptoms and Signs
The classic "textbook" description of sinusitis is aching pain, usually over the involved sinus, with congestion, foul nasal discharge, fever, and malaise, often following a recent upper respiratory tract infection. The pain is made worse by bending over and increases by late morning. Pain may also develop at night and shift from side to side with changing positions. The headache may correspond to the sinus involved, with maxillary or anterior ethmoid sinusitis presenting as facial pain, and posterior ethmoid and sphenoid sinusitis classically presenting with pain referred to the retroorbital areas or the top of the head. On examination, there may be tenderness over the involved sinus, edematous nasal mucosa, and nasal discharge.

Clinical diagnosis of sinusitis is confounded by the fact that many of the "classic" symptoms and signs do not correlate well with sinusitis; more importantly, they do not differentiate between sinusitis (for which antibiotics are indicated) and other common problems of the upper respiratory tract, such as rhinitis and upper respiratory tract infections (for

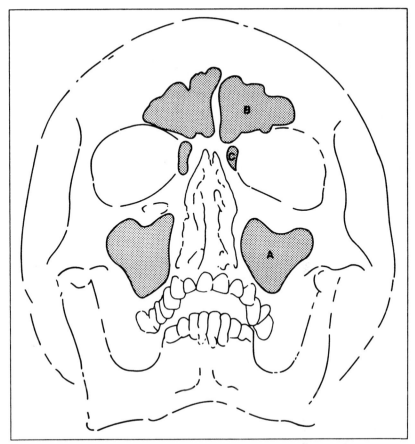

Fig. 17-1. The three pairs of sinuses seen on a Waters' view: (A) maxillary, (B) frontal, and (C) ethmoid. The sphenoid sinuses, not shown, are best seen on a lateral view.

which antibiotics usually are not indicated). Although several symptoms are found more commonly in patients with radiographically proved sinusitis than in those suspected of sinusitis who do not have the findings on x-ray, these symptoms only partially differentiate between sinusitis and other upper respiratory tract problems. Pain on mastication, fever higher than 100.4°F (38°C), pus in the middle meatus, and speech indicating "fullness of the sinuses" are each found in about 25 to 30% of patients with radiologically confirmed sinusitis, compared to less than 10% of patients with negative findings on sinus films. Preceding upper respiratory tract infection, decreased sense of smell, general malaise, and cough are each more common in patients with sinusitis (50–90%), but are also prevalent in patients without sinusitis (40–67%). Studies of the sensitivity, specificity, and predictive value of combinations of symptoms and signs have not been reported. To diagnose sinusitis by symptoms alone, therefore, is very difficult.

On examination, sinus tenderness does not differentiate sinusitis from rhinitis, but mucopurulent secretion in the nose suggests sinusitis. Using a nasal speculum, examination of the lateral wall of the nose may show pus draining from the middle meatus (maxillary and frontal and anterior ethmoid sinus drainage). Pus draining from the superior meatus (posterior ethmoid sinus drainage) is not likely to be seen. Topical decongestants may be helpful in opening the ostia at the time of the examination.

Transillumination

Transillumination of the maxillary and frontal sinuses can help establish the diagnosis of sinusitis. An attachment to the otoscope made specifically for this purpose is the best source of light. The easiest technique to examine the maxillary sinuses is to place a transilluminator over the lower orbital rim of the patient in a completely darkened room and look for a glow on the hard palate of the opened mouth. No transmission of light indicates increased likelihood of infected sinuses. In one study, 24 of 24 sinuses that showed no transillumination were found to be infected on evaluation of sinus aspirate, whereas in 15 cases in which transillumination results were clearly normal, the aspirate demonstrated no infection in all but 1. Transillumination was less helpful when findings were equivocal: of 26 sinuses in which transillumination was dull or decreased, 7 were infected as demonstrated by aspiration and 19 were not. Frontal sinuses can also be transilluminated by placing the light against the floor of the frontal sinus at the superior medial edge of the orbit. A glow should be transmitted through the anterior wall of the sinus. When interpreting this test, the clinician should remember that in approximately 5% of people, one or both frontal sinuses have not developed.

Laboratory Tests

Cultures of material swabbed from the nasal mucosa are costly and unrewarding. Several studies have shown that the results do not correlate well with those of cultures of sinus mucosa.

Short of the CT scan, plain x-rays of sinuses are the "gold standard" for the diagnosis of sinusitis in clinical practice. Comparisons of radiographic results with culture results of maxillary sinuses have shown a good correlation. In one study, 34 of 34 radiographically normal sinuses were normal on aspiration, and 30 of 31 sinuses with opaque sinuses, air fluid levels, or mucosa more than 8 mm thick were infected. The problem is cost. A full series of sinus films can cost as much as $75. In some places, a single view can be ordered. When this is possible, Waters' view is usually the most helpful: The head is tilted to prevent the temporal bone from overlapping the maxillary sinuses and, therefore, the maxillary, frontal, and ethmoid sinuses are well seen (see Fig. 17-1). Because of expense and inconvenience to patients, x-rays should not be a routine part of the evaluation of every patient presenting with possible sinusitis.

At the present time, transillumination appears to be a simple and inexpensive first step in diagnosing uncomplicated acute maxillary sinusitis; physicians should learn this procedure. Radiographic evaluation is reasonable for patients who are at high risk (e.g., patients receiving immunosuppressive drugs or with diabetes), who have suspected disease in the other paranasal sinuses, who have suspected chronic sinusitis, and/or whose illnesses do not resolve as expected.

Treatment

The most common bacterial causes of acute sinusitis are *Hemophilus influenzae, Streptococcus pneumoniae,* and various anaerobes. In chronic sinusitis, anaerobic organisms play a large role (> 50%), including *Bacteroides,* anaerobic gram-positive cocci, and *Fusobacterium* species. Less commonly, infections with *Neisseria* species, beta-hemolytic streptococcus, *Staphylococcus aureus, Pseudomonas aeruginosa,* and *Escherichia coli* are reported. Viruses account for 10% to 15% of sinusitis cases; rhinovirus is the most commonly recovered. Fungal infections are a rare cause of sinusitis in healthy persons and, when they occur, are usually caused by aspergilli. Unusual organisms causing sinusitis have been found in patients with human immunodeficiency virus (HIV) infection or other immunologically compromising conditions. Rhinocerebral mucormycosis can be fatal in the diabetic patient.

Antibiotics to which the most common organisms are sensitive have been shown by rigorous studies, including randomized, controlled trials, to be effective in treating sinusitis. Ampicillin (500 mg q6h), amoxicillin (250 mg or 500 mg tid), doxycycline (200 mg initially followed by 100 mg qd), and trimethoprim-sulfamethoxazole (2 tablets bid) all have been shown to work, without striking differences. The choice among them should be made according to convenience and cost. Because there is evidence that sinus x-rays frequently continue to be abnormal and symptoms are still present after 7 to 10 days, a 2- to 3-week course is probably best.

Topical sympathomimetic decongestants (e.g., xylometazoline [Otrivin]) are usually added. The typical dosage is several drops in each nostril every 8 hours for 3 to 5 days. The pediatric-strength decongestant reputedly protects against rebound congestion sometimes seen with adult-strength decongestants. Prescribing analgesics for symptomatic relief of pain is appropriate, and heat and steam inhalation (standing in a shower or near a steaming kettle) is often advised. If polyps coexist, nasal steroids may be added. None of these recommendations has been subjected to rigorous evaluation, but they are reasonable and inexpensive.

When to Refer

Consultation with an otolaryngologist is appropriate for patients who appear toxic, are immunocompromised, or have complications. Complications of sinusitis can be local, such as osteomyelitis, orbital (cellulitis or abscess which can progress to blindness), or intracranial (meningoencephalitis, brain abscess, or cavernous sinus thrombosis). Patients with recurrent or chronic disease that is resistant to medical management also should be referred. In those cases, a CT scan of the sinuses frequently reveals obstruction of the ostiomeatal complex and limited sinus surgery using an endoscopic technique may be indicated.

Patients with acute frontal sinusitis or persistent sphenoid sinusitis should be referred. Because the frontal sinuses drain poorly and because of the possibility of serious complications (e.g., osteomyelitis or intracranial extension leading to meningitis, subdural abscess, cavernous sinus thrombosis, frontal lobe abscess), some specialists advise that acute frontal sinusitis be considered an ear-nose-throat emergency. Hospitalization may be advised for intravenous antibiotic therapy, close observation, and surgical drainage. Persistent sphenoid sinusitis is of concern because the location of the sphenoid sinus makes it a potential parameningeal focus for seeding the brain.

Malow JB, Creticos CM. Nonsurgical treatment of sinusitis. Otolaryngol Clin North Am 1989; 22(4):809–18.
  A good, general discussion of clinical presentation, etiology, and complications of sinusitis.

Daley CL, Sande M. The runny nose: infection of the paranasal sinuses. Infect Dis Clin North Am 1988; 2(1):137–47.
  Another good general review, covering pathophysiology, etiology, clinical presentation, differential diagnosis, complications, and treatment.

Weber AL. Inflammatory diseases of the paranasal sinuses and mucoceles. Otolaryngol Clin North Am 1988; 21(3):421–37.
  A concise discussion of acute and chronic sinusitis, including complications, unusual causes such as granulomatous disease and mycotic infections, and illustrations of radiographic findings.

Axelsson A, Runze U. Symptoms and signs of acute maxillary sinusitis. ORL J Otorhinolaryngol Relat Spec 1976; 38:298–308.
  Analyzes symptoms and signs of acute maxillary sinusitis and correlates these with radiographic results. One of the few studies critically evaluating the clinical presentation of sinusitis.

Evans FO, et al. Sinusitis of the maxillary antrum. N Engl J Med 1975; 293:735–9.
  Transillumination and x-ray results correlated well with examination of maxillary antrum aspirates. Nasal swab cultures did not.

Axelsson A, et al. Treatment of acute maxillary sinusitis. Acta Otolaryngol (Stockh) 1981; 91:313–8.
  Elaborates on medical treatment of acute sinusitis.

Hamory BH, et al. Etiology and antimicrobial therapy of acute maxillary sinusitis. J Infect Dis 1979; 139:197–202.
  Discussion of etiologic agents and effective treatments.

Lew D, et al. Sphenoid sinusitis: a review of 30 cases. N Engl J Med 1983; 309:1149–54.
  A review of a rare type of sinusitis in adults.

18. SORE THROAT
Robert M. Centor and Frederick A. Meier

Sore throat is one of the four most frequent reasons for episodic outpatient care in the United States. Patients usually seek medical attention primarily for symptomatic relief; physicians typically are concerned with preventing rheumatic fever. Because sore throats caused by group A beta-hemolytic streptococci tend to be severe, predispose to rheumatic fever, and need to be treated, they become the focus of the visit. However, other causes of sore throat must also be considered. Viral respiratory infections, the most frequent cause of sore throat, require only symptomatic therapy, but infections due to some less common agents require specific evaluation and treatment.

Group A Streptococcal Pharyngitis
The benefits of diagnosing and treating group A streptococcal pharyngitis fall into four categories:

1. *Rheumatic fever prevention.* Both acute rheumatic fever and post-streptococcal glomerulonephritis are "nonsuppurative" complications that can follow group A streptococcal pharyngitis. Although the incidence of acute rheumatic fever has fallen precipitously during the past 30 years, recent outbreaks show that it still can pose a threat, especially to children and young adults in crowded living situations. Antibiotic treatment decreases the risk of acute rheumatic fever by 90%, and the protective effect of treatment can be shown even in patients who begin antibiotic therapy as long as 9 days after the onset of symptoms. Although glomerulonephritis may be linked to a prior streptococcal infection, it is a rare, strain-specific complication that usually resolves with complete restoration of normal renal function. The issue of whether antibiotics decrease the risk of post-streptococcal glomerulonephritis is unsettled.

2. *Prevention of suppurative complications.* The suppurative complications of group A streptococcal pharyngitis, such as peritonsillar abscess, suppurative otitis media, and cervical lymphadenitis, have in the past 40 years almost disappeared in North America and Western Europe, probably because of antibiotic therapy.

3. *Decreased spread to close contacts.* Antibiotic therapy has been shown in studies from the 1950s to decrease both spread of epidemic group A streptococcal pharyngitis (in schools and army barracks) and spread of endemic illness (in families).

4. *Decreased duration of disease.* Although classic early studies demonstrated that prompt treatment of Group A streptococcal pharyngitis shortened its course, this has not been considered a proven benefit until recently. Prompted by the availability of rapid antigen detection tests, several careful studies have now shown that prompt antibiotic therapy, as opposed to waiting 24 to 48 hours for culture results, decreases the duration of symptoms by about a day.

Clinical Diagnosis
To achieve symptomatic benefit, group A streptococcal pharyngitis must be diagnosed and treated at the initial visit, based on signs and symptoms and, where appropriate, antigen test results. Routine throat culture results take 24 to 48 hours, and thus provide only confirmatory information.

While a definitive diagnosis of group A streptococcal pharyngitis cannot be made from clinical data alone, the probability may be assessed from information obtained in the medical history and physical examination, coupled with knowledge of the prevalence of group A streptococcal pharyngitis in the patient population. This probability estimate provides a rationale for prescribing or withholding antibiotics in the absence of laboratory results. Significant clinical variables include: tonsillar exudates; swollen, tender anterior cervical lymph nodes; absence of a cough; and a history of fever. As the number of these variables increases from zero to four, the probability increases that a patient's sore throat is due to group A streptococci. Table 18-1 shows the probabilities of group A streptococcal pharyngitis in patients with different scores from populations with different disease preva-

Table 18-1. Probability (%) of group A streptococcal pharyngitis based on prevalence and clinical findings ("strep score")

Strep score*	Prevalence	
	In most office practices	In emergency rooms
0	1%	3%
1	4%	8%
2	9%	18%
3	21%	38%
4	43%	63%

*Strep score is derived by giving 1 point for each of the following: tonsillar exudate, anterior cervical adenopathy, absence of cough, presence of fever.

lence. Most office practices will observe an underlying prevalence of 10%, while emergency rooms see a higher prevalence, in the 20% range.

Laboratory Diagnosis

ANTIGEN TESTS. Numerous rapid antigen detection methods are available for office use. These tests are all based on identifying streptococcal antigen from throat swab material, but differ in the extraction methods and antigen-antibody identification methods used. Most commercial tests now use the acid extraction method, which is faster than enzyme extraction, although it concentrates the antigen less efficiently and is therefore less sensitive. Enzyme immunoassay is the identification technique used most often in commercial tests; the alternative, latex agglutination, requires more skill to interpret, and is therefore less specific when used by unskilled personnel. Rapid office tests based on acid extraction/enzyme immunoassay have sensitivities of about 80% and specificities of around 98%.

THROAT CULTURE. While in the past throat cultures have been the primary diagnostic test for group A streptococcal pharyngitis, they are neither perfectly sensitive nor perfectly specific. Using multiple-swab/multiple-culture techniques as a reference standard, the sensitivity for a single swab/single culture is about 90%. Studies of asymptomatic adults show a positive culture rate of 1%, so the specificity of throat culture for diagnosing streptococcal pharyngitis is 99% in adults. Test conditions can influence these test characteristics. Several studies have compared office cultures with laboratory cultures, and found sensitivities that range widely from 29 to 90% and specificities that range from 76 to 99%.

Although pediatricians sometimes attempt to interpret cultures after as few as 6 hours, most authorities hold that cultures should be read only after a minimum of 24 hours of incubation. Waiting for culture results denies patients the opportunity for symptomatic relief afforded by early antibiotic therapy, and without reliable follow-up, leaves some patients with group A streptococcal pharyngitis untreated and susceptible to its complications.

SEROLOGIC TESTS. Serologic tests, like antiDNase and antistreptolysin O (ASO) titers, confirm the diagnosis of streptococcal infection with elevated titers that appear several weeks after the pharyngitis. These tests have no role in the clinical diagnosis of group A streptococcal pharyngitis, and should be reserved for research purposes or for retrospective diagnosis of recent streptococcal infection.

Recommended Clinical Strategy

If the clinical probability of group A streptococcal pharyngitis exceeds 40%, as determined by an estimate of prevalence and the clinical indexes, the patient may be treated without performing any laboratory tests. At or above this probability, the benefits of early treatment outweigh the risks of giving antibiotics to some patients who do not have group A streptococcal pharyngitis. If the probability of group A streptococcal pharyngitis is less than 40%, but greater than 5%, an antigen test should be performed and only those patients who have a positive result should be treated. Because of the imperfect sensitivity of the rapid antigen test, cultures should be done on those patients with negative results on rapid tests, to facilitate the prevention of rheumatic fever by follow-up treatment of patients with positive culture and negative rapid antigen test results. Patients who have a probability of streptococcal infection of 5% or less almost always have a viral infection; they need not be cultured and can be treated symptomatically.

This strategy assumes culture-positive patients can always be contacted. If patients cannot be reliably contacted, treatment or reassurance must be based solely on the clinical presentation and rapid antigen test result. In circumstances of unreliable follow-up, the threshold for treatment without testing should be lowered to 16%, reserving rapid antigen testing only for patients with clinical probabilities of disease less than that threshold.

Treatment
While intramuscular penicillin produces a higher rate of bacteriologic eradication of group A streptococci from the pharynx, oral penicillin (250 mg po qid for 10 days) has also been shown to prevent rheumatic fever and shorten the course of disease. Because oral penicillin is less associated with anaphylaxis, it is usually prescribed in cases of presumed group A streptococcal pharyngitis. Erythromycin, despite its gastrointestinal symptoms, remains the agent of choice in penicillin-allergic patients. Because bacteriologic treatment "failures" have no implication for rheumatic fever prevention, "test of cure" (reculturing) after a course of therapy is unnecessary, unless the patient remains symptomatic. In persistently symptomatic patients, amoxicillin-clavulinic acid (250 mg po tid for 10 days) is a plausible second-line drug; in these patients, it has been theorized, beta-lactamase–producing flora may inactivate penicillin, preventing adequate therapy with penicillinase-sensitive agents alone.

Other Causes of Sore Throats
Most other bacterial and viral agents cause self-limited sore throats with nonspecific findings. More serious and even life-threatening pharyngeal infections, such as epiglottitis and diphtheria, have specific presentations that must be promptly recognized so that effective treatment can be initiated. Pharyngitis associated with ulcers or abscesses may also be caused by bacteria and viruses that respond to specific therapy.

Nonspecific Presentations
Viral pharyngitis typically presents as a mild sore throat accompanied by cough and coryza. Patients rarely have temperatures above 101°F (38.3°C). While the pharynx is often red, inflammatory exudates are less common and less extensive than in bacterial sore throats. Pharyngitis presenting in association with conjunctivitis is usually due to a self-limited adenovirus infection that clears in 4 to 5 days. Fevers to 103 to 104°F (39.4–40.0°C) may be present, with chills, myalgias, and tonsillar exudates. When the presentation is typical for a viral etiology, only symptomatic treatment is needed.

Epstein-Barr virus (EBV) infection may cause a subacute pharyngitis. EBV infectious mononucleosis often presents with pharyngitis, which is exudative in about half of the patients, and is accompanied by fever, prominent cervical lymphadenopathy, and fatigue. Palatal petechiae are seen in about 25%. Diagnosis is strengthened by the presence of atypical lymphocytes on a blood smear and may be confirmed by the differential agglutination "spot" test for heterophil antibodies; the latter have largely supplanted the more complicated Paul-Bunnell-Davidsohn assay (see Chap. 116). The tendency of patients with this infection to develop a rash with ampicillin therapy is a contraindication to using this drug in patients with pharyngitis. Since amoxicillin appears to behave similarly to ampicillin in causing rashes, EBV infectious mononucleosis should be ruled out when embarking on amoxicillin-clavulinic therapy for persistent sore throat.

Non–group A beta-hemolytic streptococci, especially group C organisms, may cause sore throats in adults, but have not been implicated in the pathogenesis of rheumatic fever. When compared to group A streptococcal pharyngitis, group C–associated sore throats are generally less frequent and less severe. These organisms will not be identified by rapid antigen tests and, if only group A–specific techniques are used to identify beta-hemolytic colonies on routine culture, will be lumped together in the "non–group A" category or not mentioned at all on culture reports. Although treatment has not been shown to modify the course, most non–group A organisms are penicillin- and erythromycin-sensitive, and there is no contraindication to empiric treatment.

Arcanobacterium (formerly *Corynebacterium*) *haemolyticum*, an agent that is not detected by routine culture techniques, causes a rare syndrome of pharyngitis and rash that is potentially susceptible to antistreptococcal antibiotic regimens.

Mycoplasma pneumoniae may cause pharyngitis, and is more likely to be associated with bronchopulmonary symptoms than streptococcal pharyngitis. Treatment with erythromycin or tetracycline (250 mg qid for 7–10 days) may shorten the course. Culture of this organism is difficult and impractical in clinical settings and serum IgM assays are insensitive early in the course; the decision to treat must be based on clinical suspicion.

Chlamydia pneumoniae has recently been recognized as a respiratory pathogen and has been isolated from patients with symptomatic pharyngitis without evidence of other pathogens. Diagnosis is impractical to confirm, requiring cell culture techniques. Treatment with erythromycin or a tetracycline is of unproved value, but is reasonable in a patient with pharyngitis associated with bronchopulmonary symptoms or with a persistent pharyngitis associated with negative streptococcal cultures; this regimen will cover *M. pneumoniae* as well as *C. pneumoniae*.

Neisseria gonorrhoeae has not been shown to cause symptomatic pharyngitis, so cultures for this organism need not be obtained in patients with sore throats. Throat cultures for *N. gonorrhoea* should, however, be considered in patients who have signs and symptoms of genitourinary gonorrhea, or who are contacts of persons with gonorrhea, regardless of the presence or absence of sore throat. Diagnosis requires culture on Thayer-Martin media, and differentiation of *N. gonorrhoea* from commensal upper respiratory *Neisseria*. Treatment is important because if the infection is not eradicated from the pharynx, the gonococcus may reseed genital epithelia during oral-genital intercourse. Ceftriaxone, 250 mg intramuscularly, is recommended to eliminate such colonization.

Severe Sore Throat Syndromes

EPIGLOTTITIS. *Hemophilus influenzae* can produce an epiglottitis distinct from the usual sore throat that can progress rapidly to life-threatening airway obstruction. Pain disproportionate to the degree of inflammation, pooling of saliva with associated drooling, and a soft muffled voice are typical findings. A lateral neck film is used to confirm the diagnosis; visualization of the epiglottis via indirect laryngoscopy may precipitate obstruction and should be avoided. Treatment includes close observation, usually in the hospital; maintaining an adequate airway, with intubation if necessary; and intravenous antibiotics (usually a third-generation cephalosporin such as ceftriaxone).

DIPHTHERIA. Caused by *Corynebacterium diphtheriae*, diphtheria is a pseudomembranous pharyngitis with systemic toxemia. While uncommon, outbreaks still occur in the United States, and it is estimated that 20% of adults have an inadequate immunization status. The sore throat and fever are usually mild; systemic signs include weakness, malaise, and a pulse rate that is rapid and out of proportion to the fever. The pseudomembrane is a gray-white, tenacious exudate that leaves a focally hemorrhagic raw surface when plucked from the posterior part of the pharynx. Other exudative sore throats, including Vincent's angina described below, are occasionally associated with an oropharyngeal membrane. The membranes in these cases are less extensive and systemic signs of toxemia are not present. Identification or isolation of *C. diphtheriae* requires special laboratory maneuvers, such as fluorescent antibody stains of the pharyngeal swab specimen or removed pseudomembrane, and special culture media; treatment with antitoxin and penicillin or erythromycin must therefore be initiated before diagnostic confirmation.

PERITONSILLITIS AND PERITONSILLAR ABSCESS (QUINSY SORE THROAT). Formerly a common suppurative complication of group A streptococcal infection, peritonsillitis and peritonsillar abscess are now usually associated with mixed oropharyngeal flora: *Staphylococcus aureus*, oral streptococci, and anaerobic bacteria. Presentation is usually unilateral, and characterized by severe pain, often resulting in impaired swallowing. In the past, treatment with penicillin has been successful, but recently beta-lactamase–resistant agents have been advocated; if an abscess is present, incision and drainage by an experienced clinician may be necessary.

Pharyngitis Associated with Ulcers

VINCENT'S ANGINA (TRENCH MOUTH). This disorder is a painful, ulcerative pharyngitis, gingivitis, and tonsillitis, resulting from a mixed spirochete-anaerobic bacterial infection. A foul odor is often present from the mouth. Exudate commonly forms over the ulcerated areas and is sometimes confused with the diphtherial pseudomembrane. Diagnosis can be confirmed by an experienced microbiologist or clinician, with a Gram's stain of the exudate showing corkscrew, bacillary, and coccal forms. Treatment includes saline and peroxide mouthwash and oral penicillin or erythromycin; some consultants now advocate beta-lactamase–resistant agents such as amoxicillin-clavulinic acid to cover anaerobes.

HERPANGINA. This self-limited pharyngitis is due to coxsackieviruses, usually occurring in the summer months, sometimes in epidemics. It presents with multiple small (1–2 mm) vesicles or ulcers on the soft palate. Patients with herpangina do not appear very ill, and treatment is symptomatic.

HERPES SIMPLEX VIRUS. Primary infection with herpes simplex virus can present as pharyngitis with vesicles that become ulcers. It may occur at any time during the year. The ulcers tend to be fewer and larger than those seen with herpangina, and may appear on the buccal mucosa, tongue, floor of the mouth, or posterior pharynx, rather than just the soft palate. A rapid Giemsa (Dif Quik) stain will reveal multinucleated giant cells. Patients with primary herpes simplex virus pharyngitis usually appear sicker than those with herpangina. Early treatment with acyclovir shortens the duration of symptoms.

CANDIDA ALBICANS OROPHARYNGITIS (THRUSH). This form of pharyngitis presents with inflammatory ulcers, often covered by cottony plaques that yield characteristic yeast as demonstrated by Gram's stain. It is often associated with immune deficiency states. Treatment is with clotrimazole troches or nystatin.

Symptomatic Therapy

Analgesics such as acetaminophen, aspirin, and ibuprofen decrease the pain associated with pharyngitis. Antihistamine elixirs (Benadryl) have a topical effect and may reduce pharyngeal pain when they are swished or gargled. Use should be limited to 2 teaspoons (25 mg) every 4 to 6 hours to avoid sedation or other antihistamine side effects from swallowed medication. Inflamed pharyngeal mucosa may also be soothed by saline gargles (made from ½ teaspoon of salt added to 1 cup of warm water), a variety of throat lozenges (some over-the-counter preparations even contain benzocaine or other local anesthetics), and other "home remedies."

Recurrent Sore Throat

Patients may occasionally describe either prolonged symptoms or recurrent sore throats. Several possibilities should be considered in the differential diagnosis.

As mentioned above, some patients with group A streptococcal pharyngitis will not respond to an initial course of penicillin, perhaps because of the presence of beta-lactamase–producing organisms. Patients with persistent or recurrent symptoms who have been treated for streptococcal pharyngitis should be recultured. If repeat cultures demonstrate group A streptococci, a course of amoxicillin-clavulinic acid (250 mg po tid for 10 days) is reasonable. If cultures of "therapeutic failures" do not grow group A streptococci, an alternative diagnosis should be considered.

Recurrent or chronic sore throat may also accompany an allergic condition such as rhinitis with postnasal drip, and may respond to a therapeutic trial of antihistamines. Irritants such as cigarette smoke should also be considered.

Centor RM, Meier FA, Dalton HP. Throat cultures and rapid tests for diagnosis of group A streptococcal pharyngitis. In: Sox HC Jr, ed. Common diagnostic tests: use and interpretation. 2nd ed. Philadelphia: American College of Physicians, 1990: 247–64.
Provides the evidence for the approach to group A streptococcal pharyngitis presented here.

Denny FW. Effect of treatment on streptococcal pharyngitis: is the issue really settled? Pediatr Infect Dis J 1985; 4:352–4.
A concise editorial by the dean of clinical streptococcologists.

Dajani AS, et al. Prevention of rheumatic fever: a statement for health professionals by the Committee on Rheumatic Fever, Endocarditis, and Kawasaki Disease of the Council on Cardiovascular Disease in the Young, the American Heart Association. Circulation 1988; 78:1082–6.
Current, authoritative recommendations.

Brook I. Emergence and persistence of beta-lactamase producing bacteria in the oropharynx following penicillin treatment. Arch Otolaryngol Head Neck Surg 1988; 114:667–70.
A scenario for failure of oral penicillin therapy of group A streptococcal pharyngitis.

Kaplan EL, Johnson DR. Eradication of group A streptococci from the upper respiratory tract by amoxicillin with clavulanate after oral penicillin V treatment failure. J Pediatr 1988; 113:400–3.
"Additional studies of streptococcal treatment failures must be carried out so that optimal therapy can be determined. In the meanwhile, . . . the combination of amoxicillin and potassium clavulanate can be added to the list of effective antimicrobial agents."

Cimolai N, et al. Do the beta-hemolytic non-group A streptococci cause pharyngitis? Rev Infect Dis 1988; 10:587–601.
In 1989, the answer appeared to be: yes in adults; no in children.

Meier FA, Centor RM, Graham L, Dalton HP. Clinical and microbiological evidence for endemic pharyngitis among adults due to group C streptococci. Arch Intern Med 1990; 150:825–9.
A clinical description of group C streptococcal pharyngitis.

Todd JK. The sore throat: pharyngitis and epiglottitis. Infect Dis Clin North Am 1988; 2(1):149–62.
A pediatrician reviews the most common causes of sore throat.

Hayden GF, Hendley JO, Gwaltney JM. Management of the ambulatory patient with a sore throat. Curr Clin Top Infect Dis 1988; 9:62–75.
Discusses the relative frequency, evaluation, and treatment of various causes of sore throat.

Aronson MD, Komoraff AL. Pharyngitis. Curr Ther Infect Dis 1990; 3:101–5.
A concise review of evaluation and treatment of streptococcal and other types of sore throats, including diagnostic algorithms for common, unusual, and high-risk conditions.

19. HOARSENESS
James P. Browder and Duncan S. Postma

Hoarseness is an abnormality of voice production characterized by breathiness or harshness of the voice. It results from a lack of smooth approximation of the vocal cords, either from intralaryngeal pathology or a lack of normal vocal cord mobility. Hoarseness rarely presents as a functional disorder and is usually associated with a demonstrable laryngeal abnormality. If persistent, the symptom demands definitive diagnosis because lesions such as laryngeal carcinoma require early and specific treatment.

Causes

Primary Intralaryngeal Causes

Primary intralaryngeal conditions are the most common causes of hoarseness. Viral laryngitis is characterized by the acute onset of hoarseness without dyspnea and is usually accompanied by rhinopharyngitis. The syndrome is more common in the winter months. Bacterial laryngitis is less common but can be life-threatening, as in the case of acute epiglottitis (supraglottitis), caused by *Hemophilis influenzae*. Acute epiglottitis typically produces a "muffled" voice rather than true hoarseness.

Chronic exposure to tobacco smoke, even passively, can produce irritative laryngitis with edema of the laryngeal mucosa, particularly along the free edge of the vocal cord where vibration is most intense. This trauma, plus exposure to the carcinogens in tobacco smoke, can lead to dysplasia of the laryngeal mucosa, in situ cancer, and eventually frankly invasive epidermoid carcinoma.

Voice abuse is also a common cause of vocal cord lesions. They occur in children who are habitual "screamers," cheerleaders, workers in noisy environments, singers, teachers, and lawyers. Lesions of the vocal cords include nodules ("singer's nodes"), polyps (more closely linked to smoking), and contact ulcers. The ulcers usually present as hoarseness with upper neck or pharyngeal pain, which is exacerbated by speaking or singing.

Malignant tumors are less common but should be considered in anyone with hoarseness, particularly those who smoke or abuse alcohol. The incidence is highest in the sixth and seventh decades of life, and affects men more frequently than women.

Other, less common intralaryngeal causes of hoarseness are foreign body ingestion, benign tumors, traumatic granulomas from intubation, granulomatous diseases, myxedema, and esophageal reflux.

Secondary Intralaryngeal Causes

Weakness of the intrinsic laryngeal muscles, because of myasthenia gravis or hypothyroidism or a bulbar palsy (usually associated with significant dysphagia), can cause hoarseness. Cricoarytenoid joint arthritis or fixation can also cause hoarseness and has been documented in association with rheumatoid arthritis, gout, systemic lupus erythematosus, intubation trauma, and accidental injury.

Laryngeal Nerve Damage

Laryngeal nerve damage is an infrequent cause of hoarseness. Because the left recurrent nerve has a longer course than the right, it is affected almost ten times more often. The superior laryngeal nerves are less often paralyzed than the recurrent laryngeal nerves, and their paralysis is probably less often recognized, since the effects are more subtle. The most frequently identified causes of recurrent laryngeal nerve palsy are surgical procedures of the thyroid, neck, or chest and malignancies of the thyroid, esophageal, pulmonary, or other tissues that either directly invade or compress the nerve. Other causes include diabetic or viral neuropathy. In many cases, the cause is never identified.

Functional Hoarseness

Functional hoarseness refers to changes in voice quality not attributable to any detectable organic pathology. Dysphonia plicae ventricularis ("false cord hoarseness") results from using the false instead of the true vocal cords for phonation. If often follows laryngitis and persists after the infection has resolved. Spastic dysphonia, a jerky, poorly coordinated voice with variations in pitch and intensity, may be the result of disease in the central nervous system. Aphonia (complete absence of the voice) is rarely conscious malingering, although secondary gain from the illness may play a major role in its occurrence.

Gastroesophageal Reflux

Gastroesophageal reflux is an uncommon but frequently missed cause of chronic hoarseness. It presents as mild hoarseness, often worse in the mornings, accompanied by increased amounts of phlegm and a mild-to-moderate throat pain, and sometimes a bad taste in the mouth. This condition is more likely to occur in smokers and those who use alcohol, making the precise cause of these symptoms sometimes difficult to establish. The diagnosis is confirmed by barium swallow radiograph and treated with the usual measures for gastroesophageal reflux (see Chap. 42).

Diagnosis

History

The history should focus on five important areas:

1. What was the nature of the onset of the hoarseness, and how long has it been present? An acute onset, without antecedent trauma or history of foreign body ingestion, suggests an infectious or inflammatory cause. A more chronic course is consistent with voice abuse, irritation from smoking, or neoplasia. Hoarseness that develops only late in the course of a day suggests a neuromuscular disorder (e.g., myasthenia gravis or a partially compensated recurrent laryngeal nerve palsy).

2. Is the hoarseness constant or intermittent? Constant hoarseness suggests a persisting structural change in the larynx such as those secondary to tumor, trauma, or a poorly compensated cord palsy. Functional aphonia is usually constant, although the patient can produce a normal cough on demand, demonstrating physiologic closure of the glottis. Dysphonia plicae ventricularis presents as a constantly harsh voice ("stage whisper"), but also is associated with a normal cough. Intermittent hoarseness usually implies a benign or temporary condition, and its cause may be voice fatigue, "postnasal drip," or idiopathic.

3. What are the associated regional symptoms? Sore throat, ear pain, and dysphagia with hoarseness of more than 2 weeks' duration strongly suggest malignancy. Dyspnea can also signal a cancer or, less often, bilateral vocal cord palsies. Pain can also be a prominent symptom with a contact ulcer or arthritis. A more acute course suggests infection or a foreign body; dyspnea and drooling with a muffled voice strongly suggest acute epiglottitis. Aspiration may accompany a tracheoesophageal fistula (either congenital or associated with trauma or tumor erosion) or, more commonly, unilateral vocal cord palsy, in which case the voice usually has an "especially breathy" or "raspy" quality. Reflux of acid gastric contents may result in hoarseness secondary to an irritative laryngitis, which is typically worse in the mornings.

4. What are the associated systemic symptoms? For example, is there weight loss (malignancy); cough, hemoptysis, or chest pain (intrathoracic etiology); fever (infection); or generalized weakness without weight loss (neuromuscular disorder)?

5. What are possible etiologic or contributing factors? For example, is there a history of voice abuse or trauma, including surgery and cigarette or alcohol abuse?

Physical Examination

Emphasis should be placed on the oral cavity, oropharynx, and neck. However, examination to exclude medical causes, such as myasthenia gravis or hypothyroidism, should be considered.

An indirect (mirror) examination of the larynx is usually indicated in patients complaining of hoarseness. It is mandatory in three situations: (1) if hoarseness has persisted for more than 2 weeks; (2) in patients at high risk for laryngeal cancer, that is, older people and anyone who is a heavy smoker and/or drinker; and (3) in patients with the associated symptoms of dyspnea, pain, aspiration, or dysphagia. Indirect laryngoscopy is not usually indicated in a clear-cut situation of recent voice abuse or with the typical clinical presentation of laryngitis. Prompt evaluation is necessary if hoarseness of acute onset is associated with severe sore throat, dysphagia, or dyspnea. These are the symptoms of acute epiglottitis, which is a medical emergency because it can produce early acute airway obstruction secondary to edema of the supraglottic tissues. If acute epiglottitis is suspected, care must be taken in examining the patient, lest laryngospasm and asphyxiation be induced.

The definitive diagnosis of a mucosal lesion of the larynx can often be made by indirect examination alone. Smoker's laryngitis usually appears as edematous and erythematous vocal cords, often with polypoid changes. Vocal cord nodules typically appear as bilaterally opposing "knots" at the junction of the anterior and middle thirds of the vocal cords. Polyps occur in the same location as nodules but appear as erythematous, smooth, mobile lesions, usually larger than the typical nodule. Contact ulcers appear like any ulcer; they are found at the junction of the middle and posterior thirds of the vocal cords at the tip of the vocal process of the arytenoid cartilage.

Malignancies, when advanced, present as angry, exophytic mass lesions or ulcerations, typical of epidermoid cancer. However, early cancer of the vocal cord may be subtle, presenting as a small, white plaque or an erythematous nodule. A mass or ulcer involving a vocal cord that is immobile for no apparent cause is an ominous sign and may represent occultly invasive cancer.

With laryngeal paralysis, the affected vocal cord is usually in the paramedian position (slightly lateral to the midline). With a unilateral recurrent nerve palsy, the paralysis may not be obvious for several reasons: The paralyzed cord may adduct slightly because of the action of muscles that are innervated either bilaterally or by another nerve; also, the nonparalyzed cord may cross the midline to make contact with the paralyzed cord as a compensatory maneuver, giving the impression of a normal glottis. A superior laryngeal nerve or a combined paralysis is more unusual, and the findings may be subtle. Usually the cord is slightly bowed and flaccid; with speaking, it is seen to be at a lower level than its partner.

With functional hoarseness, there are no laryngeal abnormalities on indirect inspection. Dysphonia plicae ventricularis, however, usually can be identified by demonstrating close approximation of the false cords during phonation, which obscures the true cords.

Treatment

The treatment of viral laryngitis is supportive; increased household humidity, cough suppressants, and analgesics are usually sufficient therapy. "Laryngitis" that does not improve in 7 to 10 days may indicate more significant pathology, and treatment should not be continued without a thorough diagnostic evaluation.

Early vocal cord nodules, polyps, or contact ulcers often respond favorably to strict voice rest. Ideally, this means no use of the voice at all, although in practice minimal use of the voice is usually the best one can hope to achieve. Whispering should be discouraged, since it causes nearly as much vocal strain as yelling. If the patient must speak, a soft, breathy voice is least traumatic. If hoarseness persists for longer than 2 weeks, referral to a speech pathologist or otolaryngologist is indicated.

All patients with laryngeal mass lesions persisting longer than 2 or 3 weeks should be referred to an otolaryngologist for laryngoscopy and possible biopsy. Recurrent laryngeal nerve palsy is evaluated by a careful node examination, posteroanterior and lateral chest x-ray with special lordotic views, and barium swallow if needed. With minimal symptoms and no identifiable etiology, hoarseness can be managed by waiting for 9 to 12 months. Teflon augmentation of a unilaterally paralyzed vocal cord is often very helpful and is a relatively uncomplicated procedure.

Hess CP. An approach to throat complaints. Foreign body sensation, difficulty swallowing, and hoarseness. Emerg Med Clin North Am 1987; 5(2):313–34.

A discussion of the emergency evaluation of patients presenting with these complaints, emphasizing that they may represent either one disease or several unrelated clinical problems. Treatment options available to the emergency physician as opposed to referring the patient for specialty care are presented.

Vaughn CW. The hoarse patient. When to refer. Hosp Pract April 30, 1989; 24(4A):21–24, 29.

An excellent presentation of voice abnormalities and their common causes. Specific indicators for referral are listed. Since most hoarseness is caused by local self-limiting pathology, need for referral to a specialist is unusual.

Maragos NE. Hoarseness. Prim Care 1990; 17(2):347–63.

Reviews anatomy, pathophysiology, and ear-nose-throat examination techniques, and briefly discusses medical treatment and surgical procedures.

McNally PR, et al. Evaluation of gastroesophageal reflux as a cause of idiopathic hoarseness. Dig Dis Sci 1989; 34:1900–4.

A thorough presentation of the presenting signs and symptoms of this disorder. The authors note that throat pain and nighttime heartburn are more likely to correlate with severe esophagitis in patients with hoarseness.

20. RHINITIS
W. Paul Biggers

Rhinitis is a general term for a variety of unpleasant symptoms, including nasal obstruction, discharge, itchiness, and sneezing. These symptoms result from several syndromes with characteristic presentations but differing pathophysiologic causes and varying responses to therapy. The most commonly encountered syndromes include allergic rhinitis, vasomotor rhinitis, rhinitis medicamentosa, mechanical nasal obstruction with secondary rhinitis, and the rhinitis of pregnancy. Patients often present with more than one of these syndromes or with symptoms that are not specific for any single one. Various forms of rhinitis often occur with a closely related sinusitis; the nose and paranasal sinuses share blood supply as well as autonomic and somatic neural controls.

Allergic Rhinitis

Allergic rhinitis results when inhaled allergenic particles such as pollen grains are deposited on the nasal mucosa of susceptible individuals. Such individuals have a genetic predisposition to manufacture IgE in response to antigenic proteins. When antigen and antibody bind to mast cells or histiocytes on the respiratory epithelium, histamine and a variety of other vasoactive and inflammation-mediating substances are released. These substances cause increased capillary permeability, with resulting tissue edema and nasal obstruction, as well as increased mucus production and discharge, itching of the nose and palate, and sneezing. Concomitant bronchospasm, with cough and wheezing, may occur in some individuals if allergenic particles are small enough to be deposited lower in the airway. Allergic conjunctivitis, with itching, tearing, redness, and swelling, may also occur concurrently.

Allergic rhinitis affects more than 10% of the population and can be seasonal or perennial. Seasonal rhinitis occurs at the times of year when specific allergens, which vary from region to region, are present in the environment. In general, in temperate climates these include tree and flower pollens in the early spring, grass pollens later, and ragweed and mold spores in late summer and fall. In the winter, common allergens include house dust from heating ducts, mold spores from houseplants, and other allergens trapped in poorly circulating indoor air. Seasonal rhinitis affects all age groups; symptoms usually begin in childhood or young adulthood and often become less intense with aging. Seasonal rhinitis is often associated with allergic conjunctivitis.

Perennial rhinitis occurs in response to allergens present throughout the year or, in individuals with a broad range of sensitivities, to a number of different allergens. House dust is a potent antigenic mixture, containing excretions of the house dust mite and common cockroach, dander from house pets, feathers, and synthetic fibers. Patients who are allergic to cats are often responding not to dander (shed epithelial cells) but to dry salivary proteins deposited on the cat's fur during grooming activities. Volatile paints, especially epoxy resins, and household cleaning agents are other common sensitizers. Nonimmunologic stimuli such as tobacco smoke, perfumes, newspaper print, and alcohol often increase nasal symptoms in persons with perennial rhinitis, as they do in persons with vasomotor rhinitis. Perennial rhinitis is less likely to be associated with allergic conjunctivitis than seasonal rhinitis, and affects children and young adults more than middle-aged individuals.

Food allergy is a rare cause of rhinitis, and is more likely to affect young children than adolescents or adults. The mechanism for this condition is controversial, and many subjects with skin test reactions to certain foods have no clinical symptoms when exposed to them.

Diagnosis

The diagnosis of allergic rhinitis is established primarily by the history of typical symptoms (sneezing, itchy and watery eyes, clear thin watery or mucoid nasal discharge, and/or nasal airway obstruction) after exposure to an allergen. Symptoms that occur virtually every year at the same time suggest seasonal rhinitis, whereas the fluctuating presence of year-round symptoms suggests some form of perennial rhinitis or vasomotor rhinitis, or both. It is difficult to separate vasomotor rhinitis and allergic rhinitis on the basis of history, unless the rhinitis is secondary to seasonal allergens or specific irritants.

On physical examination, the nasal mucous membrane may display several different presentations. The common and classic finding, typically seen in patients with longstanding and almost constant rhinitis, is pale, boggy, swollen turbinates. However, early in an attack, when there is a great deal of sneezing and reaction, the mucosa may be quite red and swollen. The mucosa may also have a characteristic blue (cyanotic) appearance, when vasodilatation and slow blood flow result in oxygen extraction from the capillaries.

The presence of eosinophils on a Wright's stain of nasal secretions, either in clumps or constituting more than 10% of the white cells present, indicates a probable allergic process. To obtain the best specimen, the patient should blow the nose directly onto wax paper or cellophane; the secretions thus obtained are then transferred to a glass slide. Alternatively, the nasal mucosa can be swabbed with a cotton-tip applicator, but for best results the applicator must be left in place for 2 to 3 minutes. Eosinophilia is frequently absent in the peripheral blood count specimen, even when marked allergic symptoms are present.

The allergens responsible for allergic rhinitis can often be identified by a lengthy history, which can be very time-consuming. Immunologic testing should be reserved for patients with relatively severe allergic symptoms and those not readily controlled by symptomatic medical therapy. Skin tests done by intracutaneous or scratch techniques are often helpful in identifying not only the nature of the offending allergen, but also to some degree the severity of the allergy. The identification of specific allergens by in vitro testing, using radioimmune assay techniques, is now also widely available. The most common test employed is the radioallergosorbent test (RAST), which measures the patient's level of IgE for a specific allergen. Serum samples are tested for specific allergens that have been identified by a thorough history and questionnaire. In vitro testing is less sensitive and more expensive than skin testing, and a more limited selection of antigens is available. It is helpful, however, in patients taking antihistamines, or with equivocal skin test results, or with skin conditions that make skin tests inappropriate (e.g., generalized atopic dermatitis or dermatographism, a form of enhanced skin sensitivity). Nasal provocation tests, which reproduce symptoms by spraying the suspected antigens directly on the nasal mucosa, are occasionally helpful when other test results do not correlate with the history.

Treatment

The goal of treatment should be the reduction of symptoms to tolerable levels, but patients should be reminded that total elimination of symptoms is rarely possible. The choice of regimens should be determined by the severity of the patient's complaints, the duration of symptoms, convenience, cost, and individual preference. Patients with mild seasonal rhinitis should be treated with antihistamine-decongestant regimens and topical steroids, as discussed below, during their allergic season and spared the time, expense, and other potential problems associated with skin testing and immunotherapy. Referral to an allergist for immunologic testing and treatment should be reserved for patients with relatively severe allergic symptoms and those not readily controlled by symptomatic medical therapy.

ENVIRONMENTAL MODIFICATION. In seasonal rhinitis, environmental modification can produce considerable relief. Exposure to the offending antigen can be avoided by staying indoors, filtering room air with air conditioners or electrostatic filters, and even leaving the area during peak season. For perennial rhinitis, elimination of dust traps in the house (e.g., shag rugs, overstuffed furniture, feather pillows) and sources of mold spores (e.g., houseplants, sweating windows with mold spore, damp bathroom fixtures) may help. Mold control in the home may be assisted with fungicidal disinfectants, such as Lysol or chlorine bleach, as well as by the use of a dehumidifier in damp areas. Additional measures to control dust include use of washable curtains rather than venetian blinds; minimizing dust-catching items such as books in the bedroom; and use of a water-sealed vacuum cleaner, which traps particles in a water bath and does not blow dust around. Exposure to house dust mites, both dead and alive, can be minimized by encasing mattresses, box springs, and pillows in zippered plastic covers.

Table 20-1. Antihistamines commonly used for allergic rhinitis*

Class	Sedation	Anticholinergic	Adult dose†
ALKYLAMINES			
Brompheniramine (Dimetane, others)	Mild	Moderate	4 mg q4–6h
Chlorpheniramine (Chlor-Trimeton, others)	Mild	Moderate	4 mg q4–6h
Dexchlorpheniramine (Polaramine, others)	Mild	Moderate	2 mg q4–6h
Triprolidine (Actidil, others)	Mild	Moderate	2.5 mg q4–6h
ETHANOLAMINES			
Carbinoxamine (Clistin)	Moderate	Marked	4–8 mg q4–6h
Clemastine (Tavist)	Moderate	Marked	1 mg q12h
Diphenhydramine (Benadryl, others)	Marked	Marked	25–50 mg q4–6h
ETHYLENEDIAMINES			
Pyrilamine (Various)	Mild	Very mild	25–50 mg q6–8h
Tripelennamine (PBZ)	Moderate	Very mild	25 mg q4–6h
PIPERIDINES			
Azatadine (Optimine)	Moderate	Moderate	1–2 mg q12h
PHENOTHIAZINES			
Methdilazine (Tacaryl)	Moderate	Marked	8 mg q6–12h
Promethazine (Phenergan)	Marked	Marked	12.5 mg q6h or 25 mg hs
NONSEDATING			
Terfenadine (Seldane)	Little or none	Little or none	60 mg q12h
Astemizole (Hismanal)	Little or none	Little or none	10 mg q24h

*Use antihistamines with caution in pregnant patients. Pregnancy category B = chlorpheniramine, dexchlorpheniramine, diphenhydramine, clemastine, azatadine, and methdilazine. Pregnancy category C = astemizole, brompheniramine, promethazine, carbinoxamine, terfenadine, and triprolidine. See Chap. 141 for discussion.
†Dosages of drugs vary significantly based on patient age, general physical condition, weight, past experience with this type of drug, occupation (i.e., hazardous vs. nonhazardous), use of other sedating or drying agents, condition of mucous membranes, etc. Listed doses must be interpreted with caution, according to individual patient circumstances.

DRUG THERAPY. *Antihistamines* reduce itching, sneezing, and rhinorrhea by blocking histamine receptor sites on target organs. They are more effective in preventing than reversing the actions of histamine, and thus are most effective when used in anticipation of exposure to an allergen. Antihistamines alone may provide adequate relief for many patients, but troubling side effects include drowsiness and drying of mucous membranes. Alcohol can potentiate the sedative effect. The classes of antihistamines, with representative drugs, are listed in Table 20-1. Treatment is often started with an agent in the alkylamine class, which tends to be less sedating. Newer antihistamines, such as terfenadine (Seldane) cause substantially less drowsiness, but are also less potent. The response to different drugs within the same antihistamine class tends to be similar, so patients who

Table 20-2. Commonly used adrenergic decongestants*

	Strengths available	Typical adult dose
ORAL AGENTS		
Pseudoephedrine HCL (Sudafed, Novafed, others)	30-, 60-mg tablets 120-mg slow-release (SR) capsule	60 mg q6–8h 120 mg SR q12h
Pseudoephedrine sulfate (Afrinol)	120-mg slow-release (SR) capsule	120 mg SR q12h
Phenylpropanolamine HCL (Various generics, many combinations)	25-, 50-mg tablets 75-mg slow-release (SR) capsule	25 mg q4h, 50 mg q8h 75 mg SR q12h
TOPICAL AGENTS		
Phenylephrine HCL (Neo-Synephrine, others)	0.125%, 0.25%, 0.5%, 1.0% drops	2–3 gtt of 0.25–1.0% solution q4h prn, each nostril
(Nostril Spray 0.25%, Sinex Spray 0.5%, others)	0.25%, 0.5% spray	1–2 sprays q4h prn, each nostril
Oxymetazoline HCL (Afrin, Neo-Synephrine 12 hr, Dristan, others)	0.05% solution, as drops or spray	2–3 gtt or 2–3 sprays q12h, each nostril
Xylometazoline HCL (Otrivin, others)	0.05%, 0.1% drops, 0.1% spray	2–3 gtt or 2 sprays 0.05% q8–10h
Naphazoline HCL (Privine)	0.05% solution, as drops or spray	2 gtt each nostril q3h, or 2 sprays each nostril q4–6h
Tetrahydrozoline HCL (Tyzine)	0.05%, 0.1% solution	2–4 gtt each nostril q3h
Propylhexedrine (Benezedrex inhaler)	250-mg inhaler	2 inhalations prn, avoiding excessive use

*Note: All of the above, with the exception of Novafed, are available without prescription.
†As with antihistamines, decongestant doses vary significantly based on patient age, general physical condition, past experience with the drug, condition of mucous membranes, and use of other drying agents. Listed doses must be interpreted with caution, according to individual patient circumstances.
HCL = hydrochloride; gtt = drop.

fail to respond to one drug should be switched to one in another class. Once the effective class has been determined for a patient, the selection of a drug can be based on side effects and cost. Sustained-released preparations are available for many of the antihistamines, and are especially useful for bedtime administration, to control morning symptoms.

Sympathomimetic drugs (e.g., pseudoephedrine, phenylephrine phenylpropanolamine) relieve congestion, presumably reducing mucosal edema by causing vasoconstriction. Oral and topical preparations are listed in Table 20-2. They are usually used in conjunction with antihistamines, or when nasal obstruction is the predominant symptom. Oral sympathomimetics may cause hypertension and tachycardia when used in therapeutic doses, and should be used with caution in patients with hypertension and cardiovascular disease, bladder-emptying problems, and diabetes. Antihistamine-decongestant combinations are available both over the counter and by prescription. For patients with particularly troublesome and profuse rhinorrhea, newer preparations combine small doses of atropine, sympathomimetic, and antihistamine, which because of the added anticholinergic effect, offer more drying. Saline sprays or drops may help patients who are excessively dried out by oral preparations. Sympathomimetic drugs for topical use are generally dispensed in squeeze spray bottles. Topical nasal decongestants, however, must not be used routinely, because rebound vasodilatation leads to the development of rhinitis medicamentosus (see below). Patients should be strongly advised to use them for no more than a week at a time, or episodically only when most needed for symptom relief. A dilute sympathomimetic preparation such as xylometazoline (pediatric Otrivin 0.05%) may provide sufficient relief of symptoms at night without the rebound associated with stronger topical decongestants.

Topical corticosteroids provide impressive relief to patients with allergic rhinitis whose symptoms are not controlled by, or who cannot tolerate, antihistamines and decongestants. Nasal preparations containing beclomethasone dipropionate (Beconase, Vancenase), flunisolide (Nasalide), and dexamethasone (Decadron turbinaire) are available. Triamcinalone spray has recently become available. Beclomethasone and flunisolide are preferable to dexamethasone, particularly for prolonged use, because they are more active topically and less systemically absorbed. Beclomethasone is available in an aqueous suspension (Beconase AQ, Vancenase AQ), which in contrast to the older micronized powder formulation contains no alcohol or freon; the latter substances can cause mucosal irritation. Aqueous beclomethasone is therefore preferable to the powdered form and may also be less irritating than flunisolide. The usual dose range is 1 to 2 puffs in each nostril two to three times daily; the dose may be reduced once symptoms are under control. The onset of action is gradual, so patients should be advised to allow from several days to 2 weeks for full benefit to be observed. Complications are infrequent, and include irritation of the nasal mucous membrane with bleeding and, rarely, mucosal ulceration or *Candida* infections. When mucosal edema is severe, the use of a topical vasoconstrictor for the first 2 to 3 days, applied 10 to 15 minutes before application of the topical corticosteroid, may reduce the obstruction sufficiently to allow the topical preparation to reach the mucosa. A short (3–4-day) course of systemic corticosteroids is sometimes used for this purpose. Systemic corticosteroids are, however, rarely indicated. Patients with severe seasonal allergy who have failed to respond to other measures are, in exceptional cases, treated with a 2- to 3-week tapering course, but must be followed closely for side effects and for development of sinus infection.

Cromolyn sodium, which inhibits release of vasoactive substances by stabilizing mast cell walls, is available as an aerosol for nasal administration (Nasalcrom 4%). It is generally not helpful as a treatment modality once the attack is underway, and is primarily used to prevent attacks, particularly in patients with seasonal symptoms. Cromolyn may be used alone or combined with oral antihistamine and/or decongestant preparations and topical steroids, allowing reduced doses of the other agents and potentially less severe side effects. Its disadvantage is that it must be administered at least four times a day to be effective and is moderately expensive.

IMMUNOTHERAPY. Immunotherapy (hyposensitization) is usually reserved for patients with severe allergic symptoms that cannot be controlled by other means. After IgE hypersensitivity to specific inhaled allergens is demonstrated by skin or RAST testing, diluted extracts of the offending antigen are injected weekly to monthly. This results, over a period of time, in the production of "blocking antibodies," with a concomitant drop in IgE levels, and reduced symptoms. The best response to immunotherapy (80–90% improvement) has been demonstrated in patients with seasonal pollen-induced allergic rhinitis, such as sensitivity to ragweed or other grasses, trees, and weeds. Allergic rhinitis caused by molds also responds to immunotherapy, but the success rate is lower. Other environmental antigens (kapok, feather) are of questionable value in immunotherapy. Immunotherapy is less efficacious in perennial rhinitis, in which allergens such as house dust and molds play a greater role than do pollens.

Vasomotor Rhinitis

At least half of all patients with chronic, nonseasonal rhinitis have vasomotor rhinitis. The underlying cause of this condition is obscure, but the mechanism appears to be an autonomic dysfunction of the nasal mucosa that results in an exaggerated response of the mucous membrane to a variety of environmental stimuli. Patients with vaosomotor rhinitis often have coexistent allergic rhinitis and/or frequent infections of the nasal mucosa.

Typical symptoms of vasomotor rhinitis include nasal congestion and rhinorrhea, which may be profuse. Facial discomfort around the bridge of the nose and in the area of the frontal sinuses may result from pressure on the mucosa; this discomfort is sometimes described as a headache and confused with sinusitis. Symptoms are precipitated and/or exacerbated by a variety of nonspecific stimuli: heat, cold, smoke or other fumes, cooking odors or perfume, changes in temperature, atmospheric pressure, or even light intensity, emotional stress, and sexual excitement. Sneezing paroxysms, nasal itching, and eye symptoms common in allergic rhinitis are not present.

Diagnosis of vasomotor rhinitis is made by the presence of typical symptoms and the exclusion of other causes of rhinitis. A nasal smear for eosinophils is also useful to rule out allergic rhinitis.

Treatment

Vasomotor rhinitis is less responsive to treatment than is allergic rhinitis. The most effective measure is avoidance of the irritants or situations that cause the problem, although this is often not practical. Oral decongestants may provide some symptomatic relief; nasal decongestant sprays should not be used because of their high potential for abuse in this chronic condition. Antihistamines are of limited efficacy; they may reduce rhinorrhea by their drying effect. Since the drying effect parallels the sedative effect, antihistamines are best used at bedtime. Corticosteroid sprays may be prescribed for relief of extreme exacerbations.

Surgical reduction of enlarged turbinates to mechanically improve airflow is sometimes considered in severe cases where obstructive symptoms are prominent.

Rhinitis Medicamentosa

Congestion and irritation of the nasal mucosa may result from use or abuse of a number of drugs. Overuse of sympathomimetic nasal drops or sprays is the most common cause. The topical application of sympathomimetic drugs causes profound vasospasm, with dramatic relief from nasal congestions. However, once the effect of the sympathomimetic wears off, a rebound vasodilatation occurs, with increased capillary permeability. In response to this the patient may spray even more vasoconstrictor into the nose, and a vicious cycle develops. Rebound congestion becomes responsible for a larger and larger part of the nasal symptoms. After a few weeks, raw denuded areas of mucosa are seen, with a fiery red mucous membrane, and most of the symptoms are due to medication. This problem is less likely to develop if patients use weak (pediatric) sympathomimetic preparations, follow prescribed dosage schedules, and use the drugs for no more than a week at a time. Treatment consists of explaining the cause of the problem to the patient, and withdrawing the sympathomimetic drug. A short (1–2-week) course of topical corticosteroids may also be helpful in relieving the symptoms. A dilute sympathomimetic nasal spray such as 0.05% xylometazoline hydrochloride (pediatric Otrivin) could be given at night only. The habitual application of cocaine to the nasal mucosa may also lead to profound inflammation, as well as chronic bleeding and septal perforation. Cocaine use should be considered in patients with severe rhinitis without other causes.

Other drugs associated with nasal congestion include oral contraceptives, sympathoplegic antihypertensives (e.g., methyldopa, clonidine, reserpine), and nonsteroidal anti-inflammatory drugs. Sensitivity to aspirin is part of a recognized triad, which also includes asthma and nasal polyps.

Miscellaneous Causes of Rhinitis

Rhinitis of pregnancy, an increase in nasal congestion thought to be hormonally mediated, is often exacerbated by the increased blood volume during the third trimester. Women with preexisting allergic or vasomotor rhinitis tend to have a worsening of symptoms during pregnancy, as well as with use of oral contraceptives, although a small percentage have less nasal obstruction during the course of pregnancy. The latter patients may actually develop increased patency of the nasal passages, with resulting dryness of the nasal mucosa, and increased patency of the eustachian tube with secondary autophony, an increased sensitivity to sounds of their own bodies. Such patients will complain of hearing their own respirations, reverberations of consonants, especially "m" and "n" in their ear, and exaggerated sounds of their own footsteps. Patients should be referred to an otolaryngologist for nasopharyngeoscopy and tympanometry; treatment with topical estrogens may be of benefit.

Hyphothyroidism is also reported to cause a chronic stuffy nose, but this is uncommon in adults. Deviated nasal septum, nasal tumors, and foreign bodies are anatomic causes of nasal obstruction, which is usually unilateral. Rhinitis associated with upper respiratory viral infection is common, and often more intense in patients with allergic rhinitis; the rhinorrhea may be clear initially, but become purulent, with a predominance of neutrophils on nasal smear.

Nasal Polyps

Polyps can arise in the nasal mucosa in association with perennial allergic rhinitis or chronic sinusitis, or may occur without such antecedents as part of a triad which also includes aspirin sensitivity and asthma. Polyps are usually multiple, and present as fleshy pale masses projecting into the nasal cavity. They may be asymptomatic or result in nasal obstruction and discharge. When polyps are suspected or detected, consultation with an otolaryngologist is appropriate to confirm the diagnosis, rule out neoplasm, and plan treatment.

Symptomatic nasal polyps may be treated by surgical excision and/or topical corticosteroids. Topical medication alone may be adequate to cause regression of early small polyps, but surgery is usually required for larger ones. Treatment with corticosteroids usually requires 4 to 5 months for resolution. Surgery is required if there is a recurrence, if the polyps are unusually large and do not shrink, or if the polyp occludes an ostium. Polypectomy is a safe and effective outpatient procedure, but must often be repeated every 1 to 2 years because of the tendency for polyps to recur. Topical corticosteroids are also used to retard regrowth of polyps in patients who require frequent surgeries, or whose symptoms persist after surgery because of generalized mucosal disease.

Howarth PH. Allergic rhinitis: a rational choice of treatment. Respir Med 1989; 83:179–88.
 Presents a succinct rational approach to a very common clinical problem, emphasizing clinical assessment, epidemiology, pathophysiologic mechanisms, and objective testing in vitro.

Langer HM. Allergic rhinitis: a medical insight. J Otolaryngol 1989; 18:158–64.
 A detailed discussion of the pathogenesis of allergic rhinitis and mediator release. Review of antihistamines used in treatment with a good comparison of antihistamines, corticosteroids, and other therapeutic modalities.

Spector SL. Ocular, nasal and oral cromolyn sodium in the management of non-asthmatic allergic problems. Allergy Proc 1989; 10:191–5.
 Nasal and oral cromolyn sodium use in the management of nonasthmatic allergic problems. This article discusses what is generally perceived as a very safe long-term therapeutic modality. The pharmacologic basis for therapy is emphasized.

Mikaelian AJ. Vasomotor rhinitis. Ear Nose Throat J 1989; 68:207–10.
 An excellent discussion of this entity for the nonotolaryngologist. Vasomotor rhinitis is extremely common and often exists concomitantly with allergic rhinitis.

Busse W. New directions and dimensions in the treatment of allergic rhinitis. J Allergy Clin Immunol 1988; 82:890–900.
 Emphasizes treatment techniques along with objective and subjective evaluation of efficacy and also discusses the safety of various treatment modalities in long-term use.

Naclerid RM. Allergic rhinitis. N Engl J Med 1991; 325:860–9.
 An accessible and current review, emphasizing therapeutic approaches.

V. LOWER RESPIRATORY PROBLEMS

21. ASTHMA
James F. Donohue

Asthma is an obstructive pulmonary disease characterized by narrowing of the airways, airflow obstruction, inflammation of the airway, and increased airway hyperresponsiveness. Asthma affects 4 to 7% of the American population, accounts for 4 million office visits per year, 1 million emergency room visits, 430,000 admissions, and 2 million hospital-days per year. The prevalence of, severity of, and death rate due to asthma have increased in the past decade, especially in African-Americans and Hispanics. The reason for these increases is not clear. Suggested explanations include: environmental changes, with an increase in indoor air pollution and allergens and contamination of the food chain with chemicals; changes in therapy; and poor access to health care, with widespread patient reliance on self-medication without seeking medical assistance. A major reason for death due to asthma is undertreatment resulting from an inadequate assessment of severity by either the doctor or the patient.

The Asthmatic Response
Multiple mechanisms underlie the increased airway hyperresponsiveness in asthma; these include smooth muscle abnormalities, increased vascular permeability, disordered function of the autonomic nervous system, epithelial damage, and airway inflammation. After exposure to most stimuli, there is an immediate reaction characterized by mediator release followed by a delayed response; exercise causes an immediate but no delayed response. The immediate bronchospasm and decrease in lung function resolve within 30 minutes to 60 minutes and can be blocked or shortened by beta-adrenergic drugs. The delayed or "late" response occurs 6 to 8 hours later, after an influx of polymorphonuclear cells and eosinophils into the lung, with a subsequent decrease in lung function. Airway hyperresponsiveness reflects the late asthmatic response, as do the longer-lasting chronic symptoms, which increase in severity after repetitive exposure to the stimulus.

Evaluation
Symptoms of asthma include intermittent wheezing, breathlessness, tightness of the chest, cough, and sputum production of variable intensity and duration, usually getting worse at night or early morning.

Stimuli for asthmatic attacks are multiple, and include cold air, exercise, exposure to allergens or irritants, viral upper respiratory tract infections, stress, and drugs such as beta-blockers, aspirin, and nonsteroidal antiinflammatory agents. Certain dietary chemicals, such as sulfites, and tartrazine may also cause asthma. Additional confirmation of the diagnosis is obtained if the symptoms are reversed following treatment. In two well-recognized variants, known as cough syndrome and dyspnea syndrome of asthma, patients complain of either cough or dyspnea without overt wheezing. These patients characteristically have mild obstruction and are identified by a positive therapeutic response to bronchodilators or by bronchial challenge testing. Asthma is suspected in patients with an unexplained cough of 6 weeks' duration or in otherwise healthy or young patients who have dyspnea.

Physical Examination
The physical examination confirms the presence of bronchospasm and indicates the severity of an individual attack. Patients having severe asthma attacks often speak in short sentences, sit upright, use accessory respiratory muscles, have a high resting heart rate, with inspiratory and expiratory wheezing, and are diaphoretic. The thorax generally appears hyperinflated. Wheezing, which may have been present for a long time or be absent during severe attacks accompanied by low flow rates, is not a precise sign of severity or of the response to therapy.

Laboratory Evaluation
Laboratory measurements of airflow by spirometry or peak flow meter establish the diagnosis, and are used to quantitate the severity of obstruction and assess the response to

therapy. A diagnosis of asthma is established by a decrease in expiratory flow rates that reverses or improves following the administration of bronchodilators. The diagnosis is not aided by chest x-ray except to exclude other problems. Arterial blood gases help to establish the severity of an attack. Sputum is not usually present in new-onset uncomplicated asthma, but the presence of eosinophils in sputum may help establish an allergic cause in exacerbations of chronic asthma.

The ratio of forced expiratory volume in 1 second (FEV_1) to forced vital capacity (FVC) is decreased in the obstructive pattern; a normal ratio is 75% or more. The decrease in FEV_1 is the most useful parameter in assessing severity: 65 to 80% of predicted indicates mild obstruction; 50 to 65% indicates moderate obstruction; and less than 50% indicates severe obstruction. Patients with an FEV_1 of less than 50% following acute therapy may require hospitalization.

The peak expiratory flow rate (PEFR), an inexpensive but accurate measurement of mechanical lung function, generally is not as useful in diagnosis as in monitoring the stable patient and in assessing the response to therapy. Patients can use peak flow meters at home to measure their PEFR in the morning and evening. There is a normal diurnal variation; morning PEFRs are often 20% lower than evening rates in asthmatics. Changes of 30% usually can be managed by increasing medication; changes of 50% require office or emergency room visits. Greater changes in PEFR often require hospitalization and PEFRs below 30% of predicted indicate dangerous levels of obstruction. Peak flow measurements are also essential in the emergency setting to determine the severity of attack and to establish a disposition. Hospital admission is often necessary if peak flow rates remain less than 30% or do not respond to therapy.

Objective measures are important because there is often a lack of correlation between symptoms and severity of obstruction. Even the patient's subjective impression of improvement following an attack may be deceptive; studies have shown that 15% of patients failed to detect the presence of marked airway obstruction (reduction of FEV_1 to 50% of predicted) induced by metacholine. Patients who return to the emergency room or office following initial therapy often have more severe obstruction than the physician estimated on clinical grounds. The obstruction in some outpatients involves mucosal edema, inflammation, and mucous secretions, which may require long-term therapy before pulmonary function returns to normal. Therefore, serial spirometric or peak flow measurements are necessary, particularly when evaluating therapeutic response to inhaled antiinflammatory agents, to which the response is delayed.

SPECIAL STUDIES. At times when the diagnosis is not clear or when patients present with cough or dyspnea syndromes, it may be necessary to confirm the diagnosis by provoking an asthmatic response. Referral to an allergist or a pulmonary specialist for bronchial challenge testing with methacholine or histamine or for an exercise study can be useful.

Skin testing for allergens, the radioallergosorbent tests (RASTs), and IgE level may also be useful in the asthmatic evaluation. As avoidance of allergens is becoming the cornerstone of therapy, allergy testing is being increasingly employed.

Patients with Refractory Asthma

Evaluation of a patient with refractory asthma should include inquiry into continued exposure to known causes of asthma, an estimation of compliance with treatment, and consideration of other causes of airway obstruction. The latter include functional upper airway obstruction from anxiety, which may cause the vocal cords to be abducted to the midline during inspiration; asthma from left ventricular failure or mitral stenosis, particularly in the elderly; hyperthyroidism; anatomic lesions such as carcinoid tumors, lung cancer, or aneurysms of the thoracic aorta; and sinus disease. Gastroesophageal reflex is also an important cause of continued asthma symptoms, particularly in elderly patients and those who are obese and taking medication such as theophylline. Reflux can cause asthma by direct acid aspiration into the lung and also by reflex bronchoconstriction. Finally, it should be determined whether the patient has allergic bronchopulmonary aspergillosis by examining sputum for fungi, measuring levels of serum IgE and serum precipitants, and skin testing for *Aspergillus*.

Treatment

Goals of asthma care include (1) minimal symptoms; (2) normal activities of daily living, work, school, and recreation; (3) inhaled beta-adrenergics needed for rescue not more than twice daily; (4) peak flow rates normal or near-normal at rest or after an inhaled beta-2-adrenergic agent; (5) daily variation of peak flow rate of less than 20%; and (6) minimal side effects from medication. Avoiding precipitating factors is preferred to medications, and control of airway inflammation is superior to control of airway constriction. If medical control is necessary, the smallest amount needed to maintain control and minimize side effects should be used; inhaled steroids or inhaled cromolyn sodium along with aerosol bronchodilators are preferred.

Once the diagnosis is established and initial treatment provided, a plan should be established to accomplish the above-mentioned goals. Patients should be educated and provided with a written plan for early treatment or exacerbations. The effectiveness of the treatment program should be reviewed regularly and referral to an allergist or pulmonologist considered when the diagnosis is unclear or patients do not respond.

Allergy Avoidance

Avoiding allergens and trigger agents is a permanent requirement for all asthmatics. After establishing allergies by history, skin testing, or RAST, effective measures can be undertaken for reducing exposure to house dust mites, pollens, and animal danders. The most important place to reduce dust mites is in the bedroom. Patients should encase the mattress and bedsprings in plastic covers; replace all feather with foam-rubber pillows and cover them with hypoallergenic encasings. Carpets should be removed from the bedroom and living room areas or treated with 3% tannic acid or benzyl benzoate powder, which kills the mites. Bed linen should be washed every 7 to 10 days in hot water, and vacuuming done weekly. The patient who vacuums should be instructed to wear a mask and remain out of the room for 20 minutes after vacuuming. A high-efficiency particle arrester (HEPA), filtered vacuum cleaner may be useful, as well as an HEPA portable air filter on the floor. Rooms should be kept at less than 70°F (21.1°C) and the relative humidity under 45% by using an air conditioner or a dehumidifier if necessary. These measures are usually sufficient to control house dust mites. Growth of mites is often significant on carpets that remain damp, such as those on concrete slabs. Thus, highly allergic persons should not work in the basement.

Cat and cockroach allergens are also important causes of asthma. If the cat allergies are significant, the pet must be kept outdoors; professional exterminators may be necessary to control cockroaches. Dampness and humidity control is imperative for limiting fungi. Year-round air conditioning and dehumidification are necessary, especially during pollination. Barriers may be necessary in crawl spaces. Once a month, susceptible surfaces such as window frames, bathrooms, floors, and showers should be treated with a solution containing chloride, which kills molds.

Windows and doors should be closed during the season when plants are pollinating. While antihistamines with anticholinergic properties should be avoided, the newer drugs terfenadine (Seldane) and astemizole (Hismanal) are not contraindicated in asthmatics.

Drug Treatment

AEROSOL BRONCHODILATORS. The first agents used for mild, intermittent symptoms are beta-adrenergic agonists administered as aerosol bronchodilators (Table 21-1). Inhaled beta-adrenergic agents provide prompt relief of acute symptoms and can prevent bronchoconstriction. Inhaled administration is preferred to oral administration because of rapidity of action, efficacy, and fewer side effects. Long-acting beta-adrenergic agonists with excellent beta-2 selectivity include albuterol, metaproterenol, pirbuterol, and terbutaline (below). Options for the inhaled route are metered-dose inhaler (MDI), with or without a spacer, breath-activated dry-powder aerosol, and nebulized solutions. The latter are restricted to the acute setting or for very severe cases. The spacer is an added chamber that slows the aerosol jet and facilitates evaporation; the decreased particulate size is more easily respirable.

The MDI is preferred for ambulatory patients; properly used, 10% of the drug aerosolized

Table 21-1. Beta-2 selective[a] adrenergic inhaled bronchodilators

Drug	Formulations	Onset of action (min)	Peak effect (min)	Duration of effect (hr)	Typical dose
Albuterol[b] Proventil, Ventolin	90 μg/puff aerosol	5–15	60–90	3–6	2 puffs q4–6h
Metaproterenol[b] Alupent, Metaprel	650 μg/puff aerosol	1–5	30–60	2–5	2 puffs q4–6h
Pirbuterol Maxair	200 μg/puff aerosol	within 5	30–60	4–6	1–2 puffs q4–6h
Terbutaline Brethaire	200 μg/puff aerosol	5–30	30–60	3–6	2 puffs q4–6h
Bitolterol Tornalate	370 μg/puff aerosol	3–4	30–60	5–8	2 puffs q8h
Isoetharine[b] Bronkometer	340 μg/puff aerosol	1–6	5–15	1–3	1–2 puffs q4h

[a] Isoetharine is less beta-selective than the other drugs listed, and therefore has more potential for cardiac stimulation.
[b] Also available in solution forms for use in nebulizers.

from the MDI is deposited in the lung; the rest remains in the device or the mouth where it is swallowed and inactivated. Beta-adrenergic MDIs are used either on an "as-needed" basis or regularly every 4 to 6 hours, based on the persistence of symptoms. Typical dosages are listed in Table 21-1.

Many patients for whom MDIs are prescribed use them incorrectly and must receive repeat instruction on subsequent clinic visits. For proper use of the MDI, the patient should (1) shake the MDI, (2) exhale deeply, (3) either close the lips around the mouthpiece or keep the mouthpiece 2 in. from the mouth, (4) start inhaling slowly and then discharge the inhaler, (5) breathe deeply, (6) hold the breath 4 to 10 seconds, and (7) breathe out slowly. If the patient cannot use an MDI properly, a spacer device such as InspirEase or Aerochamber should be used. Patients do not have to be as coordinated to use the spacer. The MDI with spacer is preferred for patients who require higher doses of inhaled steroids and it can be substituted for nebulized solutions even in stable inpatients.

Albuterol (200 µg per inhalation) can be given by dry powder in a breath-activated rotohaler for those who cannot use MDIs properly or for those who do not like the taste of MDIs. The effects of dry-powder aerosols are comparable to those of MDIs.

CROMOLYN SODIUM AND INHALED CORTICOSTEROIDS. Currently, the most effective agents for preventing and modifying the late asthmatic response and controlling persistent symptoms are inhaled cromolyn sodium and inhaled corticosteroids. These drugs are not used to treat acute asthma but for maintenance.

Cromolyn is preferred as a first-line agent for children and young adults but can be used in patients of any age; corticosteroids are more useful in adults.

Cromolyn prevents bronchial constriction by blocking release of mast cell mediators and the activation of inflammatory cells. Initially cromolyn should be started at a frequency of two puffs four times a day. This can be decreased, depending on symptom control. Cromolyn sodium is prescribed as an MDI, dry-powder spinhaler, or nebulized solution, depending on the patient's needs. This agent is extremely safe and is usually inhaled after bronchodilation.

Inhaled corticosteroids in the usual dose range act locally in the lung, with little or no systemic absorption or side effects. These agents have an excellent safety record that allows them to be used in any patient whose symptoms are not controlled by bronchodilators. Corticosteroids are particularly useful in patients who have subacute illness and in preventing the allergen-induced late-phase asthmatic responses associated with bronchial hyperreactivity. Inhaled steroids should be used concomitantly in all patients taking oral steroids, in an attempt to reduce the oral dose. Keys to successful use of inhaled steroids include proper inspiratory technique, a proper dose combination with oral steroids that reduces the dose of oral agents, use of a spacer device to prevent side effects, and monitoring compliance. Effects are seen within a few days and maximum effects are achieved within 1 week. Few side effects have been seen with inhaled corticosteroids. Oral pharyngeal candidiasis is frequent, although usually not significant; it can be minimized by using a spacer device and by gargling with water after using the inhaler. Local vocal cord myopathy, a rare complication, is treated by decreasing or discontinuing the inhaled steroid. Occasionally, a patient receiving beclomethasone will cough due to oleic acid in the propellant. A change to another type of inhaled steroid or pretreatment with beta-2-agonist might be useful.

The dosages for inhaled corticosteroids are: triamcinolone (Azmacort), two puffs (100 µg) four times per day; beclomethasone (Beclovent, Vanceril), two puffs (42 µg/puff) four times a day; and flunisolide (Aerobid), two puffs (250 µg/puff) twice a day. Occasionally, it is necessary to increase the dose in order to obtain proper control. At higher doses, more systemic absorption occurs. In a well-stabilized patient, efforts may be made to reduce the frequency of dosing by half (bid).

ORAL CORTICOSTEROIDS. Oral corticosteroids are used for more severe asthma due to extensive airway inflammation. Patients who are candidates for oral corticosteroids include those who no longer derive 4 to 6 hours of relief from a beta-adrenergic agonist taken by an MDI and may be using it every few hours, complain of nocturnal symptoms, and have very poor control of daytime symptoms. A short course of oral corticosteroids is used to reverse the bronchial inflammation. The goal of therapy is to use adequate doses of oral steroids for the shortest period of time, followed by alternate-day steroids and ultimately inhaled steroids, which are safe and efficacious for patients who have not previously taken steroids. For patients who rarely require oral steroids, a prednisone taper (40, 35, 30, 25, 20, 15, 10, 5 mg) may be adequate. For those known to be refractory or who have had prior treatment with steroids, a 2- to 3-week taper starting at the same dose may be necessary.

Some patients require long-term, high-dose, oral corticosteroids. Attempts have been made to lower the steroid dose by using alternative therapy including methotrexate, troleandomycin, or gold therapy. All these so-called steroid-sparing programs have significant side effects and toxicity. They may, however, be effective in selected patients with severe asthma who are not responding to very high doses of steroids. These agents should be prescribed only by specialists who are experienced in their use.

THEOPHYLLINE. The role of theophylline is changing. Previously the agent used first in the treatment of asthma, theophylline is becoming a secondary bronchodilator because of its narrow therapeutic index. Among the reasons for theophylline's wide popularity was the fear that MDIs and beta-adrenergic agents were responsible for the increased asthma-related deaths that occurred in the late 1960s. Furthermore, theophylline serum levels could be measured and long-acting preparations were available. However, despite careful monitoring of theophylline levels, there is still poor correlation between serum levels and control of symptoms, and side effects occur in the therapeutic range.

The mechanisms of bronchodilation by theophylline are unclear. Although it is a weak phosphodiesterase inhibitor and blocks adenosine receptors, neither mechanism accounts for bronchodilation.

Theophylline can be an effective bronchodilator in patients with breakthrough symptoms despite inhalant therapy and those who cannot use inhalers. To prevent caffeine-like side effects, theophylline should be started in low dosages (e.g., 100–200 mg bid) and gradually increased to maintenance level. Steady state will usually be reached by the fourth to sixth dose. The goal is symptom control with minimal side effects. Although a therapeutic level of 10 to 20 μg/ml previously has been used, a lower level, 8 to 13 μg/dl, is now recommended. Side effects such as anxiety and GI symptoms due to increases in gastric acidity and reflux can be seen at any blood level but more severe side effects are associated with high serum levels. Cardiac and CNS toxicities occur with theophylline levels well above 20 μg/dl. Important interactions occur with diet, drugs, and viral infections. Theophylline dosage often must be reduced by at least 25% in patients receiving concomitant quinolone or macrolide antibiotics, or cimetidine (but not ranitidine). Serum levels must be periodically monitored, particularly when the patient is acutely ill. Theophylline can be used as a once-daily dose with a 24-hour preparation, given at 7 PM at night in order to prevent nocturnal attacks while minimizing undue side effects. Evening usage cuts down nocturnal symptoms and restful sleep seems to improve the patient's overall asthmatic condition.

ORAL BETA-ADRENERGIC DRUGS. The indications for long-acting oral beta-adrenergic agents such as albuterol are similar to those for theophylline: incomplete control by inhalers or nighttime asthma. The major side effects are nervousness and tremor, but tolerance to the tremor usually develops. Therapy with albuterol should be started with low doses and increased to 4 to 8 mg twice a day. Shorter-acting agents such as oral terbutaline and metaproterenol are associated with a higher incidence of side effects.

ANTICHOLINERGIC DRUGS. Anticholinergic agents are less effective in asthma than in chronic obstructive pulmonary disease (COPD) and are less potent than inhaled beta-adrenergic agents. Newer agents such as ipratropium bromide are safe and do not share in the undesirable side effects (drying of respiratory secretions and increasing heart rate) of older tertiary ammonia compounds such as atropine. The combination of ipratropium and beta-adrenergics provides few side effects and a longer duration of bronchodilation. There are no predictive factors to identify the asthmatic who will respond to ipratropium, but in general, ipratropium has a role in psychogenic asthma and in treating asthmatics who have ingested beta-blockers. Older, nonatopic patients with low FEV_1 values are more likely than younger patients to benefit from anticholinergics. The usual dose is two puffs

(18 µg/inhalation) every 6 hours. Occasionally a higher dose will benefit. A closed-mouth technique should be used with any dose to avoid exposure to the eye. The major side effect is cough.

IMMUNOTHERAPY. Although it has been used for many years, immunotherapy is controversial in the treatment of asthma. The best established indication for immunotherapy is pollen allergy, particularly when complicated by unresolving asthma. There are some risks of inducing an acute asthmatic attack with the injections, particularly in those with a high degree of skin sensitivity and unstable disease.

Treatment with immunotherapy should be considered if symptoms fail to respond to allergen avoidance and drug therapy. To minimize adverse reactions, the FEV_1 should be greater than 70% of predicted before each injection. House dust mite extract should be reserved for those cases in which mites are the only sensitizing agent. Animal dander extract should be used only when exposure is unavoidable.

Special Problems

Acute Asthmatic Attack

Anxiety can be severe during an acute attack, and the patient should be reassured while the cause and severity of the asthma attack are determined. Treatment should be started with nasal oxygen, 3 L per minute. Oxygen is a bronchodilator and helps prevent the transient falls in arterial oxygen that occur with beta-adrenergics. Next, two to four puffs of aerosol beta-adrenergic bronchodilator (albuterol, metaproterenol, or terbutaline) should be administered via an MDI with a spacer; proper technique (described above) is critical. If the attack is severe, an aerosol solution instilled by an air compressor–powered nebulizer should be substituted (albuterol, 5 mg/ml, 0.5 ml in 2.5 ml of saline, or metaproterenol, 0.3 ml in 2.5 ml of saline).

If the patient's symptoms continue and if no side effects (tachycardia, change in blood pressure) occur, treatment with the beta-adrenergic aerosol should be repeated. Parenteral bronchodilators are less effective than aerosols and should not be used in patients with heart rates greater than 140 beats per minute or older than 55 years. In others, epinephrine, 0.3 ml of 1:1000 solution subcutaneously, or terbutaline, 0.25 mg subcutaneously, can be given and repeated once or twice more. If the attacks continue after 1 hour, aminophylline should be started intravenously. If the patient is already taking oral aminophylline, the maintenance dosage of 0.3 to 0.5 mg/kg/hr should be used and serum level monitored. For nonusers, a loading dose of 5 to 6 mg/kg can be started. A loading dose of corticosteroids should also be given (prednisone 60 mg po, or methylprednisolone [Solu-Medrol] 60–125 mg IV), to be followed by an appropriate tapering of doses.

The patient should be admitted to the hospital if acute symptoms and findings such as paradoxical pulse, use of accessory muscles, abnormalities in arterial blood levels, and low PEFRs persist after 1 to 2 hours. Patients with acute asthma who are already receiving oral steroids, are taking multiple medication, or have a history of coexisting medical conditions or of prior hospitalization for asthma may also need to be admitted.

Nocturnal Asthma

Nighttime exacerbations with wheezing and cough are common in asthma, occurring once nightly in 39% of patients, and at least once weekly in 74% of all asthmatics. Even in normal subjects, peak flow rates drop 8% in the early morning; in asthmatics this decline may be to 50%. Nocturnal asthma also may be an early warning of impending asthmatic exacerbation. The causes of nocturnal decline in peak flow rates include airway cooling, nocturnal gastroesophageal reflux, increased allergen exposure in the bedroom, supine position, decreased mucus clearance, increased vagal tone, and alterations in circadian hormonal rhythms, with higher histamine level and lower catecholamine, cortisol, and cyclic adenosine monophosphate (AMP) levels. The treatment of nocturnal asthma begins with achieving good daytime control and avoiding allergens, irritants, and reflux. The bedroom should be kept warm but below 70°F (21.1°C). A once-daily sustained-released theophylline preparation may be used between 5 and 8 PM. If this is ineffective or the patient has side effects, oral controlled-released albuterol, inhaled corticosteroids, or inhaled ipratropium of up to four puffs may control the symptoms. The peak flow rate should be recorded both in the early morning and in the evening to ensure adequate treatment.

Exercise-Induced Asthma
Many adult patients experience wheezing a few minutes after conclusion of exercise, particularly after running and jogging. Factors involved in exercise-induced asthma include the intensity of exercise, climatic conditions (cold, dry air, high pollen counts, or high air pollution index), and the underlying responsiveness of the patient's airways. Some patients with significant asthmatic symptoms or abnormalities in peak flow experience bronchospasm both during and after exercise; others may have normal lung function and physical findings until after they exercise. Patients with exercise-induced asthma should (1) gradually warm up over 15 minutes, (2) avoid exercising outdoors under conditions of extreme cold or high pollution and pollen counts, and (3) be pretreated with bronchodilators such as two puffs of albuterol via an MDI 15 minutes before exercise. Although less potent, cromolyn, inhaled ipratropium bromide, and oral theophylline can be used. Combining cromolyn and an inhaled beta-adrenergic drug may provide protection for up to 4 hours for asthmatics participating in longer exercises.

Asthma in Elderly Persons
Ten percent of asthmatic patients are over 65 years old. Although most have had it since childhood or early adult life, in 1% the onset of disease occurs after the age of 60. In this age group, it is essential that a correct diagnosis be made from the somewhat broader differential diagnosis that includes COPD, congestive heart failure, upper airway obstruction, lower airway obstruction due to tumors and endobronchial disease, pulmonary embolism, aspiration of gastric fluids, and psychogenic shortness of breath. Medications, particularly oral and topical beta-blockers, nonsteroidal antiinflammatory agents, and angiotensin-converting enzyme inhibitors, are an important cause of asthma in this group. Similarly, in the elderly population, the physical stresses of asthma attacks may cause congestive heart failure and worsening of other coexisting conditions.

Elderly people are also more sensitive to the side effects of medicine used to treat asthma, in particular, oral theophylline, albuterol, and steroids. Side effects must be treated empirically, by reducing doses.

Elderly patients often have difficulty with aerosol therapy due to an inability to use the devices properly. At times, a spacer device, nebulized aerosols, and breath-activated inhaled powder (cromolyn and albuterol) are useful.

Occupational Asthma
Occupational asthma may account for up to 15% of cases of asthma. Workers are exposed to a variety of sensitizing agents and the prevalence of asthma varies widely depending on the degree of exposure, the reactivity of the agent, and the hyperresponsiveness of the patient's airways. A variety of agents including cotton dust, detergents, metals such as platinum and nickel, building materials, pharmaceutical agents, food-processing agents, rubber, resins, epoxies, and plastics can cause occupational asthma. Both immediate and delayed asthmatic reactions follow occupational exposures.

The history may reveal a temporal association of symptoms, such as wheezing, cough, or tightness in the chest, to the work environment. Individuals who are both atopic and nonatopic can develop occupational asthma, but preexistent bronchial asthma may favor the development of occupational asthma.

Workup should include environmental evaluation, pulmonary function tests, and in special circumstances, bronchial challenge testing. Occasionally it may be useful to do a preshift and postshift peak flow measurement to see if there is a major decrease. Avoiding the offending agent is mandatory and pretreatment with an aerosol bronchodilator, use of self-contained masks, or respirators may help; removal of the worker from the environment is often necessary.

Mayo PH. Results of a proposal to reduce admission for adult asthma. Ann Intern Med 1990; 112:867–71.
With use of a vigorous medical regimen and patient educational program, hospital use by asthmatics was reduced.

Barnes PJ. A new approach to the treatment of asthma. N Engl J Med 1989; 321:1517–27.
Antiinflammatory agents are emphasized, with less emphasis on bronchodilators.

Lemanske R. Late-phase IgE mediated reactions. J Clin Immunol 1988; 8:1–13.
A review of the biphasic clinical response to allergens.

Barnes PJ. Effect of corticosteroids on airway hyperresponsiveness. Am Rev Respir Dis 1990; 141:570–6.
A study of the role of steroids in asthma.

Benatur SR. Fatal asthma. N Engl J Med 1986; 314:423–9.
Notes the increasing death rates in asthma and compares two patterns: rapidly fatal asthma versus slowly progressive but ultimately fatal asthma.

McFadden ER Jr. Therapy of acute asthma. J Allergy Clin Immunol 1989; 85:151–8.
A comprehensive review of therapy during acute attacks.

Sporik R, et al. Exposure to house-dust mite allergy (DerpI) and the development of asthma in childhood—a prospective study. N Engl J Med 1990; 323:502–7.
Increased exposure to dust mites and other indoor allergens contributes to the increasing prevalance of asthma.

Sears MR, et al. Regular inhaled beta agonist treatment in bronchial asthma. Lancet 1990; 336:1391–6.
A controversial report suggesting that regular use of beta-agonists may worsen asthma.

Burrows B, et al. Association of asthma with serum IgE levels and skin-test reactivity to allergens. N Engl J Med 1989; 320:271–7.
Asthma is always associated with allergic disease and there is no evidence that there are basic differences between allergic (extrinsic) and nonallergic (intrinsic) forms.

Sheffer AL, et al. Guidelines for the diagnosis and management of asthma. J Allergy Clin Immunol 1991; 88:425–534.
Recommendations of the National Asthma Education Program of the National Institutes of Health (NIH).

Erzurum SC, et al. Lack of benefit of methotrexate in severe, steroid-dependent asthma. Ann Intern Med 1991; 114:353–60.
A double-blind, placebo-controlled study did not support the use of methotrexate in severe asthma.

22. CHRONIC OBSTRUCTIVE PULMONARY DISEASE
James F. Donohue

Chronic obstructive pulmonary disease (COPD) is a heterogeneous disorder that includes emphysema, chronic bronchitis, asthmatic bronchitis, and bronchiolitis. All are characterized by obstruction or limitation of expiratory airflow that fails to reverse completely following the use of bronchodilators. *Asthmatic bronchitis* shares features such as inflammation with chronic asthma, but differs in the presence of a smoking history and an irreversible component of obstruction despite treatment. *Emphysema* is described in anatomic terms as permanent, abnormal enlargement of pulmonary acini accompanied by destructive changes. *Chronic bronchitis* is a clinical concept defined by chronic excessive mucus secretion, leading to a persistent productive cough on most days for 3 or more months per year over at least a 2-year period. Chronic mucus hypersecretion by itself with chronic cough does not necessarily result in significant airway obstruction; however, some of these patients develop chronic obstructive bronchitis, with rapid deterioration of pulmonary function and early death.

COPD affects over 10 million people in the United States, of whom 1 million have limited activity and 500,000 receive Social Security disability benefits. A recent workshop on COPD at the National Institutes of Health concluded that overall mortality rates continue to change in ways related to smoking; female rates are up while rates for men have plateaued. Fifteen percent of smokers develop COPD and 88% of all cases of COPD are caused by smoking; other factors such as occupational and environmental insults also contribute. Spirometry is a strong predictor of mortality and prognosis: patients with a forced expiratory volume in 1 second (FEV_1) of less than 39% after using a bronchodilator have a worse 10-year prognosis than those with an increase in airway responsiveness (asthmatic bronchitis). Interventions are possible for COPD but there is a need to identify the patient with COPD earlier.

Clinical Course

The clinical course of COPD is apparently affected by multiple factors, including genetic susceptibility, exposure to inhaled irritants in the workplace, environmental air pollution, and infections in the first years of life. Lung function in adults has been shown to decrease gradually throughout life at a rate of about 20 cc per year in nonsmokers and in many nonsusceptible smokers in whom clinically significant airflow obstruction never develops. However, susceptible smokers may lose up to 60 cc each year. A patient who stops smoking does not recover lost function, but the subsequent loss of FEV_1 approaches that of nonsmokers. A teenager who takes up smoking at age 13 to 14 years may attain only 80% of maximum lung function. If smoking continues, the young adult has both a lower baseline and an accelerated rate of decline in FEV_1. Lifelong smokers often lose up to 15 years of life expectancy. It is therefore imperative to emphasize the importance of preventing cigarette smoking in teenagers.

The typical smoker who develops COPD is asymptomatic for the first 10 to 20 years of smoking, except they have colds more frequently and more severe symptoms with upper respiratory tract infections. Clinical symptoms and physical abnormalities appear relatively late, after irreversible damage has occurred. After 20 to 30 pack-years of smoking, mild dyspnea is noted, on exertion, often attributed to middle age, weight, and a sedentary life-style. While patients may complain of mild morning cough at this stage, findings on physical examination and chest x-ray are normal. The patient at risk for COPD can, however, be identified by an abnormal ratio of FEV_1 to forced vital capacity (FVC).

As the susceptible smoker ages, progressive loss of function continues and dyspnea on exercise develops; morning sputum production and cough worsen and laborers often lose the ability to work. Soon the physical stigmata of overt emphysema (hyperinflation) and bronchitis (wheezes) are apparent, and are followed by respiratory failure.

With far-advanced disease, structural changes result in chronic alveolar hypoxia, which in turn produces pulmonary hypertension and cor pulmonale. These patients are described as "blue bloaters"; they have cyanosis, edema, cardiomegaly, recurrent respiratory failure, reactive airways, polycythemia (a compensation for chronic nocturnal hypoxemia), alveolar hypoventilation, and carbon dioxide retention. Patients at this stage require frequent hospitalization and have a poor prognosis.

Patients in whom emphysema predominates have severe dyspnea and are called "pink puffers" because they maintain relatively normal arterial oxygen and carbon dioxide tensions by maintaining high minute ventilation. These patients tend to be thin and barrel-chested without cyanosis or edema, until the terminal stage of the disease. Most patients fall into a "mixed" bronchitis, emphysema clinical category.

Diagnosis

Signs

Physical findings do not correlate well with early COPD. Evaluation of the chest configuration and musculature may indicate hyperinflation. The accessory muscles of respiration (scalenes, sternocleidomastoids) contract in inspiration during periods of increasing ventilation and are palpably hardened when there is overinflation of the chest and decreased flow rates. The presence of tracheal descent with inspiration, felt by resting the tip of the index finger on the thyroid cartilage, and inward costal margin movement (Hoover's sign) correlate with long-standing overinflation that causes the rib cage and diaphragm to change shape. In patients with hyperinflation, the most prominent palpable and/or auscultatory cardiac contraction is often in the epigastrium, rather than the fourth left intercostal space. Excavation of the suprasternal space and supraclavicular fossa and recession of the intercostal spaces during inspiration are due to a phase lag between the generation of large negative pleural pressures and the resultant change in lung volume because of high airway resistance. On auscultation, breath sounds are distant and augment poorly with deep breathing; end expiratory wheezes are heard on forced expiration.

The measurement of forced expiratory time is a useful, simple maneuver for evaluating the presence of airflow limitation. After a full inspiration, the patient exhales with the mouth wide open until airflow ceases, as judged by listening at the mouth or by stethoscope over the treachea. The normal duration is 3 seconds; in COPD the time is prolonged because of increased resistance to airflow or decreased elastic recoil.

Laboratory Evaluation

OFFICE SPIROMETRY. The earliest change in bronchitis and emphysema is a decrease in the maximum midexpiratory flow rate, suggesting obstruction in the small airways or loss of elastic recoil. However, wide variability in this parameter limits its usefulness in the office.

The hallmark of COPD is a FEV_1/FVC ratio that is below 70% and does not completely return to normal following therapy. The FEV_1, expressed as a percent of predicted, is the most useful parameter in assessing severity of ventilatory impairment: 60 to 80% indicates mild, 50 to 60% is moderate, and below 50% represents severe obstruction. Office spirometry with measurements of FEV_1 and the FEV_1/FVC ratio can detect clinically significant disease and is an excellent prognostic indicator.

Spirometry should be repeated 30 minutes after the patient inhales a bronchodilator; if there is a 15% or more increase in FEV_1, there is a bronchospastic component to the obstruction. Spirometry should be repeated after 2 weeks of therapy to determine the effects of therapy and to document the irreversible component of obstruction. The FEV_1 is also used in Social Security disability determinations, for prognosis, and to document both the progress of the disease and response to therapy. Roughly 50% of patients with an FEV_1 of 1.0 L per second die within 5 years, and mean survival time is less than 2 years in those with an FEV_1 of 0.5 L per second or less.

If dyspnea does not correlate with changes in FEV_1, measurement of lung volumes and diffusing capacity may characterize the type of COPD (e.g., emphysema) and estimate the degree of functional derangement more precisely.

CHEST X-RAY. The chest x-ray appears normal early in COPD and is not useful in diagnosis. Increased lung markings in the lower lobes, the so-called "dirty lungs," and peribronchial thickening are seen in chronic bronchitis. Findings in emphysema include hyperinflation (low, flat diaphragm; enlarged retrosternal space), hypovascularity, areas of hyperlucency and bullae formation, and a small cardiac silhouette.

ARTERIAL BLOOD GASES. Arterial blood gases should be measured in patients with COPD to determine gas exchange and need for oxygen therapy (arterial oxygen tension [PaO_2]), alveolar ventilation (arterial carbon dioxide tension [$PaCO_2$]), and overall acid-base balance (pH). Baseline values are useful benchmarks for comparison during subsequent exacerbations. Blood gases obtained during the early stages of COPD show only mild hypoxemia. Later, low ventilation-perfusion ratios can cause severe arterial hypoxemia and respiratory acidosis. Secondary polycythemia often results from chronic hypoxemia, which appears to be more pronounced during sleep. An elevated $PaCO_2$ (> 44 mm Hg) resulting from obstructive lung disease usually occurs with an FEV_1 of 0.8 L per second or less. In evaluating patients with dyspnea on exertion, arterial blood gases measured during exercise can identify patients with hypoxemia not apparent on samples drawn at rest.

ELECTROCARDIOGRAM. Electrocardiographic changes of COPD are nonspecific. With severe disease, changes of right ventricular hypertrophy occur; atrial arrhythmias are common during acute illness.

SERUM ALPHA-1-ANTITRYPSIN. Serum alpha-1-antitrypsin levels should be determined in patients in whom the onset of COPD occurs before the age of 45, those with clinical emphysema in the absence of a history of smoking or bronchitis, or those with a family history of young-onset COPD. Serum alpha-1-antitrypsin deficiency, a genetic abnormality resulting from a defect at the *Pi* (protease inhibitor) locus, accounts for 1 to 2% of patients with emphysema. Persons who are homozygous for the ZZ phenotype have a high incidence (60–70%) of severe emphysema, and may also develop cirrhosis of the liver. It is thought that emphysema results because the inadequate levels of alpha-1-antitrypsin, a neutralizing protein, fail to protect the lung from damage caused by proteolytic enzymes (e.g., trypsin, elastase) released from inflammatory cells.

Deficient levels of alpha-1-antitrypsin are those less than 35% of the expected normal levels of 150 to 350 mg/dl. In people who are homozygously deficient, augmentation therapy with human alpha-1-antitrypsin (60 mg/kg/week) is available; replacement therapy is provided on a biweekly or monthly basis in an attempt to keep the serum level above 11 μM (80 mg/dl). The long-term effects of this expensive therapy are being evaluated.

General Treatment Measures

The management of COPD encompasses measures to prevent exacerbations and deterioration as well as specific treatment of bronchial disease and cor pulmonale.

Avoidance of Irritants

A top priority is avoidance of irritation and temperature extremes that will further damage the tracheobronchial tree or lead to an exacerbation of symptoms. Cessation of cigarette smoking is most important and can alter the course of the disease by slowing the rate of decline, as discussed above. Smoking should not be allowed in patients' homes, and patients should avoid poorly ventilated places where others smoke. Techniques and programs available to aid in smoking cessation are discussed in Chapter 130.

Patients with COPD should be cautioned to avoid areas with high levels of air pollution, or to curtail physical activities when unavoidably confronted with air pollution. Occupational exposure to cereal grain dusts, fumes, vapors, and irritants (e.g., formaldehyde) can also cause a worsening of symptoms.

High altitude and air travel can pose problems for hypoxemic patients and extremes of temperature should be avoided. Upper respiratory tract problems, such as rhinitis and postnasal drip, can aggravate symptoms and should be treated aggressively with measures such as saline nose drops and nonsedating antihistamines (which lack anticholinergic side effects) (see Table 20-1).

Avoidance of Respiratory Infections

Most respiratory infections are viral; avoidance may be aided by refraining from contact with crowds during viral epidemics and "flu" season and by keeping away from people with colds. Each fall, patients should receive influenza immunizations with polyvalent vaccine. Amantadine hydrochloride is useful if it is started within 48 hours of exposure to influenza A and can protect highly susceptible individuals during the 2-week latency period before the vaccine is effective (see Chap. 16). Polyvalent pneumococcal vaccine should be given once. On the basis of currently available data, it seems that prophylactic antibiotic therapy is not indicated; early patient-initiated treatment of exacerbations is more effective. Respiratory therapy and oxygen equipment used in the home should be carefully cleaned to prevent bacterial colonization and subsequent infection with pathogens.

Avoidance of Potentially Harmful Drugs

Antihistamines with significant anticholinergic side effects tend to cause inspissated mucus and can even depress ventilation in the seriously ill. Likewise sedatives, tranquilizers, and narcotics prescribed for pain relief or cough suppression can cause ventilatory depression and must be used with caution in patients with COPD; these drugs are contraindicated in those with carbon dioxide retention. Beta-blockers given for concomitant angina, hypertension, or glaucoma can worsen symptoms in COPD, particularly in patients who respond to bronchodilators. Although selective beta-blockers have been given in low dosages to patients with angina and fixed irreversible obstruction to airflow, these agents are not selective at higher doses and are best avoided.

Psychosocial Stresses

Patients who are chronically short of breath experience a great deal of anxiety, which in turn can lead to an increase in oxygen consumption and an increase in the work of breathing. Training in relaxation methods and breathing techniques and counseling about self-care can increase patients' feelings of autonomy in the control of dyspnea and are useful in coping with and controlling anxiety. Because rapid breathing can lead to air-trapping, an increase in the work of breathing, and more dyspnea, the patient should be instructed to take slow, deep breaths—the most efficient breathing pattern. Progressive exercise may help decrease the unrealistic fear of activity and dyspnea. Education, support, and reassurance are essential components in the psychological management of patients with COPD. Well-informed family members and patient discussion groups are useful resources; frequent follow-up visits can consolidate gains.

Pulmonary Rehabilitation
Training programs recommended for the patient with COPD include general physical reconditioning, breathing exercises, and specific diaphragm and intercostal training.

Inactivity and deconditioning are accompanied by increased lactate production, with high ventilatory drive and dyspnea on exertion. Moderate exercise training by walking and graded-stair climbing has been shown to be useful.

Slow abdominal diaphragmatic breathing with exhalation against pursed lips helps not only to relieve subjective dyspnea but also to decrease respiratory rate and minute ventilation while increasing tidal volume, thereby improving arterial blood gas levels.

Respiratory muscle weakness (diaphragm and intercostals) leads to respiratory failure in COPD. Thus inspiratory muscle training with a resistance device (P-Flex) improves diaphragmatic strength, endurance, and recovery time.

Education about proper coughing techniques, postural drainage, and chest percussion is helpful for the patient with thick mucus.

Nutrition
Many patients with end-stage lung disease have high-energy requirements and are malnourished, with muscle-wasting that contributes to inspiratory muscle weakness. Nutritional replacement of calories and proteins in these patients can strengthen respiratory muscle function. In patients who retain carbon dioxide, high-carbohydrate loads should be avoided since these lead to increased carbon dioxide levels.

Drug Therapy

The usual sequence for drug therapy in COPD is to start with regular use of a metered-dose inhaler (MDI) aerosol with an anticholinergic bronchodilator and a beta-adrenergic agonist. The beta-adrenergic agonist can be used on a regular basis or as rescue for immediate relief. Failure of expiratory flow rates to increase after the inhalation of bronchodilators should not be interpreted as absolute evidence of nonresponsive airways. While the amount of bronchodilation may be smaller in patients with COPD compared to those with asthma, adrenergic aerosols also enhance clearance of retained secretions and decrease air-trapping, thereby relieving the sensation of dyspnea. If symptoms remain poorly controlled, oral theophylline or a short course of oral steroids may be added.

Anticholinergic Bronchodilators
Cholinergic mechanisms are extremely important in COPD, particularly in patients who have smoked for many years, and those with low FEV_1s. Ipratropium bromide, a quaternary ammonia compound, is the anticholinergic agent of choice. It differs from other anticholinergics, such as atropine, in that it is poorly absorbed systemically; does not cross the blood-brain barrier; does not adversely affect ciliary activity, mucus transport, or secretions; and is extremely safe with a wide therapeutic margin. The main side effect is a cough. Because of its relatively slow action, ipratropium bromide is not used as a single agent for acute bronchospasm. Rather it is the first-line maintenance therapy for patients with chronic bronchitis and emphysema. In direct comparisons with beta-adrenergic agents, ipratropium is often more effective in stable outpatients with COPD.

Ipratropium bromide, 18 µg per puff, can be given as two puffs four times a day and increased to four puffs four times a day. The onset of action is 15 minutes after inhalation, the peak effect is 60 to 120 minutes, and the duration is 3 to 6 hours. An ipratropium solution will soon be available. Other anticholinergics including atropine (0.05 mg/kg) can be nebulized but have undesirable side effects (dry mouth, tachycardia, urinary retention) and should be avoided.

Beta-adrenergic Bronchodilators
Beta-adrenergic agents are most effective for immediate rescue but are also effective as maintenance therapy. Numerous agents are available, (see Table 21-1); since patients with COPD are older and many have concurrent heart disease, toxicity is more likely, and it may be necessary to give these agents in lower doses. Combining anticholinergics with beta-adrenergic bronchodilators leads to a longer duration of effect and a slight increase in peak effect, without an increase in side effects.

MDIs can be combined with a spacer for those individuals who have difficulty using the medicine. For those more severely impaired, compressor-powered nebulizers are available for nebulized use with albuterol or metaproterenol solutions. The usual dose for nebulized albuterol, 5 mg/ml, is 0.5 ml in 2.5 ml of saline given every 6 hours. For metaproterenol, the dose is 0.3 ml of 5% solution in 2.0 ml of saline given every 6 hours. The main side effects of beta-adrenergic agents include tremor, increased heart rate, and apprehension.

Theophylline
Theophylline, previously used in COPD as the first-line drug, is now relegated to a secondary role for those patients with COPD who are not controlled by anticholinergics, beta-adrenergic aerosols, and avoidance of irritants. Theophylline has important extrapulmonary effects: It improves the strength of diaphragmatic contractility, improves mucociliary clearance and cardiac output, and enhances respiratory drive. There is some evidence that even in irreversible COPD, theophylline increases exercise tolerance and prevents diaphragmatic fatigue (an action blocked by calcium channel blockers).

Theophylline has substantial toxicity in patients with COPD. Elderly patients with preexistent abnormal cardiac function are at risk for cardiac arrhythmias even if levels are in the high therapeutic range. Many experts suggest that for patients with COPD, theophylline be used in modest doses at a serum level between 8 and 12 mg/dl.

Theophylline has important interactions with other drugs that are frequently used for COPD, such as erythromycin, ciprofloxacin, and cimetidine. The metabolism of theophylline may also change when the patient has an exacerbation of COPD and develops acute cor pulmonale or has a viral illness. Therefore, careful monitoring of the blood level is indicated and patients who chronically use theophylline should have serum theophylline levels monitored, usually every 2 to 3 months. The dose should be reduced if any of the agents known to interfere with theophylline metabolism are used.

Corticosteroids
The use of oral corticosteroids in stable ambulatory patients with COPD remains controversial. Although systemic steroids are effective in acute exacerbations, only 10% of outpatients with COPD show a 20% improvement in FEV_1 with steroids. Potential positive responders to steroids include patients with asthmatic bronchitis with blood and sputum eosinophilia, positive skin test results, elevated levels of serum IgE, and a history of allergy and bronchodilator responsiveness. Many responders, however, have no definite characteristics, so a therapeutic trial is necessary. After baseline spirometry, oral prednisone (40 mg qd) or methylprednisolone (32 mg qd) is given for 2 weeks and spirometry repeated. An improvement in flow rates of 15% indicates a positive response. The dose of corticosteroids should be tapered to a low-daily or alternate-day maintenance dose (7.5–10 mg daily; 15 mg every other day).

Oral corticosteroids are more effective than inhaled steroids in stable patients with COPD, but patients who have responded to oral steroids sometimes benefit from inhaled steroids and an attempt should therefore be made to switch to inhaled corticosteroids.

Mucokinetic Agents
Many patients with COPD have thick, tenacious, or excessive mucus, yet mucokinetic therapy has not been widely accepted in the United States. Thinning the secretions and increasing the volume expectorated are desired goals best accomplished by adequate hydration, bronchodilators, steroids, antibiotics, and chest physiotherapy. Inhaled bland aerosols of water, saline, or steam have not improved mucociliary clearance or expectora-

tion. Oral expectorants such as guaifenesin or terpin hydrate in the recommended doses are not effective.

Saturated solutions of potassium iodide (SSKI) (10–20 drops q6–12h PO) are somewhat effective, but are associated with numerous side effects, including rash and hypothyroidism. An iodide derivative, iodopropylidene glycerol (Organidin), 60 mg four times a day, provides a lower dose of iodide and in one large trial improved frequency and severity of cough, chest discomfort, patient's ease of expectorating sputum, as well as overall symptoms.

Treatment of Acute Infections

Acute respiratory infections in adults do not cause COPD or permanent loss of function, but are associated with increased morbidity and mortality in patients with established disease. One-third of exacerbations are noninfectious; one-third, viral; and one-third, bacterial. The usual organisms that are implicated are *Streptococcus pneumoniae, Hemophilus influenzae,* and *Moraxella catarrhalis. Mycoplasma, Chlamydia,* and *Legionella* are less frequently involved. The relationship between bacterial infection and exacerbation is confounded by frequent colonization of the tracheobronchial tree by these organisms in asymptomatic patients.

Antibiotics are frequently prescribed for exacerbations (increase in dyspnea and mucopurulent sputum), although few double-blind, controlled studies have examined this practice. Microscopic examination of the sputum is used to guide selection of antibiotics but sputum cultures are unnecessary unless the patient is taking antimicrobials, has no response after 72 hours of therapy, or has associated fever or pneumonia. Amoxicillin (500 mg qid), tetracycline (500 mg qid) or doxycycline (100 mg bid), trimethoprim-sulfamethoxazole (double-strength bid), or erythromycin (500 mg qid) is given for 10 to 14 days. The prevalence of *H. influenzae* resistant to ampicillin (12%) and tetracycline (3%) is increasing, and that of *M. catarrhalis* is very high. Clinicians must therefore be familiar with the sensitivities of organisms in their communities. The more expensive agents (cefaclor, 250 mg tid; cefuroxime axetil, 250 mg bid; and amoxicillin-clavulanate, 250 mg tid) may be necessary when resistant organisms are suspected or cultured, although trimethoprim-sulfamethoxazole is somewhat effective in those cases. If gram-negative organisms are recovered from the sputum of patients recently on therapy or hospitalized, a quinoline such as ciprofloxacin is useful. Clinicians should, however, remember that the quinolones do not cover *S. pneumoniae.*

COPD patients should be instructed to initiate oral antibiotics on their own at the first sign of increasing dyspnea or changes in sputum (increased purulence, difficulties in expectoration). Regular biweekly or monthly use of prophylactic antibiotics is rarely indicated, unless the patient has numerous infectious exacerbations.

Oyxgen Therapy

Low-flow oxygen therapy has been shown to improve survival in COPD patients. Requirements for home oxygen include (1) PaO_2 of 55 mm Hg or less, or an oxygen saturation (SaO_2) below 85%; and (2) PaO_2 of 55 to 59 mm Hg if any of the following is present—erythrocytosis (hematocrit of 56% or more), cor pulmonale (P wave $>$ 3 mm in leads II, III, and aVF), edema, or congestive heart failure. In one study, patients given low-flow oxygen for 15 hours daily had improved survival over those given no oxygen; in another study, 24 hours of oxygen was better than 12 hours.

Low-flow oxygen can be administered from a variety of sources, including stationary oxygen concentrators, compressed oxygen gas cylinders, and liquid oxygen reservoirs. Easily portable liquid oxygen containers, or the less expensive but heavier gas cylinders, or fiberglass-wound aluminum cylinders are used by ambulatory patients who have hypoxemia with exercise. The goal of therapy is a PaO_2 of 60 mm Hg or SaO_2 of 90%; this may usually be accomplished with 1 to 2 L of oxygen per minute. The patient should be re-evaluated by blood gas measurements or oximetry after 1 month, 6 months, and then yearly, or with any exacerbation. The prescription for home oxygen must include: flow rate (L/min), frequency of use (hr/d), duration of need (months), laboratory evidence (arterial blood gas levels, oximetry), diagnosis of severe lung disease (angina pectoris, vascular disease, and cancer are not accepted), and documentation that other forms of treatment have been tried but not successfully.

Treatment of Cor Pulmonale
Low-flow oxygen, bronchodilators, and antibiotics are useful in patients with acute cor pulmonale, in which pulmonary hypertension resulting from chronic respiratory disease progresses to overt failure of the right side of the heart. Digoxin is indicated if atrial tachyarrhythmia or left ventricular failure is present, but has substantial toxicity in COPD because of a prolonged half-life and increased sensitivity to the drug in the presence of hypokalemia, hypoxemia, and concomitant adrenergic therapy. Calcium channel blockers such as nifedipine are modest bronchodilators and can be used to treat tachyarrhythmia. But because these drugs block the effect of theophylline on the diaphragm and may have unexpected hemodynamic effects due to changes in systemic and pulmonary vascular resistance, they are not routinely recommended for patients with cor pulmonale unless other measures fail and the benefits and safety are documented by invasive catheterization of the right side of the heart.

Diuretics

A triad of prerenal azotemia, hyponatremia, and low cardiac output develops in cor pulmonale and should benefit from loop diuretics. Side effects of diuretics used for cor pulmonale include reduced cardiac output and metabolic alkalosis, with increased plasma bicarbonate concentration from contraction of the extracellular volume and loss of chloride. Small doses of furosemide, accompanied by potassium chloride supplements, are recommended, along with restriction of sodium and close monitoring of fluid intake.

Phlebotomy

Some patients with chronic bronchitis develop erythrocytosis to compensate for chronic hypoxemia. The consequences of polycythemia are determined by a tenuous balance between increased oxygen transport versus high viscosity and increased pulmonary artery pressure. Although phlebotomy is rarely indicated, a trial is sometimes necessary to determine its effect on heart failure. Only a moderate decrease in hematocrit is necessary; there is no reason to lower the hematocrit below 50%.

Callahan CM, Dittus RS, Katz BP. Oral corticosteroid therapy for patients with stable chronic obstructive pulmonary disease. Ann Intern Med 1991; 114:216–23.
Meta-analysis of the literature reveals that 10% of stable COPD patients have a 20% increase in FEV_1 following corticosteroid therapy.

Anthonisen NR, et al. Prognosis in chronic obstructive pulmonary disease. Am Rev Respir Dis 1986; 133:14–20.
Patients with a postbronchodilator FEV_1 of 0.8 L have poor prognosis; those with higher baseline FEV_1 had better response to bronchodilation.

Ziment I. Pharmacologic therapy of obstructive airways disease. Clin Chest Med 1990; 11:461–86.
An excellent overview of bronchodilators, mucokinetic agents, corticosteroids, and antibiotics in COPD.

Gross NJ. Ipratropium bromide. N Engl J Med 1988; 319:486–94.
Ipratropium bromide is an extremely safe yet potent bronchodilator that is complementary to beta-adrenergic agents in COPD.

Anthonisen NR, et al. Antibiotic therapy in exacerbation of chronic obstructive lung disease. Ann Intern Med 1987; 106:196–204.
The benefits from antibiotics in COPD are only modestly significant, 68% versus 55% for placebo.

Rubin LJ. Vasodilator and pulmonary hypertension: where do we go from here? Am Rev Respir Dis 1987; 135:288–93.
The narrow risk-benefit ratio of vasodilator in pulmonary hypertension.

Burrows B, et al. The course and prognosis of different forms of chronic airways obstruction in a sample from the general population. N Engl J Med 1987; 317:1309–14.
Patients with asthmatic bronchitis have a better prognosis.

Tiep BL. Long-term home oxygen therapy. Clin Chest Med 1990; 11:505–21.
A state-of-the art review of home oxygen with future developments.

Petty TC. The national mucolytic study. Chest 1990; 97:75–83.
Iodinated glycerol was effective in COPD in a randomized, double-blind study.

Fletcher C, Peta R. The national history of chronic airflow obstruction. Br Med J 1977; 1:1645–8.
A prospective epidemiologic study of London men shows the pattern of decline in FEV_1 over a lifetime.

Stubbing DG, et al. Some physical signs in patients with chronic airflow obstruction. Am Rev Respir Dis 1982; 122:549–52.
Physical signs in COPD are complementary to spirometry.

Murciano D, et al. A randomized, controlled trial of theophylline in patients with severe chronic obstructive lung disease. N Engl J Med 1989; 320:1521–5.
Theophylline improved dyspnea in COPD due to better function of the respiratory muscles.

Dillard TA, et al. Hypoxemia during air travel in patients with chronic obstructive pulmonary disease. Ann Intern Med 1989; 111:362–7.

Gong H. Advising patients with pulmonary disease on air travel. Ann Intern Med 1989; 111:349–51.
A study designed to identify and quantify the determinants of hypoxemia during air travel in patients with COPD. The accompanying editorial reviews advice to patients, particularly regarding the need for supplemental in-flight oxygen.

23. ACUTE LOWER RESPIRATORY TRACT INFECTION
C. Glenn Pickard, Jr.

The spectrum of acute infectious lower respiratory disease in adults ranges from minor self-limited acute bronchitis to severe and sometimes fatal lobar pneumonia. Traditionally, most textbooks differentiate "acute bronchitis" from "pneumonia" and present very different strategies for diagnosis and management of each. In reality, however, the difference in management is properly based on the severity of the illness as manifested by the presence or absence of high fever, dyspnea and tachypnea, shaking chills, weakness and lassitude, or mental clouding. Patients manifesting these symptoms or signs, or with underlying problems such as chronic obstructive pulmonary disease, congestive heart failure, or immunosuppression, should be hospitalized for aggressive management including intravenous fluids and parenteral antibiotics. Patients without these findings or conditions can be safely managed as outpatients.

Frequently clinicians are concerned that they will miss small areas of pneumonia on examination of the chest and will therefore request a chest x-ray in the belief that the presence or absence of pneumonia will dictate a different strategy. Differentiating "pneumonia" from "acute bronchitis" by such measures, however, is not necessary for safe effective management.

An acute lower respiratory tract infection may be the initial presenting complaint of AIDS. A strong index of suspicion, a careful history for risk factors, and other common presenting complaints (fever, night sweats, weight loss) are crucial, since missing this diagnosis can have disastrous consequences. Negative findings on chest x-ray do not rule out pneumocystis pneumonia and further studies are mandated if AIDS is suspected. (See Chap. 114 for a further discussion of respiratory infections in patients with human immunodeficiency virus [HIV] infection.)

Causes
The cause of acute lower respiratory disease in adults is difficult to determine because traditional cultures of expectorated sputum may not reflect the cause of the infection.

False-positive results of cultures occur because the normal upper respiratory passages are frequently colonized by *Streptococcus pneumoniae* and occasionally *Hemophilus influenzae*. Since expectorated sputum is almost always contaminated with nasopharyngeal secretions, it is difficult to be certain that organisms recovered in sputum represent true lower tract pathogens. False-negative results also occur. For example, in studies of patients with lobar pneumonia and blood cultures positive for *S. pneumoniae*, results of sputum cultures obtained at the same time as the blood cultures were negative approximately 45% of the time.

In an attempt to eliminate false-positives, inpatients with pneumonia were subjected to direct transthoracic lung puncture, which was shown to produce the highest yield of single pathogens. Cultures of transtracheal aspirates were also found to be superior to cultures of expectorated sputum; however, studies of expectorated sputum in which the sputum was graded based on the number of neutrophils versus the number of buccal squamous epithelial cells present showed that "high-quality" sputum specimens (numerous neutrophils and few squamous cells) gave results comparable to those for transtracheal aspiration. There are no similar studies on ambulatory adults with acute lower respiratory tract infections. One can therefore only speculate about the probable causes, using the best data available from inpatient community surveillance studies obtained by conventional techniques in patients with a diagnosis of pneumonia. The great majority of cases are probably caused by viruses, and the next most frequent cause is probably *Mycoplasma,* particularly in younger adults. The TWAR strain of *Chlamydia psittaci* is apparently also an important pathogen in younger adults. Bacteria, primarily *S. pneumoniae* and to a less extent *H. influenzae,* probably account for only a small minority of the cases.

Factors that decrease the mucociliary cleansing of the tracheobronchial tree may make patients more susceptible to lower respiratory tract infection. These include chilling, cigarette smoking, and consumption of alcohol. Preceding viral infection is also believed to make bacterial infection more likely, although this commonly held belief has been challenged.

Evaluation

General Assessment
Early in the course of lower respiratory tract infection, the general assessment of the severity of the illness may be the only clue to serious and possibly life-threatening disease. Ill-appearing patients with a fever of 102.2°F (39°C) or more, tachypnea, tachycardia, pallor or cyanosis, flaring of the alae nasi, or mental confusion should be hospitalized regardless of the findings on chest examination or chest x-ray.

History
Most patients present with an illness of less than 2 weeks' duration, characterized by low-grade fever, sore throat, rhinorrhea, mild malaise, and initially a dry, nonproductive cough. Frequently, the visit to the physician is precipitated by a slight worsening of the symptoms, with the development of a productive cough and purulent sputum.

Physical Examination
Inflammation of the nasal mucosa and pharynx is commonly present. Percussion of the chest usually results in normal responses. Coarse rhonchi that clear or shift with cough are often present. Rales over small areas of the lung may be present.

Chest X-ray
Most patients with acute bronchitis and/or small areas of pneumonia do not require a chest x-ray for safe and effective management. Chest x-ray is indicated only when patients are sicker as previously discussed or if other diagnoses such as tuberculosis or cancer are considerations.

Laboratory Tests
Routine use of Gram's stain of the sputum is not recommended. It can, however, yield useful information, particularly when an unusual or opportunistic pathogen such as a gram-negative rod is suspected.

Sputum cultures are seldom, if ever, indicated in patients with straightforward illness because cultures done in the routine manner may miss important pathogens, fail to indicate the dominant organism, and frequently reveal only "normal respiratory flora" and/or contaminates from the upper airways.

In patients with lower respiratory tract infection, white blood cell counts with or without a differential count and erythrocyte sedimentation rates have been found to distinguish poorly between bacterial and viral infection. Although cold agglutinins are frequently present in the serum of patients with *Mycoplasma* pneumonia, this test is seldom done in the ambulatory setting because it is seldom of clinical importance to distinguish mild-to-moderate *Mycoplasma* infection from other causes of bronchitis and would rarely lead to a change in treatment. Studies of cold agglutinins in *Mycoplasma* bronchitis are not reported. Serologic studies, including those for *Legionella,* can only provide retrospective confirmation of infection and are therefore primarily useful in epidemiologic surveillance studies.

Treatment

Expectorants
Oral hydration and humidification are the most effective methods to thin the mucoid sputum and aid the patient in clearing bronchial secretions. There is no evidence that any of the commonly used orally administered agents, such as quaifenesin, are efficacious. Saturated solution of potassium iodide (SSKI) and other iodides may have a slight mucolytic action, but their use is limited by the frequent development of iodide hypersensitivity with skin rash.

Cough Suppressants
The use of cough suppressants remains controversial. Although they can effectively suppress cough and produce symptomatic relief, there is concern that suppression of cough may lead to prolonged or more serious illness by interfering with the clearance of secretions. In the absence of adequate studies or clear evidence of harm, it seems reasonable to use cough suppressants when patients' sleep or other activities are disrupted by dry, hacking cough.

Dextromethorphan (DM) and codeine are effective cough suppressants when given in adequate dosages (see Chap. 16). Many clinicians favor codeine even though there is no sound evidence that it is superior. The agent in which the cough suppressant is delivered makes little difference because the primary effect is centrally mediated. Most patients, however, prefer a syrup to codeine tablets.

Antibiotics
The presence of a productive cough with purulent sputum is frequently used as an indication for the use of antibiotics in lower respiratory tract infections. Years of clinical tradition support this approach, although well-done clinical trials have produced conflicting results on the efficacy of antibiotics in uncomplicated bronchitis. Antibiotic treatment is the standard of care if there is clinical or radiographic evidence of pneumonia, even with minimal involvement. If an unusual pathogen is suspected and/or more objective data are sought on which to base the choice of antibiotic, then Gram's stain of an adequate sputum specimen may be done and used to guide therapy (Table 23-1). Most clinicians prescribe an antibiotic such as erythromycin, ampicillin, or trimethoprim-sulfamethoxazole empirically without using either Gram's stain or culture for guidance. (See Table 23-1 for dosage.)

Because common organisms can develop antibiotic resistance, physicians must keep abreast of developing patterns in their own community and modify initial treatment accordingly. Resistance of *S. pneumoniae* to penicillin and *H. influenzae* to ampicillin has been reported but is present in only a very small percentage of organisms.

The recent introduction of the quinoline antibiotics (particularly ciprofloxacin) with a wide spectrum of antibiotic activity suggests their possible effectiveness in respiratory tract disease. The cost and relative lack of activity against the pneumococcus would seem to make it a less appropriate choice.

Follow-up

Clinical improvement should begin within 24 to 36 hours. If the patient becomes completely asymptomatic, no clinical or radiographic follow-up is necessary. Patients should

Table 23-1. Antibiotic choice based on Gram's stain of sputum

Gram's stain	Antibiotic and dosage
No pathogen seen (presumably viral, *Mycoplasma*, or *C. psittaci*)	Erythromycin, 250–500 mg po qid for 10–14 d, some cases of pneumonia due to *C. psittaci* have not responded to erythromycin; *or* Tetracycline, 250–500 mg po qid for 10–14 d
Gram-positive diplococci (presumed streptococcal pneumonia)	Penicillin V, 500 mg po qid for 10–14 d *or* Ampicillin, 500 mg po qid for 10–14 d *or* Erythromycin, 250–500 mg po qid for 10–14 d *or* Trimethoprim, 160 mg, and sulfamethoxazole, 800 mg, po bid for 10–14 d
Gram-negative coccobacilli (presumed *H. influenzae*)	Ampicillin, 500 mg po qid for 10–14 d *or* Erythromycin, 250–500 mg po qid for 10–14 d *or* Trimethoprim, 160 mg, and sulfamethoxazole, 800 mg, po bid for 10–14 d

be encouraged to contact their physician promptly if they do not improve significantly or if they worsen. Persistence of symptoms beyond 2 to 3 weeks should prompt further clinical evaluation. Symptoms persisting 6 weeks mandate a chest x-ray and other studies depending on the clinical situation.

Bartlett JC. Diagnosis of bacterial infections of the lung. Clin Chest Med 1987; 8:119–34.
An excellent review of the entire subject including the evidence for the implication of microbial agents as pathogens and the techniques for collecting and processing sputum. Contains 103 references.

Rodnick JE, Gude JK. The use of antibiotics in acute bronchitis and acute exacerbations of chronic bronchitis. West J Med 1988; 149:347–51.
An excellent general review. Summarizes the results of five randomized controlled trials of antibiotic treatment of acute bronchitis which show conflicting results of therapy. Excellent recommendations concerning therapy.

Tentisso JR, et al. Nonvalue of sputum culture in the management of lower respiratory tract infections. J Clin Microbiol 1987; 25:758–62.
Report of an excellent study and review of the literature on this subject.

Luby JP. Southwestern Internal Medicine Conference. Pneumonias in adults due to mycoplasma, chlamydia and viruses. Am J Med Sci 1987; 294:45–64.
An excellent review covering all of the pertinent references. Lists 99 references.

Chow JW, Yu VL. Antibiotic studies in pneumonia. Pitfalls in interpretation and suggested solutions. Chest 1989; 96:453–5.
An excellent editorial addressing the problems associated with studies of antibiotic efficacy in the treatment of pneumonia. Most of the points made are equally relevant to similar studies in acute bronchitis.

Fine MJ, et al. Hospitalization decision in patients with community-acquired pneumonia: a prospective cohort study. Am J Med 1990; 89:713–21.
An excellent study that generally supports the approach advocated in this chapter. The population studied is, in general, sicker.

24. SOLITARY PULMONARY NODULE
Raymond F. Bianchi

A solitary pulmonary nodule (SPN), also known as a coin lesion, is round to oval and less than 4 cm in diameter; a diameter greater than 4 cm signifies a pulmonary mass. Nodules are radiographically described as homogeneous, free of infiltrate, separated from the mediastinum and pleura by lung parenchyma, and without associated adenopathy.

The SPN is usually discovered on a chest x-ray obtained in an asymptomatic patient. The dilemma for both radiologist and clinician is determining whether the lesion is benign or malignant. About 30 to 50% of nodules are malignant, 30 to 50% are granulomas, and a small number (about 4%) are hamartomas. Rare causes include pulmonary infarction, organizing pneumonia, and arteriovenous (AV) malformations. The proportion of benign disease is higher in the Midwest and Southwest, where histoplasmosis and coccidioidomycosis are endemic. Carcinoma is more likely in those with a long history of cigarette smoking. The risk of cancer increases with age, from less than 1% in those under age 35 to 25 to 50% in those over age 50.

Diagnostic Tests

Chest X-rays
A benign process is favored by distinct nodule markings and the presence of satellite lesions. However, these findings cannot clinically eliminate a diagnosis of malignancy. The only two radiographic criteria for benign lesions are absence of nodular growth and the presence of calcium within the nodule. If old chest x-rays confirm that the nodule size has been stable for at least 2 years, the lesion is considered benign. This is based on the observation that the doubling time for pulmonary malignancies is between 1 and 16 months. Doubling time refers to the change in volume: A nodule doubles in size when its radius increases by 26%.

Calcium within a nodule is nearly diagnostic of a benign process. The calcium may be deposited in concentric rings (histoplasmosis), in a popcorn pattern (hamartoma), or in a dense central nidus. Small flecks of calcium may be seen in malignant nodules, the source being either scar or granulomatous material that has been engulfed by a spreading neoplasm. Detection of calcium within a nodule by conventional radiography may be difficult, particularly when it is distributed in a homogeneous pattern. Fluoroscopy with or without low-kilovoltage spot films may assist in identifying this type of calcification.

CT Scanning
Thin-section CT scanning is excellent for measuring nodule density and determining whether calcium is present; it may also be helpful in localizing the lesion. The density of benign nodules comes from tight cellular organization and the deposition of calcium.

Cytologic Analysis
Cytologic analysis of sputum is simple and noninvasive but an insensitive means of discovering malignancy. Analysis of three or more sputum samples is positive for tumor cells in only 20 to 30% of malignant SPNs, mainly squamous cell carcinomas.

Flexible Fiberoptic Bronchoscopy
Flexible fiberoptic bronchoscopy is recommended if sputum cytologic studies are nondiagnostic. The combination of fluoroscopic-guided bronchoscopic brushings and biopsy is diag-

nostic for 28 to 64% of SPNs. The larger the nodule, the greater the opportunity for tissue diagnosis. Proximal lesions tend to be easier to obtain specimens from, but peripheral nodules larger than 2 cm have an equally good yield. Primary malignancies are most likely to be identified by bronchoscopy, because benign nodules and solitary metastases usually do not originate in the bronchus.

Needle Biopsy

If bronchoscopy is unrevealing, or if the SPN is peripheral and less than 2 cm in diameter, percutaneous needle aspiration should be attempted. The accuracy of skinny-needle biopsy is similar to that of bronchoscopy for diagnosing primary lung cancers larger than 2 cm, and is superior for dealing with smaller primary malignancies and metastases. The risk of pneumothorax is approximately 11%, with about one-half of cases requiring drainage via a chest tube. Serious morbidity (hemorrhage, air embolism) occurs in less than 2% of patients undergoing biopsies. The spreading of tumor cells or inflammatory disease along the needle tract is rare and has been associated only with larger cutting needles or with neoplasms so advanced that the seeding has no effect on the course of disease.

Thoracotomy

Thoracotomy has low mortality and morbidity, plus the benefit of early resection of a carcinomatous nodule and the peace of mind that accompanies excision of benign lesions. When the nodule is neither calcified nor demonstrated to be of stable size, resection is often the first diagnostic maneuver in patients over the age of 35 who are believed to be good operative risks.

Diagnostic Strategy

When an SPN is first discovered, it is often not possible to be certain of a diagnosis, short of an invasive procedure. The following recommendations represent a reasonable compromise between unnecessary diagnostic testing and failure to discover important disease.

First, previous chest x-rays should be compared for nodule growth. A nodule of stable size for at least 2 years can be considered benign. If old chest x-rays are not available, the nodule should be examined for calcification. Observation of the plain film and fluoroscopy are at present the easiest and most economical ways to examine for calcium. If these simple maneuvers are nondiagnostic, CT scanning is then used. The workup can stop if the calcium pattern or density indicates that the nodule is benign.

When malignancy cannot be excluded on the basis of prior films or calcium deposition, nonsmokers under the age of 35 can be followed with serial chest x-rays. One formula is to repeat the film 1 month later, and if no change is noted, request another film in an additional 2 months. If no change is again noted, the interval to repeat the film is again doubled, to 4 months, and so on, until the nodule has been stable for 2 years.

If, however, the nodule is neither calcified nor demonstrated to be stable in size, a tissue diagnosis is indicated. When the probability of malignancy is high, thoracotomy may be the most appropriate initial procedure, particularly in patients over 35 and in smokers. If considering all the relevant clinical information, it seems that immediate surgery should be avoided (e.g., poor surgical risk, significant concomitant disease, patient's refusal), a nonsurgical diagnostic approach begins with sputum cytologic studies. Positive cytologic findings can make the diagnosis, but since this test is of low sensitivity, negative findings necessitate further evaluation. Flexible fiberoptic bronchoscopy or skinny-needle transthoracic biopsy should be used for a centrally located nodule and needle biopsy for peripheral nodules or lesions less than 2 cm in diameter. Cytologic or biopsy specimens positive for malignancy indicate the need for surgery (mediastinoscopy or thoracotomy). Negative cytologic or biopsy specimens are reassuring, but the patient must still be followed carefully with serial x-rays.

Lillington GA. The solitary pulmonary nodule—1974. Am Rev Respir Dis 1974; 110:699–707.
    A frequently referenced comprehensive review, with an outline of management protocol.

Swenson SJ, et al. An integrated approach to the evaluation of the solitary pulmonary nodule. Mayo Clin Proc 1990; 65:173–186.
An excellent review article discussing noninvasive and invasive radiologic and surgical diagnostic approaches.

Khouri NF, et al. The solitary pulmonary nodule: assessment, diagnosis and management. Chest 1987; 91:128–33.
The value of CT scans in the diagnosis of the SPN is well discussed in this article.

Siegelman SS, et al. CT of the solitary pulmonary nodule. AJR 1980; 135:1–13.
Benign SPNs tend to be denser than malignancies; density can be ascertained by CT scanning. Guidelines are offered for following presumed benign nodules without invasive tissue diagnosis.

Nardich DP, et al. Solitary pulmonary nodules: CT-bronchoscopic correlation. Chest 1988; 93:595–8.
Reviews the diagnostic yield of bronchoscopy. The yield will be predictably greater when CT suggests the nodule is in or near a bronchus.

Levine MS, et al. Transthoracic needle aspiration biopsy following negative fiberoptic bronchoscopy in solitary pulmonary nodules. Chest 1988; 93:1152–5.
Discusses the role and yield of transthoracic needle aspiration biopsy in the evaluation of the SPN.

Kaga AR, Steckel RJ, Braun R. Asymptomatic peripheral lung nodule. AJR 1980; 135:417–20.
Effectiveness and relative safety of percutaneous needle biopsy are discussed. Operator and cytologist skills are emphasized.

Wallace JM, Deutsch AL. Flexible fiberoptic bronchoscopy and percutaneous needle aspiration for evaluating the solitary pulmonary nodule. Chest 1982; 81:665–71.
The combination of flexible fiberoptic bronchoscopy and needle aspiration provided a diagnosis in 88% of patients who were found to have a malignant solitary pulmonary nodule. Neither procedure was diagnostic in patients with benign nodules.

Cummings SR, Lillington GA, Richard RJ. Managing solitary pulmonary nodules. The choice of strategy is a close call. Am Rev Respir Dis 1986; 134:453–60.
Decision analysis is used to compare the average life expectancy produced by alternative diagnostic strategies, including immediate surgery, biopsy (needle aspiration or bronchoscopic), and observation with serial chest films. The more aggressive approaches have slight advantages when the probability of cancer was high or intermediate, but the differences are small, and the patient's preferences and participation in the decision-making are urged.

Hix WR, Aaron BL. Solitary pulmonary nodule: what should be included in the work-up? Postgrad Med 1989; 84(4):57–8, 63–4.
Surgeons argue that if SPN can be judged neither stable in size nor calcified in those at risk for malignancy, thorocotomy should ensue promptly.

VI. CARDIOVASCULAR PROBLEMS

25. HYPERTENSION: WHO NEEDS TREATMENT?
C. Stewart Rogers

There is no natural boundary between "normal" and "abnormal" diastolic blood pressure (DBP). The correlation between DBP and the most prevalent cardiovascular disorders (atherosclerosis, heart failure, and stroke) begins well within the normal range and continues into the range we call hypertensive. There is no clear consensus on a uniform threshold DBP at which to begin drug treatment, although most experts agree that patients with persistent DBP levels of 100 mm Hg or higher should be treated with medications. In addition to the level of DBP, factors such as age, race, gender, comorbid conditions, and the presence of other cardiovascular risk factors should be considered in making the decision.

Risks of Hypertension
Studies of the natural history of hypertension have established the following:

1. High blood pressure causes direct cardiovascular morbidity (e.g., hemorrhagic stroke, aortic dissection, congestive heart failure) and contributes to the progression of atherosclerosis, retinopathy, and renal failure in a more prolonged and indirect manner.
2. While both DBP and systolic blood pressure (SBP) are highly correlated with morbidity, SBP is the stronger predictor of morbid outcome.
3. Hypertension is multiplicative with other risk factors—especially cigarette smoking, high levels of low-density-lipoprotein (LDL) cholesterol, and diabetes—so that their risk together is greater than the sum of their individual risks. The magnitude of absolute risk varies enormously with age, gender, and the presence of other risk factors.
4. All blood pressures are labile; higher pressures are more labile than lower ones. Persons with labile hypertension are at risk; there is no evidence that a "basal pressure," usually meaning the lowest pressure one can obtain, is a better predictor of risk than is an average of several measurements. Readings obtained under conditions of uncommon stress should be discounted and repeated readings should be taken, especially in borderline cases without other evidence of hypertensive disease, before committing the patient to a lifetime of treatment. Readings at home should be obtained if it is suspected that the blood pressure is artificially high when measured in the physician's office.
5. Women do not tolerate hypertension better than men. Although symptomatic atherosclerosis in women is generally delayed beyond menopause, thereafter rates in women increase rapidly. Direct mechanical damage from hypertension is equally prevalent in men and women at any age.
6. Elderly persons do not have a special tolerance for hypertension. Instead, the relation of morbidity to blood pressure actually accelerates with advancing age. This is true of both diastolic and isolated systolic hypertension.
7. Black men and women in the United States have higher mean blood pressures than whites at every age and a higher prevalence of hypertension. Likewise, blacks have much higher rates of hypertensive complications, especially strokes, cardiac failure, and nephrosclerosis.

Benefits of Treatment
All hypertension treatment trials reported before 1991 selected subjects based on DBP, conventionally defined by the fifth-phase Korotkoff sound (disappearance of tapping). DBP is therefore the point of comparison, even though SBP may be more closely related to morbid events. Mild hypertension is defined as a DBP between 90 and 104 mm Hg; moderate hypertension, as DBP between 105 and 114 mm Hg; and severe hypertension, as DBP of 115 mm Hg or higher.

Moderate-to-Severe Diastolic Hypertension

It has long been accepted that malignant hypertension should be treated. Sound evidence on the value of treating lesser degrees of chronic hypertension became available in the late 1960s from randomized trials initiated after the development of effective oral antihypertensive drugs. The landmark placebo-controlled trial undertaken by the Veterans Administration (VA) and published in 1970 demonstrated that treatment markedly reduced morbidity in subjects entering with a DBP above 105 mm Hg. Active treatment resulted in a 75% reduction in cardiovascular events, compared to the placebo-treated group with a DBP of 105 to 114 mm Hg. Stroke, heart failure, and accelerated hypertension were observed almost exclusively in the placebo group, while the study was less conclusive for prevention of myocardial infarction. Even partial reduction of pressure conferred major benefits; in patients who were actively treated but whose DBP remained above 90 mm Hg, about 75% of the maximal benefit observed with full control of DBP was achieved. Elderly patients profited from active treatment to the same extent as did younger ones. These outcomes were confirmed by almost all subsequent studies. The drugs used (hydrochlorothiazide, reserpine, and hydralazine) were effective across the range of blood pressures and reasonably well tolerated; major side effects (including peptic ulcer and depression) were equally observed in placebo and treatment groups.

The VA study was limited to compliant men, and clear evidence of benefit was confined to those with a DBP above 105 mm Hg.

Mild Diastolic Hypertension
About 70% of all persons with hypertension have a DBP between 90 and 104 mm Hg; approximately 50% of these people have DBPs between 90 and 94 mm Hg. While people with mild diastolic hypertension are clearly at risk, the benefits of treatment are controversial. Potential benefits of treatment must be weighed against possible adverse effects of antihypertensive drugs, adverse psychological effects induced by the diagnosis ("labeling"), and the costs of treatment in terms of both money and time. Several large clinical trials that evaluated drug therapy of mild hypertension support the following general conclusions.

1. Hypertension can be controlled in most persons although many patients require two or more drugs and a substantial minority experience adverse effects.
2. The incidence of stroke is reduced by active treatment of mild hypertension; the average reduction in stroke incidence and mortality across several community-based randomized trials of drug treatment for mild-to-moderate hypertension was 40%.
3. The incidence of morbidity and mortality from coronary artery disease was not consistently reduced by hypertension therapy in studies using diuretics, reserpine, alpha-methyldopa, hydralazine, and beta-blockers; only a few subsets showed reduced rates of coronary events within the study periods.
4. Within the mild hypertensive cohorts, those whose DBP was at the higher range (95–105 mm Hg) received more benefit from active treatment than did those at the range of 90 to 95 mm Hg.
5. Remissions occur in placebo-treated mild hypertension. In 20% or more of persons whose DBP repeatedly measured 90 to 104 mm Hg, the DBP drifted down to levels below 90 mm Hg during several years of placebo treatment. This supports the use of nonpharmacologic treatment initially in patients with mild hypertension (see Chap. 26).
6. Treatment of mild hypertension prevents progression to more severe hypertension. In one study, 12% of patients on placebo manifested a rise to levels above 104 mm Hg, and it was this subset that suffered most of the excess morbidity relative to the active treatment groups.
7. Demographic variables such as gender, race, and socioeconomic status (education and income) play a role in the magnitude of benefit of treatment, with greater benefit observed in black men and women.

Treatment Decisions
In mild hypertensives, factors other than blood pressure must be weighed in making the decision to treat. Systolic hypertension, age, and cardiac and renal impairment exert an amplifier effect on the danger of elevated DBP, as do other atherosclerotic risk factors such as smoking, diabetes, and high levels of LDL cholesterol. It is reasonable to assume that treating mildly elevated DBP in persons with other risk factors is especially useful. The presence of existing atherosclerotic disease, left ventricular hypertrophy or azotemia can be taken as evidence of individual susceptibility to hypertensive injury and grounds for aggressive management. Evidence that hypertension accelerates retinopathy and renal

failure in diabetics strongly supports the recommendation that even mild hypertension should be treated in these patients. For most others with a DBP in the mildest range (90–100 mm Hg), a period of surveillance, dietary modification, and education may be pursued for several months. Thereafter, only those with a DBP exceeding 95 mm Hg would be treated with drugs, and the rest would be followed indefinitely, with that therapeutic threshold in mind.

Isolated Systolic Hypertension

Systolic hypertension usually coexists with diastolic hypertension but may be predominant or even isolated (SPB >160 with DBP < 90 mm Hg). Isolated systolic hypertension is a major pattern in older persons, reaching a prevalence of 30% in the eighth decade. Several concepts about systolic hypertension have led to its relative neglect. SBP is highly labile and is said to reflect cardiac function more than arteriolar resistance, and systolic hypertension is viewed as a result of established atherosclerosis rather than its cause. Furthermore, it is often difficult to control predominant systolic hypertension without causing orthostatic adjustments or compromising coronary or renal perfusion. These concerns are magnified because systolic hypertension so often occurs in elderly patients with varying degrees of established atherosclerosis; impaired cardiac, renal, and baroreceptor function; and concurrent therapy with other medications. The results of the Systolic Hypertension in the Elderly (SHEP) study, published in 1991, showed a 36% reduction in stroke and significant reductions in all cardiovascular endpoints among a large population of elderly patients with isolated systolic hypertension treated with chlorthalidone (plus atenolol when needed for blood pressure control), compared to placebo-treated control patients. These results achieved with relatively inexpensive and well-tolerated drugs extend the mandate to treat to include the many elderly patients with isolated systolic hypertension. Fortunately, treatment usually reduces the systolic and diastolic pressures unequally in proportion to their initial elevation; this must be monitored in individual patients to avoid an excessive drop in coronary perfusion, which depends on diastolic pressure. The advantages and potential side effects of therapeutic agents are discussed in Chapter 26.

Littenberg B, Garber A, Sox H. Screening for hypertension. Ann Intern Med 1990; 112:192–202.
Cost-effectiveness analysis of data from all trials of antihypertensive therapy, quantitating relative cost-and-benefit projections for the spectra of severity, demography, and therapeutic options. Best current analytic review of the value of treatment.

VA Cooperative Study. Effects of treatment on morbidity in hypertension. Part I (DBP 115–129 mm Hg); JAMA 1967; 202:116–22; Part II (DBP 90–114). JAMA 1970; 213:1143–52.

The Management Committee. The Australian Therapeutic Trial in Mild Hypertension. Lancet 1980; 1:1261–7.

HDFP Cooperative Group. Five-year findings of the Hypertension Detection and Follow-Up Program. JAMA 1979; 242:2562–71.

MRFIT Research Group. Multiple Risk Factor Intervention Trial. JAMA 1982; 248: 1465–77.

Medical Research Council Working Party. MRC Trial of Treatment of Mild Hypertension: principal results. Br Med J 1985; 291:97–104.
Five studies of basic drug regimens, comprising the data base of our understanding of whom to treat. An enormous editorial response analyzed this data in various ways.

Textor S. Management of mild hypertension. Mayo Clin Proc 1989; 64:1543–52.
An outstandingly concise and reasonable summary of the above studies.

Taguchi J, Freis E. Partial reduction of blood pressure and prevention of complications in hypertension. N Engl J Med 1974; 291:329–31.

Berglund G. Goals of antihypertensive therapy: is there a point beyond which pressure reduction is dangerous? Am J Hypertens 1989; 2:586–93.
Two articles from different eras addressing the question of a target blood pressure with therapy.

Mortality and morbidity results from the European Working Party on High Blood Pressure in the Elderly trial. Lancet 1985; 1:1349–54.

Treatment of hypertension in the over-60s. Lancet 1985; 1:1369–70.

The Working Group on Hypertension in the Elderly. Statement on hypertension in the elderly. JAMA 1986; 256:70–4.
Three articles on the huge problem of treating elderly hypertensives: the major available study, a most insightful commentary, and a practical overview by an expert group.

SHEP Cooperative Research Group. Prevention of stroke by antihypertensive drug treatment in older persons with isolated systolic hypertension. JAMA 1991; 265:3255–64.
The long-awaited results of the study that should now guide the approach to isolated systolic hypertension in elderly patients.

26. EVALUATION AND TREATMENT OF HYPERTENSION
C. Stewart Rogers

Once the diagnosis of persistent hypertension has been made, patient education is essential. Issues to be stressed are as follows:
1. Hypertension is, with rare exceptions, a lifelong and asymptomatic condition.
2. There is excellent evidence that treatment reduces the risk of complications.
3. The availability of multiple treatment options allows a tolerable therapeutic regimen to be found for every patient.
4. Patients play a critical role in maintaining their own health.

There are many ways to lower blood pressure using dietary, behavioral, and medical means. In recent years, the traditional "stepped-care" approach of sequentially adding medications has been challenged by new options for single-drug therapy, with some ability to match the drug to the patient. The choice among these options depends on patient-related factors that predispose to adverse effects, predict compliance, or require treatment of a coexisting condition.

Initial Evaluation
The aims of the initial evaluation are to (1) confirm the presence of important hypertension, (2) detect the occasional case of secondary hypertension, (3) select the safest and most effective management, and (4) develop a strategy to facilitate lasting compliance.

Confirming Important Hypertension
Several large trials have shown that 20 to 40% of initially hypertensive subjects become and remain normotensive with placebo treatment through years of follow-up. For this reason it is imperative to confirm the presence of true hypertension with several readings over several weeks, especially if the elevations are small or variable and there are no signs of target-organ damage. Technique is important: The sphygmomanometer must be calibrated, and the cuff must be large enough. (The inflatable bladder should be wider than one-half the circumference of the arm; if in doubt a larger cuff should be used.) The patient must be settled and free of *unusual* stress. Readings should be taken from both arms, and if values are discrepant the higher should be used. Readings should also be obtained with the patient in both seated (or supine) and standing positions, to identify orthostatic changes. Because lability is expected when blood pressure measurements are repeated, the best strategy is to average several readings. Interest in using home measurements and ambulatory recorders is increasing, but no consensus has yet been reached on using these departures from the intermittent measurements in a physician's office, on which our understanding of hypertension is based.

Detecting Secondary Hypertension
In unusual cases, increased blood pressure is a marker for an underlying disease that requires separate management or imposes special considerations in the choice of hypotensive therapy. It is estimated that secondary hypertension occurs in less than 10% of patients with hypertension; most of these cases are due to drugs, or renal parenchymal and vascular disease. Other, more unusual secondary causes of hypertension include coarctation of the aorta and endocrine abnormalities, including pheochromocytoma, Cushing's syndrome, and hyperaldosteronism. The index of suspicion should be raised by suggestive findings on history and physical examination, including family history, severe hypertension (diastolic blood pressure [DBP] > 130 mm Hg), young age at onset (< 30 years), and failure to respond to drug therapy.

Drugs that cause hypertension include alcohol, cocaine, oral contraceptives, sympathomimetics, corticosteroids, some antidepressants, and thyroid hormones. In many clinics, the most common and neglected secondary cause of hypertension is alcoholism. Whether or not alcoholism causes hypertension in an individual patient, control of blood pressure is unlikely without control of drinking. Users of oral contraceptives who develop hypertension should stop the drug and be observed for several months for remission before it is concluded that long-term medical treatment is needed. Sympathomimetics should be used sparingly or not at all if they cause or increase hypertension.

Renal failure from any cause, including essential hypertension, is the most common underlying cause of secondary hypertension, and is detected by a serum creatinine measurement and urinalysis. Renal parenchymal disease may result from congenital renal anomalies, diabetic nephropathy, obstructive nephropathy, glomerulonephritis, and tubulointerstitial disease. Renal artery stenosis (RAS) is uncommon (about 1% or less of unselected hypertensives), but presents significant diagnostic and therapeutic challenges. It is usually unilateral, caused in young adults by fibromuscular dysplasia and in older patients by atherosclerosis, and often causes severe hypertension that may prove resistant to medical treatment. Bilateral RAS can lead to progressive renal failure. Strategies for detecting this uncommon disease are controversial and subject to evolving technologies and local expertise. The traditional screening test, rapid-sequence pyelography to detect signs of differential perfusion, has a sensitivity of only about 70 to 80%; renal scan may in some centers be an equivalent or better test. Plasma renin response to the angiotensin-converting enzyme inhibitor captopril has also been used for screening. Because the prevalence of important and correctable RAS is so low among hypertensives, most positive results on screening tests are really false-positives. At present, diagnostic efficiency is improved by selecting patients with unusually severe or resistant hypertension, abrupt increases in blood pressure, progressive azotemia despite blood pressure control, and abdominal systolic and diastolic bruits. This smaller, selected population can be studied with digital imaging of the renal arteries, where available, or with arteriography. Diagnosis depends on demonstrating a 70% stenosis of a renal artery or segmental artery and increased renin secretion from the affected side. Surgical therapy is reported to substantially improve or cure hypertension in about 80% of patients with stenosis due to fibromuscular hyperplasia, and 60% of patients with atherosclerotic stenosis.

Coarctation of the aorta should be suspected if the femoral pulse is diminished or absent, and blood pressure is decreased in the lower extremities. Diagnosis is confirmed by rib notching on chest film and by aortography.

Endocrine causes of hypertension include primary or autonomous hyperaldosteronism, which is sought for the finding(s) of unprovoked (i.e., no diuretic therapy) and/or profound hypokalemia during diuretic therapy despite compliance with a low-salt diet. Muscle weakness, fatigue, polyuria, and polydipsia may be present. The diagnosis depends on the demonstration of low plasma renin activity after volume depletion and upright posture, and high plasma aldosterone levels that fail to decrease with volume expansion and recumbency. Pheochromocytoma is suggested by unusual lability of blood pressure and by symptoms of catecholamine excess, including tachycardia, palpitations, tremor, sweating, and headache, often occurring in spells, and weight loss. Both plasma and urine catecholamines and metabolites can be measured. Determining plasma catecholamine levels is the most sensitive test; tests showing borderline values should be repeated, possibly using hospitalization to safely remove the confounding effects of antihypertensive drugs. Glucocorticoid excess is sought only in those hypertensives with typical features of Cushing's syndrome.

Selecting Safe and Effective Therapy

An initial survey of the patient's existing "target-organ" damage will determine the severity of hypertensive disease, guiding urgency and certain precautions in treatment. Identifying other "risk factors" for vascular disease, such as smoking, diabetes mellitus, and elevated levels of low-density-lipoprotein (LDL) cholesterol, also helps to direct therapeutic choices. Initial physical examination should therefore include measurements of weight and height; funduscopic examination for signs of hypertensive retinopathy, such as arteriolar narrowing, arteriovenous compression, hemorrhages, exudates, and papilledema; cardiac examination for increased rate, arrhythmias, murmurs, and S_3 and S_4 sounds; vascular examination for bruits in the neck, abdomen, costovertebral angle, and groin, and diminished or absent pulsations in the legs; and palpation of the thyroid gland. Basic laboratory studies should include determinations of serum potassium and serum creatinine concentrations, dipstick urinalysis (for protein, blood and glucose) and ECG (for left ventricular hypertrophy or other signs of cardiovascular disease). Other recommended studies, most of which can be included in an automated chemistry panel, include measurements of glucose (fasting, if possible), total serum cholesterol (followed, if abnormal, with high-density-lipoprotein, plasma triglycerides, and calculated LDL cholesterol), serum calcium, and uric acid. Microscopic urinalysis may reveal cells and casts consistent with glomerular damage before abnormalities on dipstick urinalysis or in the creatinine level are evident.

Strategies for Compliance
In the great majority of cases, antihypertensive therapy must be maintained for years or decades. Remembering doses, paying for refills, keeping appointments, tolerating real and imagined side effects, and accepting the status of patienthood for an asymptomatic illness may present real impediments to continuing treatment. These factors should be considered and discussed with the patient initially and over the course of time.

A clear and plausible rationale for treatment must be provided to patients with hypertension at the outset and repeated often over the years. The initial evaluation should consider the patient's beliefs and attitudes toward illness and taking medication, as well as the financial and social resources critical to obtaining drugs, following a diet, and keeping appointments. The goals are to prescribe a regimen that the patient can follow, and identify the services that may be needed to support patients and families in following the regimen.

Nonpharmacologic Therapy

Nonpharmacologic therapy is now recommended for the treatment of all hypertensive patients, since it will be an adjunct to medication if it is not effective alone. Most patients with mild hypertension (DBP of 90–100 mm Hg) should be treated initially without drugs. Patients with moderate-to-severe hypertension and those with comorbid conditions mandating drug treatment from the outset should also be advised about nonpharmacologic approaches.

Salt restriction, reduced alcohol intake, and weight reduction (in obese patients) are the principal techniques for lowering blood pressure without drugs. In several small studies, intake of other dietary minerals (potassium, calcium), as well as fat restriction and fish oil supplements have also been examined for their potential to lower blood pressure. In general, these results have been inconsistent or disappointing. On the other hand, moderation of excess calorie and alcohol intake may enhance general health and function as well as lower blood pressure.

Salt restriction is the most widely applicable, and perhaps the single most powerful nondrug intervention. Many Americans habitually consume over 200 mEq (4 g) of sodium daily. General reduction of a few high-sodium items in the diet (e.g., packaged meats, canned soups, snack foods, pickles, canned tomato juice) will drop most diets to below 100 mEq of sodium per day (see Chap. 143). This may achieve blood pressure control for many patients without the costs and potential toxicities of drugs. Moreover, a high-sodium diet exacerbates the potassium-wasting effects of diuretics, so salt restriction is also appropriate in patients on diuretic regimens. The increasing use of drug regimens that are not diuretic-based is further incentive to control blood volume through dietary means.

Behavioral approaches to treating hypertension apart from diet include biofeedback, exercise, and meditation. These approaches have the potential to benefit patients in ways beyond blood pressure reduction and even the modest changes they may induce can save patients with mild hypertension from years of drug therapy. However, most require a trained, committed therapist, and many patients lack the mental and social resources to implement and sustain new habits and life-style. Because patients commonly drop out of such programs over time, their chief morbidity may be relapsed and untreated hypertension.

Nonpharmacologic therapy should be tried for a minimum of 3 to 6 months in patients with mild hypertension before drug treatment is initiated. If the DBP remains between 90 and 94 mm Hg, and the patient is at low risk, consideration should be given to not using any medications. Some authorities recommend raising the DBP threshold for drug treatment to 100 mm Hg for individuals without other cardiovascular risk factors, such as systolic hypertension, elevated LDL cholesterol levels, diabetes, cigarette smoking, or evidence of end-organ damage. Such individuals should be monitored for progression of hypertension with regular visits every 3 to 6 months.

Table 26-1. Drugs for hypertension

DIURETICS		
Thiazide-like drugs	Loop diuretics	Potassium-sparing diuretics
Hydrochlorothiazide, etc.	Furosemide	Triamterene
Chlorthalidone	Bumetanide	Spironolactone
Indapamide	Ethacrynic acid	Amiloride
Metolazone		

SYMPATHOLYTICS			
Peripheral	Central	Beta-blockers	
Reserpine	Methyldopa	Propranolol	Atenolol
	Clonidine	Timolol	Pindolol
	Guanebenz	Nadolol	Acebutolol
		Metoprolol	Betaxolol
Postsynaptic		Alpha- and beta-blocker	
Prazosin		Labetalol	
Terazosin			
Doxazosin			

VASODILATORS		
Direct smooth muscle dilators	Antiotensin-converting enzyme inhibitors	Calcium channel blockers
Hydralazine	Captopril	Verapamil
Minoxidil	Enalapril	Diltiazem
	Lisinopril	Nifedipine
	Fosinopril	Nicardipine
		Isradipine

For many patients, the giving and receiving of pills and the usual early decrease in blood pressure that results are strong bonding factors that establish the basis for long-term compliance. Early initiation of drug therapy is highly beneficial in these patients. Advice that is less realistically achievable or more discouraging (e.g., weight loss, smoking cessation) can then be pursued after an initial success with medications.

Drug Therapy

Antihypertensive drugs are usually grouped as diuretics, sympatholytics, and vasodilators (Table 26-1). Within each group are agents with substantially different mechanisms of action and unique clinical uses. There are five options for a first drug: diuretics, beta-blockers, calcium channel blockers, angiotensin converting enzyme inhibitors (ACEIs), and postsynaptic adrenergic blockers.

The older adrenergic blockers (reserpine, methyldopa) and direct vasodilators (hydralazine, minoxidil) could not be used without a diuretic because the initial fall in blood pressure stimulates renin, leading to fluid retention and loss of blood pressure control. The alternative monotherapies (Table 26-2) avoid this problem in several ways including renin inhibition and altered renal hemodynamics. Although each can be used alone for hypertension, their potency is enhanced by the addition of a diuretic and, indeed, most of these drugs are available in fixed combinations with hydrochlorothiazide (HCTZ). Nonetheless, part of the purpose of alternative monotherapies is avoidance of diuretic side effects, so these options will be discussed first as single agents.

Table 26-2. Monotherapy options

Drug	Special indication	Contraindication
Diuretic	Blacks Elderly Smokers Heart failure Renal failure Cost concerns	None
Beta-blocker	Young whites Nonsmokers Coronary disease (MI survivors, angina) Migraine Performance anxiety ("stage fright")	Congestive heart failure AV block Asthma Raynaud's phenomenon Diabetic on insulin Competitive athletes
Angiotensin-converting enzyme inhibitor	Whites Heart failure Diabetes (especially with early nephropathy) Unilateral renal artery stenosis	Blacks Bilateral renal artery stenosis Pregnancy
Calcium channel blocker		
Any	Older patients Angina Coronary artery disease	Heart failure
Verapamil	Supraventricular tachyarrhythmia Asthma Migraine	AV block Beta-blocker
Postsynaptic blocker	None	Special risk of falling

MI = myocardial infarction; AV = atrioventricular.

Diuretics
Diuretics used to treat hypertension include the thiazide-like drugs, the loop diuretics, and the potassium-sparing diuretics; the latter group is usually employed in combination with the other types.

Thiazide diuretics are still the most commonly employed first drugs for hypertension because they are inexpensive, are effective taken once daily, require little titration, and have few contraindications. They are effective for hypertension of any severity or in any demographic group and they prevent the renin-mediated fluid retention provoked to some degree by most other classes of antihypertensive drugs. Almost every clinical trial of the benefits of treating hypertension used thiazide-based regimens as the active treatment.

Like most single agents, a starting dose of HCTZ, 25 mg daily, will drop each component of blood pressure about 6 to 12 mm Hg. Despite a short plasma half-life, the antihypertensive effect lasts at least 24 hours. The enhanced diuresis lasts 3 to 5 hours: patients should be instructed to take pills at a convenient time. Some patients, particularly the elderly, do well on 12.5 mg/day. There is minimal added benefit to doses over 50 mg/day, and risks of associated hypokalemia increase significantly.

In general, other diuretics are more expensive without being more effective or better tolerated. The thiazide-like drugs and the loop diuretics all share most of the metabolic side effects of HCTZ: hypokalemia, hyperuricemia, and impaired glucose tolerance. Only the thiazides raise serum calcium; this effect is usually slight and transient, but may be responsible for the 30 to 50% lower incidence of hip fractures observed in patients on thiazides. Appropriate reasons for using a non-thiazide include allergy, or either cardiac or renal failure requiring a loop diuretic. Patients with creatinine clearance below 30 ml per minute (serum creatinine > 2.5 in young adult or 2.0 in older adult) should be treated with loop diuretics (e.g., furosemide) rather than thiazides.

The metabolic side effects of thiazides do not usually contraindicate their use. Asymptomatic hyperuricemia occurs (see Chap. 95) but does not require treatment and rarely leads to gout. Diuretics may provoke glucose intolerance and can unmask latent diabetes or require some upward adjustment of hypoglycemic therapy. There is, however, no evidence that diuretics cause diabetes or precipitate diabetic crises or complications. Diuretics also cause a slight increase in plasma cholesterol levels (about 10 mg/dl) in short term trials, but this does not seem to persist beyond 1 year and is of doubtful importance.

Hypokalemia is a dose-related side effect of diuretics. Most patients on long-term diuretic therapy experience some fall in serum potassium concentration (about 0.5 mEq/L), but fewer than 10% develop a potentially important hypokalemia. Since the diuretic-induced potassium-wasting is proportional to the dietary sodium level, modest attention to sodium intake can prevent hypokalemia. Hypokalemia can frequently be avoided by using thiazide doses of less than 50 mg/day. Short-term ECG monitoring studies have failed to show a consistent arrhythmogenic effect even when mild hypokalemia is provoked, and several large diuretic-based trials of antihypertensive therapy have not shown any increased risk of sudden death. On the other hand, patients taking digitalis, those at very high baseline risk of ventricular ectopic arrhythmias, and those shown to develop hypokalemia should receive supplemental treatment with either potassium chloride (KCL), 40 mEq daily, or a potassium-sparing diuretic such as triamterene. Combinations of the latter with HCTZ are generically available and may be more effective at maintaining normokalemia than potassium supplementation. These agents should be used judiciously, however, because they add cost and carry a risk of hyperkalemia, especially in patients with renal insufficiency and those taking converting enzyme inhibitors.

Beta-Blockers
Beta-adrenergic blocking agents have been a recognized single-drug therapy alternative for more than 15 years. They reduce cardiac output and suppress the renin-angiotensin system, thus lowering blood pressure despite transiently increasing peripheral resistance. The alternative agents in this class (Table 26-3) differ in their cardioselectivity (beta-1 activity), lipid solubility, and excretion; several beta-blockers have intrinsic sympathetic activity and produce less bradycardia.

Beta-blockers as a class are more effective in young white patients than in black or elderly persons, especially when the clinical picture suggests a "hyperdynamic circulation." The latter pattern of tachycardia and wide pulse pressure is often seen in early essential hypertension. Diuretics are more likely to achieve goal blood pressures in blacks,

Table 26-3. Beta-blockers

Drug	Beta-1 selective	Intrinsic sympathomimetic activity	Lipid solubility	Excretion	Dosing frequency[a] (beta blockade)
Propranolol	No	0	High	Hepatic	bid
Timolol	No	0	Low	Hepatic	bid
Nadolol	No	0	Low	Renal	qd
Pindolol	No	+ +	Moderate	Hepatic/renal	bid
Metoprolol	Yes	0	Moderate	Hepatic	bid
Atenolol	Yes	0	Low	Renal	qd
Acebutolol	Yes	+	Low	Renal	qd/bid
Betaxolol	Yes	0	High	Hepatic	qd
Labetalol[b]	No	0	Low	Hepatic	bid

[a] All dosed every day for hypertension alone.
[b] Also possesses alpha-adrenergic blocking activity.

possibly because they often have a volume-dependent, low-renin hypertension. In elderly patients beta-blockers may encroach on a marginal cardiac reserve. Smokers treated with propranolol in one large study did not achieve the same protection from cerebrovascular events as did nonsmokers; furthermore, propranolol is less effective than other drugs for blood pressure control in smokers, possibly because nicotine accelerates its metabolism. While these demographic rules should be considered in selecting a drug regimen, they are not absolute. The best reasons to select or avoid beta-blockers are the presence of comorbidities that provide an opportunity to treat two disorders with the same drug or, conversely, that contraindicate their use.

Beta-blockers may offer additional therapeutic benefits in hypertensive patients who also have angina, migraine, essential tremor, or performance anxiety ("stage fright"). In several trials, beta-blockers without intrinsic sympathomimetic activity (ISA) have been shown to improve survival after myocardial infarction; there is some evidence of a lower incidence of first events of nonfatal myocardial infarction in hypertensive patients treated with beta-blockers versus diuretics. On the other hand, beta-blockers have been associated with short-term adverse effects on lipid levels, and choice of another drug may be prudent in hypertensive patients with marked elevations of serum cholesterol.

About 25% of hypertensive patients have an absolute or relative contraindication to beta blocker therapy or will not tolerate such therapy if tried. Strong contraindications include asthma (or chronic obstructive pulmonary disease [COPD] with a clear bronchospastic element), congestive heart failure (CHF) (unless due exclusively to diastolic dysfunction), higher than first-degree atrioventricular (AV) block, Raynaud's disease, and tightly controlled or "brittle" insulin-treated diabetes (beta-blockers may mask the symptoms of hypoglycemia). Relative contraindications include lesser degrees of cardiopulmonary disease, diabetes in general, peripheral arterial disease, COPD, or depression. It is not uncommon for beta-blockers to unmask these conditions in predisposed persons. Beta-blockers reduce exercise tolerance, and are relatively contraindicated in persons dependent on a top physical performance, such as competitive athletes.

Some of the relative contraindications of beta-blockers can be accommodated by use of agents with beta-1 selectivity or ISA, or possibly, lower degrees of lipid solubility. Beta-1 selective blockers are often well tolerated at lower doses in COPD patients without bronchospasm and in patients with diabetes and peripheral vascular disease. They also may be more effective in smokers. Beta-1 selectivity is only relative, however, and is lost at higher doses (> 100 mg/day of either atenolol or metoprolol). Beta-blockers with ISA have less negative effects on cardiac rate and output as well as renal and peripheral blood flow, and have not been associated with adverse effects on lipid levels; however, they are not likely to increase survival after myocardial infarction or improve angina, and may not help control tachyarrhythmias. Adverse CNS effects of beta-blockers such as depression and sleep disturbances may be related to their lipid solubility, although the data documenting this relationship are insufficient. Propranolol's high CNS penetration may be important in its prophylaxis against migraine.

The duration of full beta-blocking effect and the route of elimination are indicated in Table 26-3. Any of these drugs can be used once daily for treatment of hypertension alone because the blood pressure rebounds very slowly even after the drug is gone. When concomitant angina, arrhythmia, or other disease is also being treated, the shorter-acting drugs must be taken more often. The route of elimination may be a consideration in patients with renal or hepatic failure, although such patients can be treated with any beta-blocker if the dose is carefully titrated against the blood pressure and heart rate. As of 1991 only propranolol was available generically, at dramatically lower cost than the other beta blockers and alternative monotherapies.

Labetalol is a beta-blocker with additional alpha-blocking properties that may be more effective in blacks and more appropriate for elderly patients than other beta-blockers. It preserves renal and peripheral blood flow and usually does not aggravate bronchospasm. Despite these advantages, its beta-1 effects are nonselective and the usual precautions apply.

Angiotensin Converting Enzyme Inhibitors
The ACEIs captopril, enalapril, lisinopril, and fosinopril block the activation of angiotensin, thus acting as vasodilators affecting cardiac preload and afterload alike. They also

block secondary fluid retention by suppressing the stimulation of aldosterone. Used alone, these drugs can normalize the blood pressure in 35 to 70% of hypertensives without affecting cardiac output or rate, renal function, or cerebral blood flow. Diuretic cotreatment markedly enhances their effect, with another 25% achieving the goal blood pressure. Similar enhancement is seen with calcium channel blockers but not with beta-blockers. Whites respond much better than blacks to monotherapy with ACEIs, but this racial difference is eliminated when diuretics are added.

There are some special advantages to these drugs and a few cautions. ACEIs actually improve survival in severe CHF and thus are indicated for concomitant heart failure and hypertension. ACEIs may delay the progression of early diabetic nephropathy by reducing the excessive glomerular filtration pressure that seems to cause proteinuria and result in nephron loss. Once renal insufficiency has become established, however, the potential benefit of ACEIs on renal function is controversial. Furthermore, ACEIs raise potassium levels by suppressing aldosterone. While this is an advantage in cotreatment with diuretics, it is a caution for patients with renal failure and a contraindication to use with potassium supplements or potassium-sparing drugs like triamterene. ACEIs must also be used with great caution in patients already volume-depleted by diuretics because marked hypotension has occurred. The major subjective side effect of ACEIs is a chronic nonproductive cough, which occurs in 5 to 10% of patients; the cause is unknown.

While ACEIs are particularly effective for unilateral RAS, they are contraindicated in bilateral stenosis because they block the angiotensin-mediated efferent glomerular arteriolar constriction needed to maintain filtration pressure, and acute renal failure may result. Converting enzyme inhibitors are also contraindicated in pregnancy because fetal wastage has occurred in animal studies.

The ACEIs have been heavily promoted on the basis of some limited information suggesting that they have fewer adverse effects on quality of life than do other antihypertensive drugs. Captopril has compared favorably with methyldopa and propranolol in such areas as sedation, mood alteration, and impotence. There are no quality-of-life data comparing ACEIs to diuretics, calcium channel blockers, or the less lipid-soluble beta-blockers. Finally, these drugs and the calcium channel blockers are very expensive.

Calcium Channel Blockers

The calcium channel blockers verapamil, diltiazem, nifedipine, nicardipine, and isradipine are direct vasodilators that can be used alone for hypertension. These drugs reduce cardiac muscle and vascular smooth muscle contractility, reducing systolic inotropic force and blood pressure. In hypertensive patients the drop in left ventricular contraction is compensated by the decrease in afterload, so that cardiac output is usually well maintained. Balanced preload and afterload reduction ameliorates the reflex tachycardia that occurs with older vasodilators like hydralazine, and the enhancement of renal blood flow promotes natriuresis and obviates the need for diuretic cotherapy.

The calcium channel blockers dilate coronary as well as systemic arteries, and were originally released for treating angina. Other special uses and precautions vary with the specific drug. The five available calcium channel blockers vary in their degree of negative inotropic effect and in their suppression of AV nodal conduction. Verapamil is the most cardiodepressant and can aggravate or unmask CHF; it most strongly slows AV conduction, which can help control supraventricular tachyarrhythmias but can also cause AV block in predisposed persons. Constipation is a potential side effect. At the other extreme, nifedipine and especially nicardipine have little negative effect on either contraction or conduction in the heart; indeed, tachycardia is a potential side effect, as are flushing and diarrhea. Diltiazem is intermediate in these properties.

The best reason to select a calcium channel blocker for monotherapy of hypertension is still coexisting angina. The vasodilating properties may also be beneficial in some patients with esophageal spasm, Raynaud's disease, or migraine. Verapamil can be used to prevent recurrent supraventricular tachycardia, to control the ventricular rate in atrial fibrillation, or to improve the hemodynamics in hypertrophic obstructive cardiomyopathy. Calcium channel blockers may also be good choices for patients with conditions that preclude or discourage the use of other agents, such as diabetes, asthma or peripheral vascular disease. The metabolic effects are minor and they do not affect lipid levels. Unlike the converting enzyme inhibitors, calcium channel blockers work equally well as monotherapy in blacks and whites with hypertension. Sustained-release preparations of verapamil, diltiazem, and nifedipine allow once- or twice-daily dosing; even the nonsustained release formulations can be given twice daily for blood pressure control but the drug level's peaks and valleys have greater potential for adverse effects (especially with nifedipine). Adding a thiazide-type diuretic enhances the efficacy of calcium channel blockers to a lesser degree than it does a beta-blocker or an ACEI. Calcium channel blockers can be combined with other antihypertensives to enhance their potency; verapamil, however, should not be used with a beta-blocker because their cardiodepressant effects are additive.

Alpha-1-Blockers
The sympatholytic agents prazosin, terazosin, and doxazosin can be used alone without diuretics. They have the possible advantage of slightly favorable effects on plasma lipids and no specific contraindications. However, initial treatment or dosage increments can cause orthostatic hypotension, which is of particular concern in elderly patients; first-dose syncope has been reported. The smallest starting dose should be used, with the smallest incremental increases; changes should be made with the bedtime dose and with careful warnings to the patient. Tachyphylaxis occurs when these agents are used to treat CHF; anecdotal data suggest that this may occur in the treatment of hypertension as well. Neither tachyphylaxis nor orthostatic symptoms have been major problems with the newer, long-acting drugs terazosin and doxazosin. Nevertheless, the 1988 update of the Joint National Committee report did not recommend this class of agent for initial monotherapy.

Other Agents
Several drugs listed in Table 26-1 are not suitable for monotherapy but work well in combinations.

RESERPINE. The oldest anti-hypertensive drug has fallen into academic neglect, although it was used in most of the trials on which our treatment rationale is based and there has never been a comparative trial in which reserpine was found inferior in potency or side effect profile. When cost is a factor, it offers a significant advantage: The combination of HCTZ, 25 mg, and reserpine, 0.1 mg, taken once daily can cost the patient as little as $20 a year. The diuretic is necessary because when used alone, reserpine leads to fluid retention and tachyphylaxis. Doses above 0.25 mg/day often cause lasting sedation, depression, increased gastric acidity, and nasal congestion; only the latter effect is common at the smallest doses. Because reserpine depletes catecholamines, its onset of action is delayed, and its effects prolonged; it should be discontinued prior to elective surgery, to permit the use of adrenergic agents as needed for blood pressure control. Reserpine should be avoided, along with most other sympatholytics, in patients with a history of clinical depression.

METHYLDOPA AND CLONIDINE. These centrally acting sympatholytics block rather than deplete catecholamines, and their effects disappear more quickly than those due to reserpine. They offer no other clear advantage to offset their much higher price. When used alone, both methyldopa and clonidine can cause fluid retention, and both cause sedation and depression in susceptible persons. Methyldopa can cause a chemical hepatitis and should be avoided in patients with potential hepatic comorbidity (e.g., alcoholics). Clonidine is an option for severe hypertension (including "urgent" and malignant hypertension), but when used in high doses for severe hypertension, there is a potential for dangerous rebound effects if clonidine is abruptly stopped. Some nephrologists prefer clonidine to beta-blockers as the step-2 sympatholytic in regimens requiring minoxidil.

HYDRALAZINE AND MINOXIDIL. These direct vasodilators are traditionally used as a third drug, along with a diuretic and sympatholytic. Used alone either one provokes fluid retention and a reflex tachycardia that can cause angina. In elderly patients with blunted baroreceptor response, however, hydralazine used with only a diuretic can lower blood pressure and improve cardiac output by unloading the left ventricle.

Hydralazine was used in the original trials of treating hypertension, and is the least expensive vasodilator on the market. At doses of over 200 mg/day, hydralazine will induce lupus, reversible on discontinuation, in 20% of patients. Headache and digestive intolerance are also common.

Minoxidil is an extremely potent antihypertensive, usually reserved for the resistant hypertension associated with renal failure where it is added to furosemide and a strong sympatholytic. Hirsutism, fluid retention despite diuretics, and pericardial effusions can occur. Numerous case reports describe excessive hypotension with minoxidil, provoking symptoms of cerebral and retinal ischemia.

Strategy for Drug Selection and Initial Resistance

Considerations in selecting or avoiding the alternative monotherapies are summarized in Table 26-2. When the first drug at full dose does not achieve the goal blood pressure, another can be substituted or added to the first. As noted, all nondiuretic drugs are enhanced by the addition of small doses of HCTZ (12.5–25.0 mg/day). Finding a well-tolerated first drug should achieve treatment goals in about 50% of patients and adding a diuretic should normalize blood pressure in another 20–30%.

Failure of the regimen is an occasion to review the diagnosis, goals, diet, and compliance before concluding that additional medication is indicated. Resistance to simple drug therapy increases (slightly) the likelihood of a surgically curable cause of hypertension, and increases greatly the value of finding it if it is there. Artifacts of measurement may occur, especially in elderly patients whose rigidly calcified vessels are not occluded by external cuff pressure. Extreme caution is required when signs of iatrogenic hypoperfusion supervene despite a stable elevated blood pressure. Another common perplexity is "white coat hypertension," wherein the blood pressure is persistently raised by the stress of a visit to the physician. Resistant hypertension may be an indication for home or ambulatory recordings. Home blood pressure measurements with a manual sphygmomanometer encourage patient participation in treatment as well as provide data.

The usual treatment goal is 140/90 mm Hg, but this should be modified at times when resistance occurs. Elderly patients with predominant or isolated systolic hypertension usually respond well to cautious implementation of standard regimens, but occasionally full control of systolic blood pressure cannot be achieved without an unacceptable fall in DBP. Since coronary perfusion occurs largely during diastole, angina or worse can develop. Similarly, proceeding too fast or pushing to full normalization of blood pressure can, in some persons, lead to cerebral hypoperfusion, especially on an orthostatic basis. At times, changing to drugs with less sympatholytic effect can preserve positional adjustments, but other patients will have to settle for partial control of blood pressure. There is some evidence that partial control confers most of the benefit of full control.

A major cause of resistance to antihypertensive drugs is inadequate control of plasma volume, either initially or after reflex fluid retention occurs on therapy. Failure of initial monotherapy is an indication to press for mild sodium restriction or to add a diuretic. For patients already taking HCTZ, serum creatinine concentration and cardiac function should be reviewed to determine a need to change to furosemide (see above).

The single largest cause of treatment failure at any step is noncompliance. Clues are missed appointments, failure to bring in medications, inability to recount dosage schedules, complaints about cost or side effects (or denial of any side effects), and no fall in blood pressure. Corrective steps include patient education about the rationale for hypertension control, eliciting patient attitudes toward treatment, coping with concerns about the financial costs and convenience of drugs and visits, and finding medications with acceptable side effects. It is clearly futile to add a third drug if the first two are not being taken; worse, it is dangerous, because the patient may suddenly comply fully and become hypotensive.

Resistant Hypertension

About 20 to 30% of hypertensive patients will not achieve reasonable blood pressure goals on the regimens defined above and will require combination therapy. All of the monotherapies can be used in combination with the exception of beta-blockers and converting enzyme inhibitors, which are not additive. It is probably most reasonable to choose agents from fundamentally different classes (see Table 26-1), and it is pointless to combine two drugs from the same subgroup (e.g., two beta-blockers or calcium channel blockers). Thus, a combination of a diuretic, a sympatholytic, and a direct vasodilator should have additive

Table 26-4. Selective stepped-care for hypertension

Patient group	Initial choice	Substitute or add	Add	Avoid*
Anyone, those with cost concerns	HCTZ	Reserpine	Hydralazine	—
Elderly	HCTZ	Vasodilator		Sympatholytic Beta-blocker
Young and white	Beta-blocker or ACEI	HCTZ	Vasodilator	—
Black	HCTZ	CCB	—	—
Coronary disease	Beta-blocker	CCB	HCTZ	Minoxidil
Heart failure	Furosemide	ACEI		Beta-blocker Verapamil Minoxidil
Renal failure	Furosemide	Clonidine or prazosin	Minoxidil	Potassium-sparing diuretics
Diabetics	ACEI	HCTZ	—	Beta-blocker

*Relative or absolute contraindications, ineffective, or problematic (see text).
ACEI = angiotensin-converting enzyme inhibitors; CCB = calcium channel blockers; HCTZ = hydrochlorothiazide.

potency while counteracting some of the mechanisms of resistance (reflex fluid retention and tachycardia).

In general, the same special advantages and precautions of single agents carry over into their use in combinations, with a few exceptions. Some of the demographic distinctions drop away when diuretics are added to other first-line drugs, with race and age becoming less important. Sometimes opposite side effects can be neutralized by combinations (e.g., hyperkalemia with ACEIs and hypokalemia with diuretics, increased heart rate with vasodilators and decreased with sympatholytics). Conversely, additive toxicity, such as cardiodepression and conduction block of both beta-blockers and verapamil, or the additive hyperkalemia of potassium-sparing diuretics and ACEIs or beta-blockers, must be avoided.

Table 26-4 suggests step-up regimens for the major demographic and clinical situations.

General Concerns

Compliance with hypertension therapy is improved by once- or twice-daily dosing; every effort should be made to avoid a third or midday dose for this asymptomatic disorder. Most of the drugs described above can be dosed daily when hypertension is the only target of therapy: the blood pressure usually rebounds slowly even after the drug is long gone. Exceptions requiring twice-daily dosing are clonidine, hydralazine, calcium channel blockers (unless in sustained-release forms), and captopril.

Combination tablets may cut cost and improve compliance. These should be considered whenever the relative dosage is close to that of the separate ingredients.

Although it is usually assumed that antihypertensive therapy is permanent, an increasing amount of literature suggests that about 20 to 30% of patients can be titrated down and even taken off medication after months or years of therapy. Many of these patients were doubtlessly diagnosed too quickly and never had sustained hypertension, and many others may have made life-style or dietary changes in the interim that controlled their blood pressure. Some patients on therapy, however, may have corrected the pathophysiology that caused their hypertension. Most stable, well-controlled patients deserve a trial of "step-down" therapy, but it is critical to avoid overselling the hope of cure and losing touch with the majority of patients who will require permanent medication.

Larson A, Strong C. Initial assessment of the patient with hypertension. Mayo Clin Proc 1989; 64:1533–42.
Clear, current overview with table of official recommendations.

Hla K, Feussner J. Screening for pseudohypertension. Arch Intern Med 1988; 148:673–6.

Zachariah P, Sheps S, Smith R. Clinical use of home and ambulatory blood pressure monitoring. Mayo Clin Proc 1989; 64:1436–46.

Mejia A, et al. Artifacts in measurement of blood pressure and lack of target organ involvement in the assessment of patients with treatment-resistant hypertension. Ann Intern Med 1990; 112:270–7.
Three approaches to the technical problems of blood pressure determination. Problems addressed include lability, noncompressible brachial artery, "white coat hypertension," and measurement artifacts causing "resistance" to therapy.

The National Blood Pressure Education Program Coordinating Committee. National High Blood Pressure Education Program working group report on ambulatory blood pressure monitoring. Arch Intern Med 1990; 150:2270–80.
Reviews the literature on ambulatory blood pressure monitoring's techniques, costs and clinical utility.

Tucker R, LaBarthe D. Frequency of surgical treatment for hypertension in adults at the Mayo Clinic from 1973 through 1975. Mayo Clin Proc 1977; 52:549–55.

Lewin A, et al. Apparent prevalence of curable hypertension in the Hypertension Detection and Follow-up Program. Arch Intern Med 1985; 145:424–7.
Two studies suggesting that surgically-curable hypertension is very rare (probably < 1% of "routine" hypertensives).

MacMahon S. Alcohol and hypertension: implications for prevention and treatment. Ann Intern Med 1986; 105:124–6.
Editorial summary of epidemiologic data linking heavy drinking with hypertension.

England W, et al. Cost effectiveness in the detection of renal artery stenosis. J Gen Intern Med 1988; 3:344–50.

Frederickson E, et al. A prospective evaluation of a simplified captopril test for the detection of renovascular hypertension. Arch Intern Med 1990; 150:569–72.

Postma C, et al. The captopril test in the detection of renovascular disease in hypertensive patients. Arch Intern Med 1990; 150:625–28.

McCarthy J, Weder A. The captopril test and renovascular hypertension: a cautionary tale. Arch Intern Med 1990; 150:493–95. (editorial)
Four articles on the elusive diagnosis of renovascular hypertension. The last three update the promising screening tool called the captopril test and discover that it is not perfect.

Young W, et al. Primary aldosteronism: diagnosis and treatment. Mayo Clin Proc 1990; 65:96–110.

Benowitz N, et al. Pheochromocytoma—recent advances in diagnosis and treatment. West J Med 1988; 148:561–67.
Two rare endocrine tumors that can cause hypertension—rarely.

The 1988 report of the Joint National Committee on Detection, Evaluation, and Treatment of High Blood Pressure. Arch Intern Med 1988; 148:1023–38.
This is the fourth periodic update of the National Institutes of Health committee that reviews the state of this art and recommends reasonable practice standards for hypertension.

Schwartz G. Initial therapy for hypertension—individualizing care. Mayo Clin Proc 1990; 65:73–87.

Gifford R. Mild hypertension: critical analysis of different therapeutic approaches. Cleve Clin J Med 1989; 56:337–45.
Two excellent summaries of the principles and details of initial drug therapy.

Moser M. Relative efficacy of, and some adverse reactions to, different antihypertensive regimens. Am J Cardiol 1989; 63:2B–7B.

Freis E. Critique of the clinical importance of diuretic-induced hypokalemia and elevated cholesterol level. Arch Intern Med 1989; 149:2640–2648.

Kaplan N. How bad are diuretic-induced hypokalemia and hypercholesterolemia? Arch Intern Med 1989; 149:2649.

Three views of the current controversies regarding the traditional diuretic-based stepped-care approach to hypertension.

Wallin JD, Shah SV. β-Adrenergic blocking agents in the treatment of hypertension. Arch Intern Med 1987; 147:654–9.

Williams G. Converting-enzyme inhibitors in the treatment of hypertension. N Engl J Med 1988; 319:1517–25.

Kaplan N. Calcium entry blockers in the treatment of hypertension. JAMA 1989; 262:817–23.

Khoury A, Kaplan N. Alpha-blocker therapy of hypertension: an unfulfilled promise. JAMA 1991; 266:394–8.

State-of-the-art reviews of the major classes of antihypertensive drugs.

Edelson JT, et al. Long-term cost-effectiveness of various initial monotherapies for mild to moderate hypertension. JAMA 1990; 263:407–13.

Moser M. Cost containment in the management of hypertension. Ann Intern Med 1987; 107:107–8; Ann Intern Med 1988; 108:777.

Two thoughtful discussions presenting the cost advantages of thiazides and propranolol over the newer drugs.

27. ANGINA PECTORIS
Mark A. Hlatky and Daniel B. Mark

Angina is the cardinal symptom of myocardial ischemia, which results from a mismatch between the supply and demand of myocardial oxygen. The correspondence between the symptom (angina pectoris) and the pathophysiologic state (myocardial ischemia) is far from perfect. Myocardial ischemia commonly occurs in the absence of symptoms (so-called silent ischemia), and typical angina pectoris may occur in the absence of detectable myocardial ischemia. In North America and Europe, myocardial ischemia due to coronary atherosclerosis is by far the most common underlying cause of angina pectoris. Other less frequent causes include various forms of valvular disease (particularly aortic stenosis), cardiomyopathies (particularly hypertrophic forms), and congenital heart disease. This chapter focuses on the patient with suspected or documented atherosclerotic coronary artery disease (CAD).

Pathophysiology

Myocardial ischemia results from a mismatch between myocardial oxygen demand and supply. This most often occurs when a primary increase in myocardial oxygen demand outstrips the supply capacity of a coronary artery narrowed by atherosclerosis. The increased demand is usually due to physical exertion, and the mismatch between supply and demand is quickly alleviated once exercise ceases. Myocardial ischemia and angina may also result from a primary decrease in myocardial blood flow, which is most often due to platelet aggregation or coronary vasoconstriction at the site of an atherosclerotic coronary artery plaque. When atherosclerosis is present, decreased oxygen-carrying capacity of the blood due to anemia or hypoxemia may also cause angina.

Myocardial ischemia may or may not produce angina, or other "angina-equivalent" symptoms. The reasons why some episodes of ischemia do not lead to symptoms remain unresolved, and "silent myocardial ischemia" is currently a focus of clinical investigation.

Clinical Evaluation

History
The clinical history contains over 90% of the information needed to estimate the likelihood that the patient's symptoms are due to coronary disease. The clinician should first listen to the patient's own description of the problem, and then pursue an active line of questioning, first with general questions such as "What makes the discomfort better?" and then with specific questions such as "What happens to the discomfort when you take a deep breath?" A common error is to ask only about "pain," since many patients with myocardial ischemia will insist they do not have "pain," only "discomfort" or "pressure." It is also important to avoid leading questions and to take enough time to obtain a complete description of symptoms.

Angina pectoris is classified according to its character, clinical course, and severity. The character of symptoms contains the most information about the likelihood of underlying CAD. *Typical angina pectoris* refers to a visceral discomfort usually located in the middle region of the chest, but also in the neck, jaw, shoulder, or arm, predictably precipitated by increased cardiac work (i.e., increased heart rate or blood pressure or both) and relieved within 5 to 10 minutes after the precipitating factor is removed or nitroglycerin is taken. Chest discomfort that lacks one or more of these features is considered *atypical angina pectoris*. The term *nonanginal chest pain* should be reserved for symptoms for which a noncardiac origin for the discomfort can be determined on clinical grounds alone (i.e., costochondritis, esophageal reflux).

The clinical course and severity of angina symptoms are the key factors in assessing prognosis and choosing therapy. *Stable angina* refers to a symptom pattern that has remained relatively constant in frequency, duration, and precipitating factors for 6 weeks or more. *Unstable angina* covers a wide spectrum of clinical syndromes, defined by a changing pattern of angina. The onset of either symptoms at rest, or prolonged pain that does not respond to nitroglycerin, or both, is a worrisome pattern associated with an increased short-term risk of myocardial infarction or sudden death. Recent onset of rest or prolonged angina merits prompt evaluation and treatment, and usually requires hospital admission. Because symptoms may be few in patients who have reduced their level of activity, the severity of angina should be assessed in light of the patient's current level of physical exertion. It is helpful to inquire whether common activities of daily living (e.g., walking a block or up a flight of stairs) cause angina.

Cardiac Physical Examination
Coronary atherosclerosis by itself (and most episodes of myocardial ischemia) produce no abnormal physical findings. Prior myocardial infarction or myocardial ischemia occurring at the time of the examination may cause mitral regurgitation, an S_3 gallop, or a palpable dyskinetic segment of myocardium. However, the physical examination in patients with chest discomfort is aimed primarily at detecting causes of symptoms other than coronary atherosclerosis. A variety of other cardiac conditions, including aortic stenosis and hypertrophic cardiomyopathy, are associated with typical angina and should be excluded because a very different approach to therapy is required. Some noncardiac causes of chest pain my also be detected by physical examination; for example, discomfort reproduced by palpation of the costochondral junctions may confirm a musculoskeletal etiology.

Probability Analysis
The clinical diagnosis of CAD is based on an assessment of probability, which varies with the patient's type of symptoms, age, gender, and coronary risk factor profile (Table 27-1). In general, the likelihood that chest discomfort is due to coronary disease is higher in older patients, and at any age the probability is higher in men than in women. More typical symptoms are also associated with a higher likelihood of CAD.

The precise probability level that is sufficient to establish the diagnosis of CAD on clinical grounds can be debated, but an 85 to 90% probability should be sufficient to initiate medical therapy on clinical grounds alone. Patients in the "gray zone" of 15 to 85% probability of disease should undergo further diagnostic testing. The need for further testing in patients with "low probability" of coronary disease (< 15%) should be based on

Table 27-1. Probability of coronary disease according to symptoms, gender, age, and risk factors

Age (yr)	No. of risk factors*			
	0	1	2	3
Typical angina				
Males				
35	29	52	73	87
45	56	73	85	92
55	80	87	91	94
65	92	93	94	96
75	97	97	97	97
Females				
35	9	25	50	76
45	19	37	59	79
55	35	52	68	81
65	55	67	76	84
75	74	77	82	86
Atypical angina				
Males				
35	3	7	17	35
45	9	16	29	46
55	23	33	46	58
65	48	55	62	69
75	74	75	76	78
Females				
35	<1	2	7	19
45	1	4	10	22
55	4	7	14	25
65	8	13	20	28
75	17	22	27	32

*Hyperlipidemia, smoking, diabetes.

factors such as the patient's occupation and level of concern, and the exact symptom profile. The probability of disease that is "too low" to merit further testing is again a matter of judgment and debate, but probabilities of less than 5% rarely require further evaluation.

Laboratory Testing

Goals

Laboratory testing in the patient with symptoms suspected to represent CAD has two aspects: diagnostic and prognostic. Diagnostic assessment attempts to answer the question "What is the likelihood that this patient's symptoms are due to atherosclerotic coronary artery disease?" Prognostic assessment, on the other hand, addresses the question "What is the likelihood that this patient will soon die or have a myocardial infarction?" Laboratory tests may be helpful for assessing either diagnosis or prognosis, or both.

Resting ECG

Every patient undergoing evaluation for angina pectoris should have a resting 12-lead ECG. Evidence of prior myocardial infarction establishes the diagnosis of CAD disease with high probability (90–95%) and also implies a worse prognosis. ST-segment depression or T-wave inversions on a resting ECG are suggestive of, but not specific for, the diagnosis of CAD; these findings are associated with a worse prognosis among patients with established CAD. The resting ECG also influences the choice of further diagnostic tests, since abnormalities of either conduction or the ST segments may make an exercise ECG uninterpretable.

Exercise Testing
The two major indications for a treadmill exercise ECG in patients with chest discomfort are (1) to provide further diagnostic information in patients with an intermediate or low probability ($< 85\%$) of coronary disease after clinical assessment, and (2) to help assess prognosis. The ST-segment response on the exercise ECG is not interpretable in the presence of left ventricular hypertrophy, left bundle branch block, or intraventricular conduction abnormalities. In addition to the amount of ST-segment shift, factors such as the exercise duration and stage, heart rate, symptoms, and blood pressure response must be considered for proper interpretation.

ST-segment depression on the exercise ECG has an average sensitivity of about 70% and an average specificity of about 85% for the diagnosis of CAD. The sensitivity of the test is higher in patients with typical symptoms and more extensive CAD; the specificity of the test is decreased at higher heart rates. Using probability analysis (e.g., Bayes' rule), exercise test data can be combined with the pretest likelihood of disease, to refine the diagnostic assessment.

An estimate of the prognostic risk can also be assessed based on exercise treadmill test findings using this exercise duration, the presence of symptoms, and the degree of ST-segment depression on the ECG. The combination of exercise-limiting angina, inability to reach stage III of the Bruce protocol, and ST-segment depression of 1 mm or greater has a very poor prognosis. Patients with adverse prognostic findings should be considered for early coronary angiography with an eye toward coronary revascularization. Patients with stable symptoms who are able to exercise into stage III or IV of the Bruce protocol without angina and with ST-segment depression of 1 mm or less generally have a good prognosis. The decision for coronary angiography or further testing in such patients should be based on the need to establish the diagnosis definitively, since the mortality rate within 2 years is low ($\leq 1\%$).

Radionuclide Studies
Thallium scintigraphy (myocardial perfusion scan) is an adjunctive test used to assess patients with suspected CAD. In this test, the patient exercises on a standard treadmill and a dose of radioactive thallium 201 is injected at peak exercise. Thallium 201 distributes through the myocardium in proportion to the coronary blood flow. Imaging using a gamma camera is done immediately after exercise (immediate images) and is repeated several hours later (delayed images). Areas of myocardium that are relatively underperfused (i.e., ischemic) take up less thallium on the immediate images, but appear normal on delayed images. In patients unable to perform an exercise test (e.g., due to intermittent claudication) thallium testing can be done using orally or intravenously administered dipyridamole (a coronary vasodilator). The sensitivity of the thallium scintigram for the diagnosis of coronary disease is higher than that of the exercise ECG at similar levels of specificity, but it is more expensive and less available than conventional treadmill testing.

Another adjunctive diagnostic procedure is to measure left ventricular function at rest and during exercise using radionuclide ventriculography. In the presence of significant myocardial ischemia, the normal rise in exercise ejection fraction is blunted, and may be reduced relative to the baseline value.

Both radionuclide studies provide information about diagnosis and prognosis. The likelihood of coronary disease is increased by a positive test result; the prognosis is closely related to the number and severity of ischemic zones on thallium scan and to the exercise ejection fraction during radionuclide ventriculography.

Neither thallium scintigraphy nor radionuclide ventriculography are first-line tests for evaluating patients with chest pain (with the exception of patients in whom an exercise ECG would be uninterpretable). Either test can be helpful in (1) following up an inconclusive exercise ECG when it would be desirable to avoid coronary angiography, or (2) providing additional prognostic information to assist in decisions concerning coronary revascularization. The choice between these two tests should be based primarily on availability and local expertise with these techniques, rather than on theoretic considerations of the relative value of assessing myocardial perfusion versus left ventricular function.

Angiography

The definitive test for the diagnosis of anatomic CAD remains the coronary angiogram. This test can be performed quite safely in the hands of experienced operators (i.e., an overall procedural complication rate of $\leq 1\%$, with a mortality rate of $< 0.1\%$). The location and severity of coronary atherosclerotic lesions can be accurately assessed only by a coronary angiogram. The physiologic significance, however, of anatomic lesions often must be assessed using a functional study, such as the exercise test. The coronary angiogram also provides a "road map" for coronary revascularization therapy.

Diagnostic Strategy

The optimal cost-effective strategy for the evaluation of chest discomfort has not been established. The following principles represent one approach to diagnosis.

In a patient with *stable* symptoms, the probability of disease should be estimated first on clinical grounds (see Table 27-1). In patients with a clinically established diagnosis of CAD, the goal is to choose the best therapy. If symptoms are mild (e.g., New York Heart Association class I or II), an exercise test can be used to stratify the patient into a category of high or low risk for myocardial infarction or death. Low-risk patients with mild symptoms need only medical therapy, while high-risk patients merit further evaluation by coronary angiography. In patients with severe (i.e., New York Heart Association class III or IV) but stable angina, coronary angiography may be ordered without prior exercise testing if coronary revascularization will be needed to improve the patient's quality of life.

We use the term *progressive angina* to refer to a patient whose angina is precipitated by progressively lesser amounts of exertion, but in whom the angina continues to be relieved promptly by rest or nitroglycerin. Patients whose angina is becoming progressively more severe, but who are without angina at rest or prolonged episodes of pain have a prognosis similar to patients with stable angina and can generally be evaluated as outpatients using the same approach outlined in the previous paragraph. Progressive angina warrants an intensive effort at medical therapy, and coronary revascularization should be strongly considered for patients whose symptoms do not respond adequately.

Patients with *new-onset angina* need a careful history to evaluate risk. Patients with new-onset angina that is always relieved within 5 to 10 minutes and that is precipitated only by exercise at a predictable level have a risk similar to that in patients with chronic stable angina. Many patients with new-onset angina have some elements of rest pain, prolonged pain, or a variable threshold, and a higher short-term risk of cardiac events. This latter group of patients should be considered to have unstable angina.

Patients with *unstable* angina require careful evaluation. The occurrence of symptoms at rest or symptoms not responsive to nitroglycerin generally requires hospital admission for stabilization of symptoms using intensive medical therapy (i.e., bed rest, aspirin, intravenous heparin and nitroglycerin, and a beta-blocker or calcium channel blocker or both). Most cardiologists now recommend that cardiac catheterization be performed in patients with unstable angina unless there are relative contraindications to coronary angiography (e.g., renal insufficiency) or there are reasons to avoid coronary revascularization (e.g., coexisting illness, patient's preference).

Treatment

Therapeutic Principles

All patients with known or suspected coronary atherosclerosis should receive optimal medical therapy, the foundation of which is risk factor modification aimed at stopping smoking, lowering cholesterol levels, treating diabetes and hypertension, and achieving ideal body weight. Risk factor modification should also be continued after coronary revascularization, to prevent disease progression.

Drug Therapy

Four major classes of drugs are used in the treatment of patients with CAD: nitrates, beta-blockers, calcium channel blockers, and antiplatelet agents.

Nitrates reduce myocardial oxygen requirements through their venous and, to a lesser extent, arterial dilatory properties, as well as by a direct coronary vasodilator effect.

Sublingual nitroglycerin (0.4 mg) remains the mainstay of therapy for an acute attack of angina; the patient should sit down and take 1 tablet every 5 minutes until the pain is relieved, or intolerable side effects develop. The patient should be told to seek medical attention if discomfort persists despite treatment with 3 to 4 nitroglycerin tablets over 20 minutes. Nitroglycerin tablets degrade when they are exposed to strong light or to heat, so fresh tablets should be purchased every few months, kept in a dark or opaque container, and extra tablets stored in the refrigerator. Long-acting nitrate preparations (including oral nitroglycerin capsules, transcutaneous nitroglycerin patches or paste, or oral isosorbide dinitrate) are effective in the prophylaxis of angina. Nitroglycerin patches are easier to use than paste, but more expensive. Most patients find oral preparations (e.g., isosorbide dinitrate, 10–40 mg po tid–qid) a more convenient form of long-acting nitrate. Emerging evidence suggests that tolerance to the effect of nitrates may develop with continuous therapy, but this may be prevented by having a nitrate-free period at night.

Beta-blocking drugs act to reduce myocardial oxygen demand by lowering the resting heart rate and blood pressure and blunting their rise during exercise. In addition to their beneficial effects on angina, beta-blockers have been shown to prolong survival after acute myocardial infarction. A wide variety of beta-blocking agents are available, with roughly equal efficacy for the treatment of angina. (See Table 26-3, Chap. 26.) The choice of a beta-blocker should be individualized based on the side effect profile and dosing interval. Cardioselective agents (e.g., metoprolol, 50–100 mg PO bid; atenolol, 50–100 mg PO qd) may be preferable, particularly in smokers, to avoid bronchospasm. Water-soluble agents (e.g., atenolol, 50–100 mg PO qd; nadolol, 40–160 mg PO qd) appear to have fewer central nervous system effects. All beta-blockers may depress left ventricular function and should be used cautiously, if at all, in patients with congestive heart failure.

Calcium channel blockers (e.g. nifedipine, diltiazem, verapamil) are effective antianginal agents, through both their direct coronary vasodilator effects and their peripheral vasodilator properties that reduce myocardial oxygen demand. Verapamil and diltiazem also reduce heart rate, reducing oxygen demand further. Nifedipine (10–30 mg po tid–qid) may cause undesirable increases in heart rate in some patients, which can be counteracted by adding a beta-blocker. Verapamil (80–120 mg po tid–qid) and, to a lesser extent, diltiazem (30–60 mg po tid–qid) may depress heart rate, cardiac conduction, or left ventricular function sufficiently to cause symptoms in some patients, particularly when used in combination with beta-blockers; nifedipine does not affect conduction and the slight myocardial depression is generally outweighed by its vasodilator properties, making it a useful agent in patients with bradycardia or left ventricular dysfunction.

Platelet active agents, particularly aspirin, have no demonstrated effect on exertional angina pectoris, but have been proved to be effective in the treatment of unstable angina and in the prevention of death after myocardial infarction.

A *stepped-care approach to drug therapy* is useful in patients with stable angina. All patients should receive sublingual nitroglycerin to treat acute attacks of angina. Most patients will also need medication to prevent anginal attacks, with either beta-blockers or long-acting nitrates used as first-line therapy. In patients without heart failure, beta-blockers are preferable, since they are the only class of medication that clearly both relieves angina and has been shown to improve survival in patients with coronary disease. The dose should be titrated according to symptoms and resting heart rate (goal, 50–60 beats/min). Long-acting nitrates can be used as initial therapy or added to a beta-blocker to improve control of symptoms. Calcium blockers are useful if symptoms cannot be controlled with beta-blockers and long-acting nitrates. The goal of medical therapy is to eliminate or significantly reduce symptomatic episodes of myocardial ischemia. While some clinicians have advocated testing to detect silent ischemia in patients whose symptoms have been controlled with medical therapy, the value of detecting and treating these episodes is currently unproved. An exercise test on therapy may be a useful adjunct to judge efficacy of therapy objectively, but it remains to be shown that routine follow-up exercise testing adds significant information to a good clinical history.

Coronary Revascularization
Two major forms of coronary revascularization are currently available, namely, coronary artery bypass graft surgery (CABG) and percutaneous transluminal coronary angioplasty (PTCA). Coronary revascularization is a rational approach to myocardial ischemia caused

Table 27-2. Medical and surgical survival probability (%) at 5 years according to left ventricular ejection fraction and no. of diseased vessels*

No. (or type) of diseased vessels	Medical	Surgical
60% Ejection fraction		
1	97	99
2	95	98
3	91	97
Left main	85	97
40% Ejection fraction		
1	94	97
2	91	96
3	87	94
Left main	77	94

*Assumes that the patient is a 53-year-old man with a 24-mo history of typical, stable angina occurring six times a week. He has a history of smoking and hypertension, but no prior myocardial infarction. The resting ECG is normal.

by obstructive atherosclerotic disease, but carries an immediate procedural risk, as well as increased costs. Selection of patients for coronary revascularization should be based on (1) the need to control symptoms, and (2) the likely effect on prolonging survival.

In all major randomized studies, coronary revascularization has been shown to be effective in controlling angina pectoris. Patients who have severe symptoms, particularly those whose symptoms cannot be adequately relieved on medical therapy, are clearly appropriate candidates for coronary revascularization. The precise form of revascularization should depend on the technical suitability of the coronary anatomy for either CABG or PTCA. In general, patients with single-vessel disease usually undergo PTCA, while patients with severe three-vessel disease or left main coronary disease usually receive CABG. Patients undergoing PTCA should be candidates for CABG in the event of abrupt vessel closure, which occurs in 3 to 5% of such patients. It is important to be familiar with the results of coronary revascularization as performed locally, since results may differ considerably among centers. There is evidence that centers with higher volumes and greater experience achieve better results.

While it is widely agreed that coronary revascularization should be used to relieve angina that does not respond adequately to medical therapy, use of revascularization primarily to increase patient survival time remains controversial. Both randomized and observational studies have shown that patients with the worst prognosis on medical therapy (i.e., those with left main coronary disease) live significantly longer after coronary revascularization. The higher the risk of death or myocardial infarction on medical therapy, the greater the consideration should be for coronary revascularization. The overall prognosis of the medically treated patient with CAD is a function of the left ventricular function, the anatomic severity of the disease, and the stability and severity of anginal symptoms. Five-year survival estimates for sample patients undergoing medical and surgical therapy are summarized in Table 27-2. Risk assessment should be performed first using readily accessible clinical information, then with noninvasive tests, and finally with angiography. The approach to a patient must be individualized based on the patient's risk and symptom profile and frank discussions with the patient concerning his or her personal preferences.

Constant J. The clinical diagnosis of nonanginal chest pain: the differentiation of angina from nonanginal chest pain by history. Clin Cardiol 1983; 6:11–6.
An excellent discussion of the nuances of history-taking.

Diamond GA, Forrester JS. Analysis of probability as an aid in the clinical diagnosis of coronary-artery disease. N Engl J Med 1979; 300:1350–8.
Outlines the approach to probability assessment of patients with chest pain.

Pryor DB, et al. Estimating the likelihood of significant coronary artery disease. Am J Med 1983; 75:771–80.
Another method of probability assessment for individual patients.

Silverman KJ, Grossman W. Angina pectoris: natural history and strategies for evaluation and management. N Engl J Med 1984; 310:1712–7.
Outlines an integrated approach to diagnosis and treatment.

Mark DB, et al. Prognostic value of a treadmill exercise score in outpatients with suspected coronary artery disease. N Engl J Med 1991; 325:849–53.
Provides a method for estimating prognosis from symptoms, exercise duration, and ST-segment changes on a treadmill test.

Shub C. Stable angina pectoris: 3. Medical treatment. Mayo Clin Proc 1990; 65:256–73.
Up-to-date overview of medical therapy.

Califf RM, et al. The evolution of medical and surgical therapy for coronary artery disease. A 15-year perspective. JAMA 1989; 261:2077–86.
An integrated approach to the survival benefits of bypass surgery.

The Veterans Administration Coronary Artery Bypass Surgery Cooperative Study Group. Eleven-year survival in the Veterans Administration randomized trial of coronary bypass surgery for stable angina. N Engl J Med 1984; 311:1333–9.
Recent report of randomized trial showing initial survival benefits in high-risk patients, but a decline in benefit after 7 to 10 years.

Alderman EL, et al. Ten-year follow-up of survival and myocardial infarction in the randomized Coronary Artery Surgery Study. Circulation 1990; 82:1629–46.

Rogers WJ, et al. Ten-year follow-up of quality of life in patients randomized to receive medical therapy or coronary artery bypass graft surgery. The Coronary Artery Surgery Study (CASS). Circulation 1990; 82:1647–58.
Latest reports of the last major randomized trial of medical and surgical therapy.

Holmes DR, Jr, Vlietstra RE. Balloon angioplasty in acute and chronic coronary artery disease. JAMA 1989; 261:2109–15.
An overview of the newest form of coronary revascularization.

28. CONGESTIVE HEART FAILURE
Laurence O. Watkins

Congestive heart failure (CHF) is a clinical syndrome that occurs as a consequence of myocardial muscle dysfunction and results in edema, fatigue, and dyspnea especially after exertion. Ischemic heart disease is the cause in 60 to 70% of patients, often but not always after recurrent myocardial infarctions. Prominent nonischemic causes include hypertension, alcohol, and valvular heart disease. The prevalence of idiopathic cardiomyopathy varies but approaches 20 to 25% in some series.

Pathophysiology
The hemodynamic characteristics of CHF are decreased cardiac output and elevated ventricular filling pressure. Low cardiac output is the basis for patients' complaints of weakness, lethargy, and easy fatigability. If left ventricular filling pressure cannot be maintained at normal levels, the pulmonary capillary wedge pressure rises, which can result in interstitial and alveolar edema and decreased pulmonary compliance. These are the basis for exertional dyspnea, orthopnea, and paroxysmal nocturnal dyspnea (PND). If the filling pressure of the right ventricle is high, the resulting elevation of central venous pressure is associated with hepatic congestion, pedal edema, and in severe cases, ascites and anasarca. The congestive symptoms result from responses in both the venous and the arterial circulations to compensate for chronic reduction of cardiac output. Decreased renal

perfusion stimulates the renin-angiotensin-aldosterone system, which results in augmented sodium and fluid retention. This mechanism serves to maintain cardiac output by increasing ventricular preload. In the early stages of CHF, increases in systemic vascular resistance (afterload) serve to maintain an adequate tissue perfusion pressure in the face of decreased cardiac output. Later, further artericlar constriction acts to preserve regional flow to the heart and brain even at the expense of reduced flow to other organs, such as the kidneys, and at the cost of increased cardiac work.

In recent years, it has been recognized that diastolic dysfunction of the left ventricle may cause symptoms of CHF, especially in patients with hypertension (and associated left ventricular hypertrophy), but also in patients with coronary artery disease and hypertrophic cardiomyopathy. The left ventricular end-diastolic pressure (LVEDP) is elevated, though not because of volume overload; exertional dyspnea and orthopnea may result.

Diagnosis

CHF is frequently misdiagnosed. On the one hand, CHF may cause only subtle complaints so that the diagnosis is not considered. On the other hand, symptoms and signs of CHF are also caused by other common diseases (e.g., obstructive lung disease, obesity, and venous insufficiency) so that a diagnosis of CHF can be made in error.

Criteria

A variety of symptoms and signs characteristic of heart failure may be used to establish the diagnosis. One large study of heart disease, the Framingham Study, used major and minor criteria for CHF that reflect current clinical judgment. Major criteria were PND or orthopnea, neck vein distention, rales, cardiomegaly, acute pulmonary edema, S_3 gallop, increased venous pressure (> 16 cm H_2O), circulation time of 25 seconds or longer, and hepatojugular reflux. Minor criteria were ankle edema, night cough, dyspnea on exertion, hepatomegaly, pleural effusion, vital capacity decreased by one-third from maximum, and tachycardia (rate $\geq$ 120/min). Weight loss of 4.5 kg or more in 5 days in response to treatment was considered either a major or a minor criterion. The diagnosis of CHF required the presence of two major, or one major and 2 minor criteria.

In a study of clinical criteria for chronic CHF in patients with coronary artery disease referred for catheterization, CHF was associated with two clinical findings: cardiomegaly (cardiothoracic ratio > 0.48 on chest x-ray) and the presence of a third heart sound (S_3). This criterion for the cardiothoracic ratio was derived from a study of predominantly white patients, and may not apply for blacks of West African descent because they have relatively smaller thoracic diameters. Dyspnea on exertion was a sensitive indicator of CHF, and the specificity of this symptom was higher if either orthopnea or PND was present. Pulmonary rales, peripheral edema, tachycardia (heart rate > 100/min at rest), and neck vein distention were present only infrequently, since many patients who might have had these signs were already being treated for CHF. However, if present, these findings were highly specific for CHF. Similarly, radiographic findings of pulmonary venous cephalization, interstitial edema, and Kerley's B lines were infrequent; they were absent if heart size was normal. Cardiomegaly, an S_3, or clinical findings of CHF correctly identified 53% of patients with an LVEDP greater than 15 mm Hg and 73% of patients with an LVEDP greater than 12 mm Hg.

In a study of patients being followed with dilated cardiomyopathy, an episode of orthopnea during the week preceding the evaluation was reported by 91% of patients with pulmonary capillary wedge pressures greater than 22 mm Hg. Similarly, a pulse pressure–systolic pressure ratio of less than 25% was a specific (91%) marker for identifying patients with a moderately reduced cardiac index.

Strategy

To establish the diagnosis of CHF, the clinician should inquire about dyspnea, decreased exercise tolerance, and peripheral edema, either current or past. Unfortunately, the patient's complaints may not reflect accurately the degree of cardiac dysfunction. There is generally poor agreement between the New York Heart Association clinical classification of patients on the basis of exertional symptoms and objective assessment of exercise performance. Because pulmonary disease often underlies exertional dyspnea, a history of cigarette smoking, chronic sputum production, wheezing, or asthma should be sought. Attempts should also be made to determine the cause of cardiac dysfunction, by seeking a history of hypertension, exertional chest pain, palpitations, rheumatic fever, murmur, excessive alcohol intake, or onset of symptoms after a viral infection or pregnancy. Physical examination should be directed particularly toward determining whether there is congestion in the peripheral or pulmonary circulation, cardiomegaly, and abnormal heart sounds (S_3, S_4) or murmurs. The presence of the latter would suggest valvular disease, either congenital or acquired.

Investigation

If CHF is suspected, a chest x-ray should be obtained, both to obtain an accurate estimate of cardiac size and to determine whether there is pulmonary vascular congestion or evidence of intrinsic pulmonary disease. An electrocardiogram may indicate specific forms of disease. Occasionally, if the cause of CHF remains unclear or if diastolic dysfunction is suspected, echocardiography with Doppler evaluation may be warranted. It is the ideal method for detecting and assessing the severity of valvular disease and cardiomyopathy (dilated, hypertrophic, or restrictive). In some patients, echocardiography will allow detection of left ventricular hypertrophy, and if combined with pulsed Doppler evaluation, detection of isolated diastolic dysfunction. In the majority of such patients, radionuclide ventriculography will confirm normal ventricular ejection fraction and reduced rates of early diastolic filling. In some patients, the presence of chest pain or murmurs may suggest that a surgically correctable lesion is present. In these cases, referral for further, invasive evaluation should be considered.

Prognosis

The prognosis of patients with CHF is poor. In the Framingham Study, of the 142 patients who developed CHF, 62% of the men and 42% of the women died within 5 years, despite treatment with diuretics and digitalis. In a study of CHF associated with coronary artery disease, 40% of those with either cardiomegaly or an S_3 died within 36 months, regardless of whether medical or surgical therapy was applied.

Treatment Measures

Many different modalities are available for the treatment of CHF. The imbalance between cardiac output and peripheral tissue demands can be corrected either by decreasing tissue demand or by altering the factors that affect cardiac output, namely preload, afterload, and myocardial contractility. The choice of therapy should be guided by the underlying cardiac abnormality and the ensuing pathophysiologic adaptations. For example, patients with pulmonary and visceral congestion and peripheral edema require different therapy from patients whose major problem is low cardiac output. If CHF is new or recently worse, precipitating causes should be sought and treated first. While the underlying cause of CHF may be myocardial contractile failure, worsening may be due to uncontrolled hypertension; arrhythmias; pulmonary infection; worsening ischemia; side effects of antiarrhythmic or other drugs; excessive salt intake; poor medication compliance; anemia; or metabolic factors such as hypoxemia, hypercapnia, acidosis, hypokalemia, or hypocalcemia.

General Measures

ACTIVITY. The ambulatory patient who experiences symptoms on mild or marked exertion should be advised to avoid isometric exercise. In more severely compromised patients, periodic bed rest will allow increased renal (instead of muscular) perfusion and consequent diuresis, with relief of congestive symptoms.

SALT RESTRICTION. For patients whose symptoms result from peripheral or pulmonary congestion, ventricular preload should be reduced. Restriction of dietary sodium to 2 g per day opposes the tendency to renal salt and water conservation and reduces intravascular volume and ventricular filling pressures.

Drugs for Preload Reduction

DIURETICS. A diuretic should be added if symptoms do not resolve with salt restriction alone.

THIAZIDES. A daily dose of a thiazide diuretic such as hydrochlorothiazide (50–100 mg) promotes sodium and water excretion if renal function is normal.

LOOP DIURETICS. If CHF is moderate or severe, or if the serum creatinine concentration exceeds 2.5 mg/dl, a more potent, loop diuretic such as furosemide (usually 40–240 mg/day; maximal dose, 1000 mg bid) may be necessary. Bumetanide (usually 1–6 mg/day) and ethacrynic acid are as potent as furosemide; there is little to differentiate them, except that furosemide and bumetanide should be avoided in patients who are allergic to sulfonamides. The natriuretic effect, and hence the dosage, of the loop diuretics depend on renal plasma flow, which varies markedly among CHF patients. The duration of action of loop diuretics is 6 to 8 hours in normal individuals but is usually prolonged in patients with CHF. In some patients, a single daily dose reduces congestive symptoms, although in others twice- or thrice-daily administration is necessary.

COMBINED REGIMENS. In patients with refractory edema, 20 to 40 mg of furosemide will enhance the maximal diuresis obtained with thiazides, and addition of furosemide, rather than substitution, may be effective. Metolazone (5–10 mg qd) is effective in patients with marked renal insufficiency. The addition of metolazone often produces brisk diuresis in patients refractory to maximal recommended doses of furosemide. If this occurs, volume status and potassium levels should be observed closely.

POTASSIUM REPLACEMENT. It is doubtful whether total body potassium depletion, other than that attributable to increased age or decreased muscle mass, is a characteristic of CHF patients treated with diuretics. Hypokalemia (serum potassium ≤ 3.5 mEq/L) is rarely observed in CHF patients treated with 50 to 100 mg of hydrochlorothiazide, or 40 to 80 mg of furosemide per day. It may occur more commonly when higher doses of potent diuretics are used, but accurate estimates of incidence are not available. It is prudent to measure serum potassium before and 2 weeks after institution of diuretic therapy and to give supplementary potassium only if hypokalemia develops. Treatment of hypokalemia is especially important when digitalis glycosides are being used, because hypokalemia makes digitalis-associated arrhythmias more likely to occur. Addition of the potassium-sparing diuretic amiloride (5–10 mg/day) is more effective than potassium chloride supplements of 40 to 80 mEq/day. Triamterene (100 mg qd–100 mg qid) and spironolactone (25–100 mg qid) also spare potassium. These agents are contraindicated in patients taking converting enzyme inhibitors, which also promote potassium retention.

NITRATES. Long-acting nitrates diminish congestive symptoms by reducing preload. They decrease venous return by inducing pooling in venous capacitance vessels; they are unlikely to be effective in patients whose severe peripheral edema restricts venous distention. Isosorbide dinitrate (5–10 mg sublingually or 20–40 mg PO q4–6h) reduces preload, causes mild arteriolar relaxation, and usually reduces systemic blood pressure. Dosage should be titrated so that the systemic blood pressure difference between the supine and the upright position is less than 20 mm Hg.

In patients whose major symptoms reflect a low output state, the aim of therapy is to increase the cardiac output. This may be achieved by either increasing myocardial contractility or decreasing afterload.

Drugs to Improve Myocardial Contractility
Myocardial contractility can be improved by a number of oral inotropic agents. Digoxin is the most commonly used. It is particularly useful when atrial fibrillation is present and should be used to decrease the ventricular response to 60 to 90 per minute. The utility of chronic oral digoxin therapy for CHF has been questioned, particularly for patients in sinus rhythm with normal cardiac size. A number of studies have shown no deterioration in function or exacerbation of heart failure when digitalis is discontinued in this population. Studies on the efficacy of digitalis in patients with ventricular dilation accompanied by moderate-to-severe left ventricular dysfunction have yielded conflicting results. In a randomized, double-blind, crossover trial, 14 (56%) of 25 CHF patients with normal sinus rhythm obtained benefit from digoxin. These patients had more severe CHF, greater left ventricle size, and an S_3. Persistence of an S_3 after maximal diuretic therapy was an

excellent predictor of response to digoxin (sensitivity 100%, specificity 90%). In patients whose renal function is normal, the usual maintenance dose is 0.25 mg/day, and a loading dose is not necessary. If renal function is impaired (e.g., serum creatinine > 1.5 mg/dl), digoxin should be reduced to 0.125 mg/day or 0.25 mg every other day.

A double-blind, placebo-controlled study that compared the effects of digoxin and the angiotensin-converting enzyme (ACE) inhibitor captopril during maintenance diuretic therapy in patients with significant ventricular dysfunction and mild-to-moderate heart failure revealed no significant improvement in exercise capacity by either drug compared to placebo. However, use of either drug, compared to placebo, reduced the need for increased diuretic therapy, number of hospital admissions, and treatment failures.

Clinically important benefits of digoxin appear to be confined to a small proportion of patients with severe heart failure and the drug should be avoided in those with diastolic dysfunction. Thus, in patients with compensated heart failure, especially when an ACE inhibitor is employed, it may be prudent to discontinue digoxin and to restart it only if decompensation occurs. In contrast, digitalis may be started in patients with advanced heart disease who remain symptomatic despite treatment with ACE inhibitors and diuretics.

Drugs for Afterload Reduction

Vasodilators such as the hydralazine–isosorbide dinitrate combination and ACE inhibitors (e.g., captopril, enalapril, and lisinopril) have been shown to improve left ventricular function and reduce mortality in patients with CHF. These agents augment cardiac output by increasing stroke volume and may act to lower ventricular filling pressure as well. As a class they are especially effective in patients with normal or elevated systolic pressure and those with mitral regurgitation. On the basis of favorable results in large-scale clinical trials, ACE inhibitors have emerged as a major mode of treatment for patients with heart failure. Enalapril has been shown to be effective even in severe CHF.

Clinical trials of ACE inhibitors have identified factors that predispose to side effects, and established a safe dose titration scheme for the initiation of therapy, which permits the use of these drugs in over 90% of patients with CHF. Hypotension and renal insufficiency may occur in patients given ACE inhibitors who have a history of recent initiation or increase in diuretic dose, gastrointestinal disturbances or other diseases that would predispose to volume depletion, or a resting systolic blood pressure of less than 100 mm Hg. Withholding or reducing diuretics and beginning therapy with small doses of ACE inhibitors will minimize side effects. The usual test dose of ACE inhibitor is 2.5 mg of enalapril given twice daily or 6.25 mg of captopril given three times daily. In patients at risk of complications who are not acutely ill, tolerance should usually be assessed for 1 week before the dose of the drug is advanced. The dose is then titrated upward until side effects are observed or a target blood pressure is attained; a systolic blood pressure of 100 to 110 mm Hg is a reasonable goal. Although dose-response relationships are difficult to establish clearly, clinical experience indicates that many patients may require 20 mg of enalapril twice a day or 50 mg of captopril three times a day for maximum benefit.

Diuretic requirements may vary after initiation of ACE inhibitors and the effects of these agents must be carefully monitored during follow-up. In patients whose diuretic dose was reduced, it may be necessary to return the dose to pretreatment levels to avoid fluid retention. However, some patients may not need to continue diuretics if the ACE inhibitor is well tolerated and salt restriction is observed. Indeed, volume depletion resulting from addition or reinstitution of diuretics may cause symptomatic hypotension or renal insufficiency at doses of ACE inhibitor that were previously tolerated. Clinical experience indicates that diuretic requirements may decrease during chronic therapy with enalapril, so that reduction in diuretic dose rather than in the ACE inhibitor may relieve orthostatic symptoms that develop in the weeks following initiation of treatment.

The expected effects of reduction in circulating angiotensin II concentrations should be considered in assessing the response to ACE inhibitors. Troublesome hypotension may be seen only with the first dose, as the circulation adjusts to the decline in angiotensin II. Reduction in blood pressure to "hypotensive" levels may occur but should not trigger dose reduction in the absence of orthostatic symptoms. A predictable rise in serum creatinine concentration of approximately 0.2 mg/dl occurs in most patients with moderate-to-severe heart failure who are treated with enalapril. In the absence of intercurrent events, renal function then stabilizes in the great majority of patients. A rise in serum potassium level is another predictable effect of ACE inhibitors; this may be used to benefit the patient who requires potassium supplementation. Hyperkalemia will often resolve with reinstitution of a diuretic at former dose levels as tolerance to the ACE inhibitor is established. Cough has emerged as a troublesome side effect, especially in patients with mild heart failure who seldom experience this symptom as a consequence of their disease. Although reduction of dose or substitution of another ACE inhibitor may help, resolution of this adverse effect usually requires discontinuing the drug.

More traditional vasodilators, hydralazine and nitrates, may be used in heart failure when ACE inhibitors are poorly tolerated or produce incomplete relief of symptoms. The daily dose of hydralazine required to improve symptoms varies widely (100–800 mg) but is usually equal to or greater than 200 mg/day. Hydralazine should be used with caution in patients with ischemic heart disease complicated by angina, but the concern that this drug might produce coronary steal is seldom realized. Hydralazine therapy should be initiated with a test dose of 12.5 to 25.0 mg and then continued as tolerated at 6-hour intervals. Dose titration to 100 to 200 mg/day as needed for relief of symptoms and reduction in blood pressure can proceed rapidly if lower doses are well tolerated.

Since hydralazine dilates systemic arterioles only, concomitant venodilating therapy with long-acting nitrates is frequently necessary to control preload adequately.

Treatment Strategy

The choice of therapy must be individualized, but should be dictated by the degree of left ventricular dysfunction and severity of symptoms. Drug therapy will likely require adjustment during follow-up. The management of patients with asymptomatic left ventricular dysfunction is in a state of evolution, but available data suggest that strong consideration should be given to initiating treatment with ACE inhibitors, especially after extensive myocardial infarction. In patients with mild heart failure and little tendency to sodium retention, ACE inhibitors and dietary restriction are an ideal choice. The presence or development of fluid retention will necessitate the addition of a diuretic, usually a loop diuretic, as left ventricular dysfunction and renal insufficiency progress. In patients with advanced left ventricular dysfunction (left ventricular ejection fraction < 0.35), digitalis and nitrates are frequently used along with diuretics and ACE inhibitors to optimize therapy. Hydralazine should be considered in patients with ACE inhibitor intolerance or when systolic blood pressure and symptoms of heart failure are not adequately controlled by these drugs. Calcium antagonists should be used with caution in patients with advanced left ventricular dysfunction but may be efficacious in patients who have persistent hypertension or anginal symptoms despite other therapy.

Stevenson LW, Perloff JK. Limited reliability of physical signs for estimating hemodynamics in chronic heart failure. JAMA 1989; 261:884–8.
Rales, edema, and jugular venous distention are often absent when pulmonary capillary wedge pressure exceeds 22 mm Hg.

Ghali JK, et al. Precipitating factors leading to decompensation of heart failure. Arch Intern Med 1988; 148:2013–6.
In urban black patients with a history of heart failure, decompensation is often precipitated by noncompliance with diet and/or drug treatment and less commonly by arrhythmia or infection.

Gerlag PGG, Joseph JN, Van M. High dose furosemide in the treatment of refractory congestive heart failure. Arch Intern Med 1988; 148:286–91.
When creatinine clearance is severely reduced, high doses of furosemide (250–4000 mg/day) can be given over long periods, without serious side effects.

The Captopril-Digoxin Multicenter Research Group. Comparative effects of therapy with captopril and digoxin in patients with mild to moderate heart failure. JAMA 1988; 259:539–44.
Both drugs improve exercise time and reduce treatment failures.

Cohn JN, et al. Effects of vasodilator therapy on mortality in chronic congestive heart failure. N Engl J Med 1986; 314:1547–52.

The first demonstration that addition of vasodilators to digoxin and diuretic therapy reduces mortality.

The Consensus Trial Study Group. Effects of enalapril on mortality in severe congestive heart failure. N Engl J Med 1987; 316:1429–35.
Enalapril in doses of 2.5 to 40 mg/day reduced mortality in patients with severe progressive heart failure.

Kessler KN. Heart failure with normal systolic function. Update on prevalence, differential diagnosis, prognosis and therapy. Arch Intern Med 1988; 148:2109–11.
Diastolic left ventricular dysfunction associated with hypertension, CHD, hypertrophic cardiomyopathy, diabetes, and other conditions may lead to elevated LVEDP causing exertional dyspnea and orthopnea.

The SOLVD Investigators. Effect of enalapril on survival in patients with reduced left ventricular ejection fractions and congestive heart failure. N Engl J Med 1991; 325:293–302.
The addition of enalapril to conventional therapy significantly reduced mortality and hospitalizations for heart failure in patients with chronic congestive heart failure and low ejection fractions.

Cohn JN. Comparison of enalapril with hydralazine-isorbide dinitrate in the treatment of chronic congestive heart failure. N Engl J Med 1991; 325:303–10.
Demonstrated greater survival benefit with enalapril compared to isorbide dinitrate. Suggests that the different physiologic effects of the two regimens might lead to enhanced benefit if they are used in combination.

29. REHABILITATION AFTER MYOCARDIAL INFARCTION
Thomas E. Kottke and Mark A. Hlatky

The aim of rehabilitation after myocardial infarction (MI) is to return patients to full productive lives. This is a major challenge, for many patients do not return to work after an MI, and often many more are needlessly restricted in less dramatic ways.

A cardiac rehabilitation program must address five problems: (1) return to physical activity, (2) concerns about sexual activity, (3) psychological adjustment, (4) return to work, and (5) prevention of reinfarction and death. A prerequisite for effective rehabilitation is control of ischemia, arrhythmias, and congestive heart failure, and modification of cardiac risk factors.

Return to Physical Activity
Since prolonged bed rest for the MI patient was abandoned in the early 1950s, mobilization has come earlier and earlier in the course of recovery. Current practice is to begin ambulation in the coronary care unit and progressively increase activity under direct supervision until discharge from the hospital. Activity recommendations after MI should be tailored to the individual patient.

To assure both patient and physician that home activities immediately after discharge can be tolerated, hospitalized patients can be readily assessed by monitoring symptoms, heart rate, blood pressure, and ECG during walking or climbing stairs. Low-level formal exercise testing is often performed prior to discharge to provide more detailed information for counseling and postdischarge exercise prescription. The patient should be carefully monitored during exercise testing for signs of ischemia, insufficient cardiac output, or arrhythmia. A heart rate at least 10 beats per minute lower than this threshold should be set as the safe maximum for activity, since it has been shown that most complications occur in patients who have marked ischemic responses and who have exceeded the threshold heart rate.

After discharge, patients should progressively resume their former levels of activity.

Formal cardiac rehabilitation programs can speed conditioning and assist psychological adjustment and risk factor modification, particularly in high-risk patients. Unsupervised progressive conditioning is suitable for selected patients, such as those with normal blood pressure response to exercise, no signs or symptoms of myocardial ischemia at heart rates below 120, no evidence of congestive heart failure, and no complex ventricular arrhythmias.

Unsupervised activity is best guided by teaching the patient to take his or her pulse and not exceed the determined safe maximum for exercise heart rate. Initially, short periods of walking two or three times daily with rest periods in between are usually well tolerated. If no symptoms occur, both higher levels and longer durations of activity should gradually be attempted.

A maximum (symptom-limited) exercise test performed 6 to 12 weeks after discharge can give both the physician and the patient an objective assessment of physical work capacity and can identify those patients who should be considered for invasive evaluation. Exercise testing is also useful for reassuring the patient about the safety of physical activity. However, if arrhythmia is suspected, the 24-hour rhythm monitor or event recorders are more sensitive than the exercise test.

Many patients who have had an MI have been sedentary and are poorly conditioned. For them, programs aimed at increasing exercise capacity may be useful. Attaining a training effect allows the same level of external work to be achieved at a lower heart rate and blood pressure, reducing the demands on the heart. Thus, activities that would otherwise precipitate angina can be performed comfortably. A conditioning program usually consists of dynamic exercise with large muscle groups (e.g., walking, jogging, swimming) at adequate heart rates (e.g., 60–80% of the maximum safe heart rate) for sufficient duration (15–60 minutes) and frequency (at least three times a week) to achieve and sustain a training effect.

Sexual Activity

The return to sexual activity is a primary concern of a large proportion of cardiac patients of all ages. In one Veterans Administration study, 49% of MI patients reported concerns about sexual activity, usually fear of chest pain, impotence, or death during intercourse. To forestall sexual dysfunction resulting from such fears and to indicate that sexual activity is an appropriate topic for discussion, the physician should make a point of inquiring whether the patient expects changed sexual activities as a result of heart disease.

The estimated peak heart rate during sexual activity is about 120 beats per minute and is sustained for only about a minute. Thus, as a guideline, the cardiac stress of intercourse can usually be tolerated if a rise in heart rate to 120 beats per minute causes no symptoms. For the patient with continued anxiety about sexual activity, Holter monitoring during intercourse may be a method of demonstrating that the activity is safe.

Symptoms can also be averted by lessening the metabolic demands of sexual intercourse, for example, by pausing intermittently, changing position, and emphasizing foreplay. Sexual activity in the morning or after a nap may be less likely to cause cardiac symptoms than after a long day or a heavy meal. Angina medications should be accessible; if angina is expected during sexual activity, nitroglycerin should be taken before starting.

Psychological Adjustment

An acute MI is usually a crisis for the patient and family. Thoughtful explanation of the nature of the illness and the expected course can help to dispel many unwarranted fears and concerns. Well-designed pamphlets are available through the state affiliates of the American Heart Association; these may be useful during a period when patients have many questions and anxieties about their illness.

Early and progressive ambulation helps combat the anxiety, depression, and low self-esteem common after an MI. Exercise testing and training may also help allay fears about activities by establishing safe limits, thus avoiding both inappropriate restrictions and dangerous excesses. Formal cardiac conditioning programs may be particularly helpful for anxious patients, who find reassurance from the structured approach and support from interaction with other post-MI patients. Additional counseling and therapy may be necessary for the occasional patient with prolonged or excessive depression or anxiety after an MI.

Return to Work
Returning the patient to gainful employment is a major goal of post-MI rehabilitation. Whether this goal is achieved is often affected by socioeconomic factors such as the patient's age, type of employment, job satisfaction, ability to control the work schedule and pace, and financial necessity for continued employment. The patient's symptoms and functional capacity certainly must dictate the feasibility of resuming work. Clearly, the physical demands of the occupation must not exceed the limits imposed by symptoms. Exercise testing may aid decision-making by providing objective evidence concerning functional capacity. Physician advice may prove decisive in borderline cases. Workers in sedentary occupations may return as soon as 3 weeks after uncomplicated MI and convalescence, while laborers may have to delay returning to work for longer periods. Because their stamina may be low, patients might wish to work part-time for the first few weeks, if possible.

The patient can be prepared psychologically for returning to the job by the physician's emphasizing, early in the course of rehabilitative treatment, that most MI patients go back to work. Physicians should also be prepared to speak with employers who may be reluctant to rehire the patient. If the patient needs to be retrained, contacting the state's vocational rehabilitation program while the patient is still in the hospital will speed this process.

Hyperlipidemia
Control of hyperlipidemia through diet, weight control, exercise, and, when necessary, medication significantly reduces progression of coronary atherosclerosis and reduces recurrent events. Evidence from randomized trials suggests that the goal low-density lipoprotein should be 2.6 mmol/L (100 mg/dl).

Prevention of Reinfarction and Death
Patients suffering an acute MI are at higher risk of death over the first year, and particularly over the first few months, following the event. Prevention of recurrent infarction and cardiac death should be an integral component of cardiac rehabilitation.

Vigorous efforts to control the cardiac risk factors should be intensified after an MI. Elevated blood pressure increases cardiac work and aggravates ischemia. Smoking has adverse hemodynamic and metabolic effects that may precipitate myocardial ischemia and sudden death. Hyperlipidemia promotes the progression of the atherosclerotic process. Obesity increases the strain of any activity on both muscles and heart. Excessive psychological stress adds further burdens to a diseased heart.

Beta-Blocking Agents
Beta-blocking agents have been shown to reduce subsequent coronary events after MI. A beta-blocker is therefore recommended for all patients. There is evidence that the improved prognosis depends on treatment being started early; most experts recommend starting patients on beta-blockers before hospital discharge. Preferred beta-blockers are those without intrinsic sympathomimetic activity, such as propranolol, nadolol, atenolol, and metoprolol. Because survival of patients who suffer a recurrent infarction while on beta-blocker therapy is better than for those who are not taking a beta-blocker, patients should continue the drug as long as possible. Contraindications include worsening congestive heart failure, bronchospasm, and exacerbation of depression on the medication.

Smoking
There is strong and consistent evidence from observational studies that smoking is an important risk factor for subsequent coronary events after MI and that stopping smoking reduces risk. Patients should be advised to stop smoking while in the coronary care unit, when they may be particularly susceptible to such advice. This advice should be repeated on follow-up visits; failure to ask the patient about smoking may imply that it is no longer an important issue. Patients who are abstinent should be congratulated and those who are unsuccessful should be encouraged to try again. Special smoking cessation programs may be effective (see Chap. 130 for advice on facilitating smoking cessation efforts).

Exercise Training
Exercise training has also been shown in several trials to reduce the mortality after MI, but because of the small numbers of patients enrolled in these studies, the differences

have not been statistically significant. Thus, recommendations regarding exercise after MI should be guided more by the expected effect on symptoms than by any potential effect on mortality. It is uncertain whether beta-blockers prevent exercise from inducing a training effect. However, it is clear that maximum exercise capacity can be increased, even on beta-blockers. Therefore, post-MI patients should be continued on beta-blockers during exercise rehabilitation.

Social Reinforcement of Risk Modification
Patients are faced daily with social and visual cues to return to their previous life-styles. Rehabilitation efforts must therefore emphasize skills, social supports, and the availability of choices to maintain behavioral changes. Dietary adherence will probably be improved by having the whole family adopt a low-sodium, low–saturated fat cuisine by learning skills in food buying and preparation and in choosing satisfactory foods while dining out. Smoking cessation will be facilitated if other household members also stop smoking and all smoking paraphernalia is discarded. The spouse should participate in the patient's walking or exercise program. In addition to making adherence easier for the cardiac patient, this strategy allows the physician to introduce other family members to healthy habits.

Greenland P, Chu JS. Efficacy of cardiac rehabilitation services. With emphasis on patients with myocardial infarction. Ann Intern Med 1988; 109:650–63.
An analysis of the effects that a practitioner can expect to achieve from various cardiac rehabilitation interventions.

Squires RW, et al. Cardiovascular rehabilitation: status 1990. Mayo Clin Proc 1990; 65:731–55.
Authoritative review of the state of the science of cardiac rehabilitation.

Hanson P, ed. Exercise and the heart. Cardiology clinics. Vol. 5 1987.
A recent compilation of articles on exercise and the heart plus guidelines for exercise prescription for patients with heart disease.

DeBusk RF, et al. Identification and treatment of low-risk patients after acute myocardial infarction and coronary-artery bypass graft surgery. N Engl J Med 1986; 314:161–6.
Provides decision rules for the management of patients after MI and heart surgery.

Wenger NK, Hellerstein HK, eds. Rehabilitation of the coronary patient. 3rd ed. New York: Wiley, 1991.
Contains much useful information, including details of rehabilitation program delivery and planning and facilitation of return to work.

McLane M, Krop H, Mehta J. Psychosexual adjustment and counseling after myocardial infarction. Ann Intern Med 1980; 92:514–9.
A review, emphasizing resumption of sexual activity after MI.

30. PAROXYSMAL SUPRAVENTRICULAR TACHYCARDIA
Ross J. Simpson, Jr.

Paroxysmal supraventricular tachycardia (PSVT) is a commonly occurring, rapid (140–220 beats/min), narrow-QRS-complex tachycardia. Episodes occur without obvious precipitating cause and often affect patients who have no obvious heart disease. Attacks may last from less than a second to several days, and the interval between episodes may vary widely.

The natural history of PSVT is not known. Except in patients with structural heart disease or Wolff-Parkinson-White (WPW) syndrome, it does not appear to shorten life. However, in patients with chronic heart disease, PSVT may precipitate angina, congestive heart failure, or syncope. Patients with WPW syndrome and a history of unusually rapid PSVT or atrial fibrillation may, in rare instances, die suddenly.

The electrophysiologic basis for the most common forms of PSVT is ultimately a congenital or acquired duplicate conducting pathway between the atrium and ventricle. The tachycardia often is initiated by a premature atrial beat that blocks in one pathway and conducts slowly down the alternate pathway. By the time the slowly conducting beat reaches the distal connection of the pathway, sufficient time has elapsed to allow reentry into the previously blocked pathway and retrograde conduction back to the atrium occurs. Conduction down the first pathway may reoccur and the cycle may be repeated indefinitely.

Approximately 50% of patients with PSVT have both the normal and abnormal pathway located within the atrioventricular (AV) node. In approximately 30% of patients, an extranodal pathway is present. If the extranodal pathway conducts antegradely from the atrium to the ventricle during sinus rhythm, the diagnosis of WPW syndrome is made. Occasionally, the extranodal pathway is not obvious during sinus rhythm and serves only as the retrograde conducting limb of the circuit. In approximately 10% of patients, PSVT occurs by reentry within the atrium or sinus node, or by non-reentrant mechanisms, as seen during ectopic atrial tachycardia.

Diagnosis

The clinical manifestations of PSVT depend on the presence or absence of structural heart disease and the rate of tachycardia. The most common clinical symptoms are the sudden onset of palpitations, light-headedness, weakness, or shortness of breath. Most patients without structural heart disease tolerate rapid PSVT without incapacitating symptoms. If preexisting heart disease is present, congestive heart failure or angina pectoris may occur as a consequence of the rapid heart rate.

Clinical Signs

At heart rates over 180 beats per minute, systolic blood pressure falls, and diastolic filling pressure rises, even in patients with normal hearts. The pulse is regular and rapid; mechanical pulsus alternans may occur if there is heart failure or a very rapid heart rate. Polyuria begins after 4 to 6 hours but is not seen in patients with mitral stenosis or chronic left ventricular failure. If the arrhythmia persists for several days, salt and water retention occurs, even in patients with normal hearts.

ECG

An ECG of the tachycardia is essential for diagnosis because paroxysms of atrial fibrillation and ventricular tachycardia can produce identical symptoms. Patients with infrequent episodes may require procedures other than a simple ECG to diagnose the cause of their symptoms. A Holter monitor rarely documents PSVT because of the unpredictable frequency of attacks, and a treadmill exercise test only rarely induces PSVT. An ECG telephone transmitter has become the standard technique used to document infrequently occurring, nonsustained arrhythmias. Patients suspected of PSVT can carry this device in a purse or briefcase. During an attack, they connect the leads, dial a central number, and use the device to transmit an ECG. If this fails, cardiac pacing techniques are successful in inducing the arrhythmia in almost all patients prone to PSVT.

In most instances, the ECG of PSVT is characteristic. The QRS complex is typically narrow (< 0.10 second in duration) and monotonously regular (except at the beginning and end of the tachycardia, when variation in the rate is expected), and there is no evidence of AV dissociation. Often, the P wave is not visible because it occurs synchronously with the QRS complex. Less frequently, a retrograde P wave (negative P wave in leads II, III, and aVF) is visible following or preceding the QRS complex.

Differential Diagnosis

Differential diagnosis of a rapid, regular narrow-QRS-complex tachycardia includes sinus tachycardia, atrial flutter with 2:1 block, rapid atrial fibrillation, and paroxysmal atrial tachycardia with block. Normal sinus P waves (upright P waves in leads I, II, and III) before the QRS complex suggest sinus tachycardia; an irregular ventricular response suggests atrial fibrillation. Atrial flutter with a 2:1 block may resemble PSVT if the flutter is atypical and the two P waves for each QRS complex cannot be readily separated from the ST segment and T waves. Paroxysmal atrial tachycardia with block is seen with digitalis intoxication and resembles atrial flutter except that the atrial rate is slower, the degree of AV block may be greater than 2:1, and escape or accelerated junctional beats may be present.

If the QRS duration is prolonged ($\geq$ 0.12 second) the rhythm is probably ventricular tachycardia. Ventricular tachycardia may be confirmed by AV dissociation and fusion or capture beats on long rhythm strips of lead II or V1. Misdiagnosis of ventricular tachycardia for PSVT with aberrant conduction or bundle-branch block may have disastrous consequences since administration of drugs such as verapamil may provoke severe hypotension or ventricular fibrillation. If a wide-QRS-complex tachycardia is strongly suspected of being supraventricular in origin, positioning an esophageal electrode or a catheter in the right atrium may be required for definitive diagnosis. An additional advantage of these invasive procedures is that the PSVT can be broken by pacing through the electrode.

Treatment

Most episodes of PSVT will terminate spontaneously. However, because episodes may last for days and cause major hemodynamic changes, termination of the tachycardia is recommended even in asymptomatic patients. The following interventions, listed in order of preference, are commonly used to interrupt PSVT.

"Vagal" Maneuvers

Because sympathetic tone can maintain the tachycardia and counteract the parasympathetic effect of vagal maneuvers, the patient should be placed in the reclining position. The Valsalva maneuver is performed by asking the patient to take a deep breath and bear down as if to have a bowel movement. The physician places a hand on the abdomen to provide opposing pressure. Carotid sinus massage is performed by providing even, firm pressure on one carotid body at the carotid artery below the angle of the jaw. This maneuver should not be done in patients with bruits in either carotid or in elderly patients. The rarely used diving reflex is performed by having the patient turn onto the side and, while holding the breath, immerse his or her face in ice water. A physician should be present during this maneuver.

Verapamil

Verapamil is administered as one or more 5-mg intravenous boluses to a maximal dose of 0.10 to 0.15 mg/kg if the arrhythmia is not broken. Verapamil is reported to be effective in over 90% of patients who have not responded to vagal maneuvers. Verapamil should not be administered to patients with wide-QRS-complex tachycardia because of the potentially disastrous consequences of a misdiagnosis of ventricular tachycardia. In addition, it may accelerate the ventricular response to atrial fibrillation in patients with WPW syndrome and therefore should be avoided in such patients. Verapamil should also not be given to patients with chronic heart failure, acute pulmonary edema, acute myocardial infarction, or hypotension.

Adenosine

Adenosine is highly effective in terminating PSVT and may be used as an alternative to verapamil. It is administered intravenously as a rapid bolus of 6 mg, followed, if necessary, by 12 mg, via a large peripheral or central vein. Adenosine's extremely brief duration of action ($<$ 1 minute) may make it safer than verapamil. On the other hand, the short half-life has disadvantages; recurrence of PSVT after initial termination may occur in up to one-third of patients. At the present time, there is limited clinical experience with adenosine and no clinical trials comparing it to verapamil. Its cost is substantially higher, and it is not clearly preferable unless verapamil is contraindicated or has failed.

Side effects of adenosine are generally transient and include dyspnea, chest discomfort, and flushing. Adenosine should not be administered to patients taking dipyridamole, which potentiates its action, and may be ineffective in patients taking theophylline, which antagonizes its effects. Adenosine should be used with caution, if at all, in patients with asthma or other forms of obstructive lung disease, because it may cause bronchoconstriction.

Other Drugs
Intravenous edrophonium (10 mg), propranolol (up to 0.15 mg/kg), or digoxin will also terminate PSVT. Digitalis has been implicated as a cause of death in patients with WPW syndrome and should not be given to these patients. If the patient is not hypotensive, vasopressor drugs like phenylephrine should not be used because of the possibility of precipitating pulmonary edema or other cardiovascular complications.

Electrical Conversion
Electrical direct current (DC) conversion synchronized to the QRS complex is also infrequently needed but is recommended if the patient appears hemodynamically unstable, is having angina, is hypotensive, or has other evidence of impaired cardiac output. Usually only 25 to 50 W-seconds is required to convert PSVT. Electrical pacing, involving catheterization of the right atrium, is safe and effective, but is rarely used because of the usual success of pharmacologic therapy.

Prevention

It is difficult to predict how the pattern of recurrence of PSVT will change with age. Infants and young children may "grow out" of their arrhythmia, while adults tend to have the propensity to PSVT for decades or for life.

Drug Therapy
Drug therapy is usually helpful in preventing recurrent episodes of tachycardia. However, patients with infrequent PSVT (e.g., < one occurrence/year) or PSVT that causes only mild symptoms may not require long-term treatment. Chronic therapy is also not recommended following the first episode of PSVT in such patients. Possible goals of long-term therapy in the treatment of PSVT are to decrease or eliminate recurrent episodes and to modify the severity or improve the ease of termination of episodes. All of the drugs outlined below may abolish frequent episodes of PSVT. However, because the frequency of occurrence of PSVT varies over time and a particular drug may increase, decrease, or have no effect on the frequency of episodes, prolonged observation, with follow-up by measuring blood levels of the drug, is necessary to establish drug efficacy or failure.

Before beginning long-term therapy, the patient's history, physical examination, chest film, and ECG should be reviewed to determine if ventricular preexcitation (WPW syndrome) from a manifest AV connection is present (shortened PR interval, widened QRS complex, and ST and T abnormalities) and to evaluate underlying structural heart disease. Hypokalemia, congestive heart failure, unexplained heart murmurs, or other medical conditions should be investigated and treated. Caffeine and nicotine may have sympathomimetic effects, but it is unlikely that stopping these drugs will have a significant effect on the frequency of occurrence of PSVT in most patients.

Drugs that prolong conduction and refractoriness in the antegrade direction of the AV node (e.g., digoxin, beta-blockers, verapamil) are particularly useful in the treatment of PSVT, because if they do not prevent PSVT, they often slow the rate of the tachycardia and aid in terminating PSVT. They also have a low frequency of side effects. These drugs are generally the standard of therapy of AV nodal reentrant PSVT. Digoxin, and probably verapamil, should not be used in patients with WPW syndrome.

Digoxin, because of its long half-life and infrequent systemic side effects, is often the initial therapy in patients who do not have WPW syndrome. If a therapeutic digoxin plasma concentration does not offer protection from PSVT or digoxin is contraindicated, a beta-sympathetic blocking drug may be used. If beta-blockers are used, the dosage is adjusted to achieve beta-blockade. Verapamil, 120 mg three times a day, may also be effective if WPW syndrome is not present. Most patients require a combination of drugs to prevent recurrences. The combination of digoxin and a beta-sympathetic blocking drug is particularly effective for patients with AV nodal reentry.

If drugs that slow the AV node are not successful in preventing attacks of tachycardia, a quinidine-like drug (e.g., quinidine, procainamide, or disopyramide) is recommended. These drugs act by slowing conduction and prolonging refractoriness in the accessory or retrograde pathway in the AV node. They may reduce the frequency of attacks but often do not change the rate of the tachycardia if it occurs. If atrial flutter or ectopic atrial tachycardia is suspected, these drugs should be administered in combination with a drug that prolongs the refractory period of the AV node, because, alone, they have the potential to increase the ventricular response rate.

Flecainide and propafenone are not recommended for routine treatment for supraventricular arrhythmia but may be useful in the management of patients who have not responded to other drugs and have no evidence of organic heart disease. Such patients should be referred to a cardiac electrophysiologist.

Diagnostic Cardiac Pacing Studies

Referral to an experienced cardiac electrophysiologist for diagnostic cadiac pacing studies is also recommended for patients who have PSVT despite adequate drug therapy, who have syncope, or who have had an episode of atrial fibrillation in the setting of WPW syndrome. Rare patients in whom drugs cannot modify the tachycardia are recommended for surgery, endocardial catheter ablation of an AV connection, or implantation of an antitachycardia pacemaker.

Wu D, et al. Clinical electrocardiographic and electrophysiologic observations in patients with paroxysmal supraventricular tachycardia. Am J Cardiol 1978; 41:1045–51.
Reviews of electrophysiology and ECG characteristics of PSVT.

Wood P. Polyuria in paroxysmal tachycardia and paroxysmal atrial flutter and fibrillation. Br Heart J 1963; 25:273–82.
Classic description of hemodynamic consequences of PSVT.

Anderson JL, Jolivette DM, Fredell PA. Summary of efficacy and safety of flecainide for supraventricular arrhythmias. Am J Cardiol 1988; 62:62D–5D.
Based on a review of the world literature, the authors conclude that flecainide was effective in two-thirds to three-fourths of PSVT patients, most of whom had not responded to standard treatment. In those studies in which side effects were reported, adverse effects were noted in 6.9% of patients, including worsened arrhythmia, conduction disturbances, congestive heart failure, paresthesias, and visual disturbances.

Brugada P, Smeets LRMJ, Wellems JJH. Spectrum of supraventricular tachycardia. Am J Cardiol 1988; 62:4L–7L.
Readable review of mechanism, ECG diagnosis, and treatment of PSVT.

Gallagher JJ, et al. The preexcitation syndrome. Prog Cardiovasc Dis 1978; 20:285–327.
Reviews Wolff-Parkinson-White syndrome.

Waxman MB, et al. Vagal techniques for termination of paroxysmal supraventricular tachycardia. Am J Cardiol 1980; 46:655–64.
Reviews effectiveness of vagal maneuvers in terminating PSVT.

Sung RJ, Elser B, McAllister RG. Intravenous verapamil for termination of re-entrant supraventricular tachycardias: intracardiac studies correlated with plasma verapamil concentrations. Ann Intern Med 1980; 93:682–9.
Effect of plasma levels of verapamil on PSVT.

Steinman RT, et al. Wide QRS tachycardia in the conscious adult: ventricular tachycardia is the most frequent cause. JAMA 1989; 261:1013–6.
Ventricular tachycardia is the most common cause of wide-, regular-QRS-complex tachycardia, especially in patients with atherosclerotic heart disease.

Wellens HJ, Brugada P, Smeets JL. Antiarrhythmic drugs for supraventricular tachycardia. Am J Cardiol 1988; 62:69L–73L.
Current recommendations for drug therapy of PSVT.

Hammill SC, Pritchett EC. Simplified esophageal electrocardiography using bipolar recording leads. Ann Intern Med 1981; 95:14–8.
Describes a useful method to detect P-wave activity during tachycardia.

Rankin AC, McGovern BA. Adenosine or verapamil for the acute treatment of supraventricular tachycardia. Ann Intern Med 1991; 114:513–515.
A thoughtful editorial that compares the two drugs and concludes that adenosine offers no clear advantage over verapamil unless its potential for improved safety is confirmed.

31. PREMATURE VENTRICULAR CONTRACTIONS
Ross J. Simpson, Jr.

Premature ventricular contractions (PVCs) can cause unpleasant symptoms and are associated with increased risk of sudden cardiac death in some patients with structural heart disease. Physicians often administer potent antiarrhythmic drugs in an attempt to suppress these arrhythmias, although there is no evidence that such treatment prevents death. Indeed, there is evidence that in patients with chronic ischemic heart disease, suppression of PVCs with encainide and flecainide increases the risk of death.

Prevalence
PVCs are found in healthy individuals as well as in patients with severe structural heart disease. In a 24-hour period, PVCs are present in 30 to 50% of patients without apparent heart disease and are found on approximately 0.8% of routine ECGs. They are more common in older people. Complex forms are not rare: In a study of 50 normal medical students, 25 had at least one PVC in 24 hours, and of these, 6 had multiform PVCs, 3 had R-on-T PVCs, 1 had a couplet, and 1 had a five-beat run of ventricular tachycardia. Although frequent PVCs are statistically associated with complex forms, ventricular tachycardia and other complex forms may commonly occur in patients with infrequent isolated PVCs.

In the presence of structural heart disease, PVCs are common. During the early phase of acute myocardial infarction (MI) virtually 100% of patients have PVCs, approximately 10% of patients have R-on-T PVCs, and 15% of patients have ventricular tachycardia. The prevalence of PVCs decreases rapidly after MI but increases again following discharge from the hospital. Patients with chronic angina pectoris or previous MI have a high prevalence of PVCs, and 5 to 10% of patients have asymptomatic, short-duration ventricular tachycardia during a 24-hour period. PVCs also occur frequently in patients with other types of heart disease, including hypertensive and valvular heart disease, idiopathic hypertrophic subaortic stenosis, sarcoidosis, and mitral valve prolapse.

Relationship to Sudden Cardiac Death
Not all patients with PVCs are at increased risk for sudden death. Factors that increase risk include the presence and type of underlying heart disease, the frequency and complexity of the PVCs (i.e., R-on-T, couplets, multiform QRS complexes, and consecutive PVCs), concurrent drug use, and the presence of other diseases. If the patient is otherwise clinically healthy, the occurrence of simple PVCs is not known to increase the risk of death.

In contrast, patients with ischemic heart disease and PVCs may be at increased risk of sudden death, particularly if ventricular contractility is decreased. For example, the combination of complex PVCs and congestive heart failure (CHF) is associated with a sixfold increase in risk of sudden cardiac death. Most deaths in the first 6 months following an MI occur in patients with a low ejection fraction (< 0.4) and complex PVCs. Prolongation of the QT interval also predisposes to ventricular fibrillation.

Drug-Induced PVCs
Drugs, including quinidine, procainamide, disopyramide, phenothiazines, tricyclic antidepressants, digitalis, and the newer antiarrhythmic drugs, such as flecainide, can cause PVCs and ventricular fibrillation. Patients who have heart disease as manifested by CHF, or who use digitalis, have hypokalemia, and have prolonged QT intervals are at greatest risk. In the setting of chronic ischemic heart disease, flecainide and encainide may be particularly arrhythmogenic. Because physicians expect patients with ventricular arrhythmias to die suddenly, an excess mortality caused by drugs may often go unnoticed.

Diagnosis

Symptoms and Signs
Patients with frequent or complex PVCs may be asymptomatic or may complain of palpitations, light-headedness, syncope, or atypical chest pain. Symptoms of ventricular tachycardia are related to the rate and the underlying mechanical reserve of the heart. Ventricular tachycardia may be a stable rhythm and some patients may be relatively asymptomatic

and feel only palpitations or light-headedness, symptoms similar to that noted in patients with paroxysmal supraventricular tachycardia (PSVT). Others, with more rapid ventricular rates or more depressed cardiac contractility, may have syncope, profound hypotension, diaphoresis, angina, and impaired tissue perfusion. On physical examination, the pulse is regular and rapid, and physical findings of atrioventricular (AV) dissociation, including venous cannon A waves and variation in the intensity of the first heart sound, may be present.

ECG

A PVC is premature, wide, and often bizarre in appearance. The ST segment and T wave are abnormal and often in the opposite direction from the QRS complex. The pause following a PVC is often fully compensatory; however, a PVC may capture the atrium retrogradely, reset the sinus node, and cause a less-than-compensatory pause. Interpolated PVCs are PVCs squeezed between two normally occurring sinus beats that occur when a PVC does not reset the sinus node or interfere with AV conduction of the subsequent, normal sinus beat. The coupling interval between PVCs and sinus beats may be fixed for brief periods such that there is less than a 0.06-second variation in the coupling intervals from the normal QRS complex to the PVC.

Ventricular tachycardia is defined as three or more consecutive PVCs. The rate varies from 100 to over 200 beats per minute, and the rhythm may be slightly irregular or as regular as with PSVT. Sustained ventricular tachycardia may be difficult to distinguish from PSVT with bundle-branch block or conduction aberration; however, AV dissociation and ventricular capture and fusion beats identify ventricular tachycardia. Occasionally, AV dissociation may be absent or incomplete because of intermittent atrial capture by the ventricles. Other, useful, but less reliable ECG features of ventricular tachycardia include a QRS duration of greater than 0.14 second, extreme left axis deviation, or certain abnormal QRS configurations (e.g., a mono- or biphasic right bundle-branch block–shaped QRS complex on lead V_1). Consecutive PVCs at a rate of less than 100 per minute are usually referred to as accelerated idioventricular rhythm.

Other Studies

Most PVCs can be diagnosed from the standard ECG. Modified precordial leads or esophageal leads may aid diagnosis by detection of the AV dissociation. If necessary, intracardiac electrodes can be inserted for definitive diagnosis. A 24-hour Holter monitor should be used if nonsustained ventricular tachycardia is suspected or if unexplained symptoms suggestive of brady or tachycardia are present.

Treatment

Deciding whether to treat PVCs is difficult since not all patients with PVCs are at risk of sudden death and treatment is often disruptive and dangerous. Moreover, the frequency of PVCs varies so greatly that very large reductions in observed PVCs on 24-hour Holter monitoring of an individual patient must be observed before it is reasonable to conclude that treatment, rather than spontaneous variation, is responsible for the change. Although a reduction in frequency or complexity of PVCs is often used as a marker of successful treatment, it is not known whether this actually prevents sudden cardiac death.

Treatment is rarely recommended for frequent PVCs or complex PVCs including triplets. Longer runs of ventricular tachycardia are generally treated by admitting the patient to a monitored setting in the hospital since treatment with antiarrhythmic drugs may worsen the arrhythmia. Hypokalemia, CHF, and coronary ischemia should be optimally treated. Cardiac drugs may be discontinued, and PVC frequency and complexity and the number of episodes of ventricular tachycardia noted. Often 48 hours of monitoring is necessary to document such frequency. The effect of exercise on the arrhythmia and an estimation of cardiac contractility by echocardiogram, nuclear angiography, or cardiac catheterization should be made. An antiarrhythmic drug is then administered, and the efficacy of the drug is evaluated by continuing ECG monitoring and peforming treadmill exercise testing. Referral to a cardiac electrophysiologist for an electrophysiologic pacing study should be done for all patients cardioverted from sustained ventricular tachycardia, in patients in whom the diagnosis of a wide-QRS-complex tachycardia is in doubt, or when there is evidence of an old, transmural infarction, or in patients who have been resuscitated from sudden cardiac death. A cardiac pacing study will often reproduce the arrhythmia and facilitate treatment of these patients.

Drug Therapy
It is best to think of the antiarrhythmic drugs according to their effect on specific characteristics of the cardiac action potential. One scheme divides the drugs into those that act like the prototype drugs: quinidine, lidocaine, flecainide, verapamil, or propranolol. Because there is considerable individual variability in drug responsiveness and half-life, therapy with these drugs should be guided by serum drug levels whenever possible.

QUINIDINE-LIKE DRUGS. Quinidine-like drugs (quinidine, procainamide, and disopyramide) are the most commonly used antiarrhythmic drugs in the treatment of chronic PVCs. They slow the upstroke of the action potential and decrease cellular excitability by depressing the rapid sodium-dependent channel. Quinidine-like drugs decrease conduction velocity in both normal and abnormal fibers. The most serious side effect of these drugs is the potentiation of life-threatening ventricular arrhythmias. This complication is most likely to occur if the QT interval is excessively prolonged prior to or during therapy.

Quinidine is available as the sulfate salt. The usual dosage is 200 to 400 mg every 6 to 8 hours. Longer-acting preparations are available as a gluconate salt or as a time-release tablet. Quinidine has negligible depressant effects on left ventricular function, but other side effects include diarrhea, tinnitus, thrombocytopenia, and hypotension. As many as 25% of patients given quinidine may have to discontinue it because of side effects.

Procainamide is available as an immediate-release preparation administered 200 to 750 mg every 3 to 4 hours or as a slow-release preparation administered every 6 to 8 hours. Nausea is not infrequent with procainamide. Antinuclear antibodies are present in a high percentage of patients, but a lupus-like syndrome occurs in only a small number of these patients. As with quinidine, the depressant effect on left ventricular contractility is small.

Disopyramide is administered as 100 to 120 mg every 6 to 8 hours. Side effects include urinary retention, dry mouth, hypotension, and exacerbation of CHF. Disopyramide is a potent depressor of left ventricular contractility and should be administered rarely, if ever, to patients with a history of CHF or cardiac ejection fraction of less than 0.3.

LIDOCAINE-LIKE DRUGS. Lidocaine-like drugs selectively depress the rapid sodium current in partially depressed fibers. This difference in effect on the action potential may partially explain the relatively low reported incidence of lidocaine-potentiated arrhythmias. Orally administered lidocaine-like drugs include mexiletine and tocainide. Tocainide is administered 400 to 600 mg every 8 hours to produce therapeutic drug concentrations of 4 to 10 μg per milliliter. The drug may cause pulmonary fibrosis, leukopenia, and thrombocytopenia and is currently infrequently used. Mexiletine is administered at doses of 200 to 300 mg every 8 hours to achieve blood levels of 1 to 2 μg per milliliter. Mexiletine may be combined with other drugs of the quinidine class and may be particularly useful in patients with a long QT interval since it generally does not prolong the QT interval. Tremor is a dose-related side effect.

FLECAINIDE-LIKE DRUGS. These drugs include flecainide and propafenone. They decrease the rate of rise of the upstroke of the action potential in a use-dependent manner, and slow conduction in all cardiac fibers but do not lengthen the duration of action potential of Purkinje fibers under normal circumstances.

Although these drugs are highly effective in suppressing PVCs, they cause excess mortality in patients with frequent PVCs in the posthospital recovery period of acute MI. These drugs should generally be reserved for the treatment of life-threatening arrhythmias including ventricular tachycardia and fibrillation, and administered under supervision of a cardiologist.

VERAPAMIL-LIKE DRUGS. Calcium blocking drugs, such as verapamil may be effective in treating certain types of PVCs and other ventricular arrhythmias, particularly in preventing the ventricular tachycardia associated with coronary artery spasm or in treating exercise-potentiated ventricular arrhythmias. They may suppress PVCs associated with hypertension-induced left ventricular hypertrophy. They have an established safety record and have minimal side effects. Verapamil is generally given in an oral dose of 80 to 120 mg three times a day. Higher doses may be required for control of exercise-induced ventricular tachycardia.

PROPRANOLOL-LIKE DRUGS. Beta-sympathetic blocking drugs are effective in controlling catecholamine-potentiated PVCs and other ventricular arrhythmias, including those induced by anesthetic agents, thyrotoxicosis, and digitalis excess and those associated with cardiac ischemia. Beta-sympathetic blocking drugs are particularly useful in treating patients with exercise-induced ventricular tachycardia.

Propranolol is administered in a dosage of 20 to 80 mg every 6 to 8 hours. Side effects include fatigue, lethargy, impotence, exacerbation of CHF, potentiation of bradyarrhythmias in patients with preexisting sinoatrial disease, and bronchospasm in patients prone to asthma. Because these drugs depress left ventricular function, the combination of propranolol and disopyramide should be avoided. The water-soluble beta-blocking drugs, including atenolol and nadolol, need less dose titration and less frequent dosing intervals.

Moss AJ. Clinical significance of ventricular arrhythmias in patients with and without coronary artery disease. Prog Cardiovasc Dis 1980; 23:33–52.
Excellent review of the prevalence and significance of PVCs in clinical practice.

Brodsky M, et al. Arrhythmias documented by 24 hour continuous electrocardiographic monitoring in 50 male medical students without apparent heart disease. Am J Cardiol 1977; 39:390–5.
Frequency and complexity of PVCs in a population free of organic heart disease.

Hiss RG, Lamb LE. Electrocardiographic findings in 122,043 individuals. Circulation 1962; 25: 947–61.
ECG abnormalities in normal subjects.

Bigger JT Jr. Relation between left ventricular dysfunction and ventricular arrhythmias after myocardial infarction. Am J Cardiol 1986; 57:8B–14B.
High prevalence of PVCs occur after infarction. Ventricular arrhythmias are related to mortality independent of life ventricular dysfunction.

The Cardiac Arrhythmia Suppression Trial (CAST) Investigators. Special Report. Preliminary report: effect of encainide and flecainide on mortality in a randomized trial of arrhythmia suppression after myocardial infarction. N Engl J Med 1989; 321:406–12.
Encainide and flecainide suppress PVCs in asymptomatic patients after MI but cause excess deaths.

Woosley RL. Pharmacokinetics and pharmacodynamics of antiarrhythmic agents in patients with congestive heart failure. Am Heart J 1987; 114:1280–91.
Easy-to-follow review of basic clinical pharmacologic principles relevant to antiarrhythmia drug treatment.

Nygaard TW, et al. Adverse reactions to antiarrhythmic drugs during therapy for ventricular arrhythmias. JAMA 1986; 256:55–7.
Clinically significant adverse reactions to antiarrhythmic drugs are common. An acceptable risk-benefit ratio is likely only in patients at high risk for serious arrhythmia.

Akhtar M, et al. Wide QRS complex tachycardia: reappraisal of a common clinical problem. Ann Intern Med 1988; 109:905–12.
Ventricular tachycardia is the most common mechanism for wide-QRS-complex tachycardia. Correct diagnosis can be made from ECG and clinical criteria.

Bigger JT, Fleiss JL, Rolnitzky LM, the Multicenter Post-Infarction Research Group. Prevalence, characteristics and significance of ventricular tachycardia detected by 24-hour continuous electrocardiographic recordings in the late hospital phase of acute myocardial infarction. Am J Cardiol 1986; 58:1151–60.
Occurrence of ventricular tachycardia related to frequency of PVCs. Ventricular tachycardia doubled risk of dying following MI.

Tchou PJ, et al. Automatic implantable cardioverter defibrillators and survival of patients with left ventricular dysfunction and malignant ventricular arrhythmias. Ann Intern Med 1988; 109;529–34.
Highly effective new treatment to prevent death from recurrent malignant arrhythmia.

32. ATRIAL FIBRILLATION
Ross J. Simpson, Jr.

Atrial fibrillation is a disorganized supraventricular rhythm characterized by a lack of effective atrial contraction and irregular, chaotic, and often rapid ventricular rates. It is probably the most common stable arrhythmia encountered in clinical practice, but its potential to cause harm to the patient is often underestimated. Even in the absence of obvious organic heart disease, atrial fibrillation may triple cardiovascular mortality. The reason for this increase in mortality is not clear, but may be partially related to a predisposition of patients to embolic stroke. Risk for embolic stroke or systemic emboli is greatest in patients with concomitant mitral stenosis, mitral insufficiency, and congestive heart failure. However, the risk is present, although very low, even in patients with lone atrial fibrillation.

Atrial fibrillation may be characterized by the rate of its ventricular response, its duration, pattern of recurrence, and its association with organic heart disease. Atrial fibrillation is referred to as rapid when ventricular rates are in excess of 120 beats per minute, as controlled for rates between 120 and 60 beats per minute, and as slow when the rate is less than 60 beats per minute. It is referred to as acute if it is present for less than 3 days, as chronic if it has been present for months, or as paroxysmal if episodes are self-terminating and recurrent. Atrial fibrillation occurring in the absence of obvious organic heart disease is referred to as lone atrial fibrillation.

Incidence, Prevalence, and Risk Factors
Approximately 2% of older adults will develop atrial fibrillation over a 20-year period. This risk increases with a person's age and deteriorating general health, with the prevalence of atrial fibrillation ranging from a low of 0.04 per thousand for young male pilots to 11.3 per thousand for older male civil servants to a 50 per thousand for fit Scotsmen over the age of 65.

Atrial fibrillation generally follows the development of congestive heart failure or obvious cardiovascular disease; coronary artery disease is the most common underlying condition. Although many patients with atrial fibrillation have nonspecific ST-segment and T-wave abnormalities or intraventricular conduction delays suggesting left ventricular hypertrophy, 3 to 11% of patients have no obvious organic heart disease.

Rheumatic mitral stenosis or insufficiency, congestive heart failure, and myocardial disorders that predispose to impaired diastolic relaxation of the left ventricle are strongly associated with atrial fibrillation. Hypertensive cardiovascular disease, especially if left ventricular hypertrophy is present, is a common antecedent of atrial fibrillation. Aortic stenosis and insufficiency are less commonly associated with atrial fibrillation except in the terminal stages of the disease. Sinus node dysfunction, acute and chronic pericarditis, thyrotoxicoses, acute alcohol abuse, and possibly chronic ventricular demand pacing also predispose to atrial fibrillation.

Atrial fibrillation occurs in acute infarction and rarely may be the initial manifestation of myocardial infarction. However, it may occur later in the hospital course of acute infarction as a consequence of concomitant congestive heart failure. It is seen in less than 10% of patients with transmural infarctions and is more likely to occur in older patients with infarctions, and those with a history of heart failure prior to admission, low systolic blood pressure on admission, wide P waves, and marked ST elevation. In addition, up to 20% of patients recovering from coronary artery bypass surgery may have an episode of atrial fibrillation.

Pathophysiology

Premature atrial beats trigger atrial fibrillation in patients with diffuse atrial fibrosis and scarring by conducting slowly or conducting through abnormal paths in the atrial myocardium. For atrial fibrillation to be sustained and not immediately self-terminating, the atrium must be sufficiently enlarged. Sustained atrial fibrillation is rare in infants and young children but is common in adults if an enlarged atrium is demonstrated by echocardiography, chest film, or a prolonged P-wave duration on the ECG.

Diagnosis

Clinical Signs

The heart rate is irregularly irregular and often associated with a pulse deficit between the radial or other peripheral arteries and the ECG or apical rate. This occurs due to variable ventricular filling and failure of some of the beats to generate sufficient pressure to perfuse, or occasionally to open the aortic valves. Symptoms are variable and depend on the age of the patient, the presence of structural heart disease, the extent of left ventricular dysfunction, and the rate. Rapid ventricular rates may cause angina pectoris in patients with coronary artery disease or left ventricular hypertrophy. In patients without serious organic heart disease, atrial fibrillation generally presents as palpitations, weakness, and light-headedness rather than syncope, severe hypotension, or pulmonary edema. However, in patients with aortic stenosis, idiopathic hypertrophic subaortic stenosis, mitral stenosis, severe left ventricular hypertrophy, or severe diastolic dysfunction, acute onset of atrial fibrillation often provokes hemodynamic decompensation, with hypotension or pulmonary edema.

ECG

The diagnosis of atrial fibrillation is made by the irregularly irregular ventricular response and the absence of obvious P waves or organized atrial activity in ECG leads II or V_1, and the presence of an undulating chaotic ECG baseline. The width of the QRS complex is generally narrow unless the patient has a preexisting bundle-branch block or accessory pathway (Wolff-Parkinson-White syndrome).

The irregularity of the ventricular response predisposes to aberrantly conducted beats referred to as "Ashman beats." The QRS complex of these beats is widened, and they often occur following a relatively long pause or long R-R interval, when the abnormal early wide QRS beat is closely coupled to a normal QRS beat. The refractory periods of the bundle branches are often not identical and are determined by the coupling interval of the conducted beat as well as the rate of the preceding beat. This pattern of a relatively long interval immediately followed by a relatively short R-R interval between beats predisposes to block in one bundle branch (usually the right bundle) and conduction through the other bundle. Ashman beats may be difficult to distinguish from ventricular ectopy.

New-onset atrial fibrillation or atrial fibrillation in the setting of pulmonary edema, thyrotoxicosis, hypoxemia, or fever is generally characterized by a rapid ventricular response. Atrial fibrillation with a slow ventricular response is more likely to occur in older patients, particularly if atrial fibrillation occurs in patients with persistent, underlying sinus node dysfunction and inappropriate sinus bradycardia. Chronic atrial fibrillation often has a controlled ventricular response and fine atrial activity reflecting less-well-organized atrial depolarization.

Evaluation

In general, most patients with the acute onset of atrial fibrillation should be hospitalized for continuous ECG monitoring. Although acute atrial fibrillation is rarely the sole manifestation of myocardial infarction or unstable angina pectoris, patients with risk factors for coronary artery disease should have serial creatinine phosphokinase measurements and ECGs performed to diagnose possible acute myocardial infarction. Even in patients in whom acute infarction is unlikely, the ECG should be monitored to evaluate the efficacy of drugs in controlling the ventricular response.

The evaluation of newly diagnosed atrial fibrillation should focus on detecting precipitating systemic or organic heart disease and assessing the potential for successful reversion to normal sinus rhythm. In addition to a history and physical examination, a chest film to evaluate cardiomegaly and thyroid function studies, particularly thyroid-stimulating hormone (TSH) level, are generally warranted. An echocardiogram will detect subclinical heart failure, pericardial effusion, left ventricular hypertrophy, valvular abnormalities, enlarged chambers, and ventricular contraction abnormalities, as seen with infiltrative disease processes or past myocardial infarction. Most importantly, the echocardiogram helps predict the success of cardioversion and the probability of maintaining sinus rhythm following cardioversion. A dilated left atrium or severe left ventricular function is associated with a high failure rate for maintaining sinus rhythm following cardioversion. The importance of echocardiography in evaluating patients with atrial fibrillation can therefore not be overestimated.

Treatment

When atrial fibrillation is diagnosed, the primary treatment decision is whether to convert the patient to sinus rhythm, to allow the patient to convert spontaneously to sinus rhythm, or to direct drug therapy at controlling the rate of the ventricular response. It is not always obvious which patients will benefit from electrical cardioversion since there is no evidence that conversion of atrial fibrillation to sinus rhythm lowers the incidence of stroke or prolongs life. Furthermore, there is little evidence that antiarrhythmic drug therapy to maintain sinus rhythm following cardioversion lowers the incidence of stroke, has a favorable impact on cardiovascular mortality, or provides long-term prevention of recurrent atrial fibrillation.

The effectiveness of verapamil in controlling symptoms by limiting the inappropriately rapid ventricular rate during exercise contrasts with the low success of restoring and maintaining sinus rhythm with other antiarrhythmic drugs. Many patients with atrial fibrillation and hemodynamically significant organic heart disease are probably best managed by effective control of the ventricular rate rather than by heroic attempts to cardiovert atrial fibrillation and maintain sinus rhythm.

Cardioversion

Most patients with new-onset atrial fibrillation generally will revert spontaneously to sinus rhythm within 24 hours of hospitalization. Patients who are hypotensive, symptomatic with angina pectoris, or dyspneic should be treated with immediate synchronized direct current (DC) cardioversion. In the absence of such symptoms, electric cardioversion should be delayed. Although the risks for complications from spontaneous cardioversion are low, patients should be monitored with telemetry of the ECG. Digitalis does not facilitate conversion, but rather aids in control of the resting ventricular response. Quinidine sulfate (200–300 mg q6h), quinidine sulfate in a time-released capsule (300 mg q8h), or quinidine gluconate (325 mg po q8h) given with digitalis may facilitate cardioversion. High-dose loading of quinidine is not recommended; however, an additional dose of quinidine given 3 hours after the initial dose may help to achieve steady-state serum levels more rapidly. Monitoring of serum drug levels and of the ECG for development of the long QT syndrome or proarrhythmic effects of the drugs is recommended. In general, quinidine should not be administered without digitalis.

If a patient does not convert to sinus rhythm spontaneously or with the combination of digitalis and quinidine within 24 hours of admission, electric cardioversion of the rhythm can be performed. If electric cardioversion is not performed at this time, it is advisable to begin anticoagulation therapy with heparin followed by warfarin sodium (Coumadin), and plan readmission to the hospital for electric cardioversion in 2 to 3 weeks. Following cardioversion, warfarin should probably be continued for an additional 2 to 3 weeks.

Stroke or systemic embolism occurs in approximately 5% of patients cardioverted to sinus rhythm and may occur days to weeks following cardioversion. Whether atrial fibrillation is paroxysmal or chronic does not appear to influence the rate of systemic embolism.

Patients who have been in atrial fibrillation for many months to a year and patients with an enlarged left atrium by echocardiogram should probably not be cardioverted.

Preventing Recurrences

Once the patient has returned to sinus rhythm, the question of maintenance drug therapy must be addressed. A prolonged P wave on ECG, a left atrial internal dimension of over 45 mm on echocardiography, left ventricular hypertrophy, mitral valve disease, and congestive heart failure predispose to recurrent atrial fibrillation. The proportion of patients who revert to atrial fibrillation following cardioversion is high and 75 to 85% of patients not maintained on antiarrhythmic drugs revert to atrial fibrillation at 1 and 2 years, respectively. Despite this high failure rate, it is reasonable to make a first attempt to maintain sinus rhythm without antiarrhythmic drugs. All of these drugs have potential toxicity, and patients most likely to maintain sinus rhythm do so without antiarrhythmic drugs. Although maintenance of sinus rhythm is improved by quinidine-like drugs, the majority of patients so treated will revert to atrial fibrillation within several years.

If an antiarrhythmic drug is used, drug levels should be followed closely and QRS width, QT interval, and any changes in ventricular ectopy monitored. If recurrent episodes cannot be prevented by quinidine, success may be achieved with flecainide, propafenone, or amiodarone. These drugs should be used in consultation with a cardiologist with electrophysiologic experience. Lone atrial fibrillation is often paroxysmal and self-terminating and may be refractory to multiple antiarrhythmic drugs.

Controlling the Ventricular Response
Digitalis is unlikely to prevent recurrences of atrial fibrillation. However, for most patients, digitalis in an oral dose of 0.125 to 0.25 mg/day supplemented by verapamil, 80 to 120 mg three to four times a day, or a beta-blocking drug such as propranolol (80–120 mg/day) is highly effective in controlling the ventricular response to atrial fibrillation. Digitalis alone is generally not effective in controlling the ventricular response to atrial fibrillation. This is particularly true if the patient is febrile, thyrotoxic, hypotensive, or under high catecholamine stimulation from any cause. Moreover, digitalis even in high doses rarely controls the inappropriate increase in ventricular response with mild exertion or exercise. In general, verapamil is better tolerated than propranolol since it preserves the patient's exercise capacity.

In patients with chronic atrial fibrillation, the ventricular response is often inadequately controlled. Commonly, the ventricular response may be controlled at rest with ventricular rates less than 100 per minute. However, ventricular rates increase rapidly, and inappropriately with trivial levels of exercise. The addition of verapamil, diltiazem, or a beta-blocking drug to the medical regimen limits this increase in ventricular rate, improves patients' symptoms, and restores exercise performance. The effectiveness of control of the ventricular response to exercise should be evaluated by exercise testing in most ambulatory patients. This evaluation may often be performed in the physician's office using a treadmill, bicycle, or other standardized exercise testing procedure.

Anticoagulation
There is considerable variation in prescribing anticoagulants to patients with atrial fibrillation. In young patients with lone atrial fibrillation, the risk of most anticoagulants is probably greater than the risk associated with embolization. However, patients with atrial fibrillation and mitral valve disease, and patients with a history of stroke, congestive heart failure, a dilated left atrium, or other forms of organic heart disease should generally receive such therapy. Moreover, since atrial fibrillation will reoccur in many patients converted to sinus rhythm, anticoagulation may be considered in patients who have a high likelihood of reverting to atrial fibrillation. Either aspirin (325 mg/day) or warfarin (to maintain prothrombin time ratio between 1.3 and 1.8 times control) is effective in short-term prophylaxis of systemic embolization. Warfarin rather than aspirin is preferred for patients with rheumatic heart disease, serious mitral valvular disease, or a history of embolization.

Atwood JE, et al. Effect of beta-adrenergic blockade on exercise performance in patients with chronic atrial fibrillation. J Am Coll Cardiol 1987; 10:314–20.
A beta-blocking drug improves rate control during exercise, but in contrast to verapamil, does not necessarily improve exercise performance.

Channer KS, et al. Towards improved control of atrial fibrillation. Eur Heart J 1987; 8:141–7.
Good review of the importance of adequate rate control in chronic atrial fibrillation.

Davidson E, et al. Atrial fibrillation: cause and time of onset. Arch Intern Med 1989; 149:457–9.
Reviews the clinical presentation, and short-term outcome of atrial fibrillation of patients presenting to a hospital emergency room.

Falk RH, et al. Digoxin for converting recent-onset atrial fibrillation to sinus rhythm: a randomized, double-blind trial. Ann Intern Med 1987; 106:503–6.
Most patients with new-onset atrial fibrillation revert to sinus rhythm spontaneously and digitalis does not aid in conversion.

Kannel WB, et al. Epidemiologic features of chronic atrial fibrillation: the Framingham Study. N Engl J Med 1982; 306:1018–22.
Etiology, incidence, prevalence, and natural history of atrial fibrillation.

Kopecky SL, et al. The natural history of lone atrial fibrillation: a population-based study over three decades. N Engl J Med 1987; 317:669–74.
Epidemiology of atrial fibrillation in the absence of organic heart disease.

Lundstrom T, Ryden L. Chronic atrial fibrillation: long-term results of direct current conversion. Acta Med Scand 1988; 223:53–9.
Most patients electrically cardioverted to sinus rhythm revert to atrial fibrillation within 1 to 2 years.

Rich EC, Siebold C, Campion B. Alcohol-related acute atrial fibrillation: a case-control study and review of 40 patients. Arch Intern Med 1985; 145:830–3.
Holiday heart syndrome: acute alcohol intoxication may predispose to atrial fibrillation.

Simpson RJ Jr, et al. The electrophysiologic substrate of atrial fibrillation. PACE 1983; 6:1166–70.
Reviews physiologic mechanism for initiation and maintenance of atrial fibrillation.

Stroke Prevention in Atrial Fibrillation Study Group Investigators. Preliminary report of the Stroke Prevention in Atrial Fibrillation Study. N Engl J Med 1990; 322:863–8.
In atrial fibrillation not due to rheumatic heart disease, antithrombotic therapy with warfarin or aspirin is effective in short-term prevention of stroke. Relative benefits of aspirin and warfarin remain unclear.

Weinberg DM, Mancini GBJ. Anticoagulation for cardioversion of atrial fibrillation. Am J Cardiol 1989; 63:745–6.
Advantages and disadvantages of anticoagulation in atrial fibrillation.

Dunn M, et al. Antithrombotic therapy in atrial fibrillation. Chest 1989; 95:118S–27S.
A review of anticoagulation.

33. PACEMAKERS
Andreas T. Wielgosz

Although the management of patients with implanted cardiac pacemakers is often supervised by a cardiologist, other clinicians must be able to recognize complications as they occur. Over 250,000 patients in the United States have artificial pacemakers, produced by some 27 companies worldwide. In spite of increasing technologic complexities, there remain three basic characteristics for each pacemaker: sensing, power, and capture. Sensing is the receiving and processing of electric signals generated by the heart. Power is the ability of the pacemaker to provide stimulation as required. Capture describes the appropriate stimulation of the heart by the pacemaker. Rate responsiveness, a relatively new function in some pacemakers, is the ability to regulate the rate, usually in response to the demand of physical activity. All pacemakers have a built-in replacement indicator, and most units implanted today are also programmable.

Complications

Local Complications

Infections around the implanted pacemaker are now very uncommon because of improved techniques. Most occur within 3 months of surgery and may present with constitutional symptoms as well as local inflammation. Tenderness and shifting or erosion at the pacemaker site can also occur without infection.

Occasionally patients with pacemakers have muscular distress. The most common syndrome is diaphragmatic stimulation, usually from phrenic nerve activation (because of its proximity to the apex of the heart). Often, the pectoralis muscle is stimulated, a problem that can be corrected in programmable pacemakers by decreasing the voltage. If muscular stimulation occurs around the pacing wires or near the pacemaker of a bipolar system, it usually indicates an electric leak.

Pacemaker Failure

About 10% of all failures (i.e., any deviation from intended function) are reported within the first week of implantation. After 1 week, only 10% of failures are accompanied by the return of symptoms; most are asymptomatic when they are first detected. In one study of 340 pacemaker failures occurring in 1705 patients over 4 years, 50% were due to lead-related problems (mainly dislodgment), 41% were battery failures, and 5% were electronic component failures. Dysrhythmias unrelated to the pacemaker occurred in 4% of failures.

Poor sensing may be due to reception of an inadequate cardiac signal, either because the lead is malpositioned or because there is an increase in threshold at the electrode-myocardial interface. Failure to sense may be accompanied by failure to capture. Usually the lead is implanted through the cephalic, subclavian, or jugular vein into the right ventricular endocardium. Fixation may be active, by screw mechanism, or passive, by barb fixation. A dislodged or fractured lead may be detected by x-ray. When no radiologic abnormalities are seen, analysis of the stimulus artifact is a sensitive way of detecting wire fracture or failure secondary to insulation disruption. Some pacemakers can be evaluated with real-time telemetry: A very low impedance suggests a break in insulation and a very high impedance suggests a fracture in the lead wire or poor connection of the lead to the generator.

Oversensing is a response of the pacemaker to undesired stimuli. The pacemaker may inappropriately sense normal cardiac electric events such as T waves, electromagnetic interference, or small potentials from contraction of the pectoralis muscle underlying the pulse generator. Myopotential inhibition of demand pacemakers can be caused by electric stimuli generated by skeletal muscle. This phenomenon has been reported in 11 to 85% of patients with unipolar lead systems and favors the use of bipolar lead systems.

Failure to capture may be due to lead interruption, exit block, subthreshold generator output, and battery exhaustion.

Power failures can be due to either disturbances in the electronic circuitry, which tend to be a random event, or battery depletion, which is usually a function of time. Beyond 5 years, battery depletion is the leading cause for pacemaker failure. A decline in rate below the fixed setting of the implanted unit is the usual indicator of power source depletion. A small or moderate decline in rate ($< 3\%$ of set rate) usually requires no intervention. However, if the decline continues, the battery needs replacement. Fluctuation in the rate usually indicates instability of the electronic circuit and should be monitored closely. Rate variations can also occur with fever, particularly in lithium-powered units. In most systems, battery depletion is indicated by alterations in pulse width and rate.

Patient Monitoring

While still in the hospital, every patient should be educated about the pacemaker. Most centers provide an instruction book. Important information, such as the model type and serial number of the implanted pacemaker unit, should either be kept in the book or be typed on a special card. This will help to identify the specific characteristics of the system that will be needed in case of complications or manufacturer recall.

After the first visit, 2 weeks after implantation, two additional visits at 3-month intervals are customary, followed by six-monthly checks. After the fifth year, patients with lithium-powered units should be seen every 3 months. Dual-chamber pacemakers (which can stimulate both atria and ventricles) may require more frequent checks. Multiprogrammable pacemakers permit noninvasive analysis of problems; this is best done by a specialist. Likewise, antitachyarrhythmia devices or implantable defibrillators require experienced specialists with sophisticated monitors capable of telemetric analyses.

Monitoring of patients with pacemakers should include inquiries about general health, signs and symptoms of heart failure, syncope, respiratory insufficiency, coronary insufficiency, skin reactions and accompanying pain, hematomas, and thrombosis. It is important to be attentive to the psychological adjustment after implantation and to provide reassurance. Following a physical examination, the patient should have an ECG taken both with and without the application of a magnet, to assess rate, sensory, power, and capture functions of the system. The magnet turns a demand pacemaker into a fixed-rhythm pacemaker.

Many specialized clinics have facilities for monitoring pacemaker systems by transmitting an audible tone by telephone. Usually the entire ECG, both with and without the magnetic mode, is relayed over the telephone. From this, pulse width and rate can be measured. Newer, more sophisticated systems provide additional electronic analyses. Telephone monitoring is used primarily to confirm the presence of pacemaker stimulation and subsequent capture and to assess the power reserve from the magnetic mode rate.

Furman S, Ayes DL, Holmes DR. A practice of cardiac pacing. 2nd ed. Kisco, NY: Futura, 1989.
Written by leading authorities in the field, this book provides an overview of pacing including current follow-up techniques.

Fearnot NE, Smith HJ, Geddes LA. A review of pacemakers that physiologically increase rate: the DDD and rate-responsive pacemakers. Prog Cardiovasc Dis 1986; 29:145–64.
A helpful introduction to the evolving technology of rate-responsive pacemakers.

Barold SS, et al. Modern cardiac pacing. Mt Kisco, NY: Futura, 1985.
More for the experts perhaps, but provides an excellent chapter on dual chamber pacemakers.

Parsonnet V, Bernstein AD. Cardiac pacing in the 1980's: treatment and techniques in transition. J Am Coll Cardiol 1983; 1:339–54.
An excellent, objective discussion of the use of pacemakers. This well-referenced article also provides a good evaluation of dual-chamber pacemakers.

Furman S. Newer modes of cardiac pacing: I. Description of pacing modes. Mod Concepts Cardiovasc Dis 1983; 52:1–5.
Describes the major stimulation modes of dual-chamber pacemakers and explains the new five-position Intersociety Commission for Heart Disease (ICHD) code.

Furman S. Newer modes of cardiac pacing: II. Intraoperative evaluation and selection of pacemakers for bradyarrhythmias. Mod Concepts Cardiovasc Dis 1983; 52:7–10.
Discusses the selection of the appropriate dual-chamber pacing system in order to restore normal physiologic, atrioventricular function.

Griffin JG, et al. Pacemaker follow-up: its role in the detection and correction of a pacemaker system malfunction. PACE 1986; 9:387–91.
Practical advice with insightful comments on patient monitoring.

34. HEART MURMURS
Park W. Willis IV

Careful auscultation in quiet surroundings frequently reveals cardiac murmurs in healthy individuals and patients without diagnosed heart disease. The distinction between an innocent and pathologic murmur can usually be made by a history and thorough cardiovascular examination. The amplitude, location, and timing of a murmur are important; however, diagnosis also depends on examination of carotid, jugular venous, and precordial pulses and heart sounds.

Systolic Murmurs

Under optimal conditions, systolic murmurs are audible with a stethoscope in 50 to 70% of normal children and adolescents. In early adulthood, systolic murmurs are less frequently detected, but the prevalence of systolic murmurs gradually increases, to reach approximately 50% in individuals over 50 years old.

Midsystolic (ejection) murmurs begin after the first heart sound (S_1), terminate before the related semilunar valve closure, and have a crescendo-decrescendo contour. These murmurs are caused by turbulence of flow as blood is ejected from the ventricle, across the aortic or pulmonic valve into a great vessel. The amplitude of a midsystolic ejection murmur varies with stroke volume; it may be diminished with premature beats and increases after long diastolic filling periods following a premature beat or during atrial fibrillation.

Pansystolic (regurgitant) murmurs are caused by turbulent flow from a high- to a low-pressure chamber. These murmurs begin with S_1 and continue through the related semilunar valve closure sound. Unlike ejection murmurs, pansystolic regurgitant murmurs often have a smooth, blowing quality and their amplitude does not change significantly with changes in diastolic filling period length.

Late systolic murmurs begin in mid or late systole and continue up to and sometimes through S_2.

Early systolic murmurs begin with S_1 and end in mid or late systole before S_2. These murmurs are caused by the same lesions responsible for pansystolic murmurs. However, because of conditions in the chamber accepting the regurgitant volume, the pressure rises to equal that in the donor chamber in late systole, decreasing retrograde flow and causing the murmur to diminish before S_2.

Innocent Murmurs

An innocent murmur occurs in the absence of any abnormality of cardiac structure of function. Murmurs associated with an abnormally large cardiac output and those caused by a selective increase in flow through a valve, such as midsystolic ejection murmurs associated with aortic regurgitation or atrial septal defect, are not considered innocent.

Innocent systolic murmurs are midsystolic and usually grade 1 to 2 of a possible 6 in amplitude. They may be louder in thin children and young adults when the stethoscope on the chest wall is close to the source of the murmur and when the cardiac output is increased by anemia, anxiety, fever, or pregnancy. Innocent murmurs are usually best heard at the left sternal edge in the second and third intercostal spaces and tend to decrease, or disappear, with upright position. A common form of innocent systolic murmur (Still's murmur) is twanging, vibratory, or grunting in quality and loudest at the lower sternal border and midprecordium. This murmur is usually found in children. In the majority of cases, it disappears during puberty but may persist into adulthood.

The cardiorespiratory murmur is an unusual type of innocent systolic murmur. It is loudest during inspiration and markedly reduced, or absent, during expiration and with breath-holding. The murmur has a high frequency and is heard best at the left sternal edge or apex. It is probably caused by the heart compressing and decompressing a portion of lung or bronchus so that the murmur is actually a breath sound.

If a systolic murmur is innocent, the carotid, jugular venous, and left ventricular apex pulses are normal; S_1 is of normal amplitude; S_2 shows physiologic splitting; and there are no abnormal extra sounds, or diastolic murmurs.

Midsystolic Murmurs in Middle and Old Age

Midsystolic murmurs in middle and old age are common and are similar to the innocent murmurs of younger individuals. The sound is maximal at the left sternal edge or aortic area but are often heard best at the apex. The amplitude frequently reaches grade 2 to 3 of 6. Because the murmurs are usually associated with some minor underlying cardiac abnormality, they are not truly innocent. Age-related thickening of the base of the aortic valve cusps (aortic sclerosis), hypertension, and dilation of the aortic root are frequent causes. In the absence of other disease, the carotid pulse is normal. When there is associated left ventricular hypertrophy, the cause of a midsystolic murmur may be calcific aortic stenosis.

Pathologic Midsystolic Murmurs
These are caused by aortic or pulmonic stenosis or atrial septal defect and may be confused with innocent murmurs in children and young adults.

Semilunar valve stenosis of mild degree is almost always associated with an ejection sound quality. These are discrete, high-frequency sounds that follow S_1 by about 0.04 to 0.06 second. Aortic ejection sounds are widely transmitted over the precordium and are usually loudest at the apex, while pulmonic ejection sounds are localized to the left sternal edge and show respiratory variation, increasing in amplitude with expiration and decreasing or disappearing with inspiration. When the degree of semilunar valve stenosis is mild, the murmurs are maximal in midsystole, similar to an innocent murmur. With increasing obstruction to blood flow, they become longer and reach maximal amplitude later in systole. Important valvular stenosis causes hypertrophy of the related ventricle, which can be detected as a sustained apical impulse or parasternal lift. S_2 is normal in mild aortic stenosis. The pulmonic component (P_2) is delayed and often diminished in amplitude in valvular pulmonic stenosis.

Although the midsystolic murmur of valvular aortic stenosis is typically heard best at the aortic area, in elderly patients it is frequently the loudest at the apex. In adults with moderate-to-severe aortic valvular stenosis, there may be no ejection sound, and the S_2 may diminish because leaflet excursion is limited by calcification. When S_2 is diminished and not well transmitted to the apex, it may be difficult to decide whether the murmur is mid- or pansystolic. When premature beats are present, a murmur that is louder after long diastolic filling periods is an important clue to outflow tract obstruction. The carotid pulse is abnormal in most patients with significant left ventricular outflow obstruction.

In the patient with a straight back due to the absence of a normal thoracic kyphosis, marked pectus excavatum, or a combination of the two, the heart is sandwiched between the thoracic vertebrae and sternum. This may narrow the ventricular outflow tracts and there is often an associated midsystolic murmur at the pulmonic area; although the heart is normal, wide physiologic splitting of S_1 and S_2 may be present. The physical examination and chest x-ray should alert the physician to this benign condition. Echocardiography may be required to exclude atrial septal defect, semilunar valve stenosis, and mitral valve prolapse.

Hemodynamically significant atrial septal defects are associated with large right ventricular stroke volumes and a midsystolic pulmonic ejection murmur that is identical in character to an innocent murmur. However, other clues to the correct diagnosis are often present. A prominent right ventricular impulse at the left sternal edge is usually palpable. S_1 is often widely split because of increased blood flow over the tricuspid valve and delayed tricuspid closure, and S_2 is usually widely split with little respiratory variation. In children and young adults with significant left-to-right shunts, a middiastolic rumble is usually audible at the lower left sternal edge.

The systolic murmur in idiopathic hypertrophic subaortic stenosis (IHSS) is midsystolic and usually loudest at the left sternal edge, rather than at the aortic area. The murmur is often associated with a sustained impulse at the left ventricular apex and an S_4. Response of the murmur to physiologic maneuvers provides specific information. The strain phase of Valsalva's maneuver, standing from a squatting position, and inhalation of amyl nitrite increase the midsystolic murmur of IHSS by causing an abrupt fall in systemic venous return, which leads to a decrease in left ventricular cavity size and augmentation of the subaortic left ventricular outflow tract gradient. The innocent midsystolic murmur decreases in amplitude with these maneuvers. Differentiation of IHSS from valvular aortic stenosis can be made by careful examination of a graphic recording of the carotid pulse. In IHSS, the carotid upstroke is brisk and usually bisferious in contour. In most cases of valvular aortic stenosis the rate of rise of the carotid pulse is slow, with a palpable systolic vibration (carotid shudder).

Other causes of midsystolic murmurs include supravalvular aortic stenosis and fibromuscular subaortic stenosis. In these variants there is no ejection sound. With infundibular pulmonic stenosis, the midsystolic murmur is maximal lower along the left sternal border and there is no ejection sound. With valvular as well as infundibular pulmonic stenosis, the pulmonic component of S_2 is delayed and soft if the outflow gradient is significant.

Pansystolic Murmurs
These are always pathologic and are usually caused by mitral regurgitation, tricuspid regurgitation, or ventricular septal defect.

A pansystolic murmur, maximal at the apex and radiating into the axilla, is evidence for mitral regurgitation. The pansystolic murmur of ventricular septal defects is usually loudest at the lower left sternal edge. Tricuspid regurgitation is most commonly a later complication of left-sided heart disease that has resulted in pulmonary hypertension. The murmur of tricuspid regurgitation is usually loudest at the lower left sternal edge, but when the right ventricle is dilated the murmur may be maximal in the fifth intercostal space in the midclavicular line. Audible only during inspiration, inspiratory increase in intensity of the murmur, an abnormal systolic wave in the jugular venous pulse, and hepatic pulsation are helpful aids in recognizing tricuspid regurgitation.

Later Systolic Murmurs
The later systolic murmur of mild mitral regurgitation, resulting from mitral valve prolapse, usually maximal at the apex, may be audible only when the patient is sitting or standing. The murmur is often associated with solitary or multiple mid or late systolic clicks.

Early Systolic Murmurs
Early systolic murmurs are uncommon. Trivial mitral and tricuspid regurgitation are two causes. In acute severe mitral regurgitation, the murmur may terminate before S_2, simulating a midsystolic ejection murmur. Echophonocardiographic studies can distinguish the murmurs when the clinical diagnosis is uncertain.

Diastolic Murmurs
Diastolic murmurs almost always indicate organic heart disease. Early diastolic decrescendo murmurs from aortic or pulmonary regurgitation begin with the appropriate sound of semilunar valve closure and are usually loudest at the left sternal edge. Mid and late diastolic murmurs are most often caused by mitral stenosis. However, they may also be caused by high volume antegrade flow over regurgitant atrioventricular valves; by premature closure of the mitral valve in severe aortic regurgitation (Austin Flint murmur); and by intracardiac shunts, especially atrial or ventricular septal defects.

Continuous Murmurs
Continuous murmurs begin in systole and persist through S_2 into diastole. The most common is the innocent venous hum, which is present in most children and many young adults. The murmur is usually loudest over the medial aspect of the right supraclavicular fossa with the patient sitting and the chin pulled upward and to the left; the murmur decreases in the supine position. Deep inspiration may increase the amplitude of a venous hum, and the murmur can be abolished by firm pressure over the ipsilateral internal jugular vein.

Pathologic continuous murmurs can result from an aortopulmonary connection. The most common of these is patent ductus arteriosus, in which the murmur is loudest at the upper left sternal edge or under the left clavicle. Other causes of continuous murmurs are congenital, traumatic, or surgically constructed arteriovenous fistulae. Coarctation of the aorta and peripheral pulmonary stenosis cause systolic murmurs, but can result in continuous murmurs, loudest in systole, when there is very severe constriction.

Evaluation
When a soft, midsystolic murmur is heard in an asymptomatic child or young adult and the remainder of the cardiovascular examination shows normal findings, there is a strong likelihood that the murmur is innocent. If the murmur disappears with standing or the strain phase of Valsalva's maneuver, the diagnosis of an innocent systolic ejection murmur is firm, and further studies are not necessary. Innocent murmurs are frequently louder with increased cardiac output caused by transient conditions such as exercise, anxiety,

fever, anemia, pregnancy, or thyrotoxicosis. Therefore, repeated examination may be helpful.

When the history, physical findings, response to physiologic maneuvers, or an unusually loud murmur suggests an organic lesion, the 12-lead ECG and chest x-ray are useful in assessing cardiac dimensions and hypertrophy. Echophonocardiography and pulse recordings are very useful when physical findings are equivocal. The greatest value of echocardiography is in the assessment of cardiac disease diagnosed by history, physical examination, chest x-ray, and ECG. Doppler echocardiography is an extremely sensitive diagnostic technique capable of detecting regurgitant flow even in the absence of an audible murmur. Trivial, physiologic amounts of tricuspid and mitral regurgitation are particularly common and when they are detected in a patient with a systolic murmur, the clinician may conclude that the Doppler findings explain the murmur. This may not necessarily be correct. Thoughtful integration of the clinical findings with anatomic information from the two-dimensional echocardiogram is required for accurate interpretation of Doppler data.

Echocardiography is useful in confirming the location and severity of clinically detected valvular lesions. This information is often valuable as part of the initial evaluation and in the follow-up of patients with heart disease.

Leatham A. Auscultation of the heart. Lancet 1958; 2:703–8, 757–65.
A two-part article presenting a classic discussion on auscultation and classification of heart murmurs.

McLaren MJ, et al. Innocent murmurs and third heart sounds in black schoolchildren. Br Heart J 1980; 43:67–73.
Of 12,050 children aged 2 to 18 years, 96.0% had physiologic S_3, 72.0% had innocent systolic murmurs, and 0.27% had innocent middiastolic murmurs.

Perloff JK. Clinical recognition of aortic stenosis: the physical signs and differential diagnosis of various forms of obstruction to the left ventricular outflow. Prog Cardiovasc Dis 1968; 10:323.
An extensive review of the subject.

Bruns DL, VanDerHauwaert LG. The aortic systolic murmur developing with increasing age. Br Heart J 1958; 20:370–8.
Systolic murmurs were present in 150 (50%) of 300 patients over 50 years old.

Barlow J, Kincaid-Smith P. The auscultatory findings in hypertension. Br Heart J 1960; 22:505–14.
Of 100 patients with hypertension, 71 were found to have systolic ejection murmurs.

Tavel ME. Innocent murmurs. In: Leon DF, Shaver JA, eds. Physiologic principles of heart sounds and murmurs. New York: American Heart Association, 1975:102–6.
An excellent discussion.

Sutton GC, Craige E. Clinical signs of severe acute mitral regurgitation. Am J Cardiol 1967; 20:141–4.
A case report and discussion of the pathophysiology underlying the clinical manifestations of acute severe mitral regurgitation.

Grimmer SFM, Tindall H, Hill JD. Diagnostic contribution of echocardiography. Lancet 1982; 1:440–1.
Only 5% of echocardiographic examinations revealed a diagnosis when there was no clinical cardiac diagnosis prior to the study.

Newburger JW, et al. Noninvasive tests in the initial evaluation of heart murmurs in children. N Engl J Med 1983; 308:61–4.
Routine ECG, chest X-rays, and M-mode echocardiography rarely improved on the diagnosis made by qualified pediatric cardiologists on the basis of history and physical examination.

Rothman A, Goldberger AL. Aids to cardiac auscultation. Ann Intern Med 1983; 99:346–53.

A *critical literature review with emphasis on the sensitivity and specificity of physiologic and pharmacologic maneuvers commonly used to aid in cardiac auscultation.*

Rahko PS. Prevalence of regurgitant murmurs in patients with valvular regurgitation detected by Doppler echocardiography. Ann Intern Med 1989; 111:466–72.
Doppler echocardiography is extremely sensitive for identifying regurgitant lesions.

Lembo NJ, et al. Bedside diagnosis of systolic murmurs. N Engl J Med 1988; 318:1572–8.
Reinforces validity of bedside evaluation.

35. MITRAL VALVE PROLAPSE
Henry J. Kahn

Mitral valve prolapse (MVP) is a condition characterized by posterior and superior displacement of the mitral valve leaflets into the left atrium during systole. Most commonly, the condition is benign, but significant complications, including arrhythmias, endocarditis, stroke, progression of mitral regurgitation, and sudden death, sometimes occur.

Abnormal valvular collagen may play a role in the pathogenesis of this condition. It has been postulated that systolic stress, when applied to the weakened valve structure, results in myxomatous degeneration, redundancy and thickening of the valve leaflets, mitral annulus dilatation, and elongation or rupture of the chordae tendineae. Conditions that are associated with abnormal collagen may also be associated with MVP; these include Marfan's syndrome, osteogenesis imperfecta, and Ehlers-Danlos syndrome.

Prevalence
The prevalence of MVP is approximately 5% when stringent diagnostic criteria are applied to large populations (such as the Framingham cohort). Early studies reported prevalences as high as 20%, especially in populations of young asthenic women. These original estimates, however, were flawed by ascertainment bias (patients referred with signs or symptoms) and by overinterpretation of echocardiogram findings.

Diagnosis

History
In the great majority of patients, MVP produces no specific symptoms and is usually detected as an incidental finding on physical examination. Symptoms of autonomic dysfunction, including palpitations, atypical chest pain, cold extremities, dizziness, fatigue, and anxiety, have been attributed to MVP (the so-called mitral valve prolapse syndrome). Recent studies, however, indicate that these symptoms are just as common in patients without MVP. In addition, patients with dysautonomia have exaggerated cardiovascular responses to autonomic stimuli, whether or not they have MVP.

Patients with a history of embolic stroke who are under the age of 45 should be evaluated for the presence of MVP since the prevalence in this group is between 20 and 40%.

Physical Examination
The classic presentation for MVP is a midsystolic click followed by a late systolic murmur. Both the click and the murmur tend to occur at the same left ventricular (LV) volume in a given patient. For this reason, both are mobile, moving earlier in systole during maneuvers that decrease LV volume (such as standing or Valsalva's maneuver) and later in systole during maneuvers that increase LV volume (such as squatting). In some patients, only a midsystolic mobile click is heard, and in some young patients only a late systolic murmur is heard. Occasionally, MVP is detected as an incidental finding on echocardiogram in a patient with no physical findings. The exact prevalence of "silent MVP" is unknown; it ranges from 8 to 22% in case series to 84% in the population-based Framingham data. Asthenic habitus, thoracic bony abnormalities, and findings suggestive of Marfan's syndrome, Ehlers-Danlos syndrome, or osteogenesis imperfecta are occasionally

noted on examination and may provide clues to the presence of MVP. It has been estimated that a systolic click and/or mitral murmur is present in 67% of echocardiographic-proved MVP, and thoracic bony abnormalities are seen in 41%. The Framingham Study showed that systolic clicks were eight times more common in women and 20 times more common in men with echocardiographic-proved MVP compared to controls. In that study, however, only 13% of the males and 8% of the females with MVP had clicks, 3% of males and 11% of females with MVP had a mitral murmur, and only 2% of females and no males with MVP had both click and murmur.

Echocardiogram
The echocardiogram is currently the "gold standard" for diagnosing MVP, although universal agreement is lacking on the exact criteria. The most widely accepted finding for diagnosis is significant (i.e., ≥ 3 mm) systolic displacement of the mitral valve leaflets into the left atrium on the two-dimensional (2D) parasternal long-axis echocardiographic view. The presence of thickened or redundant valve leaflets and the presence of mitral regurgitation are also significant since these findings are more often seen in patients with the complications of MVP. The exact incidence of thickened leaflets or mitral regurgitation in patients with "silent MVP" is unknown, but appears to be quite low. Isolated systolic displacement of the mitral valve leaflets in the apical four-chambered view without displacement noted on the parasternal long-axis view is considered a variant of normal and should no longer be used to make a diagnosis of MVP.

Complications

The most common "complication" of MVP is overmedicalization for a condition that is entirely benign for the majority of patients. Many patients experience a great deal of unfounded anxiety and fear because they believe that they have a serious cardiac abnormality. Extensive or repetitive testing may heighten those feelings and therefore should be avoided unless the test results will have a significant impact on the patient's management.

Arrhythmias commonly seen in patients with MVP include premature ventricular contractions, complex ventricular arrhythmias, couplets, and supraventricular arrhythmias. These arrhythmias, however, are also common in the general population. Although the Framingham Study showed a slight trend toward more frequent supraventricular tachycardias and premature ventricular contractions in patients with MVP when compared to matched controls without MVP, this trend was not statistically significant. The main risk factor for arrhythmias appears to be mitral regurgitation associated with MVP, especially if accompanied by evidence of left atrial enlargement or left ventricular dysfunction.

The relative risk of infective endocarditis is increased in MVP by three- to eightfold, although the absolute risk remains low (the risk of endocarditis in the general population is estimated to be 5/100,000). The major risk factor for the development of endocarditis appears to be the presence of thickened or redundant leaflets. In one study, 12 (3.5%) of 334 patients with diffuse thickening and redundancy of the valve leaflets developed endocarditis, a 70-fold increase over the baseline risk. Mitral regurgitation appears to increase the relative risk by 4- to 13-fold over the baseline risk, and males with MVP have about a sevenfold increase in the relative risk. Increased risk is also reported in patients over the age of 45, although this may be in part due to the increased prevalence of mitral regurgitation in older patients. In MVP patients without mitral regurgitation, leaflet thickening, or redundancy, the risk appears to be no higher than in the general population.

The relative risk of stroke is probably increased in MVP patients under the age of 45, although the data are conflicting. The absolute risk of stroke in the under-45 population is 3 per 100,000; the risk in patients under the age of 45 with MVP is estimated to be 1 per 6000. Isolated MVP does not appear to increase the risk of stroke in the over-45 population. Atrial fibrillation may arise as a consequence of MVP with mitral regurgitation; in that event, the risk of stroke appears related more to the presence of the arrhythmia than to the MVP.

Mitral regurgitation may progress either gradually or abruptly due to chordal rupture in some patients with MVP. Progression to severe regurgitation requiring valve replacement occurs most often in patients with thickened and redundant leaflets. In a study comparing patients with MVP and thickened leaflets to those with thin leaflets, severe regurgitation was found in 12% of patients with abnormal leaflets compared to 0% of patients with thin leaflets. Similarly, 6.6% of patients with abnormal leaflets required valve replacement, compared to 0.7% of patients with thin leaflets. In a review of the progression of regurgitation, the risk of developing regurgitation severe enough to require surgery was found to be minimal in patients below the age of 50, but rose from 0.5% at age 50 to about 4% at age 70 for men; for women the risk was less than one-half that of men.

The exact risk of sudden death in patients with MVP is unknown but appears to be extremely small. The main risk factors are moderate-to-severe mitral regurgitation, and thickened redundant leaflets, combined with frequent premature ventricular contractions.

Approach to Managing Patients

There are no universally accepted guidelines regarding the approach to patients with known or suspected MVP, and each case should be evaluated with appropriate clinical judgment rather than following a rigid algorithm. General recommendations, however, can be made based on the information presented above.

Patients who present with mild autonomic symptoms but no physical findings, or patients with an isolated click but no murmur on physical examination, need reassurance rather than an echocardiogram; these individuals are unlikely to have mitral regurgitation or thickened redundant valves, and their risk of serious complications is probably no greater than in the general population. Echocardiography is likewise not indicated for asymptomatic patients with clicks and/or late systolic murmurs. Excessive diagnostic testing may enhance the patient's perception that something is seriously wrong and is unlikely to yield information that would change management. These patients do often benefit from the assurance that (1) the symptoms do not represent serious pathology; (2) their condition will be followed periodically, and tests can always be performed at a later date should the symptoms worsen or new physical findings occur; and (3) the symptoms need not be attributed to a psychological disorder. Patients may also benefit when concerns about cardiac health are used as a reminder to follow health-related behaviors, such as smoking cessation, weight reduction, cholesterol and hypertension control, moderate exercise, and avoidance of drugs, alcohol, caffeine, over-the-counter stimulants, and decongestants.

Patients who have an incidental finding of MVP on echocardiography with no physical findings and no sign of mitral regurgitation or thickened, redundant leaflets can similarly be reassured.

Patients who have severe dizziness or syncope not due to other obvious causes may need ambulatory ECG monitoring and possibly an echocardiogram if significant dysrhythmias are noted. Beta-blocker therapy is sometimes used in such patients, although few data are available to support their efficacy.

Patients who have known or suspected MVP with the holosystolic murmur of mitral regurgitation on physical examination require an echocardiogram only if this will change the management. The same recommendation applies to patients with findings atypical for MVP but indicative of mitral regurgitation. The presence of either mitral regurgitation or thickened, redundant leaflets probably warrants the use of antibiotic prophylaxis to prevent endocarditis, although studies that prove efficacy are lacking. In patients without regurgitation or thickened leaflets, routine antibiotic prophylaxis is not indicated since the risk of adverse reaction to the antibiotic probably exceeds the risk of endocarditis. Recommended regimens for antibiotic prophylaxis are discussed in Chapter 37.

Patients with a stroke or transient ischemic attack who are under the age of 45 should be studied with an echocardiogram to determine if a high-risk MVP is present. These patients should be placed on antiplatelet therapy such as aspirin if there are no contraindications.

Patients with MVP and significant mitral regurgitation or thickened redundant valve leaflets should be followed with repeat history and cardiac examinations in order to determine whether valve surgery will be required. Periodic echocardiograms after the age of 50 may also be helpful. The optimum frequency of examinations has not been determined.

Patients with MVP who have sustained ventricular tachycardia or an episode of cardiac arrest should be considered for an electrophysiologic study and managed with appropriate antiarrhythmic therapy similar to patients without MVP.

Boudoulas H. Mitral valve prolapse: cardiac arrest with long term survival. Int J Cardiol 1990; 26:37–44.
No single finding predicts cardiac arrest consistently. Survivors had a good long-term prognosis, suggesting that ventricular fibrillation may have been an isolated event.

Deng YB. Follow-up in mitral valve prolapse by phonocardiography, M-mode and two-dimensional echocardiography and Doppler echocardiography. Am J Cardiol 1990; 65:349–54.
Retrospective study showing a higher incidence of hemodynamically significant valve abnormalities in patients with systolic murmurs, compared to those without.

Levy D, Savage D. Prevalence and clinical features of mitral valve prolapse. Am Heart J 1987; 113:1281–90.
A good general review.

MacMahon SW, et al. Mitral valve prolapse and infective endocarditis. Am Heart J 1987; 113:1291–98.
A comprehensive review of relative and absolute risks of infective endocarditis in various subgroups of patients with MVP is presented.

Marks AR, et al. Identification of high-risk and low-risk subgroups of patients with mitral-valve prolapse. N Engl J Med 1989; 320:1031–6.
Retrospective review defined low- and high-risk groups based on the absence or presence of thickened, redundant leaflets. Significant increased risk was demonstrated for endocarditis, moderate-to-severe mitral regurgitation, and need for valve replacement, but the risk of cerebrovascular accident was similar in both groups.

Nishimura RA, et al. Follow-up observations in patients with mitral valve prolapse. Herz 1988; 13:326–34.
Overall, the risk of endocarditis from MVP is low, but appears to be associated with the presence of a murmur, older age, male sex, and redundant leaflets. Other risks appear to be associated with the presence of thickened leaflets.

Perloff JK Child JS. Clinical and epidemiological issues in mitral valve prolapse: overview and perspective. Am Heart J 1987; 113:1324–32.
A review of clinical features, diagnostic criteria as suggested by the National Institutes of Health, and risk of complications.

Quill TE, Lipkin M, Greenland P. The medicalization of normal variants: the case of mitral valve prolapse. J Gen Intern Med 1988; 3:267–76.
A good discussion of the risks of overmedicalizing MVP.

Savage DD, et al. Mitral valve prolapse in the general population: the Framingham Study. Am Heart J 1983; 106:571–86.
Part 1 reviews prevalence in the Framingham cohort; part 2 reviews clinical features; and part 3 reviews dysrhythmias.

Schatz IJ. Orthostatic hypotension, catecholamines, and alpha-adrenergic receptors in mitral valve prolapse. West J Med 1990; 152:37–40.
No association between the above parameters and MVP could be demonstrated, when compared to controls.

Taylor AA, et al. Spectrum of dysautonomia in mitral valve prolapse. Am J Med 1989; 86:267.
Evidence for dysautonomia may be present in symptomatic patients, whether or not MVP is present. An exaggerated chronotropic response to isoproterenol was noted in patients with MVP, of uncertain significance.

Wilcken DE, et al. Lifetime risk for patients with mitral valve prolapse of developing severe valve regurgitation requiring surgery. Circulation 1988; 78:10–14.
Retrospective review of 50 patients in New South Wales who required valve surgery in 1982 for complications of MVP.

36. PROSTHETIC VALVES
Andreas T. Wielgosz

Prosthetic valves today are either mechanical or tissue. Mechanical valves may be described as ball-in-cage, tilting disk, or bileaflet. Tissue valves are described as porcine, homographs, or pericardial. The choice of a specific valve is usually determined by the availability and experience with that model at a given surgical center. In general, because of durability, a mechanical valve is preferred for younger patients. Designs are numerous and attempts to improve performance and minimize the risk of complications are ongoing.

Patient survival time with prosthetic valves has improved markedly in recent years. Mechanical valves should outlive the patient, and tissue valves may need replacement between 8 and 15 years.

Primary Concerns

Thromboembolism
Thromboembolism is the major complication of prosthetic valves. The introduction of cloth-covered prostheses and the use of tissue valves have substantially decreased the frequency of systemic embolization. The risk is greater with artificial mitral valves (3–5%/patient/year) than with artificial aortic valves (1–3%/patient/year). Patients with an enlarged left atrium, in atrial fibrillation, and with inadequate anticoagulation are especially at risk for embolic events.

Thrombotic material can either rest on the valve, causing dysfunction, or embolize into the systemic circulation. The former may be accompanied by the muffling or loss of prosthetic valve opening sounds or by new murmurs of regurgitation; knowledge of the character of the heart sounds in the early postoperative period may be crucial to detecting the buildup of thrombotic material.

Doppler echocardiography is being used more and more to evaluate prostheses dysfunction. In addition to a baseline reading, shortly after implantation of the valve, echocardiographic assessment should be a part of the routine follow-up at 6- or 12-month intervals, depending on the stability of the patient's condition. Technical difficulties often limit the interpretation although color Doppler may be particularly helpful in identifying paravalvular leaks. Interpretation is more accurate when baseline records taken immediately after implantation are available. When valve dysfunction from a thrombus is suspected, transesophageal echocardiography may be helpful.

All patients with mechanical valves should be treated with the anticoagulant warfarin indefinitely. Patients with tissue valves generally receive no anticoagulation therapy unless they have an enlarged left atrium, atrial fibrillation, or a history of emboli. Taking aspirin or dipyridamole in addition to warfarin has not been shown to reduce the risk of embolization, except in patients with older Starr-Edwards prostheses. Patients with mechanical prostheses, especially older models, who have an embolic episode despite adequate anticoagulation therapy should be considered for reoperation and insertion of a tissue valve.

Endocarditis
The incidence of infective endocarditis with prosthetic valves has declined over the years to an overall rate of less than 4% per year. Early infection (i.e., within 2 months of insertion) usually occurs by contamination at the time of surgery. Staphylococcus is the usual organism; fungal or gram-negative organisms are less common. Mortality remains high (65–85%).

Late endocarditis, occurring at least 60 days after insertion, is most often a streptococcal infection. Mortality is 35 to 45%. Management is the same as for endocarditis affecting natural valves. Because the symptoms of endocarditis are often nonspecific, suspicion is the key to early diagnosis. Any fever lasting more than 48 hours with a murmur (especially if new) should stimulate efforts to rule out endocarditis. Up to six samples of blood may be necessary to indicate bacteremia; the majority of positive cultures are obtained with the first two samples. In 10% of patients with endocarditis, cultures show no bacterial growth. When culture reports are negative, the decision to use antibiotics is difficult and should be made on clinical grounds.

Hemolysis
Hemolysis is uncommon with modern mechanical valves. When present, it may indicate a structural defect. Other factors contributing to hemolysis include perivalvular regurgitation and a high transvalvular pressure gradient (i.e., disproportionate valve size). Iron deficiency anemia, even when secondary to hemolysis, may aggravate the hemolytic process. When hemolysis is mild, iron and folic acid supplements may suffice. In severe hemolysis, it may be necessary to replace the valve.

Longevity and Valve Breakdown
Mechanical breakdown can occur, particularly with older valve models. The incidence of breakdown in new prostheses is less than 1% per year. Tissue valves tend to have a higher incidence of failure than mechanical valves, a factor to be considered in younger patients. The risk is greater with the valve in the mitral rather than aortic position. Other problems include ball variance found with Silastic rubber poppets, a cocked disk, fracture of balls or struts, and valve dehiscence (i.e., disruption of the suture line around the prosthesis). The resulting changes in clinical status may range from subtle (e.g., fatigue) to dramatic (e.g., acute congestive failure). Telltale findings are variations in intensity or loss of opening sounds, as thrombus accumulates on newly exposed surfaces, and murmurs of regurgitation due to incomplete closure of the valve or separation of the valve from the adjacent tissue.

Patient Monitoring

Follow-up
Follow-up of a patient with a prosthetic valve involves close monitoring not only of the valve itself, but also of the patient's overall cardiac function. Congestive heart failure, dysrhythmias, and coronary insufficiency must be treated as necessary. Patients with prosthetic valves undergoing general surgery or dental work require careful anticoagulation and bacterial endocarditis prophylaxis (see Chap. 37). During the first 3 months of pregnancy, subcutaneous heparin is recommended to avoid the teratogenic effects of warfarin; in the last 2 months, heparin is recommended to reduce the danger of bleeding. It can be stopped at the time of delivery. Bacterial endocarditis prophylaxis is recommended during the delivery.

Referral
Most large centers involved in the implantation of prosthetic valves have follow-up clinics to which patients should be referred when serious complications are suspected. Careful assessment of function and structural integrity of the valve may require diagnostic studies available only at such centers.

Silverman NA, Levitsky S. Current choices for prosthetic valve replacement. Mod Concepts Cadiovasc Dis 1983; 52:35–9.
  A succinct review of the major types of prosthetic valves, relating advantages and shortcomings to published reports as well as personal experience.

Kloster FE. Diagnosis and management of complications of prosthetic heart valves. Am J Cardiol 1975; 35:872–85.
  Deals with the major short-term and long-term complications seen in patients with prosthetic heart valves and provides recommendations for management.

Bonchek LI. Indications for surgery of the mitral valve. Am J Cardiol 1980; 46:155–8.
  Since no randomized trial has evaluated valvular operations, indications for valvular surgery are often based on the experience gained at specific centers. This article reviews the practice at the Milwaukee Regional Medical Center.

Smith ND, Raizada V, Abrams J. Auscultation of the normal functional prosthetic valve. Ann Intern Med 1981; 95:594–8.
  Reviews the auscultatory findings of the major types of prosthetic devices.

Rahimtoola SH. Valvular heart disease: a perspective. J Am Coll Cardiol 1983; 1:199–215.
An excellent, well-referenced review of valve replacement. Several associated issues including concomitant bypass surgery are discussed.

Brandenburg RO, et al. Infective endocarditis–a 25 year overview of diagnosis and therapy. J Am Coll Cardiol 1983; 1:280–91.
A description of the epidemiologic changes seen in the last 25 years. Complications and indications for surgery are well presented. The use of echocardiography is reviewed. Good references are provided.

Saour JN, et al. Trial of different intensities of anticoagulation in patients with prosthetic heart valves. N Engl J Med 1990; 428–32.
Lower doses of anticoagulants (warfarin) can provide protection comparable to more intensive therapy, but at less risk.

37. ENDOCARDITIS PROPHYLAXIS
Park W. Willis IV

Infective endocarditis is an uncommon serious complication of cardiac disease that results from microorganisms proliferating on damaged or abnormal endothelium. Despite major advances in antibiotic therapy and cardiovascular surgery, the morbidity and mortality remain significant. Therefore, it is accepted practice to administer antibiotics to susceptible patients whenever they are subjected to a procedure that may cause bacteremia.

Patients at Risk
The incidence of infective endocarditis in the general population has been estimated to be 1.1 to 3.6 per 100,000 per year. Although 20 to 30% of patients with infective endocarditis have no identifiable preexisting cardiac abnormality, many patients who are at risk of infective endocarditis and need endocarditis prophylaxis under the circumstances discussed below can be identified. These patients include those with prosthetic cardiac valves (including biosynthetic valves), most congenital cardiac malformations, surgically constructed systemic-pulmonary shunts, rheumatic and other acquired valvular dysfunction, idiopathic hypertrophic subaortic stenosis (IHSS), previous history of infective endocarditis, and mitral valve prolapse with insufficiency. Endocarditis prophylaxis is not recommended for patients with isolated secundum atrial septal defect, with secundum atrial septal defect impaired without a patch 6 months or earlier, with patent ductus arteriosus ligated and divided 6 months or earlier, or after coronary artery bypass graft (CABG) surgery.

Procedures Causing Risk
Respiratory Tract
It is important for patients at risk to receive regular dental care in order to maintain the best possible oral health. Although dental procedures are the most commonly recognized cause of transient bacteremia, poor oral hygiene and periodontal and periapical infections may induce bacteremia even in the absence of dental procedures. Edentulous patients may develop bacteremia from ulcers caused by dentures. Dental extraction is associated with bacteremia 60 to 90% of the time; periodontal surgery, fillings, and cleaning of teeth cause bacteremia less frequently. Prophylactic antibiotic therapy is recommended for all at-risk patients undergoing dental procedures likely to cause gingival bleeding. Antibiotic prophylaxis is also recommended for instrumentation and operations involving disruption of respiratory mucosa including tonsillectomy, adenoidectomy, and bronchoscopy, which may cause bacteremia. Spontaneous shedding of deciduous teeth and simple adjustment of orthodontic appliances do not present a significant risk of endocarditis and antibiotics are not recommended.

Genitourinary Tract
Urethral and prostatic manipulation often cause bacteremia. For example, at the time of transurethral prostatectomy, about 10% of patients with sterile urine have positive findings on blood culture; with infected urine the incidence of transient bacteremia is about 60%. Although data are inadequate to allow specific recommendations for the entire range of genitourinary procedures, antibiotic prophylaxis is recommended for at-risk patients who undergo cystoscopy, prostatic surgery, urethral catheterization (especially with urinary tract infection), and urinary tract surgery. Brief ("in-and-out") bladder catheterization in patients with sterile urine does not require antibiotic prophylaxis.

Uncomplicated vaginal delivery does not require antibiotic prophylaxis. In the absence of infection, antibiotic prophylaxis is not recommended for at-risk patients who undergo uterine dilatation and curettage, cesarean section, therapeutic abortion, sterilization procedures, and insertion or removal of an intrauterine device. However, patients with prosthetic heart valves or surgically constructed systemic-pulmonary shunts are at especially high risk, and it may be prudent to administer prophylactic antibiotic even for these low-risk procedures.

Gastrointestinal Tract
Bacteremia and endocarditis have been documented in association with gallbladder surgery, colonic surgery, esophageal dilation, sclerotherapy of esophageal varices, colonoscopy, upper GI endoscopy with biopsy, and proctosigmoidoscopic biopsy. Antibiotic prophylaxis for these procedures is therefore recommended for patients at risk. Upper GI endoscopy or proctosigmoidoscopy without biopsy, percutaneous liver biopsy, and barium enema have been associated with bacteremia but rarely, if ever, infective endocarditis. For these procedures, antibiotic prophylaxis is recommended only for patients with prosthetic heart valves or surgically constructed systemic-pulmonary shunts.

Other Indications
At-risk patients who undergo surgical procedures of any infected or contaminated tissues, including incision and drainage of abscesses, should be given antibiotic prophylaxis. Although clinical judgment must be exercised and regimens individualized, antibiotics effective against *Staphylococcus aureus* should be included. Even in the absence of clinically detectable heart disease, patients with a previous history of infective endocarditis are at risk, and antibiotic prophylaxis is recommended. Patients with indwelling transvenous pacemakers, arteriovenous shunt appliances for dialysis, or ventriculoatrial shunts for hydrocephalus appear to be at low risk of endocarditis but cases of endocarditis occurring in these conditions have been documented and prophylaxis may be recommended; antibiotics effective against *S. aureus* should be included.

Patients undergoing diagnostic cardiac catheterization and angiography do not require prophylaxis.

Recommendations

Infective endocarditis is rare. Even though the population at risk is large and bacteremia occurs frequently during dental and surgical procedures, the chance that a single bacteremic episode will cause endocarditis is very small. Therefore, controlled trials of the efficacy of antimicrobial prophylaxis are virtually impossible. Recommendations are based on what is known about the mechanisms of endocarditis, clinical experience and observations regarding the bacteria involved, and the efficacy of various antibiotic regimens in animal models of infective endocarditis. The antibiotic regimens outlined below have been recommended by the American Heart Association Committee on Rheumatic Fever and Infective Endocarditis.

The regimens described in Tables 37-1 and 37-2, for dental and surgical procedures of the upper respiratory tract, are directed against alpha-hemolytic (viridans) streptococci. The parenteral regimens described in Table 37-3, for GI and genitourinary tract surgery and instrumentation, are directed primarily against enterococci.

These are general recommendations. Clinical judgment is always required and individualized regimens are necessary in many cases. Patients with significantly compromised renal function may require modified doses of antibiotics. In unusual circumstances, during

Table 37-1. Recommended standard prophylactic regimen for dental, oral, or upper respiratory tract procedures in patients who are at risk[a]

Drug	Dosing regimen[b]
Standard regimen	
Amoxicillin	3.0 g orally 1 hr before procedure; then 1.5 g 6 hr after initial dose
Amoxicillin/penicillin-allergic patients	
Erythromycin *or* clindamycin	Erythromycin ethylsuccinate, 800 mg, or erythromycin stearate, 1.0 g, orally 2 hr before procedure; then half the dose 6 hr after initial dose, *or* Clindamycin 300 mg orally 1 hr before procedure and 150 mg 6 hr after initial dose

Source: Reprinted by permission from AS Dajani et al. Prevention of bacterial endocarditis: recommendations by the American Heart Association. JAMA 1990; 264:2919–22.
[a] Includes those with prosthetic heart valves and other high-risk patients.
[b] Initial pediatric doses are as follows: amoxicillin, 50 mg/kg; erythromycin ethylsuccinate or erythromycin stearate, 20 mg/kg; and clindamycin, 10 mg/kg. Follow-up doses should be one-half the initial dose. Total pediatric dose should not exceed total adult dose. The following weight ranges may also be used for the initial pediatric dose of amoxicillin: < 15 kg, 750 mg; 15–30 kg, 1500 mg; and > 30 kg, 3000 mg (full adult dose).

Table 37-2. Alternate prophylactic regimens for dental, oral, or upper respiratory tract procedures in patients who are at risk

Drug	Dosing regimen*
Patients unable to take oral medications	
Ampicillin	Intravenous or intramuscular administration of ampicillin, 2.0 g, 30 min before procedure; then intravenous or intramuscular administration of ampicillin, 1.0 g, or oral administration of amoxicillin, 1.5 g, 6 hr after initial dose
Ampicillin/amoxicillin/penicillin-allergic patients unable to take oral medications	
Clindamycin	Intravenous administration of 300 mg 30 min before procedure and intravenous or oral administration of 150 mg 6 hr after initial dose
Patients considered high risk and not candidates for standard regimen	
Ampicillin, gentamicin, and amoxicillin	Intravenous or intramuscular administration of ampicillin, 2.0 g, plus gentamicin, 1.5 mg/kg (not to exceed 80 mg), 30 min before procedure; followed by amoxicillin, 1.5 g, orally 6 hr after initial dose; alternatively, the parenteral regimen may be repeated 8 hr after initial dose
Ampicillin/amoxicillin/penicillin-allergic patients considered high risk	
Vancomycin	Intravenous administration of 1.0 g over 1 hr, starting 1 hr before procedure; no repeated dose necessary

Source: Reprinted by permission from AS Dajani et al. Prevention of bacterial endocarditis: Recommendations by the American Heart Association. JAMA 1990; 264:2919–22.
*Initial pediatric doses are as follows: ampicillin, 50 mg/kg; clindamycin, 10 mg/kg; gentamicin, 2.0 mg/kg; and vancomycin, 20 mg/kg. Follow-up doses should be one-half the initial dose. Total pediatric dose should not exceed total adult dose.

Table 37-3. Regimens for genitourinary and GI procedures

Drug	Dosing regimen*
Standard regimen	
Ampicillin, gentamicin, and amoxicillin	Intravenous or intramuscular administration of ampicillin, 2.0 g, plus gentamicin, 1.5 mg/kg (not to exceed 80 mg), 30 min before procedure; followed by amoxicillin, 1.5 g orally 6 hr after initial dose; alternatively, the parenteral regimen may be repeated once 8 hr after initial dose
Ampicillin/amoxicillin/penicillin-allergic regimen	
Vancomycin	Intravenous administration of vancomycin, 1.0 g, over 1 hr plus intravenous or intramuscular administration of gentamicin, 1.5 mg/kg (not to exceed 80 mg), 1 hr before procedure; may be repeated once 8 hr after initial dose
Alternate low-risk regimen	
Amoxicillin	3.0 g orally 1 hr before procedure; then 1.5 g 6 hr after initial dose

Source: Reprinted by permission from AS Dajani et al. Prevention of bacterial endocarditis: Recommendations by the American Heart Association. JAMA 1990; 264:2919–22.
*Initial pediatric doses are as follows: amoxicillin, 50 mg/kg; gentamicin, 2.0 mg/kg; and vancomycin, 20 mg/kg. Follow-up doses should be half the initial dose. Total pediatric dose should not exceed total adult dose.

prolonged procedures or in the case of delayed healing, it may be necessary to provide additional doses of antibiotics.

Approximately 10% of individuals with a previous history of endocarditis have a second episode; patients with prosthetic heart valves or surgically constructed systemic-pulmonary shunts are at especially high risk. Patients taking oral penicillin for secondary prevention of rheumatic fever, or for other purposes, may have viridans streptococci relatively resistant to penicillin in the oral cavity. In these cases erythromycin or one of the parenteral regimens should be used. For the same reason, patients who have recently received a therapeutic course of penicillin should have elective dental treatment delayed for 2 to 3 weeks to allow reconstitution of normal oral flora. Anticoagulation with warfarin (Coumadin) is a relative contraindication to intramuscular injections; oral or intravenous regimens should be used instead.

Dajani AS, et al. Prevention of bacterial endocarditis: recommendations by the American Heart Association. JAMA 1990; 264:2919–22.
The most recent report and recommendations of the American Heart Association Committee on Rheumatic Fever and Infective Endocarditis.

Durack DR. Current issues in prevention of infective endocarditis. Am J Med 1985; 78:Suppl 6B:149–56.
This review emphasizes the importance of relative risk according to underlying cardiac lesion, cost-benefit analysis, and other controversial issues related to endocarditis prophylaxis.

Weinstein L, Schlesinger JJ. Pathoanatomic, pathophysiologic and clinical correlations in endocarditis. N Engl J Med 1974; 291:832–7, 1122–6.
An excellent review article in two parts.

Everett ED, Hirschmann JV. Transient bacteremia and endocarditis prophylaxis. A review. Medicine 1977; 56:61–77.
A complete review of procedures causing bacteremia.

VII. PERIPHERAL VASCULAR PROBLEMS

38. CHRONIC VENOUS DISORDERS
Robert S. Grossman

Chronic venous disease includes two different but overlapping clinical syndromes: chronic venous insufficiency (CVI) and varicose veins. Both are common outpatient problems. In one middle-aged working population, some degree of CVI was found in 22%, with ulcers experienced by 1.3%, and pronounced varicosities in 4%. Venous disease results in discomfort and significant economic loss for many patients.

The leg veins and venous valves are responsible for venous return and protection of the lower extremities from high venous pressures. The three anatomic components of the system are (1) the deep veins, which carry 90% of the blood return; (2) the superficial veins, which include the greater and lesser saphenous veins and drain the superficial tissues; and (3) the perforating or communicating veins, which are valved and normally direct blood flow from the superficial to the deep system. All three systems have valves at frequent intervals that are essential to prevent retrograde flow.

Chronic Venous Insufficiency

CVI is usually caused by incompetent valves in the perforator or deep venous systems, and occasionally by chronic obstruction. The valvular incompetence may be primary, with intact, leaky valves, or secondary to previous thrombosis, with recanalization and destruction of the valves. The deep venous system is well supported by muscle and deep fascia; valvular incompetence in the deep system results in venous hypertension, even during ambulation when venous pressure normally falls dramatically. Eventually the perforator veins become dilated, with resultant valvular incompetence and retrograde flow from the deep to the superficial system. Alternatively, the perforators alone may be involved. The final common pathway involves venous hypertension transmitted to the poorly supported superficial system, and resultant edema, extravascular fibrin deposition, liposclerosis due to failure of oxygen and nutrient diffusion, and eventually skin ulceration.

CVI frequently follows thrombophlebitis; 72 to 95% of patients develop symptoms within 10 years of iliofemoral thrombosis, and 20% within 6 years of a clot confined to the calf. However, 20 to 40% of patients with CVI have no history of thrombophlebitis. In one series, venograms in 51 limbs of patients with CVI could detect evidence of old or new thrombophlebitis in only 19 limbs. Therefore, it seems that postphlebitic syndrome is not really an appropriate synonym for CVI.

Clinical Presentation
The hallmarks of CVI are edema and skin changes in the lower leg, most commonly present over the medial malleolus because it is dependent and the many perforating veins there anastomose directly with subcutaneous capillaries rather than the superficial veins. Leg ulcers are a common complication.

Edema
Edema is an early manifestation of disease and frequently responds to leg elevation. Other causes of edema, such as cardiac, renal, and liver diseases and cellulitis must be considered.

Skin Changes
The brownish pigmentation found in CVI is mainly a cosmetic problem resulting from extravasation of red blood cells and hemosiderin deposition in the skin. Dermatoses associated with CVI include eczematous eruptions, which may occasionally be generalized, and contact dermatitis resulting from topical remedies such as neomycin. A lichenified neurodermatitis may result from chronic scratching. Lipodermatosclerosis, the progressive replacement of subcutaneous tissue by fibrous tissue, results from an increased volume of interstitial fluid, tissue anoxia, and decreased fibrinolytic activity. In the chronic phase,

the dermis becomes indurated and tight, and the diameter of the lower third of the leg may actually decrease.

Ulceration of the skin may be precipitated by minor trauma. Ninety percent of leg ulcers are caused by CVI, and this etiology should be suspected in any patient with ulcers and the other stigmata of this disease. Venous ulcers, which vary in size, are frequently located over the medial malleolus and must be distinguished from ischemic ulcers, which are generally more painful and located distally on the feet and toes, as well as from hypertensive ulcers. The latter, a poorly defined but recognized unusual type of leg ulcer, follows a skin infarction on the lower leg of a hypertensive patient; the ulcers are extremely painful, commonly located on the lateral and posterior aspects of the lower leg and surrounded by a cyanotic hue.

Evaluation

The diagnosis of CVI is largely clinical. A plethora of tests is available, including bidirectional Doppler sonography to assess flow; foot volumetry to assess the change in the volume of the foot during exercise; photoplethysmography to detect the change in the blood volume in the skin; venous catheterization to measure pressures directly; and venography, which remains the gold standard. These tests are generally unnecessary before starting conservative therapy. In those rare patients for whom surgery is contemplated, venography is essential. If coexisting arterial insufficiency is suspected, this should be assessed by Doppler pressure measurements prior to the application of compressive therapy; ischemia contraindicates any form of high-compression bandaging.

Treatment

Conservative therapy for CVI will alleviate symptoms in approximately 85% of patients, although relapse is common when therapy is halted. Elevation of the ankle above the chest reduces leg vein pressures to near zero, and aids resorption of the edema fluid. Complete bed rest, with its attendant disability and risk of thromboembolism, is rarely necessary; foot elevation for 30 minutes several times daily is more practical. A footstool alone is not likely to be adequate for elevation. The ankle must be elevated higher than the hips and the hips must be higher than the heart. Patients required to stand for long periods of time should move and exercise their calf muscles as much as possible.

Ambulatory patients with edema and dermatitis may require compression stockings. Over-the-counter, low-compression stockings designed to prevent thromboembolism will not effectively treat CVI. Prescription stockings, obtained from a surgical supply store may be custom-made on the basis of measurements taken every 1½ in. along the leg, or non–custom-made relying on calf length and ankle and calf circumference for fit. One study suggests that there is no advantage to the custom-made stockings for most patients. However, for those patients with narrow ankles and large calves (which may be seen with lipodermatosclerosis), non–custom-made stockings may have an undesired tourniquet effect on the calf. The optimal pressure to prescribe is unknown, but many physicians start with 30 to 40 mm Hg; higher-pressure hose may be difficult to pull on and uncomfortable to wear. Calf-length stockings seem to be better tolerated and no less effective than longer stockings. In 1989, the cost of a pair of non–custom-made, prescription stockings was approximately $50 to $65; custom-made stockings cost the same plus a $10 fitting fee, and usually require a 2-week period for delivery. Stockings should be worn throughout the day but removed at bedtime. One unblinded study found decreased leg volume and circumference and pain on a stockinged leg compared with a nonstockinged control leg, and other studies have documented increased femoral vein flow rates, and decreased ambulatory venous pressure with compression stockings.

Skin Problems

Eczematous dermatitis will often improve with 0.025% triamcinolone cream in addition to compressive therapy. If there is extensive weeping, compresses with Burow's solution (1:32) may help dessicate the lesion.

Lipodermatosclerosis responds to compressive therapy. Stanozolol, an anabolic steroid that enhances fibrinolytic activity, was found to increase the speed of healing in one crossover study, but compression remains the most important intervention.

Venous Ulcers

Edema must be controlled in order to allow healing, usually by the application of a compressive dressing, such as Unna's paste boot. Unna's boot is a gauze bandage impregnated with a medicated paste of zinc oxide, calamine lotion, and glycerine. It is applied like an Ace wrap, but hardens to form a light cast. Unna's boot should be applied to the leg, after it has been drained by overnight elevation, directly over the skin (and ulcer), and without ointments or other dressing. Any necrotic tissue should first be débrided. Wrapping should begin at the toes and extend to the knee, and the bandage may be covered by an Ace wrap to protect clothing. Unna's boot should be changed weekly. In a prospective randomized trial, Unna boots were superior to a hydroactive dressing (Duoderm) in the healing of ulcers. Other studies suggest that compressive stockings may do as well as Unna boots; however, Unna boots require only weekly changes as opposed to daily patient compliance, and have the additional advantage of preventing scratching and the application of irritating topical remedies. Leg elevation is effective for edema control, but is impractical for most people to do long enough to allow ulcer healing; it may, however, be a necessary alternative when coexisting arterial insufficiency prohibits compression.

Ulcers accompanied by fever or lymphangitis are likely infected and should be treated with systemic antibiotics; low bacterial counts correlate with better healing. The efficacy of topical antibiotics is questionable and some agents may cause a contact dermatitis.

Surgery may be indicated for the few patients for whom conservative therapy fails. Although there are many preferred procedures, little other than series of case reports supports their use. Because patients who undergo surgery are also treated with bed rest and elevation, the lack of control groups makes assessment of surgical efficacy very difficult. More than 70% of patients have significant short-term improvement following ligation of incompetent perforator veins, although recurrence of ulceration is not uncommon even when compression stockings are used. The additional value of valve repair or transposition remains questionable. Patients with incompetent perforators and a normal deep venous system seem to respond best to surgery, whereas those with an obstructed deep system have a poor response. Split-thickness skin grafting to speed recovery should be considered for ulcers larger than 2 to 3 cm in diameter.

In a British study, treatment with the drug oxypentifylline, known in the United States as pentoxifylline (Trental), 400 mg three times a day, was shown to increase substantially the proportion of ulcers that healed in patients whose venous ulcers failed to heal after 2 months of routine outpatient therapy. While these results obviously bear replication, they offer a promising alternative treatment for difficult cases.

Varicose Veins

Varicosities occur when distending pressures are allowed into the superficial veins. They may be secondary to venous pathology elsewhere (deep or perforator system) or primary (localized to the superficial system). The cause of primary varicose veins is unclear but may be related to congenital weakness of the vein walls or incompetent venous valves.

Some degree of varicose veins can be found in 20% of the adult population. There is a 5:1 female predominance, with many women having the onset of symptoms during pregnancy. Other associated risk factors include the use of exogenous estrogen, prolonged standing, constrictive clothing, and perhaps the presence of diverticula in the colon.

Clinical Presentation

If the deep veins and perforators are normal, varicose veins are usually asymptomatic. Patients may complain of aching, cramping, heaviness, or swelling in their legs, but often request therapy for purely cosmetic reasons. The severity of symptoms in patients with primary varicose veins is generally mild compared to those with CVI. Occasionally, brisk hemorrhages can occur from minute ulcers overlying varicosities; death from exsanguination has been reported, usually in elderly patients.

Diagnosis

The diagnosis is based on the physical finding of dilated, tortuous veins most easily seen when the legs are dependent. Dilated venules may present with a cosmetically unattractive, blue, finely reticulated appearance. Although minimal tenderness may be present on palpation of the vein, severe tenderness should make one suspect a coexisting superficial thrombophlebitis. The presence of significant edema, hemosiderin deposition in the skin, or moderate-to-large skin ulcers suggests underlying deep or perforator venous disease. Generally, tourniquet and other noninvasive or invasive tests are not necessary.

Treatment

Patients should be advised to avoid prolonged standing and constrictive clothing, and to elevate their legs whenever possible. Many patients require no further treatment. In pregnant patients, symptoms will often improve following delivery. Graduated-compression stockings are useful in relieving symptoms of aching, heaviness, and edema; however, they do not remedy cosmetic concerns, and many younger patients may be unwilling to use them chronically. Only those patients who continue to have significant symptoms despite conservative therapy, or those for whom cosmetic appearance is a major concern, should be considered for more aggressive therapy.

Sclerotherapy involves the injection and subsequent compression of the dilated veins and "control points," which are thought to represent the site of incompetent perforators. Multiple injections can be made at one outpatient visit, although a series of three to eight visits is usually required. Minor complications such as phlebitis (10%) and ulceration (4%) may follow sclerotherapy but are usually self-limited.

Surgical treatment involves removal of the greater saphenous or lesser saphenous vein, at times combined with ligation of incompetent veins. Although this procedure may be done on an outpatient basis, in one study patients were hospitalized for 3.7 days on average. Typically, patients may miss 2 weeks of work during convalescence. Complications are less common but potentially more serious, and include death (0.02%), deep venous thrombosis (0.5%), bleeding, and hypesthesia.

Several randomized studies have shown that either sclerotherapy or stripping is initially effective. Two studies with longer follow-up found a substantial increase in the failure rate of sclerotherapy over time (66% at 6 years) while the benefits of surgery were longer lasting (only 20% failure at 6 years). Further subgroup analysis showed sclerotherapy to be superior for the subgroup with only superficial vein or perforator vein involvement, but when either the greater saphenous or lesser saphenous veins were involved (61% of patients), surgery was clearly superior.

Immelman EJ, Jeffrey PC. The post phlebitic syndrome: pathophysiology, prevention, and management. Clin Chest Med 1984; 5:537–50.
A scholarly and concise review of CVI, with an excellent discussion of pathophysiology.

Burnand K, et al. Venous lipodermatosclerosis: treatment by fibrinolytic enhancement and elastic compression. Br Med J 1980; 280:7–11.
A small, double-blind, crossover study of compression with and without stanozolol. Stanozolol showed a trend toward benefit in addition to the clear benefit that occurred in the stockinged group.

Johnson G Jr, et al. Graded compression stockings: custom vs. noncustom. Arch Surg 1982; 117:69–72.
A small study comparing the effect of custom-made versus non–custom-made stockings on femoral vein velocity. The authors found little difference, suggesting that non–custom-made stockings are appropriate for most mesomorphic patients.

Train JS, et al. Radiological evaluation of the chronic venous stasis syndrome. JAMA 1987; 258:941–4.
A venographic study of patients with "postphlebitic syndrome" found no evidence of old or new phlebitis in most cases.

Colgan MP, et al. Oxpentifylline treatment of venous ulcers of the leg. Br Med J 1990; 300:972–5.
In this randomized, double-blind, controlled study comparing oxpentifylline, 400 mg three times a day (equivalent to pentoxyphylline available in the United States), to placebo, approximately twice as many ulcers healed in the treatment group.

deGroot WP. Treatment of varicose veins: modern concept and methods. J Dermatol Surg Oncol 1989; 15:138–45.
A helpful description of the surgical treatment of varicose veins.

Tremblay J, Lewis EW, Allen PT. Selecting a treatment for primary varicose veins. Can Med Assoc J 1985; 133:20–5.
An excellent review comparing palatability, cost, and efficacy of sclerotherapy versus surgical stripping of varicose veins.

Sladen JG. Compression sclerotherapy: preparation, technique, complications, and results. Am J Surg 1983; 146:228–32.
Technique of compression sclerotherapy clearly explained, with helpful photographs accompanying the text.

39. ARTERIAL DISEASE OF THE EXTREMITIES
John S. Kizer

Peripheral vascular disease is a common illness. As much as 17% of the adult population aged 55 to 64 years old is afflicted by ischemic limb disease, and about one-third of these are disabled by their illness. Risk factors for the development of peripheral vascular disease include diabetes and cigarette smoking. Other risk factors for cardiovascular disease in general, such as high blood cholesterol, hypertension, and male sex, appear to be less strongly correlated with the development of peripheral vascular disease. The presence of peripheral vascular disease, on the other hand, is strongly correlated with the presence of arteriosclerotic lesions throughout the cardiovascular system.

Natural History
The short-term prognosis for patients with chronic limb ischemia is reasonably favorable. The majority of patients with claudication improve in 6 to 12 months with conservative management of diabetes and hypertension, cessation of smoking, and exercise. About 10% of patients presenting with peripheral vascular disease require amputation within 5 years; in diabetics, the rate of amputation is nearly five times higher, and for diabetic single amputees, the risk of amputation for the remaining limb is also five times higher (50% at 5 years).

Survival is reduced in the presence of peripheral vascular disease. A few patients die as a result of gangrene and sepsis. Overall cardiovascular-related mortality of patients with claudication is twice that of a comparable population without claudication. Two-year mortality rates for patients presenting with severe peripheral vascular disease may be as high as 15 to 20%.

Clinical Syndromes

Acute Vascular Insufficiency
The course of ischemic peripheral vascular disease may be complicated at any time by acute symptoms related to either an in situ thrombosis or the lodgment of an embolus, leading to limb-threatening ischemia and gangrene.

Acute limb-threatening ischemia presents as the sudden onset of severe pain in the involved leg with associated weakness and numbness. The pain may be described as a deep, continuous ache that is often excruciating. Any attempt to walk or stand aggravates the pain, and the symptoms are not relieved by rest. On clinical examination, the involved limb is cool or cold, the pulses are markedly diminished or absent in the involved portion of the limb, and the limb may be either pale or cyanotic. Often these symptoms and signs are superimposed on those of chronic ischemic arterial disease, described below. Occasional patients have aortic dissection as a cause.

Chronic Vascular Insufficiency

Symptoms of chronic ischemic vasculopathy of the extremities include pain, intermittent claudication, loss of hair, poor healing, loss of sensation, weakness, erectile failure (or dysfunction), and muscular atrophy. The level of limb involvement depends on the anatomical location of the critical arterial lesions. For example, pain in the feet and calves may result from disease anywhere in the femoral-popliteal system, whereas pain, weakness of the hip, and impotence suggest aortoiliac occlusive disease. End-stage vascular chronic disease leads to the syndrome of resting pain or pregangrenous ischemia, which is characterized by a continuous ache, incapacitating pain on exertion, and pain or rubor when the leg is dependent. Further progression of the disease leads to persistent pain at rest, muscular atrophy, skin ulcers, and eventually gangrene.

Differential Diagnosis

In evaluating the patient presenting with symptoms of arterial insufficiency, it is necessary to exclude or treat diseases simulating peripheral vascular disease, such as Raynaud's disease, erythromelalgia, or systemic vasculitis, and conditions that may exacerbate limb ischemia, such as polycythemia, hyperviscosity syndromes, anemia, and recurrent embolization from proximal sites in the vascular tree. In heavy smokers and young patients (< 40 years old), thromboangiitis obliterans should be considered (see below). It is debatable whether administration of beta-blockers or calcium channel antagonists to patients with previously stable, chronic peripheral vascular disease can increase symptoms of ischemia. Finally, before erectile dysfunction is attributed to peripheral vascular disease, antihypertensive and other medications must be excluded as a cause (see Chap. 83).

Evaluation

The diagnosis of peripheral vascular disease and evaluation of its course are ultimately based on clinical observation, the accuracy of which is not infallible. The desire of clinicians to enhance diagnostic and prognostic accuracy has led to the use of several techniques for laboratory evaluation of disease. Doppler and duplex ultrasonography are the most useful noninvasive tests for confirming obstruction and localizing areas of maximal obstruction, and both correlate well with direct arterial measurement of blood flow. Ratios of ankle to brachial artery blood pressure (ankle-brachial index [ABI]) of less than 0.35 to 0.50 as determined by ultrasound correlate well with findings of severe ischemic disease, but cannot be relied on to quantitate small degrees of improvement or decline or to correctly predict the need for surgery. Measurement of transcutaneous oxygen tension (tcO_2) has been thought to predict the failure of ischemic leg ulcers to heal when it is below 30 mm Hg and the likelihood of healing when it is above 38 mm Hg. Although calculation of the ratio of leg tcO_2 to chest tcO_2 has been suggested to improve the positive predictive accuracy of such measurements, the clinical usefulness of tcO_2 in the evaluation of peripheral vascular disease has not been convincingly demonstrated and is probably less satisfactory than ultrasound. Other noninvasive methods such as thermography are not recommended for general use.

Venous digital subtraction angiography has not been generally accepted due to poor resolution of detail, whereas arterial digital subtraction angiography provides excellent resolution for presurgical evaluation. Because arteriography adds little to the diagnostic and prognostic information provided by ultrasound, it should be reserved for patients in whom surgery or angioplasty is contemplated.

Management of Acute Arterial Insufficiency

The acute onset of limb-threatening ischemia demands immediate intervention. There is no evidence that the administration of anticoagulants, vasodilators, or experimental therapies such as prostacyclin infusion are of value in treating this condition. Depending on the nature of the anatomic obstruction as determined by arteriography, the patient may be best suited for either bypass grafting of the occluded segments, catheter embolectomy, percutaneous transluminal angioplasty, or arterial streptokinase infusion. Acute catheter embolectomy or bypass grafting may save as many as 90% of the affected extremities. However, surgical mortality as high as 15% has been reported, due to the risk imposed by the concomitant presence of coronary and cerebral vascular disease. Following successful embolectomy, many institutions recommend chronic administration of an oral anticoagulant, although firm data supporting the efficacy of such a regimen in preventing recurrent emboli from areas other than the heart do not exist. Under certain circumstances, when sepsis and serious underlying illness are present, emergency amputation is necessary.

Management of Chronic Arterial Insufficiency
The treatment of peripheral vascular disease is palliative; medical therapy is preferred over surgery in the absence of incapacitating or limb-threatening ischemia.

General Measures
In smokers, the progression of vascular disease and the rate of future amputation can be reduced by abstention from cigarette smoking (see Chapter 130). Walking should be encouraged; it is likely that a program of walking improves the clinical symptoms of claudication either through training of the affected muscles, through dilatation of collaterals, or by decreasing platelet adhesion. Although tighter control of diabetes mellitus by generally available methods may not halt the progression of peripheral vascular insufficiency, tighter glycemic control may improve nerve conduction and retard the development of peripheral neuropathy. Control of hypertension is recommended to reduce overall cardiovascular mortality; it is not clear whether control of hypertension halts the progression of peripheral vascular disease. Finally, although there is no clear relationship between diet and hyperlipidemia and the overall prognosis of peripheral vascular disease, dietary control of cholesterol intake and weight reduction may reduce overall cardiovascular mortality.

Skin Care
Attention to local skin and nail care, avoidance of trauma, and prompt attention to localized infections are of primary importance. Patients should be instructed not to soak extremities; to bathe only in warm water; to keep the extremities dry; and to wear clean, dry socks, preferably cotton. In order to prevent cracking, a hydrophilic cream such as eucerite (Eucerin) may be used daily. Where significant peripheral neuropathy is present due to obstructive involvement of the vasa nervorum such as that found in diabetics, patients must be especially vigilant to avoid thermal and physical injury. In all patients, but especially those with neuropathy, the lower extremities must be inspected frequently, searching for cracks between the toes, calluses, or pressure points. Found early, these indications of potential ulcers may be treated by keeping the feet dry or by using special shoes or inserts to relieve pressure. Calluses should be removed by a podiatrist. Shoes should be inspected for foreign objects that the patient cannot feel.

Ischemic Ulcers
Ulcers must be treated promptly with sharp débridement, and the foot elevated and wrapped in sterile, dry gauze. Débridement should be cautious and not overly vigorous since exposure of bone and deep tissues markedly decreases the likelihood of healing. Walking should be limited, and loose fitting footwear used when walking is necessary. The ulcers can be inspected and cleansed daily with half-strength hydrogen peroxide. Soaking is not advised in order to avoid overhydration of the skin and subsequent maceration of the wound.

Mild to moderate infected ulcers may be managed as above with the addition of an antibiotic. Although infected ulcers, especially those in diabetics, may contain a polymicrobial flora, recent evidence suggests that the majority of cases are due to aerobic cocci such as *Staphylococcus* and will respond to a two-week course of dicloxacillin. In some circumstances, proper treatment will require more exacting microbiologic information. The most accurate cultures are obtained from either wound biopsy or curettage, while aspirations and wound swabs are insensitive. Any ulcer eroding through to bone must be suspected of harboring osteomyelitis even in the face of negative x-rays.

Drug Therapy
Although many agents have been used to treat peripheral vascular disease, drug therapy is of limited efficacy.

PENTOXIFYLLINE. Pentoxifylline (Trental) is a drug whose mechanism of action is unknown, but is considered to favorably alter the "hemorrheologic" properties of blood possibly by increasing the in situ synthesis of prostacyclin. In controlled trials, pentoxifylline (1200 mg/day) doubled the walking time before the onset of claudication and increased both postischemic blood flow and tcO$_2$. There is no evidence that pentoxifylline delays the progression of peripheral occlusive disease

ANTICOAGULANT AND ANTIPLATELET DRUGS. Platelet microaggregates and the coagulation cascade have been implicated in the genesis of atherosclerotic lesions. However, there is no persuasive evidence, from available clinical trials, that either platelet antiaggregants or oral anticoagulants significantly alter the natural history of peripheral vascular disease. An exception is patients with recurrent arterial emboli, the majority of which originate from the left side of the heart; for these patients the administration of oral anticoagulants appears necessary to prevent recurrent distal embolization. In addition, the patient with recurrent in situ thromboses may benefit from oral anticoagulant theapy, although there is little firm information to support this approach. There is as yet no information as to the utility of ticlopidine for peripheral vascular disease.

PERIPHERAL VASODILATORS AND PROSTACYCLIN. Numerous clinical trials also provide little support for the use of vasodilators such as papaverine, isoxsuprine, cyclandelate, or nylidrin for the relief of symptoms from peripheral vascular insufficiency. Unlike the skin, muscles lack sympathetic vasoconstrictors; although pharmacologic or surgical sympathectomy may increase flow to the skin, it has little effect on blood flow to the deeper muscle bundles. Furthermore, it is likely that the arteries supplying exercising and ischemic muscles are already dilated to the fullest extent.

The role for the administration of prostacyclin or prostacyclin congeners in the treatment of advanced arteriosclerotic peripheral vascular disease has not yet been established. At this time there is also insufficient data to recommend combined therapy with PGE$_1$ derivatives and isosorbide dinitrate (a precursor of endothelial-derived relaxing factor) to prevent progression of disease, although such therapy may be effective in decreasing platelet deposition.

Surgery

In the event of limb-threatening or incapacitating limb ischemia, or nonhealing ischemic ulcers, surgical intervention must be considered. Depending on the symptoms and the nature of anatomic distribution of the arterial obstructions as determined by arteriography, the patient may be offered either bypass grafting, angioplasty of the occluded segments, or embolectomy.

Surgery is not undertaken if palliation can be achieved in other ways, such as by control of risk factors or by administration of pentoxifylline (Trental) or angioplasty. Mortality as high as 15% has been reported, due to the risk imposed by the concomitant presence of coronary and cerebrovascular disease. Complications are also common. Following surgery, attention to the modification of risk factors is again important. Cessation of cigarette smoking may improve the patency rate following bypass grafting.

Transluminal Balloon Angioplasty

This procedure may offer a reasonable alternative to surgical bypass grafting in patients unfit for surgery or with an isolated stenosis or obstruction of the femoral or iliac arteries that is less than 8 cm in length and that contains no calcium. Depending on the angiographer, primary success rates ranging from 70 to 84% and 3-year patency rates of 45 to 70% (even in the presence of total obstructions) may be obtained in the femoral arteries, and primary success rates as high as 90% and 3-year patency rates of 70 to 83% may be obtained in the iliac arteries. Patency rates following angioplasty of smaller vessels are considerably lower. These 3- to 5-year patency rates for angioplasty can be compared to the historical rates of patency of 90 to 95% following aortoiliac surgery and 70 to 75% following femoral-popliteal surgery. The role of fiberoptic laser angioplasty is as yet undefined, with perforation of the vessel wall and inability to penetrate calcified plaques looming as two major obstacles to widespread clinical use. Finally, there are no data on which to base recommendations for the use of rotary cutting angioplasty.

The precise role of transluminal angioplasty in the management of vascular disease is as yet undefined. It is not clear what proportion of patients meet the exacting criteria for transluminal dilation. Also, there have not been clinical trials comparing surgery to angioplasty for the palliation of peripheral vascular disease. It has been suggested that all eligible patients should first receive angioplasty, and then surgery if angioplasty fails. Although this treatment plan is said to offer the cheapest and safest means for avoiding operative mortality and prolonging limb survival, there are no clinical data to support its adoption. Finally, no controlled trials have indicated that postoperative or postangioplasty platelet antiaggregant or anticoagulant therapy is a useful adjuvant.

At present there is little role for vascular surgery in the treatment of impotence resulting from peripheral vascular disease. In fact, impotence may result from surgical attempts to correct obstructive or aneurysmal disease of aortoiliac junctions. For a few patients, transluminal angioplasty of the internal iliac arteries may prove useful in the treatment of impotence.

It is noteworthy that statistics have not shown a reduction in the national rate of amputation. These statistics emphasize the notion that vascular surgical intervention is only a short-term palliative procedure.

Amputation

When all else fails, surgical amputation is necessary to remove parts of extremities destined to become gangrenous. Amputation below the knee has been preferred when possible because of the common perception that rehabilitation is more often successful following below-the-knee amputation than following amputation above the knee. Recent evidence suggests, however, that the single most important factor governing rehabilitation is a healthy, well-healed stump with good sensation. In patients whose stumps do not meet these criteria, failure of prosthetic bipedal ambulation requiring stump revision is frequent. The mortality of patients leaving rehabilitation centers following amputation is 15 to 35% over 4 to 5 years.

Thromboangiitis Obliterans

When peripheral vascular disease is found in a patient under the age of 40, particularly when involving both lower and upper extremities, thromboangiitis obliterans (Buerger's disease) is suspected. This rare disease is associated with heavy cigarette smoking and occurs in men more often than women. It is characterized by focal, inflammatory lesions of small- and medium-size arteries and veins. Lesions of thromboangiitis obliterans may regress on discontinuation of smoking and recur when cigarette smoking is resumed.

Hegyeli RS, ed. Atherosclerotic reviews. Vol. 7. New York: Raven, 1980.
Excellent source for epidemiologic data concerning the prevalence and incidence of various types of atherosclerotic vascular disease.

Kammel WB, Shurtteff D. The Framingham Study: cigarettes and the development of intermittent claudication. Geriatrics 1973; 28:61–8.
Correlation of cigarette smoking with the risk of peripheral vascular disease is higher than the correlation with the risk of coronary or cerebrovascular disease.

Thompson JE, Garrett WV. Peripheral arterial surgery. N Engl J Med 1980; 302:491–503.
Overview of the field of surgical palliation of arterial vascular disease.

Ehrly AM, Saeger-Lorenz K. Influence of pentoxifylline on muscle tissue oxygen tension of patients with intermittent claudication before and after pedal ergometer exercise. Angiology 1987; 38:93–100.
Trial suggesting an improvement in oxygenation of ischemic limbs following treatment with pentoxifylline.

Stern PH. Occlusive vascular disease of lower limbs: diagnosis, amputation surgery and rehabilitation. Am J Phys Rehab Med 1988; 67:145–54.
Good review of prognosis and natural history of limb ischemia.

Lipsky BA, et al. Outpatient management of uncomplicated lower-extremity infections in diabetic patients. Arch Intern Med 1990; 150:790–7.
Infections with gram-positive cocci were most common (94% of cases; 43% of cases were pure culture). Anaerobes constituted 13% of cases but always as part of mixed aerobic-anaerobic infection. Gram-negative bacilli were present in 23% of infections (in only 8% as a pure culture).

40. THROMBOPHLEBITIS
Thomas McAfee and Christopher Bogert

Thrombophlebitis, or venous thrombosis, represents clots in the venous system. While 600,000 deep venous thromboses (DVTs) are treated each year in the United States, it is estimated that less than 25% of DVTs are diagnosed. For ambulatory care physicians, there are risks in both overdiagnosing and underdiagnosing DVTs. On the one hand, a missed DVT can lead to pulmonary embolism. On the other hand, it is unacceptable to subject a patient to the risks of anticoagulation therapy if the diagnosis of DVT is erroneous. Because clinical examination is unreliable, objective tests are required to diagnose DVT. Objective tests are also necessary to distinguish proximal thrombosis, which requires anticoagulation, from distal thrombosis, which rarely causes significant pulmonary embolus (PE) and does not require treatment.

Diagnosis

History
In addition to the classic symptoms of pain, swelling, warmth, and redness, a history of risk factors should be elicited. Major risk factors include immobility and conditions that predispose to immobility and venous stasis, such as myocardial infarction, stroke, local trauma, congestive heart failure, obesity, and surgery. Other predisposing conditions include previous DVT, malignancy, pregnancy, oral contraceptive use, vasculitis, nephrotic syndrome, inflammatory bowel disease, and polycythemia vera. Risk factors are cumulative. In a study of patients suspected of having DVT on the basis of clinical evaluation, objective measures found DVT in only 11% of patients with no risk factors, in 24% of those with one risk factor, in 36% with two risk factors, and in 50% with three risk factors. One hundred percent of patients with four or more risk factors were shown to have a DVT. Thus the presence or absence of risk factors alters the pretest probability that the patient has a DVT.

Physical Examination
The physical signs for diagnosing DVT are unreliable. While unilateral swelling and tenderness of the lower extremity are found in up to 70% of patients with proximal DVT, they are nonspecific. Other findings associated with DVT include low-grade fever, superficial venous thrombosis (SVT), diminished arterial pulses, warmth, and erythema, all of which are also nonspecific. Homans' sign or calf pain on dorsiflexion occurs in only 8% of patients with documented DVT.
Since less than 50% of patients with a clinical presentation suggesting DVT actually have a thrombosis, a large number have other disorders, which may be suggested or detected by physical examination. Disorders frequently confused with DVT include congestive heart failure, ruptured Baker's cyst, SVT, cellulitis with lymphedema, extrinsic obstruction of lymphatics, and postthrombotic syndrome.

Laboratory Studies
Venography has been accepted as a gold standard for diagnosing DVT since the 1940s. It is cost-effective, especially where it is available as an outpatient procedure. However, a study comparing venography to autopsy dissection revealed that venography was only 89% sensitive and 97% specific; thus, physicians should be aware that even the "gold standard" for diagnosing DVT is not a perfect test. Venography is invasive, can cause

local irritation, but rarely, and cannot be performed when there is massive edema. For these reasons, noninvasive methods have been sought for diagnosis.

Impedance plethysmography (IPG) is the most studied and available of the noninvasive tests. Relatively inexpensive and reliable, IPG can be performed at the bedside, in emergency rooms, or on an outpatient basis. While poor for diagnosing calf-only DVT, serial IPG is the only noninvasive test shown to provide a safe basis for withholding treatment of suspected proximal DVT. In skilled hands, it has a 98% positive predictive value for proximal DVT in symptomatic patients and a 99% predictive value for negative results. IPG cannot be used in patients who have had an amputation, leg trauma, or are currently wearing a cast, and is less accurate for patients with severe congestive heart failure, constrictive pericarditis, arterial insufficiency, hypotension, or extrinsic compression (e.g., by tumor).

Ultrasound techniques provide indirect assessment for venous thrombosis. Doppler sonography has equal specificity and sensitivity to IPG in the hands of a skilled operator and can be used successfully in the presence of many of the medical conditions that render IPG inaccurate. Like IPG, ultrasound is inexpensive, widely available, safe during pregnancy, and can be repeated frequently. Like IPG, Doppler is unreliable for detecting DVT below the knee. Doppler has not been evaluated for serial follow-up as extensively as IPG, but its equivalent sensitivity and specificity have led many to consider it an excellent alternative to IPG.

Direct visualization of the deep veins with B mode ultrasound has shown promise in diagnosing DVT, and may become an accurate and safe substitute for venography. It is a noninvasive test that directly visualizes clots and other sources of poor venous flow (e.g., hematoma or tumor). It is operator-dependent and expensive, though less expensive than venography.

Nuclear scans including ^{125}I fibrinogen uptake scanning and others have been tested but are not practical at this time. Newer *assays of cross-linked fibrinogen degradation products* (FDPs) may one day prove useful blood markers for thrombosis.

Management Strategy

If a DVT is clinically suspected, IPG or Doppler ultrasound should be performed. The choice of these tests depends on local availability and reliability. In some patients, IPG or Doppler ultrasound is inconclusive or technically impossible. In such cases, the patient can be hospitalized and anticoagulated until a venogram can be obtained. If the patient has clinical signs and symptoms suggestive of PE, a negative finding on IPG or Doppler does not rule out PE, and further tests must be done.

Thrombosis confined to the calf must be distinguished from a more proximal thrombosis. Thrombosis above the knee requires anticoagulation, whereas distal thrombosis rarely causes significant PE and does not require treatment. However, up to 20% of calf-only DVTs will subsequently extend proximally, presenting a risk for PE and postthrombotic syndrome. Patients with DVT below the knee should therefore be followed by serial IPG or Doppler every few days, but do not require anticoagulation unless the clot extends above the knee. If there is no clot, anticoagulation therapy can be withheld. The safety of serial IPG for monitoring calf thrombi for propagation has been demonstrated in four large studies, in which patients suspected of DVT with an initially normal IPG were followed with serial IPG or IPG plus ^{125}I fibrinogen uptake scanning. No patients with calf-only DVT died of PE, and IPG was shown to detect those calf DVTs that propagated. Use of serial IPG thus saves the 80% of patients with nonpropagating calf-only DVT from unnecessary treatment and its associated costs and morbidity.

Patients with a history of DVT whose symptoms recur have frequently been placed on anticoagulant therapy, based on clinical presentation alone. However, up to 70% of these patients do not have a DVT and would therefore receive unnecessary treatment. If objective studies fail to document DVT, the postthrombotic syndrome should be considered. Valvular incompetence after DVT of popliteal, femoral, or iliac veins can cause gradual onset of dependent pain and swelling. This syndrome, also called the calf pump failure syndrome, can cause symptoms of intermittent or constant aching relieved by rest and elevation.

If evaluation by history, physical examination, and objective studies cannot provide a diagnosis, one should consider "thromboneurosis." This morbid fear of PE can lead to multiple admissions for DVT treatment. Physicians frequently initiate and reinforce this fear by treating patients without objective evidence for DVT.

Treatment

The three goals of treatment for DVT are to prevent PE, decrease symptoms, and prevent postthrombotic syndrome. General measures such as elevation, immobilization, and heat have been tried without success. Although safe and early removal of the clot would seem the best management, thrombolytic agents like streptokinase have failed to meet long-term expectations and are currently recommended only for life-threatening PE and large proximal thrombi in young patients. Anticoagulation is therefore the mainstay of therapy.

Acute Treatment with Heparin

Hospitalization and intravenous heparin comprise the treatment of choice for proximal DVT. The optimal dosage is unknown, but the risk of recurrent thromboembolism is low if the partial thromboplastin time (PTT) is kept to greater than 1.5 times the patient's pretreatment value. In fact, patients with a PTT less than 1.5 times control values at any time during the first 24 hours of treatment have been associated with a 15-fold increase in thromboembolic events. Complications of heparin therapy include thrombocytopenia, which is reversible but can cause hemorrhage or thrombosis. Heparin can also cause a sensitivity rash, and infrequently leads to osteoporosis or alopecia with prolonged use.

Heparin should be started as soon as the diagnosis of DVT is made, and continued until long-term anticoagulant therapy has reached a therapeutic level. Traditionally, this maintenance anticoagulant (usually warfarin) was initiated several days after heparin was started, but recent studies show no difference in recurrence or complications when warfarin is started immediately.

Long-term Therapy with Warfarin

To prevent recurrence of DVT, long-term anticoagulation is required. Warfarin (Coumadin) is the most used long-term anticoagulant. Therapy is commonly initiated at 10 mg/day for 2 to 3 days, with daily dosage adjustments thereafter based on the results of the prothrombin time (PT). Lower initial doses are recommended for elderly or debilitated patients, because of increased sensitivity to the drug. Most patients are successfully maintained at a dose of 2 to 10 mg/day, and PT determinations are subsequently obtained at intervals of 1 to 4 weeks. The individual dose and intervals between PT determinations should be based on the patient's reliability and response to warfarin. The risk of bleeding is related to the degree of anticoagulation. Warfarin doses that achieve a PT of 1.25 times control values have been shown to be as effective as doses achieving a PT of 1.5 to 2.0 times control values, with bleeding complications decreased from 22 to 4%. The most common site of hemorrhage is the GI tract; the next most common sites are areas of wound-bleeding, vaginal-bleeding, and severe epistaxis. Serious bleeding occurs about 2% of the time, involving intracranial or GI sites. Hemorrhage can occur at any site, even when laboratory parameters are in the normal range.

Because warfarin may cause bleeding and drug interactions (Table 40-1), and requires frequent follow-up, other agents have been sought. "Mini-dose" (5000 U bid) subcutaneous heparin results in a 47% recurrence rate, but with fewer complications of bleeding than with traditional therapy. Subcutaneous heparin, in doses adjusted to raise the PTT to 1.5 times normal (average dose, 10,000 U bid), is as effective as warfarin, has fewer complications, and does not require frequent monitoring. This is particularly useful in pregnant women, as warfarin crosses the placenta, and in patients who cannot easily return for frequent follow-up.

Duration of maintenance therapy is controversial. Six weeks of anticoagulation has been shown to be as effective as the usual 3 to 6 months (i.e., with no increased risk of recurrent thromboembolism). Because more bleeding complications occur with prolonged anticoagulation, the shorter period is also safer. A first recurrence of DVT or PE requires 1 year of anticoagulation therapy. A patient with two or more recurrences or irreversible risk factors such as protein C deficiency or malignancy should receive anticoagulation therapy for life. Patients who cannot receive anticoagulation therapy or who develop DVT while undergoing therapy should have venous blockade of the inferior vena cava considered.

Table 40-1. Warfarin drug interactions

Drugs that may potentiate warfarin anticoagulation	Drugs that may inhibit warfarin anticoagulation	Foods rich in vitamin K
Allopurinol	Barbiturates	Beans
Chloral hydrate	Carbamazepine	Cauliflower
Cimetidine	Cholestyramine	Rice
Clofibrate	Colestipol	Spinach
Disulfiram	Griseofulvin	Pork
Ethanol	Oral contraceptives	Fish
Metronidazole	Phenytoin	
Nonsteroidal antiinflammatory drugs	Rifampin	
Quinidine		
Quinine		
Ranitidine		
Salicylates		
Sulfonamide		
Sulfinpyrazone		
Steroids		
Tricyclics		
Thyroid hormone		

Predisposing Conditions
After a diagnosis of DVT is made and treatment is initiated, the primary care physician should consider an underlying cause. Of patients who develop DVT with no identifiable risk factors, 5 to 15% will have a malignancy (especially lung and GI) diagnosed within 1 year. A cancer evaluation is especially important in patients whose DVTs are recurrent, multiple, treatment-resistant, or in unusual sites (neck, chest, or arm veins). Individual risk factors should guide the workup. Recurrent DVT during therapy should also alert the physician to the possibility of a rare inherited defect in coagulation (antithrombin III deficiency, protein C deficiency). These patients should be referred to a hematologist.

Prevention
The best way to avoid the morbidity and mortality associated with DVT is prevention. While prophylaxis of all ambulatory patients who are at risk for DVT is impractical, prophylaxis should be considered for high-risk patients before they undergo elective surgical procedures. Effective perioperative measures include mini-dose subcutaneous heparin and the use of electric compression stockings. Aspirin and other platelet inhibitors are not effective in preventing DVT.

Superficial Thrombophlebitis
SVT is usually a complication of varicose veins and is heralded by pain, a tender palpable cord, erythema, and warmth without generalized edema. Treatment consists of elevation, local heat, and antiinflammatory agents. Only 2.6% of patients with SVT and varicose veins have associated DVTs, while 44% of patients with SVT and no varicosities have coexistent DVT. Thus a patient with SVT and no varicose veins should be evaluated for DVT by noninvasive studies.

Browse NL, et al. Deep venous thrombosis. In: Browse NL, et al, eds. Diseases of the veins: pathological diagnosis and treatment. London: Edward Arnold, 1988; 443–556.
Extensive discussion of all phases of venous thrombosis.

Hull R, et al. Diagnostic efficacy of impedance plethysmography for clinically suspected deep-vein thrombosis. Ann Intern Med 1985; 102:21–8.
First study to show that serial IPG alone is effective for evaluating patients suspected of having DVT. Shows safety of withholding treatment if IPG results remain negative.

Philbrick J, Becker D. Calf deep venous thrombosis. A wolf in sheep's clothing? Arch Intern Med 1988; 148:2131-8.
This review of 20 papers since 1942 on the natural history of calf-only DVT found no fatal PE and no evidence that they cause chronic venous insufficiency. Up to 20% may propagate, invariably before embolizing.

Hull R, et al. Adjusted subcutaneous heparin versus warfarin sodium in the long-term treatment of venous thrombosis. N Engl J Med 1982; 306:189-94.
While low-dose subcutaneous heparin was ineffective, adjusting the dose to raise the PTT equaled warfarin's efficacy at preventing recurrence of DVT after intravenous heparin.

Petitti D, Strom B, Melmon K. Duration of warfarin anticoagulant therapy and the probabilities of recurrent thromboembolism and hemorrhage. Am J Med 1986; 81:255-9.
Retrospective review of 2422 patients showed hemorrhagic risk increases linearly with duration of warfarin therapy, and there is no increase in thromboembolic events when warfarin is taken for more than 6 weeks.

LeClerc J, et al. Recurrent leg symptoms following deep vein thrombosis. Arch Intern Med 1985; 145:1867-9.
As many as two-thirds of patients with prior DVT and recurrence of symptoms have no DVT. Thus, serial IPG may save many patients from unnecessary treatment and worry. This article also describes postthrombotic syndrome and "thromboneurosis."

Mohr D, et al. Recent advances in the management of venous thromboembolism. Mayo Clin Proc 1988; 63:281-90.
This article provides updates on several controversial issues.

Prevention of venous thrombosis and pulmonary embolism. Consensus conference. JAMA 1986; 256:744-9.
This article shows recommendations of a consensus conference on the prevention of venous thrombosis and pulmonary embolism.

VIII. GASTROINTESTINAL PROBLEMS

41. DYSPHAGIA
Eugene M. Bozymski and John W. Garrett

Dysphagia is the subjective awareness that something has gone wrong with the active mechanical transport of food from the pharynx to the stomach. Patients may describe dysphagia in a variety of ways, saying that food "sticks," "slows down," or "doesn't go down right," or they may say that they choke or regurgitate when they swallow.

Dysphagia may be suggested in the patient who complains of the constant sensation of a lump in the throat that may disappear with swallowing. This condition, globus hystericus, occurs frequently in young to middle-aged patients, often women, in whom anxiety, depression, or obsessive features are also present. By means of a careful history, globus hystericus can be distinguished from true dysphagia, and an extensive evaluation may be avoided.

"Pre-esophageal dysphagia" occurs in patients with a variety of neuromuscular disorders or cerebrovascular disease. These patients have a problem initiating the act of swallowing or transferring food from the mouth to the esophagus. Typically, such patients describe a cough or nasal regurgitation following a swallow, but they may also complain that food "sticks" in the throat.

In esophageal dysphagia, the sensation of food sticking is usually localized by the patient to be somewhere between the suprasternal notch and the xyphoid process. However, localization is not precise. The dysphagia that occurs with lesions at the lower end of the esophagus may be referred to the area of the suprasternal notch. On the other hand, it is very unusual for a lesion high in the esophagus to cause symptoms in the region of the xyphoid.

Causes

Pre-esophageal dysphagia is caused by weakness or incoordination of the pharyngeal muscles, resulting in an inability to initiate swallowing. This can be due to an inability to deliver a food bolus to the hypopharynx or to disordered pharyngeal contractions. Possible causes include mass lesions, central nervous system disease (i.e., cerebrovascular disease, Parkinson's disease, head trauma, or pseudobulbar palsy), skeletal muscle dysfunction (i.e., myasthenia gravis, muscular dystrophy, polio, dermatomyositis, and thyrotoxic or steroid myopathy).

Esophageal dysphagia may result either from obliteration or narrowing of the esophageal lumen by a structural lesion or from abnormalities of motor function. Structural lesions may be either intrinsic (i.e., esophageal carcinoma or peptic stricture) or extrinsic (i.e., mediastinal lymphoma with compression of the esophageal lumen). Diseases that cause motor failure of the esophagus include achalasia and diffuse esophageal spasm. Scleroderma involving the esophagus initially presents as a motor abnormality, but peptic strictures may supervene. Presbyesophagus is not a clinical disorder, but a term coined to describe abnormalities on barium swallows in elderly patients with various complaints. Manometric studies in these patients reveal only a slightly decreased amplitude of contraction, but no evidence of esophageal dysmotility.

Evaluation

History
The history is very important in patients with pre-esophageal or esophageal disease, and it should suggest the correct diagnosis.

Difficulty "getting it started down" is usually the description by patients with pre-esophageal dysphagia. Patients may describe nasal regurgitation or coughing with attempts to swallow, and may have a nasal quality to their voice. Pre-esophageal disease can usually be excluded when the patient has no difficulty initiating a swallow.

Progressive dysphagia is characteristic of lesions obliterating the esophageal lumen, whether intrinsic or extrinsic. Patients first notice difficulty with solid foods, which progresses to difficulty with soft foods and finally liquids. In contrast, patients with primary motor disorders may have dysphagia with liquids as well as solids from the onset. Additionally, dysphagia of motor origin tends to be intermittent, whereas dysphagia secondary to mechanical obstruction tends to be constant and relentlessly progressive. The temperature of the ingested material has no effect on the dysphagia due to obstructing lesions, but cold or iced liquids may aggravate the problem in patients with motor disorders, particularly diffuse esophageal spasm. Also, patients with mechanical narrowing of the esophagus who have an impacted bolus frequently have to regurgitate to obtain relief, whereas patients with motor disorders may pass the impacted material by "washing it down with liquids."

Physical Examination
The physical examination usually contributes little to the diagnosis. If abnormalities are present, they are unfortunately almost always manifestations of late disease, such as the systemic features of scleroderma, a palpable supraclavicular node, or recurrent laryngeal nerve involvement in inoperable or metastatic carcinoma of the esophagus.

X-ray and Other Studies
The evaluation of dysphagia should not be considered complete without barium studies or upper endoscopy with careful attention to the pharynx and esophagus, and possibly esophageal manometric studies. If a patient has difficulty initiating a swallow and pre-esophageal disease is suspected, a cine (or video) esophagram should be performed with careful attention paid to the hypopharynx (to exclude aspiration, diverticula, muscular incoordination, or a mass lesion). If esophageal disease is a possibility, a barium swallow with an upper GI series must be obtained in order to assess primary peristalsis, exclude mucosal abnormalities such as mass lesions or strictures, evaluate lower esophageal sphincter relaxation (and competence to exclude esophageal reflux), and look for mass lesions in the high fundus of the stomach. Barium studies are usually done first because they either make the diagnosis or serve to focus the attention of the endoscopist on any abnormal or suspicious area. If the x-ray study is negative, endoscopy is indicated because small mucosal lesions or Schatzki's rings may not have been visible. Esophageal manometry is always indicated when x-ray findings suggest a motility disorder, but can also be useful when evaluating patients with gastroesophageal reflux, scleroderma, and noncardiac chest pain. Manometry may also be necessary to verify and complete the investigation in patients with negative findings on x-rays and endoscopic examination, and to detect motor disorders that may have been missed by the other modalities.

Specific Clinical Conditions

Achalasia
Achalasia is a progressive neuromuscular disorder marked by a loss of ganglion cells in the esophageal body and lower esophageal sphincter; this results in absent peristaltic activity and increased lower esophageal sphincter pressure with absent or incomplete relaxation. It typically begins in middle age, although it has been diagnosed in early infancy and in the elderly. In addition to dysphagia, which is of the classic motor type, symptoms include regurgitation and occasionally chest pain and weight loss. There also may be symptoms indicative of aspiration, such as repeated bouts of pneumonitis. The physical examination is usually not helpful.

DIAGNOSIS. The chest x-ray may suggest the diagnosis of achalasia if the fluid-filled esophagus is seen as a double density with an air-fluid level behind the heart. Other findings include the absence of a gastric air bubble, probably related to the abnormal lower esophageal sphincter, and an esophagus that is not completely empty. Barium examination shows a widely dilated esophagus tapering to a beak, delayed emptying of barium into the stomach, and absence of primary peristaltic waves.
 Esophageal manometry must be performed to define the motility disorder, and demonstrates increased intraesophageal pressure (probably reflecting the retained secretions), complete aperistalsis with low-amplitude waves, and a hypertensive lower esophageal sphincter with absent or incomplete relaxation.
 Endoscopy is mandatory for exclusion of secondary achalasia resulting from a variety of other lesions, such as carcinoma of the fundus of the stomach, which can invade the

distal part of the esophagus and produce a clinical picture identical to achalasia. Also, patients with achalasia have an increased incidence of esophageal carcinoma, and should undergo repeat endoscopy if symptoms recur.

TREATMENT. Nitrates and calcium channel blockers have been used to decrease symptoms in patients with achalasia. However, effective treatment depends mainly on disruption of the high-pressure zone at the distal end of the esophagus, either by the use of the pneumatic dilator or, in certain instances, by thoracotomy and Heller myotomy. All patients suspected of having achalasia should be evaluated by a gastroenterologist who can perform endoscopy to exclude secondary achalasia and initiate treatment with medication and/or pneumatic dilatation.

Diffuse Esophageal Spasm
Diffuse esophageal spasm is a paroxysmal motor disorder of unknown cause, in which high-amplitude peristaltic contractions are intermixed with normal ones. It is more prevalent in middle-aged people and in women, but may occur in anyone. In addition to dysphagia, symptoms include prominent and distressing pain, which is often similar to the pain of angina pectoris, can be alleviated by nitroglycerin or long-acting nitrates, and at times is related to emotional stress. Because the pain is angina-like, patients are frequently evaluated for coronary artery disease. Regurgitation, weight loss, and symptoms suggesting aspiration are unusual. As in other motor disorders, dysphagia is observed during the intake of liquids as well as solids and may be aggravated by the ingestion of cold liquids. The fact that the pain can occur with swallowing (odynophagia) or can be spontaneous may be confusing, but the association of dysphagia with chest pain directs attention to the esophagus.

DIAGNOSIS. The radiologic appearance of the esophagus on barium swallow is quite characteristic of diffuse esophageal spasm; there are multiple areas of segmental spasm termed *pseudodiverticulosis of the esophagus* or *corkscrew esophagus*. If the x-ray is suggestive of diffuse esophageal spasm, the patient should be referred for esophageal manometry. Manometric results are also characteristic, demonstrating repetitive contractions in response to deglutition, as well as increased amplitude and duration of contractions. Many of the contractions are nonperistaltic; with repeated swallowing, however, some normal peristaltic contractions are seen. There also may be spontaneous activity noted in the body of the esophagus.

In many patients, the clinical presentation does not fit either the classic description of achalasia or diffuse esophageal spasm; their condition is best described as "vigorous achalasia." The term *nutcracker esophagus* is used to describe patients with central chest pain who are found to have high-amplitude, peristaltic contractions on esophageal manometry. Unfortunately, many asymptomatic patients have been found to have similar manometric findings, and it is difficult to call this a special clinical entity rather than a nonspecific motor disorder. There are many forms of the latter, and their clinical importance is uncertain.

TREATMENT. In general, patients suspected of having diffuse esophageal spasm on the basis of x-rays should be referred to a gastroenterologist for esophageal manometry. Most patients can then be managed by a primary physician using either calcium channel blockers or nitrates, which are thought to be beneficial by relaxing smooth muscle. Esophageal dilatation or a surgical myotomy can be required in severe cases, but this is very unusual.

Reflux Esophagitis with Peptic Stricture
Peptic strictures are thought to occur when repeated episodes of acid reflux lead to transmural esophageal inflammation and fibrosis with stricture formation. Most peptic strictures are found in the distal end of the esophagus and are relatively short in length.

DIAGNOSIS. Extensive evaluation of every patient with heartburn is not necessary unless the heartburn is severe or there is associated dysphagia, odynophagia, or other worrisome features. Methods of evaluating the patient with reflux symptoms include upper GI x-rays, esophageal manometry to document an incompetent lower esophageal sphincter, pH recordings to document reflux episodes, Bernstein or acid perfusion test to reproduce symptoms, esophagoscopy, and biopsy. Whether or not these are indicated is determined by the severity and chronicity of the complaints. When dysphagia is associated with esophageal reflux, a barium swallow or upper endoscopy is required. At endoscopy, all patients with peptic stricture should be biopsied to exclude Barrett's esophagus (columnar-lined esophagus, a premalignant lesion) or esophageal carcinoma.

TREATMENT. Peptic strictures are usually managed by bougienage with mercury-filled rubber dilators and aggressive medical therapy with H_2-blockers to minimize inflammation. Omeprazole (Prilosec), a proton pump blocker that almost completely suppresses gastric acid secretion, is quite useful in severe esophageal reflux and will probably become an important part of treatment in patients with peptic stricture and severe reflux.

Lower Esophageal Rings

Lower esophageal rings at the squamocolumnar junction, or Schatzki's rings, also may cause dysphagia. They may be congenital as there is no evidence of fibrosis or inflammation on pathologic specimens. When the transverse diameter of the ring is less than 12 mm, patients usually experience dysphagia. Characteristically, the dysphagia is at first intermittent, giving rise to periodic bolus impaction. These patients have long symptom-free intervals, which over the years may become shortened, until eventually symptoms are continuous. The x-ray appearance is characteristic, but the radiologist should be alerted to look for these rings, because they may be missed unless the esophagus is well distended with barium. Dilatation with mercury-filled bougies is curative.

Carcinoma

Dysphagia is the most common presenting complaint of patients with carcinoma of the esophagus. Classically, there is progressive dysphagia, initially for solids, with inexorable progression through semisolids and liquids. These symptoms are accompanied by weight loss. Odynophagia on occasion may be an initial symptom of esophageal cancer. Factors that predispose to esophageal cancer include smoking, alcohol, history of lye stricture, achalasia, tylosis palmaris et plantaris, and Plummer-Vinson web. A columnar-lined lower esophagus (Barrett's esophagus) is associated with an increased incidence of adenocarcinomas of the esophagus. The diagnosis of esophageal cancer is suggested by the characteristic x-ray appearance and confirmed by endoscopy and biopsy. If metastases have not occurred, treatment consists of preoperative irradiation followed by surgery. Unfortunately, the overall 5-year survival rate is 3 to 10%; it is higher in those patients resected for cure who have nodes that are negative for cancer.

Other Lesions

There is a long list of miscellaneous lesions that can lead to dysphagia. A partial list includes leiomyoma; mediastinal masses; radiation fibrosis; monilial infection of the esophagus; Plummer-Vinson web or upper esophageal webs, which may or may not be related to iron deficiency anemia; and thoracic aortic aneurysms.

Thorn GW, et al, eds. Harrison's principles of internal medicine. 11th ed. New York: McGraw-Hill, 1987: 169–71, 1231–9.
A classic medical presentation of GI diseases.

Sleisenger MH, Fordtran JS. Gastrointestinal disease: pathophysiology, diagnosis, management. 4th ed. Philadelphia: Saunders, 1989: 200–3, 541–658.
A comprehensive subspecialty text dealing with the esophagus in all of its aspects.

Nelson JB, Richter JE. Upper esophageal motility disorders. Gastroenterol Clin North Am 1989; 18(2):195–222.
A comprehensive review of motility disorders responsible for pre-esophageal and upper esophageal dysphagia.

Merlo A, Cohen S. Swallowing disorders. Annu Rev Med 1988; 39:17–28.
Good overview of the differential diagnosis and pathophysiology of dysphagia.

Spechler SJ, Goyal RK. Barrett's esophagus. N Engl J Med 1986; 315:362–71.
Barrett's esophagus, an acquired lesion secondary to chronic reflux, is probably more common than we appreciate. Radiographic features include high esophageal strictures and deep esophageal ulcers. The association of Barrett's esophagus with adenocarcinoma of the esophagus is discussed.

Sandler RS, Bozymski EM, Orlando RC. Failure of clinical criteria to distinguish between primary achalasia and achalasia secondary to tumor. Dig Dis Sci 1982; 27:209–13.
Three clinical criteria—onset at older age, significant weight loss, and short duration of symptoms—are reported to distinguish patients with achalasia secondary to tumor from patients with primary achalasia. Even though they are highly sensitive, they are not specific and their predictive value for distinguishing secondary achalasia from primary achalasia is exceedingly low.

Castell DO, et al. Dysphagia. Gastroenterology 1979; 76:1015–24.
A good general discussion of the topic of dysphagia centered about a case presentation.

Vantrappen G, et al. Achalasia, diffuse esophageal spasm, and related motility disorders. Gastroenterology 1979; 76:450–7.
The authors have extensive experience with esophageal motor disorders and present a compilation of their data.

Cohen S. Esophageal motility disorders and their response to calcium channel antagonists: the sphinx revisited. Gastroenterology 1987; 93:201–3.
An excellent short review of the salient features of motor disorders of the esophagus.

42. ESOPHAGITIS
Brentley D. Jeffries and Sidney E. Levinson

Esophagitis is an inflammatory process of the esophageal mucosa. The nature of injury determines the classification into subgroups of reflux, infectious, medication-induced, or physically induced esophagitis. Reflux esophagitis, by far the most common form in the ambulatory setting, is the primary focus of this chapter.

Gastroesophageal Reflux Disease
Gastroesophageal reflux disease (GERD) includes esophagitis (macroscopic mucosal ulcerations or histologic inflammation of the esophagus) as well as pyrosis (heartburn) or respiratory symptoms secondary to reflux of gastric contents above the gastroesophageal junction, even in the absence of a demonstrable esophageal lesion. It affects people of all ages, with no sex predominance. Reflux of gastric or duodenal contents into the esophagus occurs regularly in up to 10% of healthy people, and occasionally in up to 35%.

The pathogenesis of reflux esophagitis remains controversial. Many studies emphasize incompetence of the lower esophageal sphincter (LES) either intermittently or persistently, in allowing noxious mixtures of acid, proteolytic enzymes, or bile to bathe the squamous epithelial lining of the esophagus. In patients without an abnormal degree of reflux, the development of esophagitis may be related to either decreased tissue resistance or disordered peristalsis with resultant poor acid clearance. Decreased gastric emptying with a resultant increase in postprandial gastric volume may also contribute to esophagitis. Less controversial is the involvement of hiatal hernia; although not all patients with hiatal hernia have esophageal reflux, most patients with severe esophagitis have coexistent hiatal hernia.

Clinical Presentation
Most patients with esophagitis consult a physician because of heartburn, a complaint of burning discomfort behind the lower sternum or in the midepigastrium, which frequently

radiates upward. It increases soon after meals, particularly if the meals include spicy, fatty, or acidic food. It is frequently aggravated by bending, stooping, or straining. Patients may regurgitate sour or bitter fluid, or partially digested food, and may even find fluid on their pillow on awakening. Heartburn occurs with greater frequency during recumbency, and patients with severe esophagitis are likely to awaken with nocturnal pain.

Odynophagia (pain on swallowing) may occur with the passage of large boluses of hot or cold liquids through an area of inflammation. Dysphagia (difficulty in swallowing) can occur with or without structural changes within the esophagus as a result of either spasm associated with inflammation or actual impedance of passage of a bolus by a stricture. Reflux esophagitis also must be considered in patients who present with chest pain not clearly of cardiac or musculoskeletal origin.

Certain factors may help to identify patients at risk for the development of esophagitis. Pregnancy, obesity, and occupational bending or straining increase intra-abdominal pressure and predispose to reflux. Pregnant women also have reduced LES pressure secondary to elevated progesterone levels. Habitual use of acid stimulants such as caffeine, alcohol, and aspirin commonly contributes to the development of heartburn. Agents that decrease LES contraction and therefore increase reflux, such as tobacco, fatty foods, chocolate, peppermint, and excessive ethanol, also may cause heartburn. Although citrus juices or spicy foods incite symptoms by a direct irritant effect, they do not typically induce esophageal inflammation. Finally, patients with scleroderma frequently develop reflux esophagitis and patients with Zollinger-Ellison syndrome may present with refractory esophagitis.

Diagnosis

HISTORY. A typical history of heartburn is diagnostic of esophageal reflux and raises the suspicion of esophagitis. The diagnostic reliability of historical findings is increased if the pain is postprandial, postexercise, and nocturnal. Pain is typically relieved by antacids, at least temporarily, and patients frequently note more frequent symptoms when under stress.

Radiation of pain to the back, which is atypical, suggests spasm or posterior ulceration, whereas dysphagia suggests stricture. Heartburn that has been present for a long time and then decreases may herald the development of stricture, or occasionally, concomitant achalasia.

PHYSICAL EXAMINATION. Findings on examination of patients with esophagitis are usually normal. Epigastric palpation may elicit tenderness or reflux symptoms. Occult bleeding, or infrequently, melena may indicate hemorrhage from ulcerations or erosions. Weight loss and cachexia are observed in some patients with benign strictures or in association with adenocarcinoma developing within Barrett's esophagus. The latter, a premalignant metaplastic mucosal change, can develop with long-standing reflux (see Complications).

LABORATORY STUDIES. GERD is confirmed by documenting reflux, histologic inflammatory changes, or both. Mild heartburn that resolves when acid stimulants are avoided and antacid therapy is begun requires no additional evaluation. Additional studies are warranted: (1) when reflux is suspected, but the history is not characteristic of reflux esophagitis; (2) if initial measures do not completely resolve the patient's symptoms; and (3) if dysphagia, weight loss, or occult bleeding is noted.

Upper GI x-rays are often the first study obtained, in part because they are widely available and relatively inexpensive. Although relatively insensitive in detecting reflux (40%) and mild degrees of inflammation (22%), the upper GI x-rays can be considered diagnostic when evidence for reflux is seen in concert with typical symptoms. Although normal x-ray findings do not rule out reflux esophagitis, they can usually exclude other conditions, such as peptic ulcer disease, malignancy, and complications of reflux such as stricture or ulceration.

Endoscopy is a more accurate means of testing for the diagnosis of esophagitis than are upper GI x-rays, although interpretation of milder grades of inflammation is difficult. Mucosal biopsy increases the accuracy of this technique, but involves greater expense and risk. Investigation with endoscopy is warranted in patients with stricture or ulceration, with the search particularly geared toward evidence of malignancy or Barrett's esophagus. Endoscopy should be the first study performed when heartburn is seen in association with dysphagia or heme-positive stool.

The Bernstein acid perfusion test is the most sensitive nonhistologic study, the results of which are abnormal in up to 90% of patients with esophagitis. However, it is not specific, as patients with gastritis may also have a positive result. A nasogastric tube is passed a distance of 30 cm, and with the patient sitting upright, solutions of normal saline and 0.1 N hydrochloric acid are infused in a manner that allows changes to be made without the patient's knowledge. The test result is considered positive if the patient's symptoms are reproduced twice during acid perfusion and relieved during saline perfusion. Discomfort produced by acid perfusion that does not mimic the patient's symptoms should not be considered a positive result. Although the test is simple to perform, interpretation can be difficult and must employ strict criteria and is usually done by a gastroenterologist. Because the Bernstein test allows the physician and patient to compare symptoms produced by acid perfusion with those experienced spontaneously, it is most useful in patients with multiple or atypical complaints. However, it does not actually measure acid reflux, nor does it confirm the presence of mucosal inflammation, which if necessary can be verified with endoscopy.

In difficult instances, or when surgery is considered, other studies are usually performed after referral to a gastroenterologist. Esophageal manometry can delineate abnormalities of peristalsis in achalasia, esophageal spasm, or scleroderma. LES pressures of less than 8 mm Hg suggest reflux, although considerable overlap occurs between symptomatic and asymptomatic patients. The 24-hour ambulatory pH probe affords correlation of symptoms with esophageal pH. For this test a nasoesophageal probe is placed 5 cm above the LES and data are recorded via a portable monitor. Computer-assisted analysis provides a reflux score based on the degree and duration of reflux. The test is most useful in determining whether chest pain or pulmonary symptoms are related to reflux. It is easily performed, even in infants. Potential difference studies and gastroesophageal scintiscanning are less-used modalities.

Treatment

GENERAL MEASURES. The typical course of esophagitis is one of intermittent exacerbations, many of which can be managed with a combination of nonmedical methods. As this is a chronic disease with recurrence documented after completion of every medical regimen studied thus far, long-term behavioral modifications must be emphasized to the patient.

Several life-style changes can decrease the degree of reflux and reduce both symptoms and risk of esophageal inflammation. Any substances or behaviors associated with symptoms should be avoided. In particular, dietary changes and cessation of smoking should be emphasized. Nocturnal reflux may be reduced by elevation of the head of the bed 6 to 8 in. (using blocks under the frame) and avoiding food 3 hours before bedtime (because a meal stimulates acid production and increases gastric distention). Weight loss is extremely important in the obese. Avoiding large meals or recumbency after eating, frequent bending, and tight-fitting garments will decrease daytime reflux. Drugs that may exacerbate reflux by decreasing LES pressure include anticholinergics, theophylline, progesterone, alpha- and beta-adrenergic agents, diazepam, meperidine, and the calcium channel blocking agents.

DRUGS. The addition of either antacids or alginic acid (Gaviscon, which produces a foam barrier to reflux) to the measures described above effectively treats 75% of patients. For the 25% of patients who do not respond, the addition of other medicines aimed at the pathogenetic mechanisms can increase the healing of esophagitis.

Several drugs have become important additions in recent years. H_2-receptor antagonists have now become the mainstay of medical therapy for reflux esophagitis. Multiple studies have shown these drugs to be effective in relieving symptoms and improving endoscopic abnormalities; in 6 to 8 weeks, roughly 60% of patients have improved endoscopic findings with treatment versus 30% with placebo. Usual doses are cimetidine (Tagamet), 300 mg four times a day; ranitidine (Zantac), 150 mg twice a day; famotidine (Pepcid), 40 mg at bedtime, and nizatidine (Axid), 300 mg at bedtime. These drugs are generally considered equally effective. Unfortunately, many patients are refractory to standard H_2-blocker therapy and some investigators have suggested higher doses or more prolonged (3–6 month) treatment periods. Trials of reduced doses for maintenance therapy after healing have generally not been effective; 30 to 50% of patients relapse within 1 year. Long-term full-dose therapy is frequently required.

A powerful new acid-suppressing agent, omeprazole (Prilosec, formerly Losec), was recently approved in the United States for use in refractory reflux esophagitis. It acts by blocking the H^+/K^+ ATPase or proton pump, the proposed final common pathway for gastric H^+ ion secretion, and is capable of essentially complete acid suppression. In double-blind studies, omeprazole, 20 mg every day, has been shown to heal esophagitis more rapidly and in a larger percentage of patients than did ranitidine, 150 mg twice a day (85% versus 50%, respectively, at 8 weeks). Studies in rats demonstrating the development of gastric carcinoid tumors after prolonged high doses raise some concern over long-term acid suppression. Omeprazole has been approved for short-term (4–8 week) therapy of severe or refractory GERD. Unfortunately, relapse occurs rapidly when the treatment is stopped.

Prokinetic agents direct therapy at a different pathogenic defect in GERD. In theory this would offer an advantage in combination therapy with acid inhibition, but clinical studies have been disappointing. Metoclopramide (Reglan), a dopamine antagonist shown to increase LES pressure and to improve gastric emptying, has been demonstrated to achieve moderate symptomatic relief in a dose of 10 mg four times a day; one-third of patients have neurologic or psychotropic symptoms with this dose. It has not been shown to heal esophagitis. Domperidone, another dopamine antagonist, is not yet approved for use in the United States. Bethanechol, 25 mg four times a day, has been reported to increase LES pressure and improve esophageal acid clearance, but has achieved mixed success in clinical trials. Mild adverse effects are related to its cholinergic action. Cisapride, another agent not yet available in the United States, offers some promise. Like metoclopramide, it increases LES pressure and improves gastric emptying but its indirect cholinergic action is limited to the GI tract and thus is less prone to adverse CNS effects.

Sucralfate (Carafate) binds to damaged mucosa where it has a cytoprotective effect, including action as a physical barrier to mucosal irritants. In limited studies, it has been shown to be effective in symptom relief and healing. For esophagitis a 1-g tablet, suspended in 30 ml of water is given four times a day.

SURGERY. Indications for surgery include well-documented GERD that is refractory to medical therapy and associated with peptic or respiratory complications. Prospective studies have demonstrated that modern surgical procedures improve reflux and heartburn in up to 90% of patients. Recurrence of esophagitis due to operative failure is quite low at 1 year but is not unusual at 5 to 10 years. Choice of procedure depends on the experience of the surgeon; a modified Nissen fundoplication is probably the most effective and least morbid. It may be complicated by dysphagia or the gas-bloat syndrome (with the inability to belch or vomit). Pneumonia and other immediate postoperative complications are more common with procedures that use a thoracic approach, such as the Belsey Mark IV. Recent advances in medical therapy may decrease the 5% of patients with GERD that currently require surgical intervention.

Complications

Patients with long-standing erosive esophagitis are at greatest risk of developing complications. Despite a low incidence among patients with reflux, the size of the population affected makes therapy of complications a common clinical problem.

Esophageal stricture occurs in 10% of patients seeking medical attention for reflux and can cause weight loss or food impaction. Strictures may be treated with dilatation as discussed in Chapter 41.

GI bleeding from esophagitis is usually occult but can be life-threatening.

Pulmonary complications include aspiration pneumonia, laryngeal problems (hoarseness), and nocturnal asthma. There is evidence that esophageal irritation induces vagally mediated reflex bronchospasm.

Barrett's esophagus is an acquired lesion defined by a change in the mucosal lining of the esophagus from the normal squamous epithelium to a columnar-lined epithelium. It is usually limited to the distal end of the esophagus but may extend proximally and is associated with midesophageal stricture. The typical endoscopic appearance is velvety red mucosa extending proximally in tongue-like projections from the gastroesophageal junction. Barrett's esophagus is associated with a 30- to 40-fold increased incidence of adenocarcinoma of the esophagus. Although the efficacy and timing of endoscopic surveillance are controversial, some suggest frequent (every 1–2 years) biopsies.

Infectious Esophagitis

Esophageal infections occur uncommonly in immunocompetent hosts but are a serious cause of morbidity in immunocompromised patients. The vast majority of infections are caused by *Candida albicans,* herpes simplex virus (HSV), or cytomegalovirus (CMV). The first two can occur rarely in the normal host but CMV is found only in the immunocompromised, and particularly in AIDS or organ transplant patients. Diagnosis of infection is critical as specific therapies are available. Patients usually present with odynophagia, retrosternal pain, or dysphagia. Endoscopy is the procedure of choice as brushings, biopsies, and culture are required; however, double-contrast barium swallow can be suggestive in patients in whom endoscopy is contraindicated.

Candida Esophagitis
C. albicans is the most common cause of infectious esophagitis. Most affected patients have reason for at least a mild immune defect such as diabetes, malnutrition, postoperative state, treatment with antibiotics or steroids, or damaged mucosal defenses. Patients may have severe odynophagia or be asymptomatic. Oral candidiasis may accompany esophageal infection but is often absent. The typical findings at endoscopy are raised white plaques extending to the upper third of the esophagus. As *Candida* is a normal commensal organism, a positive culture or a finding of fungal forms on brushing may not be significant. Mycelial forms on brushing or invasion on a biopsy specimen is diagnostic. Treatment depends on the degree of immunocompromise and various recommendations have been given. In general, the immunocompetent patient usually responds within 7 days to nystatin oral suspension (200,000 U q2h or 500,000 U q6h) or clotrimazole lozenges (10 mg 5 times a day), with treatment continued for 2 to 6 weeks. Patients who do not respond within 7 days, or those with AIDS or moderate immune defects are treated with ketoconazole (200–400 mg qd). Those with refractory disease or severe immunocompromise receive amphotericin intravenously. The latter group also requires prophylactic therapy until recovery of immunity.

Herpes Simplex Virus
HSV is rarely a cause of self-limited esophagitis in the immunocompetent, but is more often found in the immunocompromised where it can lead to complications of bleeding, HSV pneumonia, and *Candida* superinfection. Odynophagia is the usual presenting symptom. The finding of oral or nasal HSV supports the diagnosis but confirmation requires endoscopy for tissue studies and culture. The esophageal lesions progress from vesicles to small discrete ulcers, which coalesce to larger ulcers. Cytologic and histologic studies reveal characteristic intranuclear inclusions. The immunosuppressed patient is treated effectively with acyclovir (15–20 mg/kg/day intravenously given in divided doses q8h). The immunocompetent patient requires only symptomatic therapy.

Cytomegalovirus
CMV esophagitis occurs only in the immunosuppressed patient, with odynophagia as the most prominent symptom and large shallow ulcers found on endoscopy. Cytologic or histologic studies of endoscopic biopsy specimens reveal characteristic intranuclear and intracytoplasmic inclusions and the diagnosis can again be confirmed by culture. In contrast to HSV, CMV is usually associated with widespread visceral involvement and gastric biopsy specimens are often positive for CMV as well. Therapy for CMV esophagitis has only recently become available with ganciclovir, which has appeared effective in several initial studies in AIDS patients, with the efficacy in other groups not yet well established. Long-term maintenance therapy is often required as long as immunosuppression persists.

Acquired Immunodeficiency Syndrome
The infections mentioned above often affect patients with AIDS. In addition, there are recent reports of severe aphthous ulcers of the hypopharynx and esophagus in which no infectious agents could be identified on biopsy and culture. These giant esophageal ulcers have responded to empiric corticosteroid therapy.

Medication-Induced Esophagitis
Many commonly used drugs can result in esophageal injury. A small number of medications that are believed to exert a direct injury due to prolonged mucosal contact account for the majority of cases. These include tetracycline derivatives, potassium chloride, quinidine, and emepronium bromide. Nonsteroidal antiinflammatory drugs have also been implicated. The history is often one of taking the medication in the recumbent position with an inadequate volume of fluid. Patients often present with retrosternal pain, odynophagia, and dysphagia. Most cases are self-limited and resolve in 7 to 10 days. Other medications harm the esophagus by an indirect effect. Antibiotics, immunosuppressive drugs, and chemotherapeutic agents predispose to infectious esophagitis.

Physically Induced Esophageal Injury
Ingestion of a toxic agent is a significant problem in children, alcoholics, and those with psychiatric disorders. Alkaline agents such as lye are most harmful, due to the depth of injury, and the affected patient may present with perforation or shock. Survivors face chronic complications including stricture and an increased risk of squamous cell carcinoma. Alkaline button batteries swallowed by children should be emergently removed from the esophagus.

Radiation-induced injury is not a frequent problem, as the esophagus is relatively radioresistant. At doses of 3000 rads, symptoms of odynophagia and retrosternal burning commonly occur but are usually mild and limited to the period of treatment. More severe effects are seen at doses of 4500 to 6000 rads but occur at lower doses when combined with chemotherapy, especially doxorubicin (Adriamycin). Abnormalities include abnormal motility, mucosal edema, ulceration, pseudodiverticula, fistulae, and strictures.

Richter JE, Castell DO. Gastroesophageal reflux: pathogenesis, diagnosis, and therapy. Ann Intern Med 1982; 97:93–103.
An excellent general review, with practical advice about management, but predates studies of newer agents.

Dodds WJ, et al. Pathogenesis of reflux esophagitis. Gastroenterology 1981; 81:376–94.
A thorough review of the contributory mechanism of esophageal reflux and esophagitis.

Behar J, Biancani P, Sheahan DG. Evaluation of esophageal tests in the diagnosis of reflux esophagitis. Gastroenterology 1976; 71:9–15.
The Bernstein test was more helpful than secretory studies or manometry in diagnosing esophagitis.

Chernow B, Castell DO. Diet and heartburn. JAMA 1979; 241:2307–8.
A discussion of foods that affect LES pressure and increase heartburn.

Tytgat GNJ. Drug therapy of reflux oesophagitis: an update. Scand J Gastroenterol Suppl 1989; 168:38–49.
A recent update, with discussion of omeprazole, H_2-blockers, sucralfate, and prokinetic agents.

Hetsel DJ, et al. Healing and relapse of severe peptic esophagitis after treatment with omeprazole. Gastroenterology 1988; 95:903–12.
A dose of 40 mg/day produced healing slightly more quickly than did 20 mg/day. Esophagitis recurred in 88 (82%) of 107 by 6 months.

Bozymski EM, Herlihy KJ, Orlando RC. Barrett's esophagus. Ann Intern Med 1982; 97:103–7.
Concise review of pathogenesis, pathology, and clinical features and management.

DeMeester TR, Johnson LF, Kent AM. Evaluation of current operations for the prevention of gastroesophageal reflux. Ann Surg 1974; 180:511–25.
The Nissen procedure inhibited reflux adequately, with fewer operative complications than in the Belsey procedure.

Goff JS. Infectious causes of esophagitis. Annu Rev Med 1988; 39:163–9.
A brief review with practical points on diagnosis.

Bach MC, et al. Aphthous ulceration of the gastrointestinal tract in patients with the acquired immunodeficiency syndrome (AIDS). Ann Intern Med 1990; 112:465–7.
Brief report of six cases; five responded rapidly to steroids.

Bott S, Prakash C, McCallum RW. Medication-induced esophageal injury: survey of the literature. Am J Gastroenterol 1987; 82:758–63.
Review of 127 cases found four drugs responsible for 89% of cases.

Lepke RA, Libshitz HI. Radiation-induced injury of the esophagus. Radiology 1983; 148:375–8.
Abnormal motility occurred 4 to 12 weeks and strictures 4 to 8 months after radiotherapy.

43. FUNCTIONAL DYSPEPSIA
Douglas A. Drossman

Dyspepsia is a common symptom that defies precise definition or classification. We customarily use the term to refer to "indigestion," which is an abdominal fullness or pain that can be dull, gnawing, or burning in quality, or "gaseousness," which includes belching, abdominal distention, and audible borborygmus. The discomfort is usually localized in the upper abdomen or anterior chest, and eating may aggravate or relieve the discomfort. Associated symptoms may include anorexia, nausea, or dysphoric states such as anxiety and depression.

Dyspepsia can be experienced by patients with a variety of pathologic disorders, such as esophagitis, cholecystitis, or peptic ulcer. In recent years, *Helicobacter pylori* (previously *Campylobacter*) infection has been suggested as a possible cause of dyspepsia because the presence of this organism is associated with endoscopic and histologic gastritis. Although it is reported more commonly in patients with dyspepsia, its role in producing symptoms in patients not having gastritis has not been determined. In this chapter, the term *functional dyspepsia* is used to denote symptoms in patients without structural abnormalities (i.e., with negative findings on x-ray or endoscopic studies).

The true frequency of functional dyspepsia is difficult to establish because no precise clinical criteria are established and no demonstrable structural change or physiologic aberrations exist. It is believed to occur in at least 10% of the population, but its prevalence in clinical settings varies with the type of medical practice and the willingness of the physician to use symptomatic diagnostic categories. Although the incidence in a general medical outpatient population in Great Britain was reported to be as high as 26%, this diagnosis is rarely made in gastroenterology referral practices.

The correlation between the symptoms of functional dyspepsia and specific pathophysiologic abnormalities is generally poor. Endoscopic, radiologic, and surgical evaluation of patients with chronic dyspepsia identifies structural abnormalities in 13 to 86%. This wide variation is in part explained by the lack of precise symptom definition. Furthermore, dyspeptic symptoms and disease findings are not necessarily causally related. For example, gastric biopsy specimens show inflammatory changes in 40 to 75% of patients with x-ray-negative dyspepsia, but the same proportion of asymptomatic subjects has similar pathology. Most patients and physicians believe that increased amounts of intestinal gas produce the pain and sensations of bloating and distention. However, the quantity and distribution of intestinal gas in these patients have been found to be no different from those of asymptomatic comparison groups.

Diagnosis

Dyspepsia, like pain, is accepted as present in any patient who complains of it. The physician's task is to decide whether additional diagnostic evaluation is needed to exclude specific disorders before instituting symptomatic treatment.

History and Physical Examination

The illness should be fully characterized, with attention to the diagnostic medical possibilities and the psychosocial factors influencing the experiencing and reporting of symptoms. Is the discomfort related to meals, change in bowel function, or exertion? Is it relieved by antacids or by rest? Is there dysphagia or shortness of breath? What was the setting of symptom onset? Was there associated anxiety or sadness?

Although perhaps the majority of patients presenting with dyspepsia in the primary care setting may be found to have no other pathologic diagnosis, the physician should consider in the differential diagnosis those disorders requiring specific treatment. These conditions include peptic ulcer disease (symptom is relieved by meals), cholecystitis (right-upper-quadrant pain with positive findings on ultrasound and/or hepatobiliary scan and/or abnormal liver chemistries), pancreatitis (symptom is often worse after meals), cardiac ischemia (symptom is worse during exertion), gastroesophageal reflux (symptom is worse when patient is straining or lying supine), diffuse esophageal spasm (associated with episodic dysphagia), biliary dyskinesia (associated with abnormal liver chemistries, dilated common bile duct, and delayed biliary drainage in a patient after cholecystectomy), irritable bowel syndrome (associated with changes in bowel function), and parasitic disorder such as that caused by *Giardia lamblia*. Psychological disorders to consider include anxiety (with or without panic), conversion disorder, depression with somatization, and hypochondriasis.

Additional Studies

The need for diagnostic tests is determined by the findings on the history and physical examination. It is reasonable to include a complete blood cell count and to test the stool for occult blood. If these test results are negative, additional diagnostic study is usually not needed. However, evidence for occult bleeding suggests diagnoses such as esophagitis, gastritis, peptic ulcer, neoplasia, or infectious-inflammatory bowel disease, and requires additional diagnostic evaluation. An upper GI series may be done if the patient has dysphagia, weight loss, vomiting, or a change in the pattern of symptoms with eating. These x-rays may disclose structural abnormalities (strictures, ulcers, tumor), but cannot identify esophagitis or superficial gastroduodenal erosions. Upper endoscopy, a more sensitive method for detecting mucosal abnormalities, has been recommended for evaluation of patients with continued unexplained symptoms. However, this examination does not prove cost-effective when there is no evidence for GI blood loss and the upper GI series is normal. Esophageal manometry is indicated with provocative testing (edrophonium or hot or cold liquids) only if dysphagia, regurgitation, or evidence for aspiration suggests a motor disorder of the esophagus.

Electrocardiography, possibly with exercise testing, should be considered if the symptoms are related to exertion or are associated with dyspnea. Abdominal ultrasound is of uncertain diagnostic value in the patient with dyspepsia and no other clinical findings. Among patients referred for ultrasound or oral cholecystogram, dyspepsia is equally frequent whether or not gallstones are present. Thus, if a patient complaining only of dyspepsia is found to have gallstones (within a functioning gallbladder), surgery may not be indicated. However, if the patient has symptoms also suggestive of cholecystitis, choledocholithiasis, or cholangitis (intermittent postprandial pain localized to the right upper quadrant, vomiting after meals, fever, jaundice, or abnormal liver chemistries), more thorough evaluation of the biliary system is needed, and surgical, radiologic, or endoscopic intervention is recommended if disease is found. Sigmoidoscopy and possibly examination of the stool for ova and parasites should be done if the patient reports any associated change in bowel function. Finally, more thorough diagnostic evaluation such as barium enema or colonoscopy may be needed in selected patient groups, such as patients over 45 years presenting with associated occult GI bleeding.

Treatment

If the initial history and physical examination do not indicate the need for additional tests, or if the studies ordered are nondiagnostic, the physician may give reassurance, treat the patient symptomatically, and observe over time for any changes or new clinical findings. No one medication is of proven value in relieving symptoms of dyspepsia, but each physician develops a set of treatments that seems effective in many instances. Treatment should be relatively inexpensive, safe, and tailored to the amelioration of symptoms.

Dietary Changes
Patients should avoid foodstuffs known to affect acid secretions and intestinal motility adversely. These include tobacco, caffeine, and gas-producing substances such as beans and cabbage. A low-fat diet can be recommended for patients who report increased symptoms with fatty foods. These symptoms may occur because of the associated delay in gastric emptying caused by the endogenous release of cholecystokinin. The patient with lactase deficiency should avoid milk products.

Medications
Antacids can be tried for brief periods of time. A 3- to 4-week trial of an H_2-receptor blocker (e.g., cimetidine, ranitidine) can also be done in an effort to relieve symptoms and avoid further diagnostic evaluation. There is, however, no statistical evidence that either antacids or H_2-blockers will relieve the symptoms better than placebo. Simethicone, either in combination with an antacid or as chewable tablets, can be suggested to relieve symptoms of "gas." Although this surface-acting agent disperses gas bubbles, its efficacy in relieving patient symptoms is unproved. Most of these patients are believed to have a motility disorder rather than an increased accumulation of gas. There is also a subgroup of patients who are habitual air swallowers. They are observed to swallow air and belch when experiencing stress. For these patients treatment may involve reassurance and, on occasion, a short course of benzodiazepine agents. Metoclopramide, 10 mg one-half hour before meals and at bedtime, is reported to be of some value in patients with "functional" digestive disorders. Its effectiveness may be related to its ability to improve gastric emptying, or to its centrally mediated antiemetic effect. Side effects include drowsiness, dizziness, dystonia, and on occasion, galactorrhea caused by stimulation of endogenous prolactin secretion. Other medications often used but of uncertain clinical benefit include cholestyramine and anticholinergic agents.

Thompson WG. Gut reaction. New York: Plenum, 1989.
  This well-written and enjoyable book provides a comprehensive review of functional disorders for physicians and patients.

Drossman DA. The physician and the patient: review of the psychosocial GI literature with an integrated approach to the patient. In: Sleisenger MA, Fordtran JF, eds. Gastrointestinal disease: pathophysiology, diagnosis, management. 4th ed. Philadelphia: Saunders, 1989: 3–20.
  This chapter reviews GI disorders from a biopsychosocial perspective. Included are practical suggestions for the diagnosis and care of patients with "functional" complaints.

Drossman DA, et al. Identification of subgroups of functional bowel disorders. Gastroenterol Int 1990; 3:159–172.
  The product of an international panel that developed diagnostic criteria, this article summarizes the symptoms, diagnostic studies, and physiologic data for all functional disorders, including functional dyspepsia.

Lasser RB, Bond JH, Levitt MD. The role of intestinal gas in functional abdominal pain. N Engl J Med 1975; 293:524–6.
  This important study reports no differences in the quality or composition of intestinal gas between patients complaining of gaseousness and asymptomatic persons.

Nyren O, et al. Absence of therapeutic benefit from antacids or cimetidine in non-ulcer dyspepsia. N Engl J Med 1986; 314:339–43.

In 159 patients with chronic or recurrent epigastric pain without evidence of organic disease or irritable bowel syndrome, neither antacids nor cimetidine resulted in more than a 4% improvement.

Talley NJ, Phillips SF. Non-ulcer dyspepsia; potential causes and pathophysiology. Ann Intern Med 1988; 108:865–79.
An authoritative discussion of nonulcer (functional) dyspepsia, emphasizing the importance of the history and physical examination to guide the diagnostic evaluation.

Kahn KL, Greenfield S. The efficacy of endoscopy in the evaluation of dyspepsia. J Clin Gastroenterol 1986; 8:346–58.
Reviews the disorders that cause dyspepsia, of which functional dyspepsia may be the most common, and gives a reasonable approach to diagnosis from a cost-benefit standpoint. Clinical judgment prevails; most patients with these symptoms will not require extensive evaluation.

Zell SC, Budhraja M. An approach to dyspepsia in the ambulatory care setting: evaluation based on risk stratification. J Gen Intern Med 1989; 4:144–50.
A comprehensive review of dyspepsia in a primary care setting, emphasizing the high frequency of nonulcer dyspepsia and providing a rational approach to patient care.

Jones R. Dyspeptic symptoms in the community. Gut 1989; 30:893–8.
Looks at community prevalence of symptoms.

44. PEPTIC ULCER DISEASE
Eugene M. Bozymski and John W. Garrett

Peptic ulcer disease is a common and costly medical problem. In the United States, over 4 million people have active peptic disease, with direct costs of the disease (hospitalization, physician visits, drugs) exceeding $2 billion annually. The incidence of the disease remains stable, although the number of patients hospitalized and the mortality rate have declined. Many factors have been associated with the occurrence of peptic disease: age, sex, race, nonsteroidal medication use, cigarette smoking, and family history. Although it can be effectively treated with medical therapy in an outpatient setting, peptic ulceration is a chronic disease. During the first year, relapses following adequate treatment occur in over 50% of patients.

Pathogenesis
Peptic ulcers may be regarded as resulting from an imbalance of aggressive and defensive factors.

Aggressive Factors
Of a variety of causal factors, hydrochloric acid is the most important. Duodenal ulcers virtually never occur in the absence of gastric acid, and usually heal when gastric acid output is neutralized or reduced. Nonetheless, increased acid secretion is found in only 20 to 50% of patients with duodenal ulcers. This suggests that other factors, such as proteolytic enzymes and bile acids are also important in causing peptic ulcer disease.

In addition to the standard etiologic factors, *Helicobacter pylori* (previously *Campylobacter*), a gram-negative bacteria, is thought to play a role in peptic disease, although its exact role has yet to be determined. This organism is commonly associated with active antral gastritis and investigators believe it causes that disorder. Treatment of the organism with amoxicillin and metronidazole (Flagyl) and colloidal bismuth subcitrate reverses the histologic features in a large number of cases and can lead to symptomatic improvement. Because many patients with chronic gastritis are asymptomatic and other patients remain symptomatic after treatment, the precise relationship between mucosal inflammation and dyspeptic symptoms and the eradication of the *Helicobacter* organism is unclear.

Protective Factors

Factors involved in protecting the gastroduodenal mucosa include mucus and bicarbonate secretion and mucosal blood flow, which are increased by endogenous prostaglandin production. Surface epithelial cells also play an important role in mucosal defense, both by limiting the influx of hydrogen and by restitution, a process in which the migration of epithelial cells over denuded mucosa protects the submucosa from damage.

Risk Factors

Many studies have shown that the stomach and duodenum participate in the adaptation to stress. Severe emotional tension and exacerbation of "usual" life stresses have been correlated with the onset of ulcer symptoms, and stress has been shown to cause ulcers in animals. However, no single "ulcer personality" has been defined.

Cigarette smokers are also at increased risk for duodenal ulcer disease, and are frequently resistant to medical therapy. This is probably secondary to reduced pancreatic bicarbonate output. Nonsteroidal antiinflammatory agents are capable of decreasing mucosal prostaglandin synthesis and also predispose patients to gastroduodenal ulcerations. Elderly patients in particular may be asymptomatic from peptic disease until the development of a significant complication (bleeding, perforation).

Clinical Presentation

Pain is the most frequent complaint in patients with peptic ulcer. It is described as sharp, gnawing, burning, or hunger pain, and it usually is well localized in the upper part of the epigastrium, although it may occur anywhere in the epigastric area. Frequently the patient is able to point with one finger to the area of greatest discomfort. The pain may radiate to the back, particularly when the ulcer is posterior or penetrating. It often occurs when the stomach is empty, or awakens the patient from sleep an hour or so after midnight. The pain is typically improved by ingesting food or antacids; in some patients, however, eating makes the pain worse. Ulcer pain is characteristically intermittent, with periodic exacerbations and remissions over the years.

Vomiting can occur in the absence of outlet obstruction. This appears to be more common in patients with channel ulcers and may be related to alterations in antral motility.

Complications of peptic ulcer include obstruction, GI bleeding, and perforation. Occasionally otherwise asymptomatic patients with duodenal ulcer present with anemia secondary to chronic bleeding.

Evaluation

The history should include medication usage, particularly antiinflammatory agents that are known to cause mucosal irritation. The medical history is not sufficiently specific to distinguish patients with duodenal ulcers from those with gastric ulcer, pancreatitis, "functional" dyspepsia, or gallbladder disease. It can be quite difficult to differentiate peptic disease from other abdominal problems and many patients with "classic" ulcer symptoms are not found to have an ulcer when studied by radiography or endoscopy.

Physical Examination

The physical findings are usually entirely normal in patients with uncomplicated duodenal ulcer. Sometimes there is an area of well-localized tenderness in the epigastrium. In the presence of complications, examination may disclose a tense, boardlike abdomen and peritoneal signs suggesting a perforation, or a succussion splash suggesting gastric outlet obstruction.

Laboratory Studies

Routine laboratory studies in all patients suspected of having peptic disease should include a stool test for occult blood and hematocrit determination.

There is no consensus regarding the need for upper GI x-rays or endoscopy in patients with symptoms of peptic ulcer. People under 40 years old who have symptoms consistent with uncomplicated peptic ulcer may be treated with H_2-blocker therapy or antacids as needed for pain; if the patient does well, x-ray studies need not be obtained. If the patient is older, or if there are recurrent, prolonged, or atypical symptoms, an investigation should be done.

Serum gastrin levels should be obtained in patients with severe recurrent peptic disease (to exclude gastrinoma). In patients with ordinary peptic ulcer disease, the fasting serum gastrin level is normal. If the values are in the equivocal range, a secretin stimulation test will identify patients with gastrinoma.

X-rays
An upper GI x-ray series with good air-contrast films is used to detect ulcers and identify other lesions that might masquerade as ulcers, such as gastric cancer or severe gastritis. If the duodenal bulb is markedly deformed because of previous ulcer disease, it may be impossible for the radiologist to be certain if a crater is currently present, and one must rely on symptoms to judge activity. The sensitivity of a double-contrast upper GI series is about 80 to 90% for duodenal ulcers, and approximately 60% for gastric ulcers.

Upper Gastrointestinal Endoscopy
Endoscopy provides the most accurate means of detecting the presence or absence of peptic ulcers (sensitivity of 95%). However, the procedure is not necessary when the diagnosis is otherwise clear, nor is it necessary to monitor duodenal ulcer healing by either x-ray or endoscopy; symptomatic response and stool Hemoccult tests are adequate. Gastric ulcers should be followed to healing so that nonhealing ulcers can be biopsied to exclude malignancy. Endoscopy is also necessary when evaluating patients with serious complaints and normal-appearing x-rays, patients with bleeding, or those who are being considered for peptic ulcer surgery. Endoscopy is also preferable to x-ray studies in the special instance of a pregnant woman with sufficient complaints to warrant investigation.

Gastric Secretory Testing
Although gastric acid output may be elevated in patients with duodenal ulcer disease compared to controls, routine measurement of gastric acid output is not necessary. Acid output is normally greater in men than women and decreases with age. Gastric secretory testing is useful when Zollinger-Ellison syndrome is suspected, serum gastrin levels are elevated, or a recurrent ulcer follows ulcer surgery, suggesting an incomplete vagotomy.

Complications
Hemorrhage, the most common complication of duodenal ulcer, occurs in 10 to 20% of patients. The blood loss may vary from massive GI hemorrhage to chronic, occult bleeding leading to iron deficiency anemia. Occasionally, bleeding may be the first manifestation of a peptic ulcer. Once a patient has bled from a duodenal ulcer, the chance of rebleeding is 30 to 50%. A history of duodenal ulcer disease is, however, no guarantee that the ulcer is the source of a present episode of GI bleeding.

In patients with melena, it is important to aspirate the stomach. If blood is present, the bleeding site is above the ligament of Treitz. However, the absence of blood in the gastric aspirate does not exclude bleeding from a duodenal ulcer; blood may be swept distally by peristalsis or may not have refluxed into the stomach. In the emergency room, aspiration through a nasogastric tube may detect active bleeding and help to differentiate those patients who will require urgent endoscopy and an intensive care unit bed from those who are stable and can be examined electively.

Endoscopy is the best way to identify the source of bleeding. Most patients with upper GI hemorrhage stop bleeding spontaneously. Many gastroenterologists believe that the care of the bleeding patient is improved when an accurate diagnosis has been made. Examples include bleeding from esophageal varices or the presence of a "visible vessel," which may be associated with continued bleeding, and can be found and often treated during endoscopy. This is invaluable information in the management of the patient and in planning surgery.

Penetration occurs when duodenal ulcers erode through the serosa and adjacent tissues such as the liver or pancreas. It is heralded by increasing pain that radiates into the back and may be intractable. If penetration is into the pancreas, pancreatitis may ensue. Rarely, the penetration is into a hollow viscus, resulting in a fistula. Patients should be hospitalized for stabilization and further investigation when penetration is suspected.

Perforation is a catastrophic event, accompanied by acute severe abdominal pain, rapid development of peritonitis, and rarely, bleeding. Increasing symptoms may be present for several days or weeks before the perforation. Free peritoneal air is best demonstrated on an upright abdominal or lateral decubitus film. Surgery remains the treatment of choice.

Gastric outlet obstruction is less common than hemorrhage or perforation. With the "typical" presentation, a patient with long-standing ulcer symptoms develops constant pain and then vomiting. The vomiting may be severe and lead to weight loss, dehydration, and hypokalemic (and ultimately hypochloremic) alkalosis. A splashing sound is often present when the patient's abdomen is shaken (succussion splash), indicating fluid in the stomach. Upper GI x-rays document the outlet obstruction; the cause can be confirmed by endoscopy. Obstruction may be caused by edema and inflammation or by scar. Patients with the former may respond to medical therapy, whereas those with the latter require surgery. Treatment includes hospital admission for nasogastric decompression, antacids, H_2-blockers, and avoidance of drugs that decrease gastric motility (e.g., anticholinergics).

Intractability has no strict definition. The ulcer is called *refractory* if symptoms continue or recur after 1 to 2 weeks in a patient receiving a good medical regimen, or if relapses become longer and more severe and remissions shorter. Symptoms that recur repeatedly under all but the most rigorous medical programs can also be termed refractory. Contributing causes, such as gastrinoma, antiinflammatory medications, alcohol, and psychiatric problems, should always be sought.

Medical Therapy

The goals of therapy are healing the ulcer, relieving symptoms, and preventing complications and recurrences.

Diet

Dietary therapy has not been shown to be effective in peptic ulcer disease. Although many patients find that their symptoms are aggravated by certain foods, there are no controlled studies to support any specific dietary regimen. Restriction of the use of caffeine-containing beverages and foods (e.g., coffee, tea, colas, and chocolate) and alcoholic beverages is prudent. Smoking should be curtailed because it is associated with an increased rate of peptic ulcer and decreased healing. Aspirin and nonsteroidal antiinflammatory drugs should also be avoided if possible. Milk should not be used as an antacid since it can stimulate acid secretions and is not a satisfactory buffer.

Drug Therapy

The ease of administration, lack of side effects, and therapeutic efficacy have made H_2-blockers the drug of choice in treating symptomatic acid peptic disease. Nonetheless, antacids are still useful for pain relief in peptic ulcer disease, primarily in the first days of treatment. Newer agents such as omeprazole appear quite promising.

H_2-Blockers

The H_2-receptor antagonists (cimetidine, ranitidine, famotidine, and nizatidine) are potent inhibitors of gastric acid secretion regardless of the stimulant used to increase secretion. They have been used extensively in the treatment of peptic disease and have proved to be remarkably safe. Each of these agents may be administered at bedtime or in twice-daily dosing. Cimetidine is given as 800 mg at bedtime or 400 mg twice daily; ranitidine, 300 mg at bedtime or 150 mg twice daily; famotidine, 40 mg at bedtime or 20 mg twice daily; and nizatidine, 300 mg at bedtime or 150 mg twice daily. Full-dose therapy is generally continued for 6 to 8 weeks, with healing rates of about 90% for duodenal ulcer. Failure of symptoms to respond to therapy in 5 to 7 days suggests that the diagnosis is incorrect or that the disease is complicated and the patient should be re-evaluated.

The recurrence of ulcer after stopping H_2-blocker treatment is not a rebound, but only a reflection of the natural history of peptic ulcer, which is expressed after gastric acid secretion returns to its usual rate. H_2-blockers have also been shown to reduce the recurrence rate of peptic ulcer with a smaller (one-half) dose at bedtime following a course of full-dose therapy. If ulcer disease has been severe or there have been complications, low-dose therapy for several months or even longer may be needed. Finally, some patients may use H_2-blockers during times of stress to reduce symptoms.

The side effects of H_2-blockers usually occur early in the course of treatment. H_2-blockers have been associated with CNS disturbances, elevated liver enzyme levels, diarrhea, constipation, rash, gynecomastia, renal dysfunction, and hematologic abnormalities. Cimetidine, which affects hepatic microsomal enzymes (P-450), also causes drug-drug interaction with warfarin and theophylline compounds. As data accumulate on the newer agents in this class, it is clear that the differences among them in terms of side effects is slight.

Antacids
High-dose antacid regimens have been shown in a randomized controlled trial to heal substantially more ulcers than does placebo. Important features in the choice of an antacid include neutralizing capacity, magnesium content (which causes loose stool), aluminum content (which is constipating), sodium content, taste, and cost. Calcium-containing antacids produce an acid rebound and may lead to the milk-alkali syndrome; therefore, they should be avoided. Liquid antacids are preferable to tablets because they have greater neutralizing capacity. The usual dose is 20 ml of "concentrated" antacid or 30 ml of regular antacid approximately 6 times a day. Antacids are most effective when taken 1 and 3 hours after meals, but for greater effectiveness and absorption should not be taken within 30 minutes of sucralfate or other agents such as antibiotics.

Coating Agents
Some bismuth-containing compounds (e.g., Pepto-Bismol) coat the mucosa of the stomach and duodenum. Sucralfate (Carafate), a sulfated disaccharide, binds to the proteinaceous debris in the ulcer crater and blocks penetration of acid and pepsin and also binds bile acids and enhances localized endogenous prostaglandin production. When taken 4 times a day, sucralfate has been shown to be comparable to H_2-blockers in healing duodenal ulcers. Because sucralfate acts within the lumen and there is little absorption, it is apparently very safe and has few side effects. Constipation is noted occasionally and sucralfate should not be administered with antacids or H_2-blockers. The large sucralfate tablets may be difficult to swallow, but can be dissolved in water and stirred, to make an easily swallowed slurry.

Anticholinergics
Anticholinergics are rarely used. They inhibit gastric acid secretion and decrease the contractile force of smooth muscle. They can be given with antacids or histamine H_2-receptor antagonists to patients whose ulcer is difficult to control; however, anticholinergics have been largely replaced by other agents because of lower efficacy and a high incidence of side effects.

New Agents
Omeprazole (Prilosec), a proton pump inhibitor, is capable of almost completely eliminating gastric acid secretion. This agent should be useful for the treatment of patients with refractory peptic ulcer disease at a dose of 20 mg/day.

Misoprostol (Cytotec) is a synthetic prostaglandin (prostaglandin E) that has been shown to be more effective than cimetidine in protecting the gastric mucosa from nonsteroidal-induced injury.

Decreasing the Psychovisceral Component
Physicians should develop a strong working relationship with ulcer patients and allow sufficient time for the discussion of problems. As in any chronic illness, the patient's ability to control stress is very important, and the physician can offer a great deal of support. Some patients may benefit from mild antianxiety agents or antidepressants if indicated, but a supportive physician is most important.

Helicobacter pylori
In patients with recurrent symptoms who are unresponsive to the usual medical therapy, referral for upper endoscopy with biopsies to evaluate for the presence of *Helicobacter* is indicated. Biopsy-proved *Helicobacter* may be treated with amoxicillin (250 mg tid) and metronidazole (250 mg tid) for 2 weeks and Pepto-Bismol (qid) for a month. Treatment for

this organism is not standardized and various regimens using these three drugs have been proposed. Recurrence of *Helicobacter* is common following treatment. Since it is not clear that treatment influences the natural history of the disease, treatment for *Helicobacter* cannot be recommended outside of experimental protocols.

Surgery

Today, surgery is performed on patients for whom medical therapy fails as defined by intractable symptoms or early recurrence while on an established medical regimen. When surgery is necessary, there are several options. In general, these can be divided into procedures that involve a partial gastrectomy with or without a vagotomy and those whose major emphasis is on interrupting branches of the vagus nerve. Often the choice of procedure depends on the experience of the surgeon or the technical aspects of the situation.

Soll AH. Duodenal ulcer and drug therapy. In: Sleisenger MH, Fordtran JS. Gastrointestinal disease: pathophysiology, diagnosis, management. 4th ed. Philadelphia: Saunders, 1989; 814–79.
A comprehensive review of the pathophysiology, clinical manifestations and complications, and modalities of therapy of duodenal ulcers.

Horrocks JC, DeDombal FT. Clinical presentation of patients with dyspepsia—detailed symptomatic study of 360 patients. Gut 1978; 19:19–26.
A prospective study of 360 patients with dyspepsia that contrasts textbook descriptions with patients' histories, suggesting a faulty "data base" of information with regard to peptic disease.

Dooley CP, et al. Double-contrast barium meal and upper gastrointestinal endoscopy—a comparative study. Ann Intern Med 1984; 101:538–45.
Interesting prospective study demonstrating sensitivity of x-rays versus endoscopy, and discussing the indication for each study.

Isenberg JI, et al. Impaired proximal duodenal mucosal bicarbonate secretion in patients with duodenal ulcer. N Engl J Med 1987; 316:274–9.
Feldman M. Bicarbonate, acid, and duodenal ulcer. N Engl J Med 1987; 316:408–9.
An article and an editorial that provide a good discussion of the roles of acid and decreased bicarbonate secretion in duodenal ulcer disease.

Feldman M. Mechanisms of gastric acid secretion and its pharmacologic control. Contemp Gastroenterol 1988; 1(4):8–14.
A nice review of the various components of gastric acid secretion and present medical therapy of peptic disease.

Shorrock CH, Rees WDW. Overview of gastroduodenal mucosal protection. Am J Med 1988; 84(2A):25–34.
A comprehensive review of gastroduodenal mucosal defense, including a discussion of the significance of mucosal prostaglandins.

Dooley CP, Cohen H. The clinical significance of *Campylobacter pylori*. Ann Intern Med 1988; 108:70–9.
A recent review tackling some of the major issues surrounding the importance of Campylobacter pylori in peptic ulcer disease.

Korman MG, et al. Influence of smoking on the healing rate of duodenal ulcer in response to cimetidine or high dose antacid. In: Rogers DE, et al, eds. The Yearbook of Medicine, 1982. Chicago: Year Book, 1982:381–4.
Carefully done studies indicate that there is an adverse effect of smoking on the healing rate of duodenal ulcer when treated by either cimetidine or Mylanta.

Griffin NR, Ray WA, Schaffner W. Nonsteroidal anti-inflammatory drug use and death from peptic ulcer in elderly persons. Ann Intern Med 1988; 109:359–63.
The association between nonsteroidal use and fatal peptic ulcers or upper GI hemorrhage is examined, and elderly patients are noted to be particularly at risk.

Feldman M, Burton ME. Histamine$_2$—receptor antagonists: Standard therapy for acid-peptic diseases. N Engl J Med 1990; 323:1672–1680.
An outstanding review of the pharmacology and clinical usefulness of H$_2$ blockers in the treatment and prevention of acid-peptic disorders.

Marks IN, et al. Comparison of sucralfate with cimetidine in the short-term treatment of chronic peptic ulcers. S Afr Med J 1980; 57:567–73.
Sucralfate acts primarily as a coating agent binding to the proteinaceous debris in the ulcer base, and is shown to be comparable to cimetidine in producing healing of duodenal ulcers.

Lauritsen K, et al. Effect of omeprazole and cimetidine on prepyloric gastric ulcer: double-blind comparative trial. Gut 1988; 29:249–53.
Omeprazole, a substituted benzimidazole that is a potent proton pump inhibitor, is shown to be more effective in healing and pain relief than cimetidine in the treatment of prepyloric gastric ulcer.

Walker P, et al. Life events, stress, and psychosocial factors in men with peptic ulcer disease. II. Relationship with serum pepsinogen concentrations and behavioral risk factors. Gastroenterology 1988; 94:323–30.
A discussion of the association between psychosocial factors and peptic ulcer disease.

45. IRRITABLE BOWEL SYNDROME
Douglas A. Drossman

The irritable bowel syndrome (IBS) is a physiologic disorder presumably of multifactorial etiology. The clinical course of patients with this disorder has not been well studied. Most adult patients report a long history of bowel-related difficulties going back to childhood.

The patients' complaints reflect the pattern of their bowel motility disorder: diarrhea (frequent, loose, or watery stools, usually of normal volumes), constipation (straining or infrequent, hard stools) or at different times, both. Abdominal pain is usually present and is a major factor leading to a patient's seeking health care. Pain is most often described as cramp-like and located in the mid to lower abdomen. Other nonspecific complaints include fatigue, nausea, and upper abdominal discomfort. Symptoms may be chronic and continuous or intermittent with flare-ups at times of stress, during travel, with medications, during menstrual cycles, or with dietary indiscretion—or with no apparent precipitants. There are no known complications of the disorder itself, although some patients become dependent on laxatives or narcotic analgesics.

Patients with IBS are commonly seen in primary care practices and account for 40 to 70% of referrals to gastroenterologists. Three times as many patients are hospitalized for IBS as for inflammatory bowel disease; medical costs and time lost from work because of IBS are considerable.

The physiologic disturbances underlying IBS are very common, affecting up to 17% of the population. However, most people with IBS do not seek health care for their symptoms. In this country, the disorder is most often seen in young adults, with a female-to-male ratio of 2:1. In countries in which men seek health care more readily than women, the ratio is reversed. These data suggest that sociocultural factors help determine which persons with IBS seek health care. Psychosocial factors also play a major role. Psychological stress affects bowel function in all people, and it appears that people with IBS are more susceptible. Physicians can often identify antecedent psychological and environmental events at the time of symptom onset and exacerbation. Patients with IBS who seek health care for symptoms tend to be influenced as much by life stress, poor social supports, or personality and psychiatric disorders such as depression and hypochondriasis as by their degree of altered bowel physiology. In contrast, people with IBS who have greater coping abilities and psychological stability under stress experience their illness as less disabling and are more self-sufficient in their health care.

Diagnostic Evaluation

Because no pathologic marker for the IBS exists, diagnosis depends on identifying historical data typical for the disorder. Recently, criteria for the diagnosis of IBS were established by an international team of gastroenterologists. These include the following chronic or recurrent symptoms: (1) abdominal pain relieved by defecation or associated with change in stool pattern; and/or (2) disturbed defecation (altered stool frequency or consistency, urgency or straining, feeling of incomplete evacuation, increased mucus), usually accompanied by (3) bloating or the perception of abdominal distention.

A major effort of the diagnostic evaluation is to exclude conditions that may mimic IBS. Lactase deficiency is manifested as cramp-like abdominal pain and loose, frequent stool following the ingestion of milk. If this disorder is suspected, the diagnosis can be confirmed by a breath H_2 or lactose tolerance test, but it is also reasonable to gauge clinical response to restriction of milk-containing foods. Other conditions to be considered include intestinal neoplasia, infectious or inflammatory disease, and malabsorption.

The physical examination helps mainly to exclude other medical disorders. However, localized tenderness elicited over the sigmoid colon or reproduction of the patient's pain during sigmoidoscopic examination suggests that the symptoms are bowel-related, and is consistent with IBS. An abdominal mass, rebound tenderness, and organomegaly are not typically found in the IBS.

It is difficult to know "how far to go" in the workup. The medical evaluation depends on the results of the complete history and physical examination, and must be individualized. A younger patient with a brief course of symptoms probably requires a minimum of diagnostic studies. Conversely, findings not characteristic of the IBS should prompt a more thorough workup. Such findings include the recent onset of symptoms in an older patient, reporting of blood or grease in the stool, fever, considerable weight loss, nocturnal awakening with pain, pain unrelated to changes in bowel function, or evidence suggesting metabolic disturbances. Stools should always be examined for blood; often for parasites, polymorphonuclear leukocytes, and pathogenic bacteria; and occasionally, for fat. Sigmoidoscopy (and in a patient over 40 years of age, barium enema or colonoscopy) is usually indicated. Other studies often clinically indicated include CBC, sedimentation rate, serum amylase, liver chemistries, and urinalysis.

Electrophysiologic studies of the rectosigmoid colon in patients with the IBS suggest abnormalities, such as an increased prevalence of 3-cycle-per-minute basal electrical activity when compared to the electrical pattern of healthy people. The clinical importance of this observation is uncertain, and electrophysiologic evaluation is therefore not yet recommended for diagnosis. In using a minimal diagnostic workup as suggested above, the likelihood of a missed diagnosis is small. There are now five prospective studies showing that a different diagnosis is made in only about 3% of patients followed for up to 6 years.

Treatment

Once the diagnosis is established, or it is at least determined that no additional studies are indicated, treatment should be directed toward amelioration of the symptoms, identification and modification of factors that aggravate the disorder, and encouragement of patient adaptation to what can be a chronic or relapsing condition.

General Approach

Because patients with this disorder may have chronic or recurring symptoms, an essential feature of treatment is the establishment of an ongoing physician-patient relationship. Frequent brief visits initially and during exacerbations are recommended, with the goals of reducing the patient's discomfort and providing psychosocial support. As with any chronic disorder, removal of symptoms is not always the goal of treatment. For many patients, treatment of the bowel symptoms alone may not be sufficient to produce clinical improvement; the physician must also recognize and address the contributing psychosocial factors. During periods of quiescence, the physician should set up one or two brief visits per year. This reinforces the physician's long-term commitment and, because of the patient's knowledge that there is a physician familiar with the problem, minimizes the tendency of some patients to make late-night calls or "emergency" visits.

During visits, attempts should be made to modify identified environmental stress factors or the patient's attitude toward these factors. It is usually helpful to explain that the IBS is a very real disorder in which the intestine is overly sensitive to a variety of stimuli, such as food (type or quantity), hormonal changes (e.g., menses), or stress. Patients may benefit from a discussion of the relation between altered bowel physiology (e.g., segmental spasm of the colon) and clinical symptoms (pain, constipation). Patients are also reassured to learn that the condition is not associated with malignancy or shortened life expectancy and does not require surgery. In addition, the fact that the IBS may have an important psychological component in the absence of specific physical findings should not undermine the legitimacy of the patient's very real complaints. Any implication that the problem is "emotional" is taken as a rejection by the patient.

Diet

The use of increased fiber in the form of bran ($\frac{1}{2}$ oz/day) or commercially prepared psyllium seed products (e.g., Metamucil, Effersyllium, 2 tsp bid) is strongly recommended because of their empiric effectiveness, low price, and virtual absence of side effects. Fiber has been shown to shorten the intestinal transit time, which is of benefit for patients with constipation, and may decrease symptoms in patients with IBS. The presumed mechanism is one of increasing stool bulk by hydration via bacterial breakdown of nondigestible fiber into osmotically active substrates; this minimizes the effects of the nonpropulsive segmental contractions of the colon. Patients should be informed that they may experience transient symptoms of gaseous discomfort during the first few days. (See also Chap. 144.) Food substances known to stimulate bowel action (e.g., caffeinated beverages) or produce increased intestinal gas (e.g., beans, cabbage) should be avoided. Patients with lactase deficiency who develop abdominal cramps and diarrhea when ingesting lactose should avoid milk-containing products.

Drugs

Medications are used in IBS for adjunctive control of symptoms; no single agent or class of drugs is of proved efficacy. Anticholinergic medication, such as dicyclomine (Bentyl), glycopyrrolate (Robinul), or propantheline bromide (Pro-Banthine), may reduce colonic segmental spasm and is recommended for symptomatic treatment of patients with predominant pain and constipation. It should be given $\frac{1}{2}$ to 1 hour before meals and at bedtime. No particular agent has been shown to be superior. Dosage is based on the manufacturer's recommendations, the limiting factor being the development of side effects such as dry mouth and blurry vision. Sedative tranquilizers, particularly of the benzodiazepine family, have gained much popularity. These drugs have no effect on colonic motility and may be associated with habituation. Antidepressants may be helpful with patients whose symptoms are refractory or are manifestations of depression. Other agents can be used symptomatically based on their clinical action. For example, metoclopramide can be used for symptoms of early satiety, particularly if delayed gastric emptying is documented. Imodium may be used for diarrhea, rectal urgency, or fecal soiling. Dextromethorphan (15–30 mg qid) may be used for abdominal pain; it appears to act on gut narcotic receptors without crossing the blood-brain barrier.

Physical Measures

The use of baths, hot water bottles, exercise, relaxation techniques, and periods of rest can be of benefit when individualized to the patient's needs.

Mitchell CM, Drossman DA. The irritable bowel syndrome; understanding and treatment of a biopsychosocial illness disorder. Ann Behav Med 1987; 9:13–8.
Reviews the epidemiologic, physiologic, and psychosocial aspects of the disorder, offering practical suggestions for diagnosis and patient care.

Drossman DA, et al. Psychosocial factors in the irritable bowel syndrome: a multivariate study of patients and nonpatients with IBS. Gastroenterology 1988; 95:701–8.

Documents that psychosocial factors are important determinants of which people with IBS see a physician.

Drossman DA, Lowman B. IBS; epidemiology, diagnosis and treatment. Clin Gastroenterol 1985; 14:559–73.
A general overview of IBS.

Drossman DA, et al. Identification of subgroups of functional bowel disorders. Gastroenterol Int 1990; 3:159–172.
The product of an international panel that developed diagnostic criteria, this article summarizes the symptoms, diagnostic studies, and physiologic data for all functional disorders, including IBS.

Manning AP, et al. Towards positive diagnosis of the irritable bowel. Br Med J 1978: 2:653–4.
A classic article, suggesting that a more confident diagnosis of IBS can be made when specific items are obtained from the history.

Klein K. Controlled treatment trials in the irritable bowel syndrome: a critique. Gastroenterology 1988; 95:232–41.
A critical examination of published IBS treatment trials, concluding that none offers convincing evidence for an effective therapy. Suggestions are given for essential features of much-needed, well-designed treatment trials.

Cook IJ, et al. Effect of dietary fiber on symptoms and rectosigmoid motility in patients with irritable bowel syndrome. Gastroenterology 1990; 98:66–72.
Both corn fiber and placebo were effective in alleviating symptoms. However fasting rectosigmoid pressure, which correlates with symptom severity, seemed to be reduced by fiber therapy.

Friedman G. Nutritional therapy of irritable bowel syndrome. Gastroenterol Clin North Am 1989; 18(3):513–23.
Reviews the literature on nutritional factors. While foods do not cause IBS, intolerance to some types can be identified by the dietary history. The role of fiber and "gas syndromes" are also discussed.

Shimberg E. Living with IBS. New York: Evans, 1988.
Written by a patient with IBS for other patients. Emphasizes the patient taking control over symptoms.

46. DIVERTICULAR DISEASE OF THE COLON
Douglas A. Drossman

Although almost unheard of 100 years ago, diverticular disease of the colon has now become a common, sometimes life-threatening, disorder of the elderly. Diverticulosis and diverticulitis are discussed separately because of differences in pathogenesis, presentation, and treatment.

Diverticulosis
The anatomic abnormality in diverticulosis is a pseudodiverticulum, produced by herniation of mucosa and submucosa through the serosa of the colonic wall. In the rare true diverticulum of the cecum, there is an abnormal outpouching of all wall layers. The prevalence of diverticulosis increases with age; it is found in 30% of people over age 60. However, it is estimated that only 20% of the population with diverticulosis develop symptoms. Typical symptoms include abdominal pain and tenderness and bowel irregularity, which are believed to develop from nonpropulsive colonic contractions that produce abnormally high intraluminal pressures. Patients with symptoms of diverticulosis often have thickening of the circular smooth-muscle layer of the sigmoid colon (myochosis), which is seen

radiologically as narrowing and irregular distortion of the sigmoid lumen. This appearance is at times difficult to distinguish from carcinoma or inflammatory bowel disease.

Three to 5% of patients with diverticular disease may at some time develop diverticular bleeding. The bleeding is characteristically brisk and painless, and is usually right-sided in origin. Blood loss can at times be massive and require emergency surgery, but it is more often self-limited. The chance of recurrence is approximately 20%.

The pathogenesis of diverticulosis is not yet fully established, although epidemiologic data and the results of animal studies suggest a strong association with dietary deficiency of fiber. Autopsy studies show a progressive increase in the disorder, beginning with the milling of wheat flour in the 1880s and the associated decreased consumption of crude cereal grains. Presently, the prevalence of diverticulosis is higher in Western industrialized nations, in which fiber consumption is much less than in the Third World countries. Diverticulosis has been produced in laboratory animals fed a diet deficient in fiber content. Additional studies in humans are needed to determine if eating a high-fiber diet can prevent the development of diverticulosis or its complications.

Diagnosis

In many instances, the diagnosis of diverticulosis is made incidentally during barium x-ray examination done for other reasons. Symptoms such as lower abdominal pain, localized tenderness, and episodes of diarrhea or constipation in an older patient are often attributed to diverticulosis, but may also reflect irritable bowel syndrome. Fever, leukocytosis, and/or peritoneal signs are more likely to indicate diverticulitis or other intra-abdominal infections or inflammatory conditions.

Evaluation of the older patient with recent onset of bowel disturbance should include stool examination for occult blood, complete blood cell count, sigmoidoscopy, and barium enema or colonoscopy. These are done to exclude polyps, carcinoma, inflammatory or ischemic bowel disease, or other serious medical disorders. Depending on the clinical presentation, other studies might include serum amylase, liver chemistries, and examination of the stool for inflammatory cells, bacteria, or parasitic pathogens. Recent weight loss or the presence of occult blood in the stool of a patient with x-ray–proven diverticulosis may require additional evaluation with colonoscopy to exclude carcinoma.

Diverticular bleeding should be suspected in the older patient who presents with the spontaneous passage of bright red or maroon-colored stools. The differential diagnosis includes angiodysplasia (arteriovenous malformations), polyps/carcinoma, hemorrhoids, duodenal ulcer or in the presence of pain, ischemic colitis. The diagnostic evaluation of painless rectal bleeding in the older patient depends on the rapidity of the bleeding. With massive hemorrhage, resuscitative measures and arteriographic evaluation in preparation for possible emergency subtotal or segmental colonic resection are indicated. Barium enema should not be done because the opacified colon would obscure arteriographic localization of the bleeding source. In the more stable patient with moderate bleeding, ^{99}Tc-labeled sulfur colloid, or red-cell scintiscan can help localize the site of bleeding. Colonoscopy is becoming more popular with episodic low-grade bleeding because of its greater diagnostic accuracy and therapeutic potential for heat probe or bipolar or laser coagulation. The patient who has a single diverticular bleed that stops usually does not require surgery, and the approach can be more conservative; barium enema or colonoscopy should be done to exclude other disorders. If findings are negative, no additional evaluation is needed unless another bleeding episode develops.

Treatment

A high-fiber diet has been recommended for patients with asymptomatic diverticulosis because of indirect evidence linking fiber deficiency to the disease. Bran has been shown to decrease intestinal transit time and to lessen pain in patients with diverticular disease. (See Chap. 144 for additional information on high-fiber diets.) The diet is inexpensive, may be effective in preventing progression of the disease, and has few immediate side effects. Some patients initially experience gaseous distention and nausea for several days. Patients with bowel symptoms, particularly those with pain and constipation should take 15 to 30 g of unprocessed bran per day, the dietary equivalent (2 oz of bran cereal, 10 mg of whole meal bread), or 2 to 3 tablespoons of a powdered psyllium seed preparation as a dietary supplement.

Anticholinergic drugs, such as dicyclomine (Bentyl), glycopyrrolate (Robinul), or propantheline bromide (Pro-Banthine), may be of additional benefit for treatment of pain, but are not recommended on a long-term basis. Mild analgesics can be used; narcotic agents are contraindicated, however, because of the chronic nature of the disorder. Furthermore, morphine and its cogeners increase high-pressure nonpropulsive contractions in the colon, thus possibly increasing symptoms. Some surgeons advocate sigmoid colon resection or myotomy in patients with long-standing painful diverticular disease. However, this is not generally recommended because there are no data from controlled trials that support a good clinical response.

Diverticulitis

Diverticulitis occurs in 10 to 25% of patients with known diverticulosis. It develops from a micro- or macroperforation of a diverticulum and subsequent spillage of fecal contents outside the bowel wall. The resulting inflammatory process is usually confined to the pericolic space, where it is walled off by fat, mesentery, or adjacent organs. Diverticulitis most often occurs in the sigmoid colon, possibly because of the large number of diverticula and the presence of more formed stool to produce obstruction at the diverticular neck. The severity of the clinical symptoms and signs depends on the extent of the extradiverticular inflammation. Characteristically, patients complain of acute or subacute left-lower-quadrant pain, fever, and possibly, nausea, vomiting, and constipation. In some instances, the inflammation produces symptoms of partial or complete colonic obstruction, or if the ureter is involved, may simulate a urinary tract infection. Older patients or those taking steroid preparation may present with minimal symptoms. Diverticulitis does not cause gross GI bleeding. However, on occasion the stool may be positive for occult blood.

Diagnosis
On physical examination, there is localized left-lower-quadrant discomfort and, possibly, a palpable mass or localized peritoneal signs with rebound tenderness. Rectal examination may reveal tenderness on the left or even a mass effect caused by pelvic abscess. Laboratory studies invariably show leukocytosis and, if the ureter or bladder is secondarily involved, microscopic hematuria and pyuria. Electrolyte disturbances may occur, depending on the presence of vomiting or sepsis. Flat and upright x-rays of the abdomen must be done to evaluate for a perforated viscus or intestinal obstruction. Sigmoidoscopy should be performed to exclude a distal mass or inflammatory process. The stool is usually Hemoccult-negative. Barium enema and colonoscopy are contraindicated in the acutely ill patient, particularly if free perforation is expected. With milder symptoms, barium enema or CT scan can help demonstrate the site of the disease process, identify any complications such as abscess or fistula formation, and exclude other disorders such as carcinoma, Crohn's disease, or ischemic colitis. Care should be taken to instill the barium slowly, under low pressure. Some radiologists prefer to use a water-soluble contrast medium (Gastrografin), which gives less radiographic resolution but avoids the risk of barium spilling into the peritoneum. If the patient has an abnormal urinary sediment, an intravenous pyelogram (IVP) should be done to identify possible fistulization to the ureter or bladder. Prolonged high spiking fevers, hypotension, localized peritoneal signs, and persistent leukocytosis suggest a pericolic abscess; CT scan is indicated to rule out this complication.

Treatment
The management of acute diverticulitis is directed toward bowel rest and treatment of infection. Many clinicians treat "mild" diverticulitis without hospitalization. In general these patients have little or no fever, do not appear toxic, and have minimal findings on physical examination (e.g., good bowel sounds and little or no rebound tenderness). They are treated with a low-residue or liquid diet and oral broad-spectrum antibiotics, such as amoxicillin, tetracycline, or cephalexin. This approach is often successful; however, the similarity of this clinical presentation to that of noninflammatory painful diverticular disease or irritable bowel syndrome, and the lack of adequate controlled studies of patients treated for mild diverticulitis make it difficult to be certain that treatment is responsible for the improvement. It is important for the clinician to follow the patient closely for progression of symptoms or the development of complications.

Acutely ill patients require hospitalization and should be placed at bed rest with nasogastric suction and intravenous fluid replacement. Parenteral antibiotics should be adequate to cover the normal enteric flora (*Escherichia coli,* enterococci, anaerobic bacteroids). Clindamycin and an aminoglycoside, or one of the newer broad-spectrum cephalosporins, can be used and adjusted pending the results of blood culture studies. The patient should be observed carefully with frequent abdominal examination, appropriate roentgenograms, and blood studies, so that developing complications are detected earlier. With clinical improvement, antibiotics should be continued for a total of 10 to 14 days. When the patient is clinically well, barium enema or colonoscopy is needed to confirm the diagnosis and exclude other disorders requiring additional treatment.

Surgical consultation is required for all patients who are hospitalized. Emergency surgery is recommended if a serious complication develops, such as generalized peritonitis, an enlarging abdominal mass suggesting abscess, or fistulization to the bladder or other vital organs. Thirty percent of patients with diverticulitis develop a recurrent attack, usually within the first few years. Elective surgery should be considered in this group, because recurrences are associated with increased morbidity and mortality.

Almy TP, Howell DA. Diverticular disease of the colon. N Engl J Med 1980; 302:324–31.
A complete and authoritative review.

Burkitt D. Fiber as protective against gastrointestinal disease. Am J Gastroenterol 1984; 79:249–52.
A concise discussion of the role of fiber, from the author of several classic articles on the subject.

Brodribb AJM. Treatment of symptomatic diverticular disease with high-fiber diets. Lancet 1977; 1:664–6.
Pain symptoms improved in patients treated with high-fiber diets.

Thompson WG, Patel DG. Clinical picture of diverticular disease of the colon. Clin Gastroenterol 1986; 15:903–16.
A good clinical review with an epidemiologic perspective, emphasizing the high prevalence of diverticular disease in Western society and the relatively low frequency of symptoms and complications. Management for uncomplicated disease is discussed, as are complications of diverticulitis and diverticular hemorrhage.

Chappuis CW, Cohn I Jr. Acute colonic diverticulitis. Surg Clin North Am 1988; 68(2):855–77.
Reviews epidemiology, diagnosis, and management of diverticulitis, from a surgeon's perspective.

Pohlman T. Diverticulitis. Gastroenterol Clin North Am 1988; 17(2):357–85.
A comprehensive discussion of diagnostic and therapeutic options for diverticulitis, emphasizing newer diagnostic methods reserved for the small subset of patients having serious complications. Includes a very good discussion on choice of antibiotics

47. ACUTE DIARRHEA
C. Glenn Pickard, Jr.

Acute diarrhea as discussed in this chapter is diarrhea of less than a week's duration, occurring in a nontraveling, previously healthy patient. Diarrhea may be one of the presenting complaints of human immunodeficiency virus (HIV) infections and clinicians must maintain a high index of suspicion that leads to an appropriate evaluation for HIV infection (see Chap. 114). In the United States, acute diarrhea is the second leading cause of morbidity and loss of time from work. Even though most patients with diarrhea do not visit a physician, diarrhea remains one of the most frequent diagnoses made in ambulatory care.

Acute diarrhea usually results from one of several well-known causes that present as clinically recognizable syndromes. The observations that enable one to separate the syndromes clinically are presented in Table 47-1.

Evaluation

The majority of patients with acute diarrhea present with a syndrome that resembles viral gastroenteritis. This syndrome is characterized by the abrupt onset of diarrhea, usually associated with nausea, vomiting, and crampy abdominal pain. It is more common in children and young adults and often occurs in epidemic form. The fever is usually of low grade and the diarrheal stools are loose and watery without mucus or blood.

Because diarrhea from other causes, including bacteria, parasites, and ulcerative colitis, may initially present with symptoms similar to those of viral gastroenteritis, the practitioner must decide whether to pursue any studies beyond the history and physical examination at the initial encounter. For the great majority of patients, the answer would seem to be no, for the following reasons: Most instances of acute diarrhea prove to be self-limited and resolve within several days. Few patients with acute diarrhea, regardless of the cause, are adversely affected by simple supportive treatment and observation during this initial period. Furthermore, even in those instances of known bacterial cause, current recommendations are to withhold antibacterial therapy in most mild cases.

When clinical presentation (see Table 47-1) strongly suggests a bacterial pathogen (e.g., a common-source epidemic following a community picnic, or patients presenting with high fever and bloody diarrhea), additional investigation is indicated. Diarrhea that comes only hours after eating usually comes from a preformed toxin in contaminated food. Investigation may include cultures of patient's stool and foods that are the likely source, both as an adjunct to clinical management of the patient and as a public health measure to discover the source of the epidemic. Other presentations, such as diarrhea associated with antibiotic use or diarrhea following ingestion of poorly cooked seafood containing the *Vibrio* species, are summarized in Table 47-1, and appropriate diagnostic and therapeutic measures are all well covered in the references.

Fecal Leukocyte Examination

For some patients, the clinical history does not point clearly to the cause, and the patient may appear too sick to simply treat supportively and observe. In these circumstances, the fecal leukocyte smear provides a simple, inexpensive, immediately available source of useful data to help distinguish between inflammatory diarrhea (mostly invasive bacterial infection and ulcerative colitis) and viral infection. Fecal leukocyte smears are positive in approximately 90% of patients with bacterial diarrhea and negative in about 95% of patients with viral gastroenteritis. The reported prevalence of stools positive for fecal leukocytes is 60 to 100% for *Shigella*, 36–80% for *Salmonella*, and 82 to 100% for invasive *Escherichia coli*, compared to 0 to 6% for viruses.

To examine the stool for leukocytes, 1 or 2 drops of Löffler's methylene blue is added to small flecks of mucus or stool on a clean dry slide. After thorough mixing, a cover slip is placed over the specimen, and it is examined as a "wet mount" preparation. The methylene blue stains white blood cells and enables identification of the motile trophozoites of *Giardia lamblia* and the eggs or larvae of other parasitic infections. Although there is not complete agreement on the definition of a positive result, one commonly used definition is 10 to 15 white blood cells per high-power field on five or more fields. Because stool cultures from patients with known bacterial enteritis occasionally are negative, "false-positive" results (i.e., the presence of leukocytes on a smear with a negative culture) may reflect in part problems with culture techniques. Stained smears obtained from cup specimens give a much higher percentage of positive results (95%) than do smears obtained from diapers or cotton swabs (47%).

Treatment

Fluid and Electrolytes

Management of all patients should include careful assessment of hydration and appropriate intervention with oral or parenteral fluids. Recent studies, primarily in patients with cholera, have shown that oral fluid replacement with glucose-electrolyte solutions can effectively restore hydration in most patients even when the diarrhea continues. This is possible because the intestinal absorptive capacity often remains intact at some sites in the bowel even when there is fluid secretion into the intestinal lumen at other sites.

The composition of the fluid recommended by the World Health Organization (WHO)

Table 47-1. Features of diarrhea

Agent	Source	Mode of transmission	Incubation period
Staph. aureus and Bacillus cereus (preformed toxin)	Inadequately refrigerated food contaminated with Staphylococcus	Ingestion of food containing preformed toxin	1–6 hr
Toxigenic E. coli (noninvasive)	Common cause of traveler's diarrhea; exact source unknown	Ingestion of contaminated water or uncooked fruits or vegetables	2–3 d
Shigella	Frequently found in institutional settings with poor sanitation and hygiene	Fecal-oral	1–2 d
Salmonella (nontyphoidal)	Contaminated food or water, powdered eggs, milk, poultry, pet turtles	Ingestion of contaminated food or water	8–48 hr
Campylobacter	Extensive reservoir in animals; human carriers exist	Contaminated water, contact with infected animals; probable fecal-oral human-to-human transmission	3–5 d
"Norwalk-like" viruses	Other infected patients	Probably fecal-oral	18–48 hr
Rotavirus	Other infected patients	Probably fecal-oral	48 hr
Yersinia	Often a sick dog or cat, contaminated food or water	Ingestion of contaminated food or water, fecal-oral	May be weeks
Vibrio species	Seafood	Ingestion of poorly cooked seafood	6–48 hr
Clostridium difficile	Normal flora in gut, may also be spread from environmental contamination in hospitals or nursing homes	Alteration of gut flora by fecal-oral	Usually after > 5 d of antibiotic treatment

for treating diarrhea in all age groups is 2% glucose in a solution containing sodium (90 mEq/L), chloride (75 mEq/L), potassium (15 mEq/L), and bicarbonate (30 mEq/L). However, most patients with acute diarrhea in this country do not experience the massive fluid and electrolyte loss associated with cholera, and strict adherence to this formula is unnecessary for them. Table 47-2 gives the composition of many commonly available fluids. Gatorade is the cheapest and most readily available of the fluids that contain electrolytes and therefore is recommended for the relatively more severe cases where replacement of electrolytes is important. For milder illness, fluids such as Coca-Cola and ginger ale and other fluids with low electrolyte content are adequate; it is usually recommended that carbonated drinks be "defizzed" before administration, although there is no strong evidence to support the practice. Kool-Aid and bouillon are also occasionally used and are not included in the table. Kool-Aid has no electrolyte content and is therefore comparable to soft drinks or ginger ale. Bouillon, in contrast, has a very high sodium content and can produce hypernatremia, particularly when given to children.

It is recommended that milk and milk products be avoided because some patients with diarrhea have a transient disaccharidase (including lactase) deficiency. Similarly, fats and

Table 47-1 (continued)

			Clinical features		
Age of patient	Onset	Vomiting	Abdominal pain	Fever	Characteristics of diarrhea
Any age	Abrupt	+ + + +	±	Absent	Profuse, watery, no blood or mucus
Young adults and infants	Gradual	+	+ + +	Low grade	Profuse, watery, no blood or mucus
6 mo–6 yr; sporadically in other age groups	Abrupt	−	±	High	Frequently bloody mucoid
Any age	Abrupt	+ + + +	−	Variable	Watery, occasionally mucoid
Any age	Gradual	±	+ + + +	High	Bloody mucus stool not uncommon
School children and young adults	Abrupt	+ + + +	+ + +	Low grade	Watery
Children younger than 3; occasionally older	Abrupt	+ + + +	+ + +	Moderate	Watery
Any age	Gradual	+ +	+ + + +	+ + +	Watery, less often bloody, often chronic
Any age	Abrupt	+ + + +	+ + +	+	Watery, no blood or mucus
Any age	Usually gradual	−	+ +	+	Watery, no blood or mucus

+ + + + = almost always occurs; + + + = usually occurs; + + = occasionally occurs; + = rarely occurs; ± = may or may not occur; − = does not occur.

large meals are avoided because of the clinical impression that they increase cramps and diarrhea, perhaps through gastrocolic reflex and malabsorption. There are no controlled clinical trials to support these measures, but they appear to do no harm and may well be helpful.

When fluid and electrolyte losses are severe, and particularly when they are complicated by nausea and vomiting, intravenous fluid replacement is necessary.

Antidiarrheal Drugs

Patients often request symptomatic relief from diarrhea. Although there is some controversy about their use, for most patients the advantages of using a short course of an antidiarrheal outweigh the risks.

Absorbents, such as kaolin and pectin (Kaopectate), have been used for years, despite the fact that their efficacy has not been established by clinical trials. However, they rarely if ever cause harm and are thus the least controversial alternative.

Pepto-Bismol, another commonly used proprietary agent, has recently been shown to be an effective prophylactic against traveler's diarrhea. There is speculation that the effectiveness is from the antiprostaglandin effect of salicylates.

Table 47-2. Sodium and potassium content (mEq/L) of oral liquids

Liquid	Na^+	K^+
Apple juice	1.7	26.0
Coca-Cola	1.0	0.4
Gatorade	23.0	2.5
Ginger ale	3.5	0.1
Jell-O (half strength)	15.0	0.15
Lytren	25.0	25.0
Orange juice	0.2	49.0
Pedialyte	30.0	20.0
Pepsi	0	0.6
7-Up	5.0	0.3

Note: The electrolyte values for those products that are reconstituted from local water supplies may vary slightly, depending on the electrolyte content of the water.
Source: Pietrusko RG. Drug therapy reviews: pharmacotherapy of diarrhea. Am J Hosp Pharm 1979; 36:757–67.

The greatest controversy is over opiates and similar synthetic antidiarrheals. While it has long been appreciated that these agents can decrease the frequency of stooling and hasten clinical improvement, it has been contended that this effect was at least potentially harmful because (1) it tends to mask fluid loss particularly in children, (2) it might increase "toxicity" and/or prolong the illness, and (3) it might prolong bacterial shedding. Recent well-done studies clearly seem to support the efficacy of these agents and fail to support the concerns of possible harmful effects.

The potential for drug toxicity from opiates and synthetic antidiarrheals is a serious concern, particularly in children. Central nervous system depression resulting in death was reported in a 2-year-old child who ingested only six diphenoxylate-atropine (Lomotil) tablets. Dyphenoxylate-atropine has produced hepatic coma when given to adults with chronic liver disease. The potential for abuse of opiates, such as paregoric or deodorized tincture of opium (DTO), is minor.

Dosages of the commonly used agents are as follows:

Loperamide (Imodium): 4 mg (two capsules) initially, followed by 2 mg (one capsule) after each loose stool, not to exceed 16 mg (eight capsules) in 24 hours.
Diphenoxylate-atropine (Lomotil): two tablets initially, followed by one tablet after each loose stool, not to exceed eight tablets in 24 hours.
Paregoric: 1 or 2 teaspoons of DTO orally every 4 hours; 8 to 10 drops in a glass of water every 4 hours.

The synthetic preparations, diphenoxylate-atropine and loperamide, are not pharmacologically superior to the opiates. However, many patients prefer them because of convenience of dosing. There is evidence suggesting that loperamide may be more effective and less toxic than diphenoxylate-atropine.

Antibiotics are contraindicated in the great majority of instances of acute diarrhea. There is little evidence to suggest that the course of bacterial diarrhea in mild cases is shortened by antibiotics, and there is evidence that the shedding of *Salmonella* is prolonged in antibiotic-treated patients. Antibiotics also favor the development of antibiotic-resistant bacteria. There is no rationale for the use of antibiotics in viral diarrhea.

Antibiotics have generally been thought to be indicated for severely ill patients in whom a bacterial cause is strongly suspected. Stool culture and sensitivities are necessary because no single antibiotic is certain to be effective against the various pathogens. A recent study suggests that empiric antibiotic therapy for all patients may be efficacious. If antibiotics are begun before culture results are available, common choices are ampicillin, which covers many *Salmonella* and *Shigella* species; ciprofloxacin, which covers most enteric pathogens; and trimethoprim-sulfamethoxazole (Septra), which covers most *Salmonella* species and enterotoxic *E. coli*.

Clinical Course

The majority of patients with acute diarrhea respond to symptomatic and supportive care and become asymptomatic in a week or less. In those instances in which diarrhea persists, other causes should be considered. Cultures for enteric pathogens and special cultures for *Campylobacter* should be obtained. Intestinal parasites, inflammatory bowel disease, and irritable bowel syndrome also must be considered. Malabsorption caused by pancreatic insufficiency or intrinsic bowel disease is also a consideration and usually is suspected on the basis of classic malabsorptive stools; however, in other instances the diagnosis is not suspected until a full investigation is performed, including qualitative and quantitative evaluations of fecal fat content and other studies for malabsorption. Finally, one must always consider gastrointestinal cancers as a possible cause of diarrhea—either because of obstructing lesions causing constipation followed by diarrhea or, rarely, because of secreting villous adenomas.

Goodman LJ, et al. Empiric antimicrobial therapy of domestically acquired acute diarrhea in urban adults. Arch Intern Med 1990; 150:541–6.
A well-done provocative study clearly demonstrating the efficacy of empiric antibiotic therapy in a population of patients presenting with acute diarrhea to an urban emergency room. Further studies on similar populations and, particularly, non–emergency room populations (presumably less sick) are needed.

Guerrant RL, et al. A cost-effective approach to the diagnosis and management of acute infectious diarrhea. Bull NY Acad Med 1987; 63:484–99.
An excellent clinically oriented review article offering an effective algorithm for diagnosis and treatment.

Gorbach SL. Bacterial diarrhea and its treatment. Lancet 1987; 2:1378–82.
A brief but comprehensive review. Clinically oriented and practical.

Justman F, et al. Diphenoxylate hydrochloride (Lomotil) in the treatment of acute diarrhea. Br J Clin Pract 1987; 41:648–51.
An excellent double-blind study demonstrating the efficacy of diphenoxylate and, most importantly, the lack of adverse effects in the treatment of acute diarrhea, including those cases due to bacteria. An excellent review of this controversial subject.

Koreniowski OM, Rouse JD, Guerrant RL. Value of examination for fecal leukocytes in the early diagnosis of shigellosis. Am J Trop Med Hyg 1979; 28:1031–5.
An excellent study of the role of the fecal leukocyte examination in the diagnosis of shigellosis. Includes a good brief review of previous studies.

Pietrusko RG. Drug therapy reviews: pharmacotherapy of diarrhea. Am J Hosp Pharm 1979; 36:757–67.
A superb review of the entire subject of diarrhea. Major emphasis is on the therapy, but it also includes an extensive review of pathophysiology and diagnosis. Includes 170 references.

Aserkoff B, Bennett JV. Effect of antibiotic therapy in acute salmonellosis on the fecal excretion of salmonellae. N Engl J Med 1969; 281:636–40.
An intriguing article describing a natural experiment in which approximately 1900 persons developed Salmonella enteritis as a result of contaminated turkey at a picnic. One hundred eight-five patients treated with antibiotics are compared to be a similar number of untreated subjects.

48. CHRONIC DIARRHEA
R. Balfour Sartor

Diarrhea that persists for longer than 3 weeks should be thoroughly evaluated: It is not usually caused by self-limited infectious agents, may be a symptom of significant underlying pathology, and usually has a major impact on the patient's activity. Diarrhea is defined as passage of greater than 300 g of stool per day, or more practically, as stools of liquid consistency occurring more frequently than 3 times per day or associated with urgency.

Initial Evaluation
The goal of the initial visit is to evaluate the patient's diarrhea by history, physical examination, and simple, nonexpensive laboratory tests, so that an efficient and cost-effective diagnostic evaluation can be planned. A large assortment of expensive and frequently painful procedures and laboratory tests are available to evaluate possible causes of diarrhea. It is the clinician's task to determine how each patient's symptoms can be most rapidly and efficiently evaluated and how aggressively to pursue a specific diagnosis.

History
The patient must describe what is meant by "diarrhea" and give the characteristics to the stool, such as consistency; color; odor; presence of fat, blood, or mucus; and associated abdominal pain. Symptoms that suggest a functional etiology, usually the irritable bowel syndrome, include alternating diarrhea and constipation; absence of nocturnal stools, fecal incontinence, and weight loss; and protracted symptoms with no recent change. Oily, excessively malodorous and floating stools suggest malabsorption; large-volume stools suggest a small intestinal or right colon source, while frequent small stools are associated with a distal colonic source or motility abnormalities. Fever, rectal bleeding, perianal fistulae or fissures, and extraintestinal inflammation such as migratory, nondeforming arthritis of large joints, erythema nodosum, and uveitis suggest intestinal inflammation.

History should also include drugs taken, with specific attention to magnesium-containing antacids, antibiotic therapy and laxative use, and a dietary history concentrating on artificially flavored beverages, candy (sorbitol is frequently used to sweeten candy and gum), and milk products. Other questions should include long distance running ("runner's trots"), travel in the past year, water sources (well water, camping trips), family history of chronic diarrhea or inflammatory bowel disease, concurrent diarrhea in household members, and risk factors for HIV exposure; answers may help direct the evaluation or suggest a simple trial of dietary or drug elimination therapy. Many medical illnesses may be complicated by diarrhea, especially diabetes, peptic ulcer disease (Zollinger-Ellison syndrome and antacid use), immunodeficiency syndromes, biliary obstruction, and chronic pancreatitis. Postoperative diarrhea frequently follows surgical procedures such as cholecystectomy, gastric emptying procedures for peptic ulcer disease, ileal resection, pancreatic surgery, and damage of the anal sphincter resulting from an episiotomy, hemorrhoidal resection, or repair of anal fistulae.

Physical Examination
Results of the physical examination direct further evaluation and indicate the severity of malnutrition and dehydration. Signs associated with specific causes of diarrhea include hyperpigmentation (Addison's disease, Whipple's disease), thyromegaly, postural hypotension (autonomic neuropathy or severe dehydration), lymphadenopathy (AIDS, lymphoma), digital clubbing (inflammatory bowel disease, cystic fibrosis), abdominal bruit (intestinal ischemia), peripheral neuropathy (diabetes), perianal fistulae, abscess or chronic fissures (Crohn's disease), and rectal mass or impaction. Fever, edema, anemia, abdominal tenderness or mass, or significant malnutrition or dehydration associated with diarrhea mandates a thorough evaluation. A digital rectal examination and sigmoidoscopy should be performed in all patients with chronic diarrhea and should *not* be deferred to a consultant. Stool color, consistency, mucus, and the presence of occult blood or leukocytes should be noted. Sigmoidoscopy can help differentiate inflammatory from noninflammatory causes;

diagnose laxative abuse (melanosis coli), pseudomembranous colitis, and obstructing neoplasms; and provide a means to biopsy the rectum and to efficiently collect stools for culture and parasitic examination.

Further Evaluation

For functional diarrhea suggested by history and physical examination and stool negative for occult blood, only limited measures such as ova and parasite stains, laxative screen (phenolphthalein, magnesium, and phosphorus) and trial of a lactose-free diet, to exclude simple remedial causes, are indicated. However, further evaluation is directed by a history of weight loss, large stool volumes, nocturnal stool, fecal incontinence or rectal bleeding, abnormal physical examination, or stools that contain occult blood and/or leukocytes.

Inflammatory Diarrhea

If inflammation is present, as determined by sigmoidoscopy, fecal leukocytes, occult blood, fever, abdominal tenderness, or elevated WBC, chronic infectious causes of diarrhea must be excluded. The most common cause of chronic infectious diarrhea in immunocompetent hosts is parasitic infestation. *Giardia,* usually contracted from infected water, produces protracted diarrhea, gaseous distention, and occasionally abdominal cramping. It is best diagnosed by duodenal aspiration or biopsy, but heavy infestations can be detected by stool ova and parasite examination. Amebiasis produces colitis and is best diagnosed by examination of a sigmoidoscopic mucosal scraping. *Giardia* and amoeba are commonly found in patients who have *not* traveled to other countries and are frequently transmitted by contaminated well water or contracted on camping trips. Most bacterial pathogens produce self-limited disease, but occasionally *Campylobacter* and *Yersinia* can cause protracted diarrhea of up to 2 months' duration. These organisms are easily diagnosed by stool cultures, but studies for them must be specifically requested because of their specialized growth requirements. The most common etiology of chronic bacterial diarrhea is *Clostridium difficile* toxin–induced pseudomembranous colitis, which frequently follows broad-spectrum antibiotic treatment. A *C. difficile* toxin assay should be routinely performed when a patient treated with antibiotics develops diarrhea that does not spontaneously remit within several days after stopping antibiotics or is complicated by fever or blood or if fecal leukocytes are found on fecal smear. *E. coli* 0157:H7, which produces hemorrhagic colitis and is frequently transmitted by infected ground beef or raw milk, can rarely produce protracted diarrhea (4% in a recent prospective study). *Aeromonas* species, contracted from water in summer months, also can occasionally lead to chronic diarrhea.

If an inflammatory etiology of diarrhea is suspected, but the results of stool culture, several fresh ova and parasite examinations, and the *C. difficile* toxin assay are negative, visualization of the colon and/or small bowel is required. This may be done either by colonoscopy or small-bowel barium radiography, with choice of the initial procedure guided by clinical suspicion of a colonic (bloody stools) or small-bowel (relatively large volume, grossly nonbloody) source. Colonoscopy is usually preferred over a barium enema because of better mucosal visualization of the colon and distal ileum and the ability to obtain mucosal biopsy specimens for histologic diagnosis. Because of the risk of perforation or exacerbation of colitis and possible toxic megacolon, neither a barium enema nor a colonoscopy should be performed in a patient with moderate abdominal tenderness or colonic dilation. Patients with weight loss, low serum protein levels, and possible malabsorption require small-intestinal x-rays, either an upper GI series with small-bowel follow-through or administration of contrast media directly into the duodenum via a nasogastric tube (enteroclysis), with special attention to the distal ileum. Celiac sprue (gluten-sensitive enteropathy) is best diagnosed by a peroral suction biopsy of the jejunum, although an endoscopic duodenal biopsy is more easily accomplished. Aspiration for *Giardia* and quantitative bacterial culture to diagnose small-bowel bacterial overgrowth can be done at the time of small-intestinal biopsy. The diagnosis of ulcerative colitis, Crohn's disease, sprue, and ischemic colitis can be suggested by endoscopy, x-rays, and biopsies but requires exclusion of infectious causes. Collagenous or microscopic colitis, newly described syndromes for which normal mucosa is demonstrated by colonoscopic visualization, Whipple's disease, and amyloidosis can be diagnosed histologically by specific stains.

Noninflammatory Diarrhea

If initial evaluation by sigmoidoscopy, physical examination, history, and stool examination does not suggest intestinal inflammation, a malabsorptive cause of diarrhea should be explored by obtaining a serum carotene level, prothrombin time, and qualitative stool fat staining. Also, all patients with unexplained diarrhea with no obvious inflammatory site should have fecal and urine laxative screening. Surreptitious laxative use is one of the most common causes of unexplained diarrhea. If the patient has high-volume diarrhea, a 72-hour collection to determine volume, weight, and stool fat should be performed on an outpatient basis. The determination of fecal electrolyte levels and osmolality is controversial, but has been proposed to detect osmotic diarrhea caused by ingesting poorly absorbable solutes (magnesium- or phosphate-containing laxatives) or bacterial fermentation of nonabsorbed carbohydrates. Unfortunately, many laboratories are reluctant to process fecal electrolyte specimens. An alternative means of separating secretory from malabsorptive diarrhea is the response of stool volume to 72 hours of fasting; secretory diarrheal volume will decrease by 50% or less while malabsorption volume will return to near-normal values. Fasting can only be safely done in the hospital with intravenous fluid replacement to prevent dehydration. If a secretory cause of diarrhea is documented and a laxative screen is negative, a peptide-secreting tumor should be searched for by measuring serum levels of vasoactive intestinal polypeptide (VIP), gastrin, and calcitonin and urinary levels of 5-hydroxyindoleacetic acid (5-HIAA). If malabsorption is suspected, therapeutic trials of pancreatic enzyme replacement, cholestyramine binding of bile acids, and a lactose-free diet for 1 week each are helpful and cost-effective means of establishing a specific etiology.

Special Circumstances

Male homosexual or immunosuppressed patients frequently develop infectious diarrhea. In addition to routine pathogens, *Cryptosporidium*, cytomegalovirus, *Mycobacterium avium-intracellular, herpes simplex,* and Kaposi's sarcoma must be searched for by culture and staining of endoscopic biopsy specimens in the AIDS patient with diarrhea. Two-thirds of AIDS patients with identifiable pathogens have at least transient clinical improvement of their diarrhea with specific therapy, although many have long-term diarrhea and progressive weight loss.

Postoperative diarrhea frequently responds dramatically to diagnostic and therapeutic trials of cholestyramine (after cholecystectomy or resection of < 100 cm of the distal ileum), metronidazole or tetracycline (bacterial overgrowth from loss of the ileocecal valve, enteric bypasses, partial obstruction, or gastrojejunostomy), or dietary manipulation (gastric antral resection with vagotomy, resection > 100 cm of the distal ileum, or pancreatic resection).

Some patients with chronic insulin-dependent diabetes mellitus complicated by autonomic neuropathy have refractory diarrhea that may respond to antibiotics, cholestyramine, opiates, clonidine, or a somatostatin analogue.

Treatment

Symptomatic therapy with opioid antidiarrheal agents should be avoided until a specific cause of diarrhea is discovered, as intestinal paralysis may be detrimental to severe intestinal inflammation or partial obstruction. Initial nonspecific therapy should be limited to correction of dehydration, electrolyte abnormalities, and vitamin and trace mineral deficiencies. Specific therapy is then provided when the cause of the chronic diarrhea is discovered. In appropriate clinical situations such as suspected lactose deficiency, bile acid malabsorption, postcholecystectomy diarrhea, small-bowel bacterial overgrowth, giardiasis, or pancreatic insufficiency, specific therapeutic trials may provide diagnostic information and be simpler than expensive or invasive procedures.

When to Refer

Interaction of a gastroenterologist with the primary care physician is helpful in the evaluation and therapy of secretory diarrhea, the immunosuppressed patient, and noninfectious intestinal inflammation, so that a coordinated diagnostic approach can be planned, expeditious colonoscopy and intestinal biopsies performed, and appropriate treatment plans devised for these complex patients.

Fine KD, Kregs GJ, Fordtran JS. Diarrhea. In: Sleisenger M, Fordtran JS. Gastrointestinal diseases: pathogenesis, diagnosis, management. 4th ed. Philadelphia: Saunders, 1989:280–316.
A comprehensive review of pathophysiology, classification, and differential diagnosis of diarrhea.

Smith PD, et al. Intestinal infections in patients with the acquired immunodeficiency syndrome (AIDS). Ann Intern Med 1988; 108:328–33.
A prospective search for intestinal infections in male homosexual patients with AIDS. One or more enteric pathogens were isolated from 17 of 20 patients with diarrhea, compared with only 1 of 10 patients without diarrhea; 11 of 16 patients with identified organisms clinically improved with specific therapy.

Giardeillo FM, et al. Collagenous colitis: physiologic and histopathologic studies in seven patients. Ann Intern Med 1987; 106:46–9.
A clinical and histologic study of seven middle-aged patients (six females) with chronic watery diarrhea diagnosed by biopsy specimens showing a broad band of subepithelial collagen. Five of seven patients clinically or histologically improved with sulfasalazine or steroid therapy.

Tanowitz HB, Weiss LM, Wittner M. Diagnosis and treatment of protozoan diarrheas. Am J Gastroenterol 1988; 83:339–50.
A complete review of clinical aspect of enteric protozoan diseases encountered in North America.

MacDermott RP, Stenson WF, eds. Inflammatory bowel disease. New York: Elsevier, 1991.
A recent comprehensive text on the pathogenesis, diagnosis, and management of ulcerative colitis and Crohn's disease.

49. CONSTIPATION
R. Balfour Sartor

Constipation is a symptom that has widely different meanings for both patients and physicians. It is most precisely defined as the passage of less than 35 g of fecal matter per day. In the clinical setting, a more practical definition is passage of fewer than three stools per week and/or the sensation of incomplete evacuation or straining. Because constipation is frequently the subject of myths and home remedies, the physician's advice is often neither sought nor accepted until an intractable pattern of constipation with periodic purging develops, leading to laxative abuse and dependence. Although the prevalence of constipation is not known, it is common enough to account for a $250 million laxative market in the United States. In a British survey (Connell, 1965) it was found that 16% of people 10 to 59 years old and 50% of those over 60 years old use laxatives.

Predisposing factors for constipation appear to be advancing age, immobility, drug use, and, most important, a low-fiber diet. The habit of ignoring the urge to defecate (a temporary impulse produced by stool distending the rectal ampulla) also may contribute to constipation; it results in decreased responsiveness of this reflex arc, increased volume of stool in the distal colon with subsequent rectosigmoid dilatation, and increased stool desiccation. Constipation is more frequent in women than in men. Normal women have fewer stools than men, intestinal transit time diminishes in the luteal phase of the menstrual cycle and third trimester of pregnancy, and constipation often accompanies the irritable bowel syndrome, which is more common in women than men.

Simple constipation is frequently asymptomatic; the symptoms of cramping abdominal pain, nausea, and fullness are often produced by laxatives used for perceived "irregularity," rather than by the accumulation of fecal matter within the left colon. However, long-standing constipation, usually in conjunction with laxative use, has been strongly associated with colonic diverticulosis and hemorrhoids and weakly associated with hiatal hernias. The colonic dilatation of chronic constipation predisposes patients to sigmoid volvulus.

Long-standing use of certain laxatives can produce "cathartic colon," a motility disturbance manifested by decreased propulsive activity of the right colon. Agents incriminated in this syndrome include cascara, senna, castor and croton oil, and phenolphthalein. In extreme situations, frequent purging can result in electrolyte and renal disturbances, particularly hypokalemia and hyperaldosteronism.

Evaluation

Once it has been determined that constipation is present, the goals of evaluation include detecting intrinsic gastrointestinal pathology (particularly of colonic origin), diagnosing systemic diseases presenting as constipation, and finding easily remediable causes, such as constipating drugs or poor dietary habits.

History

The history is the most important element in evaluating the constipated patient; it should focus on when and under what circumstances constipation first became a problem. The recent onset of constipation dictates a search for gastrointestinal disorders, especially carcinoma of the colon in the middle-aged or elderly patient. In contrast, a long-standing history of constipation beginning in adolescence or early adulthood without a recent abrupt change in bowel function is more compatible with a functional disorder. Many patients with short-segment Hirschsprung's disease are not diagnosed until early adulthood; these young patients have the onset of severe constipation during infancy. The history of anal surgery suggests a possible anal stricture, and laparotomies predispose to obstructing intra-abdominal adhesions. Rectal bleeding, abdominal distention, weight loss, pain, and vomiting suggest intrinsic intestinal disease with partial obstruction. Systemic medical conditions that may produce or exacerbate constipation include hypothyroidism, diabetes with autonomic neuropathy, uremia, hypokalemia, hypercalcemia, and pregnancy. A meticulous drug history of both prescribed and over-the-counter formulations should emphasize laxative use and drugs known to induce constipation. Such drugs include opiates; psychotherapeutics, including antidepressants; aluminum and calcium antacids; anticholinergics; certain antihypertensive agents; and cholesterol-binding resins. Frequently the patient is reluctant to admit the extent of laxative use or to mention the number of agents, including "home remedies," being used.

A family history may be helpful in determining the patient's attitudes toward constipation and laxative use and in identifying the rare patient with familial pseudo-obstruction.

Finally, the dietary patterns of each patient should be carefully outlined. This information helps in establishing a cause for constipation, in planning therapy through dietary manipulation, and in emphasizing to the patient the importance of dietary factors in the pathogenesis of constipation.

Physical Examination

The physical examination should be directed at identifying patients with systemic or gastrointestinal diseases that produce constipation. A careful rectal examination should include evaluation of anal sphincter tone, perianal sensory fibers, anal stricture, amount and consistency of stool in the rectal vault, rectal dilation, and the presence of a fecal impaction. The stool should be tested for occult blood. A proctosigmoidoscopy after stool evacuation with an enema is essential to search for constricting carcinomas of the lower colon, rectal distention, and melanosis coli. Melanosis coli is an apparently benign darkening of the colonic mucosa produced by pigment-engorged macrophages in the lamina propria of patients who chronically use anthraquinone laxatives (senna and cascara).

Laboratory and X-ray

The extent of laboratory or radiographic evaluation depends on the degree of clinical suspicion that an associated disorder is present. All patients should have three separate stools evaluated for occult blood. Serum calcium, glucose, and potassium concentrations, thyroid function, and BUN determinations, although not routinely indicated, are useful in patients with suspected systemic disease. Barium enemas or colonoscopy are not universally indicated but should be performed in all patients with a recent onset or abrupt worsening of constipation, weight loss, stools positive for occult blood, suggestion of bowel obstruction, or onset of constipation within the first decade of life. Radiographic abnormalities of the "cathartic colon" are usually confined to the right side and include lack of normal haustration (that mimics chronic ulcerative colitis) and bizarre contractions. Rectal manometry is useful only in the small number of patients whose constipation began in infancy or in those with fecal incontinence not related to impaction or obvious neurologic abnormalities.

Treatment

The majority of patients respond to patient re-education, a high-fiber diet, and cessation of laxatives.

Patient Re-education

The wide variation in normal stool frequency should be emphasized, as well as the fact that a stool each day is not essential for health. Life-style changes, such as increasing fluid intake and exercise, may be necessary for long-term benefits. The importance of responding to the urge to defecate at the time it first occurs should be stressed. The potential complications of laxatives should be outlined to reiterate the reasons for stopping these drugs. The benefits of a high-fiber diet should be touted, mentioning its possible preventive role in the pathogenesis of diverticular disease, hemorrhoids, hiatal hernia, and carcinoma of the colon.

High-Fiber Diets

High-fiber diets have been demonstrated in numerous studies of constipated patients, including the immobile geriatric population, to increase stool frequency, bulk, water content, and dry weight, and to decrease intestinal transit time. Many patients with mild constipation of short duration respond to dietary manipulation alone, but those whose chronic constipation is complicated by laxative dependence usually require supplemental bulk agents in dosages ranging from 10 to 20 g of dietary fiber per day. The fiber contents of common foods and supplemental bulk products, with suggestions for their use, are discussed in Chapter 144. Nearly all patients experience temporary sensations of gaseousness, abdominal distention, and cramping during the first few weeks of fiber supplementation. The physician must explain these side effects before initiating therapy, or patients will discontinue the diet before beneficial results are obtained. The beneficial effects of bran are lasting and frequently are retained with less supplementation as the colon is gradually "retrained" over a period of months. Patients with the irritable bowel syndrome may require antispasmodic drugs in addition to fiber supplementation to control abdominal pain.

Laxative Cessation

Most patients can stop the use of all laxative agents when the high-fiber diet is initiated. Laxatives should be banned on the first visit. During the 1- to 2-week adjustment period, when the high-fiber diet may not yet be completely effective, the patient will probably experience some discomfort and pass stools irregularly. During this period, Fleet or saline enemas or suppositories can be used to induce a bowel movement if none has occurred in 3 days and the patient is symptomatic. This regimen has the advantage of stimulating the rectal distention reflex while avoiding cathartics. With continued retraining and adaptation, the use of enemas and suppositories should not be necessary for the majority of patients. Some patients, especially those who are aged, institutionalized, or immobile, have unresponsive aganglionic colons from protracted laxative abuse, or have neurologic disease, do not respond to increased fiber alone. These patients may require a mild laxative with few side effects, such as milk of magnesia or lactulose (Chronulac), or occasional suppositories or enemas. Such patients should be checked regularly for fecal impactions. Numerous studies have shown decreased use of laxatives in institutionalized geriatric patients using bran therapy alone. Certain laxatives that should *not* be used chronically because of potentially serious side effects include senna (Senokot), which can cause the degeneration of the colonic myenteric plexus leading to irreversible cathartic colon syndrome; mineral oil, which can cause malabsorption of fat-soluble vitamins or aspiration producing lipoid pneumonia; dioctyl sulfosuccinate (Colace, Dialose), which can cause increased absorption of concurrently administered drugs; and those producing the cathartic colon, including cascara, castor oil, and phenolphthalein. Soapsuds enemas should never be used because of their irritant effect and the occasional production of hemorrhagic colitis.

Refractory Constipation

A minority of patients, almost exclusively women with the onset of symptoms before age 30, have severe constipation that is refractory to all forms of therapy. These patients invariably have abdominal pain and distention, which may be incapacitating, have an empty rectum on examination, usually have extremely slow colonic transit time but no colonic dilation, and may have rectosigmoid and pelvic floor neuromuscular abnormalities. These patients usually have exacerbation of abdominal symptoms with fiber supplementation and should be evaluated extensively to search for metabolic and other treatable causes of constipation and psychiatric disturbances. Colonic transit time can be measured by serial abdominal x-rays after swallowing radiolucent markers to exclude factitious constipation; normally less than 20% of markers remain in the rectosigmoid area after 5 days. Anorectal manometry may show short-segment Hirschsprung's disease or absence of rectal sensation. In extreme situations, total colectomy with ileorectal anastomosis has been advocated, but most patients continue to have abdominal pain despite increased frequency of stools.

Prevention

Prevention of constipation is easier than treatment. The relatively simple act of increasing fiber in the diet probably decreases the incidence of constipation, although experimental data have not yet been collected. There is some evidence that ingrained attitudes are beginning to change, with increased attention to dietary fiber and less fixation on bowel function. It is hoped that these attitudinal changes result in more physiologic norms in bowel function.

Bockus HL. Simple constipation. In: Bockus HL, ed. Gastroenterology. Vol. 2. 3rd ed. Philadelphia: Saunders, 1976: 936–53.
A classic, well-written, concise chapter on the pathophysiology and treatment of constipation.

Read NW, Timms JM. Defecation and the pathophysiology of constipation. Clin Gastroenterol 1986; 15:937–64.
Excellent review of the physiologic control of intestinal motility, anorectal function, and mechanisms of constipation.

Connell AM, et al. Variation of bowel habit of two population samples. Br Med J 1965; 2:1095–9.
A British survey of 1055 factory workers and 400 patients of a general medical practice, quantitating frequency of bowel movements and laxative use.

Oster JR, Materson BJ, Rogers AI. Laxative abuse syndrome. Am J Gastroenterol 1980; 74:451–8.
A review article outlining the physiologic disturbances of this psychiatric illness.

Muller-Lissner SA. Effect of wheat bran on weight of stool and gastrointestinal transit time: a meta analysis. Br Med J 1988; 296:615–7.
Analysis of 20 original articles demonstrates that bran increased stool weight and diminished transit time in each study. Although constipated patients had improved motility parameters with fiber therapy, they had a lower stool output and slower transit time after equal amounts of bran supplementation than did controls.

Hull C, Greco RS, Brooks DL. Alleviation of constipation in the elderly by dietary fiber supplementation. J Am Geriatr Soc 1980; 28:410–4.
The addition of bran to the diet of an institutionalized geriatric population prevented constipation and laxative use in 60%, with a saving of $44,000 in laxative expense per year.

Fingl E, Freston JW. Antidiarrheal agents and laxatives: changing concepts. Clin Gastroenterol 1979; 8:161–85.
A comprehensive review of the mechanisms of action and side effects of different classes of laxatives.

Reynolds JC, et al. Chronic severe constipation. Gastroenterology 1987; 92:414–20.
Two-thirds of a highly selected population referred for chronic severe idiopathic constipation had motility disturbances; 20% had isolated anal sphincter dysfunction, 24% had generalized gastrointestinal dysmotility, and 24% had an absent gastrocolic reflex.

Kam MA, Hawley RP, Lennard-Jones JE. Outcome of colectomy for severe idiopathic constipation. Gut 1988; 29:969–73.
Retrospective analysis of 44 women having colectomy for refractory constipation. Postoperatively only 50% had normal bowel function, 71% continued to experience abdominal pain and straining, and laxative use was still common.

50. ANORECTAL DISORDERS
C. Glenn Pickard, Jr.

Hemorrhoids

Hemorrhoids, the most common anorectal condition encountered in practice, are protrusions into the anal canal of stretched mucosa and underlying vascular cushions of submucosal tissues. Repeated straining to pass a small, hard stool initially produces a prolapse of rectal mucosa. Continued stretching results in redundant tissue that may prolapse outside the anal orifice with defecation. Accompanying loss of support and dilatation of the submucosal veins produce the hemorrhoidal varices responsible for the bleeding and thrombosis that are features of this condition. Internal hemorrhoids originate immediately above the dentate line, involve veins of the superior hemorrhoidal plexus, and are covered by relatively insensitive rectal mucosa. External hemorrhoids originate below the dentate line, involve the inferior hemorrhoidal venous plexus, and are covered by highly sensitive skin (squamous epithelium). This anatomic difference explains, in large part, the difference in symptoms produced by internal compared to external hemorrhoids. Stretched and redundant epithelium of the lower anal canal and perianal region appears as irregular folds or nubbins called *anal skin tags*.

The primary cause of hemorrhoids is unknown. Dietary factors are thought to be important because hemorrhoids are rare in populations that have a high-residue diet, and common in Western cultures, in which the diet is refined and low in residue. The role of heredity as a predisposing factor is difficult to assess accurately because hemorrhoids are so prevalent. The frequent occurrence of hemorrhoids during pregnancy is thought to be related to an increased venous pressure within the hemorrhoidal plexus secondary to the gravid uterus. In the patient with cirrhosis and portal hypertension, varices may develop in the hemorrhoidal venous plexus, which constitutes one of the routes of collateral circulation for the obstructed portal system.

Diagnosis

Internal Hemorrhoids
Painless bright-red bleeding with defecation is usually the first complaint of patients with internal hemorrhoids. Bleeding results from abrasion and excoriation of the hemorrhoids by passage of a hard stool or when undue straining occurs with defecation. Blood may streak the stool or drip from the anus in an amount sufficient to discolor the toilet bowl water. A lesser degree of bleeding may be detected as streaks of fresh blood on the toilet tissue or as small blood stains on underclothing. Anemia may result from recurrent hemor-

rhoidal bleeding over many months; however, hemorrhoidal bleeding should not be accepted as a cause of anemia until other potentially more serious causes of gastrointestinal blood loss have been excluded by appropriate diagnostic tests.

Prolapse of tissue with defecation may occur with hemorrhoids. Initially the prolapsed tissue retracts spontaneously when straining with defecation ceases. At a later stage, the prolapsed hemorrhoids may not spontaneously reduce and digital replacement by the patient is required. With long-standing disease, prolapse may occur with coughing, sneezing, lifting, or prolonged walking or standing until ultimately the prolapse becomes permanent. Such a constant prolapse of rectal mucosa is associated with a chronic mucus discharge, producing wetness and irritation of perianal skin and soiling of clothing.

Pain with internal hemorrhoids is uncommon; when present, it usually is not severe unless irreducible prolapse of internal hemorrhoids with venous congestion, thrombosis, and inflammation has occurred.

Internal hemorrhoids are not visible unless prolapsed and usually are not palpable on digital examination unless thrombosed. Their presence is determined by anoscopic examination. When the anoscope is introduced to its full length and slowly withdrawn, one or more variably sized reddish purple masses of tissue bulge or project into the anal canal. Rectal mucosa covering internal hemorrhoids is distinctly different in appearance from the skin lining the anal canal. The degree of prolapse can be determined by asking the patient to bear down as the anoscope is removed.

An acute irreducible (incarcerated) prolapse of internal hemorrhoids may occur following defecation or straining. Usually there is a past history of symptomatic hemorrhoids. The acutely inflamed, plum-colored protruding mass cannot be reduced because of engorgement and edema from venous congestion and thrombosis and produces an agonizingly painful condition. Inspection reveals an edematous, moist, reddish purple, often excoriated mass protruding from the anus. Attempts at manual reduction should be avoided because the swollen mass of tissue does not remain reduced and manipulation causes additional discomfort for the patient.

External Hemorrhoids

In contrast to internal hemorrhoids, external hemorrhoids frequently present with itching, burning, or pain that may be quite severe with acute thrombosis. In some patients, however, external hemorrhoids are relatively asymptomatic, and bleeding may be the only clue to their presence. The bleeding, however, is rarely as profuse as that encountered with internal hemorrhoids.

External hemorrhoids are visible on inspection without the use of an anoscope. They often are accompanied by skin tags, which may become quite extensive with resultant irritation, itching, and soiling.

Acute thrombosis of an external hemorrhoidal vein produces the sudden appearance of a painful, tender mass at the anal opening. Varying from several millimeters to several centimeters in diameter, this tense, tender swelling often contains a readily visible bluish clot beneath overlying stretched and edematous skin. Anal thrombosis usually follows a sudden episode of straining with coughing, sneezing, heavy lifting, vigorous athletic activity, defecation, or parturition. It commonly occurs in young and otherwise healthy adults and probably is related to a sudden increase in hemorrhoidal venous pressure. Although anal thrombosis may develop in patients with symptomatic hemorrhoidal disease, it is not necessarily related to internal hemorrhoids or other anal abnormalities. The key feature in diagnosis is recognition that the swelling is covered by skin and not by rectal mucosa. This observation differentiates anal thrombosis from internal hemorrhoidal prolapse.

Differential Diagnosis

Other causes for rectal bleeding include colorectal carcinoma, polyps, inflammatory bowel disease, colonic diverticulosis, and anal fissure. Sigmoidoscopy and/or colonoscopy is an important part of the routine examination for hemorrhoids, and barium-contrast study of the colon is a frequently indicated additional diagnostic test. Other anorectal conditions that require differentiation from hemorrhoids are rectal prolapse, condyloma acuminatum of the anal canal and perianal area, anal neoplasms, and prolapsed pedunculated rectal polyps. A prominent anal skin tag may indicate an adjacent anal fissure, which usually is located in the posterior midline.

Treatment

Asymptomatic hemorrhoids require no treatment. Regulation of bowel habit and avoidance of constipation by the use of psyllium-containing bulk-forming agents such as Metamucil, Effersyllium, or Hydrocil Instant may relieve hemorrhoidal symptoms and result in regression of early pathologic changes in some instances. Bleeding from internal hemorrhoids often may be controlled simply by softening the stool. Reading while sitting on the toilet should be avoided. Prolonged sitting in this manner with the anus unsupported, coupled with increased intra-abdominal pressure from the elbows-on-knees posture and repeated straining at defecation, produces venous engorgement of the hemorrhoidal plexuses and can aggravate existing hemorrhoidal disease. Hemorrhoids characteristically are intermittently symptomatic; lengthy periods of remission are common, with exacerbations often triggered by constipation or diarrhea. During symptomatic periods, anesthetic-, steroid-, and astringent-containing suppositories such as Anusol-HC and Wyanoid HC are of value.

Pain with acute thrombosis of an external hemorrhoidal vein is most intense at the outset and gradually diminishes over several days as acute inflammation subsides. Discomfort may be alleviated by warm sitz baths and local application of a topical anesthetic ointment. Shortly after the onset of acute symptoms, prompt pain relief can be obtained by evacuation of the clot under local anesthesia.

Reasons for Referral

Patients with acute thrombosis of an external hemorrhoidal vein should be referred for consideration of clot evacuation or complete excision under local anesthesia. Surgical consultation should be obtained in managing the patient with irreducible (incarcerated) prolapse of internal hemorrhoids, even though operative treatment is not advisable for the acute condition.

Patients who have recurring bleeding from internal hemorrhoids and/or extensive and bothersome prolapse should be referred for consideration of rubber band ligation, injection therapy, or hemorrhoidectomy. Rubber band ligation and injection therapy are effective treatments for mild-to-moderate internal hemorrhoids. Both procedures are most frequently done on an outpatient basis and usually produce only minor discomfort for several days with little time lost from work. Surgical hemorrhoidectomy, in contrast, should be reserved for large, far-advanced hemorrhoids. Patients are usually hospitalized for 4 to 5 days and the procedure is most often done under spinal or general anesthesia. The period of limited activity following surgery is usually 3 to 4 weeks.

Anal Fissures

An anal fissure (fissure in ano) is a superficial, longitudinal laceration or ulceration of the modified skin (squamous epithelium) that lines the anal canal just below the dentate line. Because the skin of the lower anal canal is richly innervated by sensory fibers, anal fissures are quite painful. An acute anal fissure is a laceration or tear produced most commonly by passage of a hard bolus of feces. With each defecation, the laceration is stretched again, causing severe pain that may continue for several hours. As a consequence, the patient may resist defecation, become more constipated, and experience excruciating pain with the next bowel movement.

The problem tends to be cyclic, with healing and periods of remission. Constipation initiates a new episode, with the healed fissure split open again by passage of hard feces. A chronic fissure results after several months from this process of healing and recurrent injury; it appears as an elliptic or round ulcer having an edematous and scarred base.

Evaluation

The diagnosis should be suspected from the history of pain during and following defecation. The onset of acute symptoms may be recalled as having been associated with passage of a particularly hard stool. Pain typically is severe and is characterized as cutting, tearing, or burning. Following defecation, pain may become more intense from reflex anal sphincter spasm. Bleeding may be present as a secondary complaint and usually is noted as a small amount of fresh blood on the toilet tissues.

There is usually a single anal fissure located characteristically in the posterior midline of the anal canal (except in postpartum women, in whom the fissure may be in the anterior midline). Severity of pain and tenderness and degree of sphincter spasm associated with an acute fissure often make examination traumatic and extremely painful. Because of its position in the distal portion of the anal canal, the fissure can be seen readily on external examination if traction is placed on the perianal skin to evert the anal opening gently. Because the acute fissure usually can be seen by this maneuver, anoscopic examination should be deferred until treatment makes the procedure comfortable for the patient. Digital examination is very painful and needs to be done only if the diagnosis is unclear. Digital examination usually can be accomplished after application of a topical anesthetic, with careful introduction of the gloved finger by gentle pressure on the anal verge opposite the fissure. Palpation can determine tenderness at the site of the fissure and the degree of sphincter spasm.

A chronic anal fissure commonly presents the diagnostic triad of a distal sentinel pile, a chronic ulcer in the anal canal, and a proximal hypertrophied anal papilla at the dentate level. Gentle traction on the sentinel pile—a fibrotic and edematous skin tag—everts the anus to disclose the distal portion of the chronic fissure. Topical anesthesia facilitates anoscopic examination to further visualize the fissure and the proximal hypertrophied papilla. Long-standing disease may produce enough scarring and fibrosis to result in induration and stenosis of the anal canal.

Differential Diagnosis

Other anal ulcerations that must be differentiated from anal fissure include carcinoma, chancre, ulcerations associated with blood dyscrasias, and fissures associated with granulomatous enterocolitis (Crohn's disease). These diseases have characteristic symptoms and signs, and anal ulceration associated with them should not be confused with an anal fissure. Fissures located laterally or anteriorly in men and fissures located laterally in women should arouse suspicion of another underlying disease. Anal fissures may occur concomitantly with hemorrhoids and may be overlooked if not searched for carefully.

Treatment

An acute fissure with a short history usually heals rapidly and satisfactorily with medical treatment. Pain relief can be achieved by local application of a topical anesthetic ointment before and after bowel movements and as needed otherwise for comfort. Warm sitz baths for 15 to 20 minutes following each stool provide additional symptomatic relief, resolve associated reflex anal sphincter spasm, and facilitate anal hygiene. Local application of a topical steroid cream may enhance healing. Unless an analgesic- and steroid-containing suppository is placed and held in the anal canal until it dissolves, the suppository slides immediately into the rectum where it has no influence on the fissure. Because it is practically impossible to hold a suppository in this manner, it is rarely prescribed in the treatment of fissures. Relief of constipation is essential in successful treatment of anal fissure. Proper diet, a regular bowel habit, and use of stool softeners are important features in correcting constipation.

Medical treatment is much less successful with a chronic anal fissure, although a trial of therapy is warranted. A chronic fissure may heal temporarily, only to recur several weeks or months later.

Reasons for Referral

An anal fissure that does not heal after 3 to 4 weeks of therapy, a chronic fissure with sentinel pile and hypertrophied anal papilla, and a fissure associated with anal stenosis should be referred for surgical treatment. Any fissure that is atypically located or that displays unusual features should be referred for additional diagnostic tests and appropriate therapy.

Pruritus Ani

Pruritus ani, or itching of the perianal skin, is a very common problem. It is frequently associated with hemorrhoids, but may occur as a separate unrelated problem. In addition to hemorrhoids, recognized or purported causes of pruritus ani include: anatomic lesions, such as anal fissures, polyps, and neoplasms; irritation resulting from fecal soiling, chronic diarrhea, or inadequate rectal cleansing; infections including anal condylomata and other viral, bacterial, fungal, and parasitic infections (pinworm is uncommon in the adult); and primary skin disorders with perirectal involvement, such as atopic or seborrheic dermatitis, psoriasis, and lichen planus.

A careful history and physical that includes anoscopy will usually reveal the correct etiology and treatment for many of these causes. For the many patients in whom the cause is not obvious, reasonable empiric therapy includes (1) adequate but gentle cleaning of the anus after defecation, (2) avoidance of harsh cleansing soaps or medications, (3) avoidance of tight underclothing, and (4) cautious use of nonfluorinated topical steroid creams after cleansing (such as hydrocortisone 1%).

Resistant problems probably are best managed by referral to a dermatologist.

Lieberman DA. Common anorectal disorders. Ann Intern Med 1984; 101:837–46.
An excellent, thorough, practical review. Includes 62 references.

Dennison AR, et al. The management of hemorrhoids. Am J Gastroenterol 1989; 84:475–81.
Thorough review of all treatment modalities.

Thomson WHF. The nature of hemorrhoids. Br J Surg 1975; 62:542–52.
Primarily concerned with the pathogenesis of hemorrhoids. Emphasizes the role of the submucosal "cushions."

Haas PA, Fox TA, Haas GP. The pathogenesis of hemorrhoids. Dis Colon Rectum 1984; 27:442–50.
Clear review of the pathogenesis of hemorrhoids.

Smith LE. A review of current techniques and management. Gastroenterol Clin North Am 1987; 16:79–81.
An excellent general review of pathophysiology and management.

Crapp AR, Alexander-Williams J. Fissure-in-ano and anal stenosis. Clin Gastroenterol 1975; 4:619–28.
An excellent general review.

Shub HA, Salvati EP, Rubin RJ. Conservative treatment of anal fissure: an unselected, retrospective, and continuous study. Dis Colon Rectum 1978; 21:582–3.
An excellent discussion of conservative management based on a series of 393 patients.

Jensen SL, et al. Treatment of first episodes of acute anal fissure: prospective study of lignocaine ointment versus hydrocortisone ointment or warm sitz baths and bran. Br Med J Clin Res 1986; 292:1167–9.
After 1 and 2 weeks of treatment, symptomatic relief was significantly better among patients treated with sitz baths and bran than among patients treated with ointments. After 3 weeks, there was no significant difference among the groups.

Ferguson JA, MacKeigan JM. Hemorrhoids, fistulas, and fissures: office and hospital management. A critical review. Adv Surg 1978; 12:111–53.
An excellent review including pathophysiology, diagnosis, and treatment. An extensive bibliography.

Smith LE, Henrichs D, McCullah RD. Prospective studies on the etiology and treatment of pruritus ani. Dis Colon Rectum 1982; 25:358–63.
A practical orientation to coping with this problem.

51. HEMATOCHEZIA AND OCCULT GASTROINTESTINAL BLEEDING
Robert A. McNutt and Sidney E. Levinson

Hematochezia

Hematochezia, or visible bleeding from the rectum, can originate from lesions throughout the gastrointestinal tract. The most common cause is local anal disease, usually hemorrhoids or anal fissures. Less often, bleeding is from a more proximal source, such as cancers, polyps, angiodysplasia, or diverticula.

Bleeding usually occurs with a bowel movement, although oozing and subsequent spotting of undergarments sometimes occur. Local anal bleeding frequently follows physical activities or straining at stool. The patient notes streaking or coating of the stools with fresh blood, or blood on the toilet tissue. Occasionally, blood spurts into the toilet bowl at the beginning or end of a bowel movement. Because blood can reflux proximal to the anus from oozing internal hemorrhoids, blood mixed with stool is compatible with local anal disease. The passage of blood alone or blood mixed with mucus usually represents bleeding from a more proximal source, particularly the colon.

Evaluation

Although the initial evaluation must include questioning about upper gastrointestinal problems, the history and physical examination should concentrate on the colon and rectum including questions about weight loss and change in bowel habits. Symptoms may suggest the cause of bleeding. Patients with hemorrhoidal bleeding usually have burning, itching, or aching as a result of inflammation, although hemorrhoidal bleeding can be painless. Cramping or bloating with a change in stool caliber suggests colon carcinoma or a prolapsed polyp. Bleeding from a more proximal source is usually painless. History should include a family history of inflammatory bowel disease, colonic polyps, cancer, and, in particular, familial polyposis syndromes.

In the general physical examination one should look for extraintestinal signs of inflammatory bowel disease such as iritis, erythema nodosum, or pyoderma gangrenosum. Telangiectasias or subcutaneous cysts may be associated with hereditary hemorrhagic telangiectasia or one of the familial polyposis syndromes (e.g., Peutz-Jeghers, Canada-Cronkhite).

The anorectal region must be inspected carefully for fistulae, induration, external skin tags, or prolapsed hemorrhoids. The digital rectal examination may disclose tenderness, induration, or nodularity indicating inflammation of local anal tissues or anorectal fissures. Rarely, a squamous carcinoma is palpable. Anoscopy is then performed. Anoscopy should be performed with the patient in the left lateral decubitus position and performing Valsalva's maneuver. This ensures distention of hemorrhoids that might not appear significant with the patient not straining and in the knee-chest position. Finding hemorrhoids does not preclude further workup, as hemorrhoids may be associated with proximal lesions.

After digital examination and anoscopy, the subsequent evaluation should be guided by the fact that most causes of hematochezia are local to the rectum and anus. The next step then is to perform proctosigmoidoscopy. It is reasonable, and perhaps preferable, to use a rigid sigmoidoscope because routine use of the flexible sigmoidoscope is costly and its accuracy is greatly dependent on the skills and experience of the user. Also, the anal area may be more easily examined with the rigid sigmoidoscope.

If no source of bleeding is found after proctosigmoidoscopy and anoscopy, many physicians proceed with either air-contrast barium enema or colonoscopy. The most appropriate workup strategy is debatable and is discussed in the following section on occult gastrointestinal bleeding. If air-contrast barium enema and colonoscopy fail to detect a bleeding source, it may be prudent to defer additional studies if the probability of cancer is low (i.e., young persons with no history of familial polyp syndromes), and providing that bleeding has ceased.

Other studies that may be useful include arteriography, to look for an arteriovenous malformation or tumor blush in the small bowel; technetium scans, to look for Meckel's diverticula; and upper gastrointestinal and small-bowel x-ray series. Arteriography in general should be reserved for patients with rapid, potentially life-threatening bleeding.

On occasion, arteriography is done electively in patients who present repeatedly with bleeding that requires blood replacement. It is the best clinical test for diagnosing angiodysplasia of the right colon.

Occult Gastrointestinal Bleeding

Testing for occult blood is performed in an attempt to screen asymptomatic patients or to establish the cause in patients with complaints referable to the gastrointestinal tract. While occult gastrointestinal bleeding can come from either the upper or lower gastrointestinal tract, colorectal carcinoma and polyps are found in nearly 50% of patients with occult bleeding. In the young, acid-peptic disease is the most common cause of occult bleeding. In the elderly, polyps of the colon are the most common. Besides polyps and cancer, other common causes of bleeding include angiodysplasia and local rectal disease. Diverticulosis is not a common cause of bleeding and its presence should not defer the search for cancer or polyps.

Screening

The principal reason to screen for occult blood is to detect cancer and polyps. Colorectal cancer is the second most common form of cancer in the United States and it has the second highest mortality. Because persons with early-stage cancer live longer, it has been theorized that annual screening may reduce the likelihood of dying from colorectal cancer. There is, however, no evidence that this screening leads to improved survival; if cancers are simply detected earlier, without improved survival, then the only impact on patients will be that they will live longer with their diagnosis. Indeed, the US Preventive Services Task Force found insufficient evidence to recommend for or against screening for colorectal cancer in asymptomatic patients.

Fecal occult blood testing using guaiac-impregnated paper (e.g., Hemoccult II) is the simplest and least expensive screening test. The sensitivity of this test for detecting cancer is 50 to 66%. (The digital examination is less than 10% sensitive.) Clearly, many small cancers do not bleed, or bleed so intermittently that they are difficult to detect. The sensitivity is higher for right-sided lesions, and it can be increased by rehydration of the specimen and repeat testing (two samples for 3 days). The sensitivity of Hemoccult is reduced (more false-negative results) by poor patient compliance for returning the cards (15–70% compliance), nonuniform distribution of blood in the stool, and drugs such as ascorbic acid that interfere with the test reagents. In addition, the specificity of Hemoccult is low. False-positive test results are common and can be caused by the ingestion of foods containing peroxidases (high-residue diets), iron compounds, antiinflammatory agents or other gastric irritants, or bleeding lesions other than cancer or polyps. Among all persons tested with Hemoccult II, 1 to 10% will have a positive test result, and 5 to 12% of patients with positive results will be found to have cancers. Polyps will be found in 20 to 50% of patients with positive Hemoccult results. Therefore, about half of patients will have no cause found.

Sigmoidoscopy varies in accuracy as a screening test according to the type of procedure performed and the training and experience of the examiner. The rigid sigmoidoscope is 16 to 27% sensitive and the flexible sigmoidoscope is 40 to 58% sensitive for the diagnosis of cancer. While the colonoscope is 80 to 90% sensitive for cancer, it is highly user-dependent and costly, and it carries greater risks than the flexible and rigid scopes. In addition, many patients are unwilling to undergo sigmoidoscopy or colonoscopy as a screening test.

Considering the difficulties regarding test sensitivity, specificity, cost, and safety, the US Preventive Services Task Force recommended the following screening measures:

1. *Fecal occult testing and flexible sigmoidoscopy* should be performed every 1 to 3 years in persons over the age of 50 who have (a) first-degree relatives with colorectal cancer; (b) a personal history of endometrial, ovarian, or breast cancer; (c) a previous diagnosis of inflammatory bowel disease; or (d) a history of adenomatous polyps or colon cancer.
2. *Fecal occult testing and colonoscopy* should be performed every 1 to 3 years in persons over the age of 19 who have a family history of familial polyposis or cancer family syndrome.

Screening in other individuals should be based on risk and patient preferences.

Follow-up of Positive Occult Blood Tests

The decision on how to best follow-up patients with a positive result on the occult blood test is hotly debated and depends on the trade-offs of costs and effectiveness. There are no adequate clincial trials testing competing strategies. Given the lack of clinical data, a mathematic model was developed to measure the cost and effectiveness of 22 strategies of varying intensities in the follow-up of patients with occult bleeding. The two most aggressive strategies were best, but most expensive. The best strategy was to do a barium enema; if the results are negative, a colonoscopy is done, and if this is negative the workup is stopped. If the barium enema shows positive findings, a colonoscopy should be done, and if colonoscopy reveals normal features, barium enema should be repeated. Then, if the barium enema is still positive, the colonoscopy is repeated. The next best strategy was to start with colonoscopy; if the findings are negative, a barium enema is done. If the barium enema is positive, the colonoscopy is repeated. These strategies have nearly 97% sensitivity for detecting cancer or polyps, but they cost nearly $100,000 per year of life saved (approximately 4 times the cost to save a year of a life with renal dialysis). In contrast, an alternative strategy of repeating the Hemoccult and following up only the repeat positive tests with rigid sigmoidoscopy and barium enema has a sensitivity of nearly 60% and costs only $738 per year of life saved. Clearly, the decision on how to best follow-up positive occult blood tests is unsettled. However, it is reasonable that persons with the highest likelihood of cancer such as those with a history of polyps or cancer, other cancers as described above, or ulcerative colitis should undergo aggressive searches for cancer or polyps.

Levinson SL, et al. A current approach to rectal bleeding. J Clin Gastroenterol 1989; 3:Suppl 1:9–16.
A review of causes of and approach to diagnosis and treatment of rectal bleeding.

Guide to clinical preventive services: an assessment of the effectiveness of 169 interventions. Report of the U.S. Preventive Services Task Force. Baltimore, MD.: Williams & Wilkins, 1989: 47–59.
A concise review and extensive bibliography on the issues of screening and test effectiveness.

Brandeau ML, Eddy DM. The workup of the asymptomatic patient with a positive fecal occult blood test. Med Decis Making 1987; 7:32–46.
An extensive review of varied workup strategies.

Clayman CB. Mass screening for colorectal cancer: are we ready? JAMA 1989; 261:609.
A review of trade-offs in screening.

Tedesco FJ, et al. Colonoscopic evaluation of rectal bleeding: a study of 304 patients. Ann Intern Med 1978; 89:907–9.
Describes the yield of colonoscopy in patients with a negative result on sigmoidoscopic examination and on single-contrast barium enema.

Frank JW. Occult blood screening for colorectal carcinoma: the yield and the costs. Am J Prev Med 1985; 1:18–24.
A review of costs and benefits.

Winawer SJ, et al. Progress report on controlled trial of fecal occult blood testing for the determination of colorectal neoplasia. Cancer 1980; 45:2959–64.
Among men and women aged 40 or older, 1 to 4% of Hemoccult slides are positive.

Winawer SJ, Fleisher M, Sherlock P. Sensitivity of fecal occult blood testing for adenomas. Gastroenterology 1982; 83:1136–8.
Hemoccult tests detect polyps better if they are larger than 2 cm or in the left colon.

Selby JV, et al. Sigmoidoscopy and mortality from colorectal cancer: the Kaiser Permanente Multiphasic Evaluation Study. J Clin Epidemiol 1988; 41(5):427–34.
Review of large randomized trial of early detection and suggests that decrease in colorectal cancer mortality was not due to sigmoidoscopy.

Eddy D. Screening for colorectal cancer. Ann Intern Med 1990; 113:373–84.
Another good general review and discussion of policy guidelines.

52. GALLSTONES
Michael D. Apstein

Gallstones occur in 10% of the US population, with a prevalence of 25% in women over 50 years old. Each year, 1 million patients are newly diagnosed with gallstones; half of whom undergo cholecystectomy, at an estimated annual cost of 4 to 6 billion dollars. Key issues include when to look for gallstones; which patients should be treated; and the role of the newer therapies, such as laparoscopic cholecystectomy and medical dissolution, and the experimental therapies, lithotripsy and contact solvent dissolution. Preventive measures may be useful in those who are at very high risk of gallstone formation, such as patients on very-low-calorie diets for rapid weight loss, or those receiving total parenteral nutrition (TPN) for as little as 4 weeks.

Pathogenesis and Epidemiology

Gallstones are classified by composition: cholesterol or pigment (bilirubinate salts of calcium). Patients have either one type or the other. In the United States, 80% of gallstone patients have cholesterol stones. Since only cholesterol stones potentially can be treated with dissolution therapy or lithotripsy, identifying stone type is of practical significance.

Patients who develop cholesterol gallstones typically have a "triple defect": (1) supersaturation of bile with cholesterol, due to hypersecretion of cholesterol from the liver and/or hyposecretion of bile salts; (2) accelerated cholesterol nucleation; and (3) incomplete gallbladder emptying.

Risk factors for cholesterol gallstones as a result of increased biliary cholesterol include the following: female gender; parity; obesity; rapid weight loss; increasing age; a family history; or the administration of estrogens, fibric acids, or anabolic steroids. Additionally, because of decreased gallbladder motility, patients with gallbladder stasis syndromes or spinal cord injury, or those receiving octreotide are at risk for cholesterol gallstones.

The pathogenesis of pigment gallstone is less well understood, but is related to a combination of overproduction of unconjugated bilirubin, increased amounts of biliary ionized calcium, decreased bile salt levels, and motility defects. Excess biliary ionized calcium complexes with unconjugated bilirubin, precipitates, and grows to form stones. Normally, bile salts both solubilize unconjugated bilirubin and bind to ionized calcium. Consequently, bile-salt deficiency promotes pigment stone formation by making more unconjugated bilirubin and ionized calcium available for coprecipitation.

The major risk factors for pigment gallstone formation include hemolytic disorders, hepatic cirrhosis, increasing age, ileal disease or resection, long-term TPN, and biliary infection. All except the last risk factor are associated with "black" gallbladder stones. In these hard and brittle stones, calcium bilirubinate precipitates in a sterile gallbladder and the bilirubin in the precipitate polymerizes and oxidizes. In contrast "brown" stones form when there is a biliary infection in either the gallbladder or the bile ducts; these stones have a soft, greasy consistency from the presence of calcium palmitate, dead bacteria, and mucin. Heretofore, it was believed that ileal disease or resection led to cholesterol stone formation. However, better studies now confirm that these patients are at risk for pigment, not cholesterol, stones.

Clinical Syndromes

Asymptomatic Gallstones

Most gallstone patients are asymptomatic. For unclear reasons, males have half the risk of becoming symptomatic as females. If asymptomatic gallstones ("silent stones") are diagnosed, for example, by routine ultrasonography during pregnancy, patients can be advised that the chances of developing symptoms over a lifetime are approximately 20%. If symptoms develop, they generally do so within the first 5 years of diagnosis. In more than 90% of patients who develop symptoms, the initial symptom is biliary pain (misnamed "colic") rather than a potentially life-threatening complication, such as acute cholecystitis, cholangitis, or pancreatitis.

Biliary Pain
Biliary pain typically occurs in the epigastrium or right upper quadrant, and is caused by transient obstruction of the cystic or common bile duct. It lasts from 30 minutes to several hours, is steady rather than crampy (i.e., not "colic"), and may be accompanied by nausea and vomiting. Ill-defined "dyspeptic" symptoms, such as fatty-food intolerance and postprandial bloating, indigestion, or flatulence, cannot be attributed to gallstones because they are no more common in gallstone patients than in those without gallstones.

During an uncomplicated episode of biliary pain, the findings on physical examination are usually normal. Fever, rebound tenderness, and leukocytosis are absent. If these findings are present, acute cholecystitis or other complications must be suspected and excluded.

Patients with even one episode of biliary pain do not have a benign course: 50% of these patients will experience recurrent pain during the next 20 years. Most who develop recurrent pain do so within the first 5 years. Acute cholecystitis or other complications occur at a linear rate of 1% per year. By 20 years, almost half of these patients will have had a cholecystectomy or other definitive treatment.

Complications

Acute Cholecystitis
Acute cholecystitis, inflammation of both bile and the gallbladder wall, results from obstruction of the cystic duct by gallstones. "Acalculous" acute cholecystitis, seen in seriously ill, immobilized, hospitalized patients, probably results from obstruction of the cystic duct with "biliary sludge." Acute cholecystitis begins with biliary pain that does not remit and is associated with anorexia, nausea, vomiting, fever, and abdominal tenderness and/or guarding, whose severity and localization vary with the extent of the inflammation. Diagnosis is based on clinical findings and confirmed by cholescintigraphy (hepatic iminodiacetic acid [HIDA] scan), when stones or sludge is demonstrated at ultrasonography. Chronic cholecystitis is a pathologic designation for a thickened, scarred gallbladder from repeated bouts of healed acute cholecystitis.

Common Duct Stones
Common duct stones (Choledocholithiasis) usually result from the migration of gallbladder stones; only 5% involve stones formed de novo in the common duct. The prevalence of common duct stones in individuals with gallbladder stones increases from 10% at age 30 to 50% in patients 80 years or older. The natural history of common duct stones is unpredictable; approximately 50% of patients remain asymptomatic for years and 50% present clinically with obstruction or inflammation. The clinical presentation of choledocholithiasis includes biliary pain without other complications, jaundice, potentially life-threatening cholangitis, or acute pancreatitis.

Gallstone Pancreatitis
Gallstones migrating from the gallbladder cause pancreatitis by transient obstruction of the ampulla of Vater. Risk factors are small stones, a large cystic duct, and a common channel of common bile and pancreatic ducts. Gallstone pancreatitis is indistinguishable clinically from acute pancreatitis of other etiologies.

Gallstone Ileus
Gallstone ileus is a small-bowel obstruction resulting from impaction of a large gallstone that has eroded through the gallbladder wall into the small bowel. The impacted stone is usually (60%) at the ileocecal valve. One-third of patients will have no prior clinical evidence of clinical gallbladder disease. Therefore, gallstone ileus should be suspected in any elderly patient presenting with a small-bowel obstruction, especially in the absence of prior abdominal surgery that could predispose to adhesions.

Clinical Evaluation

Since the history and physical examination are unreliable for diagnosing gallstones and only 25% of gallstones have sufficient inorganic calcium salts to be visible on KUB, confirmatory imaging studies are essential for diagnosis.

Abdominal ultrasonography is the diagnostic procedure of choice for suspected gallstones, and should be performed when patient complains of biliary pain. Since it involves no patient preparation or radiation, it should be performed immediately when acute cholecystitis is suspected. Ultrasonography has a sensitivity of 95% and a specificity of 98% when done by experts. However, in patients with fever and abdominal pain, the finding of gallstones is not diagnostic of acute cholecystitis. Acute cholecystitis can be diagnosed only rarely by ultrasonography alone when edema is demonstrated in or around the wall of the gallbladder. Confirmatory nuclear medicine imaging usually must be performed. Ultrasonography can also identify evidence of common duct stones, such as a dilated common bile duct or, less frequently, common bile duct stones themselves. Furthermore, biliary sludge, nonshadowing echo-dense material within the gallbladder lumen, can be identified by ultrasonography. Sludge, seen only occasionally in outpatients, can be responsible for the same symptoms and clinical presentation as gallstones, from pain to cholangitis, to pancreatitis.

Oral cholecystography (OCG) has nearly the same sensitivity and specificity as ultrasonography for diagnosing gallstones, but does not detect sludge. OCG requires overnight preparation of the patient and is often associated with diarrhea. Most normal gallbladders (75%) will demonstrate opacification on radiographs after a single dose of contrast medium. If opacification fails to occur, the patient should be given a second dose of contrast medium and the radiograph repeated the following day. Failure to visualize the gallbladder after a second dose predicts gallstone disease with 95% accuracy. OCG is unreliable in patients who vomit or malabsorb the radiocontrast pills, who have liver disease that prevents excretion of contrast material into the biliary tree, or who are unreliable and do not take the pills.

The OCG can provide information about gallbladder function, motility, and the number, size, and density of stones, which is not easily attained by routine ultrasonography. This information is crucial when medical dissolution of stones or lithotripsy is being considered.

Nuclear medicine imaging (cholescintigraphy) with a technetium-labeled iminodiacetic acid (IDA) derivative (i.e., diethyliminodiacetic acid [DISIDA]) is the test of choice for confirming the diagnosis of acute cholecystitis. Nonvisualization of the gallbladder is consistent with acute cholecystitis, but can occur in patients with alcoholism, in patients with healed acute cholecystitis, and in those receiving TPN. Visualization of the gallbladder excludes acute cholecystitis with 99% accuracy.

Computed tomography (CT) is less sensitive than abdominal ultrasonography for the detection of gallbladder or common duct stones. It is very useful for determining calcium content of gallstones and, in the future, may play a role in determining which patients would be most suitable for medical dissolution treatment or lithotripsy. CT is the preferred imaging technique for evaluating suspected biliary or pancreatic masses.

Endoscopic retrograde pancreaticocholangiography (ERCP) is the test of choice in evaluating patients with suspected common bile duct stones or gallstone pancreatitis. As laparoscopic cholecystectomy becomes more common, so has the preoperative use of ERCP to exclude and/or remove common bile duct stones. Not all patients undergoing laparoscopic cholecystectomy need a preoperative ERCP, but which subgroup would benefit from one remains to be determined. ERCP plays no role in the diagnosis of gallbladder stones, though endoscopic retrograde cannulation to the gallbladder (ERCG) via the cystic duct is being developed in several centers.

Diagnostic Strategy

Patients with even one episode of biliary pain should be evaluated initially with ultrasonography and treated if gallbladder stones are found (see treatment options below). OCG is indicated also (1) if ultrasonography demonstrates negative findings, but the clinical suspicion of biliary tract disease is high; or (2) if the character of the stones seen on ultrasound needs to be determined prior to bile acid dissolution therapy.

The evaluation of patients with nonspecific, vague, or so-called dyspeptic symptoms is more troublesome because the discovery of gallstones is not likely to explain these patients' symptoms. When these symptoms are troublesome or accompanied by clinical findings, a thorough evaluation of the gastrointestinal tract, including barium studies and endoscopy, is indicated. These patients may have been treated previously, with only partial success, for irritable bowel disease, gastritis, or peptic ulcer disease. The discovery of gallstones may, out of frustration, lead to surgery, urged by both patient and physician, in "hope" that the symptoms will resolve following cholecystectomy. A large percentage of patients with nonspecific abdominal symptoms fail to obtain long-term relief following cholecystectomy and are then labeled as having the "postcholecystectomy syndrome."

In patients whose symptoms and signs suggest acute cholecystitis, immediate ultrasonography followed by cholescintigraphy is indicated. Nonvisualization of the gallbladder in this clinical setting should lead to early cholecystectomy.

Even with a high degree of clinical suspicion, the diagnosis of common duct stones may be difficult. Ultrasonography and CT of the biliary tree fail to detect 50% of common duct stones. ERCP is the definitive diagnostic test, and also allows for papillotomy and stone removal. Even patients with spontaneous resolution of symptoms or elevated serum bilirubin and/or alkaline phosphatase levels, which suggest passage of a common bile duct stone, should be evaluated with an ERCP to exclude remaining asymptomatic stones.

Treatment Options

There are now several surgical, as well as medical treatment options for gallstone disease.

Cholecystectomy

Cholecystectomy is the treatment of choice for the majority of patients with symptomatic gallstones or gallstone complications. However, surgery fails to relieve symptoms in 15% of patients because of operation for inappropriate symptoms. Elective, traditional cholecystectomy via laparotomy is very safe. The morbidity and mortality are age- and sex-related: 6% and 0.2%, respectively, for women aged 30, to 10% and 3%, respectively, at age 75. Men have roughly twice the operative mortality probably because of more concomitant atherosclerotic disease. Operative mortality doubles with emergency operations and quadruples when the common bile duct is explored. One-half of the morbidity is related to the biliary tract, with the most serious injury to the bile duct occurring in 0.2% of patients.

Laparoscopic cholecystectomy has almost replaced traditional cholecystectomy worldwide, with up to 85% of elective operations being performed via this approach. However, there have been no studies comparing the safety of the two approaches. Clear advantages of laparoscopic cholecystectomy include an improved cosmetic effect (a smaller scar), reduced hospital stay (approximately 1 day compared to 4–6 days), and earlier return to normal activities (approximately 7 days compared to 42 days). Early results suggest a higher rate of bile duct injury (0.8%), compared to traditional cholecystectomy (see above). A common relative contraindication is previous abdominal surgery, which may prevent adequate abdominal-wall distention for clear visibility of the gallbladder bed. Following cholecystectomy, there is no fat malabsorption and no need for a special diet.

Chemical Dissolution

Medical dissolution treatment with the natural bile acid ursodiol (ursodeoxycholic acid [UDCA]) completely dissolves small gallstones in up to 80% of highly selected patients. The applicability of this treatment is limited critically by the character and size of the stones, and severity of the symptoms. It is an appropriate treatment option for mildly symptomatic patients with small cholesterol (but not pigment or calcified) gallbladder stones, particularly those who refuse surgery or who would tolerate surgery poorly. The major disadvantages of treatment with ursodiol are that gallstones dissolve slowly (1 mm/month) and will reform in 50% of patients within 5 years.

Ursodiol decreases biliary cholesterol secretion and desaturates bile, thereby favoring cholesterol resolubilization from gallstones. Cholesterol molecules are plucked literally one by one from the surfaces of gallstones, redissolved in bile, and then expelled into the duodenum following gallbladder contraction.

Prior to initiation of ursodiol treatment, the size, number, and calcium content of the stones need to be evaluated with ultrasonography and abdominal radiograph (KUB). If small (< 10 mm), noncalcified stones that comprise less than 50% of the volume of the gallbladder are shown, ursodiol therapy can be started at 8 mg/kg in two divided doses in the morning and at bedtime. Reassessment of stone size, either by OCG or ultrasonography, after 6 months of therapy is the only specific follow-up required. Although a nonopacified gallbladder on initial OCG is *not* a poor prognostic sign, the *development* of a nonvisualized OCG during therapy predicts failure. Therefore either the development of a nonvisualized OCG or the lack of dissolution at follow-up should prompt the physician to discontinue therapy. Ursodiol should be continued for 3 months after complete stone dissolution has been confirmed by ultrasonography, not OCG. If frequent attacks of biliary pain occur (a rare event) during therapy, a delay in definitive treatment is unacceptable and such patients require surgery.

After successful dissolution, patients should be reevaluated for recurrent gallstones only if symptoms of biliary tract disease recur. Surveillance ultrasonography for gallstone recurrence is not recommended. Ursodiol, unlike its predecessor, chenodiol, is remarkably free of all side effects. However, patients should be advised that the drug is expensive (approximately $1500/year, and not all insurers cover outpatient pharmacy costs) and that a second course of therapy for symptomatic recurrence may be required.

Lithotripsy

Extracorporeal shock wave lithotripsy (ESWL) is still investigational (Food and Drug Administration Investigational New Drug Application [IND] required). It should be viewed as adjuvant to ursodiol treatment to accelerate dissolution of cholesterol stones only. The focusing of shock waves onto gallstones fragments a large stone into myriads of small pieces, which then either migrate into the duodenum without obstruction or dissolve more rapidly. Symptomatic patients with less than three (ideally a single) lucent stones, 1 to 2 cm in size, are good candidates for combination ESWL and ursodiol therapy.

ESWL has limited overall applicability since only 15 to 25% of gallstone patients qualify. Exclusion criteria include acute complications of gallstones; an obstructed cystic or common bile duct; inability to target the gallstones without avoiding bone, lung, cysts, or aneurysms; and pregnancy. Nevertheless, those individuals with a solitary, 1- to 2-cm, radiolucent gallstone in a functioning gallbladder have an 80 to 90% chance of complete stone and fragment dissolution after ESWL followed by 1 year of ursodiol therapy.

The newer lithotriptors that employ piezoceramic technology are painless and well tolerated by patients. The procedure can be done in an outpatient setting without intravenous lines or analgesics. Side effects are related to transient obstruction of the cystic or common bile ducts resulting in biliary pain, acute cholecystitis, or pancreatitis in 35%, 4%, and 2%, respectively, usually within 48 hours of ESWL.

Treatment Strategies

Silent Stones

A recent decision analysis demonstrated that prophylactic cholecystectomy for men with asymptomatic gallstones resulted in a loss of 4 to 18 days of life, depending on age. Hence, because of their relatively benign natural history, patients with silent stones should be reassured. No specific treatment or follow-up is required. Prophylactic treatment, either medical dissolution with or without lithotripsy or cholecystectomy, for individuals with asymptomatic gallstones is appropriate only in rare situations. Individuals working temporarily in remote areas of the world where rapid access to safe surgery is a problem should have their stones dissolved or gallbladder removed as appropriate prior to relocation.

Although gallbladder cancer is associated with gallstones, only certain individuals are at a high enough risk to justify a prophylactic cholecystectomy. These include (1) females of American Indian descent with gallstones, or (2) any patient with a gallstone larger than 3 cm (only about 6% of all gallstone patients). There are other conditions associated with gallbladder cancer for which, because of their rarity, screening of patients is not indicated. However, should these conditions be diagnosed in the course of medical care, a prophylactic cholecystectomy would be appropriate. These include (1) patients with calcium in the gallbladder wall ("porcelain" gallbladder), (2) patients who after acute salmonella gastritis carry *Salmonella typhosa* in the stool, (3) patients with an anomalous pancreaticobiliary duct junction, and (4) patients with gallbladder wall polyps larger than 1 cm in diameter.

The most controversial issue regarding prophylactic cholecystectomy is its role in diabetics with asymptomatic gallstones. Certainly stone complications in diabetes are more serious than in nondiabetics, and end-organ damage, especially in the elderly, increases the surgical risk. Despite a decision analysis concluding that prophylactic cholecystectomy in diabetics of either sex resulted in a *shortened* life span by 2 to 8 months regardless of patient age, the issue remains unsettled. For now, routine prophylactic cholecystectomy for all diabetics cannot be recommended. Whether particular subgroups of diabetics may benefit from prophylactic treatment remains unresolved.

Prevention
Prevention of gallstones is possible in two groups of patients at high risk for stone formation. Prophylactic medical therapy in patients receiving TPN with daily administration of intravenous cholecystokinin-octapeptide (CCK-OP) prevents gallbladder stasis, sludge, and gallstone formation. Obese patients undergoing rapid weight loss (approximately 1–2% of body weight, 2–5 lbs/wk), either by very-low-calorie diet or gastric stapling or a similar procedure, have a 25 to 40% chance of developing gallstones within 4 months. Full-dose ursodiol (8 mg/kg) for the duration of the weight loss period completely prevents stone formation. A lower ursodiol dose or the inclusion of at least 12 g of fat per day may be effective as well. Studies to answer these questions are in progress.

Biliary Pain
After excluding acute cholecystitis, patients with acute biliary pain should be treated acutely with narcotics. Following resolution of pain, patients should be treated definitively to prevent recurrent pain and/or potential life-threatening complications. Patients with small, noncalcified symptomatic stones, which developed during weight loss, pregnancy, or the use of medications such as estrogens or fibric acids, would be ideal for ursodiol therapy. Clearly, for a proportion of these patients medical therapy will fail or accelerated symptoms that compel surgical treatment will develop.

Elective cholecystectomy is the treatment of choice for the majority of patients with biliary pain, especially young (< 50 years old) healthy individuals. Surgical risks are small but real, and must be balanced against the appreciable likelihood of recurrent pain and the 1%-per-year complication rate over the patient's life span. The operative risk is higher in older, sicker patients and it is less likely that recurrent pain and/or complications will present an uncontrollable problem before the patient succumbs to concomitant illness. Decisions in these older patients clearly must be individualized.

Acute Cholecystitis
Because acute cholecystitis requires early surgery, there is no role for medical dissolution therapy.

Supportive medical measures (antibiotics, fluid and electrolyte management) followed by early cholecystectomy (within the first 72 hours of the onset of the attack) is now the preferred treatment. In contrast to "delayed" cholecystectomy (6–8 weeks later) morbidity, mortality, and the incidence of recurrent pain and complications are all reduced. In patients who are poor operative risks, management with broad-spectrum antibiotics and temporizing procedures, such as cholecystostomy, may be an acceptable alternative.

Choledocholithiasis
Unlike expectant management of asymptomatic gallbladder stones, silent stones in the common bile duct should be removed. Although their natural history is not known, the risk of potential life-threatening cholangitis probably outweighs the small risk of their removal via endoscopic sphincterotomy.

Endoscopic sphincterotomy alone (i.e., leaving the gallbladder in situ) is adequate treatment for many patients, especially the elderly, with symptomatic common bile duct stones. The risk of cholecystitis or recurrent choledocholithiasis over a 10-year period in patients so treated is low (approximately 10%).

Gallstone Pancreatitis
Once a patient has recovered from an acute episode of gallstone pancreatitis, definitive therapy is indicated, because 25% of patients will have another attack of acute pancreatitis within a month and 50% within a year if their biliary tree is not cleared of stones. Cholecystectomy and common bile duct exploration to clear the biliary tract of stones comprise the traditional treatment. Endoscopic sphincterotomy and removal of common duct stones, leaving a diseased gallbladder in place, may be an acceptable alternative in some patients.

Gallstone Ileus

The treatment for gallstone ileus is surgical removal of the obstructing gallstone. Since the patient has adequate, albeit pathologic, biliary drainage that prevents recurrent cholecystitis or cholangitis, cholecystectomy or repair of the cholecystoduodenal fistula is unnecessary.

Problems following Cholecystectomy

Postcholecystectomy Syndrome

Patients with abdominal distress, pain, or discomfort following cholecystectomy are often said to suffer from the postcholecystectomy syndrome. This nomenclature is unfortunate because there are no known symptoms that are predictably associated with cholecystectomy. There are four possible causes of patients' symptoms: (1) A biliary stricture formed secondary to surgery, (2) stone(s) remain in the common bile duct, (3) a motility disorder of the sphincter of Oddi or the bile duct exists, and (4) the symptoms following cholecystectomy are similar to those preceding cholecystectomy and were not related to the gallstones (inappropriate cholecystectomy).

Patients with severe symptoms and/or objective findings will usually have an identifiable structural abnormality of the biliary tree that can be treated. Those with mild symptoms or dyspepsia are likely to have a normal biliary tree. These patients are usually much more difficult to treat since the origin of their discomfort is unknown.

A systematic diagnostic approach is needed to determine the specific etiology of symptoms following cholecystectomy. A careful evaluation of the biliary tree with abdominal ultrasonography and determinations of serum bilirubin, alkaline phosphatase, transaminase, and amylase levels are good screening tests. However, most patients require an ERCP to satisfactorily exclude a structural lesion in the biliary tree, despite normal findings on screening tests. Biliary manometry at the time of ERCP may be useful to diagnose real, but rare, motility disorders of the sphincter of Oddi.

Retained Common Bile Duct Stone

Gallstones in the common bile duct are overlooked during about 2 to 6% of cholecystectomies. Stones should be suspected in any patient with symptoms following cholecystectomy. The ease and safety of endoscopic sphincterotomy have made management of retained common bile duct stones much simpler. It is now the treatment of choice. Re-operation is hazardous and should be a last resort.

Biliary Stricture

Most biliary strictures are caused by damage to the bile duct during a "routine" (as opposed to "difficult") cholecystectomy. They become clinically evident within 2 years of surgery. Long-term complications of an overlooked biliary stricture are secondary biliary cirrhosis and liver failure.

Patients with a biliary stricture present with intermittent jaundice or cholangitis. It is crucial to exclude retained common bile duct stones. Abdominal CT or ultrasonography may show dilated ducts, but neither will distinguish between a stricture and a retained stone. The correct diagnosis will depend on ERCP findings.

The treatment of biliary stricture is prompt surgical repair as soon as the patient is medically stable. In patients who are not surgical candidates, balloon dilation of strictures via ERCP or transhepatically is possible, but not definitive.

Apstein MD, Carey MC. Gallstones. In: Branch WT, Jr, ed. Office practice of medicine, 3rd ed. Philadelphia: Saunders 1992. In press.
A comprehensive review on all aspects of gallstone disease: epidemiology, pathogenesis, medical treatment with ursodiol, and surgical therapy including laparoscopic cholecystectomy.

Hay DW, Carey MC. Pathophysiology and pathogenesis of cholesterol gallstone formation. Semin Liver Dis 1990; 10:159–70.
An excellent review of how cholesterol stones form.

Crowther RS, Soloway RD. Pigment gallstone pathogenesis: from man to molecules. Semin Liver Dis 1990; 10:171–80.
A recent update on formation of pigment stones.

Broomfield PH, et al. Effects of ursodeoxycholic acid and aspirin on the formation of lithogenic bile and gallstones during loss of weight. N Engl J Med. 1988; 319:1567–71.
Documents the high risk of gallstone formation during rapid weight loss in humans and offers a potential preventive therapy.

Friedman GD, Raviola CA, Fireman B. Prognosis of gallstones with mild or no symptoms: 25 years of follow-up in a health maintenance organization. J Clin Epidemiol; 1989, 42:127–36.
Good epidemiologic data on the natural history of patients with mildly symptomatic gallstones.

Ransohoff DF, Gracie WA, Wolfenson LB, Neuhauser D. Prophylactic cholecystectomy or expectant management for silent gallstones. Ann Intern Med. 1983; 99:199–204.
This decision analysis supports expectant management of silent gallstones.

Friedman LS, Roberts MS, Brett AS, Marton KI. Management of asymptomatic gallstones in the diabetic patient. A decision analysis. Ann Intern Med. 1988; 109:931–9.
A decision analysis advocating watch and wait approach for diabetics with asymptomatic stones. Although a well-done study, it is not universally accepted. (See letter by AK Diehl, Ann Intern Med 1989; 110:1033, a highly respected epidemiologist.)

Ransohoff DF, Miller GL, Forsythe SB, Hermann RE. Outcome of acute cholecystitis in patients with diabetes mellitus. Ann Intern Med 1987; 106:829–32.
Reviews the mortality from acute cholecystitis and shows it is no different in diabetics than in nondiabetics. The authors suggest reevaluating the recommendation that prophylactic cholecystectomy is necessary in diabetics with silent stones.

The Southern Surgeons Club. A Prospective analysis of 1518 laparoscopic cholecystectomies. N Engl J Med 1991; 324:1073–8.
The largest experience with laparoscopic cholecystectomy to date in the United States. The operations were evenly split between academic centers and private hospitals. It is a safe operation, but since no direct comparison was made with open cholecystectomy, just how safe is not known.

Barkun ANG, Ponchon, T. Extracorporeal biliary lithotripsy: review of experimental studies and a clinical update. Ann Intern Med 1990; 112:126–37.
A good review on the status of biliary lithotripsy.

May GR, Shaffer EH. (Editorial) Should elective endoscopic sphincterotomy replace cholecystectomy for the treatment of high-risk patients with gallstone pancreatitis? J Clin Gastroenterol. 1991; 13:125–8.
A thoughtful discussion of what can be an emotional topic (at least when gastroenterologists and surgeons discuss it).

Angelico M, De Santis A, Capocaccia L. Biliary sludge; a critical update. J Clin Gastroenterol. 1990; 12:656–62.
An excellent update on the pathogenesis and clinical importance of biliary sludge (i.e., "thick" or "inspissated" bile and maybe the cause of "acalculous" cholecystitis).

IX. URINARY PROBLEMS

53. URINARY TRACT INFECTIONS IN WOMEN
Axalla J. Hoole

Urinary tract infection is one of the most common problems in ambulatory care. Women with symptoms of infection (dysuria and frequency) comprise 5 to 15% of patients seeking attention; males present much less frequently and in them these symptoms have different and more serious implications. Infections in the male are discussed in Chapter 54. Vaginitis is found in up to 10% of women presenting with dysuria.

Urinary tract infection has been defined by urine cultures of greater than 10^5 colony-forming units per milliliter of urine. When this criterion, established by comparing patients with pyelonephritis to asymptomatic controls, is applied to an ambulatory population, no more than 50% of patients with dysuria have bacterial infection. However, in symptomatic ambulatory patients, urine specimens obtained by suprapubic aspiration frequently grow a single species of pathogenic coliform bacteria in concentrations of 10^2 to 10^4 colonies per milliliter. These data suggest that colony counts of less than 10^5 are significant in symptomatic women and increase to nearly 75% the proportion of women with dysuria who have bacterial infection of the urinary tract.

In those patients in whom no bacteria are found, the cause of symptoms is more difficult to establish. Chlamydia has been described in a number of these patients; fungi and mycobacteria are rarely implicated, but should be considered. In addition, allergies or reactions to chemicals, soaps, and deodorants and rarely, cancer of the bladder can cause dysuria; urethral spasm unaccompanied by infection has been reported.

In most cases bacteria enter the urinary tract from the vaginal introitus, which under normal conditions does not harbor pathogenic bacteria. However, colonization of the introitus by pathogenic bacteria has been shown to precede some infections. A group of women has been identified in whom introital colonization readily occurs because of a property of the vaginal mucosal cell that allows pathogenic bacteria to adhere. Although these patients have more infections than their matched cohorts, the clinical application of this observation is not clear.

The conditions under which pathogenic bacteria from the vaginal introitus enter the bladder are uncertain. Few studies have examined the relation between intercourse and infection, but the available evidence suggests that it is possible for bacteria to be introduced into the bladder during intercourse, presumably by mechanical milking of the urethra. That the bacteria so introduced lead to infection also has not been shown, but the frequency of "honeymoon cystitis" supports this possibility. Other studies suggest that women who resist the urge to urinate have more infections than those who urinate on demand.

Escherichia coli is identified in 80 to 90% of nonhospitalized women with bacterial infection. *Staphylococcus saprophyticus*, the second most frequent identified bacterium, is often discarded by laboratories as a contaminant. However, *S. saprophyticus* has been obtained by suprapubic aspiration from symptomatic patients and should not be ignored. Other gram-negative species, such as *Klebsiella* species and *Proteus* species, are infrequently found in the ambulatory patient.

Recurrent infection can be either a reinfection or a relapse. Reinfection suggests a new infection from bacteria that have freshly entered the urinary tract from the vaginal introitus; relapse suggests a focus of infection, such as a bladder diverticulum or urinary tract stones, that does not allow complete eradication of the infection.

Evaluation
Clinical problems to be considered when evaluating women with symptoms of cystitis include identification of infection, location of infection (upper or lower tract), and distinguishing between reinfection and relapse when there are recurrences.

History
Cystitis typically presents with dysuria and frequency; other common symptoms include small urinary volumes, urgency, nocturia, and suprapubic pain. A history of vaginal discharge and external urethral burning rather than internal dysuria suggests vaginitis; a

temperature greater than 99.5°F (37.5°C), systemic complaints, and flank pain suggest pyelonephritis. Patients with a history of urinary tract stones or anatomic abnormalities, diabetes, multiple infections, or immunologic diseases may have complicated infections that need to be treated more vigorously than cystitis.

Chronology of infections and results of previous cultures may help differentiate relapse from reinfection. Reinfection is a sporadic event with no clear temporal relation to previous infections; relapse frequently recurs within weeks of a previous infection or the cessation of treatment. However, there is no absolute number of infections or number per year that means relapse and demands that urologic investigation be undertaken. With reinfections, the results of cultures change with each episode, whereas in relapse the causal bacteria usually remain the same from episode to episode and retain their antibiotic sensitivities.

Physical Examination

Routine examination has limited utility in evaluating urinary tract infections; however, an examination of flanks for tenderness and the abdomen for lower-quadrant or suprapubic tenderness is appropriate. Also a pelvic examination is indicated in those patients in whom a vaginal or adnexal problem is suspected.

Laboratory Tests

Examination of urine is used at the time of the patient's visit to make the tentative diagnosis of infection. A urine culture with antibiotic sensitivities is no longer considered necessary to confirm the diagnosis and direct therapy in uncomplicated cases. There is no convenient and specific test for outpatient use that can separate upper from lower tract disease.

Urinalysis

In-and-out catheterization and suprapubic aspiration of the bladder provide the most reliably uncontaminated urine samples but are impractical on a routine basis. Therefore, every effort should be made to collect a clean, midstream bladder urine sample, even if this requires both instruction and supervision of collection. This specimen, if properly obtained, correlates well with samples obtained by catheterization. Except in patients with long-standing bladder irritation, squamous epithelial cells usually denote an improperly collected specimen. Very dilute urine obtained from cooperative patients who have forced fluids (in order to provide a specimen) may contain few cellular elements.

The urine specimen should be prepared by centrifuging 10 ml of urine and resuspending the sediment in approximately 1 ml. An unspun specimen or sediment should be examined for bacteria. A Gram-stained slide is preferred; however, methylene blue, which highlights bacteria and WBCs, may be substituted. In an unspun specimen, it is generally accepted that the presence of 2 bacteria per high-power field (HPF) has a good correlation with colony counts of 10^5 per milliliter. In a urine sediment, even small numbers of bacteria should correlate well with low colony counts.

In symptomatic patients, pyuria is a sensitive indicator of infection when low colony counts are considered significant. Although 20 WBCs per HPF have less than a 50% correlation with 10^5 colonies, 5 WBCs per HPF have a good correlation with low colony counts of a single bacterial pathogen or with positive chlamydia cultures.

A *leukocyte esterase* determination on a urine dipstick test is a sensitive indicator of the presence of leukocytes, but lacks the additional information obtained from viewing a spun sediment. This test may be used to determine which urine specimens require a microscopic examination of the sediment, or to make a presumptive diagnosis if a microscope is not available.

Urinary nitrites assessment by dipstick is only 35 to 85% sensitive for identifying bacteria. It also lacks the information obtained from examination of the sediment.

Urine Culture

The urine culture has been used routinely to verify infection, but treatment is almost always begun before the results of cultures are known. Practice surveys have shown that culture results are thereafter rarely incorporated into management of routine cases. Because bacteriuria and pyuria appear sensitive enough for identifying infection, and clinical findings can indicate those patients with lower tract disease (see Therapeutic Trial), ritual cultures seem expensive and unnecessary in most ambulatory patients in whom resistant organisms are unusual. Instances in which resistant or unusual organisms might be found and cultures indicated are marked by recurrence or other features, such as recent hospitalization, previous stones, or diabetes.

Antibody Coating of Bacteria
Parenchymal infection of the kidney, unlike superficial infections of the lower urinary tract, is frequently associated with the production of antibodies. Therefore, evaluation of bacteria for antibody coating (ABC) should distinguish upper tract from lower tract infection. Unfortunately, the sensitivity and specificity of this test are not high. Among the difficulties are false-negative results in early pyelonephritis and false-positive results in long-standing cystitis. Also, this test is rarely available on the day of evaluation. These problems reduce the usefulness of the ABC in ambulatory care.

Therapeutic Trial
Acute cystitis, because it is a superficial infection of the mucosa, should respond to almost any antibiotic that reaches a high urine concentration. A number of drugs have been evaluated in single-dose or short-term (2–3-day) regimens. In virtually 100% of patients who were known to be ABC-negative, these regimens were effective in treating the lower tract disease; when abbreviated therapy was randomly assigned, there was little difference between the relapse rate of short-term compared to traditional therapy. However, short-term therapy has been associated with slightly fewer relapses than single-dose treatment. This finding may reflect failure of the single-dose regimen to sterilize the vaginal vault; even though the urine is initially freed of bacteria, persistence of vaginal bacteria may allow immediate reinfection. These observations suggest a clinical method for differentiating lower and upper tract disease. Those who respond to short-term therapy have lower tract disease; those who do not respond or relapse within a few days need to be re-evaluated.

Management
Current evidence suggests that in uncomplicated patients, infection (bacterial or chlamydial) can be identified by urinalysis, and the location of infection predicted by response to short-term therapy.

Cystitis
Patients with suspected bacterial cystitis may be started on short-term antibiotics without culture if symptoms have persisted less than 3 days (delay > 3 days generally results in increased numbers of ABC-positive tests and corresponding failures of single-dose treatment); if vaginitis or overt upper tract infection is not present; if no complicating factors, such as diabetes, urinary tract stones, recent urinary tract instrumentation, anatomic abnormalities, pregnancy, or frequent recurrences or recent relapse, exist; and if the patient can be relied on to return for follow-up visits.

The practicality of treating appropriate patients with short courses of antibiotics without routine culture is compelling. Advantages are lower expense, fewer side effects, and better compliance. These advantages seem to hold for short-course as well as single-dose therapy.

SINGLE-DOSE AND SHORT-TERM THERAPY. Successful single-dose regimens include amoxicillin, 3.0 g, or the combination of trimethoprim, 320 mg, and sulfamethoxazole, 1600 mg (TMP-SMZ, e.g., Bactrim or Septra; four single-strength or two double-strength tablets). Amoxicillin seems to be associated with somewhat more recurrences. Short-term (3-day) regimens include two single-strength or one double-strength tablet of TMP-SMZ twice a day, or amoxicillin, 500 mg 3 times a day, or doxycycline, 100 mg twice a day. As discussed above, short-term therapy seems to be associated with slightly fewer recurrences than is single-dose therapy. Most authorities suggest that a culture is not necessary after completion of therapy. The necessity of follow-up should be emphasized to the patient; patients who relapse within several days or weeks should return to be cultured, treated with conventional therapy for at least 2 weeks, and additionally evaluated if necessary.

CONVENTIONAL DRUG REGIMENS. Patients who do not fall within the guidelines for short-term therapy but have no evidence for pyelonephritis should be treated with antibiotic therapy for 10 to 14 days, following pretreatment cultures. Regimens include the drugs and doses listed for 3-day regimens, continued for the longer period. Sulfisoxazole, 100 mg 4 times a day for 10 to 14 days, is one of the cheapest drugs available and is effective against most of the bacteria seen in ambulatory practice, but has the disadvantage of more frequent administration. Quinolones and cephalosporins should have no place in the treatment of the usual case of outpatient urinary tract infection, but should be reserved for cases of resistance or allergy to the usual antibiotics.

Chlamydial Infection
In many instances in which WBCs are present in a urinary sediment but no bacteria are found, *Chlamydia trachomatis* has been identified. For these patients a more effective regimen is tetracycline, 500 mg 4 times a day for at least 7 days, or doxycycline, 100 mg twice a day for 7 days.

Dysuria
Occasionally, dysuria occurs without bacteriuria or pyuria. This symptom may occur with many diseases or with emotional problems, or when urine samples from infected patients are dilute and contain little sediment. These patients may be given the urinary tract analgesic phenazopyridine (Pyridium) and followed while problems are evaluated.

Pyelonephritis
In most cases of acute pyelonephritis, admission to the hospital is necessary, either for initial intravenous therapy in patients unable to retain oral therapy or for more extensive evaluation of complicated presentations. Occasional patients may be treated at home with oral antibiotics, but even in these patients some authorities recommend initial therapy with intravenous antibiotics. Oral agents—cephalosporins, amoxicillin and clavulanate, or quinolones—should be given for 14 days, and cultures obtained both before and after treatment. Urologic consultation should be obtained for suggestions of obstruction, stones, or anatomic abnormality.

Prevention of Recurrences

Recurrence of infection may occur because medicine was not taken, a resistant organism was present, or there is relapse from an inadequately treated focus. Usually recurrence comes from reinfection from below, rather than from a relapse of an incompletely treated infection. In every case, reasons for recurrence should be sought, but occasionally frequent reinfection can be decreased by a trimethoprim (40 mg) and sulfamethoxazole (160 mg) combination, one-half tablet per day. Other agents, such as methenamine mandelate (Mandelamine), nitrofurantoin, and sulfamethoxazole alone, are less effective but better than placebo. In those women in whom recurrences are clearly related to sexual activity, a postcoital dose of 500 mg of sulfamethoxazole decreases the number of infections. In a recent study the same result was obtained from one tablet containing 40 mg of trimethoprim and 200 mg of sulfamethoxazole. If patients have several relapses during a year that are not clearly reinfection, then anatomic studies (intravenous pyelogram, cystoscopy) should be considered.

Fang LST, et al. Efficacy of single-dose and conventional amoxicillin therapy in urinary tract infection localized by the antibody-coated bacteria technique. N Engl J Med 1978; 298:413–6.
An essay on the effectiveness of single-dose therapy.

Thomas VL, Forland M. Antibody-coated bacteria in urinary tract infections. Int Soc Nephrol 1981; 21:1–7.
An excellent review of this test.

Savard-Fenton M, et al. Single-dose amoxicillin therapy with follow-up urine culture. Am J Med 1982; 72:808–13.
Patients were randomly assigned to groups that were treated with either single-dose or conventional therapy. There was no significant difference in the outcomes.

Stamm WE, et al. Causes of urethral syndrome in women. N Engl J Med 1980; 303:409–15.
Presentation of evidence suggesting C. trachomatis and bacteria with low colony counts as causes of dysuria.

Nicolle LE. Recurrent urinary tract infection in adult women: diagnosis and treatment. Infect Dis Clin North Am 1987; 1(4):793–806.
A good review of this topic.

Bodner DR. The urethral syndrome. Urol Clin North Am 1988; 15(4):699–704.
A good review of the causes of dysuria.

Johnson JR, Stamm WE. Urinary tract infections in women: diagnosis and treatment. Ann Intern Med 1989; 111:906–17.
Recent and thorough discussion of current directions in management of urinary tract infections.

Komaroff AL. Urinalysis and urine culture in women with dysuria. Ann Intern Med 1986; 104:212–28.
A detailed discussion of the use of urine evaluation in making diagnoses in women with symptoms of urinary tract infection.

54. URINARY TRACT INFECTIONS IN MEN
Axalla J. Hoole

Urinary tract infections occur much less frequently in adult males than females, accounting for far fewer visits to physicians. Reasons for less frequent infections in males are not clearly established, but probably are related to the longer male urethra and less colonization around the urethral meatus. Infection is less frequent in young males than older males probably because of the enlargement of the prostate gland and associated instrumentation that occur in older males. Males with symptoms suggestive of urinary tract infections most often have urethritis associated with sexually transmitted diseases (see Chap. 113), epididymitis, or prostatitis. Pyelonephritis is unusual and requires urologic consultation and investigation for anatomic abnormalities or stones, or may be associated with previous instrumentation of the urinary tract. This chapter discusses painful problems of the prostate and epididymitis.

Painful Diseases of the Prostate
Because of difficulties in obtaining cultures, syndromes that appear to be of infectious origin are often associated with urine and prostatic secretions that are sterile. Lack of clear delineation has resulted in the development of several competing classifications for prostate problems. The following is one convention for defining painful diseases of the prostate.

Acute prostatitis is a systemic, febrile disease, invariably associated with a tender prostate and frequently associated with low back and perineal pain as well as dysuria and obstructive symptoms. Although prostatic secretions may contain many leukocytes and bacteria, prostatic massage is not advisable because bacteremia and sepsis may result.

Chronic bacterial prostatitis is usually more indolent and presents with low back or perineal pain that sometimes radiates into the anterior part of the thighs, the inguinal region, or the testes. There also may be pain associated with bowel movements. Occasionally, symptoms of urinary obstruction and nonpurulent early-morning urethral discharge are present. On physical examination, the prostate is tender and boggy, and usually somewhat enlarged. Often the pain from massage mimics the original pain, referring to the same areas. Prostatic secretions contain greater than 10 to 20 WBCs per high-power field (HPF) and bacteria on smear or culture.

Chronic nonbacterial prostatitis has symptoms similar to those of chronic bacterial prostatitis and is differentiated from it by examination of prostatic fluid that contains greater than 10 to 20 WBCs per HBF but no bacteria.

Prostatodynia is associated with painful symptoms like those of chronic prostatitis, but neither WBCs nor bacteria are found on examination of prostatic secretions.

Bacterial prostatitis and abscess have been found to be more prevalent in patients with AIDS and should be considered as a source of infection in all patients with suggestive symptoms or fevers of unknown origin.

Pathogenesis

Prostate infection can occur in all males but is unusual both before sexual activity and during continued celibacy. After puberty, infections occur at all ages, with an increased incidence in the later years. Acute prostatitis may occur in young males without previous evidence of urinary tract disease; however, in older men acute prostatitis often occurs in association with symptoms of chronic obstruction and may be superimposed on benign prostatic hypertrophy. In fact, in the elderly, small areas of inflammation and infection can be found in virtually all prostate glands.

Bacteria in almost all instances ascend to the prostate through the urethra. However, there is no agreement on the bacteria that are causal. The usual gram-negative urinary pathogens (predominately *Escherichia coli*) are primary bacterial pathogens. In some studies, gram-positive bacteria (predominately *Staphylococcus epidermidis*) have been identified in a large number of patients. Many investigators believe that these organisms have not been shown not to be contaminants. With increasing age, the percentage of gram-negative pathogens increases. *Chlamydia trachomatis* and *Mycoplasma hominis* have also been identified. Using localization techniques, bacteria have been found in only 10 to 50% of patients with symptoms of chronic prostatitis. Because only small areas of the gland may be infected, obtaining bacteria by massage or biopsy is unreliable. Also, prostatic secretions contain zinc salts which act as an antibacterial factor. Prostatic fluid may therefore have an unpredictable inhibitory effect on bacterial cultures. Prostatodynia and chronic nonbacterial prostatitis are thus diagnoses of exclusion and may represent limitations of our ability to investigate the prostate. As newer techniques are employed, it is probable that fewer patients will be diagnosed as having these problems.

Diagnosis

Acute disease can be identified by the history, physical examination, and presence of WBCs and bacteria, as determined by urinalysis and urine culture.

Because the chronic painful prostate diseases present with similar symptoms, diagnosis depends on a collection of expressed prostatic fluid or urine that contains prostatic fluid. This can be accomplished by obtaining the following specimens: (1) the first 10 ml of urine (containing urethral bacteria), (2) a midstream (bladder bacteria) specimen, (3) any prostatic secretions obtained from prostatic massage, and (4) a postmassage urine (containing prostatic bacteria) if no prostatic discharge is initially obtained. Bacterial growth in the prostatic secretions or postmassage urine is most significant when compared to cultures of early or midstream urine.

Because secretions may not be readily produced by massage, a midstream urine sample should be collected before examining the patient, and the patient should be asked to retain a few milliliters of urine in the bladder. If prostatic examination and massage do not produce sufficient fluid, the patient should empty his bladder. This urine contains bacteria that have been expressed into the prostatic urethra and can be compared to urethral or bladder urine obtained earlier. If there is an obvious infection, cultures need not be done, but should be obtained if the patient has a complicated or persistent problem.

Zinc or pH levels in prostatic fluid have been suggested as markers for infection; however, neither of these has been used successfully as a diagnostic test for chronic prostatitis.

Treatment

ACUTE PROSTATITIS. Patients with acute prostatitis are usually treated on an outpatient basis. Hospitalization may be required if sepsis, nausea and vomiting, urinary retention, or other medical problems such as diabetes are present. Antibiotic therapy is begun immediately and changed according to sensitivity patterns. In acute prostatitis, most antibiotics penetrate the prostate wall. Any antibiotic to which the usual bacterial pathogens are susceptible may be used. One regimen is ampicillin and an aminoglycoside given initially followed by trimethoprim-sulfamethoxazole (TMP-SMZ, e.g., Bactrim, Septra) for 30 days.

CHRONIC PROSTATITIS. In chronic prostatitis, the treatment, like the diagnosis, is not straightforward. Oral antibiotics should be used in those in whom bacteria can be identified. However, because of the difficulty in isolating bacteria or the possible presence of other agents such as *Chlamydia* or *M. hominis,* antibiotics are frequently started on the basis of greater than 10 WBC per HPF in prostatic fluid.

Doxycycline and TMP-SMZ are the drugs of first choice because each is effective against the gram-negative urinary pathogens usually associated with bacterial prostatitis. The choice of antibiotics is limited because of poor penetration into prostatic fluid. Among the tetracyclines, which in general have poor penetration, doxycycline has been shown to have adequate lipid solubility to appear in prostate secretions. It is also effective against pathogens associated with nonbacterial prostatitis, such as *Chlamydia* and *M. hominis*. Penetration of TMP-SMZ into prostatic fluid is very sensitive to prostatic fluid pH, and the drug frequently does not reach therapeutic levels in the infected prostate. Erythromycin achieves therapeutic levels in the prostate and is effective against gram-positive organisms, *Chlamydia,* and *M. hominis;* it is appropriate therapy when the latter organisms are suspected or when there is significant gram-positive growth on urine culture. Other antibiotics do not obtain adequate levels in the prostate. Quinolones have been shown to get into the prostatic fluid in higher concentrations than in the serum which is in keeping with their pharmacologic properties. Short-term treatment has been promising, but there have been few long-term studies. In one study of only 12 patients, there was a 60% cure rate 1 year after completion of therapy in patients who had *E. coli* prostatitis. Theoretic advantages and early studies suggest that quinolones may emerge as being very useful in the treatment of prostatitis. Although few data support the optimum duration of antibiotic therapy, most prospective trials have empirically used such treatment for 6 weeks.

Other therapeutic maneuvers, such as prostatic massage, sitz baths, and antispasmodics, are mentioned in reviews but are supported by few data other than anecdotes testifying to their effectiveness. One study did show that massage decreased the size of the prostate gland, but no mention was made of change in symptoms. Practical experience suggests that massage is useful in prostatodynia but should be avoided when infection is present. Because prostatic inflammation may be associated with periurethral spasm, a variety of antispasmodics have been used. However, evidence for their efficacy is usually anecdotal. Similarly, sitz baths are a reasonable, but unproved, recommendation.

Neither alcohol nor sexual activity is contraindicated, although excretion of alcohol may burn the inflamed urethra. Sexual activity may produce contraction of the prostatic urethra on ejaculation and provide internal massage; it has been suggested that this may decrease prostatic congestion and decrease pain in patients who have prostatodynia.

In patients who relapse after 6 weeks of therapy, a second course of antibiotics may be tried. Many patients continue to have relapses. Recurrences may be suppressed by daily antibiotic therapy. If obstruction and infection persist after adequate medical treatment, urologic consultation is advisable.

Surgical treatment for chronic prostatitis is controversial. If the prostate is the cause of obstructive symptoms and changes, such as nocturia, decreased stream, large postvoid residual urine (> 50 ml), or bladder trabeculation, then surgical removal of the obstructive tissue (adenoma or benign prostatic hyperplasia) may be curative. In the absence of the symptoms and bladder changes of obstruction, surgical therapy is less likely to be beneficial. Some patients with debilitating chronic prostatitis have had total prostatectomy. This treatment causes impotence and sometimes incontinence. Clearly, potential benefit has to be weighed against these complications. The use of other procedures, such as transurethral resection of the prostate for chronic prostatitis, in the absence of obstruction, benefits only about one patient in four. The remaining patients are unchanged or become symptomatically worse.

PROSTATODYNIA. Management of prostatodynia remains difficult. Despite the fact that patients with these symptoms cannot be shown to be infected, the symptoms are consistent with prostate disease. Urologic evaluation may reveal decreased urinary flow rates and increased internal sphincter tone. Frequently, however, no lesion is identified. Prostatodynia also may be part of a complex psychosexual problem. For many patients, reassurance is all that is needed; in others, diazepam, 2 mg 3 to 4 times a day, may help relieve muscle spasm, or sitz baths and massage may alleviate symptoms. However, an occasional patient may require psychiatric counseling.

Epididymitis
Infection of the epididymus is unusual before puberty or sexual activity. In males less than 35 years old, epididymitis is usually associated with urethritis and caused by organisms of sexually transmitted diseases: *C. trachomatis* and *Neisseria gonorrhoeae* in heterosexual males and *E. coli* in homosexual males. In older males, common urinary pathogens predominate and occur in association with other problems of the urinary tract, particularly of the prostate, and are related to aging and instrumentation.

Differential Diagnosis
Epididymitis can usually be diagnosed by finding a swollen tender epididymus; however, when the scrotum is red and swollen, differentiation from torsion of the testicle may be difficult. Torsion is suggested if the testicle resides higher in the scrotum, from twisting of the spermatic cord, or if the epididymus appears rotated anteriorly. But these signs and others such as a decrease in the pain of epididymitis when the testicle is raised, or firmness of the testicle early in torsion may not be appreciated by primary care providers who see these problems infrequently. Because pyuria is found with infection but usually not with torsion, a urinalysis may be useful. For adequate evaluation, however, a technetium scan and a urologic consult may be necessary.

Treatment
Initial treatment of epididymitis can be based on epidemiologic data: doxycycline for most patients under age 35 and TMP-SMZ for homosexual males and those older than 35. Treatment should be adjusted according to results of urethral or urine cultures. In older males, urine cultures after prostate massage may be more productive. A patient who appears acutely ill should be admitted for parenteral administration of antibiotics.

Lipsky BA. Urinary tract infections in men. Epidemiology, pathophysiology, diagnosis, and treatment. Ann Intern Med 1989; 110:138–49.
A detailed overview of the subject.

Drach GW, et al. Classification of benign diseases associated with prostatic pain: prostatitis or prostatodynia? J Urol 1978; 120:266. letter to the editor.
A letter establishing a workable classification system for painful prostatitis disease.

Drach GW. Prostatitis: man's hidden infection. Urol Clin North Am 1975; 2(3):499–520.
An excellent review of the problem; however, it came from the early trimethoprim era and needs updating.

Pfau A. Prostatitis. A continuing enigma. Urol Clin North Am 1986; 13(4):695–715.
Meares EM. Acute and chronic prostatitis: diagnosis and treatment. Infect Dis Clin North Am 1987; 1(4):855–73.
Two updates on prostatitis; neither discusses quinolones.

Meares EM. Bacteriological localization patterns in bacterial prostatitis and urethritis. Invest Urol 1968; 5:492–516.
A report of research on the development of a technique for localizing bacteria from the prostate.

Fair W. Prostatic antibacterial factor. Urology 1976; 7:169–77.
The author suggests an identity for this substance.

Fair W. A reappraisal of treatment in chronic bacterial prostatitis. J Urol 1979; 121:437–41.
A discussion of the failure of trimethoprim to live up to its billing.

Weidner W, Schiefer HG, Dalhoff A. Treatment of chronic bacterial prostatitis with ciprofloxacin. Results of a one-year follow-up study. Am J Med 1987; 82(4A):280–3.
A frequently quoted study about the efficacy of quinolone treatment of prostatitis.

Berger RE, Kessler D, Holmes KK. Etiology and manifestations of epididymitis in young men: correlations with sexual orientation. J Infect Dis 1987; 155:1341–3.
This study adds data from homosexual males to previous studies by this group that indicate age-related causes of epididymitis.

55. BENIGN PROSTATIC HYPERPLASIA
J. Pack Hindsley, Jr., and James L. Fry, Jr.

Benign prostatic hyperplasia (BPH) is the growth of a benign adenoma of periurethral glands that may cause an obstruction to the outflow of urine. It is rare before the age of 40, but by the age of 80, 75% of men have BPH, increasing to 95% in men 80 years or older. The mean age at which symptoms become apparent is 65 years old for white males and 60 years old for black males. Gross obstruction from BPH occurs in 20% of men aged 50 to 60, 30% of men 60 to 70 years old, and 50% of men over 80 years old.

Etiology
The exact etiology of BPH is unclear but normal testes appear to be a necessary condition for its occurrence. Eunuchs do not develop BPH, and there is regression of BPH after castration. Also, adenomas accumulate much higher levels of dihydrotestosterone than does normal prostatic tissue. These observations suggest that adenomatous tissues use androgenic hormones differently from normal tissue; however, the intracellular changes that may result are less clearly understood and no well-controlled series show any significant difference in testosterone or its metabolites in patients with BPH compared to age-matched controls. There are also no data to show that estrogen levels or the androgen-estrogen ratio changes that occur with aging are different in patients with BPH and control groups. Although data from animal models would support the old theory of a combined role of androgen and estrogen in the development of prostatic hyperplasia, more recent work has failed to support these findings in man.

The following hypothesis for the etiology of hyperplasia of the prostate has been proposed: Androgens stimulate prostatic glandular tissue to secrete a growth factor, which causes fibrostomal hyperplasia. The enlarging stromal elements have an inductive effect on the prostatic epithelium, which results in rapid growth of the glands and hyperplasia of all three types of tissue (glandular, fibrous, and muscular), accounting for the overall enlargement and bladder outlet obstruction as is commonly seen in BPH. The adenoma formed by this process gradually displaces the "true prostate" peripherally and encroaches on the central prostatic urethra, causing obstruction. The fully developed prostatic adenoma is analogous to an orange; the adenoma represents the fleshy part of the orange, and the true prostate represents the rind.

The hyperplastic prostatic adenoma may be composed of any portion or combination of glandular, fibrous, and muscular tissues. If glandular elements predominate, the adenoma is likely to be mobile and pushed aside by the force of the urinary stream. It therefore may become quite large before symptoms of severe obstruction occur. If fibrous or muscular elements predominate, the prostatic urethra is not nearly as distensible, and a much smaller adenoma can cause severe obstruction. Thus, the size of the prostate is not as important as the architecture.

The bladder compensates for obstruction in BPH by increasing the force of contraction to expel the stored urine. As the bladder wall becomes more hypertrophic, it becomes less distensible, and a sensation of fullness occurs more quickly. The bladder also may be unable to generate sufficient pressure to expel the last quantity of stored urine, leading to postvoid residual urine. If the bladder is required to generate increasingly high voiding pressure over a long period of time, the muscle bundles may separate the inner and mucosal layers and herniate outward, resulting in bladder diverticula. When the bladder contracts, urine is forced into the diverticulum, and when the bladder relaxes, urine drains back into the bladder as postvoid residual urine. The symptoms of bladder outlet obstruction, such as frequency, decreased caliber and force of urinary stream, hesitancy, and nocturia, are readily explained by the secondary compensatory changes to outlet obstruction.

Not infrequently, a combination of circumstances may exacerbate unrecognized or clinically insignificant BPH. For instance, a 65-year-old man who develops prostatitis may have increased urethral compression resulting from the prostatic edema. If he then receives a drug with alpha-adrenergic properties, such as an over-the-counter decongestant, urinary sphincter tone is increased and he may become unable to void, necessitating catheterization. A similar effect can occur from a drug with anticholinergic properties, such as an antidepressant, which decreases the force of bladder contraction. Removal of any of the three insults would ameliorate the situation and improve his voiding function. However, such a situation is a harbinger of impending surgical problems with the prostate.

Evaluation

History
The most reliable symptoms of BPH are hesitancy and nocturia. Hesitancy implies slow or delayed starting of the urinary stream, possibly with enough obstruction to require the use of abdominal muscles to generate sufficient pressure to force open the prostatic urethra.

Nocturia, or nighttime voiding, in which the patient is awakened by the need to void two or more times at night, is a moderately severe symptom indicating that the voiding sensation is being elicited at short intervals. This implies inelasticity of the bladder wall with inadequate storage capacity, and incomplete emptying (increased postvoid residual).

Acute outlet obstruction associated with BPH may be initiated by prostatic infection, constipation, medications that affect either the detrusor muscle (anticholinergics) or the urinary sphincter (alpha-adrenergics), or instrumentation. Urinary retention may also result from spasm of the pelvic floor muscles following surgery (herniorrhaphy, hydrocelectomy, perirectal abscesses, rectal trauma, or perineal trauma). As many as 46% of patients with acute retention have resolution of the acute problem and do not require prostatic surgery.

Physical Examination
Prostatic hypertrophy may occur in some degree posteriorly, laterally, and anteriorly, as well as within the bladder (intravesicular or "medium lobe" hypertrophy). Evaluation of the prostate by rectal examination allows the examiner to palpate only the posterior and a small portion of the lateral portions of the prostate; thus the size of the gland does not always correlate with the degree of obstruction. Small fibrous glands or glands with growth medially may be more obstructive than larger boggy glands.

Percussion of the suprapubic region may reveal a distended bladder in patients complaining of abdominal pain and inability to void. These patients should be catheterized to determine the amount of postvoid residual. If the postvoid residual is greater than 100 ml of urine in a patient with urinary retention, continued catheterization under supervision of a urologist is required until the reason for the bladder outlet obstruction can be determined, particularly if the urine is infected. One of the most frequent causes of retention is from overdistention of the bladder from failure to void or from overhydration. Other frequent causes are drugs, infection, or pelvic pain, particularly after surgery.

Anatomic Studies
An anatomic study is indicated when history and physical examination suggest outlet obstruction. An intravenous pyelogram (IVP) may document hydronephrosis, bladder diverticula, large postvoid residual, trabeculation of the bladder, and J-hooking of the ureters, all of which may add to the evidence that the bladder is decompensating and in need of surgery. In patients with marginal renal function (serum creatinine concentration > 2 mg/dl) or patients at high risk for renal failure from intravenous radiopaque contrast media (diabetics), an ultrasound of both kidneys and the bladder may be obtained as an alternative. Some authors recommend urodynamic studies such as cystometrograms for all patients being evaluated for bladder outlet obstruction; however, this is controversial.

Cystoscopy

Prior to surgery, cystoscopic examination is usually performed to rule out other pathology such as urethral strictures secondary to old chlamydial or gonococcal infections, bladder tumors, and bladder stones. Cystoscopy also evaluates the size and configuration of the prostate to determine the most appropriate type of surgery and whether or not bladder decompensation has progressed to the formation of trabeculation, cellule, or diverticular formation.

Treatment

Medical Therapy

There is no proved long-term medical therapy in the treatment of BPH. Several studies have shown partial resolution of outlet obstructive symptoms with administration of exogenous estrogens and antiandrogens in some patients. These treatments cause impotence, decreased libido, and gynecomastia. Estrogen therapy also increases the risks of myocardial infarction, stroke, and thrombophlebitis.

Recently, prazosin, an alpha-1-adrenergic receptor inhibitor, was shown to decrease symptoms such as voiding frequency and nocturia, but had less effect on obstruction. These findings suggest that the mechanical obstruction from hypertrophy persists, and the dynamic changes result from effects on prostatic smooth muscle. Most authors suggest that prazosin may be a useful drug in patients awaiting surgery or too debilitated to tolerate surgery.

Surgical Procedures

All procedures for removal of the adenoma depend on identifying the dissection plane between the adenoma and the true prostate, which is compressed into an outer rim often called the *surgical capsule*. A "prostatectomy" for benign disease is an adenomectomy with the surgical capsule left in place.

Transurethral resection of the prostate (TURP) is the most frequently employed surgical procedure for relief of BPH. The major advantages of TURP over open reduction is that the operation does not require an incision, which may become infected and which may compromise the accessory respiratory muscles in patients with pulmonary diseases. The major problems of TURP come from the irrigating solutions used to wash blood and debris from the operative field during resections. Electrolyte solutions cannot be used because of electroconductivity, which would preclude electrical resection currents. Sterile water causes intravascular hemolysis. The isotonic, nonelectrolyte solutions typically used such as sorbitol or glycine are absorbed systemically through veins unroofed during the procedure and may cause dilutional electrolyte abnormalities and intravascular fluid overload. In general, these complications do not occur if the resection takes less than 1 hour. If a gland is larger than what can be resected in an hour, an open surgical procedure is indicated.

Open surgical procedures frequently employed are suprapubic prostatectomy and retropubic prostatectomy. The differences between these procedures is that in the suprapubic operation the prostate is approached through the bladder, whereas in the retropubic operation the prostate is enucleated through the anterior capsule of the prostate. Either operation can be done through a small midline or transverse incision.

The perineal prostatectomy has generally been abandoned because erectile failure usually occurs. The impotence rate with the other operations for BPH is usually reported to be 5% or less; the incontinence rate is 1% or less.

Endoscopic procedures such as transurethral incision of the prostate and balloon dilation of the prostate are currently under investigation. Both of these have the disadvantage of rapid regrowth of the prostate requiring another procedure; however, results of well-controlled series are not yet available, but should be produced in the near future.

After a patient has had a procedure for benign prostatic disease, it is important to continue rectal examinations for subsequent development of nodularity suggestive of cancer in the remaining true prostate or surgical capsule. Depending on the amount of tissue removed by TURP, a patient may expect at least 10 to 15 years or more before there is regrowth and recurrence of obstruction.

Hammond GL, et al. Serum steroids in normal males and patients with prostatic diseases. Clin Endocrinol 1978; 9:113–21.

Trachtenberg J, Bujnovszky P, Walsh PC. Androgen receptor content of normal and hyperplastic human prostate. J Clin Endocrinol Metab 1982; 54:17–21.
Two studies that look at basic hormonal properties of the prostate.

Stimson JB, Fihn SD. Benign prostatic hyperplasia and its treatment. J Gen Intern Med 1990; 5:153–65.
A very-well-referenced review that examines many of the assumptions about BPH. Includes 152 references.

Benign prostatic hyperplasia. Urol Clin North Am 1990; 17:461–688.
The whole volume is devoted to BPH and covers many areas of interest to the primary care provider.

Kirby RS. Alpha$_1$-adrenoceptor inhibitors in the treatment of benign prostatic hyperplasia. Am J Med 1989; 87(2A):26S–30S.
A well-designed study that suggests symptomatic benefit from alpha-1-adrenoceptor inhibitors. Also is a good summary of the anatomy and physiology that suggest a use for this class of drug.

56. CHRONIC RENAL FAILURE
William D. Mattern

It is not unusual in ambulatory care to discover that a patient's renal function is abnormal—that is, the overall glomerular filtration rate (GFR) is reduced enough to elevate the BUN and serum creatinine concentrations. Because there may be no history to suggest the presence of underlying renal disease, and the patient may be asymptomatic, the discovery of abnormal renal function is often a surprise to both the patient and the physician. Chronic renal failure (CRF) does not usually result in symptoms until the GFR is reduced below 15 mL per minute, a GFR that would be reflected in a normal-size adult male by a serum creatinine concentration above 8 mg/dl and a BUN above 100 mg/dl. Uremic symptoms develop gradually as the GFR falls below this level. Because of adaptive changes in residual functioning nephrons, the volume and electrolyte composition of the extracellular fluid (ECF) are remarkably well preserved even beyond this point, usually until the GFR declines to below 10% of normal.

Once the abnormality in renal function is noted, the physician is faced with several questions: (1) What is the cause of the renal insufficiency? (2) Is it acute or chronic? (3) Is there a reversible component requiring prompt detection and treatment? (4) At what point should the patient be seen in consultation? (5) What should the patient be told?

Causes
The most common causes of CRF are hypertensive nephrosclerosis, glomerulonephritis, diabetic nephropathy, and interstitial nephritis. Polycystic kidney disease is a less common cause.

Hypertensive nephrosclerosis is suggested by a long-standing history of hypertension, especially with evidence of inadequate control or poor compliance, together with an unremarkable urine sediment and a 24-hour protein excretion in the range of 1 g.

Chronic glomerulonephritis is suggested by a history of acute nephritis or of the nephrotic syndrome, along with mild-to-moderate hypertension and a 24-hour protein excretion in excess of 2 g.

Diabetic nephropathy typically is accompanied by a long-standing history of diabetes mellitus, along with a more recent history of proteinuria, a 24-hour protein excretion in excess of 2 g, and mild-to-moderate hypertension.

Interstitial nephritis can be caused by (1) analgesic excess (phenacetin); (2) other drugs, such as the nonsteroidal antiinflammatory agents; (3) lead exposure, as occurs with the ingestion of moonshine whiskey; (4) urinary reflux during childhood, usually with a history of recurrent urinary tract infections; and (5) hereditary nephritis (Alport's syndrome), usually with a family history, with males more severely affected than females. Regardless of cause, chronic interstitial nephritis may present with an unremarkable urine sediment, a 24-hour urine protein excretion in the range of 1 g, and mild-to-moderate hypertension. It may be presumed mistakenly to be hypertensive nephrosclerosis unless a careful history is taken.

Polycystic kidney disease is inherited as an autosomal dominant trait. The greatly enlarged cystic kidneys are usually palpable. History and physical examination are thus critical in diagnosis.

Evaluation

Patients with a severe abnormality, whose prior renal function is unknown, or who have had a rapid change in function should be thoroughly evaluated. Elderly patients with diabetes or hypertension who have a modest elevation of serum creatinine compatible with the serum BUN may require no additional evaluation.

The basic components of the evaluation for CRF, in addition to data from the history, are the urine sediment, the 24-hour urinary protein excretion, and the evaluation of renal size. It is also essential to rule out acute renal failure and obstruction.

Urine Sediment

The finding of broad, waxy casts in the urine sediment is typical in all patients with CRF. Striking abnormalities of the urine sediment suggest acute renal parenchymal disease of vascular, interstitial, glomerular, or tubular origin. For example, the acute necrotizing renal vasculitis of malignant hypertension or polyarteritis presents with gross or microscopic hematuria, as does the acute interstitial nephritis induced by certain drugs and the acute glomerulonephritis following streptococcal and other types of bacterial and viral infections. The findings of numerous pigmented granular casts and renal tubular cells in the urine sediment suggest acute tubular necrosis (ATN).

The 24-Hour Urinary Protein Excretion

The amount of protein excreted varies depending on the cause of the CRF. Usually patients with vascular disease (nephrosclerosis) and tubular-interstitial disease excrete 1 to 2 g of protein per day, whereas patients with chronic glomerulonephritis and diabetic nephropathy excrete more than 3 g of protein per day.

Renal Size

Although documenting reduced renal size establishes that renal failure is chronic, renal size is not reduced in all forms of CRF. Renal size is reduced in chronic interstitial nephritis and chronic glomerulonephritis, and is usually reduced in nephrosclerosis. It is often normal in diabetic nephropathy, and is greatly increased in polycystic kidney disease. Sometimes a simple x-ray of the abdomen suffices to document renal size, but if the renal outlines are not visualized, a renal ultrasound study or an intravenous pyelogram (IVP) should be obtained.

Intravenous Pyelogram

The intravenous pyelogram (IVP) provides an indication of renal function and size. When renal function is adequate, it defines renal anatomy, particularly the anatomy of the upper collecting system (the renal calyces). However, adequate visualization is usually not possible when the GFR falls below 25% of normal or the serum creatinine concentration is greater than 8 mg/dl. Furthermore, IVP dye can cause ATN in older patients, patients with multiple myeloma, and patients with diabetic nephropathy. Diabetic patients are particularly at risk for this complication, and IVP dye should be avoided if at all possible.

Acute Renal Failure

Acute renal failure should always be considered in the patient who presents with abnormal renal function, particularly if the duration of the renal insufficiency is uncertain. Acute renal failure is suggested by (1) a BUN that is increased out of proportion to the increase in serum creatinine concentration, (2) an "active" urine sediment, and (3) particular clinical settings. If the BUN–serum creatinine ratio is greater than 15:1, two possibilities should be considered: (1) prerenal azotemia, from causes such as severe congestive heart failure or acute intravascular volume depletion (e.g., caused by diuretic therapy or bleeding); and (2) urinary tract obstruction, from causes such as prostatic hypertrophy in older men or neurogenic bladder in patients with diabetes.

Although ATN is uncommon in ambulatory patients, it has been increasingly recognized in two situations: (1) following x-ray contrast media in high-risk patients, such as those with long-standing diabetes and preexisting renal insufficiency; and (2) following intense effort in the heat, typically among young athletes in training, military recruits, or construction workers. These patients may develop rhabdomyolysis with myoglobinuria, marked by a history of dark urine and a urine dipstick that is positive for blood in the absence of gross or microscopic hematuria.

Even in the patient with established CRF, it is important to consider superimposed acute renal failure, especially from readily reversible causes such as diuretic-induced intravascular volume depletion, lower urinary tract obstruction, or urinary tract infection.

Management

There are three important goals in the long-term management of the patient with mild-to-moderate CRF: (1) to reduce as much as possible the rate of progression of the renal disease; (2) to treat, as necessary, the disturbances in body fluid and electrolyte composition that develop as renal function is lost; and (3) to establish a relationship with the patient that provides reassurance during the initial stages and a therapeutic alliance as end-stage renal disease (ESRD) approaches.

Slowing the Rate of Progression

The most useful index of the rate of progression of CRF is the serum creatinine concentration; roughly speaking, it doubles each time the GFR is reduced by one-half. Thus, if the serum creatinine concentration is 1 mg/dl at a normal GFR of 120 ml per minute, a value of 2 would be expected at a GFR of 60; of 4, at GFR of 30; and of 8, at GFR of 15. However, as CRF progresses, the serum creatinine concentration may be lower than expected because muscle creatinine production declines and renal tubular creatinine secretion increases. Nevertheless, sequential changes in the serum creatinine concentration provide a convenient and reasonably reliable estimate of the rate of change in the GFR.

The rate of progression of CRF can be reduced in several ways. In patients with drug-induced chronic interstitial nephritis, the offending drug can be discontinued. In patients with diabetic nephropathy, "tight control" of the blood glucose level may contribute to the preservation of renal function.

Attention has focused recently on two more fundamental approaches to slowing the rate of progression in CRF: control of hypertension and reduction of dietary protein intake. Control of hypertension is the single most effective means to slow the rate of progression, regardless of the drugs used and the cause of the CRF. A number of studies, most of which are small and uncontrolled, suggest that dietary protein restriction will also slow progression. A large, controlled, national study of this question is currently ongoing. Most patients can comply with a reduction in protein intake to about 40 g per day; lower levels require special substitutions in the diet that few patients can sustain. Independent of any effect on the rate of progression, the reduction in protein intake consistently produces a fall in the BUN and may thus delay the onset or alleviate symptoms of uremia.

Treating the Complications

Hypertension occurs throughout the course of disease in most patients with CRF. Diuretic drugs remain the cornerstone of therapy. The thiazides are not generally effective when the GFR falls below 25 ml per minute (i.e., serum creatinine $>$ 4.0 mg/dl). The "loop diuretics," such as furosemide or ethacrynic acid, are effective at GFRs below this level. The diuretic response is dose-dependent, and the dose can be varied over a wide range as needed to obtain a response.

In recent years, both the calcium channel blockers and the angiotensin-converting enzyme (ACE) inhibitors have been used to control blood pressure in patients with CRF. Several early studies suggest that both may help to preserve renal function apart from their effect on hypertension, particularly ACE inhibitors used in patients with diabetic nephropathy. Long-term controlled studies are underway to see whether these preliminary findings can be confirmed. Both the calcium blockers and the ACE inhibitors must be used with care in patients with CRF whose renal perfusion is reduced due to severe congestive heart failure, marked volume depletion, or bilateral narrowing of the renal arteries (as may occur as a consequence of atherosclerosis). By interfering with the intrarenal mechanisms that maintain GFR when renal perfusion is decreased, the ACE inhibitors, in particular, can cause an acute fall in GFR and a concomitant rise in serum creatinine concentration.

The management of *sodium balance* (diuretic dose and dietary sodium intake) requires careful attention in patients with CRF. The normal kidney can maintain sodium balance over a wide range of sodium intakes, eliminating sodium from the urine when the intake approaches zero. In patients with CRF, the adaptive changes in tubular function permit sodium balance to be maintained only when sodium intake is in the normal range. Urinary sodium excretion cannot be reduced below 20 to 80 mEq per day, and, as a result, aggressive diuretic therapy or dietary salt restriction can lead to acute intravascular volume depletion and prerenal azotemia. On the other hand, acute oral salt loads above the normal range of intake cannot be excreted promptly. Most antihypertensive agents have a tendency to cause salt retention, and administration without adequate simultaneous diuretic therapy can lead to progressive expansion of ECF volume and edema formation, with resulting exacerbation of hypertension or precipitation of congestive heart failure.

Hypokalemia is less likely to occur as a complication of diuretic therapy in patients with CRF than in patients with normal renal function. Oral potassium supplements and potassium-sparing diuretics, such as triamterene and spironolactone (Aldactone), should be avoided because acute hyperkalemia may result.

Hyperkalemia is unusual in the course of CRF if potassium intake is normal, since distal tubular potassium secretion is well maintained until GFR is severely reduced. Hyperkalemia may occur earlier in the course of CRF under the following circumstances: (1) most commonly, as part of the syndrome of hyporeninemic, hypoaldosteronism, and type IV renal tubular acidosis (RTA) in patients with diabetes mellitus who have mild-to-moderate renal insufficiency (serum creatinine of 2–4 mg/dl); (2) as a consequence of the use of diuretic drugs that selectively interfere with distal tubular potassium secretion, such as triamterene and spironolactone; and (3) as a consequence of the use of nonsteroidal antiinflammatory drugs or ACE inhibitors, both of which, through different mechanisms, impair distal tubular potassium secretion. The hyperkalemia due to type IV RTA is usually mild (not > 5.5 mEq/L). If it is more severe, a combination of furosemide, sodium polystyrene sulfonate (Kayexalate), and/or fludrocortisone acetate (Florinef) may be necessary for control, and consultation with a nephrologist should be obtained.

Hyperphosphatemia, a relatively late complication in the course of CRF, does not usually occur until the GFR declines below 25 ml per minute. Treatment consists of the administration of aluminum-containing antacids, such as Amphojel and Basaljel, in doses titrated to maintain the serum phosphate concentration at or below 5 mg/dl. These antacids are given immediately after meals; they bind phosphate in the upper intestinal tract, preventing its absorption. The liquid forms are more effective than the tablets or capsules, but frequently are difficult for patients to take because they are not palatable or cause nausea. Constipation is a universal complication of the phosphate-binding antacids but can usually be effectively treated with sorbitol. Magnesium-containing antacids should be avoided because magnesium is absorbed, and reduced renal excretion may result in hypermagnesemia.

Azotemia develops gradually throughout the course of CRF, in parallel with the reduction in GFR. It does not require treatment until late in the course, when the BUN exceeds 100 to 125 mg/dl. At this point, patients usually experience uremic symptoms, including weakness, malaise, and morning nausea. Reduction of the BUN by dietary protein restriction is associated with marked improvement in these symptoms. Most patients are able to adapt to a 40-g protein-restricted diet, which is recommended when early symptoms of uremia develop. When the BUN exceeds 100 mg/dl and uremic symptoms recur on this diet, plans for chronic dialysis should be made.

Hypocalcemia occurs early in the course of CRF. The major contributing factor is a negative calcium balance from a decrease in the renal production of the active metabolite of vitamin D, $1,25(OH)_2D_3$. Oral calcium supplements improve the calcium balance and are routinely given as long as the serum phosphate concentration is below 6 mg/dl. A typical dosage is 500 mg twice a day, given before meals to promote absorption.

Metabolic acidosis develops in all patients with CRF, but it is usually mild and does not require specific treatment unless the plasma bicarbonate concentration falls below 15 mEq/L. In such instances, alkali supplements may be given, in the form of sodium bicarbonate tablets or as Shohl's solution, a combination of sodium citrate and citric acid that contains 1 mEq of bicarbonate alkali equivalent and 1 mEq of sodium per milliliter. In most patients the plasma bicarbonate concentration can be maintained at or above 15 mEq/L with 30 to 60 mEq/L of alkali supplement per day.

Anemia, usually normocytic, also may develop relatively early in the course of CRF because of decreased renal production of erythropoietin. The severity of the anemia generally correlates very poorly with the severity of the CRF, and in most patients, is not severe even when CRF is advanced. Hematocrits are usually in the range of 20 to 25%. The anemia does not cause overt symptoms in most patients, but does reduce exercise tolerance and may precipitate angina in patients with underlying coronary heart disease. Superimposed anemia from folic acid or iron deficiency is suspected when the mean corpuscular volume is abnormal. Human recombinant erythropoietin was approved for use in CRF and ESRD in 1989, is available for intravenous and subcutaneous administration, and is reimbursed by Medicare for patients with ESRD who are on chronic hemodialysis. Data from multicenter trials in chronic hemodialysis patients indicate that restoration of the hematocrit to levels above 30% increases energy, improves exercise tolerance, and generally improves overall health status. Blood pressure must be monitored very carefully, since significant increases in blood pressure may occur as the hematocrit rises. The decision to use erythropoietin to correct the anemia in patients with CRF should be carefully considered in view of the cost ($5000–10,000/year if Medicare coverage is not available) and the need for very careful patient monitoring.

Referral

Initial consultation with a nephrologist, although not always essential, can be helpful to verify that reversible contributing causes have been properly excluded and to establish personal contact in the event that subsequent referral for ESRD evaluation is needed. Continuing contact with the primary physician can provide valuable reassurance to the patient with CRF. This relationship may become vital as the patient begins to come to terms with the irreversible and progressive nature of the renal disease, and as referral for ESRD therapy is being considered.

Referral should be considered, in general, when the GFR falls below 25 ml per minute and the serum creatinine concentration rises above 4 to 5 mg/dl. Beyond this point, the rate of loss of function is quite variable. In patients with diabetic nephropathy, progression to ESRD may occur rapidly, often within 6 months once the serum creatinine reaches this point. Early initiation of ESRD therapy may be particularly beneficial in this subset of patients.

Bourgoignie JJ, et al. Water electrolyte and acid-base abnormalities in chronic renal failure. Semin Nephrol 1981; 1:91–111.
An excellent overview of electrolyte and acid-base abnormalities and their management.

Friedman E. Diabetic nephropathy: strategies in prevention and management. Kidney Int 1982; 21:780–91.
A superb discussion of the management of diabetic nephropathy, including CRF, dialysis, and transplantation.

Noth RH, et al. Diabetic nephropathy: hemodynamic basis and implications for disease management. Ann Diabetic Complications 1989; 110:795–813.
Good general summary.

Harkonen S, Kjellstrand CM. Exacerbation of diabetic renal failure following intravenous pyelography. Am J Med 1977; 63:939–46.
A careful study highlighting the risk of IVP dye in diabetic patients with renal insufficiency.

Bettmann MA. Guidelines for use of low-osmolality contrast agents. Radiology 1989; 172:901–3.
A subject of recent interest.

Grossman RA, et al. Nontraumatic rhabdomyolysis and acute renal failure. N Engl J Med 1974; 291:807–11.
A good clinical description of this condition.

Bennett WM, DeBroe ME. Analgesic nephropathy—a preventable renal disease. N Engl J Med 1989; 320:1269–71. editorial.
Good recent summary and interpretation.

Buckalew VM Jr, Schey HM. Analgesic nephropathy: a significant cause of morbidity in the United States. Am J Kidney Dis 1986; 7:164–8.
Excellent general review.

Torres VE. Present and future of the nonsteroidal anti-inflammatory drugs in nephrology. Mayo Clin Proc 1982; 57:389–93.
Good background information on the mechanism of action of these drugs and their multiple potential adverse effects on kidney function.

Brenner BM, Meyer TW, Hostetter TH. Dietary protein intake and the progressive nature of kidney disease. N Engl J Med 1982; 307:652–9.
The best recent article explaining how dietary protein intake may contribute to hyperfiltration and loss of renal function in diseased and normal kidneys as part of the aging process. The role of hyperglycemia as a contributing factor to hyperfiltration and loss of function in the diabetic kidney is also discussed.

Bricker NS. Sodium homeostasis in chronic renal disease. Kidney Int 1982; 21:886–97.
A good reveiw of sodium balance in chronic renal disease and its importance in relation to dietary sodium intake and the use of diuretics.

Keane WF, et al. Angiotensin converting enzyme inhibitors and progressive renal insufficiency. Ann Intern Med 1989; 111:503–16.
A comprehensive review of experimental and clinical studies on the effect of ACE inhibitors to preserve renal function, particularly in patients with diabetes mellitus.

Ihle BU, et al. The effect of protein restriction on the progression of renal insufficiency. N Engl J Med 1989; 321:1773–7.
A prospective, randomized trial in 64 patients followed for 18 months showing better preservation of renal function in the group treated with a low protein diet.

Ruilope LM, et al. Converting enzyme inhibition in chronic renal failure. Am J Kidney Dis 1989; 13:120–26.
An excellent overview of data on the progression of CRF, including comments on the role of hypertension, low-protein diet, and specific antihypertensive drugs.

Eschbach JW, et al. Recombinant human erythropoietin in anemic patients with end-stage renal disease. Ann Intern Med 1989; 111:992–1000.
The results of treatment with erythropoietin are reviewed in over 300 chronic hemodialysis patients.

Evans RW, Rader B, Manninen DL, and The Cooperative Multicenter EPO Clinical Trial Group. The quality of life of hemodialysis recipients treated with recombinant human erythropoietin. JAMA 1990; 263:825–30.
Quality-of-life assessment in the same group of hemodialysis patients shows a definite improvement in function, energy level, and health status.

57. RENAL STONES
Romulo E. Colindres and C. Richard Morris

Renal stone disease has an incidence of approximately 0.7 to 2.1 cases per 1000 persons per year in the United States. One to 10% of the population will have had a kidney stone by the age of 70. Calcium stones are the predominant type; less commonly, stones are composed of magnesium and ammonium phosphate (struvite or infection stones), uric acid, cystine, and other constituents. The recurrence rate of calcium stones is approximately 15% at 1 year and 50% at 10 years.

Renal stones are usually first detected between the third and fourth decades of life. The occurrence of stones much before that time suggests that the patient has a hereditary condition, such as primary hyperoxaluria, cystinuria, or renal tubular acidosis. Idiopathic calcium nephrolithiasis is approximately three times more common in males than in females. Renal stones caused by primary hyperparathyroidism, renal tubular acidosis, and chronic urinary infection are more common among women.

Pathogenesis

Calcium Stones

Approximately 65% of renal stones in the United States are composed predominantly of calcium oxalate or of a mixture of calcium oxalate and calcium phosphate; 8% are composed of calcium phosphate. Patients with calcium nephrolithiasis often have metabolic disorders. In a study of 460 consecutive calcium stone–forming patients, idiopathic hypercalciuria was the most common disorder, found in 21% of patients; hypercalciuria, hyperuricosuria, or a combination of both was found in 37% of patients. Less prevalent, with each affecting 1 to 6% of patients, were hyperuricemia, primary hyperparathyroidism, renal tubular acidosis, inflammatory bowel disease, medullary sponge kidney, and sarcoidosis. No disorder was found in 20% of patients.

Idiopathic hypercalciuria can be caused by increased absorption of calcium from the gut (absorptive hypercalciuria), impairment of renal tubular reabsorption of calcium (renal hypercalciuria), or an increase in the filtered load of calcium as a consequence of hypercalcemia.

Between 10 and 50% of patients with calcium stones have decreased excretion of citrate, usually idiopathic and often accompanied by a persistently acid urine (hypocitric aciduria). Hypocitraturia can also be seen with prolonged metabolic acidosis and with persistent hypokalemia. Because citrate combines with calcium to form relatively soluble complexes, and also inhibits spontaneous nucleation and crystal growth, decreased excretion of this anion may be a factor in the pathogenesis of calcium stones. Replacement with potassium citrate may prevent stone formation in patients with hypocitraturia.

Inflammatory bowel diseases are frequently associated with calcium oxalate and uric acid stones as a consequence of fluid and bicarbonate losses that lead to a persistently concentrated and acid urine. Furthermore, if malabsorption occurs, unresorbed bile acids increase the permeability of the colon to unbound oxalate, leading to hyperoxaluria and the excretion of calcium oxalate, a poorly soluble calcium salt.

Other conditions that can lead to oversaturation of the urine with calcium include acquired or congenital hyperoxaluria, a persistently low urine volume, and a decrease in the ill-defined chemical inhibitors of crystal growth and aggregation normally present in urine. In patients with hyperuricosuria, uric acid or urate crystals may serve as a nidus for the aggregation and growth of calcium crystals.

Uric Acid Stones

Five to 10% of renal stones are composed predominantly of uric acid. Hyperuricosuria or hyperuricemia is found in only 50% of patients who form uric acid stones. Only 25% of patients with gouty arthropathy form uric acid stones. In the majority of patients, uric acid stones can be attributed to the continuous excretion of a concentrated and acid urine or to a structural abnormality of the urinary tract. Because the pK of uric acid is 5.47, at a urine pH of 5 or less, the less soluble uric acid is excreted in preference to urate salts.

Uric acid stones are characteristically radiolucent on intravenous urography. As a result, they can be misdiagnosed as tumors or polyps.

Struvite (Infection) Stones
Ten to 15% of stones are composed of magnesium and ammonium phosphate (struvite or infection stones). Struvite stones are formed in the presence of a high concentration of ammonium in a urine having a persistently alkaline pH (≥ 7.5). Under normal circumstances, alkaline urine has a low concentration of NH_4^+. However, in patients with urinary tract infections caused by urea-splitting organisms, particularly *Proteus* species, the bacterial urease hydrolyzes urea to form ammonia and HCO_3^-. The resulting urine has an alkaline pH and is supersaturated with calcium phosphate. The high NH_4^+ concentration in urine leads to the formation of magnesium and ammonium phosphate crystals, which aggregate, grow, and become stones that block the movement of bacteria, making treatment of the infection very difficult. Hypercalciuria and the excretion of a small volume of very concentrated urine can contribute to the pathogenesis of struvite stones. Recurrence is common, and gradual loss of renal function often occurs. These stones are usually radiopaque and have the configuration of staghorn calculi.

Urologic dissolution of these stones is usually required. Inhibitors of bactrial urease, combined with antibiotics, have been used in patients who cannot undergo dissolution of the stones. However, there is considerable toxicity associated with these inhibitors.

Cystine Stones
Cystine stones form in children and young adults whose kidney tubules lack the ability to reabsorb cystine normally because of a congenital defect in the transport of this amino acid. The increased concentration of cystine in the urine decreases its solubility and promotes crystal aggregation and growth. Excretion of an acid and concentrated urine increases the propensity for stone formation.

Cystine stones are pale yellow and slightly radiopaque because of their sulfur content. The stones may pass into the ureter or may develop into staghorn calculi. Patients with cystinuria have frequent urinary tract infections and loss of renal function is almost invariable.

Clinical Manifestations

Renal stones first become manifest in one of the following ways:

Asymptomatic renal stones discovered fortuitously on a plain x-ray of the abdomen or on an intravenous urogram

Asymptomatic hematuria or repeated bouts of urinary infection

Acute renal colic resulting from partial or total ureteral obstruction (see Acute Renal Colic)

Nephrolithiasis is said to be "metabolically active" when there is evidence of new stone formation, stone growth, or passage of gravel in the past year; all of these conditions are manifestations of crystalluria and supersaturation of the urine with the mineral constituents of the stones. Metabolically active disease should be investigated for possible predisposing causes and treated vigorously. Stones are said to be "surgically active" when there is a history of renal colic, urinary obstruction, or infection in the past year. The presence of surgically active disease need not imply metabolically active disease, because these symptoms are the consequence of stones formed in the past.

Evaluation

The evaluation of patients with nephrolithiasis should proceed as follows:

1. In patients who have a history of renal colic and/or hematuria but who have not passed stones or gravel in the urine, the diagnosis should be confirmed, usually by intravenous urography. Forty to 80% of stones can be seen on a plain film of the abdomen. However, an intravenous urogram is usually done to identify less opaque stones; to determine the number, configuration, and characteristics of the stones more precisely; and to exclude obstruction or structural abnormalities of the urinary tract.

2. Predisposing factors that may be contributing to the formation of stones and to the

metabolic activity of the disease should be identified from the history and physical examination. Conditions that predispose to stone formation include habitually low fluid intake, prolonged immobilization (for calcium stones), a family history, associated diseases (gout, renal tubular acidosis, primary hyperparathyroidism, small-bowel disease, urinary tract obstruction, and chronic urinary infection), and use of certain drugs (large doses of vitamin D and possibly vitamin C, acetazolamide [Diamox], absorbable antacids, and triamterene).

3. The composition of stones should be determined, whenever possible, by sending them to a qualified laboratory for detailed analysis. Treatment is largely influenced by the type of stones.

4. The initial evaluation of all patients with nephrolithiasis should include measurement of the serum concentration of calcium, other electrolytes, creatinine, uric acid, and phosphorus. A urinalysis should be done to look for bacteria and crystals and to measure pH, looking for a defect in urinary acidification. A urine culture should be done to exclude associated infection. Subtle elevations of the serum calcium concentration merit investigation including an assay of serum parathyroid hormone.

5. Patients who have formed a single calcium-containing stone and who have not had previous stone episodes need not undergo a detailed metabolic evaluation unless the history, physical examination, or screening laboratory tests suggest the presence of a systemic disease or metabolic disorder. Nevertheless some experts advocate that these patients should have measurement of calcium and uric acid in a "spot" urine sample or in a 24-hour urine collection.

6. A detailed metabolic evaluation is warranted if any of the following conditions are present: (a) The patient has many stones or metabolically active disease; (b) the clinical setting and the preliminary laboratory findings suggest the presence of a systemic disease or metabolic disorder that might be causing the formation of stones; or (c) the stone recovered is not composed predominantly of calcium oxalate (such stones are seen more commonly in several metabolic disorders).

7. A detailed evaluation should not be undertaken until patients have fully recovered from an episode of renal colic (generally 3 or 4 weeks after the episode), when they are on their normal intake of fluids and food. Such an evaluation includes measurement of the excretion of calcium, uric acid, citrate, oxalate, cystine, creatinine, and volume in one or more 24-hour samples of urine. The measurement of creatinine excretion is useful to ascertain the adequacy of the collection and to calculate creatinine clearance. Normal values for excretion of these solutes are shown in Table 57-1. Additional metabolic studies are contingent on the results of the excretory studies and on the presence or absence of abnormalities in serum. Thus, one might measure calcium excretion in urine after fasting and after a calcium load in patients with severe hypercalciuria so as to distinguish between

Table 57-1. Daily urinary excretion of various solutes

Solute	Women	Men
Calcium (upper limits of normal)		
mg/24 hr	250	300
mg/g of creatinine	140	140
mg/kg of body weight	4	4
Uric acid (upper limits of normal)		
mg/24 hr	750	800
Citrate (mg/24 hr)		
Upper limits of normal	1200	865
Average excretion	700	592
Lower limits of normal	320	230–320
Oxalate (upper limits of normal)		
mg/24 hr	50	50
Creatinine (average excretion)*		
mg/kg of body weight	15–25	20–30

*Varies in proportion to muscle mass.

renal and absorptive hypercalciuria. Automated stone-risk analysis packages that permit the measurement of a variety of solutes, other than the conventional ones indicated above, are now available commercially. Whether or not such a detailed analysis of urine composition will be helpful in predicting risk and guiding treatment remains to be determined.

Treatment Principles
1. The purpose of medical treatment is to prevent the recurrence of stones and, if possible, to promote dissolution of existing stones.
2. Any underlying or predisposing causes such as urinary obstruction, urinary infection, drugs, or renal tubular acidosis should be corrected or eliminated if possible.
3. Medical treatment includes increasing urine volume, decreasing the excretion of stone constituents by dietary changes or pharmacologic therapy, and administering agents that increase the solubility of stone constituents.
4. Patients with a first, single calcium stone and no obvious systemic disease or abnormality on preliminary studies probably need no treatment beyond that necessary to ensure an increase in urine volume. Dietary restriction of calcium, purines, and oxalate is indicated if the history suggests high intake of these solutes.
5. Patients with metabolically active or recurrent stone disease, those with systemic diseases, or those who do not have calcium stones are also treated with increased fluid intake and dietary restrictions. However, they also usually require more specific therapy with drugs that decrease the excretion of stone constituents, increase the solubility of these constituents, or inhibit crystal nucleation and growth.

Treatment Modalities

Fluid Intake

Patients with stone disease should be encouraged to drink between 3 and 5 L of fluid every day to ensure a urine volume of at least 2.5 L per day and to reduce the propensity for crystallization of calcium and urate salts and the spontaneous nucleation of calcium oxalate.

Reduction of Urinary Excretion of Stone Constituents

Thiazide diuretics, in doses equivalent to 50 to 100 mg of hydrochlorothiazide divided into two doses per day, decrease the urinary excretion of calcium by 40 to 50% in both renal and absorptive hypercalciuria and reduce the formation or passage of new stones in 80 to 90% of hypercalciuric patients who are on a high fluid intake. The thiazide diuretics exert this hypocalciuric effect by increasing the reabsorption of calcium in the distal convolution of the nephron. Salt intake must be restricted because extracellular fluid volume expansion may negate this effect. Diuretic therapy may cause hypokalemia. The associated hypocitraturia predisposes to stone formation. Consequently, hypokalemia should be corrected with potassium citrate in patients on diuretics who initially have or who subsequently develop hypocitraturia.

Thiazide diuretics may also be useful in patients without demonstrated hypercalciuria. In some patients with absorptive hypercalciuria, the decrease in calcium excretion caused by the diuretics is only transient. Therefore it is necessary to ascertain that calcium excretion remains low after several months of therapy.

Patients with absorptive hypercalciuria should reduce their calcium intake. However, a low-calcium diet may be unnecessary in such patients if they are treated with diuretics. A low-calcium diet may lead to increased intestinal absorption of oxalate, thus producing hyperoxaluria. Thus, patients with severe calcium stone disease should be encouraged to follow a low-oxalate diet by avoiding leafy vegetables.

Cellulose phosphate, an agent that binds calcium in the gut, may be useful in some patients with severe refractory absorptive hypercalciuria. However this agent can lead to a negative calcium balance and osteoporosis. Therefore it probably should not be used in children and postmenopausal women. Administered in a dose of 2.5 to 5 g tid, cellulose phosphate also decreases the intestinal absorption of magnesium and increases the absorption of oxalate. Patients taking cellulose phosphate should therefore follow a high-magnesium, low-oxalate diet.

Patients with calcium stones who have hyperuricosuria can be treated with a diet low in purines by avoiding glandular meats. Those patients with severe hyperuricosuria or those who do not respond to dietary restriction may be treated with allopurinol, 100 to 300 mg/day.

Increasing the Solubility of Stone Constituents
Uric acid and cystine are more soluble in alkaline than in acid urine. The solubility of uric acid increases markedly at a urine pH of 6.5 to 7.0. Similarly, the solubility of cystine in urine increases two- to threefold at a pH above 7.5. A urine pH of 6.5 to 7.0 in a person eating a normal diet can be achieved by giving 1 mEq of bicarbonate per kilogram of body weight per day divided in three or four doses. Approximately 2 mEq of bicarbonate per kilogram of body weight per day is necessary to achieve a sustained urine pH of 7.5. Bicarbonate can be given as tablets (1 g = 12 mEq) or as Shohl's solution (sodium citrate and citric acid, 1 ml = 1 mEq). A carbonic anhydrase inhibitor such as acetazolamide (Diamox), 250 mg, can be given at bedtime. Patients should be instructed to measure their urine pH with a "dipstick" to document the adequacy of the chosen dose of bicarbonate.

Patients with cystinuria can be treated with D-penicillamine, which forms soluble complexes with cystine. This drug is toxic and should be used only after other measures have failed.

Inhibitors of Crystallization and Nucleation
Organic phosphate, prescribed as neutral phosphate at a dose of 1.5 to 2.5 g/day, may be effective in some patients with normal calcium excretion or in patients with hypercalciuria who do not respond to thiazide diuretics. Orthophosphate increases the excretion of phosphate, carbonate, and citrate and increases urine pH, leading to increased complexation of calcium, thus making it more soluble. Furthermore, pyrophosphate and citrate inhibit the formation of calcium oxalate crystals.

Potassium citrate has been approved for use in patients with calcium nephrolithiasis who have hypocitraturia. It increases complexation of calcium and it also inhibits nucleation and crystallization of calcium oxalate. Furthermore, it increases urine pH and therefore decreases the concentration of undissociated uric acid in patients with hyperuricosuria. The usual dose is 30 to 90 mEq/day divided into two or three doses. Preliminary results with this drug are very promising. There are few adverse effects. Citrate is, therefore, a potential first-line drug for the treatment of patients with metabolically active stone disease even in patients with only mild hypercalciuria.

Table 57-2 summarizes general treatment schemes for calcium nephrolithiasis according to the severity of the stone disease and to the presence of associated disorders.

Acute Renal Colic
Severe flank pain (colic) occurs when stones produce obstruction as they descend through the collecting system. Obstruction often occurs at one of four sites along the course of the ureter: the ureteropelvic junction, the point of entry into the bony pelvis, the posterior part of the pelvis (near the broad ligament in women), and the ureterovesical junction. Nonstone causes of renal colic include passage of blood clots or papillae, from papillary necrosis in patients with diabetes mellitus or phenacetin abuse.

Renal colic is abrupt in onset and typically occurs in the early morning hours; the pain reaches a crescendo over 20 to 60 minutes and may last for hours. It is often excruciating and frequently associated with nausea and vomiting. Spontaneous resolution is gradual over minutes to hours. Stones in the proximal and midureter cause flank pain that radiates to the abdomen. As stones enter the distal ureter, pain radiates to the groin and testicle in men and to the labia majora in women. Stones in the intramural segment of the vesical ureter produce symptoms of bladder irritation. Impaction of the stones at any point in the ureter results in intense local inflammation and intense pain in the area of impaction.

Evaluation
Physical findings are generally unremarkable, apart from costovertebral angle tenderness. Impaction may produce localized, deep tenderness over the area of inflammation and tenderness elicited on percussion over the obstructed kidney. *Urinalysis* reveals microscopic hematuria in 75 to 100% of cases; gross hematuria occurs in 18% of patients. Bacteria

Table 57-2. Summary of approaches used for prevention and treatment of calcium nephrolithiasis

Approach	Multiple or recurrent stones	Single stone
Increased fluid intake to ensure urine volume of 2.5 L/day	+	+
Dietary restriction: low calcium, purine, and oxalate	+ (Depending on drug therapy chosen and on severity of metabolic abnormality)	+ (If dietary history indicates need)
Drug therapy		Usually not necessary
Thiazide diuretics	a	
Potassium citrate	a,b,c(Hypocitraturia)	
Neutral orthophosphate	b,c(Absorptive hypercalciuria with phosphate leak)	
Allopurinol	c(Hyperuricosuria)	
Sodium cellulose phosphate	c(Severe absorptive hypercalciuria)	

[a] First-line drug can be used whether or not hypercalciuria or hypocitraturia is present.
[b] Second-line drug to be used in patients who do not respond to or are refractory to thiazide diuretics.
[c] To be used for special indications indicated in parentheses.

should be sought on microscopic examination, and a urine culture should be obtained. Pyuria is common, even in the absence of infection, and the urine may contain stones or stone fragments ("gravel").

Radiographic evaluation is necessary to confirm the diagnosis, to assess stone size and number, and to determine the degree of obstruction. This should be deferred until the patient is comfortable and optimal studies are possible. Stones are nearly invariably radiopaque (92%). Most stones (40–80%) are seen on plain films, but identification can be improved by evacuating the bowel, obtaining lateral and oblique views, and inspecting common points of obstruction. Intravenous pyelography should be performed in patients in whom stones are not apparent. Delay in the appearance of contrast material is the first indication of obstruction. Radiolucent stones should be suspected when filling defects are present at a point of obstruction. If radiographic studies are normal, other causes of pain and hematuria should be sought.

Treatment
Ninety percent of stones less than 5 mm in diameter pass spontaneously, but it is impossible to predict which will not. Patients can usually be managed with analgesics and observed as outpatients. During the passage of a stone, the urine should be filtered through a gauze, and stone analysis performed. It is clear that some patients have only a single stone, whereas others have frequent recurrences. The probability of recurrence after a single stone is 50% in 10 years; differences in the type of stone do not appear to determine recurrence rate. In those in whom there is recurrence, chronicity is the rule.

Indications for urologic consultation include concurrent infection, severe or increasing obstruction, deterioration in renal function, intractable pain, lack of progress down the ureter, and severe gross hematuria. Hospitalization and urologic consultation may also be required for patients who have such severe pain, nausea, and vomiting that they become dehydrated.

The extent of recovery in renal function after obstruction is inversely related to the duration and severity of obstruction. In experimental animals, recovery is usually complete if total obstruction is limited to 1 or 2 weeks. Little or no function returns after obstruction of 6 weeks' duration. Limited data from humans suggest incomplete recovery after 30 to 60 days of complete obstruction.

Urologic Approaches

Urologic intervention is indicated in some patients with acute renal colic as discussed above, in patients who have resistant infection in the presence of a stone, and in patients who have a large stone burden that is unlikely to respond to medical therapy alone, particularly if there is metabolically active disease and if there is progressive destruction of renal tissue. Urologic intervention, even nonsurgical, is probably not indicated in the treatment of asymptomatic sterile stones that are less than 0.5 cm in diameter.

Recent improvements in the urologic treatment of stones include ureteroscopy, extracorporeal shock wave lithotripsy (ESWL), and percutaneous nephrolithotomy (PNL). In most centers, less than 5% of patients with severe stone disease and renal colic require surgical treatment.

Ureteroscopy is the treatment of choice of obstructing lower ureteral stones. The success rate in this situation is approximately 98% with ureteroscopy and only 70% with ESWL. Treating obstructing midureteral stones is very difficult and the choice of method for removal must be individualized. Stones that are treatable with ESWL include those that measure 2 cm or less, particularly if they are free floating in the pelvis of the kidney or if they are located in the upper third of the ureter. The procedure is usually carried out in an outpatient setting and is devoid of many short-term complications. The long-term effects are not known. Under optimal conditions, 70 to 90% of patients will respond to ESWL, but 50 to 60% will require an ancillary procedure to remove fragments of stones that are not passed spontaneously. Percutaneous lithotripsy combined with mechanical breakup of stones, although more invasive, is associated with less recurrence of stones and better success rates (90–95%) than is ESWL. Therefore, larger stones and those that do not usually respond to ESWL, such as stones composed of cystine and struvite, are managed with percutaneous dissolution and removal. Total removal of struvite stones usually requires percutaneous dissolution alternating with ESWL. Urologic procedures are not a substitute for medical therapy to prevent the formation of new stones.

Follow-up

Patients with renal stones should be evaluated annually to assess the metabolic and surgical activity of their disease. Patients who have complications such as infections, renal colic, or loss of renal function and those being treated with drugs should be seen at shorter intervals.

Kumar R, guest ed. Medical and surgical management of nephrolithiasis. Semin Nephrol 1990; 10:1–53.
This issue is devoted almost entirely to nephrolithiasis. Several experts give an update on the pathophysiology, evaluation, and medical and surgical management of renal stones.

Coe, FL, Gillenwater JY, guest eds. Proceedings of the National Institutes of Health consensus development conference on prevention and treatment of kidney stones. J Urol 1989; 141:707–808.
An authoritative review and discussion of all types of kidney stones.

Smith LH. Urolithiasis. In: Schreir RW, Gottschalk CW, eds. Diseases of the kidney. 4th ed. Boston: Little, Brown, 1988: 785–813.
A concise, well-written, and thorough reveiw of the topic.

Coe FL. Treated and untreated recurrent calcium nephrolithiasis in patients with idiopathic hypercalciuria, hyperuricosuria, or no metabolic disorder. Ann Intern Med 1977; 87:404–410.
Reviews the metabolic and clinical disorders found in 460 consecutive calcium stone–forming patients. The author demonstrates that treatment with thiazide diuretics and allopurinol effectively prevents recurrence of calcium oxalate stones in patients with hypercalciuria and hyperuricosuria, respectively.

Pak CYC. Medical management of nephrolithiasis in Dallas: update 1987. J Urol 1988; 140:461–7.
An excellent state-of-the-art review, suggesting that high fluid intake and dietary restrictions alone may be sufficient treatment for patients with a single-stone episode or with disease of mild-to-moderate severity. The author favors choosing pharmacologic therapy

that selectively treats the underlying metabolic abnormality in patients with severe stone disease.

Prevention and treatment of kidney stones (consensus conference). JAMA 1988; 260: 978–81.
Summarizes the prevention and treatment of kidney stones as discussed at a consensus development conference sponsored by the National Institutes of Health. Important issues addressed include methods of prevention of stones and their effectiveness, the role of lithotripsy in treatment, clinical and laboratory approaches for the evaluation, and directions for future research.

Uribarri J, Oh MS, Carroll HJ. The first kidney stone. Ann Intern Med 1989; 111:1006–9.
Reviews the rate of recurrence of renal stones in patients with a single episode caused by a calcium-containing stone, and the benefits and risks of specific therapy for stone disease with thiazide diuretics and allopurinol, as compared to the benefits derived from conservative treatment with high fluid intake and dietary restrictions ("stone clinic effect"). The authors conclude that specific drug therapy is not warranted in patients with a first kidney stone and, therefore, that extensive metabolic evaluation is unnecessary under these circumstances.

Segura JW. Surgical management of urinary calculi. Semin Nephrol 1990; 10:53–63.
A detailed but succinct review of modern urologic procedures used to remove urinary calculi.

58. HEMATURIA
John E. Anderson

Hematuria may be a presenting complaint, an abnormality found during the evaluation of other symptoms, or be detected by routine urinalysis in an asymptomatic patient. Its source may be anywhere in the urinary tract, from glomerular and nonglomerular sites in the kidney to lesions in the collecting system (the renal pelvis, ureters, bladder, and urethra). The most prominent etiologies include neoplasms, nephrolithiasis, infections, and intrinsic renal disease, particularly glomerulonephritis.

Screening for hematuria, even to detect urologic malignancies in older patients, is not of established value. However, most authorities recommend that once they are detected, all episodes of hematuria be evaluated, whether the patient presents with grossly bloody urine or is totally asymptomatic with red blood cells (RBCs) found only on urinalysis. These recommendations are based on reports of serious lesions in 5 to 20% of patients who had only asymptomatic microscopic hematuria. Nonetheless, not every patient has the same risk or requires the same workup. Although lesions such as malignant neoplasms are life-threatening and require prompt detection, other causes have minimal or no impact except for the anxiety produced in the patient and provider. The challenge is to choose the appropriate evaluation for each patient.

Is It Hematuria?

The first step is to determine whether hematuria does, in fact, exist. False-positive hematuria can occur when dipsticks react to hemoglobin or myoglobin or to bleach contaminating the collection containers. Pigmenturia from a variety of foods and drugs (e.g., beets, rifampin) may color urine and be confused with gross hematuria. A microscopic examination, therefore, must be done to confirm the presence of RBCs.

Because a few RBCs are normally found in urine, the definition of hematuria on microscopic examination is somewhat arbitrary. Different urine centrifugation and RBC quantification techniques produce different results, and different diagnostic methods have been used to define a normal patient population. The reported upper limit of normal therefore has ranged from 1 to 10 RBCs per high-power field (HPF). Most authorities agree, however, that 3 to 5 RBCs per HPF is a reasonable definition of clinically significant hematuria.

Dipstick testing is sensitive to 5 to 10 RBCs per HPF; a positive test therefore correlates with the abnormal range of the microscopic examination.

Because large numbers of patients may present with modest microscopic hematuria, a repeat urinalysis to confirm the problem is often recommended. If hematuria is not found on the second urinalysis and an obvious explanation for the initial abnormality exists, such as contamination from menstrual bleeding, bacterial cystitis, recent vigorous exercise, or fever, further workup may not be required, provided the patient is not in a high-risk group and a follow-up urinalysis can be obtained in a few months.

Diagnostic Strategy

Once hematuria is confirmed, the patient's age, sex, history, physical findings, amount of bleeding, and urinalysis can be used to guide both the direction and the extent of the evaluation. In general, the goal is to determine whether the evaluation should be targeted at either urologic or nephrologic causes. The former are generally structural abnormalities such as tumors or stones, and the latter, parenchymal renal disease such as glomerulonephritis or interstitial nephritis. Although there is considerable overlap, the distribution according to age of the patients of the various etiologies, the accompanying signs and symptoms, and concomitant urinalysis findings that may differentiate glomerular from nonglomerular bleeding can help direct the evaluation.

Infections, stones, malignant neoplasms, and benign prostatic hypertrophy account for approximately 70% of hematuria episodes and are particularly common in patients older than 40 years. Consequently, the evaluation of all degrees of hematuria in older patients cannot be deferred or ignored and should emphasize the predominantly urologic causes. Urologic consultation is appropriate for most older patients since cystoscopy is needed to identify lesions such as bladder carcinoma that are frequent causes of bleeding from the lower urinary tract or to localize the site of upper tract bleeding.

Hematuria in patients under 40 years is more likely to be from infection—cystitis in females, for example—or from glomerulonephritis. The rarity of neoplasia in this age group changes the approach from a primarily urologic evaluation to a search for evidence of the many causes of glomerulonephritis and other intrinsic renal diseases. Possible exceptions to these guidelines include women with asymptomatic microscopic hematuria in whom the yield of an extensive evaluation for bladder neoplasms may be quite low. Smoking is a major risk factor for transitional cell carcinoma, and therefore may be a decisive reason for pursuing a urologic evaluation in male and female patients of all ages.

Components of the Evaluation

History

A description of the hematuria may suggest a cause. Blood clots and bright red urine are more likely to have a urologic source; dark-, cola-, or tea-colored urine suggests glomerulonephritis. Initial hematuria suggests urethral bleeding; terminal hematuria suggests bleeding from the prostate. Gross, painless hematuria throughout voiding suggests a neoplasm and requires urgent urologic evaluation and cystoscopy in any age group. Hematospermia (i.e., bloody ejaculate) is of prostatic origin and although disconcerting, requires no workup.

Accompanying symptoms are nonspecific. Suprapubic pain, urgency, frequency, and dysuria often occur with urinary tract infections, but bladder carcinoma, which usually presents as painless hematuria, can also produce the same symptoms. Nephrolithiasis typically presents with severe flank pain radiating to the abdomen and groin, but can also cause painless hematuria. Bleeding from any source can cause ureteral colic similar to stones if clots obstruct the ureter. Renal artery emboli can also cause flank pain and hematuria; they usually occur in patients with risk factors for systemic embolization, such as intermittent atrial fibrillation or dilated chambers of the heart.

In younger patients and in those older patients whose initial evaluation for common urologic causes is unrevealing, glomerular causes should be sought. A history of pharyngitis 2 weeks prior to the development of cola-colored hematuria is classic for poststreptococcal glomerulonephritis. Upper respiratory tract infections other than streptococcal pharyngitis also cause glomerulonephritis and can induce episodes of intermittent hematuria in patients with preexistent forms of glomerulonephritis such as IgA nephropathy and familial nephritis. The presence of fever, rash, or arthralgia may suggest that the cause of glomerular hematuria is a systemic illness such as a vasculitis or an infection such as endocarditis. A family history of hematuria, renal insufficiency, hearing loss, or cystic renal disease may lead to a diagnosis of familial hematuria, familial nephritis (Alport's syndrome), or polycystic kidney disease. Recent vigorous exercise can cause hematuria of apparent glomerular origin.

Drug and hematologic histories should be obtained from all patients. Many drugs, such as the ubiquitously employed nonsteroidal antiinflammatory agents, can cause interstitial nephritis and hematuria. Anticoagulation may induce hematuria but further evaluation is required because an underlying lesion is often present. Estrogen-containing birth control pills have been implicated in the loin-pain hematuria syndrome, a renal vascular disorder predominantly of young women who present with recurrent episodes of severe flank pain and hematuria. In blacks and some persons of Mediterranean origin, sickle-cell trait and sickle-cell disease can cause hematuria. Sickle-cell trait may be the most common cause of hematuria in younger blacks.

Physical Examination
Although in many cases a physical examination will not provide an answer to the cause of hematuria, it should still be carefully performed. Palpation of the abdomen and flanks for masses may detect renal tumors or polycystic kidney disease. A prostate examination may identify benign prostatic hypertrophy or carcinoma. Visual examination of the genitourinary organs may locate bleeding from urethral, vaginal, or other lesions. Clues to glomerular disease include hypertension and peripheral edema. Fevers, rashes, arthritis, and heart murmurs may be evidence of systemic illnesses such as vasculitis, connective tissue disorders, and endocarditis, all of which can cause glomerulonephritis and hematuria.

Laboratory Tests
URINALYSIS. A urinalysis with microscopic examination performed by the physician or an experienced laboratory technician is critical. It confirms the presence of RBCs in the urine, and provides significant information about the cause of hematuria. Ideally, it should be done on a fresh, concentrated morning specimen in order to prevent lysis of RBCs in hypotonic urine. The aim is the detection of proteinuria, pyuria, bacteria, RBC casts, or dysmorphic RBCs, which direct further evaluation. The following patterns of findings have particular significance:

Pyuria and bacteriuria suggest infectious causes such as cystitis, pyelonephritis, or prostatitis. Hematuria that disappears after treatment of confirmed bacterial cystitis in females may not require further evaluation.

Pyuria without bacteriuria on microscopic examination or urine culture most frequently occurs with chlamydial infections or coliform infections of low colony count, but may occur with tuberculosis of the urinary tract or an interstitial nephritis such as analgesic nephropathy.

Proteinuria, RBC casts, and dysmorphic RBCs are all evidence of intrinsic renal disease, particularly glomerulonephritis. Proteinuria of 2+ or greater on dipstick does not usually occur with bleeding of urologic origin. RBC casts are virtually always the result of glomerulonephritis. They should be assiduously sought along the edge of the coverslip where they are most commonly found. If techniques for assessing RBC morphology such as phase-contrast microscopy, supravital staining (Sedi stain), or urine RBC indices are available, it may be possible to distinguish bleeding from urologic sources (normal RBCs) from bleeding of glomerular origin (distorted, dysmorphic RBCs).

OTHER LABORATORY STUDIES. Serum creatinine concentration should be measured to evaluate renal function on all patients. Other tests of potential value include a tuberculin skin test (PPD) and urine acid-fast bacillus (AFB) cultures for patients with sterile pyuria, hemoglobin electrophoresis for those at risk of sickle hemoglobinopathies, throat culture and antistreptolysin (ASO) titers if a history of upper respiratory symptoms is obtained, and serum complements and antinuclear antibodies if evidence of a systemic illness is present. The serum lactate dehydrogenase concentration (LDH) is almost always elevated in patients with renal emboli. A 24-hour urine collection is needed to quantify proteinuria of 2+ or greater and to detect hypercalciuria, a common cause of hematuria in children that recently was also found in adults.

X-rays and Other Procedures
Intravenous pyelography (IVP) provides the best overall visualization of the renal parenchyma, collecting system, ureter, and bladder. Most stones, including radiolucent ones, many renal tumors and cysts, intrinsic ureteral lesions such as transitional cell carcinoma, and some bladder lesions are easily found with this test. Structural lesions such as obstructions, which predispose to infection and loss of renal function, can also be found. Together an IVP and cystoscopy can detect and localize most of the common urologic causes of hematuria. An IVP has little utility in younger patients with clear evidence of acute nephritis. The major risks of intravenous contrast material are nephrotoxicity and idiosyncratic reactions. Nephrotoxicity is more likely to occur in those with preexistent chronic renal insufficiency (creatinine concentration > 2 mg/dl). Age, diabetes, congestive heart failure, and volume depletion also may be risk factors for renal failure. Adequate hydration may decrease these risks. Idiosyncratic reactions range from urticaria to death from cardiovascular collapse but the incidence of the latter is 1 in 40,000 to 75,000 examinations.

Renal sonography is a good alternative to the IVP, especially in patients at risk of contrast dye toxicity. One analysis has found it to be less expensive and as sensitive for malignancy as the IVP in asymptomatic patients, with lower morbidity. This conclusion is not applicable to symptomatic patients, and is very dependent on the technical quality of the sonogram. Ureteral lesions also may be missed. Sonography can also detect renal masses not found on IVP, confirm the presence of masses suspected on IVP, and determine whether a lesion is a simple fluid-filled cyst or the solid or complex lesion of renal carcinoma. It probably should be performed in older patients when no source of hematuria was found on IVP.

Computed tomography (CT) can also detect renal masses not found on IVP or confirm and characterize suspected masses. It is a more expensive alternative than sonography in patients thought to be at risk of IVP dye toxicity.

Angiography may be the only way to detect arteriovenous malformations, and might be performed in patients with gross, painless hematuria, after other studies have been performed to rule out carcinoma and glomerular disease such as IgA nephropathy.

Cystoscopy visualizes the bladder and urinary outlet tract, areas not seen well on radiographic or sonographic procedures. Bleeding sites can be seen directly and upper tract bleeding localized to one side. Carcinoma of the bladder is the most common, serious lesion detected with this procedure. Cystoscopy should be performed early in the evaluation of most patients, particularly older patients in whom neoplasms and infections are the common serious causes of hematuria. Since the procedure is uncomfortable, particularly in young men, it should be avoided in those for whom the yield is quite low (i.e., those < 40 years old where the cause of hematuria is apparent, such as a stone or glomerulonephritis).

Urine cytology is an important, safe test that can detect transitional cell carcinoma of the bladder and collecting system missed on IVP and cystoscopy. It is much less sensitive for detecting renal cell carcinoma. It should be done routinely on 3 separate days in all patients at risk of neoplasms, especially smokers and older patients with hematuria of nonglomerular origin.

Renal biopsy is useful in certain patients, but the risks must be balanced against the benefits. The diagnosis of most cases of acute glomerulonephritis, such as poststreptococcal, does not require a biopsy. A biopsy is often required, however, to distinguish among the various idiopathic glomerulonephritides that cause hematuria. For example, the most common glomerular cause of isolated hematuria is IgA nephropathy (Berger's disease) which can only be specifically diagnosed by finding IgA on immunofluorescent stains of the glomerulus. The recently described thin-basement-membrane disorder, which may also be a common cause of isolated hematuria, can only be diagnosed with electron microscopy of the glomerular basement membrane. Diseases such as focal glomerular sclerosis and membranoproliferative glomerulonephritis, which can cause hematuria and proteinuria, have few, if any, diagnostic features short of biopsy. For most of these disorders, however, therapy either is not required or is of uncertain benefit. Renal biopsy is, therefore, often reserved for those patients with substantial proteinuria (> 1–2 g/day) or a decline in renal function, both of which can portend progressive renal damage. It is also occasionally done in patients with isolated hematuria for nontherapeutic indications such as genetic counseling, ending a cycle of unpleasant and expensive evaluations for hematuria, or for employment or insurance issues. Consultation with a nephrologist is needed in making decisions about the utility of a renal biopsy.

Follow-up

If the initial evaluation is unrevealing, as it may be in 20 to 50% of patients, follow-up is necessary. For patients over 40 years old, undetected malignancy, especially carcinoma in situ of the bladder, is the major concern. If hematuria continues, cystoscopy and urine cytologies should be repeated at 3- to 6-month intervals and an IVP at 1 year as directed by the urologist. Patients in whom glomerulonephritis is diagnosed or is likely as the cause of hematuria should have blood pressure measurements, serum creatinine determinations, and urinalysis performed yearly.

Referrals

The primary question to consider in making a referral to the appropriate specialist is whether hematuria is likely of urologic or nephrologic origin. The answer may not be clear in many cases but the following principles should be observed:

Gross, painless hematuria throughout voiding should prompt urgent urologic evaluation.
Older age, smoking, and to some extent male sex are major risk factors for urologic malignancy and should prompt urologic evaluation for all but the most clearly diagnosed cases.
Patients with unexplained hematuria of any amount (i.e., without characteristics of glomerular hematuria such as RBC casts, dysmorphic RBCs, and proteinuria) and with a nondiagnostic IVP should have a urology referral.
Hematuria of apparent glomerular origin requires nephrology referral if the serum creatinine concentration is elevated, hypertension is present, a systemic illness is evident, or there is greater than 1 to 2 g of protein in the urine.

Abeulo JG. Evaluation of hematuria. Urology 1983; 32:215–25.
Excellent, thorough review of the causes and workup of hematuria.

Benson GS. Hematuria algorithms for diagnosis. JAMA 1981; 246:993–5.
Succinct diagnostic algorithm.

Sutton JM. Evaluation of hematuria in adults. JAMA 1990; 263:2475–80.
A review that includes a diagnostic algorithm.

Carson CC. Clinical importance of microhematuria. JAMA 1979; 241:149–50.
Retrospective study of 200 patients, mostly older adults. Urges evaluation based on a 20% rate of serious lesions and 13% malignancy rate.

Golin AL. Asymptomatic microscopic hematuria. J Urol 1980; 124:389–98.
Retrospective review of 246 cases. Urges a careful follow-up protocol for those undiagnosed initially.

Froom P. Significance of microhematuria in young adults. Br Med J 1984; 288:20–2.
Retrospective study of 1000 men aged 18 to 33 found one malignancy over 15 years.

Bold R. The significance of asymptomatic microhematuria in women and its economic implications. Arch Intern Med 1988; 148:2629–32.
Suggests that the risk of neoplasms in asymptomatic women is very low.

de Caestekes MP. Localization of hematuria by red cell analyses and phase contrast microscopy. Nephron 1989; 52:170–3.
These relatively new techniques may help localize bleeding sites and are being introduced into clinical practice.

Seigel AJ. Exercise related hematuria. JAMA 1979; 241:391–2.
Reports an 18% incidence of hematuria after a marathon.

Tieboach A. Thin-basement-membrane nephropathy in adults with persistent hematuria. N Engl J Med; 320:14–8.
Another explanation for idiopathic hematuria, the clinical consequences of which are unknown.

Andres A. Hematuria due to hypercalciuria and hyperuricosuria in adult patients. Kidney Int 1989; 36:96–9.
An established condition in children, which needs further confirmation of its significance in adults.

Woolhandler S. Dipstick urinalysis screening of asymptomatic adults for urinary tract disorders. I. Hematuria and proteinuria. JAMA 1989; 262:1214–9.
Critical review finds no convincing evidence of the utility of screening.

Antolak S. Urologic evaluation of hematuria occurring during anticoagulant therapy. J Urol 1969; 101:111–3.
Found on 82% incidence of significant urologic lesions.

Corwin H. The diagnosis of neoplasia in patients with asymptomatic microscopic hematuria: a decision analysis. J Urol 1988; 139:1002–6.
Finds sonography and cystoscopy to be as sensitive as and safer than IVP and cystoscopy in this group of patients.

59. PROTEINURIA
Katherine A. Huffman

Normally the urine contains 150 mg or less of protein per 24 hours, composed of albumin (40%), immunoglobulins and other plasma proteins (20%), and protein of uroepithelial origin—Tamm-Horsfall protein—(40%).

Pathophysiology
Proteinuria occurs as a result of one of three major abnormalities: impaired function of the glomerular capillary wall or overproduction of or decreased tubular resorption of freely filterable protein. The glomerular capillary wall acts as a molecular sieve that retards the passage of large proteins such as albumin. Therefore, albuminuria reflects increased permeability of the capillary wall. Smaller proteins (e.g., myoglobin and lysozyme) are filtered across the capillary wall and resorbed by the tubule or excreted in the urine. Overproduction proteinuria results from an increased excretion of a normally filterable protein, exemplified by excretion of myoglobin or light chains. Tubular proteinuria, which is rare, occurs when the tubules have an impaired ability to reabsorb low-molecular-weight proteins. This discussion focuses on albuminuria, the most common type of proteinuria.

Detection of Proteinuria
There are two commonly used laboratory methods to detect proteinuria. The dipstick test is convenient and specific but does not detect light chains or protein at a concentration of less than 30 mg/dl. False-positive reactions are uncommon but may occur with decomposed or alkaline urine. The protein precipitation test, using 5% sulfosalicylic acid, is exquisitely sensitive, although less convenient, and gives false-positive reactions with radiographic contrast agents, tolbutamide, penicillins, and sulfisoxazole. The major advantage of the sulfosalicylic acid test is its ability to detect light-chain proteins. For routine screening in a physician's office, the dipstick method is adequate and efficient, and does not give confusing, false-positive reactions. Because the test depends on concentration, however, unusually concentrated or dilute urine gives misleading results. If clinical suspicion for light-chain proteinuria is high, the sulfosalicylic precipitation test should be used.

Diagnostic Evaluation
Proteinuria is abnormal and requires additional evaluation, except when the urine is highly concentrated or when the patient has an intercurrent acute illness or urinary tract

infection, or has been exercising heavily. In the latter instances the urinalysis should be repeated after resolution of the illness or before exercise. The initial diagnostic step is quantification of the protein lost per 24 hours and careful examination of the urine sediment. Proteinuria coupled with hematuria or pyuria represents different renal disease processes and is evaluated differently from isolated proteinuria. When cellular elements or casts are present, the patient should be referred to a nephrologist for further evaluation, which may include a renal biopsy.

If the 24-hour protein excretion exceeds 150 mg and there are no other urine sediment abnormalities, the following steps should be undertaken to establish a diagnosis:

Perform a history and physical examination, noting any family history of renal disease and any evidence for collagen vascular or other systemic illness (e.g., diabetes).

Repeat quantification of urine protein, particularly if the first sample was collected when the patient was clinically ill (febrile, severely hypertensive, or in congestive heart failure).

Evaluate for orthostatic proteinuria (see Isolated Nonnephrotic Proteinuria); if orthostatic proteinuria is diagnosed, serum urea and creatinine should be measured, but an extensive renal evaluation is not necessary.

Order laboratory studies, including CBC, serum urea, creatinine, glucose, total protein, albumin, 24-hour creatinine clearance, and urine culture.

If the patient has nephrotic-range proteinuria ($\geq$ 3.5 g/24 hr), serum cholesterol, and antinuclear antibody should be measured. Referral to a nephrologist should be made for consideration of a renal biopsy.

If polycystic kidney disease is suspected, renal ultrasound should be performed.

If paraproteinemia is suspected, serum protein electrophoresis and urinary immunoelectrophoresis are necessary.

Isolated Nonnephrotic Proteinuria

Isolated proteinuria is defined as urinary protein excretion in excess of 150 mg per 24 hours in the absence of any other urine sediment abnormalities. It is helpful and important to distinguish isolated nonnephrotic from nephrotic-range proteinuria. The former category includes functional, orthostatic, and constant proteinuria.

Functional proteinuria is defined as transient low-grade proteinuria in the absence of apparent renal disease. Congestive heart failure, fever, seizures, heavy exercise, emotional stress, hypertension, and infusion of albumin or epinephrine can cause proteinuria that resolves when the stimulus is removed. In a recent report of 313 emergency medical admissions with no known renal disease, 30 (9.5%) had proteinuria greater than 1+ on admission, which had resolved by the ninth hospital day. The major diagnoses in these patients were congestive heart failure, seizures, pneumonia, and fever. When isolated proteinuria is detected in a patient who is acutely ill, the first step is to reconfirm the presence of proteinuria after the acute stress subsides.

Orthostatic (postural) proteinuria is characterized by the appearance of proteinuria in the upright position and its disappearance in the recumbent position. The total amount of protein excreted is usually less than 1.5 g per 24 hours. It typically occurs in otherwise healthy, asymptomatic people and is detected incidentally during a routine examination. Because the prognosis and need for additional evaluation differ between orthostatic and nonorthostatic (constant) proteinuria, differentiation is important.

A quantitative method to detect the presence of orthostatic proteinuria has been established. On arising at 7 AM, the patient voids and discards the urine. Thereafter, all urine is collected in a single container until 10 PM, when the patient voids into the same bottle and immediately assumes a recumbent position. At 7 AM on the following morning (immediately on arising), the patient voids into a second bottle. If the patient has orthostatic proteinuria, the recumbent collection should contain 75 mg of protein or less, and the sum of both specimens should be 1500 mg or less. Alternatively, a qualitative test using sulfosalicylic acid can be used; the recumbent specimen should be negative, and the upright specimen should be positive.

The mechanism by which an upright posture causes proteinuria is not well understood. The appearance of proteinuria may reflect altered glomerular capillary-wall permeability, which is manifested when coupled with the hemodynamic consequences of an upright position (e.g., decreased renal blood flow). Renal histologic results from men with orthostatic proteinuria showed that 8% of patients had unequivocal evidence of renal disease, 45% had subtle but definite alterations of the glomerulus, and 47% appeared normal. Ten years after the time of diagnosis, 49% of all these individuals had proteinuria, yet none had impairment of renal function. Therefore, the prognosis of patients with orthostatic proteinuria appears to be excellent. A renal biopsy is not indicated unless there are changes in the patient's clinical picture, such as alterations in the urine sediment, serum creatinine, or amount of proteinuria. Yearly follow-up examinations are advised, including repeat urinalysis.

Constant proteinuria is an arbitrary category that includes patients whose proteinuria persists during recumbency but does not fall into the category of nephrotic-range proteinuria because less than 3.5 g of protein per 24 hours is excreted. This group is generally regarded with concern, although data on the importance and prognosis of constant proteinuria are scarce. A 40-year follow-up study of university students with proteinuria on entrance physical examinations found that the mortality rate was increased only in those who had constant proteinuria or clinically obvious renal disease. Those who had intermittent proteinuria had the same mortality rate as persons with no renal abnormalities.

If the patient has a normal creatinine clearance and no other urine sediment abnormalities, there is no reason to perform a renal biopsy. As long as there is no clue to underlying renal disease, clinical follow-up at 3-month intervals is advised initially. If renal function and urine sediment remain unchanged, less frequent clinic visits are appropriate. The appearance of hematuria, an increase in proteinuria, or a decrease in creatinine clearance warrants additional evaluation, with consideration of a renal biopsy.

Nephrotic Syndrome
Protein excretion in excess of 3.5 g per 24 hours is termed *nephrotic-range proteinuria*. The nephrotic syndrome is defined as nephrotic-range proteinuria together with its consequences: hypoalbuminemia, hyperlipidemia, and edema.

Initial evaluation of the nephrotic syndrome should include determinations of 24-hour protein and creatinine clearance. Unless the nephrotic syndrome is clearly caused by an associated systemic illness (e.g., diabetes mellitus), referral to a nephrologist for kidney biopsy is in order.

The nephrotic syndrome can be divided into two groups by cause: idiopathic and secondary. The idiopathic nephrotic syndrome is additionally classified by glomerular histopathology. Of the primary glomerulopathies, only minimal-change disease clearly responds to steroid therapy. The rate of rise of serum creatinine may be retarded by the use of corticosteroids in membranous glomerulopathy. The importance of making a histopathologic diagnosis is not only in detecting treatable disease but also in providing the patient and clinician with an appreciation for the clinical patterns and prognoses that characterize different lesions. The nephrotic syndrome may be associated with a variety of infections, malignancies, drugs, allergies, systemic diseases, and inherited disorders. If the underlying disease can be treated successfully, or if it spontaneously remits, the nephrotic syndrome also may resolve.

Angiotensin-Converting Enzyme Inhibitors
Angiotensin-converting enzyme inhibitors (ACEIs) have been shown to reduce proteinuria in diabetics and in some nondiabetics, presumably by changing intrarenal hemodynamics and possibly by changing the permeability of the glomerular filtration barrier. Angiotensin II causes efferent arteriole constriction; ACEIs cause efferent arteriole dilatation and reduce intraglomerular pressure. In addition to decreasing proteinuria, there are reports that decreased intraglomerular pressure retards the progression of renal disease, especially in diabetics.

Unfortunately ACEIs can precipitate acute renal failure in low-flow or fixed-flow states such as bilateral renal artery stenosis, renal artery stenosis to a single kidney, advanced renal disease, and severe myocardial dysfunction with low cardiac output. Also, serum potassium levels may rise as decreased angiotensin II levels result in decreased aldosterone release from the adrenal cortex.

In clinical practice, ACEIs are appropriate and probably beneficial in diabetics with proteinuria, especially early in the course of diabetic nephropathy and especially if hypertension coexists. In proteinuria of nondiabetic origin, there is insufficient evidence to make a recommendation for the use of ACEIs for the purpose of decreasing proteinuria.

Serial determinations of creatinine, potassium, and urinary protein levels are necessary during treatment to monitor efficacy and possible adverse effects.

Reuben DB, et al. Transient proteinuria in emergency medical admissions. N Engl J Med 1982; 306:1031–3.
Nine and one-half percent of emergency medical admissions had transient proteinuria that disappeared by the ninth hospital day.

Robinson RR. Isolated proteinuria in asymptomatic patients. Kidney Int 1980; 18: 395–406.
A very lucid and concise review of the mechanisms, clinical importance, and prognosis of nonnephrotic proteinuria in the asymptomatic patient.

Rytanf DA, Spreiter, S. Prognosis in postural (orthostatic) proteinuria. N Engl J Med 1981; 305:618–21.
A 42- to 50-year follow-up of six patients diagnosed by Thomas Addis. None developed renal disease or died of a renal cause.

Levitt JI. The prognostic significance of proteinuria in young college students. Ann Intern Med 1967; 66:685–96.
A retrospective study with a 37- to 45-year follow-up showing that persons with intermittent proteinuria have no increase in mortality, whereas those with constant proteinuria or clinically apparent renal disease have a definite increase in mortality.

Glassock RJ, et al. Primary glomerular diseases. In: Brenner BM, Rector FC, eds. The kidney. 4th ed. Philadelphia: Saunders, 1991: 1182–279.
A detailed, complete review of primary glomerular disease.

Brenner BM, Hostetter TH, Humes HD. Molecular basis of proteinuria of glomerular origin. N Engl J Med 1978; 298:826–33.
A review of the properties of the glomerular capillary wall that impart to it the ability to retard the passage of protein and other macromolecules.

Collaborative study of adult idiopathic nephrotic syndrome. A controlled study of short-term prednisone treatment in adults with membranous nephropathy. N Engl J Med 1979; 301:1301–6.
The most-often quoted reference to support treating membranous nephropathy with prednisone. The treated group had a less rapid rate of rise in serum creatinine.

Schrier RW, Gottschalk CW. Diseases of the kidney. 4th ed. Boston: Little, Brown, 1988: 414–29, 1971–87.
A good textbook approach to proteinuria and an in-depth discussion of the nephrotic syndrome.

Heeg JE, et al. Reduction of proteinuria by angiotensin converting enzyme inhibition. Kidney Int 1987; 32:78–83.
Lisinopril but not conventional antihypertensive therapy reduced proteinuria by 60% in patients with renal insufficiency of different causes. The antiproteinuric effect of the ACEI lisinopril appears to be a result of efferent (postglomerular) vasodilation.

Taguma Y, et al. Effect of captopril on heavy proteinuria in azotemic diabetes. N Engl J Med 1985; 313:1617–20.
Proteinuria decreased from 10.6 to 6.1 g day in 10 azotemic diabetics who were given captopril. The antiproteinuric effect appears to be due to decreased intrarenal hypertension rather than to a change in systemic blood pressure.

Reams GP, Bauer JH. Effect of enalapril in subjects with hypertension associated with moderate to severe renal dysfunction. Arch Intern Med 1986; 146:2145–8.
Enalapril was given to nine patients with hypertension and renal insufficiency: BP was controlled without significant change in renal function and proteinuria decreased.

Abraham PA, et al. Efficacy and renal effects to enalapril therapy for hypertensive patients with chronic renal insufficiency. Arch Intern Med 1988; 148:2358–62.
Enalapril reduces BP and proteinuria in hypertensive patients with chronic renal insufficiency. Serum potassium and creatinine levels can increase and should be monitored.

Bear R. Enalapril therapy in patients with renal function impairment. Arch Intern Med 1988; 148:2343–4. editorial.
Excellent summary of mechanisms of action of ACEIs.

60. URINARY INCONTINENCE IN THE ELDERLY
Mark E. Williams

Approximately 15 to 30% of elderly people living in the community have urinary incontinence; in the institutional setting, the prevalence approaches 50%. Urinary incontinence can result in substantial psychological, social, medical, and economic problems. If not effectively treated, it increases social isolation, frequently results in a loss of independence through institutionalization, and predisposes to infection and skin breakdown.

Normal Neuroanatomy and Physiology
The location of adrenergic and cholinergic neuroreceptors within the bladder and urethra influences the pathogenesis and treatment of incontinence. Alpha-adrenergic receptors, abundant in the bladder outlet, increase urethral resistance when stimulated. Beta-adrenergic receptors, predominant in the body and dome of the bladder, cause relaxation of the detrusor (the muscular layer of the bladder). Cholinergic receptors, located throughout the bladder and urethra, produce detrusor contractions. Bladder filling can be viewed as a sympathetic nervous system activity produced by detrusor relaxation and urethral resistance to outflow, while voiding is a parasympathetic activity mediated by detrusor contractions.

The following neurologic pathways are involved in maintaining continence: Stretch receptors in the bladder wall communicate the volume status to the brain. When a critical degree of bladder distention is reached, detrusor contractions occur and must be inhibited by higher cortical centers to avoid abrupt bladder emptying. Voluntary voiding is accomplished in part by increasing intra-abdominal pressure through contractions of the abdominal muscles and diaphragm, synchronized with relaxation of the urethral sphincter.

To maintain urinary continence, bladder pressure must be less than intraurethral pressure. Bladder pressure is related to intra-abdominal pressure, the amount of urine contained in the bladder, and the contractile state of the detrusor muscle. Detrusor tone is augmented by decreased CNS inhibition, cholinergic stimulation, and increased afferent stimulation; it is diminished by cholinergic inhibition, muscle relaxants, and decreased afferent stimulation.

Intraurethral pressure is maintained through periurethral striated muscle, smooth muscle of the urethra and bladder neck, and urethral muscle thickness. The external urethral sphincter, which allows voluntary cessation of urine flow, is not necessary for continence.

Smooth muscle tone of the urethra and bladder neck is an important determinant of intraurethral pressure and thus bladder outlet resistance. Factors that increase tone include prostatic hypertrophy and alpha-sympathetic stimulation. Tone is weakened by sympathetic blockade; muscle relaxants; bladder prolapse, which decreases the sphincter's mechanical advantage; and the consequences of surgical manipulation of the pelvis, bladder, or urethra. Thickness of the urethral mucosa in women is maintained by estrogens and decreases with estrogen deficiency.

Pathophysiology
The fundamental lesion in incontinence is bladder pressure sufficient to overcome urethral resistance. Five basic mechanisms, which may occur singly or in combination, are responsible: detrusor instability, overflow incontinence, sphincter insufficiency, functional illness, and iatrogenic factors.

Detrusor instability occurs when bladder contractions overcome normal urethral resistance. Synonyms include *unstable bladder, spastic bladder,* and *uninhibited bladder.* This is the most common type of incontinence, occurring in up to 70% of patients in some series. Three basic causes of this instability include: (1) defects in CNS inhibitory mechanisms, such as in bilateral frontal lobe lesions; (2) hyperexcitability of afferent sensory pathways, such as in acute cystitis, small bladder capacity, bladder wall hypertrophy, and fecal impaction; and (3) deconditioned voiding reflexes.

Deconditioned voiding reflexes may be self-induced or iatrogenic. For example, embarrassment over a single episode of incontinence can lead to frequent voiding in an attempt to avert another accident. Chronic low-volume voiding, however, may result in decreased bladder capacity, increased detrusor tone, and increased bladder wall thickness, all of which aggravate detrusor instability and can lead to future episodes of incontinence. Iatrogenic deconditioning can result when continence becomes associated with uncomfortable equipment, such as cold bedpans or toilet seats, or when incontinence is rewarded by increased physical attention.

Overflow incontinence occurs when urine flows only at large bladder volumes, and is the result of inadequate bladder contractions or elevated urethral resistance to flow. Causes include (1) bladder outlet obstruction, such as by prostatic hypertrophy, calculi, or carcinoma; (2) detrusor inadequacy, also called *atonic bladder or neurogenic bladder,* which may occur in Parkinson's disease, diabetic autonomic neuropathy, or lumbosacral spinal cord disease; and (3) impaired afferent sensation, a form of atonic or neurogenic bladder, such as in diabetes mellitus. Clinical features include a palpable or percussible bladder, often with suprapubic tenderness. A cystometrogram reveals no bladder contractions despite high pressures (> 20 cm H_2O) and high volumes (> 400 ml).

Sphincter insufficiency, or *stress incontinence,* is common in elderly women and occurs when urethral resistance to flow is reduced. The probable causes are postmenopausal changes in the urethral mucosa, related to the decline of estrogens, combined with weakness of the pelvic muscles that comes with multiparity. In addition, urinary tract infections can precipitate stress incontinence. The prevalence of symptomatic stress incontinence depends on the definition; most young nulliparous women admit occasional minor "leakage." Stress incontinence in men usually occurs only with urinary tract infection, after urologic surgery, or as a result of severe neurologic disease.

Clinical features include incontinence following coughing, laughing, straining, or other conditions that cause an abrupt increase in intra-abdominal pressure. Patients are often dry at night. Physical examination may demonstrate visible leakage of urine on coughing or during abdominal palpation to increase intra-abdominal pressure. Pelvic examination may reveal a reddened vulva or periurethral tissue (secondary to decreased estrogen), or relaxed pelvic musculature. Palpable funneling of the urethra (the Bonney-Read-Marchetti test) suggests sphincter weakness; it may be demonstrated by placing the tips of the first two fingers on each side of the urethra and extending them only 1 or 2 cm into the vagina. If an impact is felt against the fingertips when the patient coughs, then funneling is present. Laboratory studies may disclose signs of urinary tract infection.

Functional incontinence occurs in urologically normal people who cannot or will not reach the toilet in time to avoid an accident. Musculoskeletal and environmental limitations may cause incontinence in an otherwise continent person. Cognitively impaired patients may not recognize the need to void, or be able to locate and use the facilities.

Patients who become incontinent to command more attention can be a difficult management problem. This "spiteful" incontinence is intermittent and usually does not occur at night. Usually an element of depression, hostility, or anger is present.

Iatrogenic incontinence, caused by drugs or other factors, may aggravate or unmask any of the above problems. The use of potent, fast-acting diuretics or physical restraints may make it difficult for elderly people to be continent. Psychoactive medications such as sedative hypnotics or antipsychotics may create a loss of attention to bladder cues. Sphincter weakness may be precipitated by muscle relaxants, sympathetic blockers, or other agents that affect the autonomic balance in the CNS.

Evaluation

Unfortunately, there is no definitive diagnostic test to establish the cause of incontinence. Diagnosis must be based on history and physical findings, with some simple maneuvers, and selected use of laboratory studies and more sophisticated tests. The history may point to one or more of the types of incontinence described above. Information obtained should include the onset, duration, and pattern of incontinence (e.g., intermittent, continuous, morning, night, after medications); the amount of urine lost; all medications used; associated symptoms (straining, dysuria); excessive fluid intake; and relevant medical or surgical conditions, such as diabetes, pelvic or urinary tract surgery, or neurologic diseases.

The physical examination should identify neurologic abnormalities, and include pelvic and rectal examinations. During pelvic examination, stress-induced leakage may be revealed by having the patient cough or perform the Valsalva maneuver; atrophic changes of the vaginal mucosa are suggested by a thin reddened appearance, and may be confirmed by a smear for epithelial maturation, an estrogen effect. Rectal examination should be performed to detect fecal impaction, abnormalities of anal sphincter tone and contractility, and prostate nodules. Prostatic enlargement determined by rectal examination correlates poorly with the presence of obstruction; the absence of prostatic enlargement does not rule out obstruction, since encroachment on the urethra by the median lobe of the prostate may not be palpable. The bladder should be palpated and percussed for evidence of distention. Perineal sensation should be tested to determine lower spinal cord function.

Laboratory studies should include a urinalysis and, to exclude polyuric syndromes, serum glucose, calcium, electrolyte, and creatinine measurements. Postvoid residual urine volume should be determined; a volume of more than 50 to 100 ml is abnormal. Urine culture should be performed if infection is suspected.

Additional studies should be requested as needed to determine the choice of therapy or when surgery is considered. Cystometrograms may help to characterize suspected neurologic abnormalities. Urethral pressure profiles may differentiate among the causes of urethral sphincter weakness and determine the presence and severity of urethral obstruction.

The diagnosis may be simplified if the following points are kept in mind: (1) A palpable or percussible bladder usually signifies overflow incontinence. (2) The absence of signs of overflow or stress incontinence suggests detrusor instability. (3) If stress incontinence is present, particularly in older women, it may be the only lesion, or it may be mixed with detrusor instability; cystometric studies are indicated to differentiate the two.

Treatment

A positive attitude and other general supportive measures are important. Behavioral therapies and bladder training programs are especially effective for motivated patients. Biofeedback procedures require trained personnel, but have been shown to be very effective. Generally the treatment is tailored to the underlying mechanism of incontinence.

Detrusor Instability

Medications are used to decrease detrusor contractions. Imipramine has both anticholinergic actions that inhibit the force and frequency of detrusor contractions and alpha-sympathetic activity that increases urethral sphincter tone. The usual starting dose is 25 mg at bedtime, but higher dosages may be required. Alternative agents that have both anticholinergic and antispasmodic properties include drugs such as oxybutynin (Ditropan), flavoxate (Urispas), and propantheline (Pro-Banthine). The dosages of all of these drugs must be titrated. Complications of drug regimens include increased residual volumes or urinary retention and side effects such as confusion, agitation, orthostatic hypotension, dry mouth, and cardiac arrhythmias.

Nonpharmacologic interventions include bladder training programs in which a voiding schedule is established and the interval between voidings gradually extended. This may be a helpful adjunct or alternative to drug treatment.

Overflow Incontinence

A nonpharmacologic strategy is frequently the treatment of choice for overflow incontinence. Surgery is preferred in instances of mechanical outlet obstruction, such as prostatic hypertrophy, calculi, or carcinoma. When overflow is the result of an atonic bladder, the first step is to decompress the bladder with either indwelling or intermittent catheterization for a period of 10 to 14 days. If bladder function is not restored, voiding efforts may be augmented by techniques such as double voiding, or use of Credé's or Valsalva's maneuver.

Outlet obstruction can sometimes be overcome by the use of alpha-sympathetic blockers such as phenoxybenzamine or prazosin; these drugs may be helpful to delay or avoid surgery. When the cause of overflow is an atonic bladder without urethral obstruction, the cholinomimetic agent bethanecol may increase detrusor tone and contractility. The concomitant side effects at effective doses may limit its usefulness. Skeletal muscle relaxants such as baclofen and dantrolene may relieve functional outlet obstruction caused by dyssynergy between the detrusor and external sphincter.

Long-term catheterization is sometimes indicated. Infection is less likely with intermittent catheterization than with use of a continuous indwelling catheter; if the patient is unable to perform self-catheterization, it can be done by family members with minimal training.

Sphincter Insufficiency

Sphincter insufficiency in estrogen-deficient women may respond to treatment with oral or topical estrogens to restore the thickness of the urethral mucosa. Urethral sphincter tone may also be increased by the use of alpha-adrenergic agonists such as phenylpropanolamine. Imipramine, with both alpha-adrenergic and anticholinergic activity, is a good alternative choice in patients with both sphincter insufficiency and detrusor instability.

Other measures that may be helpful include exercises to strengthen pelvic floor muscles and increased ambulation; the latter augments the perception of bladder filling. In resistant situations, surgical procedures to support a prolapsed bladder may be effective. Urodynamic evaluation should be performed prior to surgery to detect nonsurgical conditions such as detrusor instability.

Functional Incontinence

Functional incontinence is best managed by a behavioral approach. Physical and environmental impediments to toileting should be recognized and corrected. To avoid paradoxically conditioning the patient toward incontinent behavior, toileting immediately after an episode of incontinence should be avoided, as should unpleasant stimuli such as bedpans or low or cold toilet seats. A toileting program should be established based on an evaluation of the patient's voiding pattern. To accomplish this, the patient is checked every 2 hours for 48 hours, and a record kept of whether the patient is wet or dry. The optimal toileting schedule should then be established to allow toilet use at a time when the bladder is most likely to be full. Successful toileting should be positively reinforced.

Palliative Measures

A variety of products are available to keep incontinent patients dry and to control odor without being excessively bulky under clothing. These include rubber or plastic pants with absorbant pads or superabsorbant chemicals, intermittent self-catheterization as discussed above, and external catheters or collecting devices. Indwelling catheters and collection systems are used only as a last resort.

Williams ME, Pannill FC. Urinary incontinence in the elderly. Ann Intern Med 1982; 97:895–907.
A comprehensive general reference that contains material not summarized elsewhere.

Ouslander JG, ed. Geriatric urinary incontinence. Clin Geriatr Med 1986; 2(4).
Excellent general reference.

Ouslander J, et al. Incontinence among nursing home patients: clinical and functional correlates. J Am Geriatr Soc 1987; 35:324–30.

Ouslander J, et al. Genitourinary dysfunction in a geriatric outpatient population. J Am Geriatr Soc 1986; 34:507–14.

Sier HC, Ouslander JG, Orzeck S. Urinary incontinence among geriatric patients in an acute-care hospital. JAMA 1987; 257:1767–71.
These three articles summarize the characteristics of older patients with urinary incontinence based on the setting in which they are examined.

Resnick NM, Yalla SV. Detrusor hyperactivity with impaired contractile function. JAMA 1987; 257:3076–81.
Describes a new syndrome that appears to be fairly common.

Resnick NM, Yalla SV. Management of urinary incontinence in the elderly. N Engl J Med 1985; 313:800–5.
Good review of management options.

Schnelle JF, et al. Management of geriatric incontinence in nursing homes. J Appl Behav Anal 1983; 16:235–41.

Hadley EC. Bladder training and related therapies for urinary incontinence in older people. JAMA 1986; 256:372–9.
These two articles primarily address nonpharmacologic therapies for incontinence.

J Am Geriatr Soc 1990; 38:263–386.
This issue contains 26 articles on urinary incontinence, including the role of urodynamic testing, diagnostic evaluation in patients with neurologic disease, initial evaluation, pharmacologic treatment, estrogen therapy, bladder training, pelvic floor muscle exercises, biofeedback, vaginal surgery and suprapubic approaches for stress incontinence, electrical stimulation, and behavioral approaches in long-term care settings.

61. URINARY CATHETERIZATION
Todd A. Linsenmeyer

Urinary catheters are used in outpatients for a variety of indications. Effective management of patients with catheters requires familiarity with catheter types and with the benefits, complications, and commonly encountered problems of each.

Urinary catheters range in size from 6 to 30F, in increments of even numbers. The French size is equivalent to the circumference of the catheter in millimeters, or approximately three times the catheter diameter. For most purposes, a 16 to 18F catheter is preferred for adult males. A narrower catheter, such as a 12F, will often buckle during attempts to pass it down the male urethra, but can be used effectively in females.

Problems with Catheter Insertion

Inadequate lubrication is a common cause of difficulty in passing urinary catheters, particularly in males. Lubricant applied to the catheter tip is frequently wiped off in passage through the first few centimeters of the urethra. Adequate lubrication for easy catheter passage may be obtained by using a Tomey or Leur-Lok Syringe to *gently* introduce 5 ml of sterile, water-soluble lubricant directly into the urethra prior to catheter insertion. Because this amount of lubricant may block the openings at the end of the catheter and prevent backflow of urine, a second syringe filled with 5 to 10 ml of sterile saline may be needed for irrigation once the catheter is correctly placed.

If the catheter cannot be passed because obstruction is met, the approach may be modified according to the suspected cause. In a male who is anxious or has a neurogenic bladder, a spastic external sphincter may be the problem. Attempts at advancing the catheter should be halted immediately; the sphincter often relaxes in 5 to 10 seconds, allowing the catheter to pass easily into the bladder. Substituting lidocaine (2% Xylocaine) gel for water-soluble lubricant also often helps to relax the sphincter. In men with prostatic hypertrophy, coudé-tip catheters may facilitate passage; they have a slightly curved end, which is narrower and more rigid than a round-tip catheter and passes more easily over the prostate and into the bladder. A larger-caliber catheter (20 to 22F) may also be effective in men with prostatic hypertrophy, because it is able to push aside the obstructing lobes. If obstruction is due to suspected urethral stricture or prostatic carcinoma, a small (12 or 14F) catheter, used with a lubricant as described above, may be able to pass through the nondistensible portion of the urethra. If these measures are ineffective, a urologist should be consulted. Excessive force should always be avoided, because of the risk of creating a false passage or perforating the urethra.

Intermittent Catheterization
Intermittent catheterization (IC), or in-and-out bladder catheterization performed several times a day, is very effective in patients with neurogenic bladder dysfunction who are unable to empty their bladders at all, or who have large postvoid residual urine volumes. It may also be used in patients with transient urinary retention. IC is preferable to indwelling catheterization for long-term or chronic use because it is associated with a substantially lower risk of urinary tract infections, bladder stones, urethral strictures, epididymitis, and penoscrotal fistulae.

Home use of IC is most effective in patients who are able to catheterize themselves; otherwise the procedure may impose a significant burden on a spouse or family member. Since only registered or licensed practical nurses are allowed to perform IC, the cost of paying for the procedure to be performed several times a day is usually prohibitive. Other limitations to the use of IC include poor vision; poor hand function; small hyperreflexic bladders with frequent emptying (< every 4 hours); poor patient acceptance or compliance; severe lower extremity spasticity, especially in females; or anatomic considerations, such as intravaginal urethra or urethral stricture.

Catheters for intermittent use in females are generally 6 to 8 in. long and 12 to 14F in caliber. Male catheters are longer and usually 16F in caliber. Some patients with impaired hand function may be able to use the Bard "Touchless" catheter. This is a single-use catheter contained within a plastic bag, which can be advanced through the bag into the bladder without being directly touched. Because the bag also serves as a reservoir to collect the urine, it may be used in patients with hemiplegia or other problems who are unable to hold both the catheter and a urine receptacle simultaneously.

While sterile technique is used for IC in hospitalized patients, clean technique is recommended for outpatients because it is easier to perform, costs less, and leads to improved compliance. Patients do not use gloves, but simply wash their hands and the catheter with soap and water before and after insertion. A single catheter may be used repeatedly and does not require any special care between catheterizations. Some patients store the folded catheter between uses in a purse or other container, such as a plastic bag; others keep it soaking in a water-peroxide solution, which is changed daily to control risk of bacterial contamination. Rotating several catheters and hanging them to dry between uses is another option. There are no guidelines on when to switch to a new catheter, but many people do so weekly.

The frequency of IC is adjusted to keep the volume of each catheterization at less than 400 ml, in order to avoid bladder overdistention. Typically this results in intervals of 4 to 6 hours, but by restricting fluid intake to 2000 ml per 24 hours, many patients require catheterization only every 6 to 8 hours. Patients with high evening or night urine volumes should restrict oral fluid intake after 4 PM and/or add an extra evening catheterization so that they may sleep through the night. The same approach is appropriate for patients with high evening and early morning volumes resulting from mobilization of dependent lower extremity edema. Patients should also add in an extra catheterization any time they have an increased fluid intake.

IC can be taught by a registered or licensed practical nurse in the hospital or home setting; a minimum of three or four sessions is usually required to teach the anatomy of the bladder and urethra and help patients build technical skill and confidence.

Complications
Introduction of bacteria into the bladder occurs, although much less frequently than with indwelling catheters. Treatment of asymptomatic bacteriuria without pyuria is controversial, particularly if the organism is resistant to oral antibiotics. *Proteus mirabilis* and other urea-splitting organisms should be treated however, because they cause an alkaline urine with an increased propensity to form stones.

Urethral trauma with a small amount of bleeding can sometimes occur, particularly in men with enlarged prostates. This problem can often be remedied by using a curved-tip (coudé) catheter. The rare problem of pubic hairs accidently being passed into the bladder via the catheter may be eliminated by proper hygiene and care at catheterization.

Indwelling Catheters

Catheters for indwelling use (Foley catheters) have inflatable balloons at the tip to maintain the catheter in the bladder. The most commonly used balloon size is 5 cc. In men who have recently undergone prostatic resection to prevent the catheter from sliding down into the prostatic urethra, 30-cc balloons are indicated. Three-way catheters have, in addition to a channel for urine and a channel to the balloon, a third channel for bladder irrigation.

Foley catheters are available in rubber, latex, and plastic materials, with or without coatings of silicone, Teflon, or other synthetic materials. The synthetic coatings reduce friction against the urethra, and thus are less likely to excite an inflammatory response: This results in less urethral irritation and less catheter encrustation.

Foley catheters may drain into either a 2000-ml bag that hangs from the bed or chair, or a bag strapped to the leg, available in sizes from 300 to 1000 ml. Leg bags are inconspicuous but require more frequent drainage; many individuals use them during the day and switch to the large 2-L bag at night.

Catheter Care

Indwelling catheters should be inserted with strict sterile technique. Before the catheter is passed into the bladder, the balloon should be tested by inflating and deflating it with sterile water or saline. This will detect the occasional defective balloon that will not deflate. Once the catheter is inserted, a free flow of urine should be obtained before the balloon is inflated. Discomfort when the balloon is inflated suggests that it is incorrectly placed in the urethra. The balloon should then immediately be deflated and the catheter advanced further into the bladder to prevent urethral injury.

In order to minimize bacteriuria, a closed drainage system should be maintained: The drainage bag and tubing should never be disconnected from the catheter, except to be changed, and the bag should never be opened, except to drain urine. The drainage bag should be kept below the level of the patient at all times, and never inverted; it should be emptied every 6 to 8 hours with care not to contaminate the spigot. The tubing should be inspected to ensure that urine is flowing freely from the bladder into the bag.

Patients should be encouraged to drink at least 2 L of fluid a day to help keep the bladder and tubing clear of debris and mucus. Instillation of 25 to 50 ml of antimicrobial agents such as hydrogen peroxide or chlorhexidine into the drainage bag may decrease bacterial contamination of the bag, but whether this reduces bladder bacteriuria is uncertain.

The urethral meatus should be gently cleaned of any encrustations once or twice daily, with water or normal saline. Cleansing with povidine-iodine or green soap has actually been shown to increase the incidence of infection when compared with no care, possibly because the detergents interfered with natural defenses. Aggressive meatal care may therefore be detrimental. Catheters in men should be taped in an upward direction, toward the abdomen rather than downward to the leg. While drainage is not quite as efficient, the risk of a penoscrotal fistula is reduced. In women, the catheter may be secured to the thigh.

Although monthly changes are often recommended for long-term indwelling catheters, there are no data to support an "ideal" interval for routine changes, and the approach can therefore be individualized. Obviously, catheters should be changed for leaking or debris and encrustations that may lead to obstruction. Routine urinalysis and culture of catheterized patients have little clinical utility, since asymptomatic infections do not require treatment and culture results correlate poorly with subsequent symptomatic infections.

When an indwelling catheter is removed and left out, the patient should be monitored with a follow-up urinalysis and culture. In patients who may have subsequent retention and bladder distention, a urine culture is recommended prior to catheter removal. Appropriate antibiotics should then be administered for 72 hours before and after removal to prevent sepsis. Urodynamic studies and/or cystoscopy may be needed for evaluation of recurrent infections, incontinence, or retention after catheter removal.

Complications

Bacteriuria is inevitable in patients with chronic indwelling catheters. Bacteria may ascend the tubing into the bladder or pass up the meatus between the catheter and urethra. The prophylactic use of antibiotics via catheter irrigation, topical application to the meatus, systemic administration, or catheter impregnation is ineffective in reducing catheter-induced bacteriuria. Antibiotic treatment of asymptomatic bacteriuria is not recommended and may result in selecting out resistant organisms. An exception to this is the presence of a urease-producing organism (e.g., *P. mirabilis, Morganella morganii,* or *Providencia stuartii*), suggested by a urine pH of 7 or higher. By increasing urine pH, such organisms induce precipitation of calcium phosphate and ammonium magnesium phosphate (struvite), which may result in catheter encrustation and blockage, as well as bladder stones.

Pyelonephritis and urosepsis are serious and potentially life-threatening complications of indwelling catheters. Patients with flank pain, fever, or other signs of systemic illness without an obvious source should be treated with appropriate broad-spectrum antibiotics pending the results of cultures.

Periurethral infections such as prostatitis, epididymitis, and scrotal abscess occur occasionally in men following prolonged catheterizations. Treatment is with antibiotics and, when indicated, surgical drainage.

Catheter debris, encrustation, or bladder stones may result from a reaction to a foreign body (catheter) in the bladder, or from colonization with urease-producing bacteria, as discussed above. Gentle irrigation of the catheter with 100 to 200 ml of normal saline will usually clear the tubing of debris. Vigorous irrigation may cause bladder distention and bacteremia from organisms colonized within the bladder. Debris and encrustation may be controlled by maintaining a dilute urine and, if possible, eradicating urease-producing organisms. Bladder stones or debris may cause catheter obstruction; removal is usually possible by cystoscopy.

Urine leakage around the Foley catheter sometimes develops, more often in women. It usually results from bladder spasms in response to infection, obstruction, or stimulation by the catheter balloon of sensory receptors in the trigone area. Urinary tract infection is the most likely cause of sudden leakage in a catheterized patient. It is important not to treat this problem with a larger catheter, which can lead to dilatation of the urethra. Instead, the catheter and balloon placement should be checked, and mechanical obstruction ruled out. The urine should be cultured, and patient treated with a 7- to 10-day course of antibiotics based on the results. If incontinence continues, an anticholinergic medication such as oxybutynin (Ditropan) (2.5–5.0 mg tid) should be tried to decrease bladder spasticity; common side effects include dry mouth and constipation.

External Catheters

External catheters should be considered for men who are able to void, but without control. Overflow incontinence must be ruled out before an external catheter is employed. External collecting devices for women are of limited utility; one type that is secured in the vagina with an adhesive is easily dislodged.

"Condom" external catheters for men are available in a variety of types, differing in the way they are attached to the penile shaft (external tape versus internal circumferential tape or glue), the thickness of the condom, and the type of tip that is connected to the leg bag tubing. Success at keeping the condom attached to the shaft of the penis is the major criterion for choice. Since each patient's anatomy and body habitus are different, a trial of several different types and sizes is often needed. External catheters are sized as pediatric/geriatric (22-mm diameter), small (25-mm diameter), medium (30-mm diameter), and large (35-mm diameter). Another device, a "drip collector" shaped like a condom catheter, can be slipped over the penis; it is made out of an absorbent material that can hold 80 ml of urine, requiring no tubing or bag.

Catheter Placement and Care

Prior to placement of the catheter, the penile skin should be washed with soap and water and dried thoroughly. Pubic hair should be moved off the penile shaft to allow a good seal between the skin and the catheter. Condom catheters should be changed daily and the penile skin inspected for breakdown.

The condom catheter can be used with a leg bag, usually most comfortable for the patient when attached to the upper inner part of the thigh. In an alert hemiplegic patient, the leg bag is best placed on the leg with feeling, so that the patient can help monitor strap tightness and bag fullness. In a cognitively impaired hemiplegic patient, the bag may be best placed on the side with decreased sensation; this gives the patient less stimulus for tampering with the appliance. In patients with no lower extremity sensory deficit, the leg bag should be alternated from one leg to the other to prevent skin breakdown around the straps. The leg bag should be emptied when it is half full, in order to keep urine from refluxing up the tubing and to prevent the bag from getting so heavy that it detaches from the tubing.

Leg bags vary in capacity from 300 ml to 1000 ml; the larger bags are usually preferred because they require less frequent emptying. At night or when the patient is at bed rest, it is recommended that the condom catheter and tubing be connected to a 2-L hanging bag.

Complications

Skin irritation or edema may be caused by a reaction to tape, allergy to soap or the condom, or a condom that is too small. The cause should be identified and corrected, and the skin treated by removing the condom and leaving the penis exposed to the air for a prolonged period. One method is to have the patient sleep with the condom off at night with a urinal between his legs.

Breakdown of skin around the base of the penis or scrotum is most commonly caused by the condom being taped on too tight, by a ridge of excess condom pressing in at the base of the penis, or by poor hygiene. If the breakdown is superficial, the measures described above may suffice. If there is no improvement or skin breakdown is severe, an indwelling catheter should be inserted and left in place until the skin heals.

Condom catheters may repeatedly fall off if they are an inappropriate size and type for the patient, or if the patient has a retractile penis. The bag may disconnect if it is allowed to overfill or if the tubing is an improper length. Older catheters made of thinner latex may twist the tubing.

Woods DR, Bender BS. Long-term urinary tract catheterization. Med Clin North Am 1989; 73(6):1441–54.
Discusses types, complications, and management of indwelling catheters.

Warren JW. Catheters and catheter care. Clin Geriatr Med 1986; 2(4):857–71.
Reviews indwelling, external, intermittent, and suprapubic catheterization, with emphasis on the infectious complications.

Warren JW. Catheter-associated urinary tract infections. Infect Dis Clin North Am 1987; 1(4):823–48.
Extensively referenced review of the spectrum of infections and infectious complications associated with urinary catheters.

Schaeffer AJ. Catheter associated bacteriuria. Urol Clin North Am 1986; 13(4):735–47.
Excellent review including both indwelling and intermittent catheterization.

Diokono AC. Clean intermittent self-catheterization. In Yalla SV, McGuire EJ, Elbadaw A, eds. Neurology and urodynamics. New York: Macmillan, 1988: 410–6.
An in-depth review of IC.

X. MUSCULOSKELETAL PROBLEMS

62. OSTEOARTHRITIS
L. Celeste Robb-Nicholson and Matthew H. Liang

Osteoarthritis, also called *osteoarthrosis* and *hypertrophic* or *degenerative joint disease*, is a generally noninflammatory arthritis seen radiographically in 90% of adults over the age of 50. It is the most common form of chronic arthritis and is responsible for pain and limitation of motion in approximately one-fourth of the adult population.

Primary osteoarthritis accounts for 90% of patients with osteoarthritis in an unselected practice. The most commonly involved joints are the distal interphalangeals (DIPs), proximal interphalangeals (PIPs), hip, knee, first metatarsal phalangeal joint (MTP), and cervical and lumbosacral spine. Some degree of degenerative change in articular cartilage is universal with increasing age, but onset, rate of progression, and severity vary greatly. If a joint is malaligned or has been traumatized or inflamed, the changes appear more rapidly. Secondary osteoarthritis results from mechanical incongruity and/or cartilage destruction, which may be caused by congenital defects, joint infection or inflammation, trauma, or endocrine-metabolic disease.

Clinical Presentation
The most common presenting symptoms in patients with osteoarthritis are pain, stiffness, joint enlargement, and limitation of joint motion. The pain of osteoarthritis begins insidiously; patients describe an aching or nagging discomfort. Morning stiffness or stiffness after prolonged immobility generally lasts less than 30 minutes. Early in the course, joint pain occurs after vigorous activity, but with deterioration and significant structural activity, pain may occur after modest or minimal activity, and eventually, even at rest. For most patients with early osteoarthritis, flares of symptoms are self-limited. It is not clear whether this is the natural course of the disease, whether the pain is caused by synovitis from hydroxyapatite crystals, or whether pain leads to resting of the joint and resolution of symptoms.

Joint enlargement results from osteophyte formation and feels hard in comparison to the spongy feel of synovial proliferation. Deformity and subluxation result from bony overgrowth, loss of cartilage, and collapsed subchondral bone and cysts. Limitation of motion results from joint surface incongruity, muscle spasm, capsular contracture, and structural blockage from osteophytes or loose bodies.

Diagnostic Evaluation
The diagnosis of osteoarthritis is based on characteristic symptoms and physical findings. X-ray evaluation is extremely helpful in the diagnosis of osteoarthritis of weight-bearing joints and the spine. The four cardinal radiologic features that must be present to make a definite diagnosis include (1) unequal loss of joint space (an early finding), (2) osteophytes, (3) eburnation (juxta-articular sclerosis), and (4) subchondral bone cysts. However, the severity of pain in osteoarthritis correlates poorly with the radiologic appearance of the joint. Because the radiographic findings of osteoarthritis are extremely common, the clinician should always consider another diagnosis, especially if the following are present: (1) The complaint is in an uncommon joint for osteoarthritis, such as the glenohumeral joint. (2) Signs and symptoms of systemic illness exist. (3) Neuromotor or vascular symptoms are present. (4) Symptoms have been present for less than a month or are of acute onset. (5) There is objective evidence of synovitis, which is unusual in osteoarthritis.

Laboratory tests are normal in primary osteoarthritis, and therefore are useful only when a diagnosis other than osteoarthritis is suggested by clinical findings.

The approach to osteoarthritis varies somewhat according to the site of involvement.

Hand
Involvement of the hand is characterized by bony proliferation and the absence of objective synovitis in the small joints of the fingers: Heberden's (DIP joints) and Bouchard's (PIP joints) nodes. Early symptoms usually include aching, discomfort, and stiffness, increased by heavy finger use. The first metacarpophalangeal (MCP) joint, the base of the thumb, is a common site and produces pain worsened by gripping and twisting movements of the

hands. Apart from this site, however, MCP joints are rarely involved, except in secondary osteoarthritis after hemochromatosis. X-ray evaluation of Heberden's and Bouchard's nodes is unnecessary.

Hip
Approximately 60% of patients with osteoarthritis of the hip complain of pain in the area of the greater trochanter and, less frequently, pain in the groin, back of the thigh, low back, or referred to the knee. The pain and stiffness associated with early osteoarthritis of the hip usually follow immobility and periods of excessive weight-bearing.

The hip is relatively inaccessible to examination by observation or palpation. The earliest abnormality is reduced internal rotation (normal internal rotation is 35–45°) and abduction (normal is 45–50°). With progression of disease, hip motion is restricted in all directions, and the hip is flexed and foreshortened.

Important negative findings include absence of abnormality in other joints and a normal neuromuscular and vascular examination. Areas about the hip should be palpated for discrete tenderness secondary to bursitis, tendinitis, or muscle spasm. If the pain is referred to the area of the greater trochanter, trochanteric bursitis may be the cause of the pain.

Unequal leg length may be a cause of osteoarthritis of the hip; a difference greater than 1 in., measured from the symphysis pubis to the medial malleolus, could cause hip pain by placing stress on the abductor muscles of the longer leg. Because the leg on the involved side is generally shortened by disease, the finding of a longer leg on the symptomatic side suggests that greater disparity existed before the onset of disease.

The earliest x-ray finding of osteoarthritis of the hip is unequal narrowing of the joint space. Minor narrowing may be detected if there is a difference in width of greater than 1 mm between the joint spaces of the normal and affected sides. If bilateral narrowing is present, unequivocal narrowing must be present before the diagnosis can be made with confidence. The joint space is probably abnormal if it is less than 4 mm in patients under age 70 or less than 3 mm in patients over 70. Osteophytes alone are not diagnostic of osteoarthritis, nor is there a relation between the presence of osteophytes and clinical symptoms.

Primary osteoarthritis of the hip may be classified into two prognostic groups by radiologic picture: superolateral and medial. With superolateral disease, persistent unilateral involvement and progressive symptoms are the rule. In the medial form of osteoarthritis, involvement is usually bilateral initially or with time, and progression is variable.

Knee
Osteoarthritis of the knee produces pain after weight-bearing, particularly climbing, descending stairs, and rising from a sitting position. The diagnosis is made by (1) eliminating other possible causes of knee pain such as pes anserinus or patellar bursitis, tendinitis, internal derangement, inflammatory joint disease, joint instability, and hip disorders; and (2) finding specific clinical and x-ray evidence of osteoarthritis. A weight-bearing film of both knees provides the most sensitive method of looking for cartilage loss and assessing the amount of varus or valgus deformity. Both anteroposterior (AP) and lateral views are necessary. Both knees should be included in the x-rays to evaluate the importance of radiologic changes.

Spine
Virtually everyone has pathologic evidence of osteoarthritis of the spine by age 70, occurring in the vertebrae or posterior diarthrodial joints. The most commonly involved areas are the lower cervical spine (C6–7) and the lower lumbar spine (L3–S1). Osteoarthritis of the spine produces poorly localized pain, which may radiate along the paraspinal areas and extend to the buttocks. Nerve root encroachment by an osteophyte or irritation by synovitis may produce neurologic symptoms. If the spinal cord is compressed, upper motor neuron symptoms may develop. Stiffness and decreased range of motion are common symptoms as well. On examination, stiffness, crepitus, local pain and tenderness, and muscle spasm may be present. In the neck, lateral flexion, rotation, and extension are usually more limited than forward flexion. Two very common syndromes occur in the cervical spine: compression of the sixth cervical nerve and compression of the seventh

cervical nerve. In the former, one may note weakness in the biceps on shoulder flexion and in the wrist extensors by testing wrist extension against resistance. There is diminished biceps deep tendon reflex and diminished sensation to the thumb and index finger. In compression of the seventh cervical nerve, one notes weakness of the triceps by testing extension against resistance, a diminished triceps deep tendon reflex, and diminished sensation to the index and middle fingers.

In the lumbar spine, L4–5 and L5–S1 are most commonly involved. Acute symptoms may be superimposed on chronic mechanical low back pain. Severe loss of spinal mobility usually does not occur until late in the disease.

Involvement of the spine requires AP and lateral and oblique x-ray views. Diagnostic findings include straightening or reversal of lordosis; narrowing of the intervertebral disk spaces with anterior and posterior osteophytes; laterally situated osteophytes on the vertebral bodies; sclerosis; and encroachment on the intervertebral foramina by osteophytes and malaligned vertebral bodies.

Treatment

In the medical management of osteoarthritis, the natural history of the disease must be kept in mind. For example, osteoarthritis of the fingers is generally not progressive and does not lead to crippling or loss of function. Although osteoarthritis of the weight-bearing joints, especially unilateral disease, is more likely to progress, one-third of cases do not.

Preservation of function and reduction in pain are the major goals of management. The therapeutic plan should begin with an evaluation of the effect of the disease on the patient's life. What necessary activities can't the patient do? Does the pain interfere with work, play, or sleep, and how much discomfort is experienced with these activities? Treatable components of joint symptoms such as bursitis and tendinitis should be identified, and biomechanical factors, which may exacerbate the degenerative process, should be reduced.

Biomechanical Factors

Early treatment in osteoarthritis of the hip or knee should be directed at correction of biomechanical problems that accelerate the degenerative process. If a discrepancy in leg length exists, a trial of therapy with a heel wedge of equivalent height may reduce symptoms considerably. Appliances such as canes and crutches are very helpful. For example, a static force of 385 pounds on one hip may be reduced to 66 pounds with a downward push of 38 pounds. Quadriceps-strengthening exercises in osteoarthritis of the knee are useful in providing additional support to the joint. Weight reduction should be recommended, although it is often difficult to achieve. In normal gait, three to five times the body weight is distributed across the knee or hip, and even a modest weight loss can reduce this force considerably.

Osteoarthritis of the cervical or lumbosacral spine may be painful because of nerve entrapment, muscle spasm, and/or joint inflammation. General measures include a cervical collar and cervical traction for cervical spine pain. For lumbosacral spine pain, useful general measures include instructions on techniques to reduce stresses on the back, isometric exercises for the abdominal muscles, and stretching of the hip flexors. A custom-made corset, available through physical therapy departments, is helpful. In acute pain, muscle spasm, or nerve entrapment, the mainstays of treatment are bed rest and analgesics.

Local Measures

In general, cold is likely to be useful in acute musculoskeletal pain and heat in subacute pain. There is no proof that deep heat is better than superficial heat. There is no advantage of one type of superficial heat over another (moist heat, hot packs, hot soaks, paraffin, hot mud). Heating pads should be discouraged because patients may fall asleep during the application and suffer first-degree burns. Relative contraindications to heat include sensory neuropathies and circulatory impairment.

In patients with osteoarthritis of the hands, avoiding excessive finger use, such as in crocheting, is sometimes all that is required for symptomatic relief. Local symptomatic relief may be achieved by soaking the hands in warm water in the morning and using nylon spandex stretch gloves at night. Osteoarthritis of the first carpal-metacarpal joint responds well to thumb splinting. Rarely is surgery necessary, but persons with refractory pain may be considered for joint osteoplasty or arthrodesis. In patients with Heberden's and Bouchard's nodes, occasionally one joint is symptomatic out of proportion to the others, and local steroid injection into the joint or mucinous cyst may offer temporary benefit.

Steroid Injections
A careful search for pes anserinus, trochanteric bursitis, or tendinitis is useful, because these conditions respond to local steroid injection. Intra-articular steroids usually have little role in osteoarthritis of the hip or knee, but can be tried if there is clinical evidence of synovitis (caused by intra-articular debris), or if the onset is abrupt. Steroid injection of the hip is a difficult procedure and should be undertaken only by a skilled rheumatologist or orthopedic surgeon under fluoroscopic guidance. Steroid injections should not be done more than six times in the life of a joint and not within 6 weeks before joint surgery.

Drug Therapy
Anti-inflammatory medication is often useful in osteoarthritis with symptoms such as swelling, stiffness, and warmth. Aspirin and most nonsteroidal anti-inflammatory drugs (NSAIDs) are comparable in their effects and can be used intermittently. For many patients, joint rest or even simpler analgesics, such as acetaminophen, may be sufficient. Recent evidence suggests that prolonged use of NSAIDs may accelerate cartilage degeneration. All the NSAIDs have similar side effects, which include peptic ulceration and bleeding, gastrointestinal intolerance, fluid retention, platelet abnormalities, and hepatic and renal dysfunction (see Chap. 64). In elderly patients, in whom osteoarthritis is particularly common, NSAID-associated gastropathy can be a major problem. Both patient tolerance to side effects and individual therapeutic response may vary from one preparation to another. Therefore, one may be effective when others fail, and, if necessary, several alternatives should be tried. For the majority of patients, flares of symptoms with inflammation are self-limited, and aggressive medication is rarely necessary. Patients should be educated to use aspirin and NSAIDs in a way that best enables them to function with their disease.

Surgery
When joint destruction is advanced and pain or disability is refractory to conservative treatment, total joint replacement should be considered. An "end-stage" joint is likely when the patient is prevented from sleep or minimal weight-bearing by pain, requires narcotics for pain, or has an unacceptable functional limitation. Other considerations include whether the damaged joint is the primary limiting condition, whether the total joint replacement will outlive the patient, and whether there are other treatment options. In the young patient with medial compartment narrowing and varus deformity of the knee, osteotomy may be recommended as a procedure to postpone total joint replacement. Contraindications to total joint replacement include youth (great physical activity may hasten loosening, requiring revision surgery), lack of motivation (recovery after total joint replacement requires vigorous physical therapy), the presence of active infection or severe neurosensory deficits, and inadequate "bone stock."

Pain relief is achieved in more than 90% of patients who undergo total joint replacement of the knee and hip. Clinical failure requiring revision surgery occurs in approximately 2% of patients. Operative mortality ranges from 0.5 to 1.9%; facilities treating 50 patients per year or fewer have a higher mortality. Morbidity is less than 2%, and complications include loosening of the prosthesis with time, deep or superficial infection, and dislocation.

For total joint replacement to be successful, the patient must have a clear understanding of goals. Physical activity is not completely normal after total joint replacement, and patients often must modify habits that place the prosthetic hip at risk of dislocation. Dental and surgical procedures associated with bacteremia should be performed with antibiotic prophylaxis (see Chap. 37). The best results in total joint replacement require careful patient selection, medical follow-up, patient education, and rehabilitation management.

Hamerman D. The biology of osteoarthritis. N Engl J Med 1989; 320:1322–30.
An excellent review of relevant cartilage biochemistry.

Brandt KD. Management of osteoarthritis. In: Kelly WN, et al, eds. Textbook of rheumatology. Philadelphia: Saunders, 1989: 1501–10.
A good general discussion of management.

Sheon RP, Moskowitz RW, Goldber VM. Soft tissue rheumatic pain: recognition, management, prevention. Philadelphia: Lea & Febiger, 1982: 172–202.
A good discussion on examination and diagnosis of soft tissue symptoms associated with osteoarthritis.

Vainionpan S, et al. Tibial osteotomy for osteoarthritis of the knee: a 5 to 10 year follow-up study. J Bone Joint Surg [Am] 1981; 63:938–46.
A review of outcomes.

Harris WH, Sledge CB. Total hip and total knee replacement. Parts I and II. N Engl J Med 1990; 323:725–31, 801–7.
A good general review of management and outcomes.

Liang MH, Cullen KE, Poss R. Primary total hip or knee replacement: evaluation of patients. Ann Intern Med 1982; 97:735–9.
A review of outcomes in total joint replacement and suggested evaluation of patients.

Jubb R. Non-steroidal anti-inflammatory drugs and articular cartilage. Curr Med Lit (Rheumatol) 1984; 3:6–8.
A review of basic research on the effects of aspirin and NSAIDs on articular cartilage.

63. RHEUMATOID ARTHRITIS
Suzanne V. Sauter

Rheumatoid arthritis (RA) is a chronic inflammatory disease of unknown cause that may affect any synovial joint and associated tendon sheath. There is no one typical presentation. It may begin as a symmetric subacute polyarthritis or as an acute asymmetric oligoarthritis or monoarthritis. Morning stiffness lasting several hours is a prominent symptom, as are pain and easy fatigability. Pain and functional impairment are modestly related to the magnitude of synovitis or deformity. Fatigability may be related to the mild-to-moderate anemia that often occurs. Many organ systems may be involved, including the lacrimal and salivary glands, pleura, pericardium, lungs, spleen, bone marrow, and nerves.

The course of RA is highly variable. Approximately 30% of patients have a mild course characterized by months to years of complete or partial remissions between periods of flares and little if any deformity. Another 10% have a single period of active arthritis lasting 6 to 12 months, followed by a long clinical remission with only occasional flares. About 50% of patients have progressive disease but only a small minority (approximately 3% of patients) have a progressive, erosive, destructive arthritis that is resistant to therapy. A poor prognosis has been associated with an insidious onset, with involvement of large proximal joints, presence of rheumatoid factor, development of rheumatoid nodules, and extra-articular manifestations of the disease.

The variable course of RA demands that therapy be tailored to each individual patient. Comprehensive management must include drug, physical and occupational therapy, and assistance with making necessary changes in life-style.

Drug Therapy

Strategy
Drug therapy is usually instituted in three steps. A first-line drug is used to control pain and decrease inflammation; it does not retard progression of disease. First-line drugs, effective in approximately 80% of patients, include aspirin and other nonsteroidal anti-

inflammatory drugs (NSAIDs). A second-line drug is used only after 3 to 6 months of adequate first-line therapy or in patients who have evidence of progressive disease. Second-line drugs are effective in an additional 15 to 20%, and include gold, penicillamine, and antimalarials. A third line of therapy, with immunosuppressive drugs, is required in only those patients who do not respond to second-line drugs or have unrelenting disease. These drugs, primarily prednisone, azathioprine (Imuran), and methotrexate (Rheumatrex), should be used only after consultation with a rheumatologist. The trend has been to use more aggressive therapy earlier in the disease process, especially within the first few years if there is evidence for ongoing disease activity such as persistent synovitis or development of extra-articular manifestations.

First-Line Drugs

Aspirin is the drug of first choice and the standard to which all other drugs are compared. Despite the proliferation of NSAIDs, in large trials none has been shown to be superior to aspirin in all parameters, all are more expensive, and long-term toxicities are not as well characterized. Aspirin should therefore be used first and a switch to another first-line drug made only after there has been no response to aspirin given at therapeutic levels for several weeks.

The anti-inflammatory dosage of aspirin is 3.5 g a day or more; up to 7.8 g a day may be needed to obtain a response. Because the absorption of aspirin is reduced by elevation in gastric pH, concomitant use of antacids decreases serum salicylate levels, and intermittent use results in fluctuating salicylate levels. When given regularly in antiinflammatory doses, small increases or decreases in aspirin dose may result in significantly higher or lower drug levels.

The therapeutic serum salicylate level is about 20 to 25 mg/dl. Tinnitus and decreasing auditory acuity, symptoms of salicylate toxicity, may occur at subtherapeutic salicylate levels in about one-half of patients. Decreasing the dose clears the symptoms but the anti-inflammatory effect may be suboptimal. Serum salicylate levels are helpful in children and older people, who may not report tinnitus or other symptoms of salicylate toxicity.

Aspirin is available in many forms: enteric-coated, microencapsulated, dispersed in a matrix, buffered, condensed, substituted, and mixed with other analgesics (Table 63-1). Enteric-coated and matrix preparations appear to reduce gastrointestinal blood loss, slow absorption, and increase plasma half-life. Condensed aspirin, or salicylsalicylic acid or salsalate, may also cause less dyspepsia and less gastrointestinal bleeding. Substituted salicylates generally are better tolerated by people with dyspepsia and other symptoms related to aspirin.

There is little to recommend one of the substituted salicylates over another. There is no evidence that substituted salicylates are less effective than aspirin. Given the higher costs of special preparations, plain or enteric-coated aspirin in therapeutic doses is the first step in therapy.

Common toxicities of aspirin include tinnitus, as discussed above, and a variety of gastrointestinal side effects (see discussion in Chap. 64). Aspirin also acetylates the platelet membrane and can prolong bleeding for the life of the platelet, or 7 to 10 days. Allergic reactions include rhinitis, bronchospasm, nasal polyps, angioneurotic edema, and urticaria. The use of aspirin in pregnancy is controversial. Although it is apparently not teratogenic, it can cause small birth weight, delayed labor, and bleeding in the mother and newborn child and should not be used in third trimester.

Diflunisal (Dolobid), a drug structurally similar to aspirin, is not metabolized to salicylate, but its clinical pharmacology and indication for use are similar to those of aspirin. Convenience of twice-a-day dosing is its main advantage.

Nonsteroidal anti-inflammatory drugs are summarized in Chapter 64, and their side effects discussed in detail. The responses to aspirin and the newer NSAIDs vary widely from patient to patient. Choosing one of the newer drugs is often based on cost, patient tolerance, frequency of dosing, and specific toxicities. If a patient does not respond to one of the newer drugs, it may be preferable to switch to a drug in another class rather than to another drug of the same class. The variability of patient response makes the selection of NSAIDs more of an art than science. The safety of nonsteroidal drugs during pregnancy has not been adequately studied. Premature closure of the ductus arteriosus is reported with NSAIDs used at term.

Combinations of two or more NSAIDs or NSAIDs and aspirin appear to be irrational. Unintentional combination therapy happens frequently as patients may be taking over-the-counter ibuprofen in addition. These drugs are highly protein-bound and use of two drugs decreases plasma levels and increases excretion. Drug interactions occur, particularly with anticoagulants, and great care must be taken when adding aspirin or a NSAID to another highly protein-bound drug.

Second-Line Drugs

None of the NSAIDs has been shown to slow the disease process in patients with progressive, destructive, erosive, polyarticular disease. A second-line drug (gold, penicillamine, or an antimalarial) is indicated in patients who have not responded after 3 to 6 months of adequate first-line drug therapy and who have evidence of progressive disease (especially the development of marginal erosions). There is equivocal radiographic evidence that gold halts joint destruction in patients with early disease. Both gold and penicillamine can improve subjective and objective disease activity, such as morning stiffness, grip strength, and number of swollen and tender joints. Sedimentation rates and titers of rheumatoid factors also are reduced. Although hydroxychloroquine can reduce symptoms of RA, there is no evidence that it can halt disease progression. All second-line drugs can improve or normalize hemoglobin and improve the subjective sense of well-being.

Parenteral gold therapy is often used before penicillamine or antimalarial drugs, largely because it is an older drug with better characterized benefits and toxicities. Although gold is indicated in active disease, it is ineffective in patients with destructive disease without synovitis, except perhaps in Felty's syndrome. Contraindications include pregnancy, history of gold toxicity, and renal insufficiency.

Gold sodium thiomalate (Myochrysine) and gold thioglucose (Solganal) are the most widely used parenteral preparations. Usually gold is given in two test doses of 10 mg and 25 mg intramuscularly before beginning a trial of 50 mg intramuscularly each week for 20 weeks. Because gold is a slow-acting drug, a 1-g trial is necessary to assess efficacy. If gold is effective after 20 weeks, it is then administered every other week until a total dose of 1.5 g is given, followed by 50 mg every 3 to 4 weeks. There are no clear guidelines to the cessation of therapy if the arthritis is inactive. Often the gold is continued for years or until it is no longer effective.

Side effects of gold have been reported in up to 75% of patients, and proteinuria in up to 25%. In drug trials, about 30% of patients drop out because of toxicity. Because of the wide range of toxicities, physicians must be very familiar with the drug before prescribing it. Toxicities include rash, stomatitis, alopecia, proteinuria, hematuria, nephrotic syndrome, eosinophilia, thrombocytopenia, leukopenia, aplastic anemia, flushing, pulmonary interstitial fibrosis, myalgias, arthralgias, hepatitis, diarrhea, and metallic taste.

Policies for monitoring gold therapy vary considerably. Some centers obtain a blood cell count, including platelet count, and a urinalysis before each injection; others obtain these before every other injection. In either situation, the patient should be queried before each injection about rash, itching, oral lesions, and metallic taste.

Auranofin (Ridaura), the oral form of gold therapy, has been available since 1985, and is better tolerated but less efficacious than parenteral gold. The toxicity profiles are similar, although renal problems and cytopenia are less common with auranofin. The overall dropout rate in drug trials averages 10%. Common adverse reactions include leukopenia (2%), thrombocytopenia (3%), glomerular damage manifested as proteinuria and hematuria (5%), rash (30%), and stomatitis (15%). Diarrhea occurs in nearly one-half of persons receiving the drug. It is managed by reducing the dose from the usual 6 mg a day to 3 mg a day or by dividing the dose to 3 mg twice a day from the usual single daily dose. With these maneuvers, very few patients need to stop the medication because of diarrhea. Auranofin should not be used in patients who have had a severe allergic, hematologic, renal, or dermatologic reaction to parenteral gold.

Like parenteral gold, auranofin is a slow-acting drug requiring at least 3 months before improvement is noticed. If there is no objective response in 6 months, the oral gold should be stopped. Blood cell counts including platelet count and urinalysis should be done monthly.

Penicillamine is used if a patient does not respond to gold or develops a toxicity. It is begun after the gold toxicity resolves; the two drugs are not given concurrently. Penicilla-

Table 63-1. Selected salicylate preparations

Type	Formulations	Dosage	Wholesale cost/day ($)	Comments
ASPIRIN (ACETYLSALICYLIC ACID, ASA)				
Plain aspirin	325-, 500-, 1000-mg tablets	3.5–7.0 g/day in divided doses	0.10–0.75	Should be taken with meals; do not use with anticoagulants
Buffered aspirin	325-, 500-mg tablets	3.5–6.0 g/day in divided doses	0.29–1.80	Buffers are magnesium and aluminum hydroxide or magnesium carbonate and aluminum glycinate; salicylate levels with equivalent doses are lower
Enteric-coated aspirin				
Easprin	975-mg tablets	2.9–3.8 g/day in divided doses	0.70–0.94	Half-life of salicylates increases as dose is increased
Ecotrin	325-, 500-mg tablets	3.5–6.0 g/day in divided doses	0.50–1.10	Enteric coating decreases fecal blood loss about 50%
Generic	325-mg tablets	3.5–6.0 g/day in divided doses	0.40–0.60	
Matrix aspirin				
Zorprin	800-mg capsules	3.2–6.0 g/day	0.94–1.65	Salicylate is released as pH rises in lower duodenum, so use of antacids or H_2-blockers results in greater gastric absorption

SUBSTITUTED SALICYLATE			
Choline salicylate Arthropan	870 mg/5 ml of liquid	3.2–6.0 g/day in divided doses	1.04–1.82
Magnesium salicylate Doan's, others	325-, 500-mg tablets	1.9–3.0 g/day, in divided doses	1.10–1.68
Magnesium choline salicylate Trilisate	500-, 750-, 1000-mg tablets 500 mg/ml of liquid	1.5–3.0 g/day, in once or twice daily dosing	0.94–2.27	Does not affect platelet aggregation
SALSALATE (SALICYLSALICYLIC ACID)			
Disalcid, others	500-, 750-mg tablets	3 g/day, in divided doses	1.48–1.73	Insoluble in gastric secretions, absorbed in small intestine; less blood loss and peptic disease; weak prostaglandin inhibitor; does not inhibit platelet aggregation
DIFUNISAL			
Dolobid	250-, 500-mg tablets	0.15–1.5 g/day, in divided doses	1.56–2.94	Used primarily for treatment of pain, although good anti-inflammatory effects

mine is well absorbed from the gastrointestinal tract but must be given on an empty stomach.

Penicillamine has a high incidence of toxic effects and should be used with great care. Side effects include leukopenia, thrombocytopenia, aplastic anemia, membranous glomerulonephritis with proteinuria and nephrotic syndrome, hematuria, rash, dysgeusia, stomatitis, and induction of autoimmune syndromes such as myasthenia gravis, Goodpasture's syndrome, and systemic lupus erythematosus. The incidence of nephrotoxicity may be increased if there has been previous nephrotoxicity to gold. Dysgeusia, the most frequent side effect, does not necessitate stopping therapy; supplementation of the diet with oral zinc often corrects the change in taste. Penicillamine can block vitamin B_6 (or pyridoxine) metabolism, and supplementation may be necessary if the diet is inadequate.

The toxicity of penicillamine is minimized by a "go slow, go low" regimen. The initial dosage of 250 mg/day is increased by 125- to 250-mg increments every 3 months, to a maximum dosage of 1000 to 1500 mg/day. Usually 2 to 3 months are needed after initiation or change in therapy before its effect can be assessed. Evaluation for side effects include a careful history, blood cell count, platelet count, and urinalysis. These tests are commonly done once every 2 weeks during the first 6 months of therapy and monthly thereafter.

Hydroxychloroquine (Plaquenil) appears to be about as effective as gold in reducing signs and symptoms. The incidence of toxic side effects is about 7%, lower than that for gold or penicillamine. Hydroxychloroquine is given orally at a maximum dosage of 400 mg/day. If the patient responds, the dosage should be reduced after approximately 8 weeks of therapy to the minimum needed to control symptoms.

The most important side effects occur in the eye—pigmentation around the macula, retinal edema, and scotomata, resulting in decreased color vision and visual acuity. Fortunately, decreasing visual acuity is rare, approximately 1 in 1000 patients a year, and blindness is very rare. Ophthalmologic examination is needed at baseline and then every 6 months. The examination should include visual acuity, funduscopy, visual fields, and slit lamp. Other side effects include rash, bleaching of hair, alopecia, leukopenia, agranulocytosis, heartburn, nausea, diarrhea, myopathy, and CNS problems.

Sulfasalazine (Azulfidine), although not FDA-approved for the treatment of RA, is being used. Several trials, including one controlled, double-blinded study comparing sulfasalazine with parenteral gold, have demonstrated that sulfasalazine is about as effective as parenteral gold but better tolerated, although 16% of the sulfasalazine-treated group was withdrawn from therapy because of adverse drug effects including rash, gastrointestinal problems, hepatitis, and leukopenia. The dose of sulfasalazine was increased weekly from 500 mg twice a day to 500 mg 4 times a day. About 10% of sulfasalazine-treated patients were withdrawn because of a lack of response after 3 months of treatment.

Third-Line Drugs

The long-term efficacy of first- and second-line drugs is disappointing in those patients with aggressive disease; some patients fail to respond to therapy, and in others drugs may be initially effective but fail after 12 or more months of therapy. Therefore the trend has been to introduce those third-line drugs with acceptable levels of toxicity earlier into the treatment regimen. Third-line drug therapy includes methotrexate (Rheumatex), azathioprine (Imuran), and several other immunosuppressives, immunomodulators, antimetabolites, and combination therapies which are used experimentally.

Methotrexate is used in patients who have failed on one or more second-line drug therapies, and also should be supervised by a rheumatologist. It has a relatively prompt onset of action, usually within 6 to 8 weeks. It may be given either orally or by intramuscular injections in doses of 5 to 25 mg weekly, 7.5 mg orally being the most common. Adverse reactions may appear in up to 65% of patients receiving the drug, but the usual dropout rate is about 15% in 26-week trials, less than that of penicillamine or injectible gold. Reactions include stomatitis, nausea, alopecia, diarrhea, herpes zoster, headache, mild leukopenia, and thrombocytopenia. The risk of developing cirrhosis of the liver remains unclear, but is probably 1 to 2%; liver biopsies are recommended after 2 years or a 1.5- to 2.0-g total dose of methotrexate. The risk of cirrhosis may be increased if there is a prior history of hepatitis, alcohol ingestion, diabetes mellitus, or obesity. The long-term efficacy and safety beyond a few years of therapy are not known. Obviously careful monitoring and patient selection are critical factors. Women of childbearing potential should not be given methotrexate until pregnancy is excluded and effective contraception is practiced.

Azathioprine (Imuran) should be used only under the supervision of a rheumatologist. An oral dose of 1 to 2 mg/k is given daily. The major toxic reaction is leukopenia, but allergic hepatitis can occur. There is a risk for increasing lymphoreticular and epithelial malignancies.

Corticosteroids are indicated for rheumatoid vasculitis, but the indications for using them in rheumatoid synovitis are unclear. Although few side effects occur when steroids are used for only 1 to 2 weeks, once a corticosteroid is started, it is often very difficult to stop because flares of arthritis occur after withdrawal of the drugs. The benefit of steroids must therefore be weighed against the long-term consequences, which include cataracts, hypertension, diabetes mellitus, myopathy, osteoporosis, cushingoid habitus, and hyperlipoproteinemia. Before steroids are begun, all other regimens such as nonsteroidal drugs, rest, and joint protection should be maximal.

Prednisone is commonly used because of its short duration of action. It should be used at the lowest possible dose, usually less than 10 mg/day, and preferably in an alternate-day schedule.

Intra-articular steroid injections have been widely used, but there are few studies of their efficacy. Benefits from a single injection of a long-acting agent such as triamcinolone hexacetonide (Aristospan) may last from a few days to months. To use repeated injections, each with only short-term benefit, is illogical, if not dangerous.

Supportive Care

Drug therapy is only one part of the management of RA. Other forms of care, such as physical and occupational therapy and surgery, are necessary to decrease pain and maintain function.

Physical Therapy

Physical therapy includes the application of heat and cold, splints, ambulatory aids, and exercises. It helps to maintain range of motion, strengthen weakened muscles, and protect joints. It is not known how much deformity can be prevented, but there is some evidence that overuse or misuse of inflamed joints may hasten deformity.

Referral to a physical therapist experienced in the treatment of arthritis should occur early in the course of disease as well as when there has been a major change in disease activity. A physical therapist can outline an exercise program as well as instruct in the use of heat, cold, ultrasound (deep heat), paraffin, contrast (heat, followed by cold), and relaxation techniques for control of pain. The therapist also can provide gait analysis and prescribe correct footwear.

Rest

During periods of acute synovitis, rest of joints decreases swelling and pain. Patients may feel more fatigued and require limited bed rest; usually 8 to 10 hours at night and 1 to 2 hours during the day are sufficient. If only a single joint, such as a wrist, is inflamed, it can be maintained in a functional position with a lightweight plastic splint. After periods of rest, active range-of-motion exercises are necessary to prevent atrophy. With chronic inflammation, pain and swelling contribute to disuse and atrophy of muscles and flexion contractures.

Heat and Cooling

Cooling is used to decrease pain during acute flares, and heat is used for chronic disease. Both modalities can be applied in several ways, best chosen in consultation with a physical therapist. Indiscriminate use of heat can cause burns, and improper use of ice can cause skin necrosis. Neither should be used if a sensory neuropathy is present. A patient can be taught the use of mineral oil–paraffin baths for hands and other joints. Most patients obtain considerable pain relief from hot showers, a heating pad, or an electric blanket.

Exercise

Range-of-motion exercises are done twice a day, preferably during a time of minimal stiffness such as following a hot shower. Strengthening exercises require increasing the number of repetitions. Weights are seldom used in exercises for RA. In general, isometric exercises are preferable to isotonic exercises because there is less stress on joints. During a flare, the number of repetitions is reduced, but the exercise program, especially range-of-motion exercises, is not stopped.

Gait Analysis
If the hips are painful or knee deformities are present, a therapist can help select an appropriate cane, crutch, or walker to improve gait and protect the damaged joint.

Footwear
RA commonly causes severe foot deformities, such as subluxation of metatarsophalangeal joints, hallux valgus deformities, cock-up or claw toes, widened forefoot, flat feet, inversion or eversion of the ankle, or development of a high longitudinal arch with weight-bearing over the lateral part of the foot. With these deformities, calluses can develop over the points of bony protrusion or painful bunions may form over a hallux valgus. A physical therapist may provide information on appropriate footwear, such as extra-depth shoes, or make appropriate modifications, such as use of molded, closed-cell foam innersoles. In general, shoes should be wide and deep enough to accommodate the wider forefoot and cock-up toe deformities. They should be made of soft and pliable material, with a strong heel counter and rubber soles. For painful metatarsal heads, a metatarsal bar can be added to the rubber sole of a shoe just behind the metatarsal heads. With severe foot deformities, a prosthetist-orthotist can design shoes to accommodate the deformity.

Occupational Therapy
Occupational therapists experienced in the treatment of patients with RA can advise patients concerning the use of lightweight splints and adaptive and assistive devices; they also can assess activities of daily living. Referral should be made early in the course of disease, to teach joint protection and energy conservation before joint deformities occur. Although some splints, such as molded plastic resting splints and gauntlet-type wrist splints, are available commercially, it is advisable to have an occupational therapist check them for proper application. Often therapists can construct either static (resting) or dynamic splints to prevent or correct mild deformities. A wide variety of assistive and adaptive equipment, such as raised toilet seat, grab bar, long-handled shoehorn, adapted bath sponge, eating utensils, combs, and button hooks, can be made or purchased. A therapist can make an analysis of daily activities and provide advice on appropriate equipment to improve function and reduce stress on inflamed joints.

The occupational therapist may need to work with a vocational rehabilitation counselor to assess employment opportunities or modifications in the current job, or to assist in job training or retraining. Educational and social support groups are available to provide information and support for arthritic patients. Some communities have resource directories for therapeutic exercise pool programs, recreational opportunities, and other resources for those with arthritis.

Disability
Patients who have severe functional disability from RA may be eligible for Social Security disability insurance (SSDI) if they have contributed to Social Security or Supplemental Security Income (SSI) if they have not. The specific medical disability criteria for active RA include a "history of persistent joint pain, swelling, and tenderness involving multiple major joints and with signs of joint inflammation on current physical examination despite prescribed therapy for at least three months, resulting in significant restriction of function of the affected joints and clinical activity expected to last at least 12 months." To this information about the clinical presentation must be added documentation of the diagnosis: positive serologic test for rheumatoid factor, or antinuclear antibodies, or elevated sedimentation rate or characteristic histologic changes in biopsy of synovial membrane or subcutaneous nodule.

Objective evidence about functional impairments can be provided in part by carefully kept records of physical, radiographic, and laboratory findings. Information in the medical record should include information about an inability to perform work task and ordinary daily activities.

If medical criteria are insufficient to determine disability, the judgment is based on "functional residual capacity"—that is, the ability to perform basic work activities, such as sitting, standing, walking, lifting, pushing, pulling, and carrying, and activities that require fine dexterity. Finally, some estimate is made of the ability to perform *any* work that may be available in the national economy. Factors included in this step are age, education, and previous work experience. No consideration is given to availability of work.

Surgery
A large number of surgical interventions are now available for correcting the deformities of RA. Because there are few absolute indications for surgery, the patient, surgeon, and primary physician must work together. Most surgery is undertaken for a combination of objective deformity or joint destruction and subjective pain or inability to function.

For some hand deformities, such as tendon tear, soft tissue surgery can be helpful. For persistent synovitis of one or two joints (e.g., elbow or knee) that have failed to respond to medical therapy, a synovectomy may be helpful; it does not slow the disease process but can relieve pain and decrease swelling for several years. Soft tissue surgery is indicated for nerve entrapment such as carpal tunnel syndrome that has not responded to conservative therapy.

Arthroscopic surgery is done for some knee problems such as meniscal tears. Arthroplasty, or total joint replacement, is now well established for the hip, knee, and metacarpophalangeal joints. Arthrodesis, or joint fusion, is still used to stabilize unstable ankles, thumbs, or proximal interphalangeal joints.

Huskisson EC. How to choose a non-steroidal antiinflammatory drug. Clin Rheum Dis 1984; 10:313–23.
Provides excellent advice on NSAIDs summarized as follows: Do not prescribe unless necessary, "beware of high risk drugs, beware of high risk patients," know the medications, and supervise patients closely.

Dromgoole SH, Furst DE, Paulus HE. Rational approaches to the use of salicylates in rheumatoid arthritis. Semin Arthritis Rheum 1981; 11:257–83.
A lengthy discussion of the pharmacology and clinical usefulness of salicylates. Side effects, toxicities, and individual preparations are discussed in detail.

Semble EL, Wu WC. Antiinflammatory drugs and gastric mucosal damage. Semin Arthritis Rheum 1987; 16:271–86.
Review of aspirin- and NSAID-induced acute and chronic damage to gastric mucosa, and its management. These medications need to be taken with food or generous amounts of liquids. H_2-blockers do not seem to reduce gastrointestinal hemorrhage. Prostaglandin E_1 analogue reduces erosion and injury but its role in preventing massive gastrointestinal bleeding is uncertain.

Abramson SB, Weissmann G. The mechanisms of action of non-steroidal antiinflammatory drugs. Arthritis Rheum 1989; 32:1–9.
Discusses prostaglandin- and nonprostaglandin-dependent mechanisms of action. Article reviews effect of NSAIDs on superoxide, phospholipase, chondrocyte proteoglycan synthesis, transmembrane confluxes, and chemoattractant binding.

Roubenoff R, et al. Effects of antiinflammatory and immunosuppressive drugs on pregnancy and fertility. Semin Arthritis Rheum 1988; 18:88–110.
Reviews pubished data on aspirin, NSAIDs, and second- and third-line drugs as they affect fetal development and fertility.

Ward JR, et al. Comparison of auranofin gold sodium thiomalate and placebo in the treatment of rheumatoid arthritis: a controlled clinical trial. Arthritis Rheum 1983; 26: 1303–15.
Recent study of parenteral and oral gold preparations. It references all the classic controlled drug trials showing efficacy of parenteral gold.

Weinblatt ME, et al. Long-term prospective trial of low dose methotrexate in rheumatoid arthritis. Arthritis Rheum 1988; 31:167–75.

Thirty-six-month open trial of methotrexate after randomized crossover trial is reported. Risk of cirrhosis in patients appeared low.

Williams HJ, et al. A controlled trial comparing sulfasalazine, gold sodium thiomalate, and placebo in rheumatoid arthritis. Arthritis Rheum 1988; 31:702–13.
The power of placebo medications can never be underestimated. Thirty-nine percent of patients studied had important improvement with placebo treatment.

Felson DT, Anderson JJ, Meenan RF. The comparative efficacy and toxicity of second-line drugs in rheumatoid arthritis: results of two metaanalyses. Arthritis Rheum 1990; 33:1449–61.
Reports the results of analyzing 66 trials of methotrexate, parenteral gold, penicillamine, sulfasalazine, auranofin, chloroquine, and hydroxychloroquine for relative efficacy. The first four drugs had no detectable differences but all the studies were too small to detect a difference. Seventy-one drug trials were analyzed for toxicity by average dropout rate. Auranofin and antimalarials had the least toxicity. Methotrexate trials had fewer dropouts than did trials of penicillamine, sulfasalazine, and gold.

Yelin E, et al. Work disability in rheumatoid arthritis: effects of disease, social and work factors. Ann Intern Med 1980; 93:551–6.
A study of 180 persons in Massachusetts and California explored factors that influenced work disability from RA. Factors that affected employment included length of illness, severity of disease, education, and autonomy at the workplace.

Meenan RF, Liang NH, Hadler NM. Disability Task Force on the Arthritis Foundation. Social Security disability and the arthritis patient. Bull Rheum Dis 1983; 33:1–7.
A summary of the eligibility criteria for Social Security disability and the process for disability determination, including information on the medical disability criteria, the appeals process, and the process of re-evaluation. There are also suggestions on the physician's role in the process of disability determination.

Challenging the pyramid: a new look at therapeutic approaches for rheumatoid arthritis. March 9–10, 1990, Miami, Florida. J Rheumatol 1990; 17:Suppl 25:1–44.
Eight articles that outline the current controversies in the management of RA, especially the use of the slower-acting, so-called disease-modifying medications. The only consensus seemed to be that these drugs should be used by a competent physician and an informed patient. The diagnosis of RA must be confirmed and the disease must be persistently active; rheumatologists are starting these drugs earlier.

64. NONSTEROIDAL ANTI-INFLAMMATORY DRUGS
Bernard Lo

Nonsteroidal anti-inflammatory drugs (NSAIDs), which have powerful anti-inflammatory and analgesic effects, are widely used for a variety of musculoskeletal conditions. They also may cause serious side effects, accounting for about 20% of adverse drug reports to the Food and Drug Administration (FDA). Both clinicians and patients need to be familiar with the risks of NSAIDs, to ensure that side effects are recognized promptly and that the benefits for a particular patient outweigh the risks.

Faced with a confusing array of new NSAIDs and claims by manufacturers, clinicians may wonder which drugs they should prescribe. No NSAID has been shown to be consistently more effective than other NSAIDs, either for acute or for chronic use. There is no way to predict which NSAID will be most effective for an individual patient: One NSAID may be ineffective or have severe side effects, while another may be both effective and tolerable. For patients with chronic illness that will require long-term usage, a therapeutic trial of several drugs may be necessary, and dosing frequency, cost, and side effects may be deciding factors. Properties of commonly used NSAIDs are described in Table 64-1.

Table 64-1. Nonsteroidal anti-inflammatory drugs*

	Strengths available	Dosage	Daily cost ($) (wholesale)	Comments
PROPIONIC ACIDS				
Ibuprofen Advil, Nuprin, Medipren, others Motrin, Rufen, others	200 mg, over the counter 300-, 400-, 600-, 800-mg tablets	200–800 mg tid–qid	0.23–1.30	Available over the counter at lowest cost Most effective with qid dosing May cause renal insufficiency at dose of 800 mg/day
Naproxen Naprosyn Anaprox	250-, 375-, 500-mg tablets 275-, 550-mg tablets 12.5 mg/5 ml suspension	200–500 mg bid	1.22–1.91	Most popular of bid dosing group
Fenoprofen Nalfon, Fenopron	200-, 300-, 600-mg capsules 600-mg tablets	200–600 mg tid–qid	1.31–2.40	Acute interstitial nephritis may be more common
Ketoprofen Orudis	25-, 50-, 75-mg capsules	50–75 mg tid–qid	1.90–2.95	
Flurbiprofen Ansaid	50-, 100-mg tablets	100 mg bid–tid, or 50 mg qid	1.70–2.50	
INDOLE ACETIC ACIDS				
Indomethacin Indocin, others	25-, 50-mg capsules 75 mg SR	25–50 mg tid 75 mg SR qd–bid	1.40–2.26	Very effective, but relatively high incidence of side effects
Tolmetin Tolectin	200-, 600-mg tablets 400-mg capsules	400 mg tid–qid	2.07–2.76	Causes false-positive sulfasalicylate test for proteinuria

Table 64-1 (continued)

	Strengths available	Dosage	Daily cost ($) (wholesale)	Comments
Sulindac Clinoril	150-, 200-mg tablets	150–200 mg bid	1.64–2.02	Renal toxicity may occur, despite claims that it is renal-sparing
PHENYLACETIC ACID				
Diclofenac Voltaren	25-, 50-, 75-mg tablets (enteric-coated)	50 mg bid–tid 75 mg bid	1.36–2.47	Manufacturer recommends following liver function tests; marked elevations (8 times baseline) occur in 1% of patients
FENAMATES				
Meclofenamate Meclomen	50-, 100-mg tablets or capsules	50–100 mg tid–qid	1.40–2.57	Diarrhea in 10–30% of patients, requiring discontinuation in 4%
OXICAMS				
Piroxicam Feldene	10-, 20-mg capsules	10–20 mg qd	1.00–1.70	Once-a-day dosing possible; elderly patients may need less frequent dosing to prevent accumulation of drug

PYRAZOLES Phenylbutazone Butazolidin	100-mg tablets or capsules	100 mg tid (recommended for short-term use, ≤ 7 days, only)	1.50	While very effective, has relatively high incidence of side effects, including agranulocytosis and aplastic anemia; potentiates effect of oral hypoglycemics and warfarin (Coumadin)
SALICYLATES Aspirin	See Table 63-1 for alternative formulations	See Table 63-1	See Table 63-1	Enteric-coated preparations reduce GI symptoms and can be given bid; may precipitate acute gouty attacks; occult salicylate toxicity may occur, especially in the elderly

*Note: Within each category, the more recently marketed drugs are listed last.
SR = slow release.

Side Effects of NSAIDs

Gastrointestinal Side Effects

GI side effects are the most common, and GI bleeding and perforation the most frequently lethal side effects of NSAIDs. There is no simple way to reduce serious GI side effects of NSAIDs.

Symptoms such as nausea, dyspepsia, and abdominal pain are common and cause about 5% of patients to discontinue NSAIDs. Patients on NSAIDs are also at increased risk for erosions and ulcers as seen on endoscopy; the incidence of new gastric ulcers found on endoscopy in patients taking NSAIDs may be as high as 13% in 1 month. The gastric mucosa probably adapts to continued ingestion of NSAIDs, and many of these endoscopic findings resolve spontaneously. The association between duodenal ulcers and NSAIDs is less clear. Symptoms and endoscopically documented lesions are poorly correlated, and ulcers associated with NSAIDs are more likely to be silent than ulcers found in the general population.

Bleeding is the most serious GI side effect, with a case fatality rate of about 10%. Of every 1000 patients taking NSAIDs, about one or two will require hospitalization for upper GI bleeding. While the relative risk for GI bleeding is low, about 1.5 in users of NSAIDs compared to nonusers, the absolute number of bleeds that occur is high because of the large number of patients taking NSAIDs. NSAIDs similarly increase the risk of GI perforation and of death related to ulcers.

Both local and systemic effects are important in the pathogenesis of ulcers. Inhibition of prostaglandin E_2 by NSAIDs causes breakdown of the gastric mucosal barrier. Claims that certain NSAIDs have less GI toxicity should be interpreted skeptically. For example, sulindac has minimal acute effects on gastric mucosa, but in the long term may actually have a higher risk of upper GI bleeding than other NSAIDs. While newer NSAIDs are touted as having fewer GI complications, one recent study suggested that piroxicam, meclofenamate, and naproxen had a higher rate of GI complications than did ibuprofen.

Risk factors for serious GI toxicity are not well defined. Current GI symptoms do not reliably identify patients at risk for serious complications because in over 50% of NSAID-associated upper GI bleeds, there are no preceding warning symptoms. Patients who previously had to stop NSAIDs because of GI side effects or who have used antacids or H_2-blockers for such side effects are at high risk. Patients on higher doses of NSAIDs and on combinations of NSAIDs, such as those who take over-the-counter ibuprofen in addition to prescribed medications, are also at higher risk for bleeding. Thus it is reasonable to use the lowest dose that is effective and to avoid combinations of NSAIDs. It is likely that patients with previous ulcer disease are at greater risk.

Prevention of NSAID-associated ulcers is complicated and controversial. If a patient taking NSAIDs develops upper abdominal pain, the first step is to consider whether NSAIDs are really needed. If so, the prostaglandin E analogoue misoprostol prevents NSAID-associated gastric ulcers, reducing the incidence from 22% to 6% in one well-designed study. A recent study found that misoprostol was more effective than sucralfate in preventing gastric ulcers in patients who continue to take NSAIDs after developing upper abdominal pain. Neither medication, however, was particularly effective in relieving dyspepsia. While it is plausible that misoprostol prevents GI bleeding associated with NSAIDs, no studies have addressed this issue. The dose of misoprostol is 100 to 200 µg 4 times a day. At these doses, 25% to 40% of patients develop diarrhea, and about 3% cannot tolerate the drug because of severe diarrhea. Misoprostol costs $25 to $50 per month.

Duodenal ulcers develop far less frequently than gastric ulcers in patients taking NSAIDs. Full doses of ranitidine protect against the development of duodenal ulcers in NSAID users but offer no protection against gastric ulcers. Misoprostol may be less effective in preventing duodenal ulcers.

If a patient with a history of serious complications of ulcer disease requires treatment with NSAIDs, it is reasonable to initiate prophylaxis concurrently. Misoprostol would be appropriate for patients with previous complications of gastric ulcer, whereas ranitidine would be appropriate if the complications were due to duodenal ulcers.

If ulcers are documented, NSAIDs should be stopped if at all possible; otherwise treatment with H_2-blockers may be less effective. Large gastric ulcers may require treatment for many months. Omeprazole may be more effective than H_2-blockers for treating gastric ulcers; moreover, continued NSAID use does not impair the effectiveness of omeprazole. The FDA, however, has not approved omeprazole for treating ulcers. Misoprostol may be effective in treating gastric ulcers if NSAIDs must be continued. There are few data to support the use of sucralfate. There is no evidence that switching to another NSAID will potentiate ulcer healing, but stopping cigarette smoking and alcohol ingestion does enhance healing.

Renal Side Effects

Renal insufficiency is the most common renal side effect of NSAIDs. Renal prostaglandins cause vasodilation and maintain renal perfusion when the renin-angiotensin system or the adrenergic nervous system is activated. By inhibiting renal production of prostaglandins, NSAIDs decrease renal blood flow and the glomerular filtration rate. Patients who are taking diuretics or who have congestive heart failure or ascites are at greatest risk. In elderly patients on diuretics, 20% of patients also taking NSAIDs may develop renal insufficiency. Patients with a baseline creatinine concentration greater than 1.5 mg/dl and patients undergoing general anesthesia are also at increased risk. Usually the decline in renal function reverses after the NSAID is stopped. It may be prudent to check a follow-up serum creatinine level in patients who fall into the high-risk categories mentioned above. For patients taking short-acting NSAIDs such as ibuprofen, the creatinine level should be checked within several days of starting therapy. For patients taking longer-acting drugs such as sulindac or piroxicam,. it should be checked 2 or 3 weeks after starting therapy.

Sulindac has been claimed to cause less renal insufficiency than other NSAIDs because it does not inhibit renal prostaglandin production in normal persons. However, in patients with baseline creatinine levels above 1.5 mg/dl or in patients with ascites, sulindac has been shown to compromise renal function.

Sodium and water retention may also result from inhibition of renal prostaglandin synthesis. Clinically this may present as edema, exacerbation of congestive heart failure, or impaired effectiveness of loop diuretics such as furosemide. In addition, NSAIDs enhance the tubular response to antidiuretic hormone, which may lead to water retention and clinical hyponatremia. Severe hyponatremia may occur shortly after initiation of NSAID therapy, particularly in patients already receiving thiazide diuretics.

Hyperkalemia may result from a hyporenin hypoaldosterone state induced by NSAIDs. This may occur both in patients with preexisting renal disease, particularly elderly patients with diabetes, and in normal persons. Patients taking other drugs that impair potassium excretion, such as angiotensin-converting enzyme inhibitors and potassium-sparing diuretics, are at increased risk and should have a follow-up potassium level checked.

Nephrotic syndrome and acute renal failure due to *interstitial nephritis* and *papillary necrosis* have also been reported in patients on NSAIDs.

Impairment of Antihypertensive Drugs

NSAIDs may blunt the effects of antihypertensive regimens, including diuretics, beta-blockers, and angiotensin-converting enzyme inhibitors. The magnitude of the effect is as high as 16/9 mm Hg in the upright position. There is little convincing evidence that any NSAID causes less hypertension, although there is a suggestion that sulindac may be preferable. There are no data to predict which hypertensive patients will be most adversely affected by NSAIDs. It is prudent to recheck blood pressures in hypertensive patients after starting long-term NSAID use.

Hepatic Toxicity

Asymptomatic elevations of liver transaminases and hepatitis have been reported. These abnormalities generally resolve when the drug is discontinued. However, fulminant hepatitis and death have been reported, most recently with diclofenac. Other drugs implicated with fatal liver disease include ibuprofen, fenoprofen, piroxicam, phenylbutazone, and tolmetin. It has been suggested that patients on long-term NSAID therapy who have other risk factors for hepatic injury, such as alcohol use and injection drug use, be monitored with liver function tests.

Other Side Effects
Central nervous system symptoms include headache, tinnitus, dizziness, drowsiness, impaired concentration, confusion, and depression, especially in elderly patients. Indomethacin causes the most CNS toxicity. Aseptic meningitis has been reported, most commonly with ibuprofen.

Hematologic effects inhibit platelet aggregation and can therefore cause bleeding. Unlike aspirin, which irreversibly acetylates platelets for their lifetime of 8 to 10 days, the inhibition caused by other NSAIDs is reversible after the drugs are stopped. Death from agranulocytosis and aplastic anemia are well recognized, most frequently with phenylbutazone. Diclofenac has also been implicated in aplastic anemia.

Allergic reactions include anaphylaxis. Patients with the aspirin hypersensitivity syndrome of asthma and nasal polyps may also react to other NSAIDs.

Dermatologic reactions include a variety of rashes, urticaria, and rarely, Stevens-Johnson syndrome.

Drug Interactions
Most NSAIDs are bound to plasma proteins. They may displace other tightly bound drugs, such as sulfonylurea oral hypoglycemic agents, warfarin, and phenytoin, and increase their activity. Through their effect on platelets, NSAIDs can potentiate the bleeding tendency caused by heparin and warfarin. In addition, drugs such as phenylbutazone and meclofenamate prolong the prothrombin time in patients taking warfarin. NSAIDs may also alter the metabolism of other drugs, with phenylbutazone being most widely implicated.

Salicylates
Aspirin is the oldest anti-inflammatory drug. When used wisely, it is both effective and inexpensive. Aspirin and other salicylic acid derivatives are available in a variety of preparations (see Table 63-1 in Chap. 63).

Clinical Pharmacology
Aspirin is rapidly hydrolyzed to salicylate, which is biologically active. Anti-inflammatory effects are achieved at serum levels of 15 to 30 mg/dl. Analgesic effects may be achieved at lower doses.

Salicylate is metabolized by the liver. At near anti-inflammatory doses (usually about 4 g/day), the two major metabolic pathways can be saturated. A small increase in the dose of aspirin can then cause a dramatic increase in serum levels. In addition, the plasma half-life of salicylate is proportional to serum levels; the higher the serum level, the longer the half-life. Thus at near anti-inflammatory doses, the dose should be increased by no more than 1 tablet a day. A steady state will occur only after the patient has been on the new dose for a week.

Side Effects
Aspirin, like other NSAIDs, causes GI symptoms, gastric ulcers, and upper GI bleeding. Enteric-coated preparations cause fewer symptoms and endoscopic abnormalities. However, there is no clear evidence that enteric-coated aspirin reduces the risk of upper GI bleeding. In fact, there is no evidence that any form of aspirin has a different risk of GI bleeding than other NSAIDs. A variety of other measures are frequently taken to reduce GI symptoms, including taking aspirin with meals, dissolving the tablets in water, or using buffered aspirin. None of these approaches, however, has been rigorously shown to reduce GI distress.

Tinnitus and hearing loss occur at serum salicylate levels between 20 and 45 mg/dl. Clinical lore advised using tinnitus to estimate serum salicylate levels; when tinnitus was reached, lowering the dose slightly would result in a therapeutic anti-inflammatory level. This approach is unreliable, particularly in elderly persons who have high-frequency hearing loss and do not experience tinnitus even at toxic serum salicylate levels.

Occult salicylate toxicity may occur, especially in elderly patients. It may present as dyspnea or tachypnea (due to the direct effect of aspirin on the respiratory center, causing respiratory alkalosis). It may also present as confusion, lethargy, ataxia, tinnitus, or hearing loss. Other features are dehydration, oliguria, and metabolic acidosis. The diagnosis may be missed, and patients in whom treatment is delayed have a higher mortality.

Aspirin must be used carefully in patients with gout. Salicylate at low doses raises serum uric acid levels, and at higher doses can lower it. In either case, gouty attacks can be precipitated.

Other side effects are similar to those of other NSAIDs.

Drug Interactions
Antacids, which are often taken to reduce the GI distress that aspirin frequently produces, lower serum salicylate levels by reducing the absorption of aspirin and enhancing the excretion of salicylate. Furthermore, if antacids are discontinued, serum levels of salicylate may rise. Corticosteroids also lower serum salicylate levels, so the salicylate level may rise if concomitantly administered steroids are discontinued.

Aspirin may enhance the therapeutic effects of warfarin and oral hypoglycemics, so that doses of these drugs may need to be lowered.

Minimizing the Risks of NSAIDs

Clinicians can take several steps to minimize the risks of NSAIDs. Consideration of the following questions may help.

Does the patient really need an NSAID? Can other drugs, such as acetaminophen, be used to relieve the patient's symptoms? Might nonpharmacologic therapies, such as heat, be effective?

Is this patient at increased risk for side effects? As discussed above, patients with preexisting ulcer disease and renal insufficiency are at increased risk. Concomitant use of corticosteroids also increases risk. Furthermore, patients who have congestive heart failure or ascites, who are taking loop diuretics, or who have impaired potassium excretion are at increased risk of renal complications.

Elderly patients whose chronic illness will require long-term therapy are at increased risk because of preexisting renal impairment, decreased drug clearance, and greater susceptibility to adverse drug reactions. In contrast, younger, otherwise healthy patients who have an acute condition that will not require long-term use are at less risk.

Are some NSAIDs more risky? Clinicians appreciate that indomethacin and phenylbutazone, while very effective, have greater risks than other NSAIDs. In addition, meclofenamate has more side effects than other NSAIDs.

There is no convincing evidence that any of the NSAIDs have fewer side effects than others. Comparing side effects of different drugs is problematic because it is difficult to control for dosage, duration of treatment, severity of illness, and comorbid conditions. As with other classes of drugs, clinicians should become familiar with a few NSAIDs, rather than trying to use the entire pharmacopeia. In general, it is better to prescribe NSAIDs with which there is greater clinical experience, rather than the newest NSAID. In recent years, several new NSAIDs have been withdrawn because of serious side effects. In 1982 benoxaprofen was withdrawn because of fatal hepatitis. In 1987 suprofen was withdrawn because of its association with a syndrome of flank pain and acute renal failure in young, otherwise healthy patients.

How can the risks be minimized? Careful monitoring and follow-up, as discussed previously, are essential. For the elderly, lower or less frequent doses may be clinically effective, while reducing the risk of GI and renal side effects.

Paulus HE. Nonsteroidal anti-inflammatory drugs. In: Kelly WN, ed. Textbook of rheumatology. Philadelphia: Saunders, 1989:765–91.
Comprehensive review of these drugs.

Hawkey CJ. Non-steroidal anti-inflammatory drugs and peptic ulcers: facts and figures multiply, but do they add up? Br Med J 1990; 300:278–84.
Superb review of the issues and controversies. Points out basic epidemiologic and clinical questions that need to be answered.

Soll AH, et al. Nonsteroidal anti-inflammatory drugs and peptic ulcer disease. Ann Intern Med 1991; 114:307–19.
Comprehensive review of the topic.

Clive DM, Stoff SJ. Renal syndromes associated with nonsteroidal antiinflammatory drugs. N Engl J Med 1984; 310:563–72.
Classic review of the topic.

Murray MD, Brater SC. Adverse effects of nonsteroidal anti-inflammatory drugs on renal function. Ann Intern Med 1990; 112:559–60.
Brief editorial review, emphasizing acute renal failure within days of starting ibuprofen.

Radack K, Deck C. Do nonsteroidal anti-inflammatory drugs interfere with blood pressure control in hypertensive patients? J Gen Intern Med 1987; 2:108–12.
Critical evaluation of the relevant literature.

Gay GR. Another side effect of NSAIDs. JAMA 1990; 264:2677–8.
Editorial review of hepatotoxicity with NSAIDs, particularly a recent report of fatal hepatotoxicity with diclofenac.

Kimberly RP, Plotz P. Salicylates including aspirin and sulfasalazine. In: Kelley WN, ed. Textbook of rheumatology. Philadelphia: Saunders, 1989:739–64.
Comprehensive review of salicylates, calling enteric-coated aspirin an almost ideal NSAID.

Diclofenac. Med Lett Drugs Ther 1988; 30:109–11.
Warns about hepatic and bone marrow toxicity associated with this drug. In general, this publication is a good source of critical information about new drugs.

65. GOUT
Kenneth E. Sack

Gout is an inflammatory joint disease induced by uric acid crystals. It occurs more commonly in men, with a peak onset between ages 40 and 60. In women, gout typically appears after menopause. Primary gout results from the overproduction or underexcretion of uric acid. Most patients, however, are underexcretors. For other causes of hyperuricemia, see Chapter 95.

The risk of developing acute gout is directly proportional to the degree and duration of hyperuricemia. Patients with higher serum urate levels generally experience their first attack of gout earlier in life. The Framingham Study showed that gout first appeared at a mean age of 39 years in patients with maximum serum urate levels of 9 mg/dl or greater, and at 50 years in those with serum urate levels of 7 to 8 mg/dl. During a 12-year observation period, gout developed in 14% of men with an initial serum urate level between 7 and 8 mg/dl and in 83% of those with a serum urate level of 9 mg/dl or more. The relatives of patients with gout are at higher risk for having the disease, even if they have normal serum urate levels; gout is particularly common in relatives of women who manifest the disease before menopause.

Acute Gouty Arthritis
Acute gout typically manifests as the sudden onset of pain and swelling in a distal joint. The involved joint is usually warm, dusky red, and exquisitely sensitive to touch. The first metatarsophalangeal (MTP) joint is the target in 50% of initial gouty attacks; eventually 90% of patients have an attack in this joint (podagra). Additional causes of podagra include joint infection, cellulitis, osteoarthritis, superficial bursitis, trauma, pseudogout, sarcoidosis, psoriatic arthritis, reactive arthritis (e.g., Reiter's syndrome), and embolic disease. Other joints commonly affected by gout are (in order of frequency): the ankle, knee, wrist, finger, and elbow. A polyarticular onset of gout occurs in 10 to 15% of patients, most often women. In these patients, the serum urate level is frequently less than 7 mg/dl. Gout may develop in a distal interphalangeal joint previously damaged by osteoarthritis, especially in elderly women who have been taking diuretics for a prolonged period.

Gout recurs within 1 year after the first episode in more than 50% of patients. Subsequently, attacks become more frequent; by 10 years, 90 to 95% of untreated patients have had recurrences.

Tophaceous Gout

Tophi are nodular deposits of uric acid that reflect the degree and duration of hyperuricemia. They rarely appear if the serum urate level is persistently below 10 mg/dl and seldom become visible until 10 years after the onset of gout.

Typical locations for tophi are the proximal ulnar surface of the forearm, the olecranon process, the Achilles tendon, and the pinna of the ear; but tophi may develop virtually anywhere including the spinal articulations. Tophi are not visible on radiographs unless they have become calcified. They characteristically produce sharply marginated erosions just proximal to the joint space, often accompanied by an overhanging rim of cortical bone. Joint space narrowing in chronic tophaceous gout, unlike that in rheumatoid arthritis, tends to occur late in the disease. Fortunately, tophaceous gout is decreasing in frequency; but it is still around, often mimicking rheumatoid nodulosis.

Diagnosis

Gout is the likely diagnosis in a patient with acute, self-limited attacks of inflammation in characteristic joints, particularly in the presence of hyperuricemia or with a history of gout in a family member. Even when clinical manifestations are typical and are accompanied by an elevated serum urate level, the diagnosis is never certain until aspiration of an affected joint demonstrates urate crystals in the synovial fluid. (Urate crystals are needle-like, slightly larger than a red blood cell, and show strong negative birefringence). If the tap is "dry," the fluid expressed from the aspirating needle may contain the diagnostic crystals. Compensated polarized light microscopy facilitates correct crystal identification. Making a definitive diagnosis avoids potentially serious errors, such as missing a mimicker of gout (e.g., septic arthritis) or instituting long-term prophylaxis inappropriately.

False-negative findings from the aspirated material can occur when the fluid comes from a contiguous uninvolved area, the crystals settle out in the joint itself or in the tube containing aspirated fluid, the crystals exist in a solely ultramicroscopic form, the examiner is inexperienced in identifying crystals, or the polarizing equipment does not have a compensator. False-positive results on synovial analysis can result when changes in temperature and pH cause crystals to form in the aspirated material or when other crystals or contaminants look like urate crystals.

Treatment

Acute Gouty Arthritis

For many years, colchicine in high doses (e.g., 0.5 mg taken orally every 1–2 hours until symptoms abate or gastrointestinal disturbance ensues) was the preferred treatment for acute gout. It served also as a maneuver to confirm the diagnosis. However, with the currently available potent and well-tolerated anti-inflammatory agents, it is rarely necessary to subject patients to the gastrointestinal side effects of high-dose oral colchicine. Additionally, patients with other forms of crystal-induced arthritis (e.g., pseudogout) and those with sarcoid arthritis or psoriatic arthritis may also respond to high-dose colchicine therapy, rendering the drug less useful as a means of diagnosing gout.

Virtually any nonsteroidal anti-inflammatory drug (NSAID) is effective in treating acute gout. Many clinicians use indomethacin as initial therapy, possibly because it was the first NSAID proved to be as effective as the more toxic phenylbutazone. Unfortunately, central nervous system side effects (e.g., migraine-like headache) preclude the use of indomethacin in some patients. But all NSAIDs have toxicities that can limit their usefulness in treating acute gout. Injury to the gastrointestinal tract is common, especially in elderly patients, and nephrotoxicity is a problem in patients with compromised renal function. See Chapter 64 for further details.

When NSAIDs are contraindicated, a short course of oral or parenteral steroid therapy can ameliorate acute gout (e.g., 30 mg of prednisone or methylprednisolone given daily for 2–3 days, then tapered over 5–7 days). Similarly, a steroid injection into the affected joint can terminate an attack of gout.

For hospitalized patients unable to take oral medications, intravenous colchicine is often effective treatment for acute gout and causes little gastrointestinal toxicity. The usual dose is 2 mg initially, followed if necessary by 1 to 2 mg 5 to 6 hours later. The colchicine is diluted in 15 to 20 ml of 5% dextrose and water or normal saline and administered slowly to avoid extravasation (colchicine is a highly irritative substance). Administering more than 5 mg of colchicine in a 24-hour period may induce bone marrow toxicity.

Prophylaxis
A single episode of acute gout does not necessarily call for long-term prophylaxis. The Framingham Study showed that during a 12-year observation period, 25% of patients with acute gout had only one episode. Usually, however, patients with a serum urate level greater than 7 mg/dl have multiple attacks, which tend to occur with greater frequency over time. Individuals with recurrent attacks require prophylaxis aimed at reducing serum urate levels to 6 mg/dl or less. For highly motivated patients who are reluctant to take medications for prolonged periods, reducing the intake of high-purine food (organ meats, sweetbreads, yeast, sardines, herring) and abstaining from alcohol can help lower serum urate levels and may reduce the frequency of gouty attacks. When patients taking diuretics suffer repeated gouty attacks, it is advisable to discontinue the diuretic and, if possible, substitute an agent that does not increase serum urate, such as a beta-blocker or an angiotensin-converting enzyme inhibitor, for control of hypertension. Alternatively, a urate-lowering agent may be added.

Lowering of serum urate levels can induce a flare of gout or prolong an ongoing attack. It is advisable, therefore, to start maintenance colchicine therapy (0.5 mg 1–3 times a day) several weeks before administering urate-lowering drugs. The rare patient who cannot take any of the urate-lowering agents may use chronic low-dose colchicine therapy alone to reduce the frequency of gouty attacks.

Choices of urate-lowering drugs include agents that augment excretion of uric acid in the urine and those that decrease the formation of uric acid during purine metabolism. Knowing the patient's creatinine clearance rate and 24-hour urinary uric acid excretion can facilitate the correct choice. The risk of developing renal calculi while taking uricosuric agents increases if urinary excretion of uric acid in 24 hours is greater than 600 mg after 3 days of a low-purine diet or 800 mg during intake of a normal diet. Moreover, uricosurics are relatively ineffective when the creatinine clearance is less than 50 ml per minute. Allopurinol, a xanthine oxidase inhibitor, is effective with low creatinine clearance rates, but the dosage should be adjusted downward to reduce the potential for toxicity.

URICOSURIC THERAPY. For patients who do not overexcrete uric acid, a uricosuric agent such as probenecid, with its excellent safety record, is the first choice for prophylaxis of gout. The starting dose of probenecid is 250 mg twice daily with hydration adequate to maintain high urine flow. The dose is gradually increased until serum urate levels are normal; urine uric acid excretion will then diminish (unless the patient has tophi), obviating the need for further vigorous hydration. The usual maintenance dose of probenecid is between 1 and 3 g/day. Side effects are rare and consist mainly of rash and gastrointestinal disturbance. Sulfinpyrazone, a phenylbutazone analogue, is another potent uricosuric agent. Its antiplatelet activity could theoretically benefit a patient with concomitant peripheral vascular disease. The maintenance dose of sulfinpyrazone is usually between 200 and 800 mg a day. Gastrointestinal toxicity is more common with sulfinpyrazone than with probenecid. Complete blood cell counts are advisable periodically for patients receiving sulfinpyrazone because of the possibility of bone marrow depression.

A year's therapy with either probenecid or sulfinpyrazone costs about $200 to $300.

Allopurinol is the agent of choice for hyperuricemic patients with profound uricosuria or depressed renal function. Most patients with tophaceous gout, even those receiving probenecid, will require allopurinol, both to speed the regression of tophi and to prevent the continued hyperexcretion of uric acid. Allopurinol requires only one dose a day because of the long half-life of its active metabolite, oxypurinol.

The side effects of allopurinol are usually mild and include rash, pruritus, and gastrointestinal disturbance. Desquamative skin rash, vasculitis, hepatitis, and renal failure occur rarely, but can be life-threatening. Prudence dictates starting treatment with a low dose of allopurinol (e.g., 100–200 mg/day) and gradually increasing the dose until the serum urate is approximately 6 mg/dl. Downward adjustment of allopurinol dosage in patients with renal insufficiency helps avoid severe reactions. Thus, a patient with completely normal renal function can usually tolerate 300 to 400 mg of allopurinol a day, whereas a patient with absent renal function needs only 100 mg every 3 days. A dose of 200 mg a day is probably the maximum for a patient with a creatinine clearance rate of 50 to 60 ml per minute.

As an xanthine oxidase inhibitor, allopurinol can greatly reduce the metabolism of azathioprine and 6-mercaptopurine. If concomitant use of these drugs is necessary, dosage of the cytotoxic drug should be reduced by approximately 75%. Allopurinol also increases the toxicity of cyclophosphamide. Ampicillin-related skin rashes are common in patients taking allopurinol.

A year's therapy with allopurinol costs $60 to $100.

Appelboom T, Bennett JC. Gout of the rich and famous. J Rheumatol 1986; 13:618–22.
Excellent account of gout through the ages. Did lead poisoning contribute to the downfall of the Roman Empire?

Becker MA. Clinical aspects of monosodium urate monohydrate crystal deposition disease (gout). Rheum Dis Clin North Am 1988; 14:377–94.
In-depth review of hyperuricemia, atypical presentations of gout, and the methods of establishing the diagnosis of gout.

Bomalski JS, Schumacher HR. Podagra is more than gout. Bull Rheum Dis 1984; 34:1–8.
The complete differential diagnosis of podagra. Also describes the use of colchicine in the diagnosis of gout.

Halla JT, Ball GV. Saturnine gout: a review of 42 patients. Semin Arthritis Rheum 1982; 11:307–14.
Fascinating historical review of lead poisoning as a cause of gout.

Lawry GV, Fan PT, Bluestone R. Polyarticular versus monoarticular gout: a prospective, comparative analysis of clinical features. Medicine 1988; 67:335–43.
A review stressing the unusual clinical features of polyarticular gout. Unfortunately, this is a Veterans Administration study and is limited to male patients.

Simkin PA. Management of gout. Ann Intern Med 1979; 90:812–6.
Superb, practical approach to the treatment of the patient with gout.

Simkin PA, Campbell PM, Larson EB. Gout in Heberden's nodes. Arthritis Rheum 1983; 26:94–7.
One of the first and best descriptions of this increasingly recognized phenomenon.

Wallace SL, Singer JZ. Therapy in gout. Rheum Dis Clin North Am 1988; 14:441–57.
An up-to-date, detailed review of urate-lowering and antiinflammatory drugs used in treating gout.

66. OSTEOPOROSIS
Philip D. Sloane and Steven R. Cummings

Osteoporosis is a general term for a variety of conditions characterized by a decrease in bone mass with an otherwise normal structural matrix. Most cases are idiopathic and occur in elderly people ("involutional osteoporosis"). Less than 10% of cases in women occur secondary to identifiable factors such as hyperthyroidism, use of exogenous corticosteroids, Cushing's disease, malabsorption, or renal tubular acidosis.

Osteoporosis increases the risk of fractures, primarily involving the hip, spine, and wrist. It leads to considerable pain and disability and contributes to thousands of deaths annually in elderly patients, as well as over a billion dollars a year in acute medical services alone.

Causes

Osteoporosis of the elderly occurs as part of normal aging. Skeletal mass peaks by age 30 in both men and women, is well maintained until approximately 45 years old, and then begins to decline by about 1% per year. In women this rate is accelerated during the first 5 years after menopause, to about 2 to 8% a year; it slows down to about 1% again after the age of 60. Because women generally begin with a smaller bone mass than men and have this period of accelerated loss, they are at increased risk of fractures. By age 80, a white woman is likely to have lost about 40% of her bone mass.

Many risk factors for osteoporosis have been proposed but few documented. Apart from age, the best established risk factors are race, thin body habitus, alcohol use, cigarette smoking, and corticosteroid therapy. White and Asian women have about a two to three times greater risk of hip fracture than do black or Hispanic women, primarily because their peak bone mass is less. Thin women have about twice the risk of fractures as obese women, possibly because they maintain lower levels of estrogen after menopause than do obese women and because obesity, by putting greater stress on bones, may lead to a higher peak bone density. Alocohol causes osteoporosis by suppressing synthesis of new bone. Women who consume more than two drinks a day have about a 25 to 50% increased risk of hip fractures and men who drink this amount double their risk of vertebral fractures. There is, however, no good evidence that consuming less than two drinks a day increases the risk of osteoporotic fractures. Cigarette smokers have lower estrogen levels than nonsmokers and may have lower bone densities. Corticosteroids interfere with calcium absorption and suppress formation of new bone, and chronic use increases the risk of fractures, particularly of the ribs and vertebrae. Less common risk factors for osteoporosis include: oophorectomy before natural menopause, prolonged bed rest, gastrectomy, and prolonged hyperthyroidism. Proposed risk factors that are controversial include a family history of osteoporotic fractures, low-calcium diet, high-protein diet, caffeine, sedentary life-style, diabetes, and antacids. Pregnancy and breast-feeding do not increase a woman's risk, and may even be protective.

Diagnosis

Differential Diagnosis
Bone demineralization and fractures also result from osteomalacia, an abnormally slow rate of bone matrix calcification caused by severe vitamin D deficiency, or rarely, tissue insensitivity to vitamin D. Although pure osteomalacia is rare in the elderly, it can coexist with osteoporosis. The distinction is important because osteomalacia can be treated with vitamin D. Patients at risk for osteomalacia might be identified by a history of malabsorption; previous gastrectomy; dietary vitamin D deficiency; prolonged ingestion of phenytoin, phenobarbital, or glutethimide; renal tubular acidosis; and severe chronic renal disease.

Presentation
Osteoporosis is often first suspected when a relative demineralization (osteopenia) of bone is noted on x-rays taken for an unrelated reason. A history of risk factors may also suggest the diagnosis long before the onset of symptoms. The onset of symptoms such as back pain or bone fractures occurs late, often after 20 to 25 years of net bone loss. Back pain occurs when there are compression fractures, usually located in the mid to low thoracic or lumbar regions; it is exacerbated by new fractures, often occurring during minor activity such as walking, making a bed, or tugging open a window. Multiple compression fractures of the thoracic spine lead to chronic backache, disability, and thoracic kyphosis. In addition to the spine, the wrist, hip, rib, and other bones may be fractured by very mild trauma.

Physical findings in osteoporosis are nonspecific unless an acute fracture is present. Height loss of up to 5 in. is found in severe cases because of compression fractures. The "dowager's hump," a thoracic kyphosis developing in middle age, may also be noted.

X-rays
X-rays are not very helpful in the early identification of patients at risk; osteopenia seems not to be evident on x-ray until bone mass has been significantly reduced. Although limited as screening tools, x-rays are valuable in diagnosing fractures. Compression fractures of

the vertebrae and cortical thinning are the major signs of osteoporosis. Pseudofractures, which appear as radiolucent bands, usually perpendicular to the bone surface, suggest osteomalacia; they are probably a consequence of trauma with an inability to repair microdamage.

Densitometry
Several accurate methods for measuring the mineral content of bone are available for clinical use. Single-photon absorptometry measures the mineral content of the forearm; dual-photon or dual x-ray absorptometry can measure the mineral content and density of the spine or hip; quantitative CT scanning measures the density of trabecular bone within the spine. Several studies have found that women with lower bone densities have a greater risk of future fractures. Densitometry may therefore be useful when decisions about long-term estrogen therapy depend on a woman's risk of future osteoporotic fractures. These measurements may also be useful in determining whether fractures or mild vertebral deformities are due to osteoporosis. Because bone density generally changes slowly (1–2%/year), densitometry is not precise enough to be used to assess rates of bone loss in normal women or to assess response to preventive therapies such as estrogen or calcium. However, serial measurements of rates of change may be useful in patients such as those treated with corticosteroids, who may be expected to have large and rapid (5–20%/year) changes in bone mass. The choice of densitometry method is controversial; their comparative accuracy in predicting various types of fractures has not been adequately studied.

Laboratory Tests
There are no laboratory findings diagnostic of osteoporosis; however, the laboratory is used to exclude other causes of osteopenia. The following tests may be helpful for patients with severe osteopenia: measurements of calcium, phosphorus, and alkaline phosphatase (all of which are normal in most cases of osteoporosis, and abnormal in osteomalacia or hyperparathyroidism); determination of albumin content (to allow interpretation of serum calcium); serum and urine protein electrophoresis (to rule out multiple myeloma); thyroxine (T_4) index and/or thyroid-stimulating hormone (TSH) (to screen for hyperthyroidism); and BUN-creatinine (to rule out chronic renal disease). If other causes of secondary osteoporosis are suspected, such as Cushing's disease, alcoholism, or cirrhosis, additional laboratory studies are needed.

Treatment
Treatment of established osteoporosis with fractures should be individualized, considering the patient's age, severity of disease, and other health problems. Patients with acute symptoms, such as back pain secondary to a compression fracture, require rest, and analgesia. Immobilization, including back braces, should be minimized because it aggravates demineralization. Acute pain usually subsides in about 4 to 6 weeks.

For all patients, rehabilitation is important. Retraining in the activities of daily living, and practice using assistive devices such as long-handled shoehorns and reachers may be useful. To reduce the risk of further fractures, risk of falling should be assessed and appropriate interventions made, such as training in the use of walking aides and modifications in the home environment (grab bars in tub or shower, removal of scatter rugs).

Referral to an endocrinologist for further evaluation and/or aggressive treatment (such as regimens involving calcitonin or bisphosphonates) is appropriate for nonalcoholic men and premenopausal women with osteoporosis, and postmenopausal women with recurrent painful vertebral fractures during treatment with estrogens.

Prevention
Because osteoporosis has a long asymptomatic phase and is often far-advanced by the time it is diagnosed, strategies begun earlier in life may prevent or delay the disease. During childhood and young adulthood, regular physical exercise and adequate calcium intake might facilitate maximum accumulation of skeletal mass. Abstinence from cigarette smoking and limiting alcohol consumption to less than two drinks a day may also be protective, and are appropriate recommendations for women in all age groups. There is some evidence

that weight-bearing exercise may slow bone loss, but that the benefit is lost after the exercise program is stopped.

Calcium alone seems to retard bone loss, especially in women who consume less than 400 mg of calcium a day. Premenopausal women require at least 1 g and postmenopausal women at least 1.5 g of elemental calcium daily to avoid having a negative calcium balance. Good dietary sources of calcium include sardines (560 mg of calcium/100 g), green vegetables (100–200 mg/100 g), cheeses (up to 1200 mg/100 g), and skim milk (1.2 g/quart). Simple and inexpensive calcium supplements include generic calcium carbonate, oyster-shell calcium, and Tums antacid (6 tablets = 1200 g of calcium). Women who are older than 65 should take their calcium supplements with meals to enhance absorption; about 10% of elderly persons have decreased production of gastric acid that can interfere with the absorption of calcium preparations taken without food.

Estrogens reduce the rate of fractures. They appear to be most effective in the few years immediately following menopause, when the rate of bone demineralization is most active; long-term use reduces the risk of hip, wrist, and vertebral fractures by about 50%. However, if a woman stops taking estrogen, her bone loss resumes at the accelerated, early postmenopausal rate; much of the protection against hip fractures may be lost within 5 years of discontinuing treatment.

To prevent bone loss, women should take at least 0.625 mg of conjugated estrogen or estrone, or 0.02 mg of ethinyl estradiol a day. Because this dose has been associated with a two- to fourfold increase in the risk of endometrial cancer, it is usually recommended that estrogens be accompanied by a progestin. Adding 5 or 10 mg of medroxyprogesterone or 0.70 mg of norethindrone acetate daily for the last 10 to 12 days of estrogen therapy each month prevents the endometrial hyperplasia thought to predispose to cancer. It also results in withdrawal bleeding, which some patients may find troublesome. Continuous regimens, using lower doses of progestin (2.5 mg of medroxyprogesterone or 0.35 mg of norethindrone) taken daily along with estrogen, have been advocated to reduce the frequency of vaginal bleeding after the first year of therapy; the effectiveness of continuous regimens in preventing endometrial cancer is not as well documented. Progestins, by decreasing serum high-density lipoprotein (HDL) levels, may also counteract the beneficial effect of estrogens on cardiovascular risk. Some women may choose to use estrogen alone to prevent osteoporosis. Annual endometrial biopsy is recommended for monitoring women on estrogen therapy alone; for women on estrogen with cyclic progestin, biopsy is not warranted unless bleeding occurs before the 12th day of progestin therapy. (See Chap. 81 for further discussion of estrogen therapy.) Women who have had a hysterectomy should receive estrogen alone.

Bisphosphonates (e.g., etidronate) bind to bone and decrease the rate of bone reabsorption. Preliminary studies suggest that cyclical intermittent treatment with etidronate slows bone loss and reduces the risk of vertebral fractures. Treatment with etidronate should be considered in patients with symptomatic vertebral fractures who are unwilling or unable to take estrogen. Cycles consist of 400 mg of etidronate daily for 2 weeks, and are repeated every 3 months; the medication should be taken at least 1 hour before or after meals or other medications. Between, but not during cycles, patients should take 1000 mg of calcium per day.

Vitamin D supplementation slows bone loss in older women in the northern United States who have low intakes of vitamin D. Use of a low-dosage supplement, such as one multivitamin tablet a day, is reasonable, especially to prevent osteomalacia in elderly persons who get very little vitamin D from sunlight or fortified dairy products. This is particularly true of the house-bound or institutionalized elderly.

Sodium fluoride, combined with calcium, has been shown to increase bone density in osteoporosis, but the new bone is not as strong as normal bone and fluoride thus has little or no effect on the future risk of spine fractures. Side effects include stress fractures, severe joint pain, and gastrointestinal symptoms. This treatment remains experimental, and should not be used outside of a randomized trial.

Calcitonin appears to increase spinal bone mass and reduce the rate of vertebral fractures, but it is not known whether its effects last longer than 2 years or whether it reduces the risk of other types of fractures. It is expensive and must be given several times a week by injection.

Thiazide diuretics decrease calcium excretion. Some, but not all, observational studies suggest that long-term use decreases the risk of fractures. Randomized trials on the effect of thiazides on bone loss are needed to confirm this finding.

Patients on Corticosteroids
Prevention of osteoporotic fractures in patients taking corticosteroids has not been well studied. Reasonable guidelines are as follows: (1) Minimize the dose and duration of steroid treatment, using short-acting or topical preparations if possible. (2) Consider baseline bone densitometry, perhaps repeated every 3 to 6 months, if results might alter management. (3) Maintain weight-bearing physical activity as much as possible. (4) Ensure adequate calcium intake. (5) Use vitamin D–containing multivitamin supplement daily. (6) Consider hormone therapy in postmenopausal women. (7) Refer to an endocrinologist if fractures or rapid bone loss develops despite these measures.

Riggs BL, Melton LJ III. Involutional osteoporosis. N Engl J Med 1986; 314:1676–86.
An excellent general review.

Marcus R. Understanding osteoporosis. West J Med 1991; 155:53–60.
An excellent review of pathophysiology and treatment.

Cummings SR, et al. Epidemiology of osteoporosis and osteoporotic fractures. Epidemiol Rev 1985; 7:178–208.
A comprehensive review of the epidemiology and prevention of osteoporotic fractures.

Resnick NM, Greenspan SL. 'Senile' osteoporosis reconsidered. JAMA 1989; 261:1025–9.
Discusses the differences between women over 70 and perimenopausal women, and the implications for prevention and treatment of osteoporosis in this older population.

Melton LJ III, Eddy DM, Johnston CC Jr. Screening for osteoporosis. Ann Intern Med 1990; 112:516–28.
A careful review with recommendations for selective use of screening.

Riis B, Thomsen K, Christiansen C. Does calcium supplementation prevent postmenopausal bone loss? A double-blind, controlled clinical study. N Engl J Med 1987; 316:173–7.
Two thousand milligrams of supplemental calcium slowed cortical, but not spinal, bone loss.

Dawson-Hughes B, et al. Effect of vitamin D supplementation in wintertime and overall bone loss in healthy postmenopausal women. Ann Intern Med 1991; 155:505–512.
400 IU of vitamin D daily slowed bone loss during the winter in women in the northern United States who had low vitamin D intake.

Holbrook TL, Barrett-Connor E, Wingard D. Dietary calcium and risk of hip fracture; 14-year prospective population study. Lancet 1988; 2:1046–8.
A small prospective study found a much lower risk of hip fractures among those taking at least 750 mg of calcium a day compared to those taking less than 500 mg.

Riggs BL, et al. Effect of fluoride treatment on the fracture rate in postmenopausal women with osteoporosis. N Engl J Med 1990; 322:802–9.
Patients who received fluoride treatment had a similar number of new vertebral fractures as the placebo group and more nonvertebral fractures.

Watts NB, et al. Intermittent cyclical etidronate treatment of postmenopausal osteoporosis. N Engl J Med 1990; 323:72–9.
Spinal bone mass was increased, and the rate of new vertebral fractures was reduced by half in etidronate-treated patients, compared to patients who did not receive etidronate.

Lukert BP, Raisz LG. Glucocorticoid-induced osteoporosis: pathogenesis and management. Ann Intern Med 1990; 112:352–64.
An extensively referenced review, with suggestions for preventive management.

Tinetti ME, Speechley M. Prevention of falls among the elderly. N Engl J Med 1989; 320:1055–9.

Discusses the identification of patients at risk for falling and interventions to minimize that risk.

67. NECK PAIN
Peter Curtis

Neck pain is a common problem that becomes more frequent with advancing age. It may present as a chronic recurring problem or as an acute problem; both may stem from the structures of the neck or be referred from the diaphragm, arm, or shoulder.

Causes of Neck Pain
The most common cause of neck pain, considering all age groups, is myofascitis or myofascial trigger points. In the elderly, degenerative change of the cervical vertebrae (spondylosis) is almost ubiquitous, but is associated with pain in only a small number of patients. Neck pain also may be a symptom of problems located in the arm or shoulder, notably carpal tunnel and outlet compression syndromes. Other causes of neck pain include lymphadenitis and infection (particularly in young patients), systemic diseases (e.g., ankylosing spondylitis and other inflammatory diseases), or metastases to the cervical vertebrae. Trauma, particularly from motor vehicle accidents, can lead to whiplash and other neck injuries. Sedentary occupations such as desk work and the driving of motor vehicles are often associated with pain, but the precise anatomic cause of pain is uncertain in many instances.

Painful Syndromes of the Neck
Myofascial pain is described in the chapter on nonarticular musculoskeletal pain (see Chap. 72).

Cervical spondylosis occurs in almost all people. As the neck ages, the cervical disks lose turgor and become somewhat less stable. Calcium is deposited along the margins of the vertebral bodies and apophyseal joints. With increasing bulk or with fortuitous positioning, the deposits can cause nerve root compression at the exit foramina or, when centrally placed, can cause compression of descending tracts. There also may be soft tissue irritation and muscle pain or spasm. Patients present either with radiculopathy suggestive of nerve root involvement, or pain and spasm of the trapezius and suboccipital muscle groups.

Whiplash injuries are hyperextension injuries of the neck usually resulting from a traffic accident. Anterior cervical structures (e.g., muscles, larynx, esophagus, temporomandibular joint, ligaments) are stretched and sometimes torn. In mild-to-moderate instances, the victims may be unaware of injury until a few hours or even a day later, when muscles become painful or when a "wry" neck develops. It is important to carry out a detailed neurologic examination and to obtain an appropriate x-ray of the cervical spine to look for fracture or dislocation.

Evaluation
The two major symptoms associated with neck disease are pain and limited motion. The pain may be in the neck or may radiate to the shoulder or down the arm. The history initially should be directed at identifying patients in whom systemic or metastatic disease is likely. Other information should include the onset of pain (sudden or gradual), the main focus of pain (arm, shoulder, back), the character of pain, or motions that cause pain. Myofascial pain may occur suddenly, often in association with new activity or mild trauma. The most common areas of pain are the lower pole of the scapula and the posterior aspect of the shoulder, radiating into the neck. Pain from nerve root compression may be aching or lancinating, depending on which portion of the root is involved, motor or sensory. If upper cervical roots are involved, pain may appear as an occipital headache; other roots may refer pain into the shoulder, arm, or thorax according to the level of involvement.

Physical examination should include detailed evaluation of the arm, shoulder, and thorax as well as the neck. Inspection may indicate swelling, spasm, or differences in position. The range of motion of the neck, both passive and active, should be tested through extension, flexion, side bending, and rotation. The first three movements have a range of 45 degrees, while rotation should be about 80 degrees from the face-forward position. Palpation determines if bone or muscle is involved. In myofascial syndromes the bellies of the muscles are tender, and trigger points may be identified. In radiculopathy, typical radiation of pain may be demonstrated by moving the neck through the normal range of motion but the area into which the pain radiates will not be tender. Tapping on the spinous processes of the vertebral body is a very nonspecific test. A positive Adson's maneuver suggests a thoracic outlet syndrome. This test is performed by placing the patient's hand, palm up, in the lap, and palpating the radial pulse. The head is rotated first to the affected side and then to the other, with a Valsalva maneuver performed in each position; obliteration of the pulse in either position is considered a positive test. However, the specificity of this test is poor. Muscular weakness, atrophy, and diminished deep tendon reflexes suggest nerve root involvement. Lesions at the C4–C5 interspace (C5 root) cause weakness of shoulder abductors; at C5–C6 (C6 root), weakness of elbow flexors, wrist extensors, and diminished biceps and brachioradialis reflexes; at C6–C7 (C7 root), decreased elbow extensors and diminished or extinguished triceps reflexes (C7 is the primary innervation of the triceps). Occasionally, central spinal cord compression affects descending tracts as well as cervical roots, causing upper motor neuron findings. In this case, there is spasticity and increased muscle tone in the lower extremity instead of flaccidity, and heightened rather than decreased deep tendon reflexes in the levels below the compression of descending tracts.

Laboratory studies are indicated only as suggested by the history. X-rays may be useful in identifying spondylosis if neurologic deficits are noted; however, the findings are often nonspecific because, at age 50, 50% of patients have radiographic evidence of cervical spondylosis and, at 65, 85% do. Radiographic evidence has to correlate exactly with clinical findings to be significant. Bony metastases, Paget's disease, myeloma, or ankylosing spondylitis also can be identified by x-ray or bone scan. In general, x-rays are recommended for all but the mildest cases of whiplash injury, since these often involve litigation, and bony injury should be ruled out. An electromyogram is necessary if entrapment neuropathy (e.g., carpal tunnel syndrome) is suspected, but it is rarely useful in the evaluation of cervical spondylosis. Nerve conduction studies are often helpful in the diagnosis of nerve root injury. If an injured or prolapsed cervical disk is suspected, CT or MRI is necessary for evaluation before surgery.

Management

Once organic disease has been excluded by history and clinical examination, acute or chronic neck pain can be managed by simple measures, such as ice or heat, analgesics, and rest, as well as by the specific therapies listed below. Usually a specialist is consulted about patients with neurologic deficits.

Therapy is directed toward reassuring and supporting the patient, relieving pain, reducing mechnical stresses, and relieving muscle spasm. Management of myofascial pain is discussed in Chapter 72. Several therapeutic modalities, such as deep massage, exercise, stretching, and vapocoolant sprays, are used to manage pain from spondylosis. Clinical studies have not definitively ascribed benefit to one therapy over another. Unfortunately, one is left to try various approaches and to make empirical choices based in part on what is most economical and simple to implement.

Supportive Management

Moist heat, usually provided by warm baths (15–20 minutes) taken just before bedtime, can help promote muscle relaxation. Other forms of heat include a heating pad and hydrocollator pack.

A soft collar, positioned to produce the least pain, allows the cervical muscles to relax. The collar is designed to relieve strain on the cervical muscles and to restrict flexion-extension movements. A collar should not be used for more than 3 weeks since it can lead to disuse and shortening of the neck muscles, and an increasing sense of dependency. Use of the collar should be progressively discontinued and not stopped abruptly. At night, the collar can be discarded and the patient advised to use one pillow only. The pillow should be thick at the center and thickened at the ends and tucked carefully around the neck. Sleeping with no pillow and a rolled towel under the neck can provide traction and extension for good relief in some patients. When undertaking activities such as typing or reading, patients should position objects to avoid flexion of the neck. Also, hyperextension of the neck for a prolonged period of time, as when working overhead, can cause neck pain. Patients with chronic severe neck pain may need to use a molded plastic collar for approximately 3 to 4 months.

Drugs

A variety of drugs have been used for relief of pain and reduction of muscle spasm. Aspirin or acetaminophen (Tylenol) is usually sufficient for pain relief; however, for severe disease a narcotic may be necessary for a few days, particularly at night. Any of the nonsteroidal anti-inflammatory drugs may be tried and in some instances may be effective. Muscle relaxants are usually of no benefit beyond their sedative effects. Antidepressants such as nortriptyline, 10 to 50 mg at night, can effectively raise pain thresholds.

Traction

Mild or chronic neck pain can be treated in outpatients by intermittent traction, either in the physical therapy department, or more economically, by using a home traction kit obtainable from the local drugstore. Home traction may be done sitting in a doorway, with the apparatus suspended from the door frame, or in bed. Traction pull should be at least equivalent to the weight of the head, about 7 pounds. Usually traction is ordered with weights of between 7 and 15 pounds. In the elderly, 2 to 3 pounds should be used. Clear instructions are needed, and it is useful for the patient to practice it one time in the presence of the provider. In a few patients, traction makes the pain worse and should be discontinued after a brief trial. Continuous traction is rarely indicated but is given to some patients suffering from intractable pain. This must be done in the hospital, and then only for a period of 3 to 4 days.

Physical Therapy

Isometric exercise programs are a useful adjunct to a collar and are performed by flexion, extension, and lateral motion against resistance of the hands. These exercises can be done three times daily with five repetitions of each movement. Mobilization and manipulation are being used increasingly in physical therapy units for chronic neck pain and as a useful preventive measure. Mobilization involves careful and gentle movement of the neck through the range of motion, often using gentle traction with the hands. It can be taught to one of the patient's family members. Manipulation is performed by many different kinds of health providers, especially osteopaths and chiropractors, and often seems successful, although its efficacy is not supported by controlled studies. Neurologic symptoms following a manipulation are a rare event but most frequently affects people between 35 and 50 years, particularly as a result of injury to the vertebrobasilar arteries. Exercises are also helpful, particularly in the late recovery phase and to prevent recurrences.

Injection Therapy

Injection therapy is based on the unproved theory that pain originates in apophyseal joints and can be eradicated by injection with a local anesthetic or corticosteroid. The procedure is undertaken with the patient prone and the neck flexed; 1 to 2 cc of 1% lidocaine (Xylocaine) is used, often with the addition of a crystalline suspension of steroid. A long (3-cm) needle is inserted 1 inch lateral to the spinous process (midline) and pushed down through the posterior ligament into the joint area. The mixture is injected at several points around the joint. More accurate injection can be performed with radiologic guidance; this is usually done in specialized pain clinics.

Surgery

A small number of patients with intractable pain or progressing neurologic deficits may be considered for surgery, usually after a failure of medical management.

Management of Whiplash Injury

Therapy for whiplash injury includes rest (a soft cervical collar), analgesics, and local ice/heat treatments. Occasionally symptoms secondary to mild whiplash injury are improved by gentle cervical manipulation or injection of local anesthetic into trigger points. If the symptoms persist for more than 4 weeks, gentle cervical traction (7–10 pounds) may help relieve pain. If root signs and symptoms appear, myelography or CT may be indicated to exclude a lacerated cervical disk. At this stage, particularly if litigation is involved, the clinical picture frequently becomes confused by "trauma neurosis." Because there is danger of neurologic damage, severe cases of whiplash should be admitted to the hospital for evaluation and referred to the neurologist or neurosurgeon.

Cloward RB. Acute cervical spine injuries. Ciba Clin Symp 1980; 32:1–32.
Good illustrated review of the emergency management of acute cervical spine injuries.

Kelsey JL. Epidemiology of the radiculopathies. Adv Neurol 1978; 19:386–98.
Useful discussion of the epidemiology of radiculopathies, particularly nerve root problems and neuritis related to cervical disk disease.

Grieve GP. Common vertebral joint problems. New York: Churchill Livingstone, 1981.
An excellent book giving comprehensive guidance on physical examination, mobilization, and manipulation techniques, and a critical look at a wide range of therapeutic modalities used in joint disease. Includes over 1300 references.

Murray-Leslie CV, Wright V. Carpal tunnel syndrome, humeral epicondylitis, and the cervical spine: a study of clinical and dimensional relations. Br Med J 1976; 1:1439–42.
Describes the clinical relationships between cervical spine disease and other soft tissue syndromes.

Kreuger BR, Okazaki H. Vertebral-basilar distribution infarction following chiropractic cervical manipulation. Mayo Clin Proc 1980; 55:322–32.
Indicates dangers of chiropractic manipulation with some useful references.

Saunders RL, Wilson DH. The surgery of cervical disk disease. Clin Orthop 1980; 146:119–27.
Reviews indications and methods of surgical management of cervical disk diseases.

Rothman RH, Simeone FA, eds. The spine. 2nd ed. Philadelphia: Saunders, 1982.
Good detailed text on spinal disorders with an especially good chapter on the management of whiplash injuries.

Leek JC, Gershwin MG, Fowler WM, eds. Principles of physical medicine and rehabilitation in the musculoskeletal diseases. Orlando, FL: Grune & Stratton, 1986.
Good review of evaluation and management of neck problems.

Bonica JJ, Caillet R. Lola AE. General considerations of pain in the neck and upper limb. In: Bonica, JJ, ed. Management of pain. 2nd ed. Philadelphia: Lea & Febiger, 1990:812–47, 848–67.
In-depth review of anatomy, neurophysiology, and mechanisms of neck pain with comprehensive review of management problems and pain relief.

Bland JH. Disorders of the cervical spine: diagnosis and medical management. Philadelphia: Saunders, 1987.
A superb book covering the spectrum of neck pathology as well as consultation for disease and trauma of the cervical spine and disability determinations. Little has been published since that adds significantly to the management of this condition.

68. SHOULDER PAIN
Peter Curtis

Shoulder pain can be excruciating but is often tolerable and associated with limited movement. Because the symptoms are often intermittent, many patients seek help only after recurrences or if the problem becomes chronic. In a population survey of rheumatic disor-

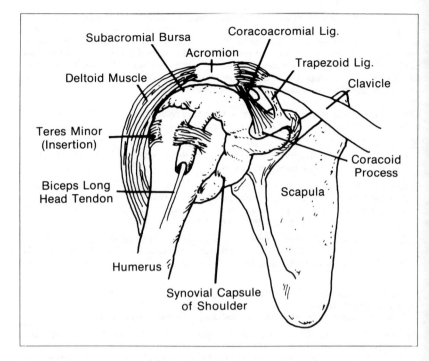

Fig. 68-1. Important structures of the shoulder joint.

ders, neck-shoulder-brachial pain was found in 9% of men and 12% of women over the age of 15.

Anatomy
The shoulder joint consists of two functioning joints (the glenohumeral and acromioclavicular) and three gliding surfaces (long head of biceps, subacromial bursa, and musculotendinous cuff). The musculotendinous or rotator cuff strengthens the capsule of the joint by the insertion into its substances of five muscles: supraspinatus, infraspinatus, teres minor, subscapularis, and long head of the triceps (Fig. 68-1).

Shoulder pain may arise from structures outside the shoulder, for example, from the cervical vertebrae, heart, lungs, or diaphragm; however, musculoskeletal disorders of the shoulder are responsible for most instances of pain. Although many specific conditions are described in orthopedic texts, most musculoskeletal problems derive either from the myofascial syndrome (fibrositis, myofibrositis, or scapulothoracic muscular syndrome) or from one of a continuum of interrelated traumatic or degenerative soft tissue processes: bursitis, tendinitis, or rotator cuff syndrome. Less frequently, well-defined conditions can be identified, such as rotator cuff tears, calcific tendinitis, or adhesive capsulitis.

General Evaluation
A history of pain or decreased mobility is the usual complaint; less frequently, swelling in or about the shoulder is noted. In myofascial disorders, the patient complains of pain that may radiate to the neck or arm or tenderness over the posterior aspect of the shoulder girdle.

The earliest and often most intense pain is felt over the deltoid muscle and may spread to the entire shoulder or radiate downward into the lateral or anterior aspect of the arm. Pain from any of the structures of the shoulder joint, except the acromioclavicular joint, is referred along the C5 dermatome, which includes the shoulder and the lateral surface of the arm to the hand. Pain from the acromioclavicular joint, which is innervated by C4, is felt directly over the joint itself. Patients with degenerative diseases often have a slow and gradual increase in the pain, although pain from bursitis or tendinitis can occur rapidly. With degenerative processes, some joint mobility usually is preserved, and the patient complains more about movement of the shoulder in a specific direction. However, movement in any direction is excruciating with infection, blood in the joint, or severe calcific tendinitis. Fever is not associated with degenerative processes and suggests other causes. Although multiple painful joints usually suggest systemic disease, several degenerative processes, such as bursitis or tendinitis, often occur simultaneously with systemic disease.

The physical examination includes examination of the neck, arm, lungs, and thorax, with careful neurologic testing for cervical disease. The shoulder is inspected for swelling and position. The patient is asked to abduct the arms (the painful arc test; as described under Shoulder Bursitis, Tendinitis, and Rotator Cuff Syndrome) to help delineate rotator cuff problems; the shoulder is palpated to pinpoint areas of tenderness, such as muscles (in the myofascial syndrome), the insertions of the rotator cuff muscles over the humeral tuberosities, the biceps insertion through the bicipital groove, or acromioclavicular joint (see Fig. 68-1). Not uncommonly, there is diffuse tenderness over several structures, which prevents specific anatomic diagnosis. The patient is asked to try to move the shoulder actively in a full range of motion. Typically, some motion is possible in degenerative problems, and the limitation of motion can be improved with gentle and slow assistance. However, with acute inflammatory processes or intra-articular bleeding and infection, limited motion (usually in all planes) is not improved by assistance. After assessing the passive range of motion, specific muscles are tested against resistance. The most frequently affected are the supraspinatus (abduction to 100 degrees) and biceps tendon (flexion of elbow).

Laboratory evaluation is not usually indicated unless specific extrinsic causes of shoulder pain are being considered. X-rays are usually not helpful in patients suspected of having degenerative disease of the shoulder; however, in selected patients with new shoulder pain, x-rays are done to search for calcium deposits and bony lesions.

Evaluation for Specific Conditions

Myofascial Syndrome

Myofascial syndrome is the most common shoulder problem seen in ambulatory care. Its cause is unknown. Often there are trigger points along the upper pole of the scapula and over the trapezius muscle where pressure stimulates referred pain. Small, tender nodules may be palpable in this area; these nodules show no specific pathologic characteristics other than local inflammation. Other findings include "scapulocostal grating" on moving the scapula or, sometimes, a "snapping" scapula caused by flicking of an osseous spur on the vertebral margin of the bone against muscle (see Chap. 71).

Shoulder Bursitis, Tendinitis, and Rotator Cuff Syndrome

The degenerative process that results in shoulder bursitis, tendinitis, and rotator cuff syndrome begins in the supraspinatus or bicipital tendons, which have relatively poor blood supply and are under stress. With time, the tendinous insertions about the shoulder become frayed and inflamed from impingement between the humoral head and the acromion. As the degeneration advances, inflammation involves other tendons and bursae and ultimately the entire capsule and acromioclavicular joint. Depending on the distribution of inflammation, patients may present with complaints of any of these structures and any of the above syndromes. It is often difficult to make an exact anatomic diagnosis, but testing of specific structures may make a precise diagnosis possible. These degenerative conditions occur most frequently in patients between the age of 50 and 60 and are more common in women and during the winter months. The disease process is unilateral in 75% of patients. Bursitis is often precipitated by minor trauma and is associated with other soft tissue disorders. The onset is often slow, and the condition may persist with exacerbations and remission for up to 2 years. Improvement is slow.

The patient with rotator cuff syndrome usually presents with aching in the shoulder, limited abduction of the arm with a painful arc of motion between 45 and 120 degrees (positive painful arc test), and loss of function of affected structures. Between about 45 and 120 degrees, the rotator cuff tendons move under the coracoacromial arch. If these tendons are swollen and inflamed, they become impinged under the arch, and pain occurs. (From 120–180 degrees, the acromioclavicular joint is used for elevation; therefore, pain that occurs only after 120 degrees abduction suggests acromioclavicular joint involvement.) There may be tenderness over the deltoid insertion at midhumerus, and the patient may complain of tingling down the arm. X-ray of the shoulder may show calcification in the rotator cuff, calcium deposits in the supraspinatus tendon, and sclerosis and cystic changes in the head of the humerus.

Rotator Cuff Rupture
By age 50 close to 25% of people have some attrition of the rotator cuff. Therefore, partial or full tears of the cuff tend to present in middle age following trauma, often a fall on the outstretched arm. The pain is acute, and the patient complains of weakness of the arm, reduced active range of motion, and pain at the limits of internal and external rotation. Partial tears are often associated with other inflammatory or degenerative disorders of the shoulder. Arthrograms are useful in confirming the diagnosis if there is no improvement after 6 weeks or if there has been obvious trauma. Early surgical repair of complete tears produces the best outcomes.

Calcific Tendinitis
Calcific deposits are present in the shoulder tissues of most people over the age of 35. Calcific tendinitis, which occurs in 2.7 to 8% of the population, has three stages: (1) an asymptomatic stage, in which calcific deposits are only detected on x-ray, (2) a chronic intermittent phase, and (3) an acute flare-up. The acute condition usually affects a relatively young and active person. The patient complains of excruciating pain, often down the arm. The surrounding muscles are acutely tender and in spasm. There is a painful arc of passive motion from 0 to 60 degrees, and the patient holds the arm splinted. The pain is caused by a calcium deposit "boil," which may subsequently rupture; this releases a toothpaste-like material and relieves the pain. The condition usually subsides within 14 days.

Adhesive Capsulitis (Frozen Shoulder)
Adhesive capsulitis results from tightening and thickening of the joint capsule with a consequent marked reduction in volume of the glenohumeral joint. The symptoms of chronic pain and generalized immobility develop over a period of several months and last up to 2 years. The peak incidence occurs between 50 to 70 years of age and is higher in women. Adhesive capsulitis is often associated with other clinical conditions, such as myocardial infarction, long-term intravenous infusions into the arm, thyroid disease, diabetes, and depression; it also can occur for only 2 to 4 weeks in situations in which there is shoulder immobilization (e.g., hemiplegia, fractures, or minor trauma and self-immobilization by the patient). Recovery is usual. Arthrography shows a marked decrease in joint space, and the humeral head may show some osteoporosis.

General Treatment
The treatment of musculoskeletal shoulder problems is usually directed toward alleviating the pathologic and anatomic cause of the disability or pain. However, because the clinical picture may not suggest a specific syndrome, management often involves an empiric sequence of therapies.

Physical Therapy
Common practice includes cooling, using ice pack applications for 20 to 30 minutes, three times daily, for the acute stage, and heating, using hot packs for 20 minutes, several times a day, for the subacute conditions.

Exercises
In the acute phase, it may be necessary to rest the arm in a sling and to treat the pain with passive range-of-motion exercises, hot-cold compresses, nonsteroidal anti-inflammatory agents, or injection of local anesthetics with or without steroids. Subsequently, active

exercises are important to increase mobility and maintain muscle bulk and flexibility. The affected arm and hand are used as a pendulum; they are swung back and forth, increasing the arc progressively. Other exercises include "wall-walking" with the fingers (gradually abducting the arm by walking the fingers up the wall), circle exercises (bending over and making ever-larger circles with the arm), and the use of overhead pulleys. Many patients have associated postural and muscle imbalance problems; attention should therefore be directed toward improving posture and providing suitable pillows or mattresses for support during rest. Exercises should be undertaken for about 5 minutes every hour during the day.

Drugs

Salicylates (600–900 mg every 6 hours) are cheap and effective. Acetaminophen and propoxyphene derivatives relieve acute pain but are not anti-inflammatory. Nonsteroidal anti-inflammatory drugs (NSAIDs) are used extensively for musculoskeletal shoulder syndromes, although there are no well-controlled studies that show significant benefits except in acute inflammatory conditions. NSAIDS may be given as a therapeutic trial for 1 to 2 weeks. No one agent is established as better than another. Commonly used NSAIDs include ibuprofen (Motrin), sulindac (Clinoril), naproxen (Naprosyn), and indomethacin (Indocin) (see Chap. 64). Because patients may respond better to one NSAID than another, different agents should be tried if there is no initial improvement. The possible side effects of these drugs (e.g., indigestion, gastric erosion, skin rash) should be reviewed with patients before prescribing.

Steroid Injections

Local steroid injections of identified tender and inflamed structures have not been shown in randomized trials to be better than physical therapy or NSAIDs; however, there is some evidence that they are useful in chronic cases resistant to other forms of therapy. Injecting lidocaine first will determine if localization is correct. In order for the injection to be made into the tendons, one should feel the needle hit bone; otherwise, the injection is made primarily into soft tissue and is more readily absorbed systemically. The dosage for periarticular injection has not been precisely defined; however, the equivalent of 40 mg of prednisone is most frequently recommended. The usual method is to mix 1 to 2 cc of 1% lidocaine with the colloidal steroid. Patients should be warned that pain in the shoulder is likely to increase over the 12 hours following an injection. This problem often can be avoided by the use of a longer-acting local anesthetic, such as bupivacaine (Marcaine), instead of lidocaine. Repeated injections of steroids into the same site produce atrophy; not more than 2 or 3 injections should be given over a 12-month period.

Treatment of Specific Conditions

Myofascial Pain

The treatment of myofascial pain revolves around identifying precipitating factors such as incorrect desk or chair height for a sedentary worker, peculiar position of body while sitting in class or movie theater, or an unusual way of doing a repetitive task such as lifting objects while working on an assembly line. This analysis may take time and some imagination to sort out, but mechanical misuse of the arm, neck, and shoulder is a major cause of pain.

Other precipitating causes of myofascial pain include sleep disturbance or depression, endocrinopathies (particularly diabetes mellitus and hypothyroidism), and other inflammatory forms of arthritis.

If no specific structures are found to be involved, the syndrome should be treated as a use-related musculoskeletal disorder with local heat, massage, active range-of-motion movements, and stretching exercises. Muscle relaxants have not proved effective. If trigger points are found, anesthesia of the area can usually be obtained by injecting 1 to 5 ml of lidocaine (Xylocaine) using a 1½-inch 22-gauge needle. If a first injection does not effect complete relief, a second injection may be used. Some authorities have recommended injecting steroids, but this practice is of questionable benefit. If there is no response to repeated injections, the diagnosis should be reassessed. Other techniques, such as local application of ethyl chloride or fluoromethane, have been tried but with less success than local anesthetic injection.

Calcific tendinitis is usually managed by orthopedic specialists. Calcific deposits can be "needled" and washed out with saline using a two-needle technique, but the benefit is questionable; however, excellent relief can be obtained by an injection of steroids and a topical anesthetic.

Adhesive capsulitis is treated initially with conservative therapy—heat, exercises, and analgesics. If there is no response, patients are referred for distention arthrography.

Scott JT, ed. Copeman's Textbook of the Rheumatic Diseases. 6th ed. New York: Churchill Livingstone, 1986.
A good general text that provides a comprehensive overview of musculoskeletal disease.

Cyriax J. Textbook of orthopaedic medicine. Vol. 1. London: Bailliere Tindall, 1978: 191–254.
Although the therapeutic portion of this two-volume textbook is somewhat outdated, the section on physical diagnosis of soft tissue lesions is excellent.

Ramamurth CP. Orthopaedics in primary care. Baltimore: Williams & Wilkins, 1981.
An excellent and practical small book providing a simple, logical approach to common problems in primary care. Short on references.

Escobar PL. Myofascial pain syndrome. Orthop Rev 1987; 16:708–13.
Good review of diagnosis and management of myofascial pain syndromes.

Birnbaum JS. The musculoskeletal manual. 2nd ed. Orlando, FL: Grune & Stratton, 1986.
An excellent, succinct, and visually stimulating book summarizing diagnosis and management.

Gray RG, Tenebaum J, Gottlieb NL. Local corticosteroid injection treatment in rheumatic disorders. Semin Arthritis Rheum 1981; 10:231–54.
An excellent review article on the indications, methods, and side effects of steroid injection therapy.

Leek JC, Genshwin ME, Fowler WB, eds. Principles of physical medicine and rehabilitation in the musculoskeletal diseases. Orlando, FL: Grune & Stratton, 1986.
Particularly useful descriptions of physical therapy approaches as well as discussions of scientific basis for therapy.

69. LOW BACK PAIN
Nortin M. Hadler and Timothy S. Carey

At least 70% of the population experiences low back pain at some time in their lives. Low back pain is a self-limited disease; approximately 40% of patients remit in 1 week, 60 to 85% in 3 weeks, and 90% in 2 months. Along with remission, low back pain is characterized by a striking likelihood of recurrence. The first attack of low back pain is usually the shortest and least severe; recurrences usually last longer. Back symptoms occur with equal prevalence in men and women, beginning in the twenties and thirties, and peaking in the forties to early fifties, although back pain syndromes can occur throughout life. Primary care physicians see back pain commonly and may view lumbar pain as intractable and difficult to treat. In reality the illness is usually self-limited.

Etiology
The cause of low back pain is undetermined in the overwhelming majority of patients. Many structures possess sensory innervation, and several are potential sources for pain that mimics the symptoms of disk herniation. Despite endless speculation on the pathogenesis of nonspecific low back pain, there is no clear-cut way to differentiate fibrositis, myositis, facet joint pain, ligamentous strain, or any other of the causes to which this regional disease has been ascribed. Seldom are we able to attribute any episode of back illness to a particular back disease.

Structural abnormalities of the disk occur early in life, frequently before age 30. In older subjects, disintegration is almost ubiquitous. Disk herniation arises in that part of the spine subjected to the heaviest mechanical stresses, usually C5–C6, L4–L5, and L5–S1. Intradisk pressure measured in various positions has shown that inappropriate standing, lifting, and sitting all increase stresses on intervertebral disks. The prevalence of serious causes of back pain in unselected back pain patients is low: approximately 2% will have a disk herniation, 0.6% will have a malignancy as a cause of their pain, and less than 0.001% will have osteomyelitis.

Evaluation

History

Information about the quality of pain, age of the patient, and presence of other symptoms will help to separate patients with low back pain of systemic cause from the vast majority with self-limited regional disease. Sciatica is a term that indicates pain radiating from the lower back down the posterior thigh. While such symptoms may be associated with disk protrusion, in the absence of neurologic signs, initial diagnostic and therapeutic plans are the same as for nonradiating mechanical back pain. Spinal stenosis classically presents not as acute back pain, but rather as pain in the buttocks and legs on exercise or prolonged standing (pseudoclaudication). The pain is relieved by rest or by assuming a forward-bending posture.

All back pain patients should be asked about changes in bowel or bladder function. Such history can be an early indication of cauda equina syndrome, which mandates rapid surgical intervention. Clinical settings that should greatly increase suspicion of systemic disease include (1) back pain in the elderly, accompanied by historical or physical signs of malignancy (pain with metastatic disease or myeloma tends to be more continuous, progressive, and prominent when the patient is recumbent); (2) back pain along with fever, which suggests infection and requires aggressive investigation; (3) back pain with five specific historical features that together are up to 95% sensitive and 85% specific for ankylosing spondylitis. These features are (1) age at onset of less than 40, (2) insidious onset, (3) duration for at least 3 months, (4) morning stiffness, and (5) improvement with exercise. Because the prevalence of ankylosing spondylitis in the back pain population is low (1–3%), the positive predictive value of these screening questions will also be low, 11% for a prevalence of 2%.

While tumor, infection, and ankylosing spondylitis do not exhaust the list of diseases that present as back pain, most of the other problems are accompanied by hints that are obvious in the history and physical examination. For example, young women with genitourinary problems such as urinary tract infections or pelvic inflammatory disease may present with an initial complaint of pain in the back, but it is usually readily apparent that the problem is not a regional musculoskeletal illness.

Physical Examination

The back and neurologic examination usually determines whether immediate surgical consultation or conservative treatment is necessary (Table 69-1). Inspection of gait and heel-and-toe walking assesses the weakness of the gastrocnemius and tibialis anterior muscles. Changes in posture, including loss of lumbar lordosis, are totally nonspecific, as are pelvic tilt, scoliosis, and degree of kyphosis or lordosis. Measurements of spinal motion are seldom useful in evaluating low back pain, but normal mobility should direct thinking to causes of pain that are other than musculoskeletal. Straight leg raising is a clinical test that is often misinterpreted. To be positive, pain should be present in the leg during the early arc of straight leg raising (< 50 degrees). A positive test suggests to some surgeons a protruding disk of the L5–S1 region affecting the fifth lumbar nerve root. Others believe that the crossed straight leg raising test (straight leg raise on the unaffected side increases symptoms on the affected side) is an even more specific sign of a herniated nucleus pulposus. Elicitation of pain by flexion of the knee with the patient prone (the femoral stretch test) is of some use in diagnosing L3 lesions. These tests, combined with neurologic testing for motor weakness and sensory deficits, are important in defining the extent of neuromuscular compromise. With minor neurologic abnormalities, emergency surgical consultation is not necessary; referral is triggered by signs and symp-

Table 69-1. Physical examination of the back pain patient

Standing
  Inspection
  Range of motion
  Palpation
  Stand on heels and toes

Sitting
  Foot strength on dorsiflexion
  Sensory examination of the foot and lower leg
  Palpation of the spine
  Knee jerk and plantar reflexes

Lying supine
  Abdominal examination
  Peripheral vascular examination
  Straight leg raising

Lying on side
  Hip abduction
  Rectal examination

Lying prone
  Femoral stretch test
  Gluteus maximus strength
  Perineal sensation

Source: H Hall. Examination of the patient with low back pain. Bulletin on the Rheumatic Diseases. 1983; 33:1–8.

toms suggesting the cauda equina syndrome. This syndrome, presenting as acute pain and loss of autonomic function, results from central herniation of a disk below L1 and L2, which in most people is opposite the lower end of the spinal cord. It is imperative to check for saddle anesthesia, rectal tone, and cremasteric reflexes in patients with severe acute back pain.

X-rays
Lumbar spine x-rays help exclude possibilities such as infection and metastasis but are an unnecessary expense in patients in whom history and physical examination generate no specific question to be answered by x-ray. Disk degeneration is a phenomenon of aging that need not give rise to any symptoms. By age 50, 80 to 95% of adults show evidence at autopsy of lumbar spondylosis (e.g., degenerative disk disease with narrowing of the disk space, marginal sclerosis, vacuum phenomenon, disk calcification); 87% of this age group have similar findings by x-ray. By age 60, radiographic disk disease is seen in 95% of asymptomatic patients. Therefore, the mere demonstration of degenerative disk disease on lumbar spine films does not confirm the cause of low back pain; it is so commonly present that it seldom provides definitive causal information.

New imaging techniques (CT and MRI) have allowed much improved definition of the anatomy of the spinal canal and nerve roots. Up to 20% of asymptomatic patients may have CT evidence of disk prolapse; therefore, radiographic findings must be carefully correlated with the neurologic examination to avoid unnecessary surgery. Imaging of the disk and nerve roots should be considered when the physical examination indicates a root lesion and the patient's symptoms, signs, and duration of illness make surgery a consideration. Many surgeons insist on direct visualization of nerve roots through a traditional myelogram or myelogram plus CT before considering a procedure.

Treatment of Acute Episodes
Approximately 40% of patients with musculoskeletal low back pain become well within 1 week, 80% within 2 weeks, and 90% within 2 months, regardless of the treatment. Therefore, the initial management of low back pain should be conservative even in the face of

mild neurologic abnormalities. Frequent contact with the patient and assurance that they will not become neurologically impaired can be very efficacious in allaying patient anxiety.

Bed Rest

The first principle of management is bed rest. Intradisk pressures are lowest in the supine and prone positions and are substantially elevated by sitting. There is no established rule for how long bed rest should be continued, but few patients require it for longer than 1 to 2 weeks. A recent study compared a recommendation of 2 days with a recommendation of 7 days bed rest and found no difference in speed of recovery, indicating that early mobilization to walking may be advantageous. Prolonged bed rest may substantially increase the effects of deconditioning and prolong the period of disability. Bed rest may be a difficult instruction for young, active individuals to follow. Appropriate modification of the home and work environment to avoid sitting and lifting, while allowing standing, may be successful. Frequent contact with both the patient and the employer is vital to the successful early mobilization of the patient with low back pain.

Drugs

Innumerable analgesic and anti-inflammatory agents, sedatives, hypnotics, and muscle relaxants have been recommended for the immediate relief of low back pain. Many agents have not been properly tested, and their efficacy or lack thereof remains unknown. There have been studies demonstrating the efficacy of drugs compared to placebo, but no drug convincingly demonstrates a greater effect than salicylates. The recommendation for most patients with low back pain is for simple salicylates or acetaminophen while awaiting the natural progress of events. The more expensive nonsteroidal anti-inflammatory agents may of course be used and provide equivalent pain relief to salicylates, with fewer pills per day. Muscle relaxants have been demonstrated to be better than placebo, but most patients can be adequately managed with analgesia and bed rest without them. Narcotic agents may be of some use for the first few days of treatment, but are not indicated for longer treatment courses.

Traction

Traction has often been recommended in low back pain. However, with the usually applied weights of only 10 to 15 pounds, neither traction to the spinal segments nor stretch to the paraspinal muscle takes place. Studies have shown that at least 25% of total body weight is required merely to overcome lower body resistance. As presently administered, 50 to 100 pounds of traction would be needed to be effective in stretching the spinal segments. Controlled studies of lumbar traction in the management of lower back pain showed no differences in outcome between groups treated with low-weight traction and a group treated with effective traction. The need for hospitalization, the extra expense to carry out the procedure, and the absence of demonstrable benefits in an already self-limited process militate against employing traction.

Other Physical Modalities

The benefit of most physical modalities, such as ultrasound, short-wave diathermy, heat, cold, or roentgen therapy, has not been convincingly demonstrated. Little is lost with a trial of local heat supplied by heating pad or hot water bottle, although the relief obtained is usually transient.

Manipulation

Manipulation is widely used in Britain and Canada by physicians and nonphysicians, often as an alternative to bed rest. In the United States, manipulation is practiced almost exclusively by chiropractors and osteopathic physicians. The effectiveness of usual care by physicians has been compared to that of manipulation in the management of low back pain. Many studies have shown no benefit attributable to manipulation, but methodologic problems have flawed many analyses. One study did show improved function from manipulation for a subset of patients whose symptoms began 2 to 4 weeks before manipulation. This benefit was present at 1-week follow-up, with the advantage over medical therapy disappearing at 2 weeks.

Corsets and Braces
Corsets are employed in an attempt to decrease intradisk pressure during normal standing through one of two possible biomechanical mechanisms: (1) unloading vertebral pressure by increasing intra-abdominal pressure, or (2) immobilizing the spine. However, studies have failed to indicate that either mechanism takes place. The usefulness of bracing is tenuous if based on these theoretical grounds, but some patients do seem to attain some symptomatic relief.

Exercises
Directed physical therapy and personal exercise programs are nearly universally prescribed for patients with low back pain who either have chronic symptoms or are in the resolving phase of an acute episode. Four basic types of exercises are commonly recommended: (1) back hyperextension exercises to strengthen the paravertebral muscles, (2) spinal mobilizing exercises (especially flexion), (3) isometric spinal flexion with secondary increased intra-abdominal pressure, and (4) general aerobic conditioning, often combined with some of the above. The goals of recommended treatment regimens vary greatly.

In two controlled studies of exercise programs in chronic low back pain, isometric exercises yielded better clinical results than the usual flexion-extension exercises. The principle behind the isometric regimen is to eliminate any exaggerated hyperextension of the lumbar spine by strengthening the trunk muscles. These isometric contractions may be performed while standing, lying down, or even walking. When exercising lying down, patients should be on their backs with two to three pillows wedged under the head and shoulders and one pillow under the knee. The sequence of active contractions is listed below.

1. Contract the abdominal muscles (pull umbilicus toward spine) as hard as possible. Relax.
2. Contract the gluteus. Relax.
3. Combine the abdominal and gluteal contractions to produce a pelvic tilt with flexion of the lumbar spine.
4. Contract the hip flexors and pelvic floor.

After the above are mastered, the contractions are held as long as possible (5–15 seconds). Progress should be made by increasing duration and number of performances.

Conditioning exercises (e.g., brisk walking, swimming) have gained favor recently as the problem of deconditioning in low back pain patients has become more appreciated.

Recurrent and Chronic Pain

An important predictor of future episodes of back pain is a history of past episodes of pain. Patients who have had substantial episodes of pain should be counseled on home treatment of their next episode. Amelioration of the patient's fears of chronic pain and work disability are often very useful in decreasing anxiety and requests for unnecessary diagnostic technology.

Chronic back pain affects fewer than 5% of the population of low back pain patients, but this unfortunate group uses extraordinary amounts of medical care. The experience of chronic pain can lead to depression and anger at employer, friends, physicians, and disability agencies. Such patients often require specialty consultation to ensure that no remediable cause of back pain has been missed; however, the continuing involvement of a primary physician coordinating care is essential. Second opinions prior to second (or third) surgical procedures should be encouraged. Multimodality pain clinics can be helpful in selected chronic pain patients. Because randomized trials of such adjunctive therapies are generally lacking, a collaborative relationship with patient and consultant can help to design reasonable, rational trials of therapy.

While almost all patients with acute episodes of low back pain return to work, disability issues can be significant for the patient and frustrating for the physician. To be eligible for workers' compensation, the back pain must have arisen during or as a consequence of employment. Because most cases of pain occur without a discrete traumatic precipitant, determining causality in a given episode of pain is difficult to do with any certainty. Back pain is, however, more common among workers who lift heavy loads, especially if lifted at a distance from the trunk of the body. Nurses' aides who lift patients have high rates of disabling back pain. No employed group is immune, however. Bus drivers have relatively high rates of pain, perhaps due to the vibration of the bus. Social Security has explicit criteria for disability related to back pain, requiring pain plus neurologic findings. Social Security disability programs require that an individual be out of work for at least 6 months despite medical care and have a disability expected to last at least 1 year. Although the application process for Social Security disability is quite long, it is aided by timely communication between patient, physician, and agency. The physician usually benefits the patient best by transmitting a complete history and physical findings, including all comorbid conditions, rather than by submitting unsupported attestations of disability.

Surgery

Most episodes of low back pain, including recurrences, are self-limited. For most patients a reasoned conservative approach to management can provide considerable palliation during an acute episode. Improvement may be judged objectively by improved straight leg raising, improved neurologic signs, and increased spinal mobility. Many surgeons claim that refractory cases requiring surgical intervention can be identified by 6 weeks; however, nearly 50% of these patients respond to additional conservative management. Thus, surgical series selected in this fashion must improve on the 50% figure before ascribing improvement to surgery.

Signs that suggest the need for immediate surgical attention are the development of new neurologic signs or the progression of motor weakness during conservative therapy. Prolonged paralysis before attempting surgery should be avoided because recovery of function is more complete if surgery is not delayed. Pain is a relative indication; surgery is more effective in eliminating radicular pain than backache. Because the results of surgery improve in the presence of prolapse, the preoperative evaluation should include myelography, with or without CT scanning. MRI shows promise as a means to visualize nerve roots without the necessity of a lumbar puncture. However, as many as one-third of normal persons may have an asymptomatic but myelographically demonstrable prolapse. In patients with classic severe sciatica with neurologic signs, approximately 10 to 20% have negative explorations. Those with negative explorations have a poorer prognosis; they are more likely to develop postlaminectomy syndrome. Therefore, in addition to the difficulties involved in improving on the natural history of low back pain by surgery, there is the possibility that the patient may be made worse.

When a prolapsed disk can be identified and removed, patients with 6 weeks of sciatica experience a shorter duration of symptoms than when treated conservatively; after 6 months, however, the results from the only randomized trial were nearly identical for conservatively and operatively treated patients. Since conservative therapy yields good results for sciatica caused by prolapse of the lumbar disk, surgical intervention should be reserved for specific indications, such as the cauda equina syndrome or progressive paralysis.

Hadler NM. Diagnosis and treatment of backache. In: Hadler N.M., ed. Medical management of the regional musculoskeletal diseases. Orlando, FL: Grune & Stratton, 1984:3–52.
A well-referenced overview of the epidemiology, diagnostic strategies, and treatment options in the treatment of mechanical back pain.

Deyo RA, ed. Occupational back pain. In: Spine: state of the art reviews. 1987. Vol. 2.
Recent multiauthor monograph on various aspects of back pain. Contains chapters on spinal manipulation, education programs, aerobic conditioning, imaging, and other topics.

Deyo RA, Diehl AK, Rosenthal M. How many days of bedrest for acute low back pain: a randomized clinical trial. N Engl J Med 1986; 315:1064–70.
Demonstrates that seven days of prescribed bed rest has no advantage, and possibly some disadvantage, over two days.

Frymoyer JW. Back pain and sciatica. N Engl J Med 1988; 318:291–300.
Excellent, if condensed, review. If you only have one reference in your file, this is a good choice.

Liang M, Komaroff A. Roentgenograms in primary care patients with acute low back pain: a cost-effectiveness analysis. Arch Intern Med 1982; 142:1108–1112.
Discusses the prevalence of the few treatable back diseases that can be detected by radiographs.

Hadler NM, Curtis P, Gillings DB, Stinnet S. A benefit of spinal manipulation as adjunctive therapy for acute low-back pain: a stratified controlled trial. Spine 1987; 12:703–06.
Demonstrates that manipulation confers some short-term benefit in acute low back pain.

Deyo RA, Loeser, JD, Bigos SJ. Herniated lumbar intervertebral disk. Ann Intern Med 1990; 112:598–603.
Excellent review of epidemiology, natural history, and therapy of disk disease.

Weber H. Lumbar disc herniation: a controlled, prospective study with ten years of observation. Spine 1983; 8:131–40.
The only randomized trial of surgery versus conservative management in disk herniation; demonstrates a slight advantage to surgery in terms of pain relief, although benefit was lost at 10 years.

70. KNEE PAIN
Axalla J. Hoole and Laurence E. Dahners

Most knee pain in ambulatory patients is caused by (1) mechanical derangements and degenerative conditions, and (2) inflammatory diseases, including infection.

Mechanical and degenerative conditions are frequently secondary to trauma and include traumatic and degenerative tears of the meniscal cartilages, tears of the cruciate or collateral ligaments, loose bodies, patellofemoral tracking abnormalities, chondromalacia patella, osteoarthritis and popliteal (Baker's) cysts. Inflammatory conditions can be either local or systemic; local conditions include bursitis in any of the many bursae about the knee and the occasional monarticular presentation of a systemic inflammatory disease. Knee pain secondary to sepsis may include gonococcal arthritis and direct infections (usually staphylococcal or streptococcal) after trauma as well as other infections more common in patients with immune compromise.

Evaluation

History
Mechanical derangements of the knee (of either intrinsic or extrinsic structures) involve a single joint that is not inflamed. Acute mechanical derangements usually are accompanied by a history of trauma while degenerative derangements may be related to an old trauma or repetitive minor traumas. Inflammatory arthritis usually involves more than one joint, but bursitis, septic arthritis, gout, or pseudogout frequently present, at least initially, in a single joint. The patient with mechanical derangements will usually complain of sudden, acute, intermittent pain as opposed to chronic aching pain with arthritic or degenerative conditions.

The patient should be asked about the following:

1. Involvement of other joints indicating systemic disease
2. Work habits (such as kneeling), leading to chronic or acute pressure to the knee that may produce bursitis
3. Painful popping or locking of the knee, which may indicate trapping of a torn meniscus or loose body between articular surfaces
4. Giving way or buckling of the knee, which may indicate subluxation (from ligament laxity) or sudden quadriceps inhibition produced by entrapment of loose bodies or meniscal fragments

5. Pain on ascending or descending stairs or jumping, which may indicate a problem in the extensor mechanism (quadriceps, patellofemoral joint, and patellar tendon)
6. Recurrent swelling occurring after acute painful episodes, which may indicate a loose body, a meniscal tear, or subluxation of the knee. If the swelling occurs spontaneously, it may indicate an inflammatory condition.

Physical Examination
Joint examination includes inspection, palpation, and mechanical testing, and examination of joints other than the knee; multiple joint involvement suggests systemic disease. Swelling, erythema, and warmth along with decreased motion may indicate inflammatory disease or infection. The noninflamed painful knee should be inspected and compared to the other side. Absence of complete extension suggests that a meniscal fragment or loose body is locked between articular surfaces. Quadriceps atrophy suggests disuse. Valgus or varus deformity suggests degenerative arthrosis. Ecchymosis indicates trauma. Swelling may indicate a large effusion or hemarthrosis (in which case it is soft and fluid) or boggy synovitis (in which case it is tender and cannot be pushed from one location to another).

Palpation of the knee detects tenderness of specific structures, local areas of enlargement, incomplete swelling, or swelling and instability. Large effusions are not difficult to detect because of the horseshoe shaped swelling about the patella, but small effusions must be sought. With the knee in extension, fluid will be visible just medial to the patella and can be milked from this area; with pressure to the lateral side of the knee, a bulge should reappear medially (Fig. 70-1). Anteriorly there may be swelling of the prepatellar bursa or tenderness of the anterior tibial tuberosity (Osgood–Schlatter disease). Posteriorly, bulging in the popliteal fossa may represent a popliteal (Baker's) cyst, characteristically found just medial to the midline. Tenderness over the joint line may indicate a problem with the underlying meniscus. Tenderness inferior to the joint line medially suggests anserine bursitis. Tears of the collateral ligaments are associated with tenderness over their course and *mechanical* instability on varus and valgus stress (Fig. 70-2). Translation of the tibia anteriorly and posteriorly on stress (the anterior-posterior drawer sign or Lachman's test (Figure 70-3)) indicates injury of the cruciate ligaments. The patient

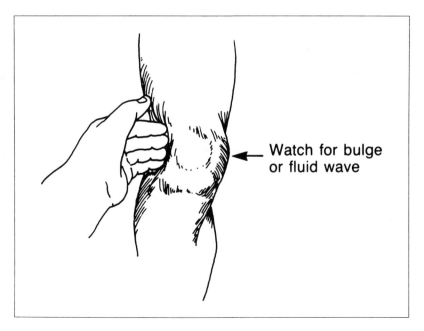

Fig. 70-1. Demonstration of knee effusion.

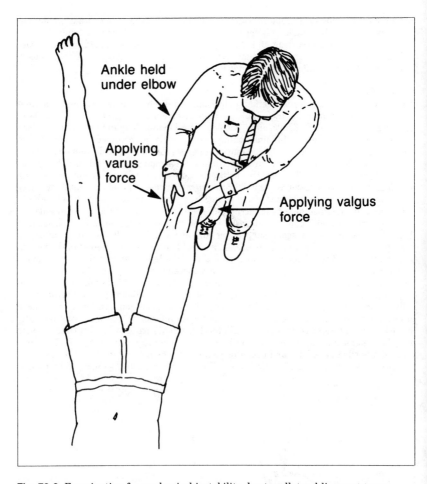

Fig. 70-2. Examination for mechanical instability due to collateral ligament tears.

should actively flex and extend the knee through its entire range of motion while the examiner palpates for crepitance in the patellofemoral joint or medial or lateral compartment.

Laboratory Tests
X-rays are indicated after trauma. Weight-bearing films can help establish a diagnosis of osteoarthritis by showing joint space narrowing and osteophytes. A CBC and sedimentation rate can be useful indicators of sepsis and inflammation. Joint fluid should be obtained from all patients who present with a knee effusion for the first time and should be sent for a Gram's stain, culture, cell count, and crystal analysis. A cell count helps differentiate infection (WBC > 20,000), inflammation (WBC 1000–50,000), and degenerative and mechanical conditions (WBC < 2000).

Management
Identification and management can be simplified by grouping problems in the following way:

1. Acute traumatic events, usually involving one knee
2. Recurrent acute painful episodes in a single noninflamed knee

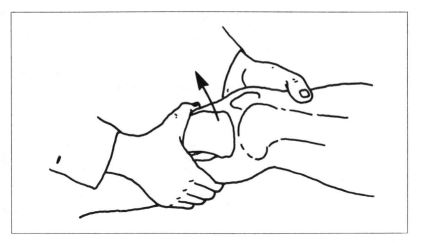

Fig. 70-3. Anterior-posterior drawer sign (Lachman's test) for cruciate ligament instability.

3. Chronic aching pain
4. Multiple or single inflamed joints. These problems require aspiration for joint fluid, frequently require inpatient management, and are not discussed further in this manual.

Acute Traumatic Events
Acute traumatic events usually involve one knee and are painful without inflammation; causes include fractures, meniscal and ligamentous tears, and patellar dislocation. To avoid displacing a nondisplaced fracture, x-rays (anteroposterior, lateral, and sunrise views) should be taken before the patient undergoes extensive examination of the knee.

Acute meniscal tears frequently present with a history of a twisting, athletic injury, with swelling that accumulates in the joint over several hours and tenderness over the affected meniscus. Patients will frequently have a loss of motion from locking of the meniscus between the articular surfaces.

Torn ligaments present with a history of an acute traumatic event to a knee that has swollen rapidly after an injury. There will frequently be loss of motion because of a tense hemarthrosis; stress of the collateral ligaments or the anterior-posterior drawer sign should demonstrate instability. Stress to injured ligaments is usually painful, but completely ruptured ligaments may sometimes not be painful on examination because there is no longer any stress applied to the nerve endings.

Acute patellar dislocations, which occur most frequently in women, are usually relocated by the time the patient reaches the doctor's office since the dislocation reduces as soon as the leg is completely extended. The patient will often state that the leg was severely deformed at the time of the injury (from patellar displacement). The patient will have a large hemarthrosis and severe pain on attempts to push the patella laterally (apprehension sign). These acute traumatic injuries should be splinted, iced, and referred to a specialist for treatment.

Recurrent Acute Painful Episodes in a Single Noninflamed Knee
Intermittent sudden acute painful episodes that resolve rapidly, but recur, may be caused by meniscal tears, loose bodies, recurrent patellar dislocation, and recurrent joint subluxations.

Meniscal tears in the young patient may be related to a past acute traumatic event, but in the patient aged 40 and above, degenerative meniscal tears may be produced without trauma. The patient frequently relates repeated locking episodes and sudden sharp pains, with or without the knee popping and/or giving way. The patient will have tenderness over the joint line. Radiographs will be normal. In some patients, typical signs and symptoms of a meniscal tear resolve upon being treated with nonsteroidal anti-inflammatory medications. This course may be tried before the patient is referred to a specialist.

Loose bodies present with similar symptoms to meniscal tears, but the patient may have felt the loose body in his knee. X-rays frequently show a defect in the medial femoral condyle typical of osteochondritis dissecans from which the loose body came. This condition requires arthroscopic treatment.

Recurrent patellar dislocation occurs most frequently in young women, aged 15 to 30, although it usually begins after an acute traumatic episode. The patient will usually report deformed appearance of the knee on flexion that resolved on extension. Treatment involves anti-inflammatory medications along with physical therapy to strengthen the vastus medialis portion of the quadriceps mechanism.

Recurrent subluxation of the knee from ligament laxity occurs more commonly in young men. Usually patients relate a history of an old traumatic twisting injury to the knee and complain of giving way; on physical examination, an anterior drawer sign or Lachman's test (usually the anterior cruciate ligament is involved) suggests ligamentous laxity. These patients require referral to an orthopedist.

Chronic Aching Knee Pain
Chronic aching knee pain is associated with chondromalacia, plica syndrome, tendinitis, degenerative joint disease, Osgood–Schlatter disease, bursitis, and popliteal cyst. Extensor mechanism pain in chondromalacia, tendinitis, and Osgood–Schlatter disease is usually exacerbated by ascending and descending stairs or inclines because of the extensive work necessary by the quadriceps during these activities. Although some asymptomatic patients also have grinding, painful grinding in the patellofemoral joint suggests a diagnosis of chrondromalacia (especially in younger women) or osteoarthritis in the older patient.

Chondromalacia patallae is thought to be caused by abnormal patellofemoral tracking. X-ray (sunrise view) may document lateral subluxation of the patella. Conservative management of chondromalacia is usually sufficient, although complete resolution of symptoms is frequently impossible. The patient must be reassured that the condition is benign and usually self-limited. Restricting athletic activity and prescribing anti-inflammatory medicines usually result in improvement. Immobilization in an acute episode and use of ice packs after exercise may also be useful. Isometric and terminal quadriceps exercises (exercising only from 10–15 degrees of flexion) may be used to strengthen the vastus medialis in order to pull the patella back medially.

Plica syndrome is caused by an inflamed fold of tissue thought to be an embryologic remnant that lies just medially to the distal pole of the patella. These patients frequently have extensor mechanism pain but may also experience popping that can be confused with meniscal tears. There should be tenderness over the medial femoral condyle and sometimes the plica can be palpated. This condition also usually responds well to anti-inflammatory medications but if necessary the plica can be removed arthroscopically.

Tendinitis can occur in any of the tendons about the knee but is most common in the patella tendon. The patient experiences pain in the region of the patella tendon that is exacerbated by climbing stairs but is most notable with jumping (jumper's knee). Patients frequently respond to several weeks of immobilization followed by several months of avoidance of jumping coupled with anti-inflammatory medication.

Osteoarthritis of the knee is very common in patients over age 40. It is frequently associated with obesity and varus deformity. Patients often complain of pain and stiffness after a period of immobilization. This pain improves with light activity; however, with continuous activity the pain worsens. Effusions are infrequent, and there should be no signs of inflammation; bony enlargement is common. Radiographs demonstrate a narrowed joint space, subchondral sclerosis and cysts, and osteophyte formation. Anti-inflammatory medications are frequently effective in providing pain relief. Quadriceps strengthening exercises, swimming as a substitute for walking (if pain worsens with walking), and local heat also may help. Patients with constant severe pain that does not respond to conservative treatment may be considered for joint replacement; however, obesity and age less than 60 are relative contraindications.

Osgood Schlatter disease is a self-limited inflammatory condition of the tibial tuberosity/apophysis (where the patellar tendon inserts on the tibia) in adolescence. Examination shows swelling and tenderness at the tuberosity, and x-ray reveals fragmentation of the apophysis. This condition usually resolves with maturity and until then, immobilization for acute episodes and curtailing exercise is usually sufficient treatment.

Bursitis frequently occurs in the prepatellar bursa in patients who spend time kneeling and also appears in other locations around the knee after mild trauma or with recurrent pressure. A large swelling that occurs in the prepatellar bursa can be differentiated from an effusion in the knee because it cannot be milked into other portions of the knee. Marked erythema and warmth may indicate septic bursitis and may require aspiration and antibiotics. Most patients respond well to wrapping, avoiding trauma or pressure to the area, and anti-inflammatory medication. Aspiration of fluid should be a last resort because of the possibility of causing a draining sinus and infection in subcutaneous bursae.

Popliteal cysts (Baker's cyst) cause a swollen tender area just medial to the midline on the posterior aspect of the knee. They are related to degeneration of the posterior joint capsule and distention of the gastrocnemius-semimembranosus bursa and usually are associated with an abnormality within the knee itself. Cysts usually resolve with treatment of the knee pathology, and, if they are asymptomatic, they do not require treatment at all. Ultrasonography is a useful test to demonstrate the cyst (and rule out tumor) in patients with large and painful cysts. Aspiration followed by instillation of steroid can produce acute resolution; however, the cysts may recur if the intra-articular pathology is not treated. Occasionally a ruptured cyst may cause pain and swelling of the calf, thus resembling a deep venous thrombosis.

Chang WS, Zuckerman JD, Pitman MI. Geriatic knee disorders, Part 1: evaluative techniques. Geriatrics 1988; 43(2):73–83.

Chang WS, Zuckerman JD. Geriatric knee disorders, Part 2: differential diagnosis and treatment. 1988; 43(3):39–42, 44–46.
These two articles discuss knee problems in the elderly in more detail.

Zarins B, Adams M. Medical progress. Knee injuries in sports. N Engl J Med 1988; 318:950–61.
An excellent summary of this subject, with several useful drawings.

Hoppenfeld S. Physical examination of the knee joint complaint. Orthop Clin North Am 1979; 10:3–20.
A very useful and understandable review of the examination.

Noble J. The painful knee. Br J Hosp Med 1979; 22:169–76.
Presents a classification and discussion of an approach to knee pain.

Wigley RD. Popliteal cyst: variations on the theme of Baker cyst. Semin Arthritis Rheum 1982; 7:1–10.
An excellent review of this problem.

Gruber MA. The conservative treatment of chondromalacia patellae. Orthop Clin North Am 1979; 10:105–15.
A good overview of the disease.

Wilson FC. Degenerative disease of the knee: clinical aspects and management. NC Med J 1978; 39:360–63.
A very brief but useful overview for initial reference.

Kellgren JH, Lawrence JS. Osteoarthrosis and disc degeneration in an urban population. Ann Rheum Dis 1958; 17:388–97.
Population study from which data on prevalence and associated findings of osteoarthrosis are usually taken.

71. TENDINITIS AND BURSITIS
Kenneth E. Sack

Tendinitis and Tenosynovitis

The terms *tendinitis* and *tenosynovitis* are imprecise. Short of surgical exploration, the degree to which a tendon or its surrounding synovial sheath is damaged or inflamed is always presumptive. Nonetheless, pain in or near a tendon usually evokes a diagnosis of tendinitis. Patients with tendinitis typically give a history of blunt trauma to the area or repetitive activity (overuse) of the affected part; they characteristically demonstrate pain on active or passive stretching of the tendon. Tenosynovitis describes the condition of swelling or crepitation occurring along the course of the tendon. Acute infectious tenosynovitis, a classic feature of gonococcal disease, causes the patient to resist even the slightest motion of the involved area. Common sites of tendinitis are described in Table 71-1.

Noninfectious tenosynovitis usually improves with joint rest or short-term therapy with a nonsteroidal anti-inflammatory drug (NSAID). For refractory cases, injection of the tendon sheath with 5 to 10 mg of a soluble steroid (e.g., triamcinolone acetonide) often speeds recovery. High resistance to injection indicates that the needle may be in the tendon itself, and injection could cause it to rupture. In this instance, the needle should simply be withdrawn slightly until the steroid can be easily injected. Frequent injections of a given structure or the use of less soluble "depo" steroid preparations (e.g., triamcinolone hexacetonide) can produce local tissue atrophy. Occasionally, persistent symptoms necessitate surgical excision of a chronically inflamed tendon sheath.

Common Tendinitis Syndromes

Carpal Tunnel Syndrome
Although not strictly a tendinitis, carpal tunnel syndrome often results from inflammation of the volar wrist tendons and surrounding soft tissues. It manifests as paresthesias or discomfort in the sensory distribution of the median nerve; occasionally pain radiates proximally as far as the shoulder. Nocturnal exacerbations often dominate the clinical picture.

Repetitive activity involving the upper extremities (e.g., gardening), synovitis of the wrist, and pregnancy can each lead to carpal tunnel syndrome; when there is no obvious

Table 71-1. Common Sites of Tendon Injury

Finger flexors (trigger finger)
Thumb extensors at the radial styloid (de Quervain's disease)
Wrist and finger extensors at the lateral epicondyle (tennis elbow)
Wrist and finger flexors at the medial epicondyle (golfer's elbow)
Supraspinatus tendon near the greater tubercle of the humerus
Hip abductors at the greater trochanter
Hip adductors at the pubis
Popliteus tendon at the lateral femoral condyle
Iliotibial band* at the lateral tibial plateau (runner's knee)
Patellar tendon (jumper's knee)
Tibialis posterior tendon near the tibia–fibula interosseous membrane (shin splints)
Foot and toe extensors
Achilles tendon at the calcaneus
Plantar fascia* at the calcaneus

*A fascial band without an associated muscle; thus, not a true tendon.

inciting event, it is important to search for possible associated conditions, such as hypothyroidism, acromegaly, and amyloidosis. Proximal nerve injury, as from cervical degenerative conditions, can render the distal nerve more vulnerable to damage (double-crush syndrome).

PHYSICAL FINDINGS. A tingling sensation in the sensory nerve distribution elicited by gently tapping the carpal tunnel at and just distal to the flexor crease near the palmaris longus tendon (Tinel's sign) or after fully flexing the patient's wrist for 30 to 60 seconds (positive Phalen's maneuver) suggests median nerve dysfunction.

Severe and long-standing damage to the median nerve can produce thenar atrophy due to involvement of the abductor pollicis brevis and opponens pollicis muscles. It can also cause decreased sensation in the median nerve distribution.

DIAGNOSTIC STUDIES. An electromyogram and a nerve conduction study help to confirm the diagnosis of carpal tunnel syndrome and to exclude a cervical radiculopathy or other neuromuscular disorder. Prolonged sensory conduction time (latency) across the carpal tunnel and a decrease in sensory signal amplitude are typical findings. Abnormal motor conduction across the carpal tunnel and electromyographic abnormalities in the thenar muscles also may occur. A normal nerve conduction study, however, does not exclude the diagnosis of carpal tunnel syndrome.

Use of a lightweight wrist splint, initially for most of the day and then only at night, often relieves the symptoms. Injection of 10 to 20 mg of a soluble corticosteroid into the carpal tunnel may provide additional benefit. (Placement of the needle on the ulnar side of the palmaris longus tendon at the distal volar wrist crease helps avoid direct injection into the median nerve.) When symptoms have been present for more than 6 to 12 months, medical treatment is frequently ineffective, and surgical release of the flexor retinaculum becomes necessary. Surgical intervention is indicated early for carpal tunnel syndrome due to trauma or to infiltrative disorders such as amyloidosis.

De Quervain's Disease

De Quervain's disease refers to swelling and tenderness over the volar portion of the "snuff box" resulting from chronic tenosynovitis of the abductor pollicis longus and extensor pollicis brevis tendons. Stretching the affected tendons by active or passive adduction of the thumb exacerbates symptoms. Pain due to degenerative disease of the first carpometacarpal joint is little affected by these maneuvers.

Therapy with a thumb splint and a nonsteroidal anti-inflammatory agent suffices in most cases, but some patients need an injection of 5 to 10 mg of a soluble steroid for lasting relief. Rarely, refractory discomfort requires surgical release of the stenosed tendon sheath.

Tennis Elbow (Lateral Epicondylitis)

Lateral epicondylitis manifests as pain and tenderness at the origin of the finger and wrist extensors when resistance is applied. This maneuver is more sensitive if done with the patient's elbow extended, but in severe cases pain occurs with a flexed elbow as well. Pathologic specimens show involvement principally of the extensor carpi radialis brevis tendon. Patients with entrapment of the posterior interosseous nerve as it passes into the supinator muscle may experience pain in the proximal forearm or near the lateral epicondyle, but this condition usually occurs in association with weakness of the finger and thumb extensors.

Conservative management of lateral epicondylitis consists primarily of splinting the wrist in neutral position, wearing a forearm band (a narrow strip of rubber and Velcro that wraps around the upper forearm), or NSAID therapy. Ultrasound treatments provide occasional benefit. When symptoms abate, a program of gradual stretching and strengthening exercises should begin. Some physicians advocate one or two injections of steroid into the involved area, but relapse of symptoms is common and the risk of soft tissue atrophy is high. In refractory cases, surgical release of the anterolateral elbow capsule and extensor tendons may become necessary. Even with optimal treatment, as many as 40% of patients with tennis elbow continue to have minor symptoms over a 5 to 6 year follow-up period.

Golfer's Elbow (Medial Epicondylitis)
A rarer syndrome than lateral epicondylitis, medial epicondylitis manifests as pain and tenderness at the origin of the flexor–pronator muscles on the medial epicondyle of the elbow. Careful neurologic examination will exclude compression of the ulnar nerve, which can become entrapped between the two heads of the flexor carpi ulnaris muscle. Treatment of medial epicondylitis is similar to that of lateral epicondylitis.

Supraspinatus Tendinitis
See Chapter 68.

Bursitis

Bursae are fluid-filled, often synovial-lined, sacs located at friction-prone areas such as bone-tendon and muscle-muscle interfaces. The human body contains at least 150 such structures, most of which are unnamed. Some bursae, such as the anserine (the combined insertion of the sartorius, gracilis, and semitendinosus tendons on the medial tibia) and the subdeltoid, are present at birth. Others, particularly the more superficial bursae, form later at areas subject to repeated friction.

Typical sites of bursal inflammation are the olecranon, subdeltoid, greater trochanter, ischial tuberosity ("weaver's bottom"), prepatella ("housemaid's knee"), anserine, calcaneus, and medial first metatarsophalangeal joint (bunion). Patients with bursitis usually give a history of repeated trauma to the involved area. Women with obese legs are prone to develop anserine bursitis.

Pain on active or passive motion of an extremity may be the only indication of bursitis. Inflammation of a superficial bursa, such as that overlying the olecranon process, often causes only painless swelling. Fever, extreme tenderness, surrounding cellulitis, or evidence of local skin trauma (particularly in an immunocompromised patient) suggests associated infection, usually with *Staphylococcus aureus*, and mandates aspiration of the bursa.

Noninfected bursal fluid ordinarily contains less than 1000 WBC/μl (range of 50–11,000), predominantly mononuclear cells. Infected fluid, however, often contains more than 50,000 WBC/μl (range of 1500–400,000), predominantly polymorphonuclear cells; the Gram's stain is positive in about 70% of these cases. Crystal-induced bursitis may cause surrounding erythema and low-grade fever, with bursal cell count ranging from 1000 to 6000 μl. Examination of the fluid with a polarizing microscope usually reveals the offending crystal.

Treatment varies with the location and cause of bursitis. Resting the involved extremity is essential for deep, musculotendinous bursitis. NSAIDs and local steroid injections are useful adjuncts. For mild superficial bursitis, local protection may be all that is necessary. More severely involved bursae usually require aspiration followed by compressive dressings and NSAIDs. When aspirating the olecranon bursa it is prudent to insert the needle from either the medial or lateral aspect rather than directly over the olecranon process; otherwise persistent drainage may ensue. Intrabursal injection of a soluble, short-acting steroid may hasten recovery and prevent recurrences, but it can also cause local skin atrophy. Most cases of infected bursitis respond to a 14-day course of oral semisynthetic penicillin (e.g., dicloxacillin).

Brody DM. Running injuries. Prevention and management. Rheumatology Rounds. Summit, NJ: Ciba-Geigy, 1987; 1–36.
Superb descriptions and illustrations of common running injuries and their management.

Ho G, Mikolich DJ. Bacterial infection of the superficial subcutaneous bursae. Clin Rheum Dis 1986; 12:437–57.
Detailed treatise on the recognition and treatment of infected bursae, from authors with extensive experience.

Larsson LG, Baum J. The syndromes of bursitis. Bull Rheum Dis 1986; 36:1–8.
Nice review of clinical evaluation and treatment of bursitis.

Pinals, RS. Traumatic arthritis and allied conditions. In: McCarty D, ed. Arthritis and allied conditions. Philadelphia: Lea & Febiger, 1989; 1371–89.
General review of tendinitis and bursitis as well as other traumatic musculoskeletal conditions.

72. Nonarticular Musculoskeletal Pain
Kenneth E. Sack

Patients with chronic, ill-defined musculoskeletal pain present a challenging clinical problem. Important diagnostic considerations in such patients include muscle disease (e.g., secondary to trauma, infection, polymyositis), neurologic disorders (e.g., neuropathy, nerve entrapment, reflex sympathetic dystrophy, Parkinson's disease), bone disease (e.g., infection, neoplasm, hypertrophic osteoarthropathy), endocrinopathies (e.g., hypothyroidism, hyperparathyroidism), infectious disease (e.g., bacterial endocarditis), drug effect (e.g., steroid withdrawal, vitamin A overuse), phlebitis, panniculitis, vasculitis, and polymyalgia rheumatica. In most cases, a careful history and physical examination will direct the clinician to the likely source of the discomfort. Laboratory studies usually add little to the evaluation of patients with this type of pain.

Differential Diagnosis

History
The following details may be important.

CIRCUMSTANCES SURROUNDING THE ONSET OF PAIN. Pertinent examples are physical trauma (especially work related) and emotional trauma (death of a friend or relative, or the anniversary of a death).

CAREFUL DESCRIPTION OF THE PAIN. Sharp, lancinating pain is often neuropathic. Dull, aching pain becoming worse at night suggests a bone tumor such as an osteoid osteoma. Constant, unvarying pain symbolizes severe injury or inflammation, but it can also herald psychogenic rheumatism.

CONDITIONS THAT ALLEVIATE OR EXACERBATE PAIN. Musculotendinous strain or inflammation causes pain that usually decreases with rest. Conversely, pain of infectious, neoplastic, or psychogenic origin ordinarily does not abate with rest.

THE MANNER IN WHICH THE PATIENT DESCRIBES THE PAIN. Emotionally charged descriptions, such as "being stabbed with a knife," or unduly vague statements, such as "I can't describe it," may suggest psychogenic syndromes.

THE MEANING OF THE SYMPTOM TO THE PATIENT. A surprising amount of useful information may come from asking the patient to speculate on the cause of his or her pain.

ASSOCIATED COMPLAINTS. Fatigue and disturbed sleep are common in patients with fibromyalgia; morning stiffness, localized temporal headache, loss of vision, or jaw claudication suggests polymyalgia–temporal arteritis complex.

CURRENT MEDICATIONS. Use of narcotics, psychotropic drugs, and agents capable of inducing pain (e.g., high doses of steroids or vitamin A) merits attention.

SOCIAL SETTING. Relevant issues may be marital discord, substance abuse, excessive physical or emotional demands of the patient's occupation, potentially injurious hobbies, and pending legal claims (e.g., for disability insurance, workers' compensation, or a personal injury lawsuit).

FAMILY HISTORY OF PAINFUL OR DEBILITATING CONDITIONS. Rheumatic diseases, neuromuscular disorders, and neoplasias, as well as multiple functional complaints, may have a familial association.

THE IMPACT OF PAIN ON THE PATIENT. How the pain affects his or her household functions, job responsibilities, and interpersonal relations provides vital information for designing a comprehensive treatment program.

Physical Examination
Physical abnormalities with potential relevance are clubbed fingers in hypertrophic osteoarthropathy, periungual infarcts and splinter hemorrhages in vasculitis, puffy hands in reflex sympathetic dystrophy, swollen and tender temporal arteries in giant cell arteritis (often associated with polymyalgia rheumatica), heart murmur and splenomegaly in bacterial endocarditis, tremor and muscle rigidity in Parkinson's disease, and dry skin and "hung-up" deep tendon reflexes in hypothyroidism.

The characteristic findings of fibromyalgia, myofascial pain, and psychogenic rheumatism are described under Chronic Musculoskeletal Pain Syndromes.

Laboratory Tests
In the assessment of patients with diffuse musculoskeletal pain, laboratory tests routinely consist of a complete blood count; erythrocyte sedimentation rate; urinalysis; liver and thyroid function tests; and serum creatinine, glucose, and calcium concentrations. If muscle weakness or sensory deficits are present, a serum creatine phosphokinase (CPK) determination, an electromyogram, and nerve conduction studies may prove helpful.

Chronic Musculoskeletal Pain Syndromes
Since the 1800s, the medical literature has been rife with articles on "muscular rheumatism." The numerous studies on this subject are nearly impossible to evaluate because valid criteria for diagnosis are lacking, proper controls are absent, and the researchers could not ensure double-blind trials. It may be best to refer to this category of illness as "pain amplification syndromes" and attempt to define subtypes that share reproducible symptoms and signs and that respond to similar treatments.

Following are summaries of the typical clinical characteristics and therapies of three common chronic pain syndromes: fibromyalgia, myofascial pain, and psychogenic rheumatism. Lumping all pain syndromes into two or three categories may be inappropriate, but splitting them excessively is equally unsatisfactory. This classification is widely accepted but somewhat arbitrary, since these entities are based on clinical rather than pathologic findings. For any given patient, a precise diagnosis may be impossible.

Fibromyalgia ("Fibrositis")
Fibromyalgia, a poorly understood syndrome of waxing and waning muscle pain and stiffness, occurs predominantly in women. Manifestations include generalized aching pain or stiffness involving at least three anatomic sites for 3 months or more; multiple tender spots at characteristic locations (upper trapezius and medial scapular borders, midbuttocks, anterior costochondral junctions, lateral elbows, medial knees); and the absence of other recognizable conditions capable of producing the pain. Also common are disturbed sleep, generalized fatigue, chronic headache, and irritable bowel symptoms. Laboratory studies are normal.

Treatment requires a consistent and trusting doctor-patient relationship, reassurances that the ailment is not crippling, and acknowledgment that the pain is real. Regularly scheduled patient visits should allow plenty of time for listening and discussion. Low impact aerobic exercise (e.g., walking, jogging, swimming, biking) at least 3 or 4 days a week can reduce pain. Biofeedback may benefit patients who have no underlying psychopathology. Low-dose tricyclics (e.g., amitriptyline, 10–50 mg hs, or cyclobenzaprine, 10–40 mg/day) are occasionally effective pain modifiers; nonsteroidal anti-inflammatory drugs (NSAIDs) and steroids are usually of no benefit.

Myofascial Pain

Myofascial pain is more regional than that of fibromyalgia. Generalized symptoms usually do not occur; men and women are affected equally. Patients often report having engaged in an activity that could cause muscle strain.

"Trigger points" are the hallmark of this syndrome. They are sites of extreme muscle tenderness (usually in the muscle belly) that on deep pressure cause referred pain of reproducible distribution and quality.

Myofascial pain, especially when treated early, tends to be self-limiting. Removal of causal factors (e.g., modifying a strenuous activity) may be the only treatment necessary. Instruction in appropriate stretching exercises and the administration of deep massage by an experienced physical therapist are useful measures. When a well-defined trigger point is present, injection of the area with 1 to 3 cc of a 0.5 to 1% solution of Xylocaine, using a 25-gauge needle, may hasten recovery. Use of vapocoolant spray provides prolonged pain relief for some patients. Fluori-Methane is preferable to the highly flammable ethyl chloride. Proper technique consists of gentle passive stretching of the involved muscle group, followed by slow parallel sweeps of the jet stream starting from the trigger point and moving toward the area of referred pain.

Psychogenic Rheumatism

Psychogenic rheumatism may be a form of somatization disorder (see Chap. 110). Patients with this ailment usually give dramatic descriptions of their pain, tend to be vague as to its site, and have numerous associated functional complaints. Pain severity often varies with the patient's emotional state. Physical examination shows multiple areas of extreme tenderness to even light touch (the "touch-me-not" syndrome), but distracting the patient almost always abrogates this response.

Effective treatment is difficult at best. It requires a sympathetic, reassuring manner on the part of the physician. At times, antidepressants may help.

Barsky AJ. Patients who amplify bodily sensations. Ann Intern Med 1979; 91:63–70.
  A concise and practical review of the psychological, social, situational, and cultural considerations in assessing the patient with chronic pain.

Bennett RM. Fibrositis: evolution of an enigma. J Rheumatol 1986; 13:676–78.
  Distinguishes myofascial pain syndrome from fibromyalgia.

Campbell SM. The regional myofascial pain syndromes. Rheum Dis Clin North Am 1989; 15:31–44.
  A review, including common locations of trigger points and reference zones, presumed pathophysiology of myofascial pain, and current treatment modalities.

Engel GL. "Psychogenic" pain and the pain-prone patient. Am J Med 1959; 26:899–918.
  A classic description of the psychodynamics of pain.

Goldenberg DL. Fibromyalgia syndrome: an emerging but controversial condition. JAMA 1987; 257:2782–87.
  A reasonably complete review including current definition of fibromyalgia, proposed pathophysiology, natural history, and treatment.

Goldenberg DL. Treatment of fibromyalgia syndrome. Rheum Dis Clin North Am 1989; 15:61–71.
  Reviews the literature on the treatment of fibromyalgia.

73. NOCTURNAL LEG CRAMPS
Laurie Dornbrand

Nocturnal leg cramps are common and troublesome, but are almost never associated with serious unsuspected disease. The major issues for the clinician are recognition of the usual presentation, differential diagnosis, and treatment options.

Nocturnal cramps usually occur in the calves, with palpable firmness and bulging of the involved muscle. Episodes may occur more than once a night and are often severe and distressing. The muscles may remain sore and tender for up to several hours. Patients sometimes attain relief by dorsiflexing the involved foot or by getting out of bed and pressing the foot firmly against the floor. Massaging the muscle is usually less effective.

Nocturnal leg cramps occur most frequently in the elderly; in younger people they are more likely to occur after unaccustomed exercise. Surveys of ambulatory patients have uncovered a history of night cramps in 40 to 50%, with the prevalence increasing to 70% in those aged 50 or over. Of course many do not seek medical attention for this condition.

Diagnosis

The diagnosis is based on a typical history and the exclusion of pathologic conditions associated with cramps. It is especially important to rule out ischemic conditions. Peripheral vascular disease is suggested by symptoms of exercise-related pain, cramps, weakness, numbness or tingling, and the findings of diminished pulses, sensory deficits, and cool or discolored skin. Diabetic neuropathy also is associated with cramps. Patients with ischemia or diabetic neuropathy do not have as good a prognosis or response to drugs as patients with uncomplicated nocturnal leg cramps, and treatment should be directed at the underlying disorder. Other conditions associated with cramps include metabolic disorders (hyponatremia, hypokalemia, uremia, hyper- or hypothyroidism), pregnancy, and partial denervation (as in amyotrophic lateral sclerosis).

There are no specific physical findings or laboratory tests to confirm the diagnosis. Explanations for nocturnal leg cramps are speculative and generally fall into two categories: metabolic and mechanical. Stimulation of leg muscles at night by accumulation of unspecified metabolites has been implicated. It also has been suggested that flaccid muscles, such as those passively plantar flexed, have an increased tendency to recoil into spasm, because there is inadequate muscle tension to limit spontaneous contractions. However, the pathophysiology of the problem remains elusive.

Treatment

Many different treatments have been suggested, including drugs, exercises, and alteration in sleeping positions. Because cramps occur at irregular intervals, adequately controlled trials are necessary to evaluate therapies and to distinguish effects of therapy from placebo effect. Most of the reports on treatment of cramps lack controls or have weaknesses of experimental design.

Quinine, 200 to 300 mg at night, is the classic therapy; its efficacy has been confirmed in a number of small placebo-controlled trials. Quinine is believed to work by increasing the refractory period and thus stabilizing the muscle membranes. It also decreases the excitability of the motor end-plate by competitively blocking acetylcholine. Relief usually occurs within the first week of treatment. Many patients remain free of cramps when quinine is discontinued and require only occasional doses of the drug thereafter. The major contraindications to its use include pregnancy, a history of quinine hypersensitivity, and G6PD deficiency. Both 200-mg and 300-mg tablets are available over-the-counter, at a cost of 10 to 15 cents per dose. The drug Quinamm, marketed specifically for treatment of nocturnal leg cramps, formerly was a combination of quinine and aminophylline but currently consists of 260 mg of quinine sulfate. It requires a prescription and costs about 45 cents a dose.

Vitamin E has been reported effective in large but uncontrolled series. The usual dosage is 400 IU per day, with the duration of therapy unspecified. It has been suggested that simultaneous administration of inorganic iron may inactivate the vitamin. Conjugated estrogens (Premarin) may counteract the effectiveness. The risks of vitamin E therapy are considered to be minimal, although there have been some anecdotal reports of associated problems including fatigue, hypertension, and thrombophlebitis, usually with dosages of more than 400 IU per day.

Other drugs with reported success in relieving cramps, usually on the basis of small and/or uncontrolled studies, include methocarbamol (Robaxin), chloroquine, verapamil, diphenhydramine (Benadryl), and carisoprodol (Soma). Although phenytoin (Dilantin) is mentioned as a therapy, no studies have been published on its effectiveness. There is little evidence to support the use of any of these drugs before quinine or vitamin E.

Calf muscle stretching exercises have been reported to relieve symptoms within 1 to 7 days. The patient stands facing a wall 2 to 3 feet away and leans forward with hands on the wall and heels remaining on the floor until a pulling sensation is felt in the calves. The stretched position should be held for 10 seconds and repeated after a 5-second period of relaxation. It is suggested that this sequence be repeated three times a day until the cramps are gone.

Sleeping positions designed to minimize involuntary plantar flexion of the foot during sleep also have been recommended, based on the theory that nocturnal cramps result from spontaneous contraction of flaccid calf muscles. Patients who sleep on their back should keep the covers loose or use a board or pillow at the foot of the bed. Patients who are prone to cramps should let their feet extend over the end of the mattress. All patients should consciously stretch their legs with feet dorsiflexed rather than plantar flexed.

In the absence of general agreement on the cause of nocturnal leg cramps or controlled studies of therapies, the practitioner may select among the alternatives discussed. Vitamin E is slightly cheaper than quinine but may require administration over a longer period of time for effective control of symptoms. Stretching exercises and modification of sleeping position are free of cost but may require unacceptable changes in habits or life-style for some patients.

McGee SR. Muscle cramps. Arch Int Med 1990; 150:511–18.
An excellent review, including pathophysiology, clinical setting, and treatment of cramps. Extensively referenced

Fung MC, Holbrook JH. Placebo-controlled trial of quinine therapy for nocturnal leg cramps. West J Med 1989; 151:42–44.
A small (8 patients) but recent study that supports the effectiveness of quinine.

Ayers S, Mihan R. Nocturnal leg cramps (systremma). *South Med J* 1974; 67:1308–12.
A report of the success of vitamin E in 125 patients.

Daniel HW. Simple cure for nocturnal leg cramps. *N Engl J Med* 1979; 301:216.
All patients with frequent nocturnal cramps treated with a simple stretching exercise reported cure within a week.

Weiner LH, Weiner HL. Nocturnal leg muscle cramps. *JAMA* 1980; 244:2332–33.
A mechanical approach to the pathophysiology and treatment.

XI. REPRODUCTIVE SYSTEM PROBLEMS

74. VAGINITIS
Jack D. McCue and Laurie Dornbrand

The diagnosis of vaginitis is based on the patient's complaints of itching, burning, dysuria, dyspareunia, or malodorous or unusual discharge, and is supported by microscopic examination of vaginal secretions. The character and quantity of normal vaginal secretions may vary considerably from one woman to another, at different times during the menstrual cycle, and with other factors, such as age, degree of sexual arousal, emotional state, use of contraceptive devices or drugs, and frequency of douching. The presence of a discharge is therefore not in itself abnormal. Normal vaginal secretions derive primarily from cervical mucus, transudation through the vaginal wall, and exfoliated cells, which are altered by anaerobic and facultatively anaerobic lactobacilli. The resulting secretions are acidic (pH 3.8–4.2), clear or white, homogeneous or somewhat flocculent, viscous, essentially odorless, and contain few polymorphonuclear leukocytes (PMNs).

Symptoms of vaginitis are nonspecific, and determination of cause from clinical findings alone is unreliable. Microscopic evaluation of the discharge is essential and should include potassium hydroxide (KOH) and saline preparations of vaginal secretions; Gram's stains are very useful in experienced hands. Detection of infection is dependent on the number of organisms present and may be impaired by recent douching.

Most of the organisms associated with vaginitis can be found in asymptomatic women, and, except for trichomoniasis, treatment is usually aimed at the relief of symptoms rather than at the eradication of organisms. In most office practices, the most frequently seen causes of vaginal symptoms include candidal vulvovaginitis (45%), bacterial vaginosis (35%), and *Trichomonas* vaginitis (10%), with other and undiagnosable causes accounting for about 10%.

Candidal Vaginitis
The prevalence of positive cultures for *Candida albicans* or *Torulopsis glabrata* in asymptomatic women with normal vaginal secretions is about 20 to 50%. Factors that predispose to colonization and infection with *Candida* include diabetes, corticosteroid therapy, pregnancy, broad-spectrum antibiotics (including metronidazole), obesity, heat- and moisture-retaining clothing (such as nylon underwear), oral contraceptives, immunosuppressant drugs, depressed cell-mediated immunity, and the acquired immunodeficiency syndrome (AIDS).

Pruritus is the most common complaint associated with candidal vaginitis. Vulvar inflammation and even edema may be quite pronounced, with resultant dyspareunia and dysuria. A dry, cottage cheese–like discharge is 90% specific for yeast and is present in about 50% of instances. The diagnosis is established by a positive KOH preparation. One or more drops of 10% KOH solution are mixed with a specimen of vaginal discharge, and pseudohyphae or budding yeast forms are sought under high-dry microscopic examination. If the preparation is done properly, vaginal epithelial cells and leukocytes are lysed with only their outlines visible. The KOH reagent tends to lose potency on standing, especially when not refrigerated, and should be replenished periodically. The KOH preparation is very specific, but to yield a positive result it requires large numbers of yeast forms to be present. The Gram's stain is more sensitive than the wet mount in identifying yeast, but it requires more time and experience to interpret. Cultures are not recommended because the growth of yeast may reflect colonization rather than infection. A positive culture in the absence of a characteristic clinical presentation is neither diagnostic nor grounds for treatment. Occasionally the clinical presentation strongly suggests *Candida* infection, but yeast cannot be demonstrated on smear or even on vaginal cultures. *Candida* can, however, be demonstrated in 55% of such women from vulvar and rectal cultures, suggesting that *Candida* infection may present as a vulvar disease without detectable *Candida* organisms in the vagina. Therefore, it may be justified to treat apparent or suspected candidal vulvitis empirically, despite a negative KOH preparation.

Treatment
The usual recommended treatment for symptomatic patients is one of the imidazole antifungal drugs, with reported cure rates of 85 to 95% at 1 week after use, and 70 to 80% at 4

weeks after use. Most clinicians prefer either topical miconazole (Monistat) or clotrimazole (Gyne-Lotrimin), in regimens ranging from a single dose to 3 or 7 days. A related drug, butaconazole cream, is given for 3 to 6 days. All are safe in pregnancy. Miconazole may be given as a 200-mg suppository every day for 3 days, or a 100-mg suppository or one applicator of vaginal cream every day for 7 days. Clotrimazole may be given as a single-dose 500-mg vaginal tablet, as two 100-mg vaginal tablets every day for 3 days, one 100-mg vaginal tablet every day for 7 days, or one applicator of vaginal cream every day for 7 to 14 days. The single-dose regimen is less effective clinically. In general, the longer regimens are recommended for more severe infections. The miconazole and clotrimazole formulations used in the longer regimens (100-mg suppositories and pills, and the vaginal creams) are available over the counter. Creams may be applied to the vulva as well as inserted vaginally, and therefore may be preferable to suppositories or tablets in women with pronounced vulvar involvement. It is recommended that these medications be inserted at bedtime to reduce leakage and to prolong contact with the vaginal mucosa; when medication is used during menses, tampons should be avoided because they may absorb the therapeutic agent. Ketoconazole, an imidazole administered orally (400 mg every day for 3–7 days) gives similar results to the topical agents, but is not safe during pregnancy and is more toxic. Fluconazole is an expensive but very effective alternative that is probably less toxic than ketoconazole.

Alternative agents to the imidazoles include nystatin vaginal tablets qd to bid for 10 to 14 days, with lower reported cure rates (76.6% at 2 weeks and 50% at 4 weeks). Other suggested treatments include boric acid powders, retention douches of potassium sorbate 1 to 3%, and a 1% gentian violet solution.

Treatment of asymptomatic male sexual partners is not indicated except possibly in some instances of recurrent candidiasis in which it is suspected that the man may harbor organisms beneath the foreskin or in the urethra. *Candida* balanitis is treated with topical nystatin, clotrimazole, or miconazole.

Recurrent yeast infections are a common and distressing problem. Although recurrent vaginal candidiasis has been strongly associated with positive stool cultures for *Candida*, simultaneous treatment with oral nystatin to eliminate the presumed gut reservoir has not proved clinically effective. Alternative treatment strategies, listed in the order in which they are usually tried, include (1) supplying the patient with a refillable prescription for short-course miconazole or clotrimazole, allowing for self-diagnosis and treatment; (2) monthly prophylactic treatment with miconazole or clotrimazole or ketoconazole 400 mg for 5 days at the beginning of menses; or (3) continuous prophylaxis with ketoconazole 100 mg daily. Predisposing factors should also be addressed, including control of diabetes, avoidance of heat- and moisture-retaining nylon undergarments, and reduction of corticosteroid and oral contraceptive estrogen dosages.

Trichomonas Vaginitis
The prevalence of trichomoniasis varies considerably in different clinical settings, ranging from 13 to 23% in women attending gynecologic clinics to 75% in prostitutes. The organism is sexually transmitted and is often found in the presence of other sexually transmitted diseases, such as gonorrhea and *Chlamydia*. Trichomoniasis may rarely be transmitted nonvenereally on moist cloths, but in most cases should be considered a sexually transmitted disease; concurrent clinically silent infection with other sexually transmitted organisms should be sought. Many women (25–44%) from whom trichomonads are cultured are asymptomatic. The long-term effects of chronic asymptomatic trichomoniasis are not known, although it has been suggested that one-third of asymptomatic women become symptomatic within a few months after positive cultures are obtained. Extragenital or disseminated trichomoniasis is unknown.

In symptomatic patients, pruritus and increased or malodorous discharge are common complaints; dysuria is reported by about 20%. The classic frothy discharge (caused by CO_2 bubbles) is 70% specific for the presence of *Trichomonas vaginalis* but is found in only 10% of instances; usually the discharge is indistinguishable from that of bacterial vaginosis. The pH of secretions is usually above 4.5, and the "sniff test" described below for bacterial vaginosis may be positive. The so-called pathognomonic strawberry cervix with punctate hemorrhages or telangiectasias is found on routine pelvic exam in only 2 to 3% of instances.

Diagnosis depends on demonstration of the organism, usually by microscopic examination of a specimen of discharge mixed with saline. Pear-shaped, motile organisms (about twice the size of WBCs) with unipolar flagella are detected in approximately 60 to 70% of infected women. Because the mobility of the organism aids in its identification, the slide should be examined as soon as possible after preparation. The specimen should be taken from the vaginal vault rather than the endocervix, where trichomonads are infrequently found.

Cultures are considerably more sensitive than saline preparation in detecting trichomonads, but are tedious to process in the laboratory; in addition, commercially available media are not all equally effective. Rapid immunofluorescent antibody assays for trichomonads are somewhat more sensitive than wet mount, and, like cultures, require much more time and expense to perform. In symptomatic women with the clinical findings described above, neither cultures nor antibody assays are needed for diagnosis; these tests are best reserved for problem cases.

Although trichomoniasis is sometimes diagnosed on the basis of endocervical cytologic findings, the reliability of the Pap smear as a diagnostic test is quite variable, depending on the way it is performed and the skill of laboratory personnel in interpreting it. Smears made from the cervix alone are less likely to contain organisms than those that include specimens from the vaginal pool.

Treatment

Many gynecologists and infectious disease experts advocate treating all patients who have detectable trichomonads. They argue that asymptomatically infected women are likely to become symptomatic and also that they should be treated as a public health measure to reduce the venereal transmission of the organism. Clinicians may prefer to individualize these treatment decisions, particularly in patients who are not sexually active. Asymptomatic patients with cellular atypia on Pap smear should be treated, because the atypia may represent an inflammatory response to the trichomonad, which often resolves with eradication of the organism.

Metronidazole (e.g., Flagyl, Protostat), given orally, is the drug of choice: a cure rate of approximately 90% is achieved by a single 2-gm dose or by 1-week regimens of 250 mg three times a day, or 500 mg twice daily. Spacing the tablets out in a twice-a-day schedule or taking them with food may minimize nausea. Patients should be warned not to drink alcoholic beverages during the course of therapy because they may experience abdominal distress, nausea, vomiting, flushing, or headache. The use of metronidazole is contraindicated during the first trimester of pregnancy and in nursing mothers, although it may be used if breast feeding is suspended for 36 to 48 hours. Several studies suggest that the drug is safe in the last two trimesters of pregnancy. Clotrimazole vaginal suppositories have been suggested for use during the first trimester. A 1-week course of therapy has been reported to relieve symptoms, although it cures only about 20% of patients.

Treatment of male sexual partners of infected women is usually recommended, especially if the single-dose regimen is used. Most men carrying *Trichomonas* are completely asymptomatic, and the organism is spontaneously eliminated from the male urogenital tract over a period of weeks. However, during this time the organism can be reinoculated into the vagina. The single-dose metronidazole regimen is the one most commonly prescribed for male contacts. Because this often requires the physician to prescribe a drug for an unseen patient, some accompany the prescription with a handout explaining the treatment and its rationale. An alternative approach is for the man to use a condom or abstain from intercourse for several weeks.

Douching with vinegar (2 tablespoons in a quart of water) twice weekly, to inhibit the growth of trichomonads by reducing vaginal pH, has been suggested as an alternative therapy. The reliability of this method has not been established.

Metronidizole-resistant *Trichomonas*, although unusual, has been documented by sensitivity testing and is increasingly being recognized. It should be considered in patients who fail to respond to treatment and whose history is inconsistent with reinfection. Treatment of resistant trichomoniasis involves high-dose metronidazole regimens (2 g every day for 5–14 days, plus a broken 500-mg tablet intravaginally) and is best managed by a clinician experienced with this problem.

Bacterial Vaginosis

Bacterial vaginosis is the currently favored term for the syndrome previously referred to as nonspecific vaginitis, as well as by the successive names for presumed *Gardnerella vaginalis* infection. This short, facultatively anaerobic gram-negative rod, formerly called *Corynebacterium vaginale* and *Hemophilus vaginalis*, is present in all cases, but can also be cultured from 30 to 70% of healthy, asymptomatic women. There is no simple etiologic explanation for bacterial vaginosis, but the condition is thought to result from a polymicrobial alteration in the normal vaginal flora. A dramatic reduction in the normally predominant lactobacilli has been noted with this syndrome, along with a marked increase (up to 1000-fold) in anaerobes, such as *Bacteroides, Peptostreptococcus,* and *Mobiluncus* species, and an increased prevalence of *Mycoplasma hominis*.

The symptoms of bacterial vaginosis are typically milder than those of candidal or trichomonal infections, and there may be little or no observable irritation or inflammation of the vagina or vulva. Indeed, the term *vaginosis* was adopted rather than *vaginitis* because of the lack of associated inflammation or white blood cells. A musty or fishy odor to the genitalia or vaginal discharge is the major and usually the only symptom. The vaginal discharge is typically thin, watery or gray, adherent to the vaginal walls, and homogeneous (i.e., does not form clumps).

The diagnosis of bacterial vaginosis is based on the presence of at least three of the following four features:

1. A typical thin, homogeneous vaginal discharge.
2. Vaginal pH greater than 4.5. The pH can be tested after removal of the vaginal speculum by dipping a piece of pH paper into secretions pooled in the speculum, preferably those in the anterior blade. Contact with cervical mucus, menstrual blood, and semen, all of which are alkaline, will invalidate the test.
3. "Clue cells," epithelial cells that have lost their sharp margins and have a granular appearance because of the adherence of bacteria over the cell surface. They may be seen on a wet preparation made with a drop of saline mixed with the discharge and examined on high-dry power through a coverslip.
4. Amine odor, a characteristic fishy smell released when the vaginal discharge is alkalinized by the addition of 10% KOH reagent. An additional criterion is a characteristic Gram's stain of the vaginal discharge, with *Gardnerella* morphotypes (smaller gram-variable coccobacilli) outnumbering lactobacilli (large gram-positive bacilli). The single most reliable indicator of bacterial vaginosis is the presence of clue cells on wet mount. Both elevated pH and amine odor can also be seen in trichomonal vaginitis. Cultures have no role in clinical diagnosis of bacterial vaginosis.

Treatment

Metronidazole is the most effective antimicrobial; depending on the regimen, cure rates of higher than 90% can be expected. The standard regimen is 500 mg twice a day for 1 week, although equal cure rates were reported in one large study with two single 2-g doses on days 1 and 3. Cure rates of 65 to 85% have been reported in several other studies of 2-g single-dose regimens. A good alternative that is safe in pregnancy is clindamycin 300 mg bid for 7 days. Administration of amoxicillin together with a beta-lactamase inhibitor such as clavulinic acid (Augmentin) might be expected to increase the 30 to 80% cure rate over ampicillin or amoxicillin alone, but efficacy data are not available. Tetracycline and topical sulfonamides are not as effective.

The treatment of sexual partners remains controversial. *G. vaginalis* has been found in the urethra of 79% of male partners of infected women, and treatment with a regimen similar to that used in women has been recommended to prevent reinfection. However, there are no data on the effect of treatment of the partner, and some clinicians prefer to treat sexual partners only when bacterial vaginosis fails to respond or recurs. It is not known whether abstinence or use of condoms affects the rate of treatment failures or recurrence.

Other Conditions

Atrophic vaginitis can cause the same symptoms as infection. On physical examination, changes consistent with estrogen deficiency are noted, including pale and dry vaginal epithelium and thin vulvar skin. Treatment is local estrogen in the form of creams or suppositories (see Chap. 81).

Infectious cervicitis, usually caused by *Neisseria gonorrhoeae, Chlamydia trachomatis,* or herpes simplex, may cause increased discharge or other discomfort. Evaluation and treatment for these organisms is discussed in Chapter 113.

Other possible causes of vaginitis symptoms include dermatologic conditions such as scabies or neurotic excoriation, trauma, herpesvirus vulvitis, pregnancy, and malignancies. Increased attention to normal vaginal discharge occurs in fewer than 5% of patients with genitourinary complaints.

Not infrequently, a specific cause cannot be demonstrated for vaginitis. If clinical findings are highly suggestive of candidal infection, a trial of antiyeast therapy is warranted despite a negative KOH preparation. If there is no reason to suspect one or another cause, metronidazole may be the most appropriate therapeutic choice. It treats bacterial vaginosis as well as a clinically similar trichomonal infection that may have been missed because of a falsely negative saline preparation. Measures that increase vaginal acidity also may be considered in this situation, on the theory that acid-tolerant organisms such as *Lactobacillus* survive at the expense of pathogenic ones. Alternative choices include vinegar douches (2–4 tablespoons white vinegar in 1 quart of water) or Aci-Jel vaginal jelly. None has been rigorously evaluated.

Mandell GL, Douglas RG, Bennett JE, eds. Principles and practice of infectious diseases. 3rd ed. New York: Churchill Livingstone, 1990.

Holmes KK, et al, eds. Sexually transmitted diseases. New York: 2nd edition, McGraw–Hill, 1990.
Both of these major textbooks have several excellent and extensively referenced chapters on vaginitis.

Hill LV, Embil JA. Vaginitis. Current microbiologic and clinical concepts. Can Med Assoc J 1986; 134:321–31.

Paavonen J, Stamm WE. Lower genital tract infections in women. Infect Dis Clin North Am 1987; 1:179–98.

McCue JD. Evaluation and treatment of vaginitis. An update for primary care practitioners. Arch Int Med 1989; 149:565–68.
Three well-referenced review articles summarizing accepted approaches to vaginitis.

Addison LA. The role of the office laboratory in the diagnosis of vaginitis. Prim Care 1986; 13:633–46.
Detailed step-by-step illustrated explanations of the procedures that should be done as part of the routine office evaluation of vaginitis.

Eschenbach DA, Hillier SL. Advances in diagnostic testing for vaginitis and cervicitis. J Reprod Med 1989; 34:Suppl 8:555–65.
Compares traditional office tests and new immunoassays.

Schaaf MV, Perez–Stable EJ, Borchardt K. The limited value of symptoms and signs in the diagnosis of vaginal infections. Arch Intern Med 1990; 150:1929–33.
Confirms the nonspecific nature of presenting symptoms and signs, as well as the difficulties of precise diagnosis in the primary care setting, even when cultures are used.

Robertson WH. A concentrated therapeutic regimen for vulvovaginal candidiasis. JAMA 1980; 244:2549–50.
In a double-blind placebo-controlled study, the 3-day double-dose regimen was as effective as a 7-day single-dose schedule.

Sobel JD. Recurrent vulvovaginal candidiasis. A prospective study of the efficacy of maintenance ketoconazole therapy. N Engl J Med 1986; 315:1455–58.
Continuous ketoconazole (100 mg daily) prevented recurrent candidal vaginitis best, although cyclic clotrimazole or ketoconazole also gave good results.

Sobel JD. Pathophysiology of vulvovaginal candidiasis. J Reprod Med 1989; 34:Suppl 8:572–80.
Discusses the factors contributing to Candida *infection and recurrences. Treating sexual partners and suppressing the gastrointestinal reservoir have failed to reduce attacks.*

Hager WD, et al. Metronidazole for vaginal trichomoniasis. Seven-day vs. single-dose regimens. JAMA 1980; 244:1219–20.

The authors report an 86% cure rate with a 2-g dose (16% nausea/vomiting) versus 92% with the standard regimen (8% nausea/vomiting).

Thomason JL, Gelbart SM. Trichomonas vaginalis. Obstet Gynecol 1989; 73 (number 3, part 2):536–541.

Reviews microbiology, transmission, diagnosis, and treatment, including trichomoniasis refractory to standard treatment.

Amsel R, et al. Nonspecific vaginitis: diagnostic criteria and microbial and epidemiologic associations. Am J Med 1983; 74:14–22.

A careful and innovative examination of the reliability of the diagnostic criteria for bacterial vaginosis in 397 unselected symptomatic and asymptomatic university students. In this group, 25% met the criteria, half of whom were asymptomatic.

Eschenbach DA. Bacterial vaginosis: emphasis on upper genital tract complications. Obstet Gynecol Clin North Am 1989; 16(3):593–609.

Reviews the microbiology, diagnosis, and treatment of this syndrome in asymptomatic, pregnant, and prehysterectomy patients, and in those with multiple recurrences. Discusses the evidence for association of bacterial vaginosis with various types of upper genital tract infection.

Eschenbach DA, et al. Diagnosis and clinical manifestations of bacterial vaginosis. Am J Obstet Gynecol 1988; 158:819–28.

Gram's stain, as a single test, correlated best with the diagnosis of bacterial vaginosis; elevated pH and a positive sniff test were least specific.

Thomason JL, et al. Statistical evaluation of diagnostic criteria for bacterial vaginosis. Am J Obstet Gynecol 1990; 162:155–60.

In a comparison of various rapid clinical criteria, used singly and in combination, the presence of clue cells on wet mount was the single most reliable indicator of bacterial vaginosis. The best two combinations were clue cells and a positive sniff test, which were slightly more specific, although less sensitive than clue cells alone. Gram's stain criteria were less accurate predictors.

Jerve F, et al. Metronidazole in the treatment of non-specific vaginitis. Br J Vener Dis 1984; 60:171–74.

Patients (429) with bacterial vaginosis were given a variety of metronidazole regimens. The regimens with the best cure rates (94%) were with 2 g on days 1 and 3 and 1.2 g daily for 5 days.

Swedberg J, et al. Comparison of single-dose vs one-week course of metronidazole for symptomatic bacterial vaginosis. JAMA 1985; 254:1046–49.

Single-dose (2 g) metronidazole produced significantly inferior symptomatic cure results (47%) compared with 7 days of 500 mg twice daily (83%).

Greaves WL, et al. Clindamycin vs metronidazole in treatment of bacterial vaginosis. Obstet Gynecol 1988; 72:799–802.

The same cure rate was obtained with both drugs.

Hammill HA. Unusual causes of vaginitis (excluding trichomonas, bacterial vaginosis, and Candida albicans). Obstet Gynecol Clin North Am 1989; 16(2):337–45.

Discusses unusual infectious (e.g., ameba, mycoplasma) and noninfectious (e.g., allergic, contact, iatrogenic) causes of vaginitis.

75. BIRTH CONTROL
Axalla J. Hoole

Many methods of birth control are used throughout the world; the success of these methods is expressed as both *method effectiveness*—the idealized effectiveness of the methods used properly—and *use effectiveness*—the actual effectiveness found in practice. The method effectiveness of condoms is about 98%; however, the use effectiveness varies from 60 to 97% depending on the skill of the group being surveyed. Any method, including coitus interruptus, may work for careful couples, but no method is effective unless practiced by people dedicated to its success (see Table 75-1).

For any broad group one method of birth control is usually preferred; but the individual requires several methods as conditions change during reproductive life. While the choice of method should be individualized, surveys show preferences by age group; teenagers accept condoms, but not other barrier methods and most often do not seek postcoital contraception. For those teenaged females who are able to plan, birth control pills (BCPs) are the preferred method. From ages 19 to 30, BCPs tend to be the chosen method of contraception and planned conception; for those for whom spacing of children is not so important, the relative security of IUDs or barrier methods is sufficient. After age 30, couples with stable relationships often switch to barrier methods or intrauterine devices

Table 75-1. Typical and lowest reported failure rates during the first year of use of a method in the United States.

Method	Percent of women experiencing an accidental pregnancy in the first year of use	
	TYPICAL	LOWEST REPORTED
Chance	85	43.1
Spermicides	21	0.0
Periodic abstinence	20	
Calendar		14.4
Ovulation method		10.5
Symptothermal		12.6
Postovulation		2.0
Withdrawal	18	6.7
Cap	18	8.0
Sponge		
Parous women	28	27.7
Nulliparous women	18	13.9
Diaphragm	18	2.1
Condom	12	4.2
IUD	3	
Progestasert		1.9
Copper T380A		0.5
Pill	3	
Combined		0.0
Progestogen-only		1.1
Injectable progestogen		
DMPA	0.3	0.0
NET	0.4	0.0
Implants		
Norplant (6 capsules)	0.04	0.0
Norplant 2 (2 rods)	0.03	0.0
Female sterilization	0.4	0.0
Male sterilization	0.15	0.0

Source: Adapted from RA Hatcher, et al. Contraceptive Technology 1990–1992, 15th revised ed. New York: Irvington Publishers, Inc., 1990:134.

(IUDs); however, BCPs are relatively safe to age 45 in women who do not smoke and who are not obese or hypertensive. Contraception should be continued until 6 months after periods cease; note, however, that perimenopausal conjugated estrogens do not reliably inhibit ovulation and thus should not be used for contraception.

Natural Family Planning

Natural family planning includes a variety of methods that are based on predicting the time of ovulation. Among these are the calendar method (useful only for women with regular menses), the temperature method (daily measurement of basal temperature to identify the increase in temperature that occurs with ovulation), the cervical mucous method (change of mucus with ovulation), and the symptothermal method (combines the above measures of identifying ovulation). Although these techniques dramatically reduce the number of pregnancies, the chance of conception is too high for anyone who is seriously trying to prevent pregnancy.

Barrier Methods

Diaphragm

The diaphragm that fits snugly between the inferior rim of the symphysis pubis and the posterior vaginal fornix acts as a barrier to cervical entry by spermatozoa. Before insertion, contraceptive cream or jelly must be applied to the side of the diaphragm that comes in contact with the cervix. Additional cream or jelly may be applied to the rim of the diaphragm to create a seal of spermicide. The diaphragm should remain in place at least 6 hours after the last act of intercourse. Additional contraceptive cream or jelly may be inserted for coitus within 6 hours.

The diaphragm must be fitted by a health professional and a prescription given for one of the three basic types of diaphragms, the arcing spring, the coil spring, and the flat spring. The arcing spring diaphragm provides firm pressure on the lateral vaginal walls for women with poor vaginal muscle tone; in addition, the arcing shape of the folded rim facilitates insertion. The Koro-flex, Milex, and Bendex brands have two opposing hingelike springs in the rim and fold at these two points only; the Allflex folds at any point and holds its shape somewhat less firmly than the others. The coil spring diaphragm has a coil spring rim that folds flat for insertion; its spring strength is somewhat less firm than the arcing spring diaphragm, providing comfort to parous women with good vaginal muscle tone. That flat spring diaphragm has a thin bandlike rim that folds at any point in a single plane; its gentle spring strength is best suited for nulliparous women and women with a shallow pubic arch. For women with allergies to latex, the Milex diaphragm made of silicone can be prescribed; it is available in arcing and coil spring models.

Sponge

The vaginal contraceptive sponge consists of polyurethane foam impregnated with an aqueous solution of the spermicidal agent nonoxynol-9. The sponge should be moistened with water and squeezed gently before insertion in the vagina. Much like a diaphragm, the sponge acts both to block the cervix and to absorb ejaculate into the spermicide. It is used for a maximum of 24 hours, regardless of frequency of intercourse, and then discarded.

The contraceptive sponge comes in a universal size and requires no prescription or fitting by a medical professional. The effectiveness of the sponge is in the range of other vaginal contraceptives.

Cervical Cap

The cervical cap has been approved for use as a barrier contraceptive and is comparable in effectiveness to the diaphragm. The cap must be fitted and comes in four sizes. Spermicidal cream or jelly must be placed inside the cap before each use. It is not necessary to reapply spermicide upon repeated intercourse, and it can remain in place for up to 48 hours. Clinical trials with the cervical cap among motivated women reported first-year failure rates of about 9%.

During the NIH clinical trials, about 4% of users, after using the cap for 3 months, experienced conversions of Pap smears from Class I to Class III, compared to 1.7% of diaphragm wearers. Women for whom the cervical cap is prescribed should have a repeat Pap smear after the first 3 months of use. Beyond 3 months of use, conversion rates of Pap smears were similar to diaphragm users.

Condoms

Condoms have gained popularity in recent years, not only as a contraceptive, but also in the prevention of venereal diseases, particularly those caused by the human immunodeficiency virus, herpesvirus, and *Chlamydia trachomatis* bacteria. Condom use should be encouraged in individuals with multiple sexual partners. As a contraceptive, the condom is highly effective in couples with sufficient motivation. Failure may result from the condom breaking, sliding down, or coming off during intercourse. The condom must always be applied before intromission and held in place for removal; it is most easily used with lubricant. The failure rate reported in several studies is about 4% per year.

Oral Contraception

Birth control pills (BCPs), taken by millions of women throughout the world, include combination pills, progestogen-only pills, and "morning-after pills." Most women use combination pills; only a small number take progestogen-only "mini-pills."

Combination Pills

Combination pills contain estrogen, either mestranol or ethinyl estradiol, and one of several progestogens. The estrogens have approximately equal hormonal potency, but the progestogens vary widely in their hormonal properties. Norethindrone, used in the majority of BCPs, has progestational activity that lies between norgestrel, the most progestogenic, and norethynodrel, the most estrogenic of the progestogens.

Prevention of ovulation by suppression of follicle-stimulating hormone and luteinizing hormone requires both estrogen and progestogen. Progestogen alone can prevent implantation by providing an inhospitable endometrium, but contraception is less certain than with combination pills. For most BCPs the progestogen has the predominant effect on the endometrium. Triphasic birth control pills are combination pills in which the amount of progestogen varies throughout the cycle. These formulations have been shown to have slightly less effect on serum lipid values than the monophasic preparations; however, there is a slightly higher risk of breakthrough bleeding with the triphasic preparations.

RISKS OF VASCULAR PROBLEMS. Several large studies have shown that the estrogen component of BCPs is associated with a dose-related risk of thromboembolism. Risk decreases with decreasing estrogen to 35 µg; below this level, additional decreased risk has been difficult to demonstrate.

The increase in risk for both thromboembolic disease and stroke dramatically increases after age 35 and with cigarette smoking. However, in the nonsmoker low-dose BCPs (1/35) continue to be safer than pregnancy, even after age 40.

Progestogens, particularly the more androgenic ones, increase low-density lipoprotein (LDL) cholesterol and decrease high-density lipoproteins (HDL); in some patients triglycerides may also be elevated. Triphasic BCPs seem to have less effect on the lipid profile. The contribution made by progestogens to increased risk of myocardial infarction is unclear.

RISK OF CANCER. The major body of evidence from several large studies supports no increased risk of *breast cancer* in users of oral contraceptives, although there is evidence that suggests otherwise for some subgroups in the populations studied. Risk of *cervical cancer* is related to factors, other than oral contraceptives, that occur in women of childbearing age. When these are taken into account there is no good evidence that cervical cancer is more frequent in users of oral contraceptives. Endometrial and ovarian cancer occur less frequently in oral contraceptive users. This effect is greatest in women of low parity; the protective effect extends to 15 years after the cessation of the pills.

CONTRAINDICATIONS. Combination pills are contraindicated in women over age 35 who smoke and in women with a past history of thromboembolic or vascular disease. Other contraindications include active liver disease, abnormal liver function tests, undiagnosed breast masses, pregnancy, uterine bleeding of unknown origin, second amenorrhea, and known or suspected estrogen-dependent breast neoplasia.

Relative contraindications include hypertension, migraine headaches, diabetes mellitus, hypercholesterolemia, active gallbladder disease, and sickle cell anemia. A small percentage of patients taking BCPs develop hypertension that resolves when the pill is stopped. Some patients with migraine headaches develop an increase in headaches while on BCPs and should thereafter not use oral contraception; however, many have no change in migraine pattern. Because it is impossible to predict those in whom headaches will develop, patients with a history of migraine headaches may be started on low-dose BCPs. Some researchers have found a lowering of glucose tolerance among users of BCPs. Patients with abnormal glucose tolerance may take BCPs if they are aware of the potential change in glucose tolerance.

PILL SELECTION. Because the major serious side effects are believed to be dose related and caused by estrogens, the primary goal has become to administer the lowest possible estrogen dose. Because of the effects of progestogens on lipids, it would seem prudent to choose a less androgenic progestogen such as norethindrone over a more androgenic one such as norgestrel. Attempts to balance the clinical features of individual patients by selecting BCPs with estrogenic or progestogenic progestogens (e.g., giving hirsute women a BCP containing an estrogenic progesterone) have largely been abandoned.

The combination pills most frequently prescribed contain 30 to 50 µg of ethinyl estradiol. There are more bleeding complications at 30 µg but possibly less risk of cardiovascular complications. The most commonly used low-dose pills and their estrogen and progestogen content are listed in Table 75-2.

The initial evaluation of patients desiring BCPs should include a menstrual history, a history to disclose any of the above contraindications, and a physical examination that includes blood pressure and breast and pelvic examinations. The only laboratory evaluations necessary are a Pap smear and measurement of glucose or liver function when indicated. A lipid panel may be useful in identifying patients with increased cholesterol in whom BCPs should be used more cautiously.

Even if pills are begun on the first day of the period, alternate contraception is needed and should be used for at least the first 14 days of the first cycle.

MANAGEMENT OF SIDE EFFECTS. Reductions in the estrogen dose have greatly reduced the common side effects, such as nausea, bloating, fatigue, and fluid retention, but because of decreased support for the endometrium, breakthrough bleeding and amenorrhea have increased. Patients should be warned that menstrual periods diminish in flow and duration. Breakthrough bleeding may occur during the first several periods after starting at a low dose, when changing to a lower dose pill, or sporadically. The bleeding that occurs when starting pills is usually self-limited and often can be managed by reassurance; however, both initial and sporadic bleeding respond to additional estrogen (20 µg of ethinyl estradiol daily for 7 days). Following this therapy, sporadic breakthrough bleeding frequently does not recur. Switching to a pill with more estrogen, 30 to 50 µg, may be effective, but a dose greater than 50 µg exposes patients to increased risk. Primary care physicians should consult a gynecologic specialist if withdrawal bleeding does not occur for two or more periods and a pregnancy test is negative.

Acne may occur in patients taking combination pills with a highly progestogenic progesterone such as norgestrel. In such instances, a pill with a less progestogenic progesterone may be substituted.

A number of other unpleasant symptoms have been reported among BCP users, including depression, change in libido, nausea, and weight gain. The same symptoms are prevalent among potential BCP users and have been shown to be common among women given placebo BCPs.

Drug interactions between oral contraceptives and other medications are listed in Table 75-3.

ROUTINE FOLLOW-UP CARE. Routine examination for patients taking BCPs is recommended on an annual basis for blood pressure, breast examination, and Pap smear. A cholesterol panel is indicated, especially in those with a family history of cardiovascular disease.

Progestogen-Only Pills
Progestogen-only pills (mini-pills) are infrequently used in this country. The usual dose of progestogen is either 0.350 mg of norethindrone or 0.075 mg of norgestrel daily, much less than is in the combination pills. Effectiveness is equal to or better than barrier methods used correctly but not as good as combination pills. Breakthrough bleeding is common, and an increased incidence of ectopic pregnancies has been reported. However, there are none of the side effects of estrogens, and because of the low dose there are decreased progestogenic side effects. Advocates of progestogen-only pills suggest their use in breast-feeding mothers (breast feeding does not reliably provide contraception, and progestogen does not affect the volume of breast milk) and in patients who cannot use combination BCPs because of side effects or contraindications.

Postcoital Contraceptive Pills
Postcoital contraceptive pills (morning-after pill) are useful for women who have had unprotected intercourse and have compelling reasons for not becoming pregnant (e.g., following rape or when psychiatric problems would follow conception). The standard regimen is a combination pill containing 0.1 mg ethinyl estradiol and 1.0 mg of dl-norgestrel (Ovral). Two doses, 12 hours apart, should be given as soon as possible, but within 72 hours after unprotected intercourse. With this regimen the failure rate is only 0.16%; however, patients should be advised that if these regimens fail to prevent pregnancy, therapeutic abortion is recommended because of possible adverse effects on the fetus from the hormonal therapy. If circumstances warrant, a VDRL, gonococcal culture, and human immunodeficiency virus counseling are appropriate.

Intrauterine Device

The intrauterine device, although difficult to obtain in some parts of the country, is preferred by many women and can be an acceptable method of contraception for women who cannot tolerate BCPs or who are at high risk for complications with oral contraceptives. Such women, for example, those over 35 who smoke or have a history of thrombophlebitis or other pre-existing disease, may be candidates for an IUD.

Carefully selecting the patients for whom IUDs may be recommended is important. The contraindications are pregnancy, uterine anomalies, uterine or cervical malignancy, genital bleeding of unknown origin, acute cervicitis, presence or history of pelvic inflammatory disease, venereal disease, ectopic pregnancy, postpartum endometritis, or an infected abortion. Relative contraindications to IUD use include hypermenorrhea, severe dysmenorrhea, multiple sexual partners, congenital or valvular heart disease, and nulliparity.

IUDs produce a sterile inflammatory reaction within the endometrial cavity. An increase in polymorphonuclear cells, plasma cells, macrophages, and foreign-body giant cells appears near the IUD. Lysis of polymorphonuclear cells liberates a cytotoxin that is toxic to the sperm, oocyte, and blastocyte. These inflammatory cells also phagocytize sperm and possibly the blastocyst. Good evidence now suggests that the mechanism of action of IUDs is primarily to prevent fertilization and not to act as an abortifacient.

Insertion of an IUD is best performed at the time of menses. Uterine perforation is a known risk with IUD insertion. The perforation rate varies with the experience of the individual performing the insertion, ranging from 1 to 3 per 1000 insertions.

Pregnancy with an IUD occurs in 3 per 100 women-years of use. If the pregnancy is desired, removal of the IUD while the string is visible is the procedure of choice. The risk of miscarriage with IUD removal during pregnancy is 25%, and 50% if the IUD is left in utero.

An increased risk of pelvic inflammatory disease (PID) associated with IUD use has been reported. The risk of infection is highest in women who have more than one sex partner or a sex partner with multiple consorts, or in the first few months after IUD insertion (due to possible introduction of pathogenic organisms from the endocervix into

Table 75-2. Commonly used oral contraceptives

Drug	Estrogen (μg)	μg per month	Progestin (μg)[a]	μg per month
COMBINATION				
Loestrin 1/20 21, 28—Parke-Davis	ethinyl estradiol (20)	420	norethindrone acetate (1)	21
Loestrin 1.5/30 21, 28—Parke-Davis	ethinyl estradiol (30)	630	norethindrone acetate (1.5)	31.5
Nordette 21—Wyeth-Ayerst[b]	ethinyl estradiol (30)	630	levonorgestrel (0.15)	3.15
Levlen 21, 28—Berlex	ethinyl estradiol (30)	630	levonorgestrel (0.15)	3.15
Lo/Ovral 21—Wyeth-Ayerst[b]	ethinyl estradiol (30)	630	norgestrel (0.3)	6.3
Triphasil-21—Wyeth-Ayerst[b]	ethinyl estradiol (30, 40)	680	levonorgestrel (0.05, 0.075, 0.125)	1.925
Tri-Levlen 21, 28—Berlex	ethinyl estradiol (30, 40)	680	levonorgestrel (0.05, 0.075, 0.125)	1.925
Brevicon 21, 28—Syntex	ethinyl estradiol (35)	735	norethindrone (0.5)	10.5
Modicon 21—Ortho[b]	ethinyl estradiol (35)	735	norethindrone (0.5)	10.5
Genora 0.5/35 21, 28—Rugby	ethinyl estradiol (35)	735	norethindrone (0.5)	10.5
Nelova 0.5/35 21, 28—Warner Chilcott	ethinyl estradiol (35)	735	norethindrone (0.5)	10.5
Norinyl 1+35 21, 28—Syntex	ethinyl estradiol (35)	735	norethindrone (1)	21
Norethin 1/35 21, 28—Searle	ethinyl estradiol (35)	735	norethindrone (1)	21
Nelova 1/35 21, 28—Warner Chilcott	ethinyl estradiol (35)	735	norethindrone (1)	21
Genora 1/35 21, 28—Rugby	ethinyl estradiol (35)	735	norethindrone (1)	21
Ortho-Novum 1/35 21—Ortho[b]	ethinyl estradiol (35)	735	norethindrone (1)	21
Tri-Norinyl 21, 28—Syntex	ethinyl estradiol (35)	735	norethindrone (0.5, 1.0)	15

Ortho-Novum 7/7/7 21—Ortho[b]	ethinyl estradiol (35)	735	norethindrone (0.5, 0.75, 1.0)	15.75
Ortho-Novum 10/11 21—Ortho[b]	ethinyl estradiol (35)	735	norethindrone (0.5, 1.0)	16
Nelova 10/11 21, 28—Warner Chilcott	ethinyl estradiol (35)	735	norethindrone (0.5, 1.0)	16
Ovcon 35 21, 28—Mead Johnson	ethinyl estradiol (35)	735	norethindrone (0.4)	8.4
Demulen 1/35 21—Searle[b]	ethinyl estradiol (35)	735	ethynodiol diacetate (1)	21
Norlestrin 1/50 21, 28—Parke-Davis	ethinyl estradiol (50)	1050	norethindrone acetate (1)	21
Ovcon 50 21, 28—Mead Johnson	ethinyl estradiol (50)	1050	norethindrone (1)	21
Genora 1/50 21, 28—Rugby	ethinyl estradiol (50)	1050	norethindrone (1)	21
Norlestrin 2.5/50 21, 28—Parke-Davis	ethinyl estradiol (50)	1050	norethindrone acetate (2.5)	52.5
Demulen 1/50 21—Searle[b]	ethinyl estradiol (50)	1050	ethynodiol diacetate (1)	21
Ovral 21—Wyeth-Ayerst[b]	ethinyl estradiol (50)	1050	norgestrel (0.5)	10.5
Norinyl 1+50 21, 28—Syntex	mestranol (50)	1050	norethindrone (1)	21
Ortho-Novum 1/50 21—Ortho[b]	mestranol (50)	1050	norethindrone (1)	21
Norethin 1/50 21, 28—Searle	mestranol (50)	1050	norethindrone (1)	21
Nelova 1/50 21, 28—Warner Chilcott	mestranol (50)	1050	norethindrone (1)	21
PROGESTIN ONLY				
Ovrette—Wyeth-Ayerst	none		norgestrel (0.075)	2.1
Nor-Q D—Syntex	none		norethindrone (0.35)	9.8
Micronor—Ortho	none		norethindrone (0.35)	9.8

[a] Different progestins cannot be compared on a milligram basis.
[b] Also available in 28-day regimens at slightly higher cost.
Source: Adapted from Choice of contraceptives. The Medical Letter, 1988; 30:106.

Table 75-3. Interactions of oral contraceptives with other medications

Interacting drugs	Adverse effects (probable mechanism)	Comments and recommendations
Acetaminophen (Tylenol and others)	Possible decreased pain-relieving effect (increased metabolism)	Monitor pain-relieving response
Alcohol	Possible increased effect of alcohol	Use with caution
Anticoagulants (oral)	Decreased anticoagulant effect	Use alternative contraceptive
Antidepressants (Elavil, Norpramin, Tofranil, and others)	Possible increased antidepressant effect	Monitor antidepressant concentration
Barbiturates (phenobarbital and others)	Decreased contraceptive effect	Avoid simultaneous use; use alternative contraceptive for epileptics
Benzodiazepine tranquilizers (Ativan, Librium, Serax, Tranxene, Valium, Xanax, and others)	Possible increased or decreased tranquilizer effects including psychomotor impairment	Use with caution. Greatest impairment during menstrual pause in oral contraceptive dosage
Beta-blockers (Corgard, Inderal, Lopressor, Tenormin)	Possible increased blocker effect	Monitor cardiovascular status
Carbamazepine (Tegretol)	Possible decreased contraceptive effect	Use alternative contraceptive
Corticosteroids (cortisone)	Possible increased corticosteroid toxicity	Clinical significance not established
Griseofulvin (Fulvicin, Grifulvin V, and others)	Decreased contraceptive effect	Use alternative contraceptive

Guanethidine (Esimil, Ismelin)	Decreased guanethidine effect (mechanism not established)	Avoid simultaneous use
Hypoglycemics (tolbutamide, Diabinese, Orinase, Tolinase)	Possible decreased hypoglycemic effect	Monitor blood glucose
Methyldopa (Aldoclor, Aldomet, and others)	Decreased antihypertensive effect	Avoid simultaneous use
Penicillin	Decreased contraceptive effect with ampicillin	Low but unpredictable incidence; use alternative contraceptive
Phenytoin (Dilantin)	Decreased contraceptive effect Possible increased phenytoin effect	Use alternative contraceptive Monitor phenytoin concentration
Primidone (Mysoline)	Decreased contraceptive effect	Use alternative contraceptive
Rifampin	Decreased contraceptive effect	Use alternative contraceptive
Tetracycline	Decreased contraceptive effect	Use alternative contraceptive
Theophylline (Bronkotabs, Marax, Primatene, Quibron Tedral, Theor-Dur, and others)	Increased theophylline effect	Monitor theophylline concentration
Troleandomycin (TAO)	Jaundice (additive)	Avoid simultaneous use
Vitamin C	Increased serum concentration and possible increased adverse effects of estrogens with 1 g or more per day of vitamin C	Decrease vitamin C to 100 mg per day

Source: RA Hatcher et al. Contraceptive technology 1990–92. 15th rev ed. New York: Irvington Publishers, Inc., 1990.

the uterus during insertion). Should symptoms of PID develop, appropriate bacteriologic studies should be performed, antibiotic treatment instituted, and the IUD removed.

Product liability issues that have evolved over the past few years have left women with the choice of two IUDs, the Progestasert intrauterine contraceptive system and the ParaGard T380A Intrauterine Copper Contraceptive. The Progestasert, containing a steroid hormone (progesterone) that is released locally (65 µg progesterone/day), is effective for one year and must be replaced annually. The ParaGard copper T contains 380 mm^2 of copper and may be used for four years.

Permanent Contraception

Permanent contraception may be obtained by out-patient vasectomy or tubal ligation. Both are about 99% effective, but are associated with psychosexual disturbances. Reanastomosis is unreliable; successful reanastomosis of both fallopian tubes or vas deferens occurs in 50 to 60% cases. Among men who have had vasectomies, 50 to 60% develop antibodies to sperm that can cause sterility.

Michell DR, Jr. Contraception. N Engl J Med 1989; 320:777–87.
An excellent review with 125 references.

Hatcher RA, et al. Contraceptive technology 1990–92. 15th rev ed. New York: Irvington Publishers, Inc., 1990.
A superb comprehensive update.

Alvarez F, et al. New insights on the mode of action of intrauterine contraceptive devices in women. Fertil Steril 1988; 49:768–72.
Research that suggests the mode of action of an IUD is not by destruction of embryo.

Eichhorst BC. Contraception. Prim Care 1988; 15(3):437–59.
A very comprehensive review.

Food and Drug Administration. Cervical cap approved for contraception. FDA Drug Bull 1988; 18:18.
History and cautions on use of cervical cap.

Burkman RT. Lipid and lipoprotein changes in relation to oral contraception and hormonal replacement therapy. Fertil Steril 1988; 49:39–49.
A critical review of lipid and lipoprotein metabolism in relation to oral contraception.

Krauss RM. The effects of oral contraceptives on plasma lipids and lipoproteins. Int J Fertil 1988; 33:35–42.
Discussion of the estrogen/progestogen impact on lipoprotein physiology, favoring low-dose, low-impact formulation.

Corson SL, et al. Fertility control. Boston: Little, Brown, 1985.
A reference on all forms of fertility control and the statistical interpretation of data.

Wahl P, et al. Effect of estrogen/progestin potency on lipid/lipoprotein cholesterol. N Engl J Med 1983; 308:862–67.
A large multicenter study that shows a relation between progestogenic potency and LDL cholesterol. This work suggests a role for progestogens and estrogen/progestogenic balance in the risk for thromboembolic disease carried by BCPs.

Ling WY, et al. Mode of action of dl-norgestrel and ethinyl estradiol combination in postcoital contraception. Fertil Steril 1979; 32:297–302.
Suggests the mechanism of contraception of postcoital hormones.

Vessey MP, et al. Mortality among women participating in the Oxford Family Planning Association Contraceptive Study. Lancet 1977; 2:731–33.

Vessey MP, et al. Mortality among oral contraceptive users. Royal College of General Practitioners Oral Contraceptive Study. Lancet 1977; 2:727–31.
Two of the earliest large studies to show the risks of oral contraception.

76. ABNORMAL UTERINE BLEEDING
Deborah J. Dotters

Abnormal uterine bleeding is one of the most frequent gynecologic complaints of reproductive-age women. Menstrual norms for women in the United States are listed below.

	RANGE	MEAN
Age of menarche	9.1–17.7 years	12.8 years
Age at menopause	48–55 years	51.4 years
Cycle length	21–35 days	28 days
Duration of flow	2–8 days	4.6 days
Blood loss	20–80 ml/per cycle	35 ml/cycle

By definition, values outside of these ranges are abnormal. Any marked change from a patient's usual pattern should also be considered abnormal. Determining amounts is difficult; any bleeding that is abnormal for the patient or causes anemia should be investigated.

The following terms are often used to describe the abnormal bleeding pattern:

Amenorrhea (secondary)	The absence of bleeding for 6 months in a previously menstruating woman
Oligomenorrhea	Infrequent, irregular episodes of bleeding, occurring at intervals of greater than 35 days
Intermenstrual bleeding	Bleeding of variable amounts in between regular cycles
Menorrhagia (hypermenorrhea)	Excessive bleeding (> 80 ml or > 7 days) occurring with regular menses
Spotting	Very light, intermittent bleeding, usually not requiring a pad or tampon

Causes and Treatment

The causes of abnormal uterine bleeding may be classified into organic and dysfunctional causes. Organic causes encompass genital lesions and systemic diseases that may cause bleeding. Dysfunctional causes are related to irregularities in the neuroendocrine system. The differential diagnosis of abnormal bleeding varies with the age of the patient. Therefore, the diagnostic evaluation and treatment of abnormal bleeding is discussed by age group.

Adolescents

The most common cause of abnormal bleeding in adolescents (ages 11–16) is anovulation. Fifty-five to 85% of menstrual cycles in the first 2 years after menarche are anovulatory; 30 to 50% during the third and fourth years and less than 20% of cycles during the fifth and sixth years after menarche are anovulatory. When ovulation does not occur, there is continued stimulation of the endometrium by estrogen, but no progesterone is produced. The endometrium becomes increasingly thick and hypertrophic, until irregular shedding and heavy bleeding results. The typical patient is a frightened 12-year-old who has had one to two irregular periods and presents with profuse vaginal bleeding.

The next most frequent causes of menorrhagia in adolescents are coagulopathies and complications of pregnancy. A study of 59 adolescents hospitalized for severe menstrual bleeding reported a 19% incidence of coagulation disorders, including idiopathic thrombocytopenic purpura, von Willebrand's disease, Glanzmann's disease, thalassemia major, and Fanconi's anemia. *Pregnancy should be ruled out regardless of the patient's stated sexual activity or her parent's statements.* In general, anovulatory bleeding is painless, while accidents of pregnancy are usually associated with pain. Pregnancy complications associated with bleeding may include threatened, incomplete, or missed abortion, ectopic pregnancy, or gestational trophoblastic disease.

Less common causes of abnormal bleeding in this age group are lower genital tract conditions (vaginitis, cervicitis, foreign body), malignancy (clear cell carcinomas, ovarian germ cell tumors), and systemic diseases (renal failure, hypothyroidism, diabetes).

Evaluation of the abnormal bleeding in adolescents should include clotting studies, a CBC, and a serum or urine beta-human chorionic gonadotropin (β-HCG) assay for pregnancy determination. Evaluation of thyroid-stimulating hormone (TSH) and a urinalysis are occasionally helpful. If physical exam and laboratory analysis are unhelpful, anovulation should be suspected. A history of irregular periods strongly supports this diagnosis.

If the bleeding is mild to moderate, oral contraceptives containing 50 μg of ethinylestradiol are effective in stopping bleeding. (See Table 75-2 in Chapter 75). The patient should take one pill every 2 hours until the bleeding appreciably diminishes. The next day, after the bleeding slows, she should take one less than the total number of pills taken the day before and continue to take one less pill each day. Doses should be divided because giving more than one pill at a time causes nausea; thus, if the total is four, the pills should be taken four times a day, followed by three times a day, twice a day, and once a day. After one pill per day is reached, the patient should take one tablet for 21 days. Withdrawal bleeding should occur within 2 to 5 days of stopping the pill. For the next 3 months, the patient will make her own estrogen and will not need supplemental estrogen. Medroxyprogesterone acetate (e.g., Provera) 10 mg orally, should be given on cycle days 12 to 25 for 14 days. The patient will have a predictable period shortly after completing the progestational agent. If the patient desires contraception, oral contraceptives containing 35 μg of estrogen may be used instead. Oral contraceptives are begun on cycle day 5 or on the first Sunday after bleeding begins.

Severe hemorrhage can usually be stopped by administering intravenously 25 mg of conjugated estrogens (Premarin) over 30 minutes. This may be repeated twice if necessary. It should be followed with 2.5 mg of conjugated estrogen orally three times per day together with 10 mg of medroxyprogesterone acetate daily for 10 days. For the next three cycles, give medroxyprogesterone acetate 10 mg alone for 14 days, from cycle days 12 to 25, or substitute a 35-mg oral contraceptive.

Medical management of anovulatory bleeding in adolescents is the treatment of choice. A dilatation and curettage (D and C) is indicated only if the patient is hemorrhaging and hypovolemic and if intravenous conjugated estrogens are unsuccessful in stopping the bleeding. The latter presentation is the exception.

Reproductive-Aged Women

Pregnancy and its complications are the most common cause of abnormal bleeding in reproductive-aged women (ages 18–40). A sensitive blood or urine β-HCG assay (one that can read concentrations of < 50 MIU/ml) should always be obtained in any patient in this age group who has a menstrual aberration. If the β-HCG is positive, vaginal-probe ultrasound may be helpful in establishing the exact diagnosis. The differential diagnosis includes threatened, incomplete, or missed abortion, ectopic pregnancy, and gestational trophoblastic disease.

Other frequent causes of abnormal bleeding in reproductive-aged women are anovulation, leiomyomas, and infections (endometritis or pelvic inflammatory disease). Less commonly, endometrial polyps, endocervical polyps, and cervicitis may cause irregular bleeding. Cervical and endometrial cancers are infrequent, but need to be ruled out.

The correct diagnosis is usually suggested by the history and physical. Anovulatory cycles are characterized by a delay in menses followed by heavy, unpredictable flow. Anovulatory patients often complain of "a period every two weeks." Anovulation is common in obese and very thin women, in women with rapid changes in weight, and in women under stress. Leiomyomas tend to present with heavy, prolonged menses and an irregular, enlarged uterus on pelvic examination. Tenderness, mucopurulent cervicitis, and/or fever suggest infection. The bleeding associated with endometritis tends to be light, irregular, and prolonged.

A Pap smear should be obtained on all patients with bleeding who have not had a negative Pap in the last 6 months. Postcoital bleeding, in particular, suggests cervical cancer. Any suspicious cervical lesion should be biopsied. If no lesion is seen in a patient with postcoital bleeding, referral to a gynecologist for colposcopically directed biopsy should be considered.

Other useful diagnostic adjuncts include endovaginal ultrasound, hysteroscopy, and endometrial biopsy. An endovaginal ultrasound can be obtained by a generalist and can assess uterine size and contour, the number and location of fibroids (subserous versus submucous), and can identify polyps or other masses within the endometrial cavity. Hysteroscopy is usually the initial examination performed by gynecologists or is done if the ultrasound is negative to find polyps or submucosal fibroids. Endometrial biopsy is a simple and inexpensive office procedure with a diagnostic accuracy equal to a D and C. Biopsy will rule out endometrial hyperplasia or malignancy, and if performed in the second half of the cycle will establish whether ovulation has occurred.

The treatment of anovulatory bleeding is determined by the reproductive desires of the patient. Acute bleeding can be stopped, as described previously, with intravenous conjugated estrogens, or oral contraceptives given in a decreasing cascade, depending on the severity of the bleeding. After the acute episode, women desiring contraception are best managed with birth control pills. Induction of ovulation with clomiphene citrate is indicated in women wishing to become pregnant. Medroxyprogesterone acetate (e.g., Provera) 10 mg PO from cycle days 12 to 25, is a third alternative for anovulatory women who neither desire pregnancy nor contraception. It may be used indefinitely to promote cyclical endometrial shedding, or patients may choose to stop medroxyprogesterone acetate and wait for normal cycles. If no bleeding occurs in 2 months, medroxyprogesterone acetate should be restarted to prevent endometrial buildup.

If endometritis or PID is clinically apparent (see Chap. 79), antibiotics (doxycycline 100 mg PO bid for 10 days and metronidazole 500 mg PO qid for 10 days) should be given. Intrauterine devices should be removed if endometritis is suspected.

Nonsteroidal anti-inflammatory drugs (ibuprofen 400 mg PO tid or mefenamic acid 500 mg PO tid) have been shown to reduce menorrhagia by 30 to 50% in ovulating women and in women with IUD-related menorrhagia.

A D and C is rarely needed, but is the treatment of choice to stop the bleeding in women who present with hypovolemia or hypotension. However, a D and C is rarely curative. Most women will revert to their previous bleeding pattern within two cycles after a D and C.

Perimenopausal and Postmenopausal Women

The likelihood that abnormal bleeding is due to malignancy increases with the patient's age. Vulvar, vaginal, cervical, tubal, and ovarian cancer occur in older women in their fifth to seventh decades and must be strongly considered in the differential diagnosis of abnormal bleeding in this age group. Approximately 5% of perimenopausal and 20% of postmenopausal women with abnormal bleeding will have endometrial carcinoma; cervical cancer accounts for 4 to 5%.

Atrophic endometrium is the most common benign cause of postmenopausal bleeding and is seen in approximately 25% of cases. Endometrial polyps (15–20%), endocervical polyps/cervicitis (6–14%), and atrophic vaginitis (10%) are other common etiologies. Endometritis, urethral caruncle, and submucous myomas are less common causes.

The cause of bleeding can sometimes be diagnosed by physical examination or Pap smear, but endometrial biopsy should always be done in perimenopausal women with irregular bleeding of over 2 months duration and in all postmenopausal women. Patients should almost always be referred to a gynecologist, even if a Pap smear done by a generalist is negative. Hysteroscopy has been shown to add appreciably to the diagnostic accuracy of endometrial biopsy in this age group. An adnexal mass also may require evaluation by CT or ultrasound. Because patients occasionally mistake rectal bleeding or hematuria for vaginal bleeding, other sources of bleeding need to be considered.

Mishell DR, et al. Menorrhagia—a symposium. J Reprod Med 1984; 29:763–82.
  A thorough review of the etiologies, diagnosis, and management of menorrhagia.

Grimes D. Diagnostic dilation and curettage: a reappraisal. Am J Obstet Gynecol 1982; 142:1–6.
  Presents a strong case for the use of endometrial biopsy rather than the traditional D & C.

Claessens EA, Cowell CA. Dysfunctional uterine bleeding in the adolescent. Pediatr Clin North Am 1981; 28(2):369–78.
Reports on the causes of bleeding in this population.

Choo YC, et al. Postmenopausal uterine bleeding of nonorganic cause. Obstet Gynecol 1986; 66:225–28.
A recent series looking at the causes of postmenopausal bleeding.

Makarainen L, Ylikorkala O. Primary and myoma-associated menorrhagia: role of prostaglandins and effects of ibuprofen. Br J Obstet Gynecol 1986; 93:974–78.
Fascinating study examining the role of prostaglandins in menorrhagia and the use of prostaglandin inhibitors in treating this problem.

Droegemueller W, et al. (eds). Abnormal uterine bleeding. In: Comprehensive gynecology. St. Louis: CV Mosby, 1987:953–64.
Excellent chapter in gynecology textbook reviewing the subject of abnormal bleeding.

Speroff L, Glass RH, Kase NG (eds). Dysfunctional uterine bleeding. In: Clinical gynecologic endocrinology and infertility. 4th ed. Baltimore: Williams & Wilkins, 1989:265–82.
A concise and thorough approach to the pathophysiology, diagnosis, and treatment of irregular bleeding.

77. DYSMENORRHEA
Nancy Milliken

Dysmenorrhea, which literally means "difficult monthly flow," is crampy lower abdominal or pelvic pain that occurs before and during menstruation. Pain may radiate to the lower back and thighs and may be associated with gastrointestinal symptoms of nausea, vomiting, bloating, and diarrhea. It may also be accompanied by weakness, fatigue, headache, and, rarely, syncope.

Dysmenorrhea is commonly categorized as either primary or secondary. Primary dysmenorrhea begins shortly after menarche and has no associated pelvic pathology. Secondary dysmenorrhea is usually acquired later in life and is caused by organic pelvic disease such as endometriosis, pelvic inflammatory disease (PID), postsurgical adhesions, myomas, polyps, cervical stenosis, congenital uterine anomalies, and the use of an intrauterine device (IUD).

Primary dysmenorrhea is common. It is estimated that 50 to 60% of women will suffer from moderate to severe dysmenorrhea at some point in their reproductive lives, and that 10% of these women will be incapacitated for 1 to 3 days of each cycle. Untreated dysmenorrhea can therefore result in a significant loss of time from school or work. Fortunately, successful treatment for this problem is readily available.

Etiology
Primary dysmenorrhea is believed to be caused by prostaglandins, which produce high-intensity uterine contractions with an associated reduction in uterine blood flow. The pain is thought to be ischemic, reflecting decreased tissue perfusion. Another theory is that the pain results from a prostaglandin-induced increase in sensitivity of nerve terminals. Prostaglandins may also cause the associated gastrointestinal symptoms. The clinical finding of improved dysmenorrhea after childbirth is consistent with the ischemic pain theory, since pregnancy induces a permanent increase in uterine vascularity.

Evidence supporting the role of prostaglandins includes the finding of higher concentrations of prostaglandins in secretory as compared to proliferative endometrium. Women who have dysmenorrhea have been found to have higher levels of endometrial prostaglandins and higher serum levels of prostaglandin metabolites than do women without dysmenorrhea. In addition, menstrual-like cramps and associated gastrointestinal symptoms have been reproduced by the intravenous administration of prostaglandins.

Evaluation

It is important to elicit a history of dysmenorrhea in any woman of reproductive age. Patients may be unaware of treatment options and thus fail to report symptoms because they assume that little can be done. In addition to preventing needless suffering, inquiring about dysmenorrhea will identify patients with secondary dysmenorrhea and prompt a search for the underlying cause.

Primary dysmenorrhea typically begins about 6 to 12 months after menarche, when ovulatory cycles are usually established. Pelvic pain, as well as the associated symptoms of headaches, dizziness, nausea, vomiting, and diarrhea, usually begin with the onset of flow, but may also start before the onset of menses. The duration of symptoms ranges from hours to days. Women often note relief of symptoms while using oral contraceptives or after childbirth. The pelvic examination is normal.

Secondary dysmenorrhea should be suspected when a woman reports a change in character, duration, location, or intensity of pain. Occasionally secondary dysmenorrhea may present in a young girl prior to her first menses because a uterine or vaginal anomaly has caused outflow obstruction.

The most commonly encountered causes of secondary dysmenorrhea are endometriosis and PID. Less common causes are postsurgical adhesions, uterine myomas (fibroids), the presence of an IUD, adenomyosis, and endometrial polyps. Patients with secondary dysmenorrhea should therefore be questioned about current or former IUD use, history of gonorrhea, chlamydia, or PID, prior abdominal or pelvic surgery, infertility, and abnormal bleeding patterns. Symptoms of rectal pain, dyspareunia on deep penetration, or infertility suggest endometriosis. Pain that persists throughout the cycle suggests PID.

Pelvic exam can provide clues to the organic pathology. Endometriosis is suggested by a uterus that is normal-sized but fixed in the pelvis, with or without adnexal masses; uterosacral nodularity is characteristic of this condition. PID and its sequelae are indicated by a normal-sized uterus with thickened adnexal masses. Myomas are suggested by an enlarged, firm, irregular, and mobile uterus; adenomyosis by a slightly enlarged and boggy uterus.

The accurate diagnosis of secondary dysmenorrhea may require the use of specialized studies such as ultrasound, hysterosalpingogram, laparoscopy, hysteroscopy, or dilatation and curettage. When pelvic pathology is suspected, referral to a gynecologist for evaluation is appropriate.

Treatment

Prostaglandin inhibitors, such as the nonsteroidal anti-inflammatory agents, are the treatment of choice for most women with primary dysmenorrhea. In well-designed, placebo-controlled studies, they have been found to be effective in relieving symptoms in 61 to 100% of cycles.

Drugs that have been approved for use in the treatment of dysmenorrhea, and their recommended doses, include ibuprofen (e.g., Motrin, Advil, Nuprin, Rufen), 400 to 600 mg four times a day; naproxen (Naprosyn), 250 mg four times a day; naproxen sodium (Anaprox), 275 mg four times a day; and mefenamic acid (Ponstel), 250 mg four times a day to 500 mg three times a day. Studies have shown no advantage to beginning treatment before the onset of menses. Unless symptoms begin premenstrually, it is recommended that treatment be initiated with the onset of menses to avoid the possible ingestion of medications in early pregnancy. While approved for the purpose, aspirin is not recommended for treatment of significant dysmenorrhea because it is the weakest of the antiprostaglandins and has been found to be no more effective than placebo unless started 2 to 3 days before the onset of menses.

At the recommended doses, the side effects of these prostaglandin inhibitors are minimal. When they occur, they are usually gastrointestinal, similar to the side effects of aspirin. Women who do not respond to one antiprostaglandin often respond to another. If pain relief is not experienced after a trial of one antiprostaglandin for two consecutive cycles, an alternative drug should be tried. Most women with primary dysmenorrhea will obtain relief with one of the available prostaglandin inhibitors. Oral contraceptives are also very effective in reducing the pain of primary dysmenorrhea. Relief is obtained in 90% of women using any of the low-dose combination oral contraceptives. The mechanism of action is the inhibition of ovulation, with the subsequent reduction in the development of prostaglandin-containing endometrium. Oral contraceptives may be the treatment of choice for women with dysmenorrhea who also desire contraception and have no contraindications to the use of hormonal medication.

Antiprostaglandin drugs and oral contraceptives may be combined in women who fail to respond to either drug alone. If both of these modalities fail, a calcium channel blocker (e.g., nifedipine, 10 mg tid) may be effective. Potential side effects include transient facial flushing, moderate increase in heart rate, headaches and palpitations. When relief is not obtained by the use of these medications, secondary dysmenorrhea must again be considered, and the patient should be referred to a gynecologist for a more complete evaluation.

Secondary dysmenorrhea pain may respond to the same drugs used in primary dysmenorrhea, but treatment should be directed at the underlying cause. Prostaglandin inhibitors may relieve the increased dysmenorrhea associated with IUD use, allowing the device to remain in place if it is the preferable method of contraception. If alternative contraceptive methods are acceptable to the patient, or if prostaglandin inhibitors are ineffective, removal of the device may completely relieve the dysmenorrhea. The IUD should definitely be removed if there is any suspicion of a pelvic infection.

Secondary dysmenorrhea that fails to respond to medication or that is associated with suspected pelvic pathology or abnormal menstruation should be referred to a gynecologist for evaluation.

Rosenwaks Z, Seegar-Jones G. Menstrual pain: its origin and pathogensis. J Reprod Med 1980; 25:207–12.
A good review of concepts on the etiology of primary dysmenorrhea and the pharmacology of prostaglandins.

Sobcyzk R. Dysmenorrhea: the neglected syndrome. J Reprod Med 1980; 25:198–201.
A useful article that reviews the total impact of dysmenorrhea on women and society.

Dingfelder R. Primary dysmenorrhea treatment with prostaglandin inhibitors: a review. Am J Obstet Gynecol 1981; 140:874–79.
A summary of published reports on the effectiveness of prostaglandin inhibitors.

Dawood MY. Nonsteroidal anti-inflammatory drugs and changing attitudes toward dysmenorrhea. Am J Med 1988; 84(5A):23–33.
A review of the clinical problem of dysmenorrhea, the effectiveness of nonsteroidal antiinflammatory therapy agents, and their nonmedical benefits.

Fedele L, et al. Dynamics and significance of placebo response in primary dysmenorrhea. Pain 1989; 36(1):43–47.
Double-blind study of placebo versus antiprostaglandins showing only a transient response to placebo over four cycles (84%, 29%, 16%, 10%) compared with prolonged response (80%, 85.7%) to pirprofen and naproxen.

Anderson KE. Calcium antagonists and dysmenorrhea. Ann NY Acad Sci 1988; 522: 747–56.
A review of the effects of calcium antagonists on uterine activity and dysmenorrhea.

78. PREMENSTRUAL SYNDROME
Linn Parsons and Laurie Dornbrand

Premenstrual syndrome (PMS) is a constellation of symptoms occurring during the luteal phase of the menstrual cycle. It is sometimes referred to in the psychiatric literature as late luteal-phase dysphoric disorder (LLPDD). Common manifestations of PMS include headache, breast tenderness, abdominal bloating, edema of the extremities, fatigue, depression, irritability or tension, acneiform eruptions, constipation, increased thirst or appetite, and craving for sweet or salty foods. The symptoms begin 2 to 12 days before and subside with the onset of menstruation. Dysmenorrhea is not a part of this syndrome, although many patients suffer from both problems. Some investigators have differentiated PMS into a number of syndromes characterized by clusters of symptoms, such as mood or behavior disturbances, autonomic reactions, water retention, and pain. There has been little consistency or usefulness in such classifications.

The reported prevalence of recurrent premenstrual symptoms has ranged from 25 to 100%, with considerable variation in the operational definition of the syndrome and in the methods used to obtain this information. The consensus of questionnaire data is that 70 to 90% of reproductive-aged women are affected, with as many as 30 to 40% reporting that their symptoms are severe enough to be mentally or physically incapacitating. The costs of absenteeism and work inefficiency are considerable, and severe forms of PMS have been linked with accidents, child abuse, marital discord, criminal behavior, and suicide.

Despite the prevalence of this syndrome, little is known about its causes, and there is no consistently effective treatment. Although many causes and therapies have been explored, the evidence is contradictory and inconclusive. Most of the trials of therapeutic agents have been uncontrolled, and interpretation of the data is additionally complicated by the occurrence of a significant placebo effect.

Possible Causes

Hormones

Researchers have not been able to support a number of possible hormonal causes for PMS, including relative estrogen excess, progesterone deficiency, a reaction to withdrawal from either estrogen or progesterone, elevated luteal-phase prolactin, or increased activity of the renin-angiotensin-aldosterone system.

Neurotransmitters

Cyclic decreases in levels of CNS dopamine and serotonin have been blamed for irritability and depression, anxiety, disturbance of sleep cycles, and the carbohydrate cravings of PMS. Because dopamine is known to have a natriuretic effect on the kidney, it is possible that a deficiency is linked to premenstrual fluid retention as well.

Vitamin Deficiency

It has been suggested that premenstrual estrogens cause a relative deficiency of available vitamin B_6, which acts as a coenzyme in the biosynthesis of dopamine and serotonin. This deficiency thereby results in decreased levels of these neurotransmitters.

Fluid Retention

Symptoms of abdominal discomfort, headache, and mastalgia have been attributed to selective "fluid shifts," presumably as the result of estrogen-mediated sodium retention. However, the majority of studies have failed to correlate fluid retention with severity of PMS symptoms, and the response to diuretics has been unpredictable and often no better than to placebo.

Hypoglycemia

Increased luteal-phase insulin response to an oral carbohydrate load has been proposed to account for symptoms of nervousness, sweating, and craving for sweets. However, PMS symptoms are rarely limited to times when hypoglycemia is likely to be maximal, nor are they reliably relieved by the ingestion of food.

Psychological Factors

Although psychological and emotional factors may modulate the perception, expression, and severity of PMS symptoms, they cannot explain all the physiologic changes that have been demonstrated in women with the complaint. Tricyclic antidepressants, tranquilizers, and lithium all have been used in the treatment of PMS, but none has been shown to be more effective than placebo.

Management

Having the patient keep a diary of the presence and severity of symptoms for 2 or more months will help in the diagnosis of PMS. If the symptoms appear during the last 2 weeks of the cycle, subside with the onset of menstruation, and are absent for at least a week afterward, a diagnosis of primary PMS is reasonable. Patients may be reassured to learn that their symptoms are part of a recognized disorder. Symptoms may help guide the choice of interventions but in general it is best to begin with the simplest and safest interventions and proceed to potentially more toxic ones only if necessary.

Learning to manage stress may alleviate PMS symptoms, particularly mood disturbances. Relaxation techniques, biofeedback, and aerobic exercise may benefit individual patients.

Reducing sodium and concentrated sweets in the diet may alleviate symptoms related to fluid retention and hypoglycemia. Vitamin B_6 (pyridoxine), 500 mg daily, may be more effective than placebo in improving both mood and physical symptoms, although studies have yielded conflicting results. Patients should not exceed this dose because ataxia and sensory neuropathy have been associated with daily dosages above 2 g.

Spironolactone, 25 mg four times a day, given on days 18 to 26 of the menstrual cycle, was effective in reducing weight gain and relieving psychological symptoms in one placebo-controlled trial. Other diuretics, such as the thiazides, are widely used, even though their efficacy has not been demonstrated.

Treatment of cyclic mastalgia, a relatively uncommon manifestation of PMS, is discussed in Chapter 80.

Oral contraceptives have been recommended for patients with PMS, in part because a number of surveys have indicated that premenstrual symptoms were fewer or less severe in users compared to nonusers. Higher progestin doses correlated with fewer depressive symptoms, whereas headache or swelling was unchanged and, in some patients, even worse with oral contraceptive medication. Women who are willing to use oral contraceptives, who have primarily depressive symptoms, and who have no contraindications (see Chap. 75) may respond.

Progesterone therapy for PMS has been recommended on the basis of uncontrolled studies but was found to be no better than placebo in several double-blind controlled trials. It is usually given as the natural hormone, which is not available in oral form and must be administered daily, either intramuscularly (50–100 mg, in oil) or by suppository (100–400 mg rectally or intravaginally), from midcycle to the onset of menstruation. Both alternatives are expensive.

Other drugs that have been reported to be of therapeutic value in double-blind, placebo-controlled, clinical trials with crossover designs include the benzodiazepine alprazolam and the oral opiate antagonist naltrexone. Because of its addictive potential, alprazolam should be used with caution and only after other measures have failed. Over-the-counter preparations promoted for treatment of PMS are typically combinations of acetaminophen, a mild diuretic, and an antihistamine; the manufacturer of one such preparation reports its greatest efficacy is in reducing cramps and backache, which are generally less prominent symptoms of PMS.

Keye WR. The premenstrual syndrome. Philadelphia: Saunders, 1988.
An extensive resource on all aspects of premenstrual syndrome.

Reid RL, Ten SSC. Premenstrual syndrome. Am J Obstet Gynecol 1981; 139:85–104.
Comprehensive review of theories of etiology and therapy with complete reference list. A classic!

Rubinow DR, Roy-Byrne P. Premenstrual syndromes: overview from a methodologic perspective. Am J Psychiatry 1984; 141:163–72.
An extensively referenced review of the evidence on the nature, cause, and treatment of PMS.

Lurie D, Borenstein R. The premenstrual syndrome. Obstet Gynecol Surv 1990; 45(4):220–28.
A terse but well-referenced review of proposed causes and treatments of PMS.

Abplanalp JM. Psychologic components of the premenstrual syndrome: evaluating the research and choosing the treatment. J Reprod Med 1983; 28:517–24.
A discussion of the methodologic problems that impede the evaluation of PMS, with particular emphasis on its psychological components.

Smith S, et al. Treatment of premenstrual syndrome with alprazolam: results of a double-blind, placebo-controlled, randomized crossover clinical trial. Obstet Gynecol 1987; 70:37–43.
   A study demonstrating therapeutic benefit of alprazolam over placebo in PMS.

Chuong CJ. Clinical trial of naltrexone in premenstrual syndrome. Obstet Gynecol 1988; 72:332–36.
   Double-blind, placebo-controlled, crossover study showing benefit of naltrexone, an oral opiate antagonist, over placebo in treatment of PMS.

Benedek EP. Premenstrual syndrome: a view from the bench. J Clin Psychiatry 1988; 49(12):498–502.
   Reviews the use of PMS as a legal defense in the United States, explaining why it has not been successful.

Osofsky HJ, Keppel W, Kuczmierczyk AR. Evaluation and management of premenstrual syndrome in clinical psychiatric practice. J Clin Psychiatry 1988; 49(12):494–98.
   Emphasizes the importance of assessment over time in PMS and the need to individualize treatment strategy to the patient's history and clinical presentation. This journal issue is devoted to PMS and contains several other articles on its biology, epidemiology, and clinical aspects.

Freeman E, Rickels K, Sondheimer SJ, et al. Ineffectiveness of progesterone suppository treatment for premenstrual syndrome. JAMA 1990; 264(3):349–353.
   The largest and most recent of the controlled trials demonstrating progesterone's ineffectiveness in PMS; an accompanying editorial follows on page 387.

79. PELVIC INFLAMMATORY DISEASE
John S. Kizer

Pelvic inflammatory disease (salpingitis, salpingo-oophoritis, or acute adnexitis) is an acute or subacute ascending genital tract infection. Although there is nearly always an associated endometritis, the hallmark of pelvic inflammatory disease (PID) is an acute infectious suppuration of the fallopian tubes and ovaries. Frequently, peritonitis with or without perihepatitis (Fitz-Hugh-Curtis syndrome) also occurs.

PID is one of the most important sexually transmitted diseases in the United States for several reasons:

1. The prevalence is high (1% during the childbearing years, 2% in women aged 20–24) and has been increasing over the past decade. It is estimated that nearly 2.5 million outpatient visits and 300,000 hospitalizations are attributable to PID each year.

2. The acute symptoms are often disabling.

3. There are a number of important chronic complications, including pelvic pain, dispareunia, infertility, and ectopic pregnancy.

Risk Factors
The most important risk factor for PID is multiple sexual partners, with the risk increasing as the number of sexual partners increases and as the age at initiation of coitus decreases. The risk of both PID and the associated tubal infertility is substantially reduced by the use of barrier or chemical contraceptives. Diaphragms are the most effective, followed by condoms and spermicides. The use of either a diaphragm or a condom with a spermicide is synergistic and results in a risk reduction of nearly 70%. Although studies have suggested a protective effect of oral contraceptives, especially for PID caused by *Neisseria gonorrhoeae*, this association is not universally accepted. In fact, in some studies, use of oral contraceptives with a high content of estrogen has been associated with increased rates of tubal infertility.

The presence of an intrauterine device (IUD), instrumentation of the cervix (e.g., hysterosalpingography, uterine curettage, or attempted abortion), cervical ectropion, and vaginal douching also increase the risk of PID. Following a first-trimester abortion, the incidence of PID ranges from 4 to 12%. Women with evidence of concurrent bacterial vaginosis may be especially predisposed to this complication.

The increased risk of PID in sexually active teenagers compared to the risk in sexually active adults appears to be more related to the greater number of sexual partners than to any known physiologic difference between the two groups, although a greater frequency of cervical ectropion is present in the younger age group.

There is no evidence that community-acquired PID is followed by a lower incidence of acute or chronic complications than is secondary PID (following instrumentation).

Bacteriology

A number of presumed pathogens have been isolated from the fallopian tubes of patients with PID including *Neisseria gonorrhoeae* (20–50%), *C. trachomatis* (12–40%), anaerobes (89–90%), *Gardnerella vaginalis* (15–50%), *Mycoplasma* and *Ureaplasma* species (15–20%), herpes simplex (1–5%), and gram-positive and gram-negative aerobes such as *Escherichia coli* and Lactobacillus species. The enterococcus is recovered rarely, if ever. There is no firm evidence, however, that consideration of this varied microbiologic profile is clinically important in choosing an antibiotic regimen for the treatment of acute PID.

In community-acquired PID, it has been traditionally assumed that *N. gonorrhoeae*, *C. trachomatis*, and perhaps other sexually transmitted pathogens degrade the normal microbial defenses of the fallopian tube, permitting the secondary invasion of other organisms often found in the vaginal flora, and thereby causing clinical PID. This view has been criticized, however, and the exact role of each of these organisms in causing clinical PID is unknown. For example, antimicrobial therapy that does not include antibiotics active against anaerobes is as clinically effective as regimens that do. In addition, acute PID responds equally well to regimens with or without antimicrobials directed against *C. trachomatis*. It seems likely that in many circumstances PID may be a disease of polymicrobial synergism occurring in the setting of conditions that predispose to ascending infection of the endometrium followed by infection of the tubes and ovaries. These conditions could include douching, gonococcal or chlamydial infection, instrumentation, or a change in the bacterial flora of the vagina as reflected by the association of PID with bacterial vaginosis. Tuberculous salpingitis, which was at one time relatively common, is currently a medical rarity.

The microbiologic profile of PID varies according to the clinical setting and the criteria used for case definition. For example, gonococcal infection is more common among patients evaluated in emergency departments than in those seen in outpatient departments, presumably because of the more acute clinical symptoms associated with gonococcal infection. The gonococcus is also isolated more frequently from the adnexa of patients with classical symptoms of PID. Organisms other than *N. gonorrhoeae* are more likely to be isolated in second and third infections. The frequency with which the gonococcus is isolated diminishes with the age of the patient; this organism is present in only a small proportion of patients aged 30 to 39. It is not known whether acute gonococcal PID causes chronic changes in the genital tract that promote infection with other organisms in the absence of concurrent gonococcal infection or whether the failure to observe *N. gonorrhoeae* in later adult life is caused by partial immunity.

Laparoscopic follow-up suggests that the sequelae of PID, such as tubal adhesions and scarring, may be more often related to an infection harboring *Chlamydia,* possibly because the course of infections harboring these organisms is often relatively indolent and patients may delay or eschew evaluation. The higher frequency of tubal damage may also result from pathologic factors unique to *Chlamydia* species.

Evaluation

Clinical Findings
Patients suspected of having PID present with a wide range of symptoms, varying from mild lower abdominal pain and tenderness to the acute onset of pelvic pain following menses, with fever and exquisite adnexal tenderness ("classic" PID). Unfortunately, clini-

cal findings provide an unreliable means of diagnosis. For example, in one study laparoscopy was performed on patients who had lower abdominal pain and two or more of the following complaints: fever, vomiting, menstrual irregularity, symptoms of proctitis, tenderness of bimanual examination, probable adnexal mass or swelling, and erythrocyte sedimentation rate (ESR) greater than 15 mm per hour. Of these patients, 65% had visual evidence of salpingitis, 23% had no abnormal findings, and 12% had other problems such as acute appendicitis, ectopic pregnancy, pelvic hemorrhage, or endometriosis. The only symptoms that occurred with greater frequency in patients with salpingitis than in those with normal adnexa were fever (49% of the salpingitis group and 19.6% of the negative group) and symptoms of proctitis (6.9% versus 2.7%). Patients with abnormal vaginal discharge, an increased ESR, tenderness on bimanual examination, and pelvic pain were the most likely to have adnexitis, but this combination was found in only 20% of the patients.

Despite the variability of clinical findings, PID remains a clinical diagnosis. In an attempt to refine the diagnosis, the following criteria have been frequently proposed: (1) a history of lower abdominal pain, (2) lower abdominal tenderness (preferably rebound), (3) tenderness with movement of the cervix, and (4) adnexal tenderness. In addition, one or more of the following has been considered necessary: (1) fever, (2) leukocytosis, (3) elevated Westergren ESR, (4) inflammatory adnexal mass on physical exam or sonography, and (5) culdocentesis revealing bacteria and white blood cells in peritoneal fluid. It must be emphasized, however, that this constellation of clinical findings lacks sensitivity, and any case finding that relies on these clinical criteria will overlook a significant number of patients with PID, especially those with indolent chlamydial infection and its presumed higher frequency of infertile sequelae.

Important historical clues to the diagnosis of PID include intercourse with a new sexual partner in the past 2 months, exposure to a partner with known gonorrhea or chlamydial infection, failure to use barrier or chemical contraceptives, multiple sexual partners, drug abuse, a past history of PID, and absence of treatment with a potentially effective antibiotic in the past 2 weeks. PID in pregnant women with intact membranes is rare.

Laboratory Tests
Laboratory tests should include a WBC, Westergren ESR, a qualitative test for β-HCG to determine the likelihood of an intrauterine or ectopic pregnancy, and a VDRL test for syphilis. Identification of gram-negative diplococci on a smear of cervical mucus or the presence of mucopurulent cervicitis as defined by more than 10 to 20 neutrophils per high-power field (hpf) may increase the probability of PID to 70% or more. Similarly, demonstration of *Chlamydia* in cervical mucus by rapid antigen screening (sensitivity and specificity > 90%) also greatly increases the suspicion of PID.

Laparoscopy
Laparoscopy is considered to be the gold standard for the diagnosis of PID and should be used where the diagnosis is crucial, for example, to rule out appendicitis or ectopic pregnancy. Some physicians have advocated laparoscopy in suspected PID as a routine procedure; however, for most cases, laparoscopy is impractical and should be reserved for patients with an uncertain diagnosis or recurrences. In addition, routine laparoscopy would be prohibitively expensive in view of the nearly 3 million cases per year.

Ultrasonography
Ultrasonography, preferably endovaginal, is an extremely sensitive and specific procedure (> 95%) for tubo-ovarian abscess, especially in those cases in which physical examination suggests an adnexal mass. Ultrasound is also useful in those few patients who fail to improve within 48 hours of initial treatment.

Treatment
The management of PID is directed at treatment of the acute symptoms as well as prevention of the long-term sequelae. Although not rigorously established, there is some evidence that infertility may follow salpingitis less frequently when treatment is started within 2 days of the beginning of symptoms. This supposition and the frequent severity of clinical symptoms suggest that treatment should be started immediately even if the diagnosis is

uncertain. Sexual contacts should be advised to seek medical advice. Although most clinicians remove an IUD in patients with PID after the initiation of antibiotic treatment, the therapeutic value of this procedure is unknown.

Antibiotics

Culture results are not helpful in deciding on an antibiotic because of the polymicrobial nature of the infection and the uncertainty of the pathogenetic significance of the isolates. Because of the varied bacteria associated with PID, many authorities have recommended initiation of therapy with broad-spectrum antibiotics. In all recommendations, special attention has been given to include coverage for *Chlamydia* and for resistant *N. gonorrhoeae* (now sufficiently prevalent as to preclude treatment with antibiotics that are not resistant to β-lactamases).

The current recommendations of the Centers for Disease Control for the outpatient treatment of PID are ceftriaxone (250 mg IM) or cefoxitin (2 g IM plus 1 g probenecid PO) plus doxycycline (100 mg PO twice daily for 10–14 days) or tetracycline (500 mg PO qid). Ceftriaxone may be preferred because it is the only known therapy that will cure gonococcal infection of all anatomic sites. Preparations of erythromycin equivalent to 500 mg free base given four times daily may be substituted in pregnant patients or in those who cannot tolerate doxycycline. These recommendations are merely guidelines for therapy and alternative regimens are also acceptable. Other antibiotic regimens that have been found to be equally effective in treating PID on both an inpatient and outpatient basis include cefotaxime (2 g IV q8h); cefoxitin (2 g q6h); clindamycin plus gentamicin; clindamycin alone; metronidazole plus gentamicin; ticarcillin/clavulanate; ampicillin/sulbactam; ciprofloxacin (200 mg IV q12h for 2 days followed by 750 mg PO for 12 days); and amoxacillin/clavulanate (with or without doxycycline). Several of these may be used in patients allergic to cephalosporin or penicillin. Although spectinomycin (2 g IM) is recommended as an alternative for the treatment of resistant *N. gonorrhoeae*, it has not been recommended for treatment of PID. Interestingly, benzathine penicillin and doxycycline have also been shown to cure 97% of cases of PID proven by laparoscopy. In the treatment of pregnant women, both the quinolines and the tetracyclines should be avoided.

The effectiveness of these different antibiotic regimens, even though they do not cover all of the theoretical pathogens that may be found in PID, implies that PID is a synergistic polymicrobial infection. There is also no evidence that any one of these regimens is superior to the others in the treatment of secondary PID (associated with instrumentation) or in the treatment of complicated PID (presence of tubo-ovarian abscess or severe illness). Finally, there are no clinical data to indicate that any of these various regimens result in fewer post-PID sequelae.

Although inclusion of an antibiotic active against *Chlamydia* is not necessary for the resolution of acute PID, subsequent treatment specific for *Chlamydia* is probably essential to reduce the frequency of recurrent PID and to prevent chronic infertile sequelae. Thus, it is advisable to add doxycycline or erythromycin to any regimen that is considered inadequate for *Chlamydia,* such as ciprofloxacin. Although not confirmed, recent evidence suggests that both amoxacillin (500 mg PO q8h) and clindamycin (450 mg PO q8h) may also have significant activity against chlamydial PID.

Hospitalization

Hospitalization is appropriate when the differential diagnosis includes a surgical emergency. The Centers for Disease Control recommend inpatient therapy for patients with uncertain diagnoses, toxicity, pregnancy, inability to tolerate or follow an outpatient regimen, lack of response to outpatient therapy, or suspected tubo-ovarian abscess; it is also recommended if follow-up after 48 to 72 hours cannot be arranged. Hospitalization may also be appropriate for patients with a temperature greater than 38°C (100.4°F) or with peritoneal signs. More controversial are recommendations for inpatient therapy for all adolescents and for women with an IUD in place. There are no clinical trials on the efficacy of inpatient versus outpatient management of PID.

Sequelae

Chronic pelvic pain and dyspareunia occur in 20 to 25% of patients following PID. In these patients, laparoscopy may reveal dense perigenital adhesions, which are presumed to be the cause of pain; however, in many patients the pelvis is entirely normal. The success of surgery in alleviating these symptoms is disappointing, and the pain often persists in those who have had a technically successful operation.

In women who have had PID, the risk of subsequent ectopic pregnancy is increased 10-fold; the cumulative incidence is about 5%. PID is the underlying cause of about 40 to 50% of ectopic pregnancies, with the current rate of ectopia being 1 in 48 pregnancies.

After one bout of PID, 15 to 25% of women are infertile; after three episodes, approximately 75% are infertile. Post-PID damage is thought to be the cause of 30 to 40% of all infertility cases, resulting from post-PID scarring and distortion of the adnexa and fallopian tubes. Microsurgery may restore fertility in 30 to 60% of highly selected patients.

Prevention
Prevention of PID depends on avoidance of risk factors. Oral contraceptives should not be counted on to decrease the likelihood of PID or tubal infertility. Barrier methods such as condoms, cervical caps, or diaphragms when combined with spermicides may decrease the risk of PID by as much as 70%.

St. John RK, Brown ST, eds. International symposium on PID. Am J Obstet Gynecol 1980; 138:845–1109.
More than 40 articles of viewpoints on etiology, epidemiology, and sequelae of PID.

Westrom L. Incidence, prevalence, and trends of acute pelvic inflammatory disease and its consequences in industrialized countries. Am J Obstet Gynecol 1980; 138:880–92.
Discusses the epidemiology of PID, including risk factors and predictors of long-term sequelae.

Stamm WE. Diagnosis of *chlamydia trachomatis* genitourinary infections. Ann Intern Med 1988; 108:710–17.
Useful discussion of laboratory and clinical methods for diagnosis of chlamydial PID and cervicitis.

Cramer DW, Goldman MB, Schiff I, et al. The relationship of tubal infertility to barrier method and oral contraceptive use. JAMA 1987; 257:2446–50.
Discussion of relative risks of PID and its sequelae relative to methods of contraception.

Adler MW. The epidemiology of sexually transmitted diseases in the West. Semin Dermatol 1990; 9:96–101.
Review of modern epidemiology of pelvic inflammatory disease.

Peterson HB, Galaid EI, Zenilman JM. Pelvic inflammatory disease: review of treatment options. Rev Infect Dis 1990; 12:Suppl 6:S656–S664.
Discussion of Centers for Disease Control recommendations in light of current knowledge.

Martens MG, Faro S, Hammil H, et al. Comparison of cefotaxime, cefoxitin, and clindamycin plus gentamicin in the treatment of uncomplicated and complicated pelvic inflammatory disease. J Antimicrob Chemother 1990; 26:Suppl A:37–43.
Provides informative modern data on bacteriology of PID.

80. BREAST LUMPS, BREAST PAIN, AND NIPPLE DISCHARGE
William H. Goodson III

Breast Lumps
Breast lumps are common, occurring in up to 50% of premenopausal women. Although most lumps are benign, they are a cause of concern for both physicians and patients; ruling out breast cancer may require mammography and fine-needle aspiration or biopsy.

Definitions

Terms used to describe breast lumps are often confusing. Benign breast disease designates nonmalignant breast lumps. The trend today is to use the term *benign breast disease* for clinically detected abnormalities, and the term *fibrocystic condition* for nonmalignant changes found on biopsies.

Over 90% of biopsied lesions are fibrocystic conditions and fibroadenomas. Histologically, a variety of lesions are found, including cysts, fibrosis, adenosis, duct ectasia, hyperplasia, and papilloma. Women with a fibrocystic condition on biopsy frequently have clinical nodules, which often increase in size or tenderness just before menses. Such lesions are usually symmetrically distributed in both breasts, but may present as solitary nodules. The incidence of these clinical changes increases with age, peaks at menopause, and then declines. Clinical changes do not correlate with degrees of fibrocystic condition found histologically.

Fibroadenoma usually presents as a solitary, firm, rubbery, smooth, and mobile mass. It is most common in women younger than 30.

Some pathologic changes found on benign breast biopsies indicate a higher risk of subsequent breast cancer. Atypical lobular or ductal hyperplasia is associated with a 15% risk of subsequent breast cancer after 20 years. These changes are found in about 2 to 4% of all biopsies. Hyperplasia, papillomas, and sclerosing adenosis are associated with a slightly increased risk of breast cancer, but less so than the atypical lesion.

Clinical Evaluation

The goal of clinical evaluation is to decide if breast lumps are suggestive of breast cancer. Risk factors for breast cancer should be sought, including a previous history of breast cancer and a family history of breast cancer. If the patient has noted the lump on self-examination, she should be asked how long it has been present and whether it changes in size or becomes tender with the menstrual cycle; the presence of cyclic symptoms suggests benign disease. The breast exam should be done or repeated between day 7 to 10 of the menstrual cycle, since some lumps will regress or disappear then. The examination should include inspection and palpation of the breasts, and palpation of the regional lymph nodes. Normal breasts tend to be symmetric, although sometimes one side (usually the left) is slightly larger than the other. Areas of increased tissue density most commonly occur in the upper outer quadrant, where there is more glandular tissue; a dense area in one breast usually has a counterpart in the other. Perceived lumpiness may also result from normal tissue overlying ribs and from isolated supporting structures that are palpable after swollen breasts shrink after weight loss or childbirth. On examination, most women with lumpy breasts do not have discrete areas that warrant a further workup. A discrete lump should be evaluated with tissue sampling, but it is reasonable to follow subtle changes over two or three menstrual cycles. Multiple bilateral symmetric nodules that wax and wane with the menstrual cycle suggest benign breast disease. A dominant mass that is clearly larger, firmer, or asymmetric requires further evaluation. Breast lumps that are hard, irregular, or fixed suggest breast cancer.

Diagnostic Evaluation

Useful diagnostic procedures include mammography, fine-needle aspiration, excisional biopsy, and occasionally ultrasound.

Mammography is useful to confirm the clinical finding of a mass and also to detect other nonpalpable suspicious lesions that might require evaluation. It has *no* role in determining whether a palpable area or lump is benign. Because mammography is falsely negative in about 20% of women with palpable breast cancer, a negative mammogram does not preclude tissue sampling of a clinically detected breast mass.

Fine-needle aspiration (FNA) is a simple, rapid, and accurate procedure when done by experienced personnel. It takes about 5 minutes, it is no more painful than venipuncture, and results are available in 24 to 48 hours. When an experienced pathologist reads the specimen as benign, the false-negative rate is about 1.4%. This rate is similar to the false-negative rates for excisional biopsy and frozen section. The false-positive rate of slides read as malignant approaches zero. When the cytology is reported as suspicious, further evaluation is needed.

Excisional biopsy is required when expert FNA and cytological evaluation are not available. Excisional biopsy is also indicated if the physical examination or mammography is suspicious for cancer. The procedure is generally done under local anesthesia as an outpatient procedure. The surgeon attempts to remove the entire mass if it is small, or a portion of the mass if it is very large.

Ultrasonography reliably distinguishes cystic from solid breast masses. Because simple breast cysts (with no internal echoes) are virtually always benign, no further evaluation is needed. Generally, FNA is preferred, since it is less expensive and provides diagnostic information if the mass is solid.

Follow-up is important. A cytologic or pathologic diagnosis of malignancy requires surgical consultation. If FNA is benign and the mammogram normal, the woman should be reevaluated in 6 months. Further cancer screening should be done as indicated in Chapter 131.

Breast Pain

Premenstrual breast tenderness and engorgement are physiologic responses to cyclical variations in hormone levels; the pain typically intensifies during the last few days of the menstrual cycle and resolves with the onset of menses. Some women also experience symptoms at midcycle, presumably in response to the burst of estrogens that occurs at ovulation. Breast pain is not associated with breast cancer, and most women do not require any treatment of cyclic breast pain. A breast examination should be performed to identify any discrete areas of abnormality that require evaluation for malignancy as discussed above, and to rule out potential musculoskeletal causes, such as injury or costochondritis.

Occasionally, cyclic pain is severe enough to require symptomatic therapy. Most treatments are aimed at decreasing tissue engorgement or decreasing the effects of hormones on breast tissue. Simple and safe measures should be tried first. A firm supporting brassiere, such as one with cotton straps or of the type designed for joggers, may help by minimizing pulling and tugging from the movement of the breast on the chest wall. Salt restriction during the 1 or 2 weeks before menstruation may reduce engorgement and stretching of the breast tissue. (To prescribe an effective low-salt diet, see Chap. 143). Mild diuretics such as hydrochlorothiazide (25 mg daily for 3 days) may also be used at the time of maximal discomfort; the response rate for this approach has not been documented. Acetaminophen or nonsteroidal anti-inflammatory agents may also provide symptomatic relief.

Abstinence from methylxanthines (e.g., tea, colas, coffee, chocolate, theophylline) has been reported to reduce breast tenderness and lumpiness within 1 to 6 months. A response rate of 65% was reported in an uncontrolled study, but a subsequent controlled study found only a minor response rate. Nevertheless, the intervention is benign and may be an appealing first step for women who wish to avoid medication.

Vitamin E has received much attention, but, unfortunately, controlled studies have not shown any benefit.

Rarely, women may have disabling pain for which drugs with more serious side effects might be considered.

Danazol, a synthetic androgen that blocks estrogen synthesis, is the only hormonally active drug currently approved by the FDA for use in benign breast disease or fibrocystic condition. Doses of 100 to 400 mg per day for 3 to 6 months improve pain in 54 to 99% of women. Tenderness and pain usually respond within the first month, but lumpiness and density are slower to regress. Benefits of therapy may last a year or more, but symptoms often recur after that. Usefulness of this drug is severely limited by its side effects, including menstrual irregularities or amenorrhea, decreased libido, facial hair, acne, voice changes, headaches, and weight gain.

Bromocriptine, a dopamine analogue, blocks release of prolactin, which normally has a permissive effect on breast growth. In two very small controlled studies, it relieved cyclic breast pain in 75 percent of subjects. The dose was 2.5 mg daily for the first week of the menstrual cycle followed by 2.5 mg twice a day until menstruation. Side effects included nausea, dizziness, and malaise, which were severe enough to cause some patients to discontinue medication. In a crossover trial, patients preferred bromocriptine to danazol. The drug has not been approved for this use in the United States.

Tamoxifen also reduces breast pain, but side effects from estrogen blockade are even more severe than with danazol.

Subcutaneous mastectomy has been used to control breast pain, but it is difficult to justify.

Nipple Discharge

Nipple discharge is only rarely due to malignancy. It can be elicited from up to 65% of white women, 40% of black women, and 35% of Oriental women in their childbearing years. Discharge lasts up to 10 years after childbirth in at least one-third of women. Nipple discharge has also been reported with oral contraceptives, in both hypothyroid adolescents and hyperthyroid adults, and in women with anovulatory syndromes.

A discharge can be elicited or spontaneous, come from one or multiple ducts, be clear to green in color, and milky or bloody in consistency. The characteristics of the discharge can be reassuring. In general, only spontaneous, single-duct discharges warrant attention. Discharges that are not spontaneous require no further evaluation. Yellow-green to dark-green discharges are usually benign. Discharges from multiple ducts are usually physiologic; the exception is a spontaneous milky discharge from multiple ducts, which may be caused by a prolactin-secreting pituitary adenoma. A serum prolactin level should be obtained in patients with spontaneous milky discharges; levels above 25 µg per deciliter are abnormal, but adenomas usually have levels near 100, or higher.

Although patients are usually more alarmed by bloody discharge, a bloody discharge is more likely to be benign than malignant. In most cases for which a specific cause is found, either duct ectasia or papillomatosis is identified. A totally clear discharge is more typical of cancer, particularly with an extensive intraductal component.

If the discharge is spontaneous (e.g., noted on underwear or night clothes), the physician should seek any lumps and try to identify the duct that produces the discharge. The patient is examined with her ipsilateral hand behind her head. Firm pressure is applied around the nipple and areola at various positions until a point is found at which pressure produces a discharge. If a single duct repeatedly produces a discharge, surgical biopsy and excision are appropriate for diagnosis. Ductograms are redundant because any lesion will be excised for diagnosis, and a biopsy is indicated even if the ductogram is negative. Although cytology is frequently performed, it is usually negative even in the presence of cancer. Spontaneous discharge from multiple ducts is unusual and is best referred for specialized evaluation.

Grady D, Hodgkins ML, Goodson WH III. The lumpy breast. West J Med 1988:226–9.
An excellent review, with a primary care perspective.

Ernster VL, Mason L, Goodson WH III, et al. Effects of a caffeine-free diet on benign breast disease: a randomized trial. Surgery 1982; 91:263–67.

Parazzini F, La Vecchia C, Riundi R, et al. Methylxanthine, alcohol-free diet, and fibrocystic breast disease: a factorial clinical trial. Surgery 1986; 99(5):575–81.
Two randomized trials that found no benefit from a low-caffeine/methylxanthine diet.

Mansel RE, Wisbey JR, Hughes LE. Controlled trial of the antigonadotropin danazol in painful nodular benign breast disease. Lancet 1982; 1:928–30.
A good crossover trial evaluating the effects of danazol. Note that a marked improvement was also noted in placebo groups!

Goodson WH III, Miller TR, Sickles EA, et al. Lack of correlation of clinical breast examination with high-risk histopathology. Am J Med 1990; 89:752–56.
A lack of correlation was found between density and nodularity in physical examination and the presence of histopathology in underlying breast tissue; that is, a general physical examination does not predict the risk of breast cancer.

Wapnir I, Rabinowitz B, Greco R. A reappraisal of prophylactic mastectomy. Surg Gynecol 1990; 171(2):171–84.
A review concluding that this procedure isn't justified.

Vorherr H. Fibrocystic breast disease: pathophysiology, pathomorphology, clinical pictures, and management. Am J Obstet Gynecol 1986; 154:161–79.
An excellent review with many insights, although its final conclusions are not universally accepted.

Goodwin PJ, Neelam M, Boyd NF. Cyclical mastopathy: a critical review of therapy. Br J Surg 1988; 75:837–44.
Classifies bromocriptine, danazol, evening primrose oil, tamoxifen, and reduction of dietary fat as "definitely effective," sometimes on slim evidence.

Boyd NF, Shannon P, Krinkov V, et al. Effect of a low-fat, high-carbohydrate diet on symptoms of cyclical mastopathy. Lancet 1988; 2:128–32.
Randomized trial with a small number (21) of subjects.

Progress Symposium. Benign breast disorders: fibrocystic disease? non-disease? or ANDI? World J Surg 1989; 13:667–761.
A recent symposium, with 23 different articles on all aspects of benign breast disease. (Note: ANDI, a term used more in the British and European literature, signifies "Aberrations of Normal Development and Involution.")

Leis HP Jr. Management of nipple discharge. World J Surg 1989; 13:736–42.
One of the articles in the above symposium, discussing types of breast discharges and their evaluation and management.

81. MENOPAUSE
Thomas C. Keyserling and Robert H. Fletcher

Menses cease at an average age of about 50 years; it is unusual for menopause to begin before age 45 or later than age 55 years. During the years just before menses cease altogether, there is often an increase in variability of cycle length and a diminished menstrual flow. An underlying disease such as endometrial cancer should be considered if, during these years, there are heavy periods or bleeding between periods.

In the United States, roughly one-third of women have hysterectomies before natural menopause. For those who have oophorectomies as well, the symptoms of menopause (other than bleeding) occur rapidly and are relatively severe unless replacement estrogens are given; osteoporosis and coronary heart disease are also believed to be more common in these women.

Symptoms
Women experience a variety of symptoms associated with estrogen deficiency during the perimenopausal period. Common concerns include hot flashes, urogenital symptoms, and psychological changes. Although these symptoms are not life threatening, they may be disruptive and are often of great concern to patients.

Hot Flashes
Hot flashes occur in three-quarters of perimenopausal women, and about 30% of women complain that their hot flashes are severe. Most women who report hot flashes experience them for more than 1 year, and some experience them for more than 5 years. Hot flashes are typically brief episodes of flushing and sweating; they may, when they occur at night, disturb sleep. While the precise mechanism of hot flashes is unknown, symptoms occur at a time of estrogen deficiency and are relieved by exogenous estrogens. There is also a close temporal association between hot flashes and pulses of luteinizing hormone (LH) secretion.

TREATMENT. Because hot flashes are self-limited and often mild, treatment other than reassurance is generally unnecessary. For some women, however, hot flashes cause considerable discomfort, and treatment is desired. If estrogen replacement is not contraindicated, it is the treatment of choice. The efficacy of estrogens in relieving hot flashes has been supported by placebo-controlled trials, and the response to therapy is dose-related. A 50 to 60% reduction has been reported with daily doses of 0.625 mg of conjugated equine estrogens, and an 80 to 100% reduction with daily doses of 1.25 to 2.50 mg. Treatment with estrogens does not produce an immediate effect on hot flashes; a decrease in the frequency of episodes is seen after 2 to 4 weeks. (See Estrogen Regimens.) Progestins, clonidine, and Bellergal-S (which contains ergotamine tartrate, belladonna alkaloids, and phenobarbital) have also been shown to reduce the frequency of hot flashes in controlled trials. However, these agents are less effective than estrogens and their use is often limited by side effects.

Estrogens given only for the treatment of hot flashes can be discontinued after a few years of treatment or when physician and patient agree. The patient should be monitored for return of symptoms. If hot flashes recur, they usually do so within days to weeks after hormones are discontinued. Patients should be warned of this possibility and reassured that hormones can be resumed if desired. If hormone replacement therapy is desired for prevention of osteoporosis or coronary heart disease, withdrawal is not necessary.

Urogenital Atrophy
Urogenital atrophy is experienced to some degree by all women after menopause because urogenital tissues are estrogen dependent. The onset and severity of this effect are extremely variable. Vulvar atrophy results in thin, dry, easily traumatized genital tissues, which can lead to cracking, vaginitis, and dyspareunia. Urethral atrophy may cause urgency, frequency, and dysuria. It is not known if urinary incontinence is associated with menopause or if it is primarily related to advancing age.

TREATMENT. Exogenous estrogens given orally reverse atrophic vaginitis in 4 to 6 weeks and alleviate urgency, frequency, and dysuria caused by estrogen deficiency. Some reports suggest urinary incontinence improves when estrogens are given. Topical estrogens may also be used; they are absorbed through the vaginal mucosa in amounts similar to those absorbed from orally administered estrogens. While some women find the topical preparations inconvenient, an advantage is that once atrophy has been reversed, it may be possible to maintain the effect with infrequent doses (e.g., 1–2 per week), with the patient using her own symptoms as a guide.

Psychological Changes
The association of psychological symptoms with menopause remains controversial. Although nonspecific symptoms such as mood fluctuations, insomnia, headache, anxiety, depression, and decreased libido have been associated with menopause in some studies, this association has been refuted by others. These conflicting results may be due in part to methodological differences between the studies as well as by the fact that symptoms attributed to menopause are influenced by social and cultural factors and therefore are likely to vary according to the population of women surveyed and when the survey was done. Most randomized placebo-controlled trials of estrogen replacement in postmenopausal women have found estrogens to have a beneficial effect on psychological function, suggesting an hormonal basis for some of the psychological symptoms associated with menopause. Some investigators have proposed that the improved psychological function results from the better sleep patterns associated with estrogen use. Others have suggested that improved function occurs because symptoms such as hot flashes and vaginal dryness improve. In sum, psychological changes associated with menopause may occur in some women and not in others and are likely due to interactive effects of endocrine changes, social and cultural factors, and individual psychological characteristics.

TREATMENT. Because nonspecific psychological symptoms associated with menopause may be due to other medical or psychiatric conditions, the initial approach to these complaints should include appropriate medical and psychiatric evaluation. If no specific diagnosis is apparent, it is important to explore the patient's beliefs and concerns about menopause. Patient education and reassurance can be very effective in helping patients deal with these symptoms and often are all that is necessary. If symptoms persist, a trial of estrogen therapy is warranted. If the patient improves, estrogen treatment should be continued; if not, further evaluation is indicated.

Long-term Risks Associated with Estrogen Deficiency

Osteoporosis
Women achieve maximal bone mass in their late twenties. Bone mass is well maintained until menopause, at which time there is a rapid increase in the rate of bone loss. Because

women attain a smaller bone mass than men and experience accelerated bone loss after menopause, they are more likely to develop osteoporosis and consequently fractures (particularly of the hip, spine, and radius) than are men of similar age. A 50-year-old white female has about a 15% lifetime risk of suffering a hip or Colles' fracture and about a 32% risk of developing a vertebral fracture.

Treatment with exogenous estrogens has been shown to prevent both osteoporosis and fractures. The accelerated decline in bone mineral content after menopause can be blocked by daily estrogen administration. Studies show that about one-third to two-thirds of fractures can be prevented by regular use of exogenous estrogens, beginning about the time of menopause. The reduction in fractures appears to be greater when estrogens are begun within 5 years of menopause. Protection increases with the duration of estrogen therapy but becomes substantial and statistically significant only after 6 years and declines within 5 years after stopping estrogens. (See Chap. 66 for further discussion.)

Coronary Heart Disease
Coronary heart disease (CHD) is the leading cause of death for American women and men. While CHD is uncommon in premenopausal women, the incidence of this disease increases markedly in the postmenopausal years. The lifetime risk of death due to CHD for a 50-year-old white woman is 31%; in comparison, the risk of death for the same woman due to hip fracture is 3%, due to breast cancer is 3%, and due to endometrial cancer is 0.05%.

Because CHD rates increase in women after menopause, there is a great deal of interest in the effect of postmenopausal estrogens on rates of CHD. More than 20 epidemiologic studies have addressed this topic, and most have shown that estrogen use is associated with a reduction in CHD of 30 to 70%. Of 11 prospective cohort studies, the only one to identify an increased risk associated with estrogen use (relative risk = 1.76) is the Framingham study of Wilson and colleagues. This increased risk was for all cardiovascular endpoints: cerebrovascular disease, CHD defined as myocardial infarction and angina, and congestive heart failure. A reanalysis of the Framingham data using the more specific endpoint of CHD excluding angina showed a trend toward a protective effect associated with estrogen use among women ages 50 to 59.

The protective effect of estrogens on CHD appears to be mediated, at least in part, by its favorable effect on blood lipids. Conjugated equine estrogens affect lipoproteins in a dose-dependent fashion. The degree of lipoprotein change has varied in reported studies, but by combining the data, a reasonable estimate is that 0.625 mg/day increases high-density lipoprotein (HDL) by 10% and decreases low-density lipoprotein (LDL) by 4%, while 1.25 mg/day increases HDL by 14% and decreases LDL by 8%. Unfortunately, the addition of commonly recommended doses of progestins to postmenopausal estrogen regimens attenuates the beneficial effects of oral estrogens on HDL.

Estrogens are usually given with progestins. As there is little information on the effects of estrogens plus progestins on rates of CHD, the assessment of benefits and risks of a combined regimen is largely hypothetical.

Estrogen Therapy: Risks and Side Effects
Estrogen therapy provides clear benefits both for symptoms associated with menopause and for the prevention of osteoporosis and CHD. There are also risks associated with this treatment as well as significant side effects. The decision to initiate therapy and the choice of regimen must be based on an understanding of the risks and benefits as well as on the concerns and preferences of the individual patient.

Endometrial Cancer
Risk of endometrial cancer is several times greater for women taking estrogens without concomitant progestins than for those who do not. The studies have been controversial, but disagreement has been over the size of the risk rather than over its existence. Most studies report a four- to sevenfold increase. Risk appears to be related to both dose and duration of estrogen treatment—there may be a small risk after a few years of use, but risk is certainly present after about 5 years. Endometrial cancers in estrogen users are, on average, found at earlier stages and therefore may have a better prognosis and greater likelihood of effective treatment. The increased risk of endometrial cancer in estrogen-treated women may result from the endometrial hyperplasia caused by estrogens. Preven-

tion of endometrial hyperplasia can be achieved in most women by adding progestins for 10 to 12 days of the cycle. The effectiveness of other regimens, such as adding a progestin less frequently (i.e., every 3 months), has not been demonstrated.

Breast Cancer

Because breast tissue is estrogen dependent, exogenous estrogen is suspected of being a risk factor for breast cancer. The evidence from clinical studies is, so far, inconclusive. However, two large studies and a meta-analysis recently reported an increased risk of breast cancer among postmenopausal estrogen users. One of these studies, done in Sweden, evaluated the association of estrogen use and breast cancer among 23,244 women who had estrogen prescriptions filled and were followed for an average of 5.7 years. Although the overall relative risk of breast cancer was 1.1, the relative risk increased with the duration of treatment, reaching 1.7 after 9 years. In this study, the increased risk of breast cancer was associated with the use of estradiol and not conjugated equine estrogens. The other study followed more than 23,000 postmenopausal U.S. nurses for up to 10 years. Unlike the Swedish study, a large majority of users in this study took conjugated equine estrogens. Among current users, the risk of breast cancer was significantly elevated (relative risk 1.36; 95% confidence interval 1.11 to 1.76). Past users were not at increased risk for breast cancer. The meta-analysis reported a small but statistically significant increased risk for breast cancer (relative risk 1.07 among postmenopausal estrogen users compared to controls). Most data suggest that the relative risk, if increased at all, is small.

Gallbladder Disease

Because estrogens increase the cholesterol content of bile, they are suspected of causing gallbladder disease. One large study found a twofold increase in recognized gallbladder disease, but this has not been confirmed by other studies.

Uterine Bleeding

Postmenopausal women on hormone replacement therapy experience a high rate of uterine bleeding, which is classified as breakthrough when it occurs during treatment days and withdrawal when it occurs during treatment-free periods (typically, days 26–30 of each cycle). Patterns of bleeding correlate with type of hormonal replacement regimen. A recent prospective study compared bleeding patterns in women taking different doses (0.625 mg or 1.25 mg on days 1–25) of conjugated equine estrogens alone or with 5 mg of medroxyprogesterone on days 15 to 25. All women on the combined regimens experienced uterine bleeding: withdrawal bleeding was more common (86%) than breakthrough bleeding (14%). Of the women taking 0.625 mg of conjugated equine estrogen alone, 59% had no bleeding and 41% experienced breakthrough bleeding. In contrast, only 4% of women taking 1.25 mg of conjugated equine estrogens had no bleeding, 70% had breakthrough bleeding, and 26% experienced withdrawal bleeding.

Uterine bleeding is a major concern of patients taking estrogen; in one survey, having periods was noted as the most negative factor influencing a woman's decision to use hormonal replacement. It also increases the cost of care. Unscheduled bleeding requires diagnostic evaluation and among women taking unopposed estrogens; there is an increased rate of hysterectomy.

Other Risks and Side Effects

Up to 40% of women taking postmenopausal estrogen note breast tenderness, which is usually mild. Less common side effects are nausea and headache. Progestins can cause premenstrual-like symptoms, including bloating, irritability, edema, and breast tenderness. Although oral estrogens increase the synthesis of renin substrate, there is no evidence that taking estrogen increases blood pressure. Oral estrogens may also increase concentrations of fibrinogen and fibrinopeptides, but there is no evidence that postmenopausal women taking conjugated estrogens have increased rates of thrombophlebitis or other thrombotic events.

Estrogen Regimens

There are few absolute contraindications to estrogen therapy. Most experts agree that women with a history of endometrial cancer or breast cancer as well as women with acute,

Table 81-1. Recommended Starting Doses for Common Estrogen and Progestin Preparations

Generic	Trade Name	Dose Recommended (mg/day)
ESTROGENS		
Oral, natural		
Conjugated equine estrogen	Premarin	0.625
Piperazine estrone sulfate	Ogen	0.625, 1.25
Micronized estradiol	Estrace	1.0
Esterified estrogen	Estratab, Menest	0.625
Oral, synthetic		
Ethinyl estradiol	Estinyl	0.02
Transdermal		
17β estradiol	Estraderm	0.05
Vaginal		
Conjugated equine estrogen	Premarin Cream	0.625
PROGESTINS		
Medroxyprogesterone acetate	Provera, Amen, Curretab, Cycrin	5.0, 10.0
Norethindrone	Micronor, Nor-Q D	0.35
Norgestrel	Ovrette	0.075

severe liver disease should not be given estrogen. While a history of thromboembolic disease and chronic liver disease have been listed as contraindications, these recommendations are based on experience with oral contraceptives and are probably not applicable to postmenopausal hormone replacement.

Estrogens are available in a variety of formulations, both natural and synthetic. Common estrogen and progestin preparations and typical starting doses are given in Table 81-1. Although estrogen formulations differ in potency and route of administration, there is no evidence that one preparation is superior to others. When oral estrogens are given in doses that produce similar levels of circulating estrogens, the different preparations produce similar biologic effects. A transdermal estrogen patch (estradiol) has recently been marketed in the United States. Because estrogen given in this fashion enters directly into the systemic circulation, there is no first-pass effect; thus, the increased synthesis of hepatic proteins associated with oral estrogens does not occur. The patch is effective for treating symptoms of the menopause as well as for maintaining bone mass. However, it does not increase HDL cholesterol.

No one estrogen regimen has been shown to be superior to others in clinical trials. Women who have had a hysterectomy should receive estrogen alone. For a woman with an intact uterus, most experts recommend a regimen of estrogen plus progestin because combined therapy does not increase the incidence of endometrial carcinoma. As more data become available on the association of combined regimens with breast cancer and CHD, this recommendation may change.

A common regimen is to take estrogen (conjugated equine estrogens 0.625 mg/day, ethinyl estradiol 0.02 mg/day, or 17β-estradiol patch 0.05 mg/day) on days 1 to 25; a progestin (medroxyprogesterone 5–10 mg/day or norethindrone 0.35 to 0.70 mg/day) on days 14 to 25; and no hormones on the remaining days of the month. Because there is no evidence that a 5- to 6-day "rest" every month is of any benefit (and hot flashes may return after 3–5 days), many experts are now recommending continuous estrogen treatment with a progestin given on days 1 to 12 of each month. On this regimen, withdrawal bleeding occurs midmonth. A newer approach to replacement therapy involves administering a low dose of progestin daily (medroxyprogesterone 2.5–5.0 mg/day or norethindrone 0.35–0.70 mg/day). The effect of daily progestin administration on cardiovascular risk is not known.

All women who have breakthrough bleeding should have an outpatient endometrial biopsy, whether or not progestins are used. For women who take only estrogen, an endometrial biopsy should be considered before treatment is initiated and then annually for as long as treatment is continued. For women taking progestin cyclically, a biopsy is not recommended if bleeding starts on or after the twelfth day of progestin therapy. If bleeding starts earlier, a biopsy may be worthwhile, and the patient may need a longer cycle of progestin to prevent hyperplasia.

Withdrawal bleeding and other concerns about hormonal replacement therapy limit compliance, which in some studies has been as low as 30 to 50%. In one study, the factor most favorably influencing a woman's decision to use estrogen was a recommendation from her physician. Improved communication between patient and physician on risks, benefits, and side effects has the potential to significantly improve compliance with hormonal replacement.

Estrogens: Benefits Versus Risks

Estrogens are highly effective in treating the menopausal symptoms of hot flashes and urogenital atrophy. They should be offered to symptomatic patients with the understanding that relief of symptoms can be achieved with minimal risk. Because long-term administration of estrogens decreases the risk of osteoporotic fractures and CHD, estrogens should be considered for asymptomatic women. The potential cardiac benefits of oral estrogens given alone outweigh the increased risk of endometrial carcinoma and the possible small increases in the rate of breast cancer. Progestins given in adequate doses to prevent endometrial carcinoma attenuate the favorable lipid changes associated with oral estrogens and may negate some or all of the cardioprotective effect of oral estrogens.

Whether long-term postmenopausal estrogens do more harm than good in an individual patient depends mainly on her risk of fractures and CHD and her preferences regarding uterine bleeding after menopause, relief of menopausal symptoms, and the inconvenience of this therapy. In prescribing long-term postmenopausal estrogens, the challenge is to adequately assess the risk of osteoporosis and CHD and then to convey to the patient these risks and potential benefits of treatment, allowing her to make an informed decision.

Am J Obstet Gynecol 1989; 161:1825–68.
A collection of good reviews on various aspects of estrogen replacement therapy.

Gelfand MM, Ferenczy A. A prospective 1-year study of estrogen and progestin in postmenopausal women: effects on the endometrium. Obstet Gynecol 1989; 74:398–402.
A randomized blinded trial reviewing bleeding patterns and endometrial morphology in women taking estrogen with or without medroxyprogesterone.

Cummings SR, Black DM, Rubin SM. Lifetime risks of hip, Colles', or vertebral fracture and coronary heart disease among white postmenopausal women. Arch Intern Med 1989; 149:2445–48.
Reviews the risk of postmenopausal women developing important conditions that might be influenced by the use of hormone replacement therapy.

Bush TL, Barrett-Connor E, Cowan LD, et al. Cardiovascular mortality and noncontraceptive use of estrogen in women: results from the Lipid Research Clinics Program follow-up study. Circulation 1987; 75:1102–09.
In this large prospective study, women taking estrogens had a 60% lower risk of cardiovascular mortality. The protective effect of estrogen appeared to be substantially mediated through increased HDL levels.

Bush TL, Miller VT. Effects of pharmacologic agents used during the menopause: impact on lipids and lipoproteins. In: Mishell DR Jr, ed. Menopause: physiology and pharmacology. Chicago: Year Book, 1987:187–208.
Reviews the effects on lipids and lipoproteins of hormonal agents used during the menopause.

Stampfer MJ, Colditz GA, Willet WC, et al. Post-menopausal estrogen therapy and cardiovascular disease: Ten-year follow-up from the Nurses' Health Study. N Engl J Med 1991; 325:756–62.
This prospective study followed 48,470 postmenopausal women for up to 10 years. Current estrogen users had about half the risk of major cardiovascular disease compared with

women who never used estrogen. Among users there was also a significant reduction in cardiovascular mortality.

Colditz GA, Willett WC, Stampfer MJ, et al. Menopause and the risk of coronary heart disease in women. N Engl J Med 1987; 316:1105–10.
This large cohort study shows an increased risk for CHD in women with bilateral oophorectomy, prevented by estrogen replacement therapy.

Stampfer, MJ. Smoking, estrogen, and prevention of heart disease in women. Mayo Clin Proc 1989; 64:1553–57.
A concise review of the literature on the relationship between postmenopausal estrogen use and coronary heart disease.

Wilson PWF, Garrison RJ, Castelli WP. Postmenopausal estrogen use, cigarette smoking, and cardiovascular morbidity in women over 50: The Framingham Study. N Engl J Med 1985; 313:1038–43.
The original Framingham report suggesting an increased risk of cardiovascular morbidity among women taking estrogen.

Bergkvist L, Adami HO, Persson I, et al. The risk of breast cancer after estrogen and estrogen-progestin replacement. N Engl J Med 1989; 321:293–97.
A large cohort study suggesting a slight increased risk of breast cancer among women taking estradiol compounds. Risk increased with the duration of treatment and in women who took estrogen and progestin in combination.

Colditz GA, Stampfer MJ, Willett WC, et al. Prospective study of estrogen replacement therapy and risk of breast cancer in postmenopausal women. JAMA 1990; 264:2648–53.
In this large cohort study, current users of postmenopausal estrogens experienced a slight increase in the risk of breast cancer (relative risk 1.36). There was no increased risk among past users of replacement therapy.

Dupont WD, Page DL. Menopausal estrogen replacement therapy and breast cancer. Arch Intern Med 1991; 151:67–72.
A meta-analysis of breast cancer risk and estrogen replacement therapy, suggesting a slight increased risk of breast cancer associated with postmenopausal estrogen use.

Henderson BE, Paganini-Hill A, Ross RK. Decreased mortality in users of estrogen replacement therapy. Arch Intern Med 1991; 151:75–78.
In this prospective study of 8881 postmenopausal women followed for 7.5 years, women with a history of estrogen use had 20% lower age-adjusted all-cause mortality compared with lifetime non-users (95% confidence interval, 0.70–0.87). Current users with more than 15 years of estrogen use had a 40% reduction in all-cause mortality. Although encouraging, the results of studies reporting decreased mortality among estrogen users should be interpreted with caution. While some studies have adjusted for known risk factors, women willing to take estrogens are likely to have some characteristics that are different from non-users. Furthermore, most women currently taking estrogens also take progestins, and the influence of progestins on all-cause mortality is not known.

Ferguson KJ, Hoegh C, Johnson S. Estrogen replacement therapy: a survey of women's knowledge and attitudes. Arch Intern Med 1989; 149:133–36.
This survey assesses women's attitudes about estrogen replacement therapy and suggests that systematic education could favorably influence women's willingness to take estrogens.

Greenwood S. Menopause naturally: preparing for the second half of life. Volcano, CA: Volcano Press, 1989.
An excellent book for patients interested in learning more about menopause. It is comprehensive and gives sound advice on estrogen replacement therapy as well as alternative treatments.

82. FEMALE SEXUAL DYSFUNCTION
Cheryl F. McCartney

In recent years, women have become increasingly aware of the importance of their sexuality, for their own pleasure as well as for their expression of affection for partners. Although surveys have indicated that more than half of American adult women have a sexual problem, many women hesitate to initiate discussion of sexual concerns with their physicians. Because such problems are often easily reversible, primary care providers can make a valuable contribution to their women patients' quality of life by detecting sexual dysfunctions, adjusting medical therapy to minimize sexual side effects, offering limited sex education, and by preparing patients to accept referral to competent therapists.

Types of Dysfunction
Because sexual problems may have multiple dimensions, patient evaluation is based on systematic review of problem areas. Dysfunction may be caused by ignorance about the range of normal sexual functioning as well as by psychological or organic factors. Disruption may occur in one or more of the three phases of the sexual response cycle: *desire, arousal,* and *orgasm. Coital pain* and *mismatch within a couple* on preferences for frequency and variety of sexual activity may also be factors. Qualifying information, such as substance abuse, marital distress, or preference for same-sex partner should be obtained to amplify the description of a problem.

Desire phase disorders have recently been subclassified into hypoactive sexual desire (abnormally low or absent sex drive) and sexual aversion disorder (panic or active revulsion from sexual stimulation).

Impaired female arousal is reflected by partial or complete failure to achieve or maintain vaginal lubrication and swelling of genital tissues and can occur in women with normal desire and ability to have orgasm. This problem can result in painful intercourse.

Orgasmic function is quite variable. Approximately 8% of American women have never had orgasm. Others require stimulation of varying intensity to reach orgasm, ranging from those few who can climax in response to fantasy, kissing, or breast stimulation to those whose only orgasms occur during clitoral masturbation. Although disagreement exists on the definition of dysfunction along this range, women who need additional clitoral stimulation to reach orgasm with a partner generally are considered normal, while those with anorgasmia or lack of orgasm with a partner should be offered treatment. However, the woman's choice about the need for treatment should be respected.

Coital pain problems include dyspareunia (which can be psychogenic or the result of a medical condition), vaginismus (involuntary spasm of the muscles of the outer third of the vagina that prevents penetration), and reduced genital sensation.

Detection and Evaluation
Detection of sexual problems correlates with both the physician's comfort in discussing sexual matters and whether questions on sexual function are routinely included in the system review. It is important that the physician initiate questions about sexual function because some patients are reticent to introduce the subject and some are not consciously aware of their sexual concerns and may present with vague somatic complaints (e.g., abdominal pains or headaches) or mood disturbances (e.g., anxiety or depression). Once a problem is recognized as a sexual disorder and its dimensions defined, detailed questioning should pinpoint whether it is secondary (function was normal at one time) or primary (function was never normal), and whether it is general (happens always) or situational (occurs under specific circumstances or with a specific partner). Medical, psychiatric, interpersonal, and cultural factors contributing to the problem should be explored. Interviewing the patient together with her partner may elicit further details about the problem and is especially helpful in defining its impact on the relationship. The physician's interview should provide patients with the opportunity to reveal problems with same sex as well as opposite sex partners. Although homosexual women often have committed relationships, they fear that physicians will disapprove of their life-style; thus, they are guarded until they feel that the physician is understanding and nonjudgmental.

Organic Causes

Drugs

Because drug-related effects on sexual function are easily reversed by discontinuing the medication, or sometimes by reducing the dosage, any woman with sexual dysfunction should be routinely questioned about her drug use history. Most drugs that affect female sexual function influence the desire phase. These include central nervous system depressant drugs, such as alcohol, sedative-hypnotics, antianxiety agents, narcotics, and antipsychotics. Beta-adrenergic blocking agents, such as propranolol, can also cause loss of libido. Cancer chemotherapy drugs reduce sexual desire by damaging the ovaries and by causing general debilitation. Cimetidine reduces desire by acting as an antiandrogen (androgens stimulate desire). Ranitidine, a related drug, also has this effect, but to a lesser degree. Stimulant drugs, such as cocaine and amphetamines, have been reported to enhance desire, although their chronic use reduces it. Mixed effects on desire are reported for hallucinogens and marijuana.

The orgasm phase can be delayed in women taking high doses of antianxiety or antidepressant agents. Orgasm is often lost by women taking centrally acting sympatholytic antihypertensives such as clonidine or methyldopa, monoamine oxidase inhibitor antidepressants, or high doses of cocaine or amphetamines.

Aging

Though some surveys have indicated a decline in sexual interest with age, this finding may be due to comparing people of differing age cohorts. Earlier generations tend to hold more conservative sexual attitudes than the present group of young people. Actually, sexual interest and frequency in later life usually follow the pattern set during midlife. The end of a woman's sexual life is often decided by her male partner: she adjusts to his loss of interest or function, or she loses him because of divorce or death. Although menopause does not uniformly exert a negative influence on a woman's sexuality, the discomfort of hot flashes and the dyspareunia related to estrogen loss can result in reduced desire for some women. Older women notice that vaginal lubrication occurs more slowly and that they require more stimulation than when they were younger. Orgasmic contractions are weaker. Estrogen cream or lubricant preparations may be helpful treatments; lubricants should be water soluble, such as Astroglide, rather than petroleum jelly (Vaseline), which is not.

Physical Illness

Physicians should inquire about sexual function in women with any gynecologic condition, ranging from normal pregnancy and childbirth, to infertility treatment, benign hysterectomy, or gynecologic cancer. Women with serious or chronic illness also frequently have sexual problems. In addition to somatic changes caused by the condition itself, the illness may have psychological effects on the woman, her partner, and thus on their relationship.

Somatic effects on sexual function result from conditions or treatments that disrupt the woman's genital anatomy (such as gynecologic cancer, hysterectomy, radiation therapy), sensory or motor nerve function (such as diabetes, multiple sclerosis, traumatic paraplegia), circumvaginal circulation (such as pelvic radiation), or levels of circulating estrogen (such as oophorectomy). Sensation, lubrication, vaginal elasticity, and orgasmic contractions may be compromised, and the resulting dyspareunia can lead to a secondary loss of desire. Illnesses that affect respiration or joint function can also disrupt sexuality. In addition, physical debilitation from any severe, systemic illness and its treatment may lead to reduced sexual desire. Women may become concerned that small changes in their body function during sexual activity signal deterioration of their health, and these anxieties can interfere with arousal.

Psychological effects of physical illness on sexual dysfunction may take many forms. Adjustment to ostomies is particularly troublesome. Problems with reproductive organs or breasts often have special meaning and thus may affect a woman's sense of her femininity. Some women simply don't know that sexual function can be preserved despite removal of reproductive organs. It has been shown that the most significant determinant of posthysterectomy sexual dysfunction is the incorrect preoperative expectation of sexual alteration. With the disruption of body image, the woman's sense of attractiveness and desirability may be damaged. Guilt about past sexual activities (masturbation, premarital and extra-marital sex, venereal disease, abortion, multiple partners) and trauma from past sexual abuse can also be evoked by treatments to sexual body sites. Also, the mood disturbances that frequently occur in medically ill patients reduce sexual desire.

Difficulty with partners may occur as a result of surgery or chronic illness. Partners may be uncomfortable with the changes in the patient's body or by her new identity as a patient and may be unable to adjust sexually. The partner may also resent any loss of normal function. Some relationships are so intolerant of such stress that they dissolve. However, a supportive partner can help a woman adapt to her illness and thus hasten her return to enjoyable sexual activity.

Intervention

Ambulatory care physicians should attempt to treat sexual dysfunctions at their level of expertise. Skills range in complexity from giving permission, through basic sex education and suggesting specific modifications in sex practices, to performing intensive therapy. The decision to treat or refer can be made after an initial evaluation of the patient determines the level of therapy needed. Chart notes must respect the sensitive nature of this material, since patient records are often seen by staff other than the treating physician, or by the patients themselves.

Permission

Some women need only confirmation that they are normal to relieve guilt about erotic thoughts, feelings, fantasies, dreams, and desires. They may need permission to initiate sex, to ask for more stimulation to get aroused, to ask for specific kinds of stimulation, or to refuse sex when they are not interested. If the physician's attitude conveys that a woman is entitled to sexual satisfaction she may be able to adopt this attitude herself.

Information

Sexual problems may be caused by lack of information. For example, couples who do not know that the excitement phase in men is shorter than in women may try penetration before the woman has adequate lubrication, resulting in painful intercourse, anorgasmia, and sexual avoidance because of anticipation of dyspareunia. "Mythology" can be equally damaging, such as the belief that masturbation is abnormal or that orgasm should occur simultaneously in the man and woman during intercourse. Actually, coital anorgasmia is *not* considered a dysfunction. In addition to suggesting reading material (see list at end of chapter), physicians can educate patients about sexual anatomy, physiology, and behavior. For example, a woman's genital anatomy can be demonstrated to her (and her partner) with the aid of a mirror during her pelvic examination.

Specific Suggestions

Simple solutions to sexual problems may emerge from the evaluation of the dysfunctional couple. For example, couples with young children may notice that lack of privacy inhibits their responsiveness. The simple suggestion of locking the bedroom door or leaving children with relatives for a short visit may alleviate the problem. Women with physical impairments should be encouraged to work with their partners to change or modify their usual sexual repertoire. Simply changing the time of sexual encounters from bedtime to morning may allow partners the energy they need to enjoy sex. In general, they should allow more time for arousal to develop. The pleasures of physical closeness rather than the goal of orgasm should be emphasized. Patients should be encouraged to return to the physician to describe the effects of a change in technique. Sometimes the original suggestion does not quite work, but a subsequent modification does, or it may become clear that referral for more intensive therapy is needed.

Intensive Therapy

If the problem persists after these measures have been tried, referral to a specialist for evaluation and possible intensive therapy should be considered. The majority of patients can be significantly helped with recently developed techniques that combine psychodynamic and behavioral therapies. Qualified therapists may be identified through a local medical school, physician colleagues, or the American Association of Sex Educators, Counselors, and Therapists (AASECT). Qualified therapists have graduate degrees in the medical or behavioral sciences and special training and supervised experience in therapy for sexual dysfunctions. Because psychological or marital problems may coexist with sexual dysfunctions, therapists must be skilled in recognizing such disorders and modifying the treatment accordingly. Patients should be directed *away* from "therapists" who engage in intercourse (or any direct sexual behavior) with patients. This unethical conduct is an abuse of the power of the professional relationship. It results in a profound sense of traumatization, anger, and distrust in the patient, which is difficult to repair because of the patient's reluctance to form a new therapeutic relationship.

For the Patient

Kaplan H, Witkin MH. Sexuality: Better Homes and Gardens women's health and medical guide. Des Moines, IA: Meredith, 1981.
A basic, illustrated introduction to female sexuality and related topics.

Boston Women's Health Book Collective. Our bodies, ourselves. 3rd ed. New York: Simon & Schuster, 1984.
Clearly written coverage of sexual anatomy, physiology, development, feelings, and fantasies, with a specific discussion of masturbation.

Barbach LG. For yourself: the fulfillment of female sexuality. A guide to orgasmic response. Garden City, NY: Anchor Press, Doubleday, 1984.
Details a self-help program for anorgasmic women using masturbation training to achieve orgasm.

For the Physician

Schover LR, Jensen SB. Sexuality and chronic illness, a comprehensive approach. New York: Guilford Press, 1988.
Practical applications for clinicians of comprehensively reviewed literature about sexuality. Provides a model for sexual assessment that considers the effects of aging, of specific chronic illnesses, and of relationships. Includes an important section on training providers of sexual health care and on ethical and professional issues in treatment.

Kaplan HS. The psychosexual dysfunctions. Michels R, Cavenar JO, eds. In Psychiatry. Philadelphia: Lippincott, 1988. Vol 1, 1–19.
Textbook chapter summarizes current knowledge on psychosexual disorders with clinical descriptions of the disorders, discussion of etiology and evaluation, concepts and practice of sex therapy, and outcome studies.

Kaplan HS. The new sex therapy: active treatment of sexual dysfunctions. New York: Brunner/Mazel, 1974.
An excellent description of the basic concepts of human sexuality and of psychoanalytic and sex therapy techniques used in treating sexual dysfunctions.

Kaplan HS. Disorders of sexual desire. New York: Brunner/Mazel, 1979.
Introduces and discusses the more complex sexual dysfunction, desire phase disorder.

Kaplan HS. The evaluation of sexual disorders: Psychological and Medical Aspects. New York: Brunner/Mazel, 1983.
Describes disease states and drugs that may impair sexual function and diagnostic methods to delineate their role. Helpful tables summarize key information, and case studies demonstrate problems as they present in clinical practice.

Drugs that cause sexual dysfunction. Med Lett Drugs Ther 1987; 29(744):65–8.
An updated listing of drug effects on sexual function.

83. MALE SEXUAL DYSFUNCTION: ERECTILE FAILURE
Todd A. Linsenmeyer and Laurie Dornbrand

Sexual dysfunctions in men include loss of libido, impaired ability to achieve and maintain erections, and orgasmic difficulties such as premature or absent ejaculation. Erectile dysfunction, often referred to as impotence, is by far the most common complaint and the focus of this chapter.

Most men experience at least one episode of erectile failure, defined as the inability to maintain an erection adequate for intercourse, at some point in their lives. Recurrent or persistent erectile dysfunction affects about 1.9% of 40-year-old men, 25% of 65-year-old men, and 50% of 75-year-old men. The prevalence in diabetic men is estimated at 35 to 50%. While erectile failure is common, it is underreported to physicians. In a survey of 1180 consecutive patients seen in a Veterans Administration medical center general medicine clinic, 34% reported erectile dysfunction; while almost half of these men requested evaluation of the problem, only 6 (1.5%) had discussed it with their primary physician. Clinicians should therefore become familiar with the causes, initial workup, and available treatments for erectile failure and incorporate questions about erectile function into routine exams; otherwise patients who are inhibited about mentioning the complaint or who have a fatalistic attitude, thinking that "nothing can be done," may miss the opportunity for effective treatment.

Erectile Physiology
Penile erections are often classified as reflexogenic or psychogenic. "Tactile" afferent impulses into the sacral cord (S2–S4) and parasympathetic outflow from this region are responsible for reflexogenic erections. Psychogenic erections are thought to originate from the anterior hypothalamic area of the brain, with impulses modulated through thoracolumbar (T10–T12) sympathetic outflow to the penis. The precise interaction between the parasympathetic and sympathetic outflow is not known, but it has been established that the sympathetic system can either facilitate or inhibit erections. At a local level, erections occur when there is vasodilatation of the penile arteries causing distention of the spongy erectile tissue in the penis. This causes compression of the venous system within the penis, decreasing blood outflow and thereby helping to sustain the erection.

Causes of Erectile Dysfunction

Age
While erectile failure is more common in older men, this reflects more the prevalence of other causes of erectile dysfunction in this age group rather than the aging process itself. Normal age-related changes in sexual function include increased time and stimulation needed to reach full erection, fewer and less intense genital spasms, decreased volume of ejaculate, and longer refractory period. These changes should not be viewed as signs of impending erectile failure. The complaint of erectile failure should not be dismissed as an inevitable consequence of normal aging, nor should older men be discouraged from pursuing an evaluation.

Drugs
Many drugs have been reported to cause erectile dysfunction, most of them implicated by case reports rather than controlled studies. While the mechanism of action is often unknown, it is usually presumed to involve interference with central neuroendocrine or local neurovascular control of penile smooth muscle. Antihypertensive medications are, as a class, among the most common culprits. Erectile dysfunction has been associated with diuretics (thiazides, spironolactone), centrally acting sympatholytics (methyldopa, clonidine, reserpine, guanethidine), beta-blockers (propranolol) and alpha blockers (prazosin). Antihypertensive agents rarely associated with dysfunction include angiotensin converting enzyme inhibitors (e.g., captopril, enalapril), vasodilators (hydralazine, minoxidil), and calcium channel blockers (e.g., nifedipine, verapamil). Other commonly used drugs associated with erectile failure include cimetidine (an antiandrogen), phenothiazines, anti-

cholinergic drugs (e.g., antidepressants, antihistamines, propantheline), metoclopramide, clofibrate, estrogens, digoxin, narcotics, and alcohol.

Diabetes
Erectile dysfunction occurs at a much earlier age and with greater frequency in diabetic men than in the general population and may be an early manifestation of diabetic neuropathy. Libido is intact. Secondary neuropathic and vascular changes are presumed responsible for the problem but the precise role of each of these factors is still under investigation.

Vascular Impairment
Large vessel disease affecting the common iliac, hypogastric, or pudendal vessels usually, but not always, presents with other signs of arteriolar insufficiency, such as claudication. Atherosclerotic disease of the smaller vessels of the hypogastric-cavernous arterial bed results in decreased perfusion pressure and arterial flow to the lacunar spaces of the penis; this decreases the rigidity of erections and lengthens the time to maximal erection. Similar changes may occur when vessels are occluded as the result of pelvic trauma or irradiation. A pelvic steal syndrome secondary to an arteriovenous fistula from perineal trauma, or to atherosclerotic disease with borderline collateral penile vessels, may allow an initial erection followed by detumescence when active movements begin. Failure of venous channels to close may impair penile rigidity, even when the arterial supply is intact; with newer evaluation methods such as cavernosonography, the latter disorder is being increasingly recognized.

Endocrine Causes
Hypogonadism secondary to abnormal hypothalamic-pituitary function or to end-organ testicular failure may cause erectile failure, which is often associated with decreased libido. Similar symptoms are associated with hyperprolactinemia, which may be caused by medications, pituitary adenoma, or chronic renal failure, and which is occasionally idiopathic. Unusual endocrine causes of erectile failure include hypothyroidism, hyperthyroidism, adrenal insufficiency (Addison's disease) or excess (Cushing's disease), and acromegaly.

Neurologic Causes
Impairments of either the central or the peripheral nervous system may cause erectile dysfunction. Specific central nervous system diseases that have been implicated include Alzheimer's disease, Parkinson's disease, cerebrovascular accidents, and temporal lobe epilepsy. Spinal cord disorders that may produce erectile dysfunction include injuries, tumors, herniated disks, and transverse myelitis. Amyotrophic lateral sclerosis (ALS), multiple sclerosis, peripheral neuropathies from a wide variety of etiologies, and surgical interruption of the autonomic nerves supplying the pelvis in radical prostate, colon or bladder procedures are additional causes.

Urologic Causes
Peyronie's disease, a fibrosing disorder of the penis of unknown etiology, causes curvature of the erect penis that may be painful and/or associated with erectile failure. Fibrosis resulting from priapism, either idiopathic or associated with sickle-cell anemia, may also cause impaired erectile function, as can other anatomic disorders, such as phimosis. Inflammatory conditions such as balanitis, prostatitis, urethritis, and seminal vesiculitis may cause dysfunction secondarily, because of pain.

Medical Illness
Any systemic disease can potentially cause a decrease in well being and libido, with secondary erectile dysfunction. Specific diseases often implicated include cirrhosis, renal failure, and congestive heart failure. Apart from the abnormal estrogen-testosterone metabolism resulting from cirrhosis, alcohol consumption may cause erectile failure through associated peripheral neuropathy and central nervous system sedation. In addition to the low output state associated with congestive heart failure, patients with cardiovascular disease are often on drugs that may cause erectile failure. They also might fear that sexual activity will precipitate chest pain or myocardial infarction.

Psychological Causes
A wide variety of psychological concerns can be associated with erectile problems. The most commonly reported are anxiety disorders, including specific fears about sexual performance, anxiety about relationships in general, and anxiety as a result of traumatic sexual experiences. Depression also can reduce sexual desire, leading to erectile failure; decreased self-esteem or doubts about one's sexual function can also affect desire and/or erection. More severe psychopathology, such as manic-depressive disorder or psychosis is associated with a wide variety of sexual problems, which can include erectile failure. Furthermore, the medications used to treat these conditions may cause decreased desire, reduced erections, and absent or retrograde ejaculations. In many cases mild physiologic problems combine with psychological distress to create a significant erectile problem. For example, a patient with some reduction in blood flow due to atherosclerosis may develop performance anxiety when he notices a slight reduction in erectile response, turning a minor problem into total inability to obtain or maintain an erection.

Diagnosis

History
The type, severity, and chronicity of the disorder should be elicited in the history, and potential contributing factors identified. The medical history should focus on current medications, use of alcohol and other drugs, acute or chronic systemic illness, previous hospitalizations, and genitourinary injuries or surgical procedures. The sexual history should include the following: (1) the patient's description of the problem, and whether libido and ability to ejaculate are affected; (2) whether the onset of the disorder was sudden or gradual, and any recognized precipitating factors; (3) whether erections occur under any circumstances, either with stimulation, spontaneously, or during sleep; (4) the patient's assessment of the maximum firmness of erections currently obtainable, as a percentage of what he considers "normal"; and (5) any relationship issues or sources of stress.

Physical Examination
The physical examination focuses on endocrine, neurologic, and vascular function. Body habitus, secondary sexual characteristics (beard, body hair, and testicular size and consistency), and gynecomastia should be assessed. A normal testis should measure 3.5 to 4.0 cm. Vascular exam should include auscultation for abdominal and inguinal bruits and peripheral pulses. Neurologic exam should include deep tendon reflexes and sensory motor examination of the lower extremities. The penis should be examined for phimosis, balanitis, or inflammatory lesions. The penile shaft should be palpated for corporeal plaques in patients describing deviation of the erect penis consistent with Peyronie's disease; the absence of such plaques does not, however, contradict the diagnosis. The prostate should be examined for size, nodularity, tenderness, or inflammation, and during rectal examination the sacral plexus is evaluated by perianal sensation (S2–S4), anal sphincter tone (S4–S5), and the bulbocavernosus reflex (S2–S4). The latter may be performed by asking the patient to squeeze the glans penis during the rectal exam; when the reflex is present, the anal sphincter contracts.

Laboratory Studies
Serum testosterone should be measured; if testosterone is abnormal, luteinizing hormone (LH), and follicle stimulating hormone (FSH) levels help distinguish primary hypogonadism from hypothalamic-pituitary dysfunction. Although mean testosterone levels decline with age, the range of values in elderly men is so wide that a low level cannot be ascribed to "normal aging." Other tests frequently recommended to rule out contributing medical conditions include a chemistry panel with a fasting or 2-hour post-prandial blood glucose and a thyroid profile (free thyroxine [T_4] index or thyroid-stimulating hormone [TSH]). Prolactin levels are routinely obtained in referral settings; they are particularly helpful if there is any suspicion of a pituitary tumor, or if the patient is on a medication known to elevate prolactin.

Other Tests
The presence of nocturnal penile erections, which normally occur 3 to 5 times per night, during REM sleep, has been used as an indicator that physiologic mechanisms are func-

tioning well enough to initiate erection. Unfortunately, nocturnal erections are imperfect discriminators between physiologic and psychological causes of erectile failure and must be interpreted in the context of a more complete evaluation. Techniques available to assess presence and quality of nocturnal erections include the Snap-gauge band, which is attached to the base of the penis at bedtime and examined in the morning for breakage of three plastic filaments, each designed to snap at a different force. A more sophisticated (and costly) test, the Rigi-scan, uses two strain gauges attached to the penis and connected to a portable recorder, worn for three consecutive nights, and analyzed by computer.

Determination of penile blood pressure by Doppler technique has been used as a screening test for vascular causes. A penile-brachial ratio of less than 0.7 suggests but does not establish arterial insufficiency. More accurate and sophisticated tests use intracavernous injection of a vasoactive substance (such as papaverine), which may be used in conjunction with Doppler ultrasound of the penile arteries, measurement of intracavernous pressures with contrast infusion, and/or pudendal arteriography. The latter are highly specialized tests used in referral settings, particularly when vascular reconstruction procedures are being considered.

Treatment

Treatment is based on the underlying cause of the dysfunction, the importance of the problem to the patient, and his preferences about potential interventions. Including the patient's regular sexual partner in diagnosis and treatment planning helps to avoid misinformation and inappropriate expectations.

When a drug has been identified as a possible cause or contributing factor, a trial of 4 to 6 weeks off the agent may be necessary to assess its role. When alcohol abuse as a cause of sexual dysfunction is suspected, abstinence is likely to reverse the problem unless signs of estrogenization are present, such as testicular atrophy, palmar erythema, or spider angiomas.

Testosterone therapy is appropriate in patients with documented hypogonadism; its efficacy in patients without decreased testosterone levels has not been established, and it subjects them to potential side effects. Parenteral testosterone preparations are used; oral preparations do not achieve normal serum testosterone levels, have a higher incidence of associated cholestatic jaundice, and associated hyperlipidemia has been reported. A typical dosage regimen is 200 mg of testosterone enanthate every 2 to 3 weeks. Alternatively, testosterone cypionate may be used, but it has a slightly shorter duration of effect. Exogenous androgens may stimulate the growth of adenocarcinomas of the prostate and are contraindicated in men who have a suspicious rectal examination or known prostate cancer; men on testosterone replacement should be monitored with periodic rectal examinations. Androgens also stimulate red blood cell production; hematocrits should be checked periodically in patients with baseline values at the upper limits of normal.

Patients found to have elevated prolactin levels should have their medications reviewed for possible contributing agents, such as reserpine, methyldopa, phenothiazines, and metoclopramide (Reglan). In the absence of these and other miscellaneous causes, such as chronic renal failure and hypothyroidism, pituitary adenoma should be ruled out with a CT scan; consultation with an endocrinologist is appropriate for both evaluation and treatment.

Apart from withdrawal of drugs and treatment of endocrine problems, medical therapy for erectile dysfunction has not proved successful. Yohimbine hydrochloride, an alpha-adrenergic blocking agent, has been used but was found to be ineffective in placebo-controlled trials in patients with organic causes of erectile failure. Somewhat better results have been reported in patients without organic etiology, suggesting a placebo effect.

Penile prosthesis insertion by a urologist is the traditional surgical management. Both semirigid and inflatable types are available; the latter usually require more complex surgery and are more subject to mechanical failure, sometimes requiring reoperation. A recent alternative to penile prostheses has been intracavernous injection of vasoactive medications directly into the corpus cavernosa by the patient to stimulate erections. The most commonly used medication has been papaverine hydrochloride, a smooth muscle relaxant that results in decreased penile arterial resistance. It is used alone or in combination with phentolamine, an alpha blocker. Side effects include prolonged erections (in 2.3–15% of patients); painless fibrotic nodules within the corpus cavernosa, related to duration of treatment (1.5–60%); liver function test abnormalities; and transient hypotension. Prostaglandin E_1, an alternative agent, appears to have a lower risk of priapism, fibrosis, and systemic side effects, but more frequent penile pain and burning. These drugs are not FDA approved for intracavernous administration. Treatment with any of these agents should be closely supervised; patients must be warned to go immediately to the emergency room or their urologist if their erection lasts for more than 4 hours.

Vacuum constriction devices are another new alternative to surgical treatment. Erections are induced by a vacuum created in a plastic cylinder held over the penis, and maintained during intercourse by a constriction band placed around the base of the erect penis to impede venous outflow; this band may be kept in place for no more than 30 minutes at a time. Reported complications are usually transient and/or minor and include initial penile pain, ejaculatory difficulty, and minor penile ecchymosis and petechiae.

Surgical procedures of limited applicability include arterial reconstruction of the penile arteries to bypass obstruction. Appropriate candidates for these procedures are younger men with discrete arterial lesions rather than older men with diffuse arterial disease. Venous procedures designed to decrease excessive venous outflow from the penis in the erect state are under investigation in a number of centers; long-term follow-up studies of these procedures are not available.

Psychological treatment has traditionally been used with patients for whom no physiologic factors were known to be etiologically involved. Success rates with such cases have been variable, but generally high, especially for patients with a history of successful function prior to the development of an erectile problem. Many centers now combine psychological counseling with medical or surgical intervention. Before deciding on treatment, counseling can clarify goals of both the patient and his partner, work out conflicts, and provide psychosexual education. During treatment, counseling is typically designed to ensure that relationship problems and/or performance anxiety do not maintain the presenting problem after its physiologic causes have been addressed.

Referral

The initial evaluation will help to guide appropriate referrals to an endocrinologist, urologist, vascular surgeon, or sex therapist. Patients with erectile failure due to one or more drugs that are medically necessary and cannot be discontinued, those with irreversible organic causes, such as diabetes, and those with long-standing functional impotence that does not respond to counseling, or with a combination of these factors, may be candidates for prostheses or vacuum tumescence devices. It is highly desirable to choose centers that offer the patient a spectrum of options rather than a single choice and that consider the psychological as well as the physical impact of the choice.

Krane RJ, Goldstein I, Saenz de Tejada I. Impotence. N Engl J Med 1989; 321(24):1648–58.
An extensively referenced review of anatomy, physiology, pathophysiology, diagnosis, and treatment.

Cooke M. Evaluation of impotence. West J Med 1986; 145:106–10.
A primary care perspective on evaluating patients with erectile dysfunction.

Slag MF, et al. Impotence in medical clinic outpatients. JAMA 1983; 249:1736–40.
Reports on screening 1180 men in a VA medical outpatient clinic: 34% reported erectile dysfunction, and of these almost half chose to be examined for the problem. Of the 188 men evaluated, a medical cause was identified in nearly 80%, most commonly diabetes and other endocrine dysfunctions (38%), and medication effects (25%).

Lue TF, Tanagho EA. Physiology of erection and pharmacological management of impotence. J Urol 1987; (137):829–36.
Reviews specialized evaluation techniques and drugs used for intracavernous injections.

Drugs that cause sexual dysfunction. Med Lett Drugs Ther 1987; 29(744):65–8.
A referenced list of drugs associated with sexual dysfunction, and the adverse effects reported for each.

Wein AJ, Van Arsdalen KN. Drug-induced male sexual dysfunction. Urol Clin North Am 1988; 15:21–3.

Reviews the mechanisms of drug-induced sexual dysfunction and the role of specific agents.

Nelson, RP. Non-operative management of impotence. J Urol 1988; 139:2–5.
A concise review.

Sidi AA. Vasoactive intracavernous pharmacotherapy. Urol Clin North Am 1988; 15(1):95–100.
Discusses mechanisms, technique, and complications of intracavernous injections.

McClure RD. Endocrine evaluation and therapy of erectile dysfunction. Urol Clin North Am 1987; 15(1):53–64.
Androgen deficiency states and hormone replacement are discussed.

Witherington R. Vacuum constriction device for management of erectile impotence. J Urol 1989; 141:320–22.
In a questionnaire given to 1517 users of vacuum devices, 92% of respondents achieved erections satisfactory for intercourse, and no serious side effects were reported.

XII. ENDOCRINE AND METABOLIC PROBLEMS

84. DIAGNOSIS OF DIABETES MELLITUS
John T. Gwynne and Jorge J. Gonzalez

Diabetes mellitus is a syndrome characterized by abnormal carbohydrate and lipid metabolism. It is associated with small vessel changes in the kidney, eye and nerves, and accelerated atherosclerosis. There are two major types of overt diabetes mellitus, type I or insulin-dependent (IDDM) and type II or noninsulin-dependent (NIDDM). Patients with type I diabetes account for fewer than 10% of all diabetic patients but greater than 90% of those are less than 20 years old. Diabetes that has its onset during pregnancy is termed *gestational diabetes mellitus* (GDM) and is considered a separate entity. The term *secondary diabetes* denotes overt glucose intolerance resulting from other diseases. For epidemiologic and prognostic purposes, two other categories of abnormal carbohydrate metabolism are recognized: *impaired glucose tolerance* and *previous abnormality of glucose tolerance*. The prevalence of diabetes varies with age, race, gender, and body weight. Prevalence increases from less than 4% in those under 20 to greater than 20% in those over 65. The prevalence of diabetes, primarily NIDDM, is two to four times greater in blacks, Hispanics, and some Native Americans than in whites. In these minorities, the prevalence is nearly twice as great in women as in men. The prevalence of NIDDM is two times greater in individuals who are more than 120% of ideal body weight and four times greater in individuals more than 140% of ideal body weight than in individuals of normal weight.

Perhaps as many as 50% of patients with NIDDM remain undiagnosed for many years during which complications, which may have been prevented, are developing. Early diagnosis and intervention might significantly reduce complications and their associated psychosocial and economic costs. The economic burden of diabetes in the United States is estimated to be 11.7 billion dollars a year.

Screening
Individuals who are members of high-risk ethnic groups or who have other risk factors such as obesity, previous or potential abnormality of glucose intolerance, or a history of gestational diabetes should be screened for NIDDM biennially by measurements of fasting blood glucose. A fasting blood glucose greater than 115 mg/dl is a positive screen and suggests further evaluation. Because of fetal morbidity accompanying hyperglycemia, all women should be screened for GDM by measurement of fasting blood glucose (FBG) between weeks 24 and 28 of pregnancy.

Diagnostic Criteria
The diagnosis of diabetes can only be made by measurement of blood glucose. Standardized criteria for diagnosing diabetes on the basis of glycosylated hemoglobin or fructosamine are not yet available. Because blood glucose levels are not bimodally distributed in the population, diagnostic "cutpoints" have been based on epidemiologic and practical considerations. The following criteria, suggested by the National Diabetes Data Group (NDDG), are widely accepted. For nonpregnant adults, at least one of the following criteria must be met:

1. Presence of classic symptoms (e.g., polyuria, polydipsia, weight loss, ketonuria) together with random blood glucose > 200 mg/dl
2. Fasting plasma glucose > 140 mg/dl or fasting venous whole blood > 120 mg/dl or fasting capillary whole blood > 120 mg/dl *on more than one occasion*
3. Abnormal oral glucose tolerance test (OGTT)

Intercurrent illness, trauma, or use of numerous medications (particularly proprietary cold remedies containing phenylephrine or related compounds, glucocorticoids, estrogens, sympathomimetic drugs, and potassium-wasting diuretics) may increase plasma glucose. If one of the first two criteria is met, an oral glucose tolerance test should *not* be performed. An FBG less than 115 mg/dl virtually excludes the diagnosis of diabetes. In a survey of diabetes prevalence, 54% of patients meeting one or more of the above criteria were detected by measurement of FBG alone, whereas the remainder exhibited an FBG less than

140 but had a positive OGTT. Fewer than 3% of patients whose FBG exceeded 140 failed to meet the criterion for a positive OGTT.

The OGTT may be used to make the diagnosis of diabetes when FBG is greater than 115 but less than 140 mg/dl. While OGTT is essential for epidemiologic studies, there are only a limited number of clinical settings in which it is of value. These include: (1) identifying high-risk patients for intensive dietary treatment, (2) establishing the diagnosis in patients who present with classical findings or established complications and who have FBG less than 140 mg/dl, and (3) pregnancy. The conditions for the OGTT are different in pregnant and nonpregnant adults. The NDDG recommends the following conditions for oral glucose tolerance testing: (1) a 75-g glucose load, regardless of weight and (2) measurements of blood glucose every 30 minutes for 2 hours. Measurements of glucose for up to 5 hours may be made to diagnose reactive hypoglycemia but are not necessary for diagnosing diabetes. A positive diagnosis requires that both the 2-hour sample and one other sample between 0 and 2 hours exceed 200 mg/dl. The conditions of testing must be standardized (e.g., adequate prior carbohydrate intake, initiated fasting in the morning) if the results are to be interpreted.

Type I and Type II Diabetes

Once the diagnosis of diabetes has been established, it is important to determine the type of diabetes because therapy differs according to the clinical class. Several clinical and biochemical features distinguish type I from type II diabetes.

The most significant difference between type I and type II diabetes is dependence on insulin. Patients with type I diabetes require insulin to sustain life and develop ketoacidosis in its absence. In contrast, patients with type II diabetes do not require insulin to sustain life and, except under extraordinarily stressful conditions (e.g., auto accident, surgery, febrile illness, or death of a spouse), do not develop ketoacidosis. Type I diabetes generally has its onset before the age of 35 whereas type II generally presents after the age of 35. The prevalence of type II increases with increasing age and varies with race and sex, being particularly prevalent (> 10%) in black women over 50 years of age. At the time of diagnosis, circulating anti–islet cell antibodies are present in almost all patients with type I but are no more frequent in those with type II than in the general population (approximately 10–15%).

When the type of diabetes is in doubt, measurements of glucose-stimulated serum insulin or C-peptide levels may be helpful. In type I diabetes, fasting insulin levels are low and respond poorly to glucose challenge; on the other hand, in type II diabetes, fasting levels are generally elevated and respond well to glucose and glucagon challenge.

Other Types of Glucose Intolerance

Gestational Diabetes

Gestational diabetes develops during pregnancy in a previously normal woman and occurs in 1 to 2% of all pregnancies. All women should be screened for diabetes by measurements of FBG between weeks 24 and 28 of pregnancy. Findings that should prompt earlier screening include glycosuria; diabetes in a first-degree relative; morbid obstetrical history such as previous stillbirth, spontaneous abortion, fetal malformation, or infant weighing more than 9 pounds at birth; maternal obesity; maternal age over 30 years; and parity of 5 or more. The presence of more than one factor further increases risk. The criteria for diagnosis of gestational diabetes by OGTT are more restrictive than those for nonpregnant adults: 100 grams of glucose is administered, and glucose levels are measured every hour for 3 hours. Venous plasma glucose must exceed two or more of the following values to confirm the diagnosis: Fasting—105, 1 hour—190, 2 hour—165, and 3 hour—145 mg/dl. Early recognition and treatment of even mild glucose intolerance during pregnancy prevent perinatal morbidity and mortality and decrease fetal morbidity.

Ten to fifteen percent of women with gestational diabetes remain diabetic postpartum, and another 30% of those with normal postpartum glucose tolerance develop diabetes in the next 15 years. Women with gestational diabetes who have normal glucose tolerance after childbirth should be reclassified as having previous abnormality of glucose tolerance and should be reevaluated biennially for the development of asymptomatic overt diabetes.

Impaired Glucose Tolerance
Individuals who have an FBG less than 140 but an OGTT intermediate between normal and overt diabetes are classified as having impaired glucose intolerance (IGT). This is not a diagnosis of disease but a definition of potential risk. Findings on OGTT include a 2-hour blood glucose less than 200 mg/dl but a blood glucose greater than 200 mg/dl on at least two intermediate times. These patients are at increased risk for developing atherosclerotic cardiovascular diseases but do not develop characteristic diabetic microangiopathy in the absence of further deterioration in glucose tolerance. Prevention of macrovascular complications depends on control of risk factors, such as hypertension, hypercholesterolemia, obesity, and smoking. Between 1 and 5% of patients with IGT develop overt diabetes each year. Such patients should be screened biennially by FBG for development of diabetes.

Potential Abnormality of Glucose Tolerance
The term *potential abnormality of glucose tolerance* is applied to people who have never exhibited abnormal glucose tolerance but are at increased risk of overt diabetes on the basis of biochemical, genetic, or epidemiologic considerations. The NDDG has noted, in decreasing order of importance, the following specific risk factors for type I diabetes: the monozygotic twin of a type I diabetic (concordance approximately 50%); siblings of a type I diabetic, "especially one with identical HLA haplotype"; offspring of a diabetic; and people with islet cell antibodies. For type II diabetes, risk factors include the monozygotic twin of a type II diabetic (concordance rate over 90%); all first-degree relatives of a type II diabetic; mothers of neonates over 9 pounds; obese people; or members of certain racial or ethnic groups (in the United States, some Native Americans, particularly the Pima).

The degree of risk associated with these factors is not well established. Based on the 1977 U.S. government diabetes survey, the sibling of any diabetic who had the onset of diabetes before the age of 19 years is 10 to 14 times more likely to develop some form of diabetes than the siblings of nondiabetic controls. The risk declines to two- to fourfold as the age of onset of the proband increases. The offspring of any diabetic who developed diabetes before the age of 19 is 20- to 40-fold more likely to develop diabetes at some time during his or her lifetime than are the offspring of nondiabetic patients; the risk to the offspring declines as the age of onset of the proband increases.

Secondary Diabetes
Glucose tolerance and overt diabetes mellitus can result from a large number of diseases, either directly or by unmasking latent diabetes. Causes of secondary diabetes include pancreatic disease, endocrinopathies such as Cushing's syndrome, pheochromocytoma, and acromegaly, and a number of genetic defects. Common medications that increase blood glucose include phenylephrine-containing proprietary cold remedies, glucocorticoids, sympathomimetic drugs, and potassium-wasting diuretics. In general, patients with secondary diabetes develop microvascular complications similar to those occurring in other diabetics. It is important to consider these possibilities in every newly recognized diabetic because glucose intolerance frequently improves with treatment of the underlying illness.

Diabetes in America. Diabetes Data Compiled 1984. National Diabetes Data Group NIH Publication No. 85-1468. US Dept. of Health and Human Resources, PHS, NIH, NIADDKD, August 1985.
A comprehensive collection of statistics describing the incidence and prevalence of diabetes and its complications.

West, KM. Epidemiology of diabetes and its vascular lesions. New York: Elsevier, 1978.
The definitive work in the evolving field of diabetes epidemiology.

National Diabetes Data Group: Classification and diagnosis of diabetes mellitus and other categories of glucose intolerance. Diabetes 1979; 8:1039–57.
The consensus report of an international group of diabetologists convened by the NIH to update methods and criteria for diagnosing diabetes.

Singer DE, Samet JH, Coley CM, et al. Screening for diabetes mellitus. Ann Intern Med 1988; 109:639–49.

Review of relevant literature, concluding that general population screening is not cost effective but "might be reasonable for particular patients, for example, obese persons. . . ."

U.S. Preventive Services Task Force. Screening for diabetes. In: Guide to clinical preventive services. Baltimore: Williams & Wilkins, 1989:95–103.
A well-referenced review of the evidence for efficacy of screening tests and effectiveness of early detection. Recommends oral glucose tolerance test for all pregnant women between 24 and 28 weeks of gestation. Does not recommend routine screening for nonpregnant adults, but suggests that periodic fasting plasma glucose measurements may be appropriate for high-risk persons, such as the markedly obese, persons with a family history of diabetes, or women with a history of gestational diabetes.

O'Sullivan JB, Mahan CM. Criteria for the oral glucose tolerance test in pregnancy. Diabetes 1964; 13:278.
Established criteria for interpretation of OGTT during pregnancy.

O'Sullivan JB. Long-term follow-up of gestational diabetes. In: RA Camorine-Davolos and HS Cole, eds. Early Diabetes in Early Life. New York: Academic, 1975: 503–19.
These studies, which determined the frequency of persistent and subsequent overt diabetes in women with gestational diabetes, indicate the need for contained reevaluation of glucose tolerance in this population.

Hockstra JB, et al. C-peptide. Diabetes Care 1982; 5:439–46.
An overview of C-peptide metabolism and the potential usefulness of serum and urine C-peptide measurements in the diagnosis and management of diabetes.

85. MANAGEMENT OF TYPE I DIABETES
John T. Gwynne and Jorge J. Gonzalez

The goals of therapy for both type I and type II diabetes are the same: to improve patient well-being and to prevent acute and chronic complications. There are two approaches to achieving these goals: controlling blood glucose levels and ameliorating risk factors. In general, animal, cellular, and biochemical studies indicate that maintaining desirable blood glucose levels helps prevent microvascular complications. Good glycemic control should be started at the time of diagnosis since clinical studies suggest that, once established, retinopathy and nephropathy may progress despite improved glycemic control. The Diabetes Control and Complications Trial (DCCT), a prospective, randomized clinical trial in patients with insulin-dependent diabetes mellitus (IDDM), is designed to test the hypothesis that "tight" glycemic control prevents diabetic microvascular complications. The results of this trial, now underway, should be reported in 1995. The prevalence and incidence of atherosclerotic cardiovascular diseases are increased in type I diabetes compared to nondiabetics. While epidemiologic evidence indicates that hyperglycemia identifies patients at risk, direct evidence that tight glycemic control will prevent macrovascular complications is lacking. However, available data suggests that the more normal the blood glucose levels are, the less likely macrovascular complications are.

Goal blood glucose levels in patients with type I diabetes should be individualized, taking into account the risk of hypoglycemia, the patient's abilities, and the psychosocial costs. Fasting blood glucose levels of 140 +/− 40 mg/dl and postprandial levels less than 200 mg/dl can be achieved in most type I patients without undue constraints on daily life. Meeting these goals requires either multiple daily insulin injections or continuous subcutaneous insulin infusion and self-blood glucose monitoring. During pregnancy, blood glucose levels should be maintained between 60 and 90 mg/dl at all times, even if this requires hospitalization. Almost all patients, if properly educated and motivated, have the ability to achieve tight glucose control.

It is important to educate patients about the risks and benefits of tight control so that they can make an informed decision. The benefits of tight glycemic control include improved sense of well-being, decreased polyuria and nocturia, decreased incidence of vaginal and other infections, and protection from diabetic complications. The major risk of tight control is increased incidence of hypoglycemia. In most patients with disease of less than 10 years duration, hypoglycemia produces catecholaminergic symptoms such as sweating, palpitations, and anxiety and stimulates gluconeogenesis. These symptoms are premonitory to neuroglycopenia, have no known long-term sequelae, and indicate to the patient the need for oral carbohydrates. The associated gluconeogenesis prevents further decline in blood glucose for several hours. These events usually precede the onset of neuroglycopenia and changes in consciousness that can produce long-term deficits. In patients with disease of greater than 10 years duration, the loss of pancreatic alpha-cell function and loss of catecholamine responsiveness can lead to profound hypoglycemia. Such patients, who lack gluconeogenic reserve or do not mount a gluconeogenic response, are not candidates for meticulous blood glucose control. Such patients lack premonitory symptoms and usually have a history of hypoglycemia sufficiently severe to require intervention by another person.

Four interventions should be used to control blood glucose levels in type I diabetes: diet, exercise, insulin, and education. Insulin is also required by all type I patients to prevent ketoacidosis and to sustain life.

Diet

Dietary management of type I diabetes should conform to the patient's particular likes, dislikes, and life-style. Aids to meal planning, such as "The Exchange List for Meal Planning," are available through the American Diabetes Association and the American Dietetic Association. It is unrealistic to expect even the most sophisticated patients to adhere to complex instructions, such as exchange lists, without individual instruction and feedback from a trained dietitian or nutritionist. Thus, when available, dietary counseling should be provided by an individual with special expertise in this area and sufficient time to answer patient questions and provide adequate follow-up. In communities in which these resources are not available, designating and specially training an office nurse is one solution. The main issues in dietary management of the type I patient are quantity of calories, macronutrient composition of diet, and distribution of calories throughout the day.

Quantity of Calories
Table 85-1 summarizes one method of calculating total calories to achieve and maintain ideal body weight.

Composition of Diet
Fats should not comprise more than 30% of the daily caloric allowance; total carbohydrate, primarily fruits and starch, should comprise 50 to 65% of caloric allowance; and protein should comprise the remainder. Dietary composition can be usefully quantitated in most offices by microcomputer analysis of 3-day food diaries. This analysis offers one means of assessing actual food intake in terms of nutritional recommendations. Translating such recommendations into actual food selections requires a technique such as an exchange list or the services of someone dedicated and trained for this task. Because cardiovascular disease is the major cause of death in diabetics, a "prudent diet" (low in saturated fats and cholesterol) is desirable. Concentrated, refined carbohydrates should be discouraged because they induce wide glycemic "swings." Dietetic sweetners (fructose, mannitol) have nearly the same caloric value as glucose but induce less fluctuation of the blood sugars and are slightly sweeter, per unit weight, than sucrose.

There is evidence that consumption of vegetable fiber blunts postprandial glycemic excursions. The precise mechanism by which fiber produces this effect is uncertain, but a diminished rate of nutrient absorption seems likely. Inclusion of 25 to 35 grams of fiber per day generally produces benefits without undue discomfort or risk. Enhanced fiber consumption can be most easily achieved by substituting whole wheat for white bread and increasing the fruit and vegetables in the diet.

Table 85-1. Calculation of caloric requirement based on ideal body weight

Estimate of ideal body weight (IBW)
Women: 100 lb for height of 5 feet + 5 lb per inch over 5 feet
Example: 5'6" = 100 + (5 × 6) = 130
Men: 106 lb for height of 5 feet + 6 lb per inch over 5 feet
Example: 5'11" = 106 + (6 × 11) = 172 lb
For small frame, subtract 10%; for large frame, add 10%
Calculation of caloric requirement
Basal requirement = 10 cal/lb of ideal body weight
Activity allowance
Sedentary: add 20–30% of basal requirement
Moderately active: add 50% of basal requirement
Active: add 100% or more, depending on activity
Example: 5'4" women—sedentary, medium frame
IBW = 120 lb; basal req. = 120 × 10 = 1200 cal
Activity allowance = 30% × 1200 cal = 360 cal
Final diet = 1200 cal + 360 cal = 1560 cal
Calculation of caloric requirement for weight loss
Decrease daily caloric intake by 500 cal to obtain 1–1.5 lb of weight loss per week.
Add 500 cal per day to obtain 1–1.5 lb weight gain per week.

Distribution of Calories

The temporal distribution of caloric consumption should be related to the type and amounts of insulin used as well as the patient's life-style and pattern of exercise. Peak calorie consumption and peak insulin action should occur at the same time. Patients with labile blood glucose or patients with high caloric intake benefit from spreading intake over six meals or more a day.

Exercise increases insulin sensitivity by increasing insulin receptor activity and cellular glucose uptake. Exercise programs should be individualized and coordinated with diet and insulin so that adequate calories are available to prevent hypoglycemia; mild to moderate sustained exercise, such as walking or jogging, is preferable to brief strenuous exercise. Exercise should be encouraged only when hyperglycemia is well controlled. Exercise in the uncontrolled, insulin-dependent diabetic may induce a disproportionate counterregulatory hormone response, worsen hyperglycemia, and induce ketosis. Without additional insulin, exercise should not be undertaken if the blood glucose exceeds 300 mg/dl.

Hypoglycemia associated with exercise should be prevented by the prior ingestion of extra carbohydrates. Although exact planning is difficult, rough estimations can be made knowing that mild to moderate exercise results in an extra energy expenditure of 4 to 6 calories per minute. Thus, an hour-long brisk walk might require from 240 to 360 extra calories to prevent hypoglycemia. Exercise of an extremity markedly increases the absorption of the subcutaneous insulin injected in that extremity. Abdominal injections may therefore be preferable for someone who intermittently exercises the extremities.

Insulin Therapy

Many types of insulins, differing in source (beef/pork or human) and pharmacokinetics, are available in this country. When first introduced, human insulin was recommended primarily for patients with insulin resistance, high insulin antibody titers, local or systemic insulin allergies, and for patients receiving intermittent insulin treatment, such as gestational diabetes. As the price of human recombinant insulin has approached or, in some cases, become less than that for insulin of animal origin, human insulin has become the insulin of choice for almost all patients. The total dose of insulin should be decreased by approximately 10% when substituting human insulin for insulin of animal origin. Further adjustments should be made on the basis of self–blood glucose monitoring (SBGM). Human insulin may peak slightly sooner than animal insulin. The mean onset, peak, and duration of action of commonly employed insulin preparations are shown in Table 85-2. Considerable variability exists in individual responses.

Table 85-2. Onset, action, and duration of commonly used insulins

Type of insulin	Onset	Action (hrs)	Duration (hrs)
Regular crystalline	Rapid	2–4	5–7
Semilente	Rapid	2–4	12–16
Lente	Intermediate	6–12	24–28
NPH	Intermediate	6–12	24–28
Ultralente	Prolonged	14–24	36+

In general, regular crystalline and semilente insulin can be interchanged, as can NPH and lente. If injected immediately after withdrawal into the syringe but not after standing for greater than a few hours, the lente series of insulins can be mixed. If left mixed for greater than a few hours, the pharmacokinetics of lente insulins will be altered. Currently available human NPH and regular insulin can be mixed prior to injection without changes in the pharmacokinetics of the individual insulins. In fact, premixed insulins (NPH/Reg 70/30) are now commercially available.

Many factors in the individual patient may alter insulin kinetics, including site of injection, exercise, and insulin antibodies. Abdominal administration generally results in slower kinetics than injection into an extremity.

Insulin Regimens

The complexity of the insulin regimen needed for adequate glucose control depends in part on residual beta-cell function. Type I diabetes with some pancreative reserve tends to be "easy" to control, whereas those with no residual beta-cell function tend to be unstable ("brittle") and require more complex insulin regimens.

In a nondiabetic, 70-kg man, total daily insulin secretion is approximately 50 units. Half is secreted to maintain a constant basal circulating level, and the remainder is secreted in response to meals. Currently employed insulin regimens attempt to mimic this pattern. Improved control need not always be achieved by changes in insulin therapy; frequent changes in diet and exercise are more appropriate.

The most appropriate insulin regimen must be selected in collaboration with the patient and will depend on the patient's life-style, understanding of diabetes, and therapeutic goals. Establishing the appropriate timing and dosage can be done only through the use of an accurate monitoring technique. Possible insulin regimens are discussed in the following sections:

ONE DAILY INJECTION OF INTERMEDIATE INSULIN. In a small minority of patients with type I diabetes ($< 10\%$), there is sufficient islet cell reserve to allow adequate blood glucose control to be achieved with one injection alone. However, when tight control is sought, a single daily injection of intermediate insulin is rarely adequate. Intermediate and regular insulin given once a day have insufficient duration to control blood glucose for 24 hours, whereas ultralente alone does not provide adequate postprandial peaks.

SPLIT-MIXED INSULIN. Both an intermediate and short-acting insulin are administered from 30 to 60 minutes before breakfast and again 30 to 60 minutes before the evening meal. Generally, the total daily insulin dosage is distributed as follows:

⅔ intermediate	⅔ before breakfast
	⅓ before evening meal
⅓ short-acting	½ before breakfast
	½ before evening meal

Twice-daily intermediate insulin sustains the basal levels, whereas regular insulin before meals provides increased levels for clearing ingested nutrients.

Because of early-morning hyperglycemia (the dawn phenomenon), it may be preferable in some patients to administer the evening dose of intermediate insulin at 10:00 to 11:00 PM instead of concurrently with the regular insulin dose before the evening meal. This is perhaps the most widely used intensified insulin regimen, and it achieves satisfactory control in patients whose routines vary little from day to day. It requires fewer injections than treatment with regular insulin alone and does not have the risk of sustained hypoglycemia accompanying the use of ultralente. On the other hand, it does not offer quite as much flexibility for self-management as is available with the other two regimens.

ULTRALENTE PLUS REGULAR INSULIN AT MEALTIME. A single daily injection of long-acting ultralente insulin provides the basal background. The usual ultralente dose is in the range of 8 to 20 units a day. Regular insulin is administered 30 to 60 minutes before each major meal. Although this regimen gives greater flexibility than mixed-split insulin, the sustained duration of action of ultralente may lead to hypoglycemia as a result of cumulative insulin effect. Because ultralente is relatively peakless, the onset of hypoglycemia may be gradual, not heralded by the customary acute symptoms of anxiety, tremor, and diaphoresis, and therefore difficult to recognize.

REGULAR INSULIN WITH MEALS (TID) PLUS INTERMEDIATE INSULIN AT NIGHT. Because regular insulin has a duration of action from 6 to 8 hours, administration before each main meal provides both a sustained basal level and increases at each meal during the day while intermediate insulin (NPH or lente) provides basal coverage at night. The amount of insulin administered on each occasion must be determined empirically for each patient based on self-measured blood glucose. This regimen offers considerable flexibility but demands constant attention because of the frequency of insulin administration.

CONTINUOUS SUBCUTANEOUS INSULIN INFUSION. Several different types of miniaturized pumps for continuous subcutaneous administration of regular insulin are commercially available. They provide a continuous dose of regular insulin and deliver on demand a preprogrammed dose at mealtime. The criteria for patient selection are not well defined; however, patients who have difficulty complying with an intensified conventional regimen are also likely to have difficulty with an insulin pump. Implantable open-loop insulin pumps remain experimental and are available at only a limited number of research institutions.

Initiation of Insulin Therapy
Intensive insulin therapy is best managed by a multidisciplinary group, including a physician, nutritionist, and nurse educator, and can be initiated in either an inpatient or outpatient setting. Because of the high cost of hospitalization, there is a strong trend to outpatient initiation of insulin treatment. In only a few states, however, is outpatient diabetes education reimbursed by third-party payers. If teaching and nursing resources are available, hospitalization may be useful, even in nonketotic patients, because the initiation is easier to accomplish, and the hospital provides an opportunity for intensive patient education. It is hoped that intensive outpatient programs will become widely available in the future.

The simplest way to begin insulin therapy, in either outpatients or inpatients, is by administering 10 units of intermediate insulin in the morning and 5 units in the afternoon, or ultralente (0.2 to 0.5 units/kg) in the morning. The dosage should be increased gradually (2–3 units/day) based on self-measured blood glucose levels. Alternating split-mixed insulin treatment may be initiated at a dose of 0.5 to 0.7 units per kg ideal body weight in an adult. Total basal insulin requirements for newly diagnosed patients with type I diabetes generally are 0.2 to 0.5 units/kg/day. Subsequent adjustments are made on the basis of blood glucose measurements.

Monitoring
Measurements of urine ketones and blood glucose are both employed to monitor response to therapy and to alter insulin dose. Urine glucose testing is unreliable in IDDM. Urine glucose concentrations correlate poorly with blood glucose levels. They are usually effective in detecting marked hyperglycemia but are not useful for guiding tight control. Urinary ketones should be determined during an intercurrent illness.

Self-blood glucose monitoring has become an easy but expensive technique for monitoring control and adjusting insulin dosages. Fingerstick blood sugar measurements correlate well with venous plasma glucose determinations. Obtaining multiple daily blood sugars allows patients to change their insulin dosages and redistribute both the amount and timing of their meals to promote optimal control.

The aims of the program, including the risks and benefits, should be explained to the patient. Several algorithms have been developed to help patients adjust insulin dosages. Although specific instructions will vary, several guidelines can be offered:

1. Improvement in blood glucose control, either reduction of hyperglycemia or amelioration of hypoglycemia, can sometimes be more readily achieved through alterations of diet and exercise than through alterations of insulin.
2. In general, blood glucose levels should be measured at the times of maximum expected insulin action. When insulin treatment is started blood glucose should be measured seven times per day; before and 2 hours after each meal and at bedtime. Blood glucose should also be measured occasionally between 2 and 3 AM to look for unperceived nocturnal hypoglycemia. Control of fasting blood glucose levels is sought first, followed by control of postprandial hyperglycemia. Once suitable insulin doses are established, the frequency of SBGM may be decreased. At a minimum, patients taking split mixed insulin should measure their blood glucose fasting daily, both before dinner and at bedtime.
3. In all cases, except to prevent hypoglycemia, changes in insulin should be made gradually (1–3 units) at 2- to 5-day intervals. While initiating SBGM, patients should have a member of the team available 24 hours a day.

Hemoglobin A_1 values are a representation of the glycemia during the previous 6 to 8 weeks. This test is valuable for assessing the overall degree of control and the long-term effect of therapeutic maneuvers, but it provides little information regarding day-to-day blood glucose levels. Measurement of fructosamine, primarily glycosylated albumin and immunoglobin, is analytically more accurate than hemoglobin A_1 by column chromatography but reports mean blood glucose level for a shorter time (6–10 days) than hemoglobin A_1.

Metabolic Complications

Fasting Hyperglycemia (Somogyi Phenomenon versus the Dawn Phenomenon)
In some type I patients it is impossible to keep fasting blood glucose (FBG) at an acceptable level by increasing the amount of intermediate insulin before the evening meal. Insulin resistance varies diurnally in all patients and in nondiabetics as well. Insulin resistance increases from 4 to 5 AM until 8 to 9 AM in the morning, probably as a result of increased pulsatile growth hormone secretion. This early-morning increase in insulin resistance, the dawn phenomenon, can often be overcome and FBG controlled by delaying administration of intermediate-acting insulin from before the evening meal until bedtime. The peak of intermediate-acting insulin action will then coincide with the nocturnal increase in insulin resistance. It has been previously suggested that fasting hyperglycemia, particularly when accompanied by nightmares, wide fluctuations in glucose levels, or morning headaches, is a response to unperceived nocturnal hypoglycemia, the Somogyi phenomenon. It is unlikely that this mechanism accounts for a significant amount of fasting hyperglycemia. The triad of symptoms, nightmares, morning headaches, and wide fluctuations in FBG, originally described by Somogyi are, nonetheless, useful indicators of nocturnal hypoglycemia and should be sought during evaluation of patients on insulin.

Treatment of Hypoglycemia
DIET. Patients with type I diabetes or type II diabetes treated with insulin or oral hypoglycemic agents should always have available a source of 10 to 20 grams of simple carbohydrates for rapid treatment of hypoglycemic symptoms. This may be consumed in the form of prepackaged commercially available tablets or solutions of dextrose, 4 ounces of orange juice, or 6 ounces of nondiet soft drink. If blood glucose has not increased within 15 minutes, an additional 10 to 20 grams of glucose should be consumed. Too-vigorous treat-

ment of hypoglycemia, such as consumption of a 12-ounce soft drink, usually leads to marked hyperglycemia and renders subsequent regulation difficult.

DRUGS. Patients who cannot take glucose orally should be given intravenous glucose (25–50 g immediately) if feasible. Alternatively, such patients can be treated with intramuscular or subcutaneous glucagon by an informed family member. Glucagon for this use is available in individual vials accompanied by a syringe and needle. Patients who do not have premonitory symptoms or who have a history of decreased consciousness from hypoglycemia are candidates for glucagon therapy. A family member or individual living with the patient should be instructed in the use of parenteral glucagon.

Ketoacidosis
Ketoacidosis should always be treated in the hospital where careful monitoring is available. Patients with type I diabetes should be instructed in the use of test strips that detect ketone bodies in the urine. They should be instructed to test their urine for ketones and to call if they are unable to take oral intake; if they suspect ketosis or develop symptoms of ketosis such as rapid breathing; if they have unusually high blood glucose (e.g., > 300 mg/dl for more than 6–8 hours); or if they contract an infection or encounter other major stress.

Follow-up
Patients with type I diabetes should be seen at least every 4 to 6 months. At each visit, a written record of blood glucose should be brought for review. The routine physical examination should include blood pressure measurements; fundoscopic examination; foot examination; brief neurologic exam including testing of peripheral light touch, pin prick, proprioception, vibratory sensation, and deep tendon reflexes; as well as cardiac examination and assessment of peripheral pulses and bruits. It is unusual for Achilles tendon reflexes to remain normal when there is loss of peripheral sensation. In patients with duration of disease greater than 10 years, annual ophthalmologic examinations and measurement of serum creatinine are essential. Urine should be tested for protein excretion. The patient's understanding of insulin and diet should be periodically reviewed, and at each visit the patient should be given a nondirected opportunity to ask questions. Family planning and contraception should be reviewed with all female patients at the time of diagnosis or postpubertally, because meticulous blood glucose control is essential to prevent congenital fetal anomalies.

Prevention of type I diabetes by immunotherapy, generally cyclosporine C, remains experimental. Pancreatic transplantation should currently be reserved for selected patients who have established complications and a strong motivation for this mode of therapy. Pancreatic transplantation should be done in established centers with considerable experience under careful investigative protocols.

Krolewski AJ, Warren JH, Rand LI, et al. Epidemiologic approach to the etiology of Type I diabetes mellitus and its complications. N Engl J Med 1987; 317:1390–98.
Provides a thorough review of pathogenesis of type I diabetes, as well as information about the incidence and prevalence of complications and their relationship to glycemic control.

Unger RH. Meticulous control of diabetes: benefits, risks and precautions. Diabetes 1982; 31:479–83.
Points out the potential detrimental effects of meticulous control and the need to identify patients at unusual risk of frequent, severe, or prolonged hypoglycemia.

Nuttall FQ. Diet and the diabetic patient. Diabetes Care 1983; 6:197–207.
An instructive discussion of the deficiencies in our data base for formulating optimal diabetic diets. Points out the need for flexibility and individualization in dietary prescriptions.

ADA Committee on Food and Nutrition. Fructose, xylitol, and sorbitol. Diabetes Care 1980; 2:399–402.
Official ADA statement regarding so-called nonnutritive sweeteners.

Anderson JW, Midgley WR, Wedman B. Fiber and diabetes. Diabetes Care 1979; 2:369–79.
Observations on and discussion of dietary fiber in the management of diabetes by the major contributor in this field.

Lodewick PA. Think fast. Diabetes forecast 1983; May–June: 29.
Practical guidelines for dietary response to hypoglycemia.

Zinman B. The physiologic replacement of insulin—an elusive goal. N Engl J Med 1989; 321:363–70.
The major important issues in insulin administration including rationale, goals, insulin pharmacokinetics, practical algorithms, and future possibilities are discussed.

Berger M, et al. Absorption kinetics and biological effects of subcutaneously injected insulin preparations. Diabetes Care 1982; 5:77–91.
A comprehensive, revealing investigation of important practical modifiers of insulin kinetics, including site of injection, exercise, and temperature.

Mecklenburg RS, Benson EA, Fredlund PN, et al. Acute complications associated with insulin pump therapy. JAMA 1984; 252:3265–69.
Report of experience in 161 patients.

Service FJ, Nelson RL. Characteristics of glycemia stability. Diabetes Care 1980; 3:59–62.
A description of normal insulin physiology and its application to understanding current principles of insulin administration.

Skyler J. Type I diabetes: regimens, targets, and caveats. Diabetes Care 1982; 5:547–52.
One algorithm for altering insulin dosage in response to self–blood glucose measurements.

American Diabetes Association Policy Statement. Indication for use of continuous insulin delivery systems and self-measurement of blood glucose. Diabetes Care 1982; 5:140–42.
A consensus opinion that is still in effect.

Schmidt MI, et al. The dawn phenomenon, an early morning glucose rise: implications for diabetic instability. Diabetes Care 1981; 4:579–85.
In some patients nocturnal increases in insulin resistance may necessitate late evening administration of intermediate-acting insulin to obtain normal fasting blood glucose and to prevent nocturnal hypoglycemia.

Armbuster DA. Fructosamine structure, analysis, and clinical usefulness. Clin Chem 1987; 33:2153–63.
A complete description of this new tool for assessing short-term glycemic control.

Boden G, et al. Monitoring metabolic control in diabetic outpatients with glycosylated hemoglobin. Ann Intern Med 1980; 92:357–60.
Hemoglobin A is an accurate indicator of time-averaged blood glucose.

Zinman B, Zuniga-Guajardo S, Kelly D. Comparison of the acute and long-term effects of exercise on glucose control in Type I diabetes. Diabetes Care 1984; 7:515–9.
A small study documenting an acute drop in glucose with exercise, but no change in fasting glucose or glycosylated hemoglobin.

86. MANAGEMENT OF TYPE II DIABETES
John T. Gwynne

Type II diabetes, also known as non–insulin-dependent diabetes mellitus (NIDDM) (formerly "adult onset"), is characterized pathophysiologically by insulin resistance and impaired insulin secretion in response to glucose. The hyperglycemia of NIDDM is due to increased hepatic gluconeogenesis and decreased peripheral glucose clearance. The former predominates during nocturnal fasting while the latter predominates during the diurnal postprandial period. Hereditary predisposition plays a large role in the development of type II diabetes. In most cases, NIDDM is believed to be due to an inherited predisposition combined with environmental factors that precipitate hyperglycemia such as obesity. Prospective studies in Pima Indians, the only group for which such studies are available, indicate that insulin resistance precedes the onset of abnormal insulin secretion. Type II diabetes may be one extreme manifestation of a spectrum of metabolic disorders characterized by insulin resistance, obesity, hypertension, and atherogenic lipid changes including high triglyceride levels and low levels of high-density lipoprotein (HDL) cholesterol.

Ketoacidosis does not occur in NIDDM except with severe stress, and insulin is not required to sustain life. Exogenous insulin is not ordinarily required to prevent ketoacidosis but may be required to control hyperglycemia. The microvascular complications of diabetes—retinopathy, nephropathy, and neuropathy—occur in patients with type II diabetes but their prevalence is lower than that in patients with type I diabetes. Approximately 15% of patients with type II diabetes develop nephropathy after 15 years duration of disease. Although it is likely that good glycemic control will have the same beneficial effects in preventing microvascular complications in type II as it does in type I diabetes, no prospective trials of "tight" glycemic control in patients with type II diabetes have been conducted. However, the majority of experimental evidence suggests that "tight" control will retard the development of microvascular complications. No conclusions regarding the effects of tight control on macrovascular complications are yet possible.

There are three major elements in the treatment of type II diabetes: (1) glycemic control, (2) risk factor management, and (3) specific efforts to retard and treat complications. The latter are covered in Chapter 87. The major modalities for blood glucose control in type II diabetes are diet, exercise, hypoglycemic drugs (oral sulfonylurea, insulin), and education. A reasonable goal for blood glucose control in type II diabetes is a fasting blood glucose concentration in the range of 100 to 160 mg/dl and a postprandial glucose concentration of less than 200 mg/dl.

Diet

The objectives of dietary treatment of type II diabetes are to (1) decrease insulin resistance and (2) delay the onset of atherosclerotic cardiovascular diseases. The means to these ends are achievement of ideal body weight and amelioration of atherosclerotic risk factors. Obesity and excess caloric consumption cause insulin resistance. In a significant portion of the more than 80% of type II diabetics who are obese, clinical remission can be achieved by weight reduction. Such patients continue to exhibit abnormal insulin secretion and develop clinical disease if they regain weight. However, in most patients, sustained weight loss appears to prevent overt diabetes indefinitely. The approach to weight reduction in type II diabetics not receiving hypoglycemic drugs is the same as in nondiabetics (see Chap. 3). In type II diabetics treated with insulin or oral hypoglycemic agents, medication doses must be reduced and often discontinued during periods of caloric restriction or weight loss. The appropriate doses can best be judged by a review of the patient's records of blood glucose measurements. As a general rule of thumb, medication should be decreased by at least 50% for a daily intake of less than 1800 calories and discontinued for a daily intake of less than 1000 calories.

The diet prescribed for patients with type II diabetes should be low in total fat (< 40% of calories) and saturated fat (< 10% of calories) and high (55–65% of calories) in carbohydrate. Starches such as potatoes, bread, pasta, and rice should comprise the bulk of carbohydrate calories. Diets high in sucrose will increase plasma triglyceride levels, which have an independent predictive value for coronary heart disease in diabetics. Inclusion of fiber will decrease postprandial glycemic excursion and may improve fasting blood glucose and plasma lipid levels. Whether the effect of fiber is direct or secondary to accompanying changes in other diet constituents is uncertain. Cholesterol consumption should be restricted to less than 300 mg/day. Achieving dietary modification requires persistent effort by the physician, nutritionist, and nurse over an extended period of time, at least 2 to 6 months. Individualized dietary counseling by a trained nutritionist is more likely to succeed than is the distribution of standard printed materials. Important clinical improvements result from changes in dietary fat and cholesterol consumption even if total caloric consumption does not decrease.

In type II diabetics not taking hypoglycemic drugs, caloric intake may be spread conveniently throughout the day. In patients with type II diabetes who are taking insulin or oral hypoglycemic drugs, caloric intake must cover the periods of peak pharmacologic action, as in type I diabetics.

Hypoglycemic Drugs

Either oral agents or insulin can be used for patients in whom glycemic control is not adequate with diet alone. Because the majority of obese type II diabetics will respond to diet therapy if successfully implemented, when to treat a patient in whom diet therapy fails (because of an inability or unwillingness to change dietary habits) is a difficult question for which no uniform answer exists. In general, hypoglycemic drugs should be used if professionally supervised, dietary intervention fails to result in an acceptable weight reduction or improvement in blood glucose control after at least 6 months of persistent effort. The choice of hypoglycemic drugs—insulin or oral agents—depends on the patient's preference and response.

Oral Hypoglycemic Drugs
Sulfonylureas, the only oral hypoglycemic drugs currently available in the United States, decrease insulin resistance and hepatic gluconeogenesis and increase insulin secretion. Pancreatic islet beta cells possess specific, high-affinity, sulfonylurea receptors, which when occupied decrease resting membrane potential by increasing intercellular potassium concentration. This lowers the threshold for glucose stimulation. Whether similar specific receptors are present in other tissues is still under investigation. In peripheral tissues, sulfonylurea treatment increases the number of insulin receptors and decreases postreceptor resistance. The molecular mechanics are not known.

Considerable controversy has surrounded the use of sulfonylureas. The University Group Diabetes Program (UGDP), a randomized prospective trial, suggested that tolbutamide increases cardiovascular events. This trial has been vigorously criticized and defended. Two subsequent studies failed to show an increase in cardiovascular events in type II diabetics treated with sulfonylureas. Extrapolation of the UGDP results to second-generation sulfonylureas or to diabetics with severe glucose intolerance may not be warranted.

Table 86-1 presents the dosage range and duration of action of first- and second-generation sulfonylureas. The sulfonylureas largely are catabolized by the liver, with the resulting products largely excreted in the urine. Therefore, these agents should not be used in patients with impaired liver function or in those with renal failure in the case of chlorpropamide, acetohexamide, and tolazamide, whose active metabolites are renally excreted. Many commonly used medications either potentiate or antagonize the effects of sulfonylureas. Drugs that may enhance the hypoglycemic effects of sulfonylureas include, but are not limited to salicylates, phenylbutazone, dicumarol, chloramphenicol, and pyrazolon derivatives. Drugs that may antagonize sulfonylureas include, but are not limited to, thiazides, furosemide, phenytoin, propranolol, alcohol, and barbiturates. Several mechanisms that account for these drug interactions include interference with hepatic catabolism and displacement from albumin-binding sites. Prescribing information should be consulted to identify potential interactions.

Oral sulfonylureas are not always effective; the primary failure rate is 10 to 30% and many patients (30–60%) experience secondary failure as well. Sulfonylureas are most effective in younger diabetic patients. However, it is this group in whom the greatest risk of accelerated atherosclerosis exists, because they are at increased risk for the greatest period of time.

During weight loss, the dosage of oral hypoglycemics or insulin should be reduced or even discontinued, depending on the degree of caloric restriction.

Insulin
Insulin may be required to control blood glucose in some type II diabetics. The use of insulin for meticulous blood glucose control in type II diabetes is subject to the same considerations as in type I diabetes. (See Chap. 85 for information on routine insulin use.) Two additional modes of insulin administration have been used in type II diabetes: once-a-day, morning, intermediate- or long-acting insulin; and insulin in combination with an oral agent. Improved blood glucose control can be achieved with once-a-day morning

Table 86-1. Oral hypoglycemic agents

	Available tablet sizes (mg)	Equivalent doses (mg)	Dosage range (mg/day)	Duration of action (hr)	Doses/day
First generation					
Tolbutamide (Orinase, others)	250, 500	1000	500–3000	6–12	2–3
Chlorpropamide (Diabinese, others)	100, 250	250	100–500	60	1
Tolazamide (Tolinase, others)	100, 250, 500	250	100–1000	12–24	1–2
Acetohexamide (Dymelor, others)	250, 500	500	250–1500	12–24	1–2
Second generation					
Glipizide (Glucotrol)	5, 10	5	2.5–40.0	12–24	1–2
Glyburide (Diabeta, Micronase)	1.25, 2.5, 5	5	1.25–20.00	12–24	1–2

NPH, lente, or ultralente insulin. While this may not normalize blood glucose levels, it is more effective in type II than in type I diabetics. Combination therapy with insulin and oral hypoglycemic agents may decrease the dose of either one alone but in general does not provide any better glycemic control than does insulin alone. The use of "bedtime insulin and daytime sulfonylureas (BIDS)" is theoretically appealing since insulin will suppress enhanced nocturnal gluconeogenesis and sulfonylureas will decrease peripheral insulin resistance and increase diurnal glucose clearance. Evidence that BIDs improved glucose control compared to insulin alone is lacking. Since insulin has an independent predictive value for coronary heart disease, some have advocated using insulin alone or in combination only as a last resort in type II diabetes. However, clinical evidence that insulin administration increases the risk of coronary heart disease in type II diabetes is lacking.

Blood Glucose Monitoring

Assessing the response to hypoglycemic therapy in type II diabetes can be accomplished by several methods. Semiquantitative urinary glucose measurements are frequently misleading and are not suitable for assessing glycemic control. A single fasting blood glucose level is a more accurate measure of mean glycemic response in type II than in type I diabetes. Glycosylated hemoglobin (HbA_{1c}) or fructosamine measurements provide the most accurate means of assessing average blood glucose levels over a 60- and 5- to 7-day period, respectively. Self–blood glucose monitoring using fingerstick capillary blood and either visual or meter readings is indicated in type I diabetics taking insulin and can be a useful adjunct in other type II diabetics as well. For type II diabetics not taking insulin, self–blood glucose monitoring need not be nearly as frequent as in insulin-treated patients. Fasting measurements 2 to 3 times per week and as needed based on symptoms and activities will provide a general indication of the level of glycemic control.

Boyd AE. Sulfonylurea receptors, ion channels, and fruit flies. Diabetes 1988; 37:847–50.
Recent investigation has uncovered naturally occurring sulfonylurea-binding proteins and their role in mediating sulfonylurea effects on the pancreatic beta cell.

Johnson KH, et al. Islet amyloid, islet-amyloid polypeptide, and diabetes mellitus. N Engl J Med 1989; 321:513–8.
A review of the possible role of increased insulin secretion in the pathogenesis of type II diabetes.

Eriksson J, et al. Early metabolic defects in persons at increased risk for non-insulin-dependent diabetes mellitus. N Engl J Med 1989; 321:337–43.
A report providing further evidence for a hereditary cause of type II diabetes.

Gerich JE. Oral hypoglycemic agents. N Engl J Med 1989; 321:1231–45.
A thoughtful and comprehensive review of oral hypoglycemic agents and their role, risk, and benefits in the management of type II diabetes.

Olefsky JM, et al. Insulin resistance and insulin action. Diabetes 1981; 30:148–62.
A review of the role of insulin resistance in the etiology of type II diabetes. Different insulin response curves can be expected, depending on the site of insulin resistance (receptor versus postreceptor).

Genuth S. Supplemental fasting in the treatment of obesity and diabetes. Am J Clin Nutr 1979; 32:2579–86.
A dramatic but effective program for achieving weight loss and associated improved glycemic control or even amelioration of diabetes.

The University Group Diabetes Program VIII. Evaluation of insulin therapy: final report. Diabetes 1982; 31:Suppl 5:1–81.
Includes investigators' evaluation of the UGDP study.

Seltzer HS. A summary of criticisms of the findings and conclusions of the University Group Diabetes Program (UGDP). Diabetes 1972; 21:976–9.
A succinct review that places the criticisms into several general categories.

Kilo C, Miller JP, Williamson JR. The Achilles heel of the University Group Diabetes Program. JAMA 1980; 243:450–7.
Raises questions about the randomization used in conducting the UGDP study.

Rifkin H, ed. Physician guide to the care and management of type II diabetes. New York: American Diabetes Association, 1984
A concise, practical manual that presents the current consensus of opinion in this area.

Bogardus C, et al. Effects of physical training and diet therapy on carbohydrate metabolism in patients with glucose intolerance and non-insulin-dependent diabetes mellitus. Diabetes 1984; 33:311–8.
Notes the effects of exercise in reducing insulin resistance and provides guidelines for the therapeutic use of exercise in managing type II diabetes.

87. MANAGEMENT OF COMPLICATIONS OF DIABETES
John T. Gwynne

In addition to therapy to maintain good glycemic control, specific interventions to prevent, retard, and treat diabetic complications are an essential part of the optimal diabetic care and will both improve the quality of life and extend longevity. Routine surveillance for early detection of complications should be part of every clinical encounter with patients with type I or type II diabetes. The complications of diabetes are generally divided into two categories: microvascular, including retinopathy, neuropathy, and nephropathy; and macrovascular, including coronary, peripheral, and cerebral atherosclerosis. Cardiovascular diseases are the major cause of death in diabetics, occur earlier, and are 2 to 4 four times more prevalent than in nondiabetics. Microvascular complications are more prevalent in type I than in type II diabetes but because of the disproportionate number of type II diabetics, the absolute numbers of microvascular complications are greater in type II than in type I diabetes. Efforts to prevent microvascular complications are as important for type II as for type I diabetics. Conversely, cardiovascular disease risk factor management is as important for type I as for type II diabetics.

Microvascular Complications

Retinopathy
Diabetic retinopathy is the leading cause of new adult blindness in the United States. There are approximately 5800 new cases each year. Background retinopathy, comprised of microaneurysms and dot hemorrhage, occurs in nearly everyone who has had diabetes for longer than 10 years but does not impair vision unless it involves the macula. Proliferative retinopathy, neovascularization with retinal detachment and vitreous hemorrhages, occurs in up to 60% of type I and 30% of type II diabetics and can lead to blindness. Prospective controlled clinical trials in patients with advanced background or proliferative retinopathy have shown that panretinal laser photocoagulation reduces vision loss by 60%. Routine ophthalmoscopic examination fails to detect diabetic retinopathy as much as 50% of the time. Consequently, every patient with type II diabetes should have an ophthalmologic examination by a trained ophthalmologist at the time of diagnosis and annually from 10 years after the onset of disease. This allows for early intervention and prevents vision loss. Another important element in preserving eyesight is aggressive control of hypertension. The rate of progression from background to proliferative retinopathy can be decreased significantly by keeping systolic blood pressure (BP) less than 140 mm Hg and diastolic BP less than 85 to 90 mm Hg. Finally, vitrectomy may restore lost vision in some patients with vitreous hemorrhages.

Nephropathy
In type I diabetes, the incidence of nephropathy begins to increase after 15 years duration of disease and occurs in approximately 50% of all patients with type I diabetes. The onset of nephropathy is also related to the duration of disease in type II diabetics but less

predictably than in type I because of the difficulty in dating the onset of type II disease. Ultimately, nephropathy affects approximately 25% of type II diabetics. Diabetic nephropathy is responsible for almost one-third of all patients in chronic renal dialysis.

Untreated diabetic nephropathy follows a predictable course. The first clinical indication of nephropathy is an increase in albumin excretion. Subsequently, hypertension ensues, followed by a decline in serum creatinine and creatinine clearance. Several of these hallmarks require clinical responses. Urinary protein excretion should be determined by a dipstick test at least annually in patients with disease of long duration. Microalbuminuria ($< 100–200$ μg/24 hr) is strongly predictive of renal failure and of overall mortality in diabetes. Moreover, some evidence suggests that albumin excretion plays an etiologic role in diabetic glomerulosclerosis. Recent evidence suggests that low-protein ($< 10\%$ of calories) diets retard the progression of nephropathy. Angiotensin-converting enzyme (ACE) inhibitors decrease microalbuminuria in diabetics and may be particularly valuable in treating hypertension in diabetics. Clinical trials are underway to determine whether ACE inhibitors retard renal failure if such treatment is initiated at the onset of microalbuminuria before hypertension appears. However, ACE inhibitors are not generally indicated for the treatment of albuminuria in the absence of hypertension. The use of beta-blockers should be avoided in treating hypertension in the diabetic since they may block signs and symptoms of hypoglycemia and impair insulin secretion in type II diabetics.

Hemodialysis, chronic ambulatory peritoneal dialysis (CAPD), and renal transplantation have all been used in the treatment of diabetic end-stage renal disease (ESRD). The mortality rate of patients undergoing hemodialysis for diabetic ESRD is 20 to 35% at 1 year. In contrast, this figure is reduced to 8% for patients treated by CAPD and 15% for patients undergoing transplantation. Early transplantation improves survival. Thus, creatinine levels should be measured at least annually after 10 years duration of disease and all patients with creatinine concentrations higher than 2.0 mg/dl should be referred for consideration and planning of later (creatinine > 4.0 mg/dl) renal transplantation.

Neuropathy
Diabetic involvement of the nervous system can present in frequently puzzling ways; usually other causes of neurologic deficit must be ruled out to conclude that diabetes is responsible. Involvement of the autonomic nervous system can affect almost any organ system. Diabetic gastroparesis and nocturnal diarrhea are the most common presentations of gastrointestinal neuropathy. Cardiovascular presentations include tachycardia and bradycardia. Increased orthostatic BP changes as well as a failure to change the heart rate with the Valsalva maneuver are early "subclinical" manifestations of autonomic neuropathy and provide useful diagnostic tools. Life expectancy is diminished with the onset of autonomic neuropathies, although the neuropathy, which is often self-limited, is not usually the cause of death. Metoclopramide may be useful in treating gastroparesis. Erythromycin may help control nocturnal diarrhea.

The most common presentation of sensory neuropathy is burning pain in the soles of the feet, usually greater at night than during the day. Sensory neuropathy is almost always accompanied by loss of the Achilles tendon reflex. Diabetic mononeuropathies may also present with pain. They may be confused with many other types of pain and usually are diagnosed only by excluding other causes. Treatment of painful diabetic neuropathy is often frustrating. Numerous treatments have been advocated on the basis of findings from inadequately controlled clinical trials. The combination of fluphenazine (Prolixin), 1.0 mg every morning or twice a day, and amitriptyline (Elavil), 25 or 75 mg at bedtime, may reduce the pain through actions in the central nervous system. A substance P inhibitor (capsaicin), applied to the overlying skin for at least 3 weeks, may also reduce pain. Aldose reductase inhibitors, which increase *myo*-inositol levels, increase nerve conduction velocity but have not convincingly decreased pain. None are currently available and some that have a phenytoin-like structure result in significant toxicity.

Bilateral muscle weakness and wasting, often of the interosseous muscles of the hands or proximal muscles of the lower extremities, can also occur as a result of diabetes. No specific therapy is available.

Macrovascular Complications
The reason atherosclerosis occurs at an accelerated rate in diabetes is not known. However, coronary events are concentrated in those diabetics with traditional risk factors. Thus,

aggressive management of risk factors is indicated in diabetics. A recent consensus panel report suggested that the goal cholesterol level in all diabetics should be lower than 130 mg/dl. Because hypertriglyceridemia has an independent predictive value in diabetics that is not observed in the general population, efforts should be made to maintain triglyceride concentrations below 350 mg/dl. Dietary restriction of saturated fat and refined carbohydrates is the principal therapy. In selected patients, those with established disease in the absence of other risk factors or with a family history of early coronary heart disease, fibric acid derivatives may be indicated to lower triglyceride levels. Omega-3 fatty acid supplements also lower triglyceride levels but may cause a substantial deterioration of glucose control.

Pharmacologic treatment of high cholesterol levels poses unique problems in the diabetic patient. Bile acid–binding resins (cholestyramine, colestipil) may increase triglyceride levels. Nicotinic acid causes a deterioration of blood glucose control and fibric acid derivatives (gemfibrozil) may actually increase low-density lipoprotein cholesterol levels in some hypertriglyceridemic patients. HMG-CoA reductase inhibitors (lovastatin) are as effective in the diabetic as in the nondiabetic and do not appear to involve any additional risk.

"Diabetic Ulcers" and Foot Care

It is estimated that 50% of all amputations in the diabetic can be prevented. "Diabetic ulcers" occur in patients with sensory neuropathy and impaired circulation. Contrary to widely held precepts, small-vessel disease is not primarily responsible for the poor circulation in the diabetic foot. Atherosclerosis in the lower extremities in diabetics is more often distal to the trifurcation than that in the nondiabetic and can be treated surgically by distal bypass grafting. Thus, patients with ulcers or symptoms of claudication should undergo Doppler flow studies and differential arterial pressure measurements.

Simple measures are perhaps the most effective in preventing amputations. Every diabetic with sensory neuropathy should be instructed to inspect his or her feet every day, and inspection and sensory examination of the feet should be conducted at every physician visit. Ulcers develop at sites of unperceived injury. Maldistribution of weight-bearing, because of either sensory neuropathy or traumatic deformity, can be treated by orthotics. Podiatric care for the treatment of corns and calluses and prescribing orthotics are extremely valuable adjuncts in managing diabetic patients and preventing limb loss.

Raskin P. Blood glucose control and diabetic complications. Ann Intern Med 1986; 105:254–63.
Reviews the important adverse effects of hyperglycemia and the role of heredity in the development of complications. Concludes that "tight" glycemic control will reduce but not eliminate diabetic complications.

Brownlee M, Cerami A, Vlassara H. Advanced glycosylation end products in tissue and the biochemical basis of diabetic complications. N Engl J Med 1988; 318:1315–21
Describes one mechanism by which hyperglycemia may cause diabetic complications and new therapeutic approaches that may arise from these observations.

Clinical Practice Recommendation American Diabetes Association 1990–91. Diabetes Care 1991; 14:Suppl 2.
This supplement consists of a compilation of position statements from the American Diabetes Association, with detailed recommendations for the management of all aspects of diabetes and its complications. Includes specific recommendations for the treatment of microvascular complications as well as foot care, and the prevention of macrovascular complications.

Merimee TJ. Diabetic retinopathy. N Engl J Med 1990; 322:978–83.
Reviews the pathophysiology of retinopathy and discusses the therapeutic implications of these observations.

The Kentucky Diabetic Retinopathy Group. Guidelines for eye care in patients with diabetes mellitus. Arch Intern Med 1989; 149:769–70.
Brief consensus guidelines for the management of retinopathy.

Davis MD. Diabetic retinopathy: a clinical overview. Diabetes Metab Rev 1988; 4:291–322.
Reviews the pathophysiology, relationship to glycemic control, and clinical findings of diabetic retinopathy. Presents specific recommendations for detection, follow-up, laser photocoagulation, and vitrectomy as well as other sight-saving measures, and justifies them on the basis of results of clinical trials.

Selby JV, et al. The natural history and epidemiology of diabetic nephropathy. Implications for prevention and control. JAMA 1990; 263:1954–60.
A "state-of-the-art review" of the natural history and the risk factors for the progression of diabetic kidney disease, with recommendations for preventive strategy.

Rosenstock J, Raskin P. Early diabetic nephropathy: assessment and potential therapeutic interventions. Diabetes Care 1986; 9:529–45.
Focuses attention on early referral and control of hypertension.

Mogensen CE. Microalbuminuria predicts clinical proteinuria and early mortality in maturity onset diabetes. N Engl J Med 1984; 310:356–60.
Microalbuminuria has emerged as an important predictor of increased mortality in diabetes.

The Working Group on Hypertension in Diabetes. Statement on hypertension in diabetes mellitus. Arch Intern Med 1987; 147:830–42.
Reviews the risks and benefits of various antihypertensive therapies in patients with diabetes.

Geitz FC, Kjellstrand CM. The treatment of diabetic kidney disease. Diabetologia 1979; 17:267–81.
Compares the advantages, disadvantages, and outcomes of various approaches to managing renal failure in the diabetic.

Amair P, et al. Continuous ambulatory peritoneal dialysis in diabetics with end-stage renal disease. N Engl J Med 1982; 306:625–30.
A promising method of management with a surprisingly good outcome.

Harati Y. Diabetic peripheral neuropathies. Ann Intern Med 1987; 107:546–59.
A comprehensive overview of the manifestations of diabetic neuropathy and practical suggestions for management.

Feldman M, Scheller LR. Disorders of gastrointestinal motility associated with diabetes mellitus. Ann Intern Med 1983; 98:378–84.
Autonomic neuropathies can present in a wide variety of ways.

David JL, et al. Peripheral diabetic neuropathy treated with amitriptyline and fluphenazine. JAMA 1977; 238:2291–3.
The initial description of the effectiveness of this treatment for painful neuropathies.

88. HYPOGLYCEMIA
Rebecca A. Silliman

Almost 60 years have passed since hypoglycemia was first implicated as a cause of physical distress, yet controversy about the condition persists. There is little question that insulinomas and other tumors, alcohol intake in malnourished people, and excessive exogenous insulin in diabetics can lead to profound symptomatic hypoglycemia. On the other hand, whether or not reactive or functional hypoglycemia is a pathologic entity is more problematic. An emotion-charged literature has served to fuel the debate. Because many people have vague symptoms of malaise, fatigue, or headache that they or others believe are caused by hypoglycemia, clinicians are often called on to decide whether or not symptoms have resulted from low blood sugar.

Case Definition

Symptoms of hypoglycemia can be attributed to either adrenergic excess or insufficient central nervous system glucose. In general, symptoms caused by the former are accompanied by a rapid drop in blood glucose and those caused by the latter, by a more gradual fall. Symptoms are nonspecific but may be the major clues to the presence of an underlying process. Adrenergic symptoms include sweating, tremor, hunger, anxiety, palpitations, and tachycardia. Neuroglycopenia can cause irritability, headache, personality changes, confusion, lethargy, seizures, stupor or coma.

The level at which a relatively low blood glucose is responsible for symptoms is controversial, particularly for functional or reactive hypoglycemia. Historically, the diagnosis of hypoglycemia was made by a 5-hour oral glucose tolerance test (OGTT). A blood glucose nadir of less than 70 mg/dl, regardless of associated symptoms, defined reactive hypoglycemia. Later, it was asserted that the diagnosis could be made from symptoms alone. However, neither of these definitions is consistent with the evidence. From 10 to 50% of normal asymptomatic people have glucose levels that are at times less than 50 mg/dl. In addition, some patients experience their symptoms with normal plasma glucose levels (ranging from 73 to 153 mg/dl in one study). These same inconsistencies have been found with oral glucose tolerance testing. Patients may have no symptoms with a glucose nadir less than 50 mg/dl but report symptoms at normal plasma gucose levels. The rate of change of plasma glucose concentration does not seem to be a relevant factor.

Because of these inconsistencies, a Mayo Clinic group has recommended that the OGTT not be used for the diagnosis of reactive hypoglycemia. Rather, they consider the diagnostic gold standard to be a plasma glucose level of less than 45 mg/dl obtained at the time of spontaneous symptoms. However, this information is often difficult to obtain.

Despite the fact that there is lack of agreement on case definition and uncertainty as to the value of the OGTT, the symptomatic patients must be approached with two goals in mind: (1) to recognize a serious cause of hypoglycemia, if it is present, and (2) to provide symptomatic relief. The causes, symptoms, and treatment of hypoglycemia are considered in three categories: fasting, iatrogenic, and postprandial.

Fasting Hypoglycemia

It is important to make the distinction between fasting and postprandial hypoglycemia, because the former has much more serious implications. Fasting hypoglycemia is a rare condition. Patients who have it usually have serious underlying disease and manifest neuroglycopenic symptoms, which can progress to permanent brain damage if untreated. A history of symptoms beginning during fasting and exacerbated by exercise points to this category of hypoglycemia. Patients report alterations in personality, behavior, or intellectual functioning, and seizures, sweating, and blurring of vision most frequently occurring in the late afternoon or in the early morning before breakfast. These disturbances also may accompany exercise. However, distress can occur at irregular intervals, confusing the picture.

Tumors of the pancreatic islet cells (insulinoma) are the most common cause of fasting hypoglycemia. Other tumors are unusual causes of hypoglycemia, including large mesenchymal tumors, hepatomas, adrenocortical neoplasms, and a wide variety of other neoplasms including bronchogenic carcinoma, carcinoid tumors, and carcinoma of the breast. Nontumor causes of fasting hypoglycemia include pituitary and adrenal insufficiency, alcohol ingestion, severe liver disease, and right-sided heart failure. Impaired gluconeogenesis appears to be the mechanism in most instances. Both chronic alcoholics and binge drinkers experience hypoglycemia. Diagnosis may be difficult because symptoms often mimic acute intoxication or withdrawal; the presence of hypothermia may be an important clue. Severe liver disease, such as acute necrosis, or right-sided congestive heart failure may cause hypoglycemia. However, because of the considerable functional reserve of the liver, it is unusual for these conditions alone to be causative.

In the approach to the symptomatic patient, the absence of complaints associated with fasting excludes the diagnosis of fasting hypoglycemia. In the few patients in whom the relation is less clear, the likelihood is increased by findings consistent with one of the underlying causes. If fasting hypoglycemia is suspected from the information, confirmation by means of laboratory investigation, with the patient in the hospital, is necessary. This includes such tests as simultaneous glucose and immunoreactive insulin determinations and a prolonged fast (up to 72 hours).

"Iatrogenic" Hypoglycemia

Excess exogenous insulin or sulfonylureas may cause iatrogenic hypoglycemia. Usually the cause is clear, but in the case of surreptitious use it is not. Patients usually are health care workers with access to hypoglycemic drugs. Symptoms have no definite pattern and are not related to the fed or fasting state. The recent development of an assay for circulating C peptide has helped to exclude other causes, such as insulinoma. This "connecting peptide" is a component of the human insulin precursor and reflects endogenous insulin production. A low blood glucose, high concentration of immunoreactive insulin, and suppressed C peptide suggest surreptitious insulin injection. Similarly, when inappropriately high immunoreactive insulin and high C peptide levels suggest an insulinoma, sulfonylurea blood levels should be obtained to confirm the suspicion of abuse.

The sulfonylureas have a propensity to induce unanticipated hypoglycemia even at usual doses. Older patients and those with hepatic or renal impairment are particularly at risk. In addition, a wide variety of drugs can potentiate sulfonylurea action, including propranolol, phenylbutazone, salicylates, and clofibrate.

Postprandial Hypoglycemia

There is considerable controversy about the three principal types of postprandial hypoglycemia; alimentary, early diabetic, and functional hypoglycemia. This controversy has been perpetuated by problems with case definition. Nonetheless, many people are plagued by adrenergic symptoms occurring 2 to 5 hours after eating.

A history of gastrointestinal surgery suggests alimentary hypoglycemia. The physiologic explanation is that rapid carbohydrate absorption is followed by an excessive outpouring of insulin. This may be associated with any procedure that causes rapid delivery of a glucose load into the duodenum, such as subtotal gastrectomy, pyloroplasty, gastrojejunostomy, and vagotomy. Symptoms coincident with a blood glucose nadir appear 2 to 3 hours after meals. Carbohydrate restriction, smaller and more frequent feedings, and anticholinergic agents (e.g., propantheline 7.5 mg PO 30 minutes before meals) seem to ameliorate symptoms in many.

Postprandial hypoglycemia can occur before the onset of overt diabetes mellitus. The defect is thought to be a delayed and increased insulin release, resulting in symptomatic hypoglycemia 3 to 5 hours after eating. Treatment includes weight reduction if obesity is present and dietary modification including carbohydrate restriction (60–100 g/day) and increased protein (100–200 g/day) divided among three meals and three snacks.

If other causes of postprandial hypoglycemia have been excluded, functional hypoglycemia must be considered. It is essential not to attribute disease to those with vague symptoms because labeling can lead to additional symptoms and dysfunction. The nature of the complaints and their relation to meals must be assessed carefully. Exploration of possible emotional disturbances should be included as part of a thorough medical evaluation. Depression, anxiety, or other emotional disturbances may be operant or, in fact, the underlying problem.

Although the shortcomings of the OGTT must be recognized, this test can be useful in two ways. The fact that the vast majority of symptomatic patients do not have reactive hypoglycemia can be demonstrated effectively by the OGTT. In the small percentage of patients whose symptoms coincide with the plasma glucose nadir of the OGTT and who are not symptomatic at other times, dietary changes similar to those recommended for alimentary and early diabetic hypoglycemia may be beneficial.

Exercise-Induced Hypoglycemia

In recent years there has been much interest in hypoglycemia induced by prolonged exercise. Carbohydrate loading before competition and the ingestion of glucose- and electrolyte-containing fluids have become part of the runner's armamentarium. Although hypoglycemia has been known to occur in both marathon runners and bicyclists, the relation of this to fatigue and performance is less clear. For example, in a study of healthy men exercising to exhaustion, there was no difference in endurance between those in whom hypoglycemia developed and those in whom it was prevented by the ingestion of glucose solutions. There is no sound evidence that hypoglycemia is responsible for symptoms that ordinarily occur during exercise or that ingesting sugar prevents these symptoms.

Nelson RG. Hypoglycemia: fact or fiction? Mayo Clin Proc 1985; 60:844–50.
A review that outlines the approach to the patient with symptoms suggestive of hypoglycemia.

Felig P, et al. Hypoglycemia during prolonged exercise in normal men. N Engl J Med 1982; 306:895–900.
A study examining the role of hypoglycemia in exercise endurance. Hypoglycemic men performed as well as euglycemic men.

Butler PC, Rizza RA. Regulation of carbohydrate metabolism and response to hypoglycemia. Endocrinol Metab Clin North Am 1989; 18(1):1–25.

Field JB. Hypoglycemia. Definition, clinical presentations, classification and laboratory tests. Endocrinol Metab Clin North Am 1989; 18(1):27–43.

Arky RA. Hypoglycemia associated with liver disease and ethanol. Endocrinol Metab Clin North Am 1989; 18(1):75–89.

Daughaday WH. Hypoglycemia in patients with non-islet cell tumors. Endocrinol Metab Clin North Am 1989; 18(1):91–102.

Seltzer HS. Drug-induced hypoglycemia: a review of 1418 cases. Endocrinol Metab Clin North Am 1989; 18(1):163–83.

Hofeldt FD. Reactive hypoglycemia. Endocrinol Metab Clin North Am 1989; 18(1):185–201.

Horwitz DL. Factitious and artifactual hypoglycemia. Endocrinol Metab Clin North Am 1989; 18(1):203–10.
These articles, all from the same issue of Endocrinology and Metabolism Clinics of North America *devoted to the subject of hypoglycemia, review various aspects of the disorder.*

89. EVALUATION OF THYROID FUNCTION
Robert D. Utiger

Thyroid function can be reliably and inexpensively evaluated by measuring serum thyroxine (T_4), free T_4, and thyroid-stimulating hormone (TSH, thyrotropin) levels. These tests can be used to screen for thyroid disease, evaluate patients suspected of having thyroid disease, and confirm clinical diagnoses of hyperthyroidism or hypothyroidism. Additional tests are rarely needed. It is important to remember that abnormalities in thyroid function tests occur not only in patients with thyroid, pituitary, and hypothalamic disease, but also in patients with abnormalities in serum thyroid hormone–binding proteins, those who have nonthyroidal illness, and those taking any of a number of drugs.

Thyroid Function Tests

Serum Thyroxine and Free Thyroxine
Serum T_4 measurements indicate the total T_4 concentration, which includes both the amount that is protein-bound ($> 99.9\%$) and the much smaller ($< 0.1\%$) amount that is unbound or free (FT_4). It is the free hormone that enters cells and accounts for the hormone's biologic activity. Serum T_4 concentrations are therefore abnormal not only in patients with hyper- or hypothyroidism but also in those with increased or decreased levels of the various serum thyroid hormone–binding proteins. Measurements of serum free T_4 allow one to distinguish between abnormalities of thyroid secretion and abnormalities of thyroid hormone binding.

Serum free T_4 usually is determined indirectly as the serum free T_4 index, which is the product of the serum T_4 and the triiodothyronine (T_3)-resin uptake. The latter, which may be expressed as a percentage or a ratio, provides an estimate of the degree of saturation of the thyroid hormone–binding proteins in serum. Serum free T_4 also may be measured directly by radioimmunoassay or equilibrium dialysis.

The most common causes of abnormal serum T_4 binding are abnormalities in serum thyroxine-binding globulin (TBG) concentrations. TBG is the most important of the thyroid-binding proteins, about 70% of the T_4 in serum being bound to it, and it has the highest affinity for T_4. Serum TBG levels are increased during pregnancy, by exogenous estrogen, during acute or subacute hepatitis, by drugs such as clofibrate and fluorouracil, and as a result of an inherited increase in TBG production. The effect of estrogen requires a substantial dose, so that most combined estrogen-progesterone contraceptives now in use do not raise serum T_4 levels above the normal range. Serum TBG levels are decreased by exogenous androgen and anabolic steroid hormones, an inherited decrease in TBG production, high-dose glucocorticoid therapy, and chronic illness. Large doses of salicylate and furosemide lower serum T_4 concentrations by inhibiting T_4 binding to TBG.

The other thyroid-binding proteins are thyroxine-binding prealbumin (TBPA, also known as transthyretin) and albumin. T_4 binding to TBPA and albumin is decreased in patients with many acute and chronic nonthyroidal illnesses. T_4 binding to albumin is increased in the syndrome of familial dysalbuminemic hyperthyroxinemia. Lastly, some patients with autoimmune thyroid disease have serum immunoglobulins that bind T_4. In nearly all of these situations, serum free T_4 index values are normal, regardless of whether the serum T_4 concentrations are high or low. The exception is familial dysalbuminemic hyperthyroxinemia, because in that disorder T_3 does not bind to the abnormal albumin; the T_3-resin uptake, therefore, does not reflect the presence of increased binding protein, and the serum free T_4 index value consequently is high.

The serum free T_4 index is a generally reliable indicator of the level of thyroid function, being low in most hypothyroid patients, high in most hyperthyroid patients, and normal in most patients with abnormal T_4 binding. However, low serum free T_4 index values may be found in patients receiving large doses of glucocorticoids and in those with severe nonthyroidal illness. High serum free T_4 index values are found in three groups of euthyroid patients: those with familial dysalbuminemic hyperthyroxinemia; those with generalized thyroid hormone resistance, a rare disorder characterized by tissue resistance to thyroid hormone and compensatory T_4 and T_3 overproduction; and some who are taking drugs, such as amiodarone, which slow T_4 clearance.

Serum TSH Concentrations

Serum TSH determinations provide a very precise indication of the amount of thyroid hormone available to the pituitary and other tissues. Serum TSH concentrations in normal subjects range from about 0.5 to 4.0 mU/L; the minimum detectable value is 0.1 to 0.2 mU/L. TSH assays with such sensitivity, compared with the sensitivity limits of 1 to 2 mU/L for older assays, are now widely available, and only sensitive assays should be used. The improvement in TSH assay sensitivity, which allows ready identification of subnormal serum TSH concentrations, has rendered thyrotropin-releasing hormone (TRH) stimulation tests obsolete. While there are both pulsatile and circadian TSH rhythms, the fluctuations in serum TSH concentrations are small and thus blood for TSH assay can be collected at any time.

Serum TSH concentrations are normal in patients with all types of abnormal serum T_4 binding, as well as those with generalized thyroid hormone resistance and nearly all patients with nonthyroidal illness encountered in an outpatient setting. The concentrations are elevated in patients with even small decreases in thyroid secretion, many of whom have few or no symptoms of hypothyroidism and serum T_4 concentrations within the normal range, and usually are markedly elevated in patients with symptomatic primary hypothyroidism. A normal or low serum TSH concentration in a hypothyroid patient indicates the presence of hypothalamic or pituitary disease. Serum TSH concentrations are undetectable or low in patients with hyperthyroidism, except for the very rare patient who has TSH-induced hyperthyroidism. They also are low in euthyroid patients with autonomous thyroid secretion, because the autonomously secreted thyroid hormones inhibit TSH secretion (see Chap. 92), and in some patients with acute, severe nonthyroidal illness.

Serum Triiodothyronine (T_3)
Serum T_3 measurements are useful only to confirm the diagnosis of T_3 hyperthyroidism, that is hyperthyroidism characterized by increased serum T_3 but normal serum T_4 concentrations. T_3 hyperthyroidism should be suspected in clinically hyperthyroid patients who have low serum TSH but normal free T_4 index values.

Serum T_3 concentrations are low in most hypothyroid patients. However, they are also low in most patients with acute or chronic nonthyroidal illness, resulting from decreased extrathyroidal conversion of T_4 and T_3.

Thyroid Radioisotope Tests
Measurement of thyroid radioiodine uptake is not a useful test of thyroid function. However, it can be used to differentiate hyperthyroidism due to excess thyroid hormone secretion, as occurs in Graves' disease, from that due to thyroiditis or exogenous thyroid hormone intake. The thyroid radioiodine uptake is increased in the former and decreased in the latter two situations. Thyroid radioisotope scans provide information about regional but not overall thyroid function; they are used to evaluate patients with solitary thyroid nodules (see Chap. 92).

Evaluation Strategies

Screening for Thyroid Disease
A strong case can be made for screening asymptomatic patients older than 50 or 60 years for thyroid disease, since in such individuals the frequency of thyroid dysfunction approaches 10%.

The best single test to screen for thyroid dysfunction in outpatients is measurement of the serum TSH concentration. If it is normal, the patient is almost certainly euthyroid, regardless of the serum T_4 and T_3 concentrations. If it is abnormal, the patient most likely has some thyroid, pituitary, or hypothalamic dysfunction. Because TSH secretion is so sensitive to small changes in thyroid secretion, abnormal serum TSH values may not indicate the presence of clinically important thyroid disease. If a screening serum TSH measurement is abnormal, the serum free T_4 index should be measured to determine the type and extent of the thyroid dysfunction. Patients with high or low serum TSH concentrations who are asymptomatic and have normal serum free T_4 index values are considered to have subclinical hypothyroidism or subclinical hyperthyroidism, respectively. These situations are discussed further in Chapters 90 and 91.

Evaluation of Suspected Hypothyroidism
In a patient suspected to have hypothyroidism, serum T_4, free T_4 index (or free T_4), and TSH should be measured. Low serum free T_4 index and high serum TSH values confirm the diagnosis of primary hypothyroidism. Normal serum free T_4 index and high serum TSH values indicate some thyroid deficiency (subclinical hypothyroidism), although the patient may be asymptomatic. If the serum TSH value is normal or low in a patient who has a low serum free T_4 index, the diagnosis is secondary hypothyroidism. Other studies of pituitary function, such as measurement of the serum prolactin concentration, assessment of pituitary-adrenal and pituitary-gonadal function, and neuroradiologic studies then should be done.

Evaluation of Suspected Hyperthyroidism
In a patient suspected to have hyperthyroidism, serum T_4, free T_4 index (or free T_4), and TSH should be measured. High serum free T_4 index and low (usually undetectable) serum TSH values confirm the diagnosis. If the serum free T_4 index is normal and the serum TSH value is low, the patient may have T_3 hyperthyroidism. This possibility can be confirmed by a serum T_3 assay. Alternatively, the patient could have considerable thyroid autonomy, whether due to Graves' disease, an autonomously functioning thyroid adenoma, or a multinodular goiter, but not clinically important hyperthyroidism (subclinical hyperthyroidism). A normal serum TSH value is compelling evidence that the patient does not have hyperthyroidism, except for the very rare patient who has TSH-induced hyperthyroidism. Patients with high serum free T_4 index values due to familial dysalbuminemic

Table 89-1. Effects of some pharmacologic agents on thyroid function

1. Drugs causing primary hypothyroidism (serum T_4 low, free T_4 index low, TSH high)
   a. Lithium carbonate
   b. Inorganic iodine
2. Drugs altering serum thyroid hormone–binding proteins
   a. Increase in binding (serum T_4 high, free T_4 index normal, TSH normal)
      1. Estrogen
      2. Clofibrate
      3. Heroin, methadone
      4. Fluorouracil
   b. Decrease in binding (serum T_4 low, free T_4 index normal, TSH normal)
      1. Androgenic and anabolic steroids
      2. Glucocorticoids
      3. Salicylate
      4. Furosemide
3. Drugs altering thyroid hormone metabolism
   a. Inhibition of extrathyroidal T_3 production (serum T_4 normal, free T_4 index normal, T_3 low, TSH normal*)
      1. Propranolol and related drugs
      2. Glucocorticoids
      3. Amiodarone
      4. Oral cholecystographic agents
      5. Propylthiouracil
   b. Decrease in thyroxine clearance (serum T_4 high, free T_4 index high, TSH normal)
      1. Amiodarone
      2. Oral cholecystographic agents

*Unless the patient is hyperthyroid initially.

hyperthyroxinemia, generalized thyroid hormone resistance, or amiodarone or other drugs have normal serum TSH concentrations.

Thyroid Function Abnormalities in Nonthyroidal Illness
Many abnormalities in pituitary-thyroid function occur in patients with nonthyroidal illness. A low serum T_3 concentration, due to impaired extrathyroidal conversion of T_4 to T_3, is a very common finding in such patients, whatever their illness. Decreased production of one or more of the thyroid hormone–binding proteins or inhibition of T_4 binding to them may occur as a result of illness or drug use. In patients with severe, acute illness, serum free T_4 concentrations also may fall; serum TSH concentrations are normal or low, suggesting that TSH secretion is inhibited.

While there is usually no reason to look for thyroid function abnormalities in patients with nonthyroidal illness, it is important to be able to interpret such abnormalities correctly when they are found. A normal serum TSH value excludes the diagnosis of primary hypothyroidism in patients with low serum total and free T_4 values. Binding protein abnormalities should be identified by T_3-resin uptake tests done in conjunction with serum T_4 measurements. Treatment with T_4 is not indicated in patients with illness-induced reductions in serum T_3 and T_4 concentrations; indeed, the decreased thyroid hormone concentrations minimize the catabolic effects of illness, and thus are likely beneficial adaptations to illness.

Effects of Drugs on Thyroid Function Tests
As indicated above, a variety of drugs alter serum thyroid hormone and TSH concentrations in several ways. Table 89-1 lists the more important of these drugs and the ways in which they alter thyroid function or thyroid function test results.

Utiger RD. Evaluation of abnormal thyroid function. In: Kelley WN, ed. Textbook of internal medicine. Vol. 2. 2nd ed. Philadelphia: JB Lippincott, 1992: 2085–2089.
A general discussion of the various tests available for assessing thyroid function, the factors that affect them, and the evaluation of patients with different types of thyroid disease.

Surks MI, et al. American Thyroid Association guidelines for use of laboratory tests in thyroid disorders. JAMA 1990; 263:1529–32.
Guidelines recommending that measurement of serum free T_4 and TSH be utilized as the principal laboratory tests in patients with suspected thyroid disease.

Toft AD. Use of sensitive immunoradiometric assay for thyrotropin in clinical practice. Mayo Clin Proc 1988; 63:1035–42.

Ehrmann DA, Weinberg M, Sarne DH. Limitations to the use of a sensitive assay for serum thyrotropin in the assessment of thyroid status. Arch Intern Med 1989; 149:369–72.
Two articles describing the advantages and limitations of measuring serum TSH concentrations as the initial test of thyroid function.

Helfand M, Crapo LM. Screening for thyroid disease. Ann Intern Med 1990; 112:840–9.
A review of the results of studies of thyroid function in the community and in various medical settings. The authors conclude that community screening programs are not indicated because of low yield and high cost. Case finding in a clinic setting has a higher yield and lower cost, especially among older women.

Griffin JE. The dilemma of abnormal thyroid function tests: is thyroid disease present or not? Am J Med Sci 1985; 289:76–88.
A thorough and lucid review of the effects of abnormal thyroid hormone–binding proteins, drugs, and nonthyroidal illness on thyroid hormone production, transport, and metabolism.

90. HYPERTHYROIDISM
Robert D. Utiger

Hyperthyroidism is a rather common disorder. A community survey in Great Britain revealed a prevalence rate of 19 per 1000 women and 1.6 per 1000 men, and an estimated incidence of 2 to 3 new cases per 1000 women per year.

Clinical Manifestations
The manifestations of hyperthyroidism reflect the accelerated function of various organ systems or the inability of an organ system to meet the demands imposed by hyperthyroidism. The diagnosis also should be considered in patients with thyroid enlargement or infiltrative ophthalmopathy. Although the clinical manifestations are independent of the cause of hyperthyroidism in an individual patient, their frequency and severity are influenced by the rate of onset, the patient's age, and the vulnerability of various organ systems to excess thyroid hormone. The term *apathetic* or *masked hyperthyroidism* is used to describe elderly patients who have cardiac failure, atrial fibrillation, muscle weakness, or weight loss but not the nervousness, heat intolerance, hyperphagia, and hyperactivity that are so common in younger patients.

Psychological Symptoms
Nervousness, physical hyperactivity, emotional lability, anxiety, and distractibility occur often. These changes result in an impairment of work or school performance and disturbances in home and family life.

Neuromuscular System
Weakness and easy fatigability are common complaints. The former usually develops gradually, is progressive, and may be accompanied by muscle wasting. A fine tremor is often evident in the hands and fingers, and performing skills requiring fine coordination becomes difficult.

Skin
The skin is warm and its texture smooth or velvety. Erythema and pruritus may be present. Hyperhidrosis is a common complaint. Hair may become thin and fine, and hair loss occurs.

Eyes
An excess of thyroid hormone itself causes lid retraction and lid lag. Lid retraction results in apparent proptosis, but not in forward protrusion of the eyes, and is often accompanied by symptoms of conjunctival irritation. Infiltrative ophthalmopathy, a manifestation of Graves' disease, is discussed below.

Thyroid Gland
Enlargement of the thyroid gland is very common. In Graves' disease, both thyroid lobes are usually moderately, more-or-less symmetrically enlarged, but thyroid enlargement may be absent, especially in elderly patients. Thyroiditis results in slight or moderate diffuse thyroid enlargement; the thyroid is painful and tender in subacute thyroiditis. Toxic multinodular goiters are large and asymmetric. A thyroid adenoma causing hyperthyroidism is usually at least 3 cm in diameter.

Cardiovascular System
Cardiovascular dysfunction is common and, in some patients, the only manifestation of hyperthyroidism. Heart rate and cardiac output are increased, and peripheral resistance is decreased, resulting in palpitations, sinus tachycardia or atrial fibrillation, and cardiac failure. Examination reveals a prominent apical impulse, bounding arterial pulsations, accentuated heart sounds, systolic ejection murmur, and occasionally cardiac enlargement. Other than arrhythmias, electrocardiographic changes are limited to nonspecific ST- and T-wave abnormalities.

Respiratory Function
Abnormalities of respiration include decreased vital capacity, decreased pulmonary compliance, and respiratory muscle weakness. These abnormalities result in dyspnea and hyperventilation during exercise and sometimes at rest.

Gastrointestinal System
Increased caloric expenditure is almost always present. It results in increased appetite and food intake. Compensation is usually inadequate, so that modest weight loss occurs, but it may reach 40 to 50 lb., especially in older patients. Increased gastrointestinal motility may result in an increased frequency of bowel movements and even frank diarrhea, and minor abnormalities in hepatic function are common.

Hematopoietic System
Some patients have a modest anemia, caused by a mild deficiency in one or more hematopoietic nutrients or by increased plasma volume. Mild granulocytopenia and thrombocytopenia also may be present.

Energy and Intermediary Metabolism
Because of increased energy expenditure, energy production must be augmented; this is accompanied by increased oxygen consumption and heat production. In patients with diabetes mellitus, the requirements for exogenous insulin increase because insulin catabolism is accelerated.

Endocrine System
In women, hypomenorrhea or amenorrhea may occur, although usually menstrual function does not change. Men may have a loss of libido and impotence.

Hypercalcemia is an occasional finding; it is usually neither severe nor symptomatic. It is caused by increased bone resorption, and serum parathyroid hormone concentrations are low. Clinical osteopenia is rare.

Laboratory Diagnosis

Serum Thyroid Hormone and Thyroid-Stimulating Hormone (TSH, Thyrotropin) Concentrations
In most hyperthyroid patients, serum total and free thyroxine (T_4) and triiodothyronine (T_3) concentrations are increased, although occasionally only serum T_3 concentrations are increased (T_3 hyperthyroidism). Serum TSH concentrations are invariably low or undetectable, except in the very rare patient with TSH-induced hyperthyroidism. When hyperthyroidism is suspected, serum T_4, free T_4 index (or free T_4), and TSH should be measured. If the serum T_4 and free T_4 index values are normal, serum T_3 can be measured. Low serum TSH values alone indicate the presence of subclinical hyperthyroidism; most such patients are clinically euthyroid but they may be hyperthyroid. Recognition of the presence of hyperthyroidism in such patients must be based on clinical judgment; additional thyroid testing is of little value. Subclinical hyperthyroidism reflects the presence of thyroid autonomy and may be due to any of the disorders that cause hyperthyroidism. Patients who have elevated serum T_4 concentrations due to increases in T_4 binding in serum have normal serum TSH concentrations (see Chap. 89).

Radioiodine Uptake
Most patients with hyperthyroidism have increased thyroid radioiodine uptake. Important exceptions include patients with subacute thyroiditis, painless thyroiditis, or exogenous hyperthyroidism. The indications for measuring thyroid radioiodine uptake are to confirm a suspected diagnosis of thyroiditis or surreptitious thyroid hormone administration in a hyperthyroid patient, and as a prelude to iodine 131 (^{131}I) therapy, but *not* to diagnose hyperthyroidism. Thyroid radioisotope scans are useful in determining regional, but not overall, thyroid function, and therefore are not a test for hyperthyroidism. They may be helpful in identifying a thyroid adenoma or multinodular goiter as a cause of hyperthyroidism.

Causes of Hyperthyroidism

The underlying cause of hyperthyroidism should be identified, because the causes differ in their natural history and therefore require different therapy. The cause of hyperthyroidism in an individual patient usually can be identified by history and physical examination, with particular reliance on the duration of symptoms and the presence or absence of thyroid enlargement and of the extrathyroidal manifestations of Graves' disease. Graves' disease is the cause in roughly 90% of patients; the next most common causes are the various forms of thyroiditis.

Graves' Disease
Graves' disease occurs most often in young women, but it may occur in men and at any age. It consists of one or more of the following: hyperthyroidism, diffuse goiter, infiltrative ophthalmopathy, localized myxedema, and thyroid acropachy. Most patients with Graves' disease have both hyperthyroidism and goiter. The two usually develop concurrently and are caused by the production of thyroid-stimulating immunoglobulins (TSIs). Most patients also have ophthalmopathy, although it is clinically evident in only about 40%. Localized myxedema and thyroid acropachy are rare. Graves' disease also is characterized by spontaneous remissions, so that some patients remain euthyroid after antithyroid drug therapy is discontinued. The proportion of patients who have a remission after 1 year of antithyroid therapy varies from 40 to 60%, and it is higher when the duration of treatment is longer.

Subacute Thyroiditis
Clinical manifestations of hyperthyroidism occur in about 50% of patients with subacute thyroiditis, but this disorder is dominated by the nonspecific systemic inflammatory manifestations of the illness and by thyroid pain and tenderness. Hyperthyroidism lasts from a few weeks to a month or so and then subsides, often followed by transient hypothyroidism; ultimate recovery is the rule.

Painless Thyroiditis
Hyperthyroidism without pain or tenderness caused by thyroiditis also is short-lived. These patients have only modest thyroid enlargement and modest hyperthyroidism, from both the clinical and the biochemical points of view. Thyroid radioiodine uptake is low. Recovery occurs in a few weeks or months and may be preceded by transient hypothyroidism.

Exogenous Hyperthyroidism
Iatrogenic or factitious hyperthyroidism is likely to occur during the administration of T_4 in doses of 200 μg/day or more, T_3 in doses of 75 μg/day or more, or desiccated thyroid in doses of 120 mg/day or more. In euthyroid patients with autonomous thyroid function, smaller doses may cause hyperthyroidism. Important clues to the presence of exogenous hyperthyroidism are the absence of thyroid enlargement, normal or low serum T_4 concentrations (in patients taking T_3), and low thyroid radioiodine uptake. There have been two small epidemics of hyperthyroidism due to thyroid contamination of ground beef, and hyperthyroidism can be induced by the administration of iodide or iodine-containing drugs, such as amiodarone, in patients who have a multinodular goiter.

Toxic Nodular Goiter
Toxic nodular goiter may result in hyperthyroidism late in its natural history. Most affected patients have a long history of gradually increasing thyroid enlargement and hyperthyroidism develops insidiously. There is no ophthalmopathy or localized myxedema.

Toxic Uninodular Goiter (Thyroid Adenoma)
Hyperthyroidism occurs in some patients with an autonomously functioning thyroid adenoma, clinically manifested as a solitary thyroid nodule. Although thyroid adenomas occur in adults of all ages, most patients with hyperthyroidism are in the older age groups. The thyroid scan shows intense isotope uptake in the location of the palpable nodule and nearly complete absence of uptake elsewhere.

Other Causes
Rare causes of hyperthyroidism include iodine-induced hyperthyroidism, TSH-secreting pituitary tumors, trophoblastic tumors, and ectopic hyperthyroidism (struma ovarii).

Treatment Options
Ideal therapy for a hyperthyroid patient would be elimination of the cause so that normal pituitary-thyroid function can be restored. For most patients, however, the fundamental cause of their hyperthyroidism is not known, and no truly curative treatment is available.

Antithyroid Drugs
Methimazole (MMI) and propylthiouracil (PTU) are effective inhibitors of thyroid hormone biosynthesis, and the latter also inhibits extrathyroidal T_4 conversion to T_3. The usual initial daily dosage of MMI is 10 to 20 mg once daily, and that of PTU is 300 to 450 mg in divided doses. Some improvement usually occurs after 2 to 3 weeks of MMI treatment, and it is usually substantial after 4 to 6 weeks; the response to PTU is considerably slower. Failure of antithyroid drug therapy to control hyperthyroidism results from an inadequate dosage and/or noncompliance. As improvement occurs, the dosage should be reduced by 25 to 50% at 1- to 2-month intervals. If the patient with Graves' disease remains euthyroid while taking 5 mg of MMI or 50 mg of PTU daily for 1 to 2 months, the drug should be discontinued. Decisions about drug dosages are made largely on clinical grounds, supported when necessary by serum T_4 and TSH determinations. Recurrence may be treated

with an antithyroid drug again, although many patients choose ablative therapy. Of the two drugs, MMI is preferable not only because its antithyroid action is more rapid, but also because it can be given once daily, it does not have a bitter aftertaste, the number of pills required per day is less, and it may have fewer side effects.

Toxic reactions to the usual dosages of either drug occur in about 5% of patients, and are dose-dependent. Most are dermatologic reactions, such as pruritus or urticaria, which subside without treatment or with symptomatic therapy. More serious reactions include fever, arthritis, hepatitis, anemia, thrombocytopenia, and agranulocytosis; agranulocytosis occurs in approximately 0.1% of patients. Because these reactions usually develop rapidly, monitoring blood cell counts is not helpful. Patients should be carefully warned of the symptoms of such reactions and instructed to discontinue therapy and contact the physician immediately if any occur. Although a toxic reaction to one drug does not preclude use of the other, it is wiser to give ^{131}I therapy after a serious toxic reaction.

Drugs to Ameliorate Thyroid Hormone Effects
Some manifestations of hyperthyroidism are ameliorated by adrenergic antagonist agents. Propranolol, in dosages of 60 to 180 mg daily, results in rapid (24–48 hours) diminution of some common symptoms of hyperthyroidism, most notably palpitations, tachycardia, tremor, and anxiety, but it does not ameliorate the catabolic effects of hyperthyroidism. Propranolol is of little added benefit when given with an antithyroid drug, but it can be helpful in managing patients given radioiodine therapy, in whom improvement occurs more slowly, or in those with hyperthyroidism due to thyroiditis.

Radioactive Iodine Therapy
^{131}I therapy is effective for hyperthyroidism due to Graves' disease. The major advantages of ^{131}I therapy are that usually only a single dose is needed and it is safe. Its major disadvantage is that amelioration of the hyperthyroidism usually requires several months. For very symptomatic patients, a period of antithyroid drug therapy before ^{131}I therapy is advisable. Iodides should not be given, and care should be taken to avoid the use of iodide-containing drugs or contrast agents if ^{131}I therapy is planned. The usual dosage is 8 to 15 mCi.

There are only two important untoward effects of ^{131}I therapy: persistent hyperthyroidism and hypothyroidism. Acute temporary exacerbations of hyperthyroidism, caused by radiation-induced thyroiditis, are rare. Persistent hyperthyroidism results from inadequate therapy and is more common when smaller doses of ^{131}I are given. Hypothyroidism occurs within the first year after therapy in most patients, and it ultimately occurs in nearly all. Many physicians are reluctant to use ^{131}I therapy in children and young adults, because it might cause thyroidal or other neoplasms or gonadal damage or because the patient might be pregnant. However, ^{131}I therapy is not a proven risk factor for thyroid or other neoplasms and the gonadal radiation dose after ^{131}I is less than that which results from diagnostic radiologic procedures. Pregnancy is an absolute contraindication to its use, because ^{131}I crosses the placenta and so can destroy the fetal thyroid gland.

Surgery
Because of the simplicity, safety, and economy of antithyroid drugs and ^{131}I therapy, the only indications for subtotal thyroidectomy are hyperthyroidism during pregnancy or very large goiters.

Treatment of Specific Conditions

Graves' Disease
Antithyroid drugs or radioactive iodine (^{131}I) are both safe and effective forms of antithyroid treatment. Neither results in cure, and both require long-term observation of the patient. The choice depends on several considerations. An antithyroid drug is given in the hope that the patient will have a remission of the Graves' disease, so that hyperthyroidism does not recur after the drug is withdrawn. Although this goal is not always achieved, an antithyroid drug, preferably MMI, is the initial treatment of choice for most patients. It is the only form of therapy whereby the patient has some chance of having normal, physiologically regulated thyroid function in the future. Use of an antithyroid drug does

not preclude the use of ^{131}I should the patient have some toxic drug reaction or fail to have a remission of the Graves' disease. The beneficial effect of ^{131}I therapy is slower, and nearly all patients subsequently require T_4 therapy. Antithyroid drug therapy also is less expensive than is ^{131}I therapy.

Thyroiditis
Both subacute and painless thyroiditis are transient, and the hyperthyroidism accompanying them is usually mild. If treatment is needed, propranolol is the agent of choice. Salicylates or prednisone effectively relieves neck pain and tenderness in patients with subacute thyroiditis.

Toxic Multinodular Goiter
Ablative therapy with ^{131}I is the treatment of choice for this disorder, because it is permanent. Large doses of ^{131}I, and sometimes multiple doses, should be used, because thyroid ^{131}I uptake is usually only slightly increased and persistent hyperthyroidism is to be avoided in these elderly patients. Hypothyroidism rarely develops following treatment, because the thyroid gland contains suppressed tissue that can regain function.

Thyroid Adenoma
Because thyroid adenomas also cause permanent hyperthyroidism, ablative therapy with ^{131}I is most appropriate. The dosage used should be large (20–25 mCi) so that the nodule is effectively destroyed. There is a small risk of permanent hypothyroidism because the suppressed extranodular tissue recovers function as the production of T_4 and T_3 by the nodule declines.

Extrathyroidal Manifestations of Graves' Disease

Infiltrative Ophthalmopathy
Clinically evident ophthalmopathy occurs in approximately 40% of patients with hyperthyroidism due to Graves' disease. It usually develops gradually, along with hyperthyroidism, but it occasionally first appears months or years earlier or later. The symptoms include pain in the eyes, lacrimation, photophobia, diplopia, and blurring or loss of vision. The major signs are proptosis (exophthalmos), periorbital and conjunctival congestion and edema (chemosis), and limitation of ocular mobility. The diagnosis of infiltrative ophthalmopathy when hyperthyroidism is or recently was present is not difficult. The diagnosis is less certain if the patient is not or never was hyperthyroid (euthyroid Graves' disease). Orbital ultrasonography and computed tomography are the best procedures to confirm the diagnosis of ophthalmopathy due to Graves' disease and to exclude other causes of ophthalmopathy, such as orbital tumor or pseudotumor.

Ophthalmopathy is at its worst in most patients before their hyperthyroidism is treated. With antithyroid treatment, noninfiltrative eye signs (lid retraction, stare), local irritative symptoms, and subjective diplopia often improve; in most patients there is little change in proptosis or ophthalmoplegia. When progression occurs, it is usually in the first 1 to 2 years after antithyroid treatment. There is no satisfactory treatment. For many patients, assurance that lid retraction and stare will improve with treatment of their hyperthyroidism and that progression is unlikely is adequate therapy. Periorbital and eyelid edema may improve if patients sleep with their head elevated, and diuretics may be tried. Eye irritation and pain can be treated with 1% methylcellulose eye drops. Patients with marked inflammation or threatened vision should be treated aggressively with corticosteroids or orbital decompression. Both are reasonably effective, and there are no established criteria for selecting one over the other.

Utiger RD. Disorders of the thyroid gland. In: Kelley WN, ed. Textbook of internal medicine. Vol. 2. 2nd ed. Philadelphia: JB Lippincott, 1992: 1992–2001.
A discussion of all aspects of hyperthyroidism.

Tibaldi JM, et al. Thyrotoxicosis in the very old. Am J Med 1986; 81:619–22.
Among 25 patients aged 75 years or older with hyperthyroidism, the most common cause was Graves' disease (80%). The most common symptoms were weight loss, palpitations,

and weakness. Most patients had only a few symptoms, and many did not have thyroid enlargement.

Cooper DS. Antithyroid drugs. N Engl J Med 1984; 252:1353–62.
This article provides a detailed summary of the actions and side effects of MMI and PTU.

Shiroozu K, et al. Treatment of hyperthyroidism with a small single daily dose of methimazole. J Clin Endocrinol Metab 1986; 63:125–8.

Okamura K, et al. Reevaluation of the effects of methylmercaptoimidazole and propylthiouracil in patients with Graves' disease. J Clin Endocrinol Metab 1987; 65:719–23.
These two articles provide data indicating that MMI in doses of 15 or 30 mg daily more rapidly ameliorates hyperthyroidism than does PTU at 300 mg/day (mean, 5–7 weeks versus 17 weeks). Furthermore, single daily doses of MMI were as effective as divided doses.

Sridama V, DeGroot LJ. Treatment of Graves' disease and the course of ophthalmopathy. Am J Med 1989; 87:70–3.
Among 218 patients with hyperthyroidism due to Graves' disease who had clinically evident ophthalmopathy, it worsened in approximately 20%, did not change in 65%, and improved in the remainder when their hyperthyroidism was treated. Among 288 hyperthyroid patients who did not have ophthalmopathy, it developed in approximately 5%. The results were independent of the type of antithyroid therapy used.

91. HYPOTHYROIDISM
Robert D. Utiger

The spectrum of hypothyroidism is broad, ranging from a few nonspecific symptoms to overt hypothyroidism to myxedema coma. The biochemical spectrum is even broader as it includes patients who are asymptomatic and have normal serum thyroid hormone concentrations but elevated serum thyroid-stimulating hormone (TSH, thyrotropin) concentrations (subclinical hypothyroidism).

The most common cause of hypothyroidism is primary thyroid disease, but occasionally it results from pituitary or hypothalamic disease (hypothyrotropic hypothyroidism). Hypothyroidism occurs in 3 to 6% of the adult population, but is symptomatic only in a minority of affected individuals. It occurs several times more often in women than in men, and with increasing frequency with age, especially in women.

Clinical Features

The major symptoms and signs of hypothyroidism reflect slowing of the physiologic function of one or more organ systems. The onset usually is gradual, and the severity varies considerably and correlates poorly with the biochemical changes. Because many of the symptoms and signs of hypothyroidism are nonspecific, the diagnosis is particularly likely to be overlooked in patients with other illnesses and in the elderly.

Behavioral and Neurologic Symptoms

Most hypothyroid patients complain of fatigue, loss of energy, and lethargy. They become less active, both mentally and physically. Inattentiveness, decreased intellectual function, and sometimes overt depression may occur. Neurologic symptoms include hearing loss, ataxia, paresthesia, and carpal tunnel syndrome.

Skin

Hypothyroidism results in dry, thick, and scaly skin, which is often cool and pale. Less commonly, there is nonpitting edema of the hands, feet, and periorbital regions (myxedema). Pitting edema also may be present. Hair may become coarse and brittle, hair growth slows, and hair loss may occur.

Cardiovascular System
Hypothyroidism results in a cardiomyopathy characterized by bradycardia, diminished cardiac contractility, increased cardiac wall thickness, and sometimes pericardial effusion. These findings, along with peripheral edema, may simulate congestive heart failure, but in most hypothyroid patients cardiac function increases appropriately during exercise. Increased peripheral resistance may result in hypertension. The electrocardiogram may show low voltage and/or nonspecific ST- and T-wave changes. High serum cholesterol levels are common, although whether or not there is an increased prevalence of ischemic heart disease is controversial. Angina pectoris, when present, characteristically occurs less often after the onset of hypothyroidism, probably because of decreased activity, and it may be exacerbated by thyroxine (T_4) therapy.

Respiratory System
Dyspnea on effort is common. This complaint may be caused by enlargement of the tongue and larynx, causing upper airway obstruction, or by respiratory muscle weakness, interstitial edema of the lungs, and/or pleural effusions. Hoarseness and symptoms of sleep apnea may be prominent complaints.

Gastrointestinal System
Hypothyroidism does not cause obesity, but modest weight gain from fluid retention and fat deposition often occurs. Appetite decreases. Gastrointestinal motility is decreased, leading to constipation and abnormal distention; the latter may result from ascites as well.

Musculoskeletal System
Aches, pains, and stiffness of muscles and joints are common; less frequent are objective myopathy and joint swelling or effusions. The relaxation phase of the tendon reflexes is prolonged. Serum creatine kinase and alanine aminotransferase activities are often increased, probably attributable as much to slowed enzyme clearance as to increased muscle release.

Hematopoietic System
Anemia, caused by decreased red blood cell production, occurs in about 25% of hypothyroid patients, probably as a result of the decreased need for peripheral oxygen delivery rather than a hematopoietic defect. Most patients have no evidence of iron, folic acid, or vitamin B_{12} deficiency.

Endocrine System
Women with hypothyroidism may have menorrhagia, infertility, or secondary amenorrhea or galactorrhea. The latter is due to hyperprolactinemia. Pituitary-adrenal function is usually normal. Pituitary enlargement from hyperplasia of the thyrotropes occurs occasionally in patients with primary hypothyroidism; such enlargement also may be caused by a primary pituitary tumor, with resulting TSH deficiency. In patients with diabetes mellitus, hypothyroidism results in increased insulin sensitivity.

Laboratory Diagnosis
The diagnosis of primary hypothyroidism is established by the findings of low serum total and free T_4 and elevated serum TSH concentrations (see Chap. 89). The combination of normal serum T_4 and increased TSH concentrations is generally referred to as subclinical hypothyroidism. Such patients have some degree of thyroid deficiency; clinically, they may be asymptomatic, have some symptoms of hypothyroidism, or have only thyroid enlargement. Low serum T_4 and low or normal TSH concentrations (secondary hypothyroidism) indicate the presence of pituitary or hypothalamic disease. Further evaluation of hypothalamic-pituitary function and anatomy then is mandatory. This evaluation should include neuroradiological studies, measurement of serum prolactin levels, and assessment of pituitary-adrenal and pituitary-gonadal function.

Causes of Hypothyroidism
Attention should be given to the cause of hypothyroidism since it may be transient and therefore not require therapy. The cause usually is evident from the history and physical examination.

Primary (Thyroidal) Hypothyroidism
Primary hypothyroidism usually results from the destruction of thyroid tissue by autoimmune mechanisms, irradiation, or surgery, but it may be caused by genetic or drug-induced inhibition of thyroid hormone biosynthesis. Chronic autoimmune thyroiditis is the most common cause of hypothyroidism. It may be goitrous (Hashimoto's disease) or nongoitrous (atrophic thyroiditis). Radioactive iodine (^{131}I) therapy for hyperthyroidism results in hypothyroidism in most patients within the first year after therapy and it occurs gradually thereafter in the remainder. Hypothyroidism also results from external neck irradiation therapy in doses at 2000 rads or more, such as are used in the treatment of malignant lymphoma and laryngeal carcinoma. Hypothyroidism is expected to occur after total thyroidectomy for thyroid carcinoma; its occurrence after subtotal thyroidectomy is variable, but common. Rare causes of primary hypothyroidism include inborn errors of thyroid hormone biosynthesis and infiltrative disease such as scleroderma and amyloidosis. In all the above situations, hypothyroidism is permanent.

Transient Hypothyroidism
Drugs that block thyroid hormone synthesis and secretion, such as propylthiouracil, methimazole, lithium carbonate, amiodarone, and iodine, can cause transient hypothyroidism. Iodine can cause a substantial reduction in thyroid secretion in patients with autoimmune thyroiditis or patients who have had ^{131}I therapy, but not in normal subjects. Transient hypothyroidism also occurs in the first months after ^{131}I therapy or subtotal thyroidectomy, during recovery from subacute thyroiditis or painless thyroiditis, in the postpartum period, and following discontinuation of thyroid hormone therapy in a euthyroid patient. In situations in which hypothyroidism is expected to be transient, therapy should not be initiated unless symptoms are marked. It then should be withdrawn within 6 to 8 weeks and the patient followed for several months thereafter.

Secondary (Hypothyrotropic) Hypothyroidism
Secondary hypothyroidism is far less common than is primary hypothyroidism. TSH deficiency usually occurs along with other anterior pituitary hormone deficiencies, and is most often caused by a pituitary tumor. Other causes include pituitary infarction, infiltrative processes, trauma, and idiopathic hypophysitis. Many of the same processes may involve the hypothalamus and thereby cause thyrotropin-releasing hormone (TRH) deficiency.

Treatment

Patients with symptomatic hypothyroidism should be treated with L-thyroxine (T_4), unless their hypothyroidism is expected to be transient. Amelioration of all clinical and biochemical manifestations of hypothyroidism can usually be achieved by administering T_4 in dosages of 75 to 150 µg daily; rarely is a larger dose required. In young adults the initial dosage should be 100 µg daily; if necessary it can be increased in 25-µg increments at 4- to 6-week intervals. Improvement in energy and activity is usually evident within 1 to 2 weeks after the initiation of therapy, but objective manifestations diminish more slowly. In older patients, lower initial doses (25–50 µg) and more gradual increments are indicated. Cautious replacement is particularly warranted in patients with a history of ischemic heart disease, because angina pectoris or cardiac arrhythmias may be precipitated by T_4 therapy.

The adequacy of therapy can be assessed by clinical and biochemical means. Relief of symptoms requires dosages of T_4 that raise the serum T_4 concentration to within the normal range, although slight TSH hypersecretion may persist. While a larger T_4 dosage may have little clinical effect, it seems theoretically desirable to restore the serum TSH concentration to normal as well. Administration of dosages of T_4 sufficient to reduce serum TSH concentrations to below normal, even though serum T_4 concentrations remain within the normal range, should be avoided; prolonged therapy with such dosages of T_4 may accelerate bone mineral loss and/or have deleterious cardiovascular effects. These considerations make measurements of serum TSH the best test to use for following treatment in hypothyroid patients. Subsequent dosage adjustments are rarely indicated, and the patient can be examined at 6-month or yearly intervals. Such visits are needed mainly to reinforce the need for continued therapy, since discontinuation of T_4 therapy is an important complication of treatment. Once the patient has become clinically and biochemically euthyroid, follow-up laboratory tests are not necessary unless some symptoms or signs of over- or undertreatment occur.

Patients with subclinical hypothyroidism probably should be treated. Some may have vague and/or unrecognized symptoms and hence may benefit immediately from therapy. Also, symptomatic hypothyroidism may develop as time progresses. If such a patient is not treated, periodic re-evaluation is mandatory because of the risk of progression to overt hypothyroidism.

Thyroid preparations other than T_4, such as T_3, desiccated thyroid extract, and mixtures of T_4 and T_3, should not be used. All are more expensive than T_4. Since they all contain T_3, serum T_4 measurements in patients taking these preparations underestimate the amount of hormone being given. Therefore, the risk of iatrogenic hyperthyroidism is greater unless patients are followed using serum TSH measurements.

Utiger RD. Disorders of the thyroid gland. In: Kelley WN, ed. Textbook of internal medicine. 2nd ed. Vol. 2. Philadelphia: JB Lippincott, 1992: 1992–2001.
A discussion of all aspects of hypothyroidism.

Griffin JE. Hypothyroidism in the elderly. Am J Med Sci 1990; 299:334–45.
This review article describes the changes in thyroid function that occur during aging and the natural history and manifestations of hypothyroidism in the elderly.

Becker C. Hypothyroidism and arteriosclerotic heart disease: pathogenesis, medical management and the role of coronary artery bypass surgery. Endocr Rev 1985; 6:432–40.
This article presents a thoughtful discussion of the problem of angina pectoris in patients with hypothyroidism, the risks of precipitating angina with T_4 therapy in such patients, and its management.

Watts NB. Use of a sensitive thyrotropin assay for monitoring treatment with levothyroxine. Arch Intern Med 1989; 149:309–12.
In this study of 100 T_4-treated hypothyroid patients, 59% of those with normal serum T_4 concentrations had low serum TSH concentrations. Among the patients with elevated serum T_4 concentrations, 71% had low serum TSH concentrations. These results indicate that overtreatment is best monitored by TSH measurements.

Nystrom E, et al. A double blind cross-over 12-month study of L-thyroxine treatment of women with subclinical hypothyroidism. Clin Endocrinol 1988; 29:63–76.
T_4 therapy resulted in subjective improvement and improved psychometric function in about 25% of patients in this study.

92. THYROID NODULES
Robert D. Utiger

The term *thyroid nodule* refers here to a single thyroid nodule (solitary nodule) in a euthyroid patient whose thyroid gland is otherwise normal. Such a nodule is usually a thyroid adenoma, a thyroid cyst, or an adenomatous nodule that is part of an otherwise unrecognized multinodular goiter. It may also be a papillary, follicular, or medullary thyroid carcinoma, or rarely, a lymph node or other nonthyroid mass. Of these, only thyroid carcinoma needs to be identified; the other lesions pose no important risk to the patient.

Solitary thyroid nodules are common. They can be found in 2 to 3% of adults, and they occur 3 to 4 times more often in women than in men. Thyroid carcinoma is unusual; its incidence in the United States is 10,000 new cases each year. The key issue in dealing with a patient who has a thyroid nodule is to identify the nodule that is a carcinoma.

Clinical Findings

An asymptomatic neck mass is the presenting feature in most patients who have a thyroid nodule, whatever its cause. An occasional patient describes neck discomfort, hoarseness, dysphagia, or rapid nodule growth.

Risk factors for thyroid carcinoma include young age, male sex, a history of head and neck irradiation in childhood, and a family history of medullary thyroid carcinoma, occurring either alone or with pheochromocytoma and/or hyperparathyroidism (multiple endocrine neoplasia [MEN], type II). Thyroid nodules are more likely to be malignant in children or men not because thyroid cancer is common in these groups, but because they have benign thyroid nodules less often than do women. Both benign and malignant thyroid nodules occur about fourfold more often in patients who had head and neck irradiation in childhood. The threshold radiation dose is low and the risk is proportional to dose up to about 2000 rads; the latent period ranges from about 5 to at least 30 years.

Physical findings that increase the likelihood that a nodule is a carcinoma include fixation of the nodule to underlying tissue, cervical lymphadenopathy, and hoarseness due to vocal cord paralysis.

Diagnostic Studies

Laboratory studies should include measurements of serum thyroxine (T_4), free T_4 index, and thyroid-stimulating hormone (TSH, thyrotropin (see Chap. 89). If hyperthyroidism is present, the nodule is an autonomously functioning thyroid adenoma, and no further studies are necessary. However, many of these patients and virtually all of those who have other types of thyroid nodules are euthyroid, and further evaluation then is necessary. Serum calcitonin levels should be measured in all patients who have a family history of medullary thyroid carcinoma or other components of type II MEN.

Procedures used to determine the function and nature of a nodule in an attempt to identify carcinoma include thyroid radioisotope scanning, fine-needle aspiration biopsy, and ultrasonography.

Thyroid radioisotope scanning is done with technetium 99m (^{99m}Tc-pertechnetate) or iodine 123 (^{123}I–iodide). The results are comparable, but the former is more convenient since the image is obtained 20 to 30 minutes after administration of the radioisotope, whereas iodide imaging requires a second visit 24 hours after isotope administration. Approximately 5% of solitary nodules prove to be hyperfunctioning (hot), 85% are hypofunctioning (cold), and 10% are isofunctioning (warm). Thyroid carcinomas usually concentrate these isotopes less efficiently than does normal thyroid tissue, and thus appear hypofunctioning, but some are isofunctioning. Most benign nodules also are hypofunctioning. Therefore a thyroid scan does not establish a diagnosis of thyroid carcinoma. The principal values of a radioisotope scan are (1) recognition of a hyperfunctioning nodule, which is almost always a benign autonomously functioning thyroid adenoma; and (2) identification of other nodules in addition to the one palpated, which indicates the presence of a nontoxic multinodular goiter.

Fine-needle aspiration biopsy is a simple and reliable way to identify thyroid carcinoma and is indicated in most patients with iso- or hypofunctioning nodules; some advocate needle biopsy as the initial step in the evaluation of any patient who has a thyroid nodule. A thyroid radioisotope scan then is done only if examination of the biopsy specimen reveals hyperplastic thyroid epithelial cells, since they may indicate the presence of either an autonomously functioning thyroid adenoma or a carcinoma. Cystic nodules are readily identified by needle aspiration, and sufficient material for cytologic study is obtained in over 90% of patients with solid nodules. Approximately 15% of hypofunctioning and 10% of isofunctioning solid nodules prove to be carcinomas. False-positive or false-negative cytologic diagnoses occur in about 5% of patients.

Ultrasonography can be used to determine whether a hypofunctioning nodule is a cystic nodule, which is usually benign. However, the availability of fine-needle aspiration biopsy has rendered ultrasonography unnecessary.

Diagnostic Strategies

A patient whose radioisotope scan reveals a hyperfunctioning nodule and whose serum T_4 concentration is normal need only to be re-examined periodically. But because most thyroid nodules are iso- or hypofunctioning, most patients are referred for fine-needle aspiration biopsy. Alternative strategies are to limit needle aspiration to those patients who have risk factors for thyroid carcinoma, those whose nodule increases in size during a period of observation, or those whose nodule does not decrease in size after treatment with 100 to 150 μg of T_4 daily for several months. Few thyroid carcinomas are likely to be overlooked by these more conservative approaches, but early cytologic study offers reassurance to both patient and physician.

For patients with a history of irradiation who have no palpable thyroid abnormalities, only yearly neck examinations are necessary.

Specific Types of Thyroid Nodules

Thyroid cysts probably result from necrosis and liquefaction of some type of solid thyroid nodule. A thyroid cyst is treated by fine-needle aspiration, with cytologic examination of the fluid to rule out the possibility that the nodule is a cystic thyroid carcinoma. Aspiration results in regression or disappearance of the cyst in most patients. Fluid reaccumulates in some patients; if desired by the patient, re-aspiration may be performed but is not necessary. T_4 therapy does not reduce the likelihood of the cyst fluid reaccumulating.

Autonomously functioning thyroid adenomas are benign tumors that concentrate iodide and synthesize and secrete thyroid hormones. The autonomously secreted thyroid hormones inhibit TSH secretion and hence the function of the normal thyroid tissue is reduced; the nodule thus appears hyperfunctioning. Most patients with these adenomas are euthyroid, but when the nodules are 3 cm in diameter or larger, hyperthyroidism may be present. Patients who are euthyroid do not require treatment; a later increase in nodule size and/or in thyroid secretion is uncommon. In a study of 159 patients followed for up to 15 years, 86% had no change in nodule size and 9% became hyperthyroid. If the patient desires treatment for cosmetic reasons or local discomfort, ^{131}I should be given. This therapy effectively destroys the nodule, and there is little risk of posttherapy hypothyroidism because the suppressed thyroid tissue resumes function as nodule function declines.

Hypofunctioning benign nodules are most commonly follicular adenomas, papillary adenomas, or colloid (adenomatous) nodules. All are well encapsulated and usually compress adjacent tissue. Surgical excision of the nodule may be indicated for those patients whose nodules cause local symptoms or in whom the nodule enlarges. T_4 therapy, although widely used, does not often result in a reduction in nodule size or reduce the likelihood of the development of new nodules after surgery.

Three types of *thyroid carcinoma* (papillary, follicular, and medullary) commonly present as a slow growing, asymptomatic solitary nodule. All are treated surgically. Anaplastic carcinomas and lymphoma usually occur in patients with preexisting nontoxic multinodular goiter or Hashimoto's disease, respectively.

Papillary carcinoma, the most common thyroid carcinoma, accounts for 60 to 80% of cases. The carcinomas in patients who had head and neck irradiation in childhood are of this type. Papillary cancers occur at any age, but most often in the third and fourth decades. They are unencapsulated tumors that spread by invading the surrounding thyroid tissue or lymphatics. About 50% of patients have cervical node metastases at the time of initial surgery. This tumor has a very slow growth rate; although recurrences after initial therapy occur in 10 to 20% of patients, death from cancer is very rare.

Follicular carcinoma accounts for 10 to 20% of thyroid carcinomas and also occurs most often in the third and fourth decades. These are well-differentiated, encapsulated tumors that metastasize to the lungs and bones by blood vessel invasion. Follicular carcinoma is also a very slow growing tumor.

Medullary carcinoma is a tumor of thyroid parafollicular, rather than follicular, cells. It accounts for approximately 10% of thyroid carcinomas and occurs sporadically and in two familial forms. In one form, affected family members have only medullary carcinomas; in the other, the affected individuals may have pheochromocytoma and hyperparathyroidism as well (MEN type II). Medullary carcinoma is often multicentric and is somewhat more malignant than is papillary or follicular carcinoma. Because all medullary carcinomas secrete calcitonin, serum calcitonin measurements are valuable both to indicate the presence of this tumor and to monitor the course of disease.

Rojeski MT, Gharib H. Nodular thyroid disease: evaluation and management. N Engl J Med 1985; 313:428–36.

Griffin J. Management of thyroid nodules. Am J Med Sci 1988; 296:336–47.

Mazzaferri EL, de los Santos ET, Rofagha-Keyhans S. Solitary thyroid nodule: diagnosis and management. Med Clin North Am 1988; 72:1177–211.

Each of these three review articles describes the epidemiology and clinical manifestations of thyroid nodules, and the diagnostic and therapeutic options available for managing patients with such nodules.

Gharib H, et al. Suppressive therapy with levothyroxine for solitary thyroid nodules. A double-blind controlled clinical study. N Engl J Med 1987; 317:70–5.

T_4 therapy for 6 months was no more effective than was placebo in reducing nodule size in patients with thyroid nodules.

Hamburger JI. The autonomously functioning thyroid nodule: Goetsch's disease. Endocr Rev 1987; 8:439–47.

This article reviews the pathophysiology, manifestations, and management of autonomously functioning thyroid adenomas.

Hamburger JI. Evolution of toxicity in solitary nontoxic autonomously functioning thyroid nodules. J Clin Endocrinol Metab 1980; 50:1089–93.

These nodules were found to change in size or function in only a minority of a large group of patients followed for up to 15 years.

93. GOITER
Robert D. Utiger

Visible and/or palpable thyroid enlargement occurs in 3 to 8% of adults living in areas in which iodine intake is adequate. Virtually all of these patients are clinically and biochemically euthyroid.

Thyroid enlargement may take the form of (1) a diffuse goiter, in which both thyroid lobes are more or less equally enlarged and their surfaces relatively smooth; (2) a multinodular goiter, in which both lobes are irregularly enlarged; or (3) a solitary thyroid nodule. In large groups of patients with nontoxic goiter, roughly two-thirds have diffuse or multinodular goiter and one-third have solitary nodules. The evaluation and management of the patient with a solitary nodule are discussed in Chapter 92.

Diffuse goiter and multinodular goiter are distinguished primarily by physical examination. Serum thyroxine (T_4), free T_4 index, and thyroid-stimulating hormone (TSH, thyrotropin) should be measured to document that the patient is euthyroid (see Chap. 89). Thyroid antibody tests identify those patients with diffuse goiter who have chronic autoimmune thyroiditis. Thyroid radioiodine uptake measurements and thyroid radioisotope scans provide little information beyond that gained by palpation of the thyroid gland and should not be done routinely in patients with goiter.

Chronic Autoimmune Thyroiditis (Goitrous Autoimmune Thyroiditis, Hashimoto's Disease)

Clinical Characteristics

The goitrous form of chronic autoimmune thyroiditis is the most common cause of diffuse goiter. Most patients are women between 30 and 50 years old. The thyroid enlargement is typically moderate and symmetric, and gland surface is slightly irregular or occasionally nodular, and its texture is firm. Most patients are clinically euthyroid and have normal or slightly decreased serum T_4 concentrations and normal or slightly increased serum TSH concentrations, but some patients have overt hypothyroidism.

Pathogenesis
Goitrous autoimmune thyroiditis is a disorder of both antibody- and cell-mediated immunity. The responsible autoantibodies include cytotoxic antibodies, antibodies that inhibit TSH binding to its receptor, and antibodies that inhibit thyroid peroxidase. There is intrathyroidal accumulation of T and B cells, and decreased suppressor T-cell activity. Variations in the nature and degree of these abnormalities in serum and cellular immunity probably explain the variations in functional impairment and response to therapy found in patients with Hashimoto's disease.

Diagnosis
The diagnosis is most readily confirmed by positive results of serum tests for antithyroid microsomal antibodies; these antibodies are present, usually in high titer, in most patients with Hashimoto's disease. Positive results for antithyroglobulin antibodies are somewhat less frequent, and so tests for them are less useful. Thyroid antibodies may also be found in patients with other thyroid diseases, especially Graves' disease, and in normal individuals, but when positive, the antibody titers are much lower in these groups. Thyroid radioisotope scans show either uniform or heterogeneous patterns of isotope uptake, but at times the pattern is so varied that it resembles that of a multinodular goiter.

Prognosis
The disease usually progresses slowly over a period of months or years to the development of overt hypothyroidism. Thyroid enlargement persists, although remissions occur in some patients with small goiters and normal or near-normal thyroid function.

Treatment
To reduce the size of the thyroid gland and prevent hypothyroidism, T_4 therapy, in dosages of 75 to 150 µg daily, is recommended, except perhaps for those patients who have only slight thyroid enlargement and normal serum T_4 and TSH concentrations. The patient should be re-examined after 2 to 3 months of therapy, and semiannually or annually thereafter. In the majority of patients, thyroid size gradually diminishes. Less often, the reduction occurs rapidly and is nearly complete, or there is no change. Withdrawal of therapy is almost always followed by recurrent thyroid enlargement and/or hypothyroidism; therapy therefore should be lifelong.

Sporadic Diffuse Goiter (Simple Goiter)

Clinical Characteristics
Sporadic diffuse goiter is defined as thyroid enlargement in a euthyroid patient that does not result from an inflammatory, infiltrative, or neoplastic process. Patients with sporadic diffuse goiter are usually young women, ranging in age from 10 to 30 years. The thyroid gland is usually only moderately enlarged and is soft in consistency. Serum T_4 concentrations are normal, and serum TSH concentrations occasionally are slightly increased.

Pathogenesis
Sporadic diffuse goiter is a descriptive term, applied to a finding on physical examination. Such goiters are in fact heterogeneous when studied histologically; they contain both small hyperplastic and larger quiescent thyroid follicles. These goiters are believed, at least in their early stages, to be caused by slight TSH hypersecretion secondary to very small decreases in thyroid hormone secretion. Postulated causes of the decreased thyroid secretion include mild inherited thyroid biosynthetic defects, environmental goitrogens or drugs, and iodide excess; however, firm evidence implicating any of these factors is sparse and rarely obtained in an individual patient.

Diagnosis
This diagnosis may be made when tests for antithyroid antibodies are negative in a clinically and biochemically euthyroid patient with diffuse thyroid enlargement.

Treatment

Although treatment is not required, if thyroid enlargement concerns the patient, T_4 therapy may be given. Treatment results in some reduction in thyroid enlargement in the majority of patients and may limit the evolution from diffuse to nodular goiter.

Nontoxic Nodular Goiter

Clinical Characteristics

Nontoxic multinodular goiter is a common type of thyroid enlargement, especially in women above the age of 30 to 40 years. Such goiters may be discovered incidentally or found in patients with a long-standing history of thyroid enlargement. The patient is usually asymptomatic but may have local symptoms of thyroid enlargement, such as neck fullness, difficulty swallowing, or coughing. Both thyroid lobes are irregularly, asymmetrically enlarged; it may be possible to palpate discrete nodules of varying size and consistency. Rarely, a multinodular goiter reaches sufficient size to produce thoracic inlet obstruction or respiratory symptoms. Acute hemorrhage into a nodule may occur, resulting in a sudden increase in its size and neck pain; the pain usually subsides in a few days and the swelling subsides in several weeks.

Diagnosis

Thyroid secretion and serum thyroid hormone concentrations in patients with nontoxic multinodular goiter are, by definition, within normal limits, but such patients may have decreased serum TSH concentrations, indicating some degree of thyroid autonomy. Thyroid radioisotope scans reveal a spectrum of abnormalities, ranging from a heterogeneous uptake pattern to discrete hyperfunctioning or hypofunctioning areas that often correlate poorly with palpable nodules. From the practical point of view, the diagnosis is made by palpation. Euthyroidism should be confirmed by serum T_4 and TSH measurements; other tests are not usually indicated. In the absence of obvious nodules, tests for antithyroid antibodies serve to rule out goitrous autoimmune thyroiditis (Hashimoto's disease).

Pathogenesis

Nontoxic multinodular goiter is thought to evolve from diffuse goiter (see previous section) by progressive enlargement of local areas of autonomous hyperplasia. The growth of the palpable nodules that form as a result of this process often does not correlate with their function, so that they are seen as either hyper- or hypofunctioning on thyroid radioisotope scans, depending on whether or not they transport iodide. In time, some nodules become necrotic, cystic, or fibrotic.

Prognosis

The natural history of nontoxic multinodular goiter is one of very gradual thyroid enlargement. Continued growth of one or more autonomous hyperplastic nodules may result in hyperthyroidism, although this is rare, even in patients with large multinodular goiters. This disorder does not result in hypothyroidism. Carcinoma in a nontoxic multinodular goiter is rare, but should be suspected if a nodule is very hard and enlarges rapidly.

Treatment

If the multinodular goiter is small and there are no pressure symptoms or cosmetic problems, treatment is unnecessary. If treatment is indicated or desired by the patient, T_4 therapy may be tried. T_4 in daily doses of 100 to 150 µg modestly reduces the thyroid enlargement in about 50% of patients; rarely if ever is the normal thyroid size regained. Therapy should be given for 6 to 12 months before being abandoned as ineffective. T_4 therapy is not without hazard; it may cause hyperthyroidism in patients whose endogenous thyroid secretion is largely autonomous, as indicated by a low serum TSH concentration. If treated with T_4, the patient should be re-examined and the serum T_4 and TSH concentrations determined after several months of therapy. The development of clinical evidence of hyperthyroidism and/or a rise in serum T_4 concentration mandates the discontinuation of therapy. Very large multinodular goiters causing pressure or obstructive symptoms require surgical removal. Iodides in any form should not be administered to patients with multinodular goiter because they may induce hyperthyroidism.

Utiger RD. Disorders of the thyroid gland. In: Kelley WN, ed. Textbook of internal medicine. Vol. 2. 2nd ed. Philadelphia: JB Lippincott, 1992: 1992–2001.
This chapter includes short discussions on chronic thyroiditis and nontoxic diffuse and nodular goiter.

Hamburger JI. The various presentations of thyroiditis: diagnostic considerations. Ann Intern Med 1986; 104:219–24.
This article describes the several forms of thyroiditis and the evaluation of patients with goiter.

Hayashi Y, et al. A long term clinical, immunological and histological followup study of patients with goitrous chronic lympholytic thyroiditis. J Clin Endocrinol Metab 1985; 61:1172–8.
Among 43 patients followed for 10 to 20 years, thyroid size diminished in 57% of the T_4-treated patients and in 13% of the untreated patients, and hypothyroidism developed in 38% of the untreated patients. Thyroid histology changed little in either treated or untreated patients.

Studer H, Gerber H, Peter HJ. Multinodular goiter. In: DeGroot LJ, ed. Endocrinology. Vol. 1. 2nd ed. Philadelphia: WB Saunders, 1989: 722–32.
A succinct review of the pathogenesis and management of multinodular goiter.

94. HYPERCALCEMIA
Robert H. Fletcher

Hypercalcemia can cause obvious symptoms or can be a complication of a serious underlying disease, such as cancer or sarcoidosis. Usually, however, hypercalcemia is asymptomatic and discovered by accident on a serum chemistry panel performed as part of a general health examination or as an investigation of problems unrelated to hypercalcemia.

Definition
Serum calcium is ordinarily measured as the concentration of the total ionized and bound calcium. Because most calcium is bound to serum albumin, total serum calcium levels may vary with concentration of serum albumin. As a rule of thumb, serum calcium levels rise or fall 0.7 mg/dl per 1 g/dl of albumin. Ionized serum calcium assays have the theoretic advantage of measuring the physiologically active form of calcium. However, in ambulatory patients, assays for ionized calcium provide little additional information. Levels of ionized and total calcium (corrected for albumin concentration) are highly correlated. Also, while ionized calcium assays can detect subtle abnormalities better, this information is rarely useful in patient care.

Hypercalcemia is usually defined as a serum calcium concentration above 10.5 mg/dl (2.62 mmol/L). The precise definition of the upper limit varies from one laboratory to another according to the analytic method used, the reference population, and the choice of a cutoff point between normal and abnormal.

The prevalence of persistently elevated serum calcium levels in asymptomatic adults in the general population is in the 1/100 to 1/1000 range, depending on the criteria for abnormality and the population studied. The prevalence rises with age in women but not in men.

Judgments about the presence of hypercalcemia should not be based on single determinations. Elevations are usually small (< 1.0 mg/dl), and there is broad overlap between normal levels and levels in people with disease causing hypercalcemia. In one study, for example, 42% of patients with documented hyperparathyroidism had a mean serum calcium concentration of 10.5 mg/dl or less. Many people with a serum calcium level above 10.5 mg/dl on one determination have lower levels when the test is repeated. Therefore, serum calcium should be considered elevated only after several high levels are obtained, unless the initial levels are very high, hypercalcemia was strongly suspected before the test, or there is an associated disease that might be a cause (e.g., multiple myeloma) or a complication (e.g., renal stones) of hypercalcemia.

Symptoms
Serum calcium concentrations in the 10.5- to 11.0-mg/dl range usually are not symptomatic. In general, the faster the rise in serum calcium, the more severe the symptoms at a given serum concentration.

The classic symptoms of hypercalcemia include, in descending order of frequency, fatigue, polydipsia, mental confusion, anorexia, polyuria, nausea and vomiting, muscle weakness and constipation. Other manifestations are related to the underlying cause or to complications: bone pain, renal stones, pancreatitis, and rarely, peptic ulcer disease. Hypertension may be more prevalent in patients with hypercalcemia.

It is often difficult to detect hypercalcemia by symptoms alone. Relatively few patients have the pronounced hypercalcemia syndrome. Because the symptoms are nonspecific and common, they are easily overlooked or attributed to other diseases. Similarly, if elevated serum calcium is known to be present, it may be difficult to know, without a trial of treatment, whether it is causing symptoms.

Causes
The majority of people with mild, persistent hypercalcemia in the general population have hyperparathyroidism; approximately 90% of those identified in a general hospital have primary hyperparathyroidism or cancer. Other conditions causing hypercalcemia are less commonly encountered, and the elevations are usually not sufficiently severe or protracted to cause major complications.

Primary hyperparathyroidism is twice as common in women as in men. Until recently, primary hyperparathyroidism was usually discovered because of complications: renal stones, painful bone disease, peptic ulcer disease, or overt hypercalcemia syndrome. Now, because of widespread use of serum chemistry panels that include measurement of serum calcium, many patients (about half in one study of a community) are discovered to have primary hyperparathyroidism because of small elevations in serum calcium. Most remain asymptomatic and without detectable complications for many years after diagnosis.

Cancer often causes hypercalcemia, with carcinomas of the breast and bronchus most common. A wide variety of other malignancies can also be responsible. Multiple myeloma usually causes hypercalcemia at some time in its course. Usually the neoplasm is overt. In one series, 75% of patients had obvious bone metastases at the time the elevated serum calcium was discovered. However, hypercalcemia can occur in malignancy without metastatic bone lesions; a protein related to parathyroid hormone factor appears to be responsible for most cases of humoral hypercalcemia of malignancy. Most malignant hypercalcemia is slight and only mildly symptomatic. Renal stones and nonmetastatic bone disease are uncommon, presumably because the duration of disease is too short for metabolic complications to occur.

Thiazide diuretics decrease renal excretion of calcium and elevate mean serum calcium slightly. In approximately 2% of patients, thiazides cause hypercalcemia. In some patients, serum calcium falls after withdrawal of thiazides, usually within a month. However, most of these patients have persistent hypercalcemia when thiazides are stopped and have parathyroid adenomas found at surgery. Chlorthalidone has the same effects but other diuretics (e.g., furosemide, ethacrynic acid, spironolactone) do not cause hypercalcemia.

Vitamin D in pharmacologic dosages (as little as 50,000 IU twice a week) causes hypercalcemia by increasing intestinal absorption. This problem is found in "food faddists" and patients treated overzealously with vitamin D.

Paget's disease occasionally causes hypercalcemia in ambulatory patients. More often hypercalcemia is precipitated by a period of immobilization, in which bone deposition is decreased and the effects of abnormally high resorption are unmasked.

Sarcoidosis is associated with hypercalcemia at some time in its course, in as many as 10% of patients. The degree of hypercalcemia follows the activity of the disease and is rarely severe.

Lithium carbonate therapy, given for bipolar (manic-depressive) illness, apparently causes a small increase in parathyroid hormone secretion and is associated with small elevations in serum calcium concentrations, and rarely, overt hypercalcemia.

Thyrotoxicosis occasionally causes elevations in serum calcium, but rarely does it cause the symptoms and complications of hypercalcemia.

In the *milk-alkali syndrome,* hypercalcemia is found in association with renal insufficiency, usually in patients with peptic ulcer disease who ingest large amounts of milk and absorbable antacids (e.g., bicarbonate of soda). It is now rarely seen, perhaps because newer approaches to ulcer therapy and other forms of antacids are widely available.

In *secondary hyperparathyroidism,* patients with physiologic causes of low serum calcium concentrations (e.g., renal failure or malabsorption) have adaptive increases in parathyroid function, with return of serum calcium toward normal. It has been suggested that stimulated glands occasionally become autonomous after the hypocalcemic stimulus is removed (tertiary hyperparathyroidism), for example, after renal transplantation, but the evidence for this is not conclusive. Hypercalcemia rarely occurs under these circumstances, and if it does, calcium homeostasis returns to normal spontaneously.

Familial hypercalcemia is uncommon. Two types have been described. Familial hypocalciuric hypercalcemia resembles primary hyperparathyroidism in clinical presentation, and rarely causes complications. It is characterized by autosomal dominant inheritance and low renal excretion of calcium. Multiple endocrine neoplasia type I (MEN I) is also inherited as an autosomal dominant and is characterized by neoplasia and autonomous endocrine activity of the pituitary and parathyroid glands and the pancreas, and, in addition, peptic ulcer disease.

Other causes of hypercalcemia include *acute adrenal insufficiency, vitamin A intoxication,* and *phosphorus depletion.*

Evaluation

Faced with newly recognized hypercalcemia, the clinician should briefly consider the evidence for each possible cause. Most of the causes—but not hyperparathyroidism—can be detected or ruled out by a simple set of observations.

Primary hyperparathyroidism, in its classic form, is manifested by repeatedly elevated serum calcium concentrations, depressed serum phosphate, and hyperchloremic acidosis (e.g., serum $Cl^- > 102$). There may be elevated serum alkaline phosphatase levels, bone changes, and subperiosteal resorption, best seen by x-ray in the finger tufts; all these are signs of late and/or severe disease. In practice, the disease is often mild and the evidence equivocal. A number of assays for parathyroid hormone (PTH), reacting to different determinants of the PTH molecule, are available. PTH levels are interpreted in relation to serum calcium levels. In general, the sensitivity of these assays for detecting hyperparathyroidism is in the 50 to 95% range and the specificity in distinguishing hyperparathyroidism from the hypercalcemia of malignancy is 50 to 90%, depending on the assay. However, large elevations in individual patients can be definitive. Often the presumptive diagnosis of hyperparathyroidism is made by excluding other causes of hypercalcemia. The only definitive evidence for hyperparathyroidism is the finding of one or more pathologic parathyroid glands at surgery.

Drugs that can cause hypercalcemia should be inquired about; these include a thiazide, vitamin D, lithium, or vitamin A. If the patient is a "food faddist," and the history of vitamin D ingestion is difficult to elicit, elevated serum $1,25(OH)_2\text{-}D_3$ levels are diagnostic. If any of these drugs is responsible, serum calcium levels should fall within weeks of withdrawal. Also, ask if the patient ingests large amounts of sodium bicarbonate or calcium carbonate (e.g., Tums, Titralac). It is estimated that about 2 dozen doses (e.g., tablets) per day for weeks are necessary to develop milk-alkali syndrome.

Cancer is usually obvious from the history and physical examination, with particular attention to bone pain and common primary sites (breast and lung). Multiple myeloma usually has concomitant anemia or proteinuria.

Paget's disease should be considered in elderly, immobilized patients with elevated serum alkaline phosphatase. X-rays of the hips, spine, or skull (according to symptoms) confirm the diagnosis.

Sarcoidosis may be associated with few chest symptoms, but there is usually chest disease that is easily seen on x-ray. Response to a therapeutic trial of corticosteroids supports sarcoidosis as a cause, although many patients with other causes of hypercalcemia also respond.

Thyrotoxicosis is usually overt, except in the elderly. When in doubt, a serum thyroid panel settles the issue.

Previous chronic severe hypocalcemia from renal failure or malabsorption is clear from the medical history. In renal failure a normal serum calcium suggests increased parathyroid activity.

In practice, *familial hypocalciuric hypercalcemia* is recognized by a family history and/or a failure to respond to parathyroidectomy. MEN I is established by family history and/or evidence of autonomous activity of one of the other endocrine glands ordinarily involved (pituitary and pancreas) or the presence of peptic ulcer disease.

Management

Mild, asymptomatic hypercalcemia, of whatever cause, need not be treated. If there are no symptoms or complications, it is reasonable simply to observe patients with hyperparathyroidism, particularly if serum calcium elevations are small (e.g., < 11.5 mg/dl), the patient is at high surgical risk, or there is reason to believe the patient will not live many years. There must be reliable surveillance for changes in serum calcium concentrations or the onset of complications. Re-evaluation every 4 to 6 months is usually appropriate; most cases do not progress. It is common practice to treat hypercalcemia if serum calcium is consistently above 12.0 mg/dl; some physicians set this level as low as 11.0 mg/dl.

The following summarizes the various means of controlling chronic hypercalcemia in nonhospitalized patients. The treatment of hypercalcemia emergencies is not discussed.

Hydration and activity are the mainstays of management. Fluid intake should be at least 3 L per day, and dehydration should be avoided at all times. Inactivity reduces the rate of calcium deposition in bone and should also be avoided. For patients who might have increased calcium absorption from the gut (e.g., some patients with hyperparathyroidism or sarcoidosis), dietary calcium is often restricted. Ordinarily, this amounts to avoiding dairy products.

Drugs that aggravate hypercalcemia—thiazides and vitamin D—should be withdrawn. Several drugs have been used to lower serum calcium concentrations. Furosemide and ethacrynic acid increase renal calcium excretion but at the expense of a negative calcium balance, which in the long term may increase the rate at which bone disease develops. Corticosteroids lower serum calcium in some patients with malignant hypercalcemia and most with sarcoidosis. The onset of action is within several days. Other drugs that have been suggested and may be useful under certain circumstances include oral phosphates, estrogens, calcitonin, diphosphonates, beta-blockers and histamine blockers.

Marcus R, ed. Hypercalcemia. Endocrinol Metab Clin North Am 1989; 18(3):601–832.
An entire issue devoted to hypercalcemia. Among the articles are reviews of primary hyperparathyroidism: clinical presentation and factors influencing clinical management (pp. 631–46), laboratory diagnosis of primary hyperparathyroidism (pp. 647–58), unusual causes of hypercalcemia (pp. 753–64), and treatment of hypercalcemia (pp. 807–28).

Fradkin JE. Diagnosis and management of asymptomatic primary hyperparathyroidism. National Institutes of Health consensus development conference statement. Ann Intern Med 1991; 114:593–7.
Presents the findings of an expert panel.

Palmer M, et al. The prevalence of hypercalcemia in a health survey: a 14 year follow-up study of serum calcium values. Eur J Clin Invest 1988; 18:39–46.
A follow-up of 16,401 people in Sweden; 176 (1%) had persistent hypercalcemia.

Lufkin EG, Kao PC, Heath H III. Parathyroid hormone radioimmunoassays in the differential diagnosis of hypercalcemia due to primary hyperparathyroidism or malignancy. Ann Intern Med 1987; 106:559–60.
Shows serum PTH levels for 20 normal persons, 20 patients with humoral hypercalcemia of malignancy, and 14 patients with hyperparathyroidism, as assayed by five different laboratories.

Gray TA, Paterson CR. The clinical value of ionized calcium assays. Ann Clin Biochem 1988; 25:210–9.
Reviews evidence for the clinical value of ionized calcium assays and finds that they may be useful in specific situations: multiple myeloma, massive citrate infusion, renal failure, and severe illness.

Bonjour JP, et al. Management of hypercalcemia in relation to pathophysiology. Bone 1987;8:Suppl 1:S29–S33.
Describes the management of hypercalcemia according to the underlying cause and mechanism.

Bilezikian JP. The medical management of primary hyperparathyroidism. Ann Intern Med 1982; 96:198–202.
A review of the various modalities available to manage primary hyperparathyroidism when patients are asymptomatic and surgery is not done.

Heath H III, Hodgson SF, Kennedy MA. Primary hyperparathyroidism. N Engl J Med 1980; 302:189–93.
A description of the incidence of hyperparathyroidism in a defined population (Rochester, Minn.), by age and sex, for 1965 to 1974.

Gordon DL, et al. The serum calcium level and its significance in hyperthyroidism: a prospective study. Am J Med Sci 1974; 268:31–6.
Mild hypercalcemia was found in 17% of patients with hyperthyroidism.

Wong ET, Freier EF. The differential diagnosis of hypercalcemia. An algorithm for more effective use of laboratory tests. JAMA 1982; 247:75–80.
An algorithm for determining the cause of hypercalcemia, based on experience with hospitalized patients.

95. ASYMPTOMATIC HYPERURICEMIA
Kenneth E. Sack

The normal serum urate level, determined enzymatically, is less than 7.0 mg/dl, the level at which monosodium urate is saturated in serum. Most laboratories measure serum urate colorimetrically. By this method, urate levels are 0.5 to 1.0 mg/dl higher and may be falsely elevated in patients taking xanthines, methyldopa, L-dopa, or ascorbic acid.

Serum urate levels normally rise in males at puberty and in females at menopause. This rise from the average prepubescent level of 3.5 mg/dl is due largely to the decrease in urate excretion that begins in men at puberty and in women at menopause.

Increased serum urate concentrations result from either overproduction or underexcretion of uric acid concentration. Some individuals produce too much uric acid by virtue of an increased de novo purine biosynthesis. Another mechanism for overproduction is the increased nucleic acid turnover associated with myeloproliferative diseases, hemolytic anemias, and psoriasis. Hyperuricemia can result also from the increased breakdown of adenosine triphosphate (ATP) that sometimes accompanies severe illness, strenuous exercise, excessive alcohol consumption, and type I glycogen storage disease. Underexcretion of uric acid can occur in patients with chronic renal insufficiency or those with decreased tubular secretion but normal renal function. Organic acids, thiazides, nicotinic acid, and aspirin (in low doses) induce hyperuricemia by inhibiting the renal tubular secretion of uric acid.

Risks
Most patients with hyperuricemia never develop symptoms. Though several prospective studies describe the complications of prolonged hyperuricemia, no study has provided data

on the duration of pre-entry hyperuricemia. The potential consequences of hyperuricemia are acute and chronic gout, renal calculi (composed of either uric acid or calcium oxalate), gouty nephropathy, and acute uric acid nephropathy.

Gout
In the community-based, prospective Framingham Study, the risk of having an attack of gout during a 12-year period rose with increasing elevations in serum urate level. Gout developed in 2% of patients whose maximum serum urate level was less than 7.0 mg/dl. For a urate level between 7.0 and 7.9 mg/dl, the risk was 17%; and for levels between 8.0 and 8.9 mg/dl, the risk was 25%. Nine of the 10 patients with a serum urate level greater than 9.0 mg/dl developed gout. Of 179 women with serum urate levels greater than 6.0 mg/dl, only 5% developed gout. In a shorter-term study, only 3 of 69 men whose serum urate levels were greater than 9.0 mg/dl developed gout over a 4-year period. Thus, most patients with hyperuricemia never develop gout and do not require therapy. Some patients with a serum urate level persistently over 9 mg/dl will eventually have an attack of gout, but many will not. It is prudent, therefore, to avoid urate-lowering therapy until symptoms occur.

Renal Stones
The prevalence of uric acid nephrolithiasis in patients with gout reportedly increases in proportion to the degree of urinary uric acid excretion. In an often quoted study, uric acid calculi occurred in 11% of patients who excreted less than 300 mg of uric acid in 24 hours; they occurred in 50% of those who excreted greater than 1100 mg in 24 hours. (Stones were also more prevalent in patients with a urine pH < 5.6.) The study population, however, consisted of symptomatic patients seen at a highly specialized facility. In an analysis of 124 asymptomatic hyperuricemic patients, only one renal calculus (composed of calcium oxalate) occurred during a 6-year period. Mean 24-hour uric acid excretion in 49 of these patients was between 600 and 700 mg $\pm$ 230 mg. Presumably, hyperuricosuria, low urine pH, and dehydration contribute to the formation of uric acid calculi; but the available data do not support treating asymptomatic hyperuricemia to prevent renal calculi.

Gouty Nephropathy
Gouty nephropathy refers to the deposition of urate crystals in the renal interstitium, often with an accompanying giant cell reaction. Renal concentrating defects, proteinuria, and hypertension are sometimes attributed to this lesion. Several long-term studies, however, do not confirm that hyperuricemia by itself causes significant loss of renal function.

Acute Uric Acid Nephropathy
The acute hyperuricemia and hyperuricosuria that occur during the treatment of lymphoproliferative and myeloproliferative disorders (and occasionally with disseminated carcinoma) can cause acute renal failure, presumably due to the intraluminal precipitation of uric acid in renal collecting ducts. Therefore, it is essential to administer allopurinol and to maintain adequate hydration before and throughout chemotherapy for these conditions.

Accompanying Conditions
Numerous studies indicate an association of hyperuricemia with hypertension, diabetes mellitus, and hyperlipidemia. These latter conditions are probably responsible for the known link between hyperuricemia and cardiovascular disease. Treating hyperuricemia, however, does not reduce the risk of developing cardiovascular disease.

Treatment
Asymptomatic hyperuricemia requires no treatment. As noted previously, an elevation in serum urate level per se presents little risk to the kidneys; and the occurrence of gout is unpredictable, even at high serum urate levels. By contrast, all patients scheduled to receive chemotherapy for lymphoproliferative and myeloproliferative disorders should be given pretreatment allopurinol to prevent acute uric acid nephropathy.

Becker MA. Clinical aspects of monosodium urate monohydrate crystal deposition disease (gout). Rheum Dis Clin North Am 1988; 14:377–94.
 A detailed, understandable review of the mechanisms of hyperuricemia.

Brand FN, et al. Hyperuricemia as a risk factor of coronary heart disease: the Framingham Study. Am J Epidemiol 1985; 121:11–8.
This large, prospective study showed that the serum urate level is not an independent risk factor for the development of coronary heart disease.

Faller J, Fox IH. Ethanol-induced hyperuricemia. N Engl J Med 1982; 307:1598–602.
Ethanol, in addition to decreasing the renal excretion of uric acid, enhances urate production by increasing the turnover of adenine nucleotides.

Fessel WJ, Barr GD. Uric acid, lean body weight, and creatinine interactions: results from regression analysis of 78 variables. Semin Arthritis Rheum 1977; 7:115–21.
The nonadipose portion of body weight correlates best with serum urate levels. Elevated serum urate levels alone have little effect on renal function.

Fessel WJ. Renal outcomes of gout and hyperuricemia. Am J Med 1979; 67:74–82.
This long-term prospective study showed that hyperuricemia alone does not substantially increase the risk of developing azotemia or urolithiasis. According to these data, a theoretic cohort of patients followed for 40 years would not develop clinically important azotemia if serum urate levels were below 13 mg/dl for men and 10 mg/dl for women.

Hall AP, et al. Epidemiology of gout and hyperuricemia. Am J Med 1967; 42:27–37.
The Framingham data correlate serum urate level with the risk of developing gout. Note, however, that the criteria for gout excluded patients with normal serum urate levels.

Langford HG, et al. Is thiazide-produced uric acid elevation harmful? Arch Intern Med 1987; 147:645–9.
Five-year follow-up of 3693 patients participating in a hypertension study showed no effect of serum urate level on subsequent renal function.

Wooliscroft JO, Colfer H, Fox IH. Hyperuricemia in acute illness: a poor prognostic sign. Am J Med 1982; 72:58–62.
Six of 16 patients admitted to a coronary care unit died. Their mean baseline serum urate level was 11.1 mg/dl (peak = 20.7 mg/dl) compared to the 10 survivors (mean baseline level = 6.8 mg/dl, peak = 7.1 mg/dl). The authors postulated that tissue hypoxia leads to accelerated tissue nucleotide degradation with subsequent increased urate production.

Yu TF, Gutman AB. Uric acid nephrolithiasis in gout. Ann Intern Med 1967; 67:1133–48.
This often-quoted study showed a positive correlation of urinary uric acid excretion with the risk for developing renal calculi. The importance of increased urine acidity in causing the precipitation of uric acid in the urinary tract is discussed. The known interest of these authors in disorders of urate metabolism generated an enormous patient selection bias.

96. CORTICOSTEROID THERAPY AND WITHDRAWAL
David R. Clemmons

Corticosteroids are among the most effective and potentially dangerous drugs commonly prescribed. Their safe use requires an understanding of their physiologic effects and side effects.

Adrenal Physiology

Cortisol secretion by the adrenal gland is controlled by pituitary corticotropin (ACTH) release, which varies from minute to minute. This results in a pulsatile secretory pattern in plasma cortisol levels, but when these values are integrated the mean hormone concentration characteristically shows a pattern of diurnal variation. Under nonstressed conditions, cortisol is secreted at a rate of 15 to 20 mg/day, with a mean plasma 8 AM concentration of 10 mg/dl (range, 6–20 mg/dl), and a mean 10 PM concentration of 2 µg/dl. The cortisol secretory rate is increased during periods of stress, pregnancy, and many illnesses.

Stress is the most powerful stimulus to corticotropin secretion; it will override the normal basal corticotropin pulsations and diurnal variation.

Pharmacology of Glucocorticoids

Synthetic analogues of cortisol have enhanced biologic potency compared to cortisol, with less sodium retention at equivalent anti-inflammatory doses. They have a longer duration of action (e.g., cortisol, 8–12 hours; prednisolone, 12–36 hours; dexamethasone, 36–54 hours). Table 96-1 lists several corticosteroid preparations with their relative potencies and approximate equivalent dosages. The anti-inflammatory effect of each compound is proportional to its biologic half-life. The most commonly administered corticosteroids—prednisone, prednisolone, methylprednisolone, and triamcinolone—have intermediate half-lives. They are useful for alternate-day therapy because the hypothalamic-pituitary-adrenal (HPA) axis suppression is, in general, not apparent on the day on which no steroid is given. The salt-retaining effects of different preparations vary greatly; cortisone has the greatest mineralocorticoid activity, whereas dexamethasone has the least.

HPA Axis Suppression

Exogenous administration of glucocorticoids suppresses the HPA axis. Acute administration of glucocorticoids does not block the stress-mediated increase in cortisol secretion, but long-term administration is associated with considerable suppression. The exact time interval required to induce suppression is unknown, but it generally is believed to be between 2 weeks and 2 months, depending on the dosage, frequency of administration, and the type of steroid. Administration of 50 mg of prednisone for 5 days has been shown to suppress the HPA axis for a few days, usually without clinically important consequences. However, continued therapy with glucocorticoid dosages greater than 20 to 30 mg of prednisone per day results in continuous 24-hour suppression of corticotropin secretion and leads to loss of the stress response after about 2 to 4 weeks. Equivalent doses of short- or intermediate-acting corticosteroids cause less suppression when given in the morning rather than in the evening and as a single dose rather than in divided doses, because there is less inhibition of normal diurnal cortisol secretion.

Recovery of the HPA axis occurs in phases. The pituitary secretion of corticotropin returns first, followed by the adrenal secretion of cortisol, and finally the stress response returns. Recovery of normal corticotropin and cortisol levels may take 5 to 9 months, but recovery of the response to stress may require a full year if suppression has been profound (e.g., several months of prednisone therapy).

Therapeutic Regimens

Short-Term, High-Dose Therapy

Conditions such as poison ivy and asthma exacerbations will respond to acute, short-term administration of corticosteroids (e.g., 60 mg of prednisone/day). The duration of therapy should be limited and the therapeutic end point determined at the outset. Often only a few days of treatment is required. If the duration of treatment is less than 2 weeks, therapy can be stopped abruptly without tapering, unless this is likely to exacerbate the underlying disease. Complications of short-term corticosteroid therapy include ulceration of the gastric mucosa, hyperglycemia, sodium retention, mood changes, acute psychosis, burning and itching of mucous membranes, and masking of signs and symptoms of underlying inflammation, such as acute appendicitis.

Prolonged Therapy

Long-term administration of corticosteroid therapy is used for a variety of inflammatory and other conditions. Doses of 80 mg/day or more of a hydrocortisone equivalent (e.g., 20 mg of prednisone) predictably cause Cushing's syndrome, with its complications of obesity, hypertension, glucose intolerance, myopathy, and osteoporosis, as well as impaired wound-healing, predisposition to infection, reactivation of tuberculosis, psychiatric problems, and aseptic necrosis of bone. The incidence of complications is variable and less predictable at lower corticosteroid dosages, but they can occur. In general, their frequency and severity are related to the duration of therapy, age of the patient, and presence of preexisting conditions such as osteoporosis. The association of corticosteroid therapy and

Table 96-1. Glucocorticoid preparations

USP name	Trade name	Tablet size (mg)	Relative anti-inflammatory potency	Relative mineralocorticoid potency	Approximate equivalent dose (mg)
Short-acting (biologic half-life 8–12 hr)					
Hydrocortisone (cortisol)	Cortef Solu-Cortef*	5, 10, 20	1.0	1.0	20.0
Cortisone		5, 10, 25	0.8	0.8	25.0
Intermediate-acting (biologic half-life 18–36 hr)					
Triamcinolone	Aristocort Kenacort	1, 2, 4, 8, 16	5.0	0	4.0
Paramethasone	Haldrone	1, 2	10.0	0	2.0
Prednisone	Deltasone Meticorten	1, 2.5, 5, 10, 20, 50	4.0	0.8	5.0
Prednisolone	Delta-Cortef Meticortelone	5	4.0	0.8	5.0
Methylprednisolone	Medrol Solu-Medrol*	2, 4, 8, 16, 24, 32	5.0	0.5	4.0
Long-acting (biologic half-life 36–54 hr)					
Dexamethasone	Decadron Hexadrol	0.25, 0.5, 0.75, 1.5, 4	25.0	0	0.75
Betamethasone	Celestone	0.6	25.0	0	0.6

*Parenteral forms: dosages of oral and parenteral preparations are generally comparable.

peptic ulcer disease is controversial. Multiple studies have produced conflicting results, but from pooled data it appears that the incidence of this complication is increased from 1% in control subjects to 2% in patients taking corticosteroids. It is not known whether concomitant treatment with antacids, H_2-receptor antagonists, or sucralfate reduces this risk.

For patients who have been on prolonged therapy, tapering must be done slowly, usually over several months' time, because the HPA axis is suppressed and the stress response is impaired. Steroid withdrawal is discussed in further detail below.

Alternate-Day Therapy
In order to avoid or lessen many complications of chronic steroid use, alternate-day therapy has been advocated. This is based on the presumption that the anti-inflammatory effects of corticosteroids last longer than the metabolic actions. Prednisone and prednisolone are used for this purpose because they have an intermediate half-life and usually do not cause HPA axis suppression on the day on which no steroid is given. In general, when suppression of the underlying disease is studied, alternate-day regimens compare favorably with daily therapy. However, some diseases, such as temporal arteritis and occasionally ulcerative colitis or pemphigus vulgaris, do not respond.

For optimal alternate-day therapy, it is important that the steroid be administered in the morning as a single dose. Otherwise, the effects of doses later in the day may persist into the alternate day and also will interfere with the nocturnal increase in corticotropin secretion. Transition to an alternate-day regimen must be done with great care in patients who have been taking steroids daily for several months and have consequently developed HPA axis suppression. Such patients may have no effective circulating glucocorticoid toward the end of the second day, and cannot respond to stress. In order to avoid this hazard, the patient's total dose should gradually be reduced as much as possible prior to the transition, and given as a single daily dose. Then the steroid dose on alternate days should be gradually reduced, with this dose added to the dose on the treatment day. For example, if the daily dose of prednisone is 20 to 40 mg, the dose on the first day should be increased by 5 mg, and the dose on the second day decreased by 5 mg. If the daily dose is 20 mg or less, the doses could be adjusted in 2.5-mg increments. At the end of the transition period, the patient will be taking the entire 2-day dose on the first day.

Withdrawal from Steroid Therapy

Problems
When a patient stops chronic steroid therapy, several problems may occur. First, the underlying disease may flare, requiring the re-institution of steroids. Second, adrenal insufficiency may occur, with arthralgias, fatigue, weakness, anorexia, nausea, and vomiting. Since secretion of mineralocorticoids is usually unimpaired by glucocorticoid-induced suppression of the HPA axis, dehydration, hyponatremia, and hyperkalemia are uncommon. Third, the "steroid withdrawal syndrome" may occur, characterized by the presence of symptoms similar to those of adrenal insufficiency in patients with normal serum glucocorticoid levels. Such patients may either be receiving physiologic (or supraphysiologic) doses of corticosteroids or have been recently withdrawn from steroid therapy, with normal HPA axis function. The most common clinical features of the withdrawal syndrome are anorexia, lethargy, malaise, nausea, weight loss, desquamation of the skin, headache, and fever. When such symptoms are severe or persistent, returning to the previous level of steroids and tapering more slowly are indicated. Increasing the dose to greater than previous levels will only increase steroid dependency.

Withdrawal Regimens
For patients who have been on long-term steroid therapy, the dose should be gradually tapered, for example, with a decrease of 5 mg of prednisone per week. When the patient has been weaned to "physiologic" doses (i.e., 5 mg of prednisone or prednisolone, 20 mg of hydrocortisone), adrenal function should be assessed. An 8 AM plasma cortisol level of 10 µg/dl or greater (with the blood sample drawn prior to the administration of the daily steroid dose) is indicative of normal basal cortisol secretion. But because cortisol secretion is pulsatile, physiologic variations in cortisol secretion make a single test result difficult

to interpret; multiple samples may be necessary for the reliable assessment of adrenal function. A more efficient approach is to measure cortisol after the administration of corticotropin, which also provides an assessment of adrenal response to stress. Since adrenal mass returns after pituitary secretion of corticotropin resumes, the function of the entire HPA axis can be inferred from the ability of the adrenal to respond appropriately to stimulation. The short corticotropin test can be performed at any time of day. Twenty-five units of synthetic corticotropin (cosyntropin) is given intravenously or intramuscularly, and a blood sample for cortisol is drawn at 30 or 60 minutes. A normal response is a stimulated value of 18 μg/dl or greater. If this is not present, the patient should be switched to 20 mg of hydrocortisone per day for 1 month. The daily dosage can then be decreased by 2.5 mg per week until a dosage of 10 mg/day is reached. This is maintained until a normal corticotropin response is obtained, at which time maintenance therapy is stopped.

Steroid Coverage for Stress
When the ability of the HPA axis to respond to stress is questionable or impaired, increased dosages of steroid are needed for illness, trauma, or surgery. The patient should carry medical alert information, as well as a prepackaged syringe containing 4 mg of dexamethasone to be administered in the event of unconsciousness or vomiting. For major surgery or trauma, 100 mg of hydrocortisone given parenterally every 6 to 8 hours is needed until the stress is resolved, usually in 3 or 4 days. The dosage is then tapered to physiologic levels, usually over a week. For other illnesses, such as influenza, gastroenteritis, or minor surgical procedures such as endoscopy or dental work, an additional 100 mg of hydrocortisone per day is needed, usually given in two doses.

Axelrod L. Glucocorticoid therapy. Medicine 1976; 55:39–63.
An excellent, exhaustive review that covers steroid pharmacology, withdrawal symptoms, and short- and long-term complications of steroid therapy.

Melby JC. Systemic corticosteroid therapy: pharmacology and endocrinologic considerations. Ann Intern Med 1974; 81:502–12.
A comprehensive discussion of the treatment modalities available and the pharmacology of each drug.

Byyny RL. Withdrawal from glucocorticoid therapy. N Engl J Med 1976; 295:30–2.
A succinct description of the withdrawal regimens and the required testing during steroid withdrawal.

Meikle AW, Tyler FH. Potency and duration of action of glucocorticoids: effects of hydrocortisone, prednisone, and dexamethasone on human pituitary adrenal function. Am J Med 1977; 63:200–7.
A detailed comparison of the pharmacologic potency, duration of action, and HPA axis–induced suppression of the major glucocorticoids.

Dixon MA, Christy NP. On the various forms of corticosteroid withdrawal syndrome. Am J Med 1980; 68:224–7.
Three cases that illustrate the variety of symptoms and clinical courses that may be manifested during steroid withdrawal.

Fauci AS, Dale DC, Balow JE. Glucocorticosteroid therapy: mechanisms of action and clinical considerations. Ann Intern Med 1976; 84:304–15.
A detailed discussion of the anti-inflammatory potency of several steroid preparations and the mechanism of action of each.

MacGregor RR, et al. Alternate-day prednisone therapy. N Engl J Med 1969; 280:1427–38.
A detailed discussion of the anti-inflammatory response to alternate-day therapy and the probability of avoiding severe chronic glucocorticoid-induced complications with this treatment.

Messer J, et al. Association of adrenocorticosteroid therapy and peptic ulcer disease. N Engl J Med 1983; 309:21–4.
A meta-analysis of 71 controlled clinical trials.

XIII. BLOOD PROBLEMS

97. ANEMIA
Peter C. Ungaro

Anemia, or low blood hemoglobin concentration, is a sign of disease rather than a disease in itself. The blood hemoglobin concentration below which anemia is considered to exist has been defined by the World Health Organization as 13 g/dl in men and 12 g/dl in adult, nonpregnant women (hematocrits of about 38 and 35%, respectively); other authoritative bodies have chosen similar levels. These levels are arbitrary and do not correspond to symptoms or risk of serious underlying disease.

Table 97-1 summarizes the distribution of hematocrit and hemoglobin levels in the general population. Lower levels in women are explained in part by the prevalence of iron deficiency, in addition to their lack of androgen-stimulated hematopoiesis. On the average, hematocrit levels rise about 2 "hematocrit points" in postmenopausal women.

Detection

History

The symptoms attributed to anemia (fatigue, generalized weakness, dyspnea on exertion, and light-headedness) are also common among people in general; moreover, many of the diseases that cause anemia, such as cancer, are themselves responsible for these same symptoms. Although there is strong evidence that hemoglobin levels above 10 g/dl do not produce an excess of symptoms, symptoms clearly do occur when anemia is severe. Rapidly acquired anemia, such as that which occurs with blood loss or destruction (hemolysis), is more often symptomatic than comparable anemia of gradual onset caused by a production defect, such as iron deficiency or pernicious anemia. Also, anemias are better tolerated by people who do not engage in vigorous activity. The history is more helpful, however, in determining the cause of anemia. Family history of anemia, history of chronic illness, previous blood counts, dietary habits, and pica may all give important clues to the cause. Also, a change in stool color, history of blood loss or hemorrhoids, gastrointestinal complaints, or the use of aspirin, nonsteroidal anti-inflammatory drugs, or corticosteroids may suggest bleeding.

Physical Examination

Examination of the conjunctivae, mucous membranes, nail beds, and palmar creases for pallor will detect only severe anemia (i.e., hematocrits < 25%). As with the history, the physical examination is better suited for detecting clues to the cause of anemia, rather than the anemia itself.

Laboratory Tests

It is not recommended that anemia be sought routinely on periodic examination or screening. The search for anemia usually is prompted by the finding of a condition known to cause anemia, such as excessive menstrual bleeding, gastrointestinal blood loss, or guaiac-positive stoool. The presence of anemia is confirmed by hematocrit or hemoglobin determinations, or by a Coulter counter complete blood count. Once anemia is found to be present, a precise cause must be sought.

Approach to Diagnosis

The diagnostic workup for anemia begins with a complete blood count, a calculated mean corpuscular volume (MCV), and a reticulocyte count. The reticulocyte count must be adjusted to the hematocrit by calculating the reticulocyte index (normal value is 1–3%):

$$\text{Reticulocyte count} \times \frac{\text{actual hematocrit}}{\text{normal hematocrit}} = \text{reticulocyte index}$$

The information from these readily available, inexpensive laboratory tests categorizes the anemia, thereby limiting the number of possible diagnoses and directing the subsequent evaluation.

In Table 97-2, the most common causes of anemia are characterized by reticulocyte

Table 97-1 Hematocrit and hemoglobin in a normal population

	Male	Female (nonpregnant)
Hematocrit (%)	44 (39–50)*	39 (33–45)
Hemoglobin (gm/dl)	15 (12–17)	13 (11–15)

*Mean and 95% confidence limits are given.

Table 97-2 Characterization of anemia by reticulocyte count and mean corpuscular volume (MCV)

Anemia with reticulocytopenia (reticulocyte index < 1%)
   Microcytic—MCV 82 fL
     Iron deficiency
     Thalassemia (often reticulocytosis)
     Sideroblastic anemia
     Anemia of chronic disease (sometimes)
   Macrocytic—MCV 100 fL
     B_{12} deficiency
     Folate deficiency
     Chronic liver disease
     Myxedema
   Normocytic—MCV 82–100 fL
   (anemias that are macrocytic or microcytic are normocytic when detected early)
     Anemia of chronic disease (usually)
     Bone marrow infiltrate or failure
Anemia with reticulocytosis (reticulocte index 3%)
   (MCV is often not helpful because reticulocytosis causes macrocytosis)
   Macrocytic
     Acute blood loss (sometimes)
     Acute hemolysis (sometimes)
     Postsplenectomy
   Microcytic
     Microangiopathic
     Certain hemoglobinopathies
   Normocytic
     Acute hemorrhage (usually)
     Acute hemolysis (usually)

count and MCV. The great majority of patients with anemia fall into one of the diagnostic categories in the table. Because the MCV has been shown to be the most useful red blood cell (RBC) index, the other traditional RBC indices—mean corpuscular hemoglobin (MCH) and mean corpuscular hemoglobin concentration (MCHC)—are not included in this table.

Additional helpful information can sometimes be obtained from the RBC distribution width (RDW). The RDW is particularly helpful when it is used along with MCV in evaluating reticulocytopenic anemias. The RDW becomes elevated before the MCV becomes abnormal in early iron, folate, and vitamin B_{12} deficiency states. The RDW is particularly helpful in differentiating iron deficiency anemia from other causes of microcytic anemia, such as the anemia of chronic disease and heterozygous β-thalassemia.

Microcytic Reticulocytopenic Anemia

Most adults with a microcytic reticulocytopenic anemia have iron deficiency, although early iron deficiency is often normocytic. It is generally thought that hemoglobin must fall 2 g/dl for the microcytosis of iron deficiency to be detectable. The RDW becomes wide before microcytosis develops. The majority of patients with microcytic reticulocytopenic anemia are menstruating women, many of whom have had multiple pregnancies, and who have iron loss in excess of their iron intake. Menstruating women lose an average of 2 mg of iron per day, whereas the average adult diet contains only 15 to 18 g of iron, of which only 10% is absorbed (1.5–1.8 mg/day). This imbalance is often compounded by previous, full-term pregnancies, which, even when uncomplicated, cause the loss of an additional 500 to 1000 mg of iron.

In contrast, iron loss in the adult man and postmenopausal woman occurs primarily through the shedding of epithelial cells in the gastrointestinal tract and amounts to only about 1 mg of iron per day. Therefore, iron deficiency in these patients requires an additional explanation. Usually the cause is blood loss from gastrointestinal bleeding; occasionally, it is iron malabsorption.

Dietary habits may contribute to iron deficiency. Some women do not eat adequate amounts of major sources of iron, such as liver, red meats, apricots, peaches, prunes, apples, grapes, raisins, spinach, and eggs. However, even the poorest of diets provides adequate iron for men and postmenopausal women. Laundry starch, clay, and ice sometimes eaten in large quantities because of an insatiable craving (pica) are symptoms that suggest iron deficiency. It is questionable whether significant iron is bound by these materials.

Evaluation
Menstruating women who have microcytic anemia with reticulocytopenia and no evidence of occult gastrointestinal blood loss usually have iron deficiency anemia and seldom require additional evaluation. In other instances of suspected iron deficiency, serum iron level, iron-binding capacity, and percent saturation may be obtained (iron/total iron-binding capacity [Fe/TIBC]). Characteristic of iron deficiency are a low serum iron level, elevated iron-binding capacity, and saturation of less than 16%. Unfortunately, there are many false-positives and -negatives. The level of serum ferritin, a large iron-storage protein compound found primarily intracellularly, is more useful than Fe/TIBC. A low ferritin level is highly diagnostic of iron deficiency. False elevations can occur with diseases such as hepatitis that affect storage sites. Thus, a normal level does not exclude iron deficiency. The "gold standard" for diagnosing iron deficiency is the demonstration of trace or no stainable iron on a bone marrow aspiration specimen. However, the clinical picture and laboratory evaluation are usually sufficient, and a bone marrow aspirate is seldom necessary.

Once a diagnosis of iron deficiency is confirmed in an adult man or postmenopausal woman, a diligent search for the source of blood loss must be made. Gastrointestinal blood loss should be considered the cause until proved otherwise. One should never assume that dietary iron has been inadequate, nor should iron therapy be given without a thorough search for the bleeding source.

Treatment
The treatment of choice for iron deficiency anemia is ferrous sulfate, 300 mg (60 mg of iron) 3 times a day with meals. It is inexpensive, effective, and tolerated by most patients. Unfortunately, ferrous iron causes mucosal irritation. While many expensive iron preparations are advertised as better tolerated than ferrous sulfate, tolerance is accomplished by providing less iron or less contact with the absorptive surface and, therefore, decreased iron absorption. Ferrous gluconate tablets (300 mg, containing 30 mg of iron) are less irritating, primarily because each of the tablets contains less iron. Enteric-release tablets are also less irritating but prevent the ferrous iron from coming in contact with the absorptive mucosa of the proximal gastrointestinal tract and, therefore, result in decreased absorption.

A number of simple measures may improve compliance with ferrous sulfate therapy. Taking iron with meals reduces absorption but makes the treatment more tolerable. Gastrointestinal side effects also seem to be reduced by starting with a single ferrous sulfate tablet daily and building up to two and then three tablets per day over a period of many days. Patients should not take antacids and iron at the same time because the hydrochloric acid in the gastric secretions promotes absorption by helping to maintain iron in solution.

It is rare that patients cannot take adequate amounts of oral iron if these precautions are taken.

In the absence of continued blood loss, effective iron therapy should result in a reticulocytosis, seldom exceeding 10%, by the 10th day of treatment. After 3 weeks of therapy, the hemoglobin levels should rise by more than half the difference between the initial level and the normal level for that patient. Once normal hemoglobin levels are achieved (usually in 6–8 weeks), iron must be continued for approximately 4 to 6 months to replenish the body stores of iron. The failure to respond to oral ferrous sulfate is most often due to not taking the medication or inhibition of the absorption caused by the innovative methods patients sometimes find to reduce gastrointestinal irritation. Because iron turns the stool black, ingestion can be monitored. Additionally, it is reasonable to confirm that the original diagnosis of iron deficiency was correct.

In rare cases of patients with gastrointestinal absorption problems or severe iron deficits, parenteral iron is needed. It is given as iron dextran (Imferon), administered as either a single intravenous infusion or as a series of intramuscular injections, with the dose calculated to replace the patient's estimated iron deficits. Side effects include severe pain and staining of the skin at the site of intramuscular injections and fever; anaphylaxis has been reported. The Z-tract injection technique is helpful in preventing skin staining. Intravenous infusions must be started at a very slow rate, to minimize the risk of reaction.

Macrocytic Anemia

Anemia with reticulocytopenia and macrocytosis is often associated with liver disease in the absence of folate or vitamin B_{12} deficiency. Folate deficiency may be from an inadequate intake, often encountered in alcoholics, and increased utilization, as may occur with pregnancy. Vitamin B_{12} deficiency occurs in pernicious anemia, malabsorption, or blind loop syndrome. The anemias of vitamin B_{12} and folate deficiency are normocytic early in the course of disease. Widening of the RDW generally precedes the development of macrocytosis.

Physical Examination

Vitamin B_{12} deficiency classically produces subacute degeneration of the dorsal columns of the spinal cord, with a decrease in proprioception; however, a symmetric peripheral polyneuropathy and/or dementia frequently occur. The neurologic abnormalities may precede the development of hematologic abnormalities. Surgical scars suggest gastrectomy, blind loop syndrome, and ileal resection as causes of vitamin B_{12} deficiency.

Laboratory Tests

Assessment should begin with an evaluation of the peripheral blood smear. In patients with vitamin B_{12} or folate deficiency, oval macrocytes, hypersegmented polymorphs, and giant platelets may be found. Macrocytosis associated with hypothyroidism and liver disease presents without the above-mentioned abnormalities and with a lower MCV; the formation of target cells results from increased membrane lipids.

Characteristically, patients with vitamin B_{12} deficiency have a low serum B_{12} concentration and RBC folate level, whereas patients with folic acid deficiency have low RBC folate and normal B_{12} studies. Occasionally, folate deficiency causes low B_{12} levels. Moreover, folic acid determinations are sometimes misleading for other reasons. The serum folate level is sensitive to reductions in vitamin ingestion, even in the presence of normal body stores; dietary restriction causes the serum folate level to fall before anemia or megaloblastic changes occur. On the other hand, the RBC folate level is less sensitive but more specific, because it may fall only after anemia or megaloblastic changes have occurred. Because of these problems, some advocate obtaining serum and RBC folate and B_{12} levels in all patients who have megaloblastic anemias. A careful examination of the peripheral smear and a bone marrow examination may be necessary to clarify the diagnosis.

After a diagnosis of vitamin B_{12} deficiency is established, testing for achlorhydria or performing the Schilling test is helpful in determining the cause of the deficiency if the clinical picture is unclear. Antibodies to intrinsic factor strongly suggest a diagnosis of pernicious anemia.

Treatment

Vitamin B_{12} deficiency anemia is treated with parenteral vitamin B_{12}, usually given in a dosage of 1000 µg once a month for life. This dosage is in excess of what is required, but the excess is excreted. Most experts recommend more frequent initial doses in the presence of neurologic disease (e.g., daily injection for 2 weeks, followed by injections every 2 weeks for 6 months, then once a month for life).

Folate deficiency, which is usually caused by inadequate dietary intake, is treated by folate, 1 mg orally every day for 3 weeks or until the cause of the deficiency is corrected. Vitamin B_{12} deficiency must be ruled out before folate is administered, because folate alone can partially correct the anemia of vitamin B_{12} deficiency while the neurologic manifestations progress.

Normocytic Reticulocytopenic Anemia

Most normocytic anemias with reticulocytopenia are associated with chronic disease. Almost any severe chronic disease can result in anemia; the more common ones are chronic inflammatory diseases, such as rheumatoid arthritis, certain endocrine disorders, such as hypopituitarism, and neoplastic diseases. This anemia, which takes 1 to 2 months to develop, reflects changes in iron metabolism and the marrow response to erythropoietin that are not well understood. It is generally thought that anemias of chronic illness take 1 to 2 months to develop. Renal insufficiency results in a similar anemia caused by multiple mechanisms that include decreased erythropoietin synthesis. The diagnosis of the chronic, underlying disease is usually not difficult, but occasionally, as in abdominal lymphoma, a thorough search is needed to identify the cause.

In general, the severity of the anemia parallels the severity and chronicity of the underlying illness. The anemia is usually in the moderate range with hemoglobin levels between 7 and 11 g/dl. The serum iron and iron-binding capacity are both also reduced, and there is either low or normal percent saturation. If the anemia is disproportionately severe, other causes must be considered; in particular, the anemia of chronic disease may be complicated by folate or iron deficiency. The serum ferritin and folate levels can help sort this out; however, the laboratory evaluation of combined processes can be difficult, and bone marrow examination is often necessary. An exacerbation of a chronic anemia requires a search for a concomitant deficiency state.

Occasionally, a low hemoglobin with normal indices is encountered in those who engage in strenuous, physical exertion. This is the result of an expansion of the plasma volume, which produces anemia without a reduction in RBC mass.

Anemia with Reticulocytosis

The two common causes of anemia in which a reticulocytosis is present are acute blood loss and hemolysis. Usually the indices are not particularly helpful, especially since reticulocytes are large cells that cause the MCV to be increased.

Diagnosis

The diagnosis of hemolysis may be supported by results of additional laboratory tests. The serum haptoglobin is often depressed because of the formation of hemoglobin-haptoglobin complexes. However, if the hemolytic process is mild or extravascular, the serum haptoglobin value may be normal. Also, haptoglobin is an acute reactant that may be elevated in inflammatory states. When the binding capacity of haptoglobin is exceeded, hemoglobinuria results. Elevated serum bilirubin and lactate dehydrogenase (LDH) values provide additional evidence of hemolysis.

If there is no evidence of blood loss and the diagnosis of hemolysis is uncertain, it may be useful to observe the patient for several weeks, periodically checking for persistent reticulocytosis and anemia. When the diagnosis is uncertain, a radionuclide RBC survival study may be required to document decreased RBC survival.

Establishing a Specific Cause

A peripheral smear should be examined, particularly for spherocytes or schistocytes. Spherocytes suggest congenital spherocytosis, although they can also be encountered in immune hemolytic anemias. Schistocytes suggest a microangiopathic process or heart valve hemolysis.

Certain patients, particularly blacks or Mediterraneans, may have a glucose-6-phosphate dehydrogenase (G6PD) deficiency. Drug-induced hemolysis in these patients affects only older, enzyme-deficient cells; the younger cells have adequate enzyme levels to resist the oxidant stress. Therefore, results of enzyme screening tests are normal immediately after hemolysis, and diagnosis may require repeat determination of the enzyme level when the older cells are once more present in the circulation. A variety of drugs can cause hemolysis by other mechanisms.

If the history, review of old records, race, or ethnic origin suggests that the process may be inherited, a sickle cell preparation, hemoglobin electrophoresis, and quantitative determination of hemoglobin A_2 and F levels are indicated. The quantitative hemoglobin A_2 and F levels are helpful in detecting sickle β-thalassemia or suggesting hereditary persistence of hemoglobin F. In addition, citrate agar is needed to separate hemoglobin S from hemoglobin D, because they migrate together on routine electrophoresis.

Thalassemia

Thalassemia occurs predominantly in Mediterraneans and blacks. The most important clue to this diagnosis is microcytosis in the absence of iron deficiency; reticulocyte levels may or may not be elevated. Elevations of the quantitative hemoglobin A_2 and F levels confirm the diagnosis of β-thalassemia. α-Thalassemia has been a diagnosis of exclusion supported by the presence of microcytosis in other family members. However, a leukocyte genome probe for alpha chains will soon be available. In acquired hemolytic anemias, the direct antiglobulin (Coombs') test can help identify autoimmune erythrocyte destruction. A search for splenomegaly is needed since hypersplenism may be an important factor. Usually physical examination will suffice, but scans may be needed.

Beutler E. The common anemias. JAMA 1988; 259:2433–7.
Recent advances in the understanding of thalassemia, iron deficiency, and the anemia of chronic disease are reviewed.

Djulbegovic B, Hadley T, Pasic R. A new algorithim for the diagnosis of anemia. Postgrad Med 1989; 85:119–22.
An approach designed to avoid excessive testing is described.

Herbert V. The nutritional anemias. Hosp Pract 1980; 15:65–89.
The presentation, diagnosis, and therapy of patients with nutritional anemias are presented in a concise informative fashion.

Lindenbaum J, et al. Neuropsychiatric disorders caused by cobalamin deficiency in the absence of anemia or macrocytosis. N Engl J Med 1988; 318;1720–8.
Patients with neuropsychiatric disorders and no anemia or elevation of the MCV are described. The patients responded to therapy with vitamin B_{12}.

Westerman MP. Bone marrow needle biopsy: an evaluation and critique. Semin Hematol 1981; 18:293–300.
This review evaluates the role of the bone marrow examination, particularly the biopsy, in multiple disease states.

Krause JR. The bone marrow in nutritional deficiencies. Hematol Oncol Clin North Am 1988; 2:557–66.
In addition to bone marrow morphology, the diagnosis and treatment of B_{12}, folate, and iron defiency are described.

Schreiber AD. Immunohematology. JAMA 1982; 248:1380–5.
The pathophysiology of autoimmune hemolytic anemia and immune thrombocytopenia purpura is succinctly reviewed.

Brewer GJ. Inherited erythrocyte metabolic and membrane disorders. Med Clin North Am 1980; 64:579–96.
This comprehensive review provides the practical information needed for effective patient evaluation.

Shapiro BS. The management of pain in sickle cell disease. Pediatr Clin North Am 1989; 36:1029–45.

This comprehensive discussion of vaso-occlusive crisis applies to adults as well as children.

Cook JD. Clinical evaluation of iron deficiency. Semin Hematol 1982; 19:6–18.
This review article provides a detailed assessment of the testing procedures used to diagnose iron deficiency.

Fischer SL, Fischer SP. Mean corpuscular volume. Arch Intern Med 1983; 143:282–3.
The authors support the MCV as the only RBC index of clinical usefulness.

Selby GB, Eichner ER. Endurance swimming, intravascular hemolysis, anemia, and iron depletion: a new perspective on athlete's anemia. Am J Med 1986; 81:791–4.
Various mechanisms for anemia in athletes are discussed.

Karand A, Poskitt TR. The automated complete blood count. Use of the red blood cell volume distribution and mean platelet volume in evaluating anemia and thrombocytopenia. Arch Intern Med 1985; 145:1270–2.
The clinical usefulness of the RDW and MPV are described.

98. ABNORMAL BLEEDING
Katherine A. High and Robert H. Fletcher

Normal hemostasis requires platelets, coagulation factors, and normal vasculature. Defects in any of these can result in a bleeding diathesis. Major defects, such as hemophilia A and B or acute idiopathic thrombocytopenic purpura (ITP), are generally well recognized and unlikely to have their initial presentation in an adult ambulatory care setting. Mild bleeding disorders, or complaints about what patients perceive as abnormal bleeding or bruising, are much more commonly seen in outpatient settings.

Patterns of Abnormal Bleeding
The pattern of bleeding can suggest which element of the hemostatic system is at fault. Mucosal bleeding (epistaxis, menorrhagia) generally implies platelet defects or von Willebrand's disease (vWD). Most factor deficiencies are associated with bleeding into deeper structures (e.g., joints, soft tissue, or muscle). Because the defect is not with the initial platelet plug, but with the subsequent generation of the fibrin clot, bleeding may begin hours to days after an injury, and may recur after it has initially stopped. Vascular defects generally result in purpuric lesions; most of these encountered in a general practice (senile purpura and purpura simplex) are not associated with a true bleeding diathesis.

Causes of Abnormal Bleeding

Coagulation Factor Deficiencies
Among adults presenting with mild bleeding symptoms, vWD is by far the most common defect. In one series of patients referred for workup of mild bleeding disorders, vWD was present in 27 of 120 patients, or nearly 25%; since no diagnosis was made in 57 patients, vWD was found in 43% patients in whom a disorder could be defined. The condition is caused by a reduction in either the quantity or biologic activity of von Willebrand factor (vWF), which is necessary for mediating platelet adhesion to vascular subendothelium. The clinical manifestations are therefore mucocutaneous bleeding typical of platelet disorders.

Most patients with vWD have a mild form and thus may reach adulthood without having been diagnosed. A history of a normal labor and delivery should not exclude a diagnosis of vWD, since levels of von Willebrand factor rise markedly during the third trimester in both normal women and women with vWD. These women often weather delivery well but give a history of postpartum hemorrhage beginning several days after delivery. Since vWD is transmitted as an autosomal dominant disorder, identification of a patient means that the patient's parents, siblings, and children also need to be screened. The absence of a family history does not exclude the diagnosis, because penetrance is variable and because a number of cases arise from de novo mutations in the gene.

Most patients with vWD can be managed during surgery or trauma with the synthetic hormone arginine vasopressin (DDAVP) and do not require blood products at all. Failure to make the diagnosis before surgery or major trauma is likely to result in unnecessary treatment with blood products.

Any patient whose bleeding history is at all suspicious should be screened with activated partial thromboplastin time (aPTT) and bleeding time measurements. If a patient has either an elevated aPTT or a prolonged bleeding time, further studies, including factor assays and activity, are indicated. In contrast to other factor deficiencies where factor levels in an individual patient tend to be stable over time, factor levels vary greatly in a single patient with vWD. Thus, it is not uncommon to test a patient with a suggestive history as many as 4 or 5 times before a diagnosis is made. Since there are also variant forms of the disorder, it is appropriate to involve a hematologist in the evaluation and treatment of patients with this disorder.

The other congenital coagulation factor defects, which can all be screened for with an aPTT determination, are either much less common than vWD, or much less likely to present in an adult ambulatory care setting. Hemophilia A, for example, is nearly as prevalent as vWD, but most patients with hemophilia A have severe disease and are diagnosed in early childhood.

Thrombocytopenia and Platelet Disorders

Thrombocytopenia as a cause of bleeding is ruled out by platelet counts of greater than 100,000 per microliter. Between 100,000 and 20,000 per microliter, platelet count correlates in an inverse fashion with prolongation of the bleeding time; thus, at a count of 20,000 per microliter approximately 100% of individuals will have an abnormal bleeding time. Below 20,000, the risk of bleeding due to thrombocytopenia rises sharply, although the risk may be modified somewhat by the cause of the thrombocytopenia, for example, bleeding at a count of 20,000 per microliter is less likely in ITP than in preleukemia. In addition to hematopoietic disorders (e.g., leukemia, aplastic anemia, bone marrow invasion by tumor), thrombocytopenia may also be associated with viral infection and drugs (Table 98-1).

Congenital platelet defects such as Glanzmann's thrombocytopathy and Bernard-Soulier syndrome are exceedingly rare and virtually always diagnosed in childhood. These defects are characterized by normal platelet counts but defective platelet function, with prolonged bleeding times.

Defective platelet function most commonly results from drug-induced thrombocytopathy. Frequently used oral medications that may impair platelet function are listed in Table 98-1. A patient taking any of these medications who is facing surgery, or who complains of easy bruising, should be screened with a bleeding time. This includes patients who have ingested aspirin within 2 weeks prior to an invasive procedure. In most individu-

Table 98-1. Drugs that affect platelets

Impair function	Decrease number
Aspirin	Quinidine
Nonsteroidal anti-inflammatory agents	H_2 antagonists (cimetidine, ranitidine)
Tricyclic antidepressants	Sulfonamides
Clofibrate	Ethanol
Sulfinpyrazone	Phenytoin (Dilantin)
Dipyridamole	Valproic acid
Propranolol	Barbiturates
Some antihistamines*	Thiazides

*Azadatine, brompheniramine, clemastine fumarate.

als, prolongation of the bleeding time (e.g., from 4–8 minutes) can be detected within an hour of a single 325-mg dose of aspirin, but normalizes within 24 hours. In approximately 5 to 10% of otherwise normal persons, however, prolongation of the bleeding time with aspirin is marked (bleeding time > 15 minutes) and of much longer duration (10–14 days). Surgery or trauma after aspirin ingestion may result in severe bleeding in these individuals. Provided the blood salicylate level is zero, bleeding can be corrected with platelet transfusions. Thus, a patient who has ingested aspirin within the previous 2 weeks should not be barred from invasive procedures, but should have the bleeding time checked first.

Vascular Lesions

Medical conditions associated with vascular causes of bleeding (e.g., adrenocortical hyperfunction, dysproteinemias, amyloidosis, vasculitides) are generally easily recognized, but must be kept in mind. Vascular disorders that are much more common but do not cause serious bleeding are senile purpura and purpura simplex. Senile purpura occurs in elderly or debilitated patients, most commonly on the extensor surfaces of the forearms; other typical sites are the face, neck, and dorsum of the hands. Lesions are up to 1 cm in diameter and often occur in clusters of two or three. The etiology is thought to be decreased vascular support due to collagen loss.

Purpura simplex, or simple easy bruising, is a relatively common, benign condition that occurs mainly in women. Patients describe recurrent bruising with minor trauma (or no trauma). Results of coagulation screening tests are normal, and the condition is not associated with excessive operative bleeding; these patients require only reassurance.

Tests for Abnormal Bleeding

History

The best screening test for the presence of a bleeding disorder is a thorough history, which is sensitive, but nonspecific. Most patients with abnormal bleeding can therefore be predicted on the basis of history alone, although it is not uncommon for patients with a positive history to have normal hemostatic function. Of all the elements sought in the history, the ability to withstand a surgical challenge is the single best measure of an intact hemostatic system. Any history of prolonged bleeding following surgery, bleeding severe enough to require transfusion, or bleeding beginning 1 to 2 days postoperatively should prompt a complete evaluation. Among the other elements sought in a bleeding history, severe bleeding after dental extraction was associated with a coagulopathy in 52% of patients in one series, whereas easy bruising was less likely (30% of patients) to be associated with disease. Medical conditions predisposing to abnormal bleeding should be identified; these include liver disease, malignancy, primary hematologic disorders such as the chronic leukemias and polycythemia vera, and malabsorption syndromes. Particular attention should be paid to an accurate record of medications, in order to identify those that may affect platelets (see Table 98-1).

Laboratory Tests

If the history is suggestive, or if a major surgical procedure is planned, the hemostatic system can be assessed through a battery of four tests: the platelet count, prothrombin time (aPTT), and bleeding time. These four tests detect everything except factor XIII deficiency, a rare disorder.

Platelet counts normally range from 200,000 to 400,000 per microliter. Counts can also be estimated from a Wright stain smear; several platelets per oil-immersion high-power field, or one platelet per 10 to 20 red blood cells correspond to normal levels. Provided the platelets have normal function, a count of 100,000 per microliter is adequate to provide normal hemostasis. Platelet counts between 20,000 and 100,000 per microliter may provide adequate hemostasis; this can be assessed by checking the bleeding time.

The *aPTT* assesses the function of the intrinsic and common pathways. Thus, it is abnormal in most factor deficiencies and acquired inhibitors. Normal ranges for aPTT vary greatly from one laboratory to another; some laboratories use a very tight range (e.g., 23–32 seconds) and thus some patients with abnormal results will have no detectable defect on further workup. Other laboratories use a broader range (e.g., 25–45 seconds) and in this case some patients with disease, such as mild vWD, will consistently have an aPTT only at the upper range but not outside the normal limits. In order to interpret results, one must be familiar with the laboratory being used.

A *bleeding time* reflects three major components: platelets, vasculature, and vWF. For most widely used methods, a normal bleeding time ranges between 3 and 9 minutes. A prolonged bleeding time in a patient with a platelet count higher than 100,000 suggests a qualitative platelet defect, a vascular defect, or vWD. The major indications for performing a bleeding time are to screen for vWD in a patient with a suggestive history, or to assess the effect of medicines on platelet function.

The *PT* measures function in the extrinsic and common pathways. It is prolonged in two commonly encountered situations: patients taking warfarin (Coumadin) and patients with severe liver disease. Both of these situations are generally readily apparent; the PT has very little use as a routine screening test for bleeding disorders.

Strategy for Detecting Abnormal Bleeding

The intensity of an evaluation for abnormal bleeding should be based on the degree of suspicion raised by the history. The following scheme, abbreviated from that proposed by Rapaport, will serve for most situations in which hemostasis is in question. If the results of the screening tests are abnormal, or if the clinician suspects a bleeding disorder despite normal test results, a hematology consultation is appropriate to select and interpret more specific studies.

Level I

If the screening history is negative and a major local challenge to hemostasis (e.g., major surgery) is not present, no additional tests are necessary, even though there have been no previous surgical tests of hemostasis.

Level II

If the history is negative, including previous surgical tests of hemostasis, but a major challenge to hemostasis (e.g., major surgery, trauma) is present, an aPTT and platelet count should be done.

Level III

If the screening history raises the possibility of a hemostatic defect, or the history is negative but an unusual challenge to hemostasis is present (e.g., cardiac surgery, prostatectomy, major trauma) or bleeding would be unusually risky (e.g., central nervous system surgery), then a full evaluation is recommended: platelet count, bleeding time, aPTT, and PT. An assessment of clot stability is also recommended.

Level IV

If the screening history leaves the physician very suspicious or certain of a hemostatic defect, a variety of tests may be done in addition to those listed for level III. These include an in vitro test of platelet function, specific factors assays, and thrombin time, to detect dysfibrinogenemia or weak heparin-like anticoagulants.

Rapaport SI. Preoperative hemostasis evaluation: which tests, if any? Blood 1983; 61:229–31.
  This article proposes broad guidelines in which the intensity of the laboratory evaluation depends on the likelihood of a bleeding disorder, based on a screening history.

Wallerstein RO. Laboratory evaluation of a bleeding patient. West J Med 1989; 150(1):51–8.
  This article reviews the use of laboratory studies in patient evaluations.

Bolton-Maggs P, Wilkinson LS. Mild bleeding disorders: review of 120 patients. Clin Lab Haematol 1984; 6:247–56.
  A bleeding diathesis was defined in 53% of the patients presenting with mild bleeding. In nearly half of these, the diagnosis was vWD.

Suchman AL, Mushlin AI. How well does the activated partial thromboplastin time predict postoperative hemorrhage? JAMA 1986; 256:750–3.

Dividing patients into low- and high-risk groups on the basis of history alone, the authors showed that aPTT was a predictor of hemorrhagic complications in the high-risk group but not in the low-risk patients.

Barber A, et al. The bleeding time as a preoperative screening test. Am J Med 1985; 78:761–4.
At a hospital where bleeding times are part of routine preoperative screening, 110 of 1941 patients had a prolonged bleeding time. Prolonged bleeding time could be predicted on the basis of history alone in 83 of 100 patients. The authors concluded that bleeding time should not be used for routine preoperative screening.

Suchman AL, Griner PF. Diagnostic uses of the activated partial thromboplastin time and prothrombin time. Ann Intern Med 1986; 104:810–6.
The authors argue against routine preoperative PT and aPTT if the patient has a negative screening history.

Kitchens CS. The purpuric disorders. Semin Thromb Hemost 1984; 10:173–89.
The author reviews the pathophysiology, clinical characteristics, and approach to the patients.

Coller B. Von Willebrand's disease. In: Coleman RW, et al., eds. Hemostasis and thrombosis: basic principles and clinical practice. Philadelphia: JB Lippincott, 1987:60–96.

Miller JL. von Willebrand disease. Hematol Oncol Clin North Am 1990; 4(1):107–28.
Two reviews of the types of vWD and clinical and laboratory evaluation.

Carvalho ACA, Rao AK. Acquired qualitative platelet defects. In: Coleman RW, et al., eds. Hemostasis and thrombosis: basic principles and clinical practice. Philadelphia: JB Lippincott, 1987:750–71.
A good reference on this subject.

Schafer AI. The hypercoagulable state. Ann Intern Med 1985; 102:814–38.
The pathophysiology, differential diagnosis, and outline of a workup for patients with primary and secondary hypercoagulable states are presented.

99. POLYCYTHEMIA
James A. Bryan II

Definition
The literal definition of polycythemia is "too many cells." The term is usually applied to any condition in which the number of red cells, as measured by a hematocrit or hemoglobin concentration, exceeds the statistical norm. By this definition, the upper limit of "normal" hematocrit values in adults at sea level is accepted as 54% for men and 52% for women. However, the judgment of "too many" red cells should be put in the context of the patient's physiology or pathophysiology. For example, acclimatized people living at 15,000 feet normally have hematocrit values of about 60% and do not have a disease. On the other hand, a hematocrit of 60% in a person at sea level usually indicates disease.

Causes
Polycythemia can occur either because too many red blood cells are produced (absolute erythrocytosis, either primary or secondary) or because of a reduction in the amount of plasma in which the red cells are suspended (relative or pseudoerythrocytosis). The causes of polycythemia are listed in Table 99-1.

The prevalence of primary polycythemia is approximately 2 per 100,000 persons; the relative frequencies of the various causes of polycythemia are not known.

Pathophysiology
Primary polycythemia (polycythemia vera) is usually associated with increased white cell and platelet counts and splenomegaly. It is considered a primary myeloproliferative disor-

Table 99-1. Causes of polycythemia

Primary polycythemia (polycythemia vera)
Secondary polycythemia
  Pulmonary disease
  Heart disease with right-to-left shunts
  Hypoventilation syndromes
  Renal disease
    Polycystic disease
    Hypernephroma
  Tumors
    Ovarian thecoma
    Large uterine leiomyoma
    Cerebellar vascular tumors
  Congenital hemoglobinopathies
  Cigarette smoking
Decreased plasma volume
  Gaisböck's syndrome
  Diuretics
  Dehydration

der that can evolve into acute leukemia, myelofibrosis, or even plasma cell dyscrasia syndrome (POEMS). Acquired von Willebrand disease has also been recognized in patients with polycythemia vera. Early in the course, the coexistence of normal and abnormal stem cells can be demonstrated.

Secondary polycythemia is associated with conditions that lead to low tissue oxygen tension: lung disease, hypoventilation syndrome, and congenital heart disease with venous to arterial vascular shunting. Cigarette smoking, which increases carboxyhemoglobin levels, causes a moderate polycythemia. Abnormal hemoglobins that are associated with high oxygen affinities can also lead to low tissue oxygen tensions and polycythemia. About 60 different abnormal hemoglobins have been identified, but all are rare. When systemic oxygen tension is reduced, erythropoietin is released, possibly from the kidney, and red cell production is stimulated. If iron, vitamin B_{12}, folic acid, and protein are available, more red cells and hemoglobin are made. Other causes of secondary excess red cell production are listed in Table 99-1. The mechanisms by which they are associated with polycythemia are unknown, although erythropoietin may be the unifying factor.

Decreased plasma volume causes high hemoglobin concentrations and hematocrits, with normal total body red cell mass. When there is no apparent dehydration, the condition is called "Gaisböck's syndrome." The biologic mechanism for the syndrome is not known, but the condition is usually found in men who smoke, are under stress, are overweight, and have hypertension. The hematocrit values rarely, if ever, exceed 58%. Chronic use of diuretics is responsible for small decreases in plasma volume; the resulting hematocrit rarely exceeds 54%.

Complications
It has been difficult to establish a level of hematocrit above which symptoms or complications occur. As hematocrit values rise, viscosity rises, flow diminishes, and oxygen transport is impaired. This can translate into increased work for the heart, with heart failure and/or a tendency toward vascular occlusions, particularly stroke. These complications occur more frequently in patients with primary or secondary polycythemia, particularly at hematocrits above 55%. Some physicians believe that a concomitant elevation in platelet counts increases the risk from hyperviscosity in polycythemia vera compared to other causes of polycythemia. Cerebral blood flow apparently also is reduced by high hematocrits. In one study, only 2 of 19 patients with hematocrits above 50% had normal cerebral blood flow, whereas only 3 of 21 patients with hematocrits below 46% had abnormal cerebral blood flow. Polycythemia vera often evolves into myelodysplastic syndrome.

Evaluation
If a high hematocrit (> 52%) is found, a sequence of simple maneuvers helps to sort out the many possible causes.

History
In polycythemia vera there may be a variety of nonspecific symptoms, including headache, weakness, pruritus, and dizziness; however, none occurs in more than 50% of patients. In secondary polycythemia, symptoms are from the underlying disease, unless symptoms of hyperviscosity intervene. Diuretic or cigarette use may be associated with a mild polycythemia.

Physical Examination
Usually there are few physical findings except for a ruddy complexion and splenomegaly in polycythemia vera, the findings of an underlying pulmonary cardiovascular disease, or a mass associated with a tumor in secondary polycythemia.

Laboratory Evaluation
If polycythemia is mild (hematocrit 52–54%) and the patient is otherwise normal, additional workup is unnecessary, provided there is a likely explanation such as a history of smoking or diuretic use. Although measuring carboxyhemoglobin may identify patients whose polycythemia is caused by smoking, the same information can be obtained by repeating hematocrit values a few weeks after smoking has been stopped.

For patients with more pronounced polycythemia (hematocrit > 55%), a minimal objective laboratory evaluation should include a complete blood count with smear examination for white cell, red cell, or platelet structural abnormalities, as well as a platelet and reticulocyte count. Qualitative or quantitative abnormalities in the cellular elements of the blood imply a primary myeloproliferative process, particularly if there is a palpable spleen. Other studies include a urinalysis, looking for hematuria (i.e., kidney pathology); chest radiograph, for heart or lung disease; and arterial oxygen saturation, looking for occult deoxygenation states. Second-level studies such as computed tomography scans or pulmonary function tests including nocturnal blood gas evaluation are obtained in those in whom pulmonary problems seem likely or an occult malignancy is possible. Hemoglobinopathies are detected by hemoglobin electrophoresis.

Radioisotope studies of red cell mass discriminate between increased numbers of red cells and diminished plasma volume. Although many experts suggest beginning with this study, it is an expensive test and is often unnecessary because causes of polycythemia can be found by history, physical examination, or inexpensive screening tests. It is necessary only after secondary causes have been ruled out, and the discrimination is between polycythemia vera and Gaisböck's syndrome.

Treatment
Polycythemia vera, or primary polycythemia, is treated by phlebotomy and/or agents such as hydroxyurea or recombinant interferon alfa. The use of P_{32} and alkylating agents has been discontinued as these have been associated with myelodysplastic transformation. Vascular occlusive episodes can be reduced considerably by reducing hematocrit from over 55% to below 48% (and platelets to below 400,000/mm^3).

Treatment of *secondary polycythemia* is directed at the management of the underlying primary disease. If the primary condition cannot be controlled, one is forced to deal with the secondary polycythemia as well as the primary disease. In these instances, it is generally believed to be beneficial to maintain the hematocrit below 55%. This can be accomplished by regular phlebotomy, usually 500 ml of blood with normal saline replacement on a weekly basis until a lower hematocrit is obtained. In some patients, improvement in oxygenation through low-flow oxygen administration also aids in controlling the polycythemia.

Russell RP, Conley CL. Benign polycythemia: Gaisböck's syndrome. Arch Intern Med 1964; 1143:734–40.
A descriptive article on the clinical findings and course.

Dinterfass L. A preliminary outline of the blood high viscosity syndromes. Arch Intern Med 1966; 118:427–35.
A review of the effects of blood viscosity in various diseases.

Hurtado A. Some clinical aspects of life at high altitudes. Ann Intern Med 1960; 53:247–58.
A fascinating description of high-altitude physiology and pathophysiology.

Thomas DJ, et al. Cerebral blood flow in polycythemia. Lancet 1977; 2:161–3.
Convincing data on keeping hematocrits low to improve functional integrity of the brain.

Pearson TC, Weatherly-Wein G. Vascular occlusive episodes and venous hematocrit in primary proliferative polycythemia. Lancet 1978; 2:1219–22.
The relationship between the incidence of occlusive episodes and the hematocrit and platelet count shown in a retrospective study.

Smith JR, Landow SA. Smoker's polycythemia. N Engl J Med 1978; 298:6–10.
Red blood cell volume is increased and plasma volume reduced with increased mean hematocrits in 22 of 54 smokers.

Cates P, et al. Determination of serum immunoreactive erythropoietin in the investigation of erythrocytosis. N Engl J Med 1986; 315:283–7.
In polycythemia vera, the mean erythropoietin was below normal, but in 61% of the cases it was in the normal range.

Berk PD, et al. Increased incidence of acute leukemia in polycythemia vera associated with chlorambucil therapy. N Engl J Med 1981; 304:441–7.
All moieties affecting cell replication can induce "leukemia," some more than others.

Shamdas GJ, et al. Myelodysplastic transformation of polycythemia vera: a case report and review of the literature. Am J Hematol 1991; 37(1):45–8.
A good review.

Silver RT. A new treatment for polycythemia vera: recombinant interferon alfa. Blood 1990; 76:664.
Recombinant interferon alfa was found to have an effect in controlling red cell mass.

Beutler E. Problems in the diagnosis of the hemoglobinopathies and polycythemia. Mayo Clin Proc 1991; 66:102–4.
An editorial briefly discussing problems in the differential diagnosis of polycythemia.

XIV. NERVOUS SYSTEM PROBLEMS

100. HEADACHE
Robert W. Eckel and J. Douglas Mann

It is estimated that almost 80% of the population suffers from at least one headache each year. Of these, perhaps 50% have severe or recurrent headaches, and 10 to 20% consult physicians for the pain. Ninety percent of patients suffering from headache have common primary headache syndromes including tension headache, cluster, migraine, or some combination of the three. While these syndromes may be quite disabling, they are not life-threatening and are generally not progressive. In roughly 10% of patients with headache, the pain is secondary to an underlying "organic" or structural cause. Subdural hematoma, subarachnoid hemorrhage, brain tumor, and meningitis can present as headache, sometimes with few other symptoms or signs. Other, more common and less threatening conditions that should be considered include sinus inflammation, dental pathology, temporomandibular joint (TMJ) dysfunction, cervical spondylosis, glaucoma, temporal arteritis, new-onset hypertension, hypoglycemia, and posttraumatic headache.

Common Headache Syndromes

Tension Headache
Tension is probably the most common cause of headache, accounting in one study for 40% of the patients referred to a headache clinic. In nonspecialty clinics, the prevalence may be even higher. Women are affected 3 times more frequently than men, and there is often a family history of headache, including migraine. The clinical picture is that of bilateral, dull, constant pain in a tight band around the head, with associated face, jaw, or neck pain secondary to chronic muscle contraction in those areas. Tension headache precipitated by stress often occurs in the latter part of the day. Headaches may occur daily for years. The headache may be associated with abdominal bloating and mild nausea and is frequently accompanied by depression or anxiety. However, atypical cases exist. The pain can be throbbing rather than constant, and in 10 to 20% of patients the pain is unilateral.

Tension headache and migraine often coexist, and vascular factors seem to operate in tension headaches. Moreover, the high proportion of important psychological factors in both migraine and tension headaches and the overlapping family history have led some authors to suggest that the two conditions are the extremes of a single disorder.

Migraine
Upward of 15% of the population suffers from migraine, with a 3:1 female predominance. Migraine onset usually occurs between the ages of 10 and 30 years; only 10% begin after the age of 40. In 20 to 50% there is a family history, but the genetics of inheritance is unclear. About 60% of patients had motion sickness as children, and some patients may have recurrent attacks of vomiting and abdominal pain of unexplained origin. Headaches typically occur at intervals of 1 to 2 months, but attacks may vary from infrequent to daily. Although attacks may occur at any time, they most often happen in the early morning hours, either awakening the patient from sleep or occurring shortly after waking.

Classification of migraine is based in part on the characteristics and timing of the aura, a transient neurologic disturbance. Classic migraine headache is preceded by an aura; in interposed migraine, the aura occurs after the onset of headache; in common migraine, there is no aura; in migraine equivalent, the aura occurs without a headache; and in complicated migraine, the neurologic deficit associated with the aura becomes permanent. The aura is usually a visual disturbance, but virtually any neurologic deficit can occur. Frequently described visual disturbances include flashes of color, zigzag lines, "heat waves," dark spots with bright borders, or loss of whole sections of the visual field in one or both eyes.

In classic migraine, the head pain begins about 10 to 15 minutes following the onset of the aura and builds up relatively slowly over the course of 30 to 90 minutes. Occasionally the buildup is more rapid. In all forms of migraine, throbbing is described by 50% of patients as a dominant pain feature; in some patients, sharp, brief, ice pick–like pains may be superimposed on the more constant pain. Although usually unilateral, migraine headaches are bilateral at least 40% of the time. There is pain on motion of the head and tenderness of the scalp develops over hours. Photophobia and nausea with or without vomiting occur frequently, and diarrhea may be a symptom in some patients. Partial relief comes with lying in a quiet, darkened room. In over half of episodes of migraine, the pain lasts for less than 24 hours. Typically, classic migraine is associated with a 4- to 12-hour duration while common migraine may last many days. When migraine lasts for longer than 3 days, there is the distinct possibility of coexisting severe head pain due to muscle contraction, which may require specialized treatment.

Common migraine accounts for the majority of cases and classic migraine for less than one-third. Other forms are relatively rare. For any patient, the pattern of headache may not remain the same over years and may, for instance, evolve from classic migraine in the teens to common migraine or ice pick–like pain in middle age. About half the patients with migraine have other kinds of headache, usually tension headaches occurring between the migraine attacks.

Physicians commonly underdiagnose migraine. The majority of headaches associated with gastrointestinal disturbances and photophobia are vascular, despite the lack of aura, hemicranial pain, or pulsatile pain. Though fewer than 30% of patients with migraine have classic migraine, aura symptoms can be subtle, consisting of mood changes, an unsteadiness on the feet, nonspecific dizziness, or a sudden clarity of vision.

Precipitating factors important in migraine include stress, menstruation, contraceptive use, fatigue, lack of sleep, drop in barometric pressure, and foods, especially chocolate, alcohol, nuts, some seafoods, and dairy products. Migraine may either increase or decrease during pregnancy. Some patients report a complete cessation of migraine during pregnancy while others report an increase, particularly during the first trimester and/or right after delivery.

The causes of neurologic symptoms and headache in migraine are not well understood. Most evidence implicates a chain of biochemical events involving the trigeminal vascular system and/or abnormalities of platelet homeostasis. Serotonin seems to play a role, perhaps by stimulating local release of vasoactive and pain threshold–lowering substances.

Cluster Headache

Cluster headache is relatively rare. It occurs most often in men (85% of cases), with an onset between the ages of 20 to 50 years. The headaches are excruciatingly painful and are associated with restlessness and agitation. In contrast to the migraine patient who goes to bed, the patient with cluster headache usually is up and about, pacing. The pain is orbital or periorbital and associated with ipsilateral nasal stuffiness, lacrimation, chemosis, and Horner's syndrome. Painful episodes rarely last more than 2 hours but may occur once to several times per day. Nausea and vomiting occur with up to 40% of attacks. The term *cluster* refers to the fact that headaches occur daily or many times per day for periods of 4 to 12 weeks at a time, separated by several weeks or months with no symptoms. The headaches most typically occur in the spring and/or fall, giving rise to theories of allergic precipitants. Occasionally, patients experience a cluster of headaches followed by 1 to 2 years of headache-free time before the next cluster begins. During times when headaches are frequent, alcohol may be a precipitating factor.

Variant forms of cluster headache, such as chronic cluster, have been described. In chronic cluster, headaches are typical of cluster but the long periods of remission are absent. Headaches occur throughout the year. Another variant, paroxysmal hemicrania, affects women more frequently than men and is characterized by frequent painful attacks occurring without remissions, often without the associated symptoms and signs of cluster. This syndrome may be related more to migraine than to cluster.

Although elevated serum histamine levels have been found during cluster headache, treatment with antihistamines is rarely successful. No clear-cut changes in scalp or intracranial blood flow have been noted. The etiology of the syndrome remains obscure.

Headache Associated with Human Immunodeficiency Virus Infection

Head pain as a complaint in patients with human immunodeficiency virus (HIV) infection should trigger a thorough search for infection and malignancy. This is particularly true with new-onset headache or a major change in an established headache pattern. The extensive differential diagnosis includes toxoplasmosis, fungal or tuberculous meningitis, brain abscess, central nervous system (CNS) lymphoma, and infections of soft or bony tissues of the head and neck. Magnetic resonance imaging (MRI) is more sensitive than computed tomography (CT) with contrast material for identifying brain lesions in patients with acquired immunodeficiency syndrome (AIDS), particularly toxoplasmosis, and if not specifically contraindicated by the presence of an intracranial mass or marked cerebral edema, is usually followed by lumbar puncture. (See Chap. 114.)

Posttraumatic Headache
Headache occurs in up to 80% of patients with head injuries, ranging in severity from those associated with brain damage to injuries with only minor concussion. Posttraumatic headache develops most commonly following accidents at the workplace or in motor vehicles and develops more frequently in patients who were premorbidly considered "nervous" or "neurotic." The probability of developing posttraumatic headaches is not affected by the presence or absence of brain damage, nor is it correlated with the duration of loss of consciousness. Such headaches occur concurrently with objectively identifiable deficits in attention span and memory, reductions in the rate of information-processing, an increase in irritability, and occasionally abnormalities on electrophysiologic testing.

The posttraumatic headache, resembling either tension of vascular headache, often occurs within hours after the injury, but may be delayed by weeks or rarely months. Vertigo and light-headedness occur in a high proportion of patients, but syncope occurs in only 10%. Disturbed sleep patterns are often reported and patients are not easily reassured, often seeing multiple physicians in a search for the cause of their pain. Scalp injuries tend to result in localized pain superimposed on a background of muscle contraction headache. Headaches occur frequently and tend to worsen for a few weeks or months before improving. The problem is self-limited and resolves in less than 1 year in 70% of patients and in less than 3 years in 85%.

Because there is often litigation and because patients may have multiple complaints in the absence of findings, there is a tendency for physicians to dismiss patients with posttraumatic headaches as hysterics or malingerers. The cognitive deficits in this syndrome are not fully assessable by the usual clinical examination, and an unsympathetic attitude on the part of the physician may contribute to the development of anxiety, depression, or other psychiatric problems. It is often difficult to determine whether psychiatric components are primary or secondary.

Late sequelae of head injury include hydrocephalus, seizures, and chronic subdural hematoma, each of which may present with only subtle neurologic signs but require prompt, specific treatment. Neurologic consultation may therefore be indicated for patients with persistent posttraumatic headache.

Evaluation

History
For almost all patients with headache, the diagnosis and treatment are based on the history. Certain key points distinguish the more common primary headache syndromes from less common secondary headaches. It is often difficult to make the distinction at the time of the patient's very first headache. (See Table 100-1 for a summary of the historical features of headache syndromes.)

TIME COURSE. Primary headache syndromes such as tension, vascular, and cluster headache frequently are present for many years in a chronic/recurrent pattern. While there are exacerbations and periods of relative remission, the pattern does not change rapidly over time. If the headache has been present for years and the patient is consulting the physician for the first time, it is very important to establish why the patient is seeking care. A change in the pattern of the headache may be the result of new life stresses, the superimposition of a new type of headache on the pattern of chronic/recurrent head pain, or an exacerbation of the old headache.

The subacute onset of new headaches can be associated with underlying organic disease, particularly in the older patient. Attacks that become increasingly frequent and painful suggest intracranial mass or chronic meningitis. Brain tumor causes headache in 50 to 70% of cases and is the presenting symptom in 30%; brain tumors account for less than 1% of all headaches.

Table 100-1. Headache syndromes

Syndrome	Location of pain	Time course	Associated signs and symptoms
Primary headaches			
Migraine	Unilateral or bilateral temporal/parietal pain	Onset often in early AM; lasting 2–24+ hr; occurring infrequently or daily	Varied neurologic symptoms during aura; nausea, vomiting, photophobia
Tension (muscle contraction)	Bifrontal and/or occipital	Daily or frequent; worse later in the day	Associated anxiety and stress
Cluster	Orbital area, unilateral	Onset at night, waking from sleep, or during day; lasting 15–120 min; occurring daily for weeks to months	Ipsilateral tearing, rhinorrhea, Horner's syndrome
Trigeminal neuralgia	Facial, one or more of 5th nerve dermatomes, unilateral	Lancinating pain; 1–5 sec repetitive bouts	Trigger area, lack of neurologic findings
Psychogenic	Vertex, localized or generalized	Often constant pain; unresponsive to drugs	Associated psychosis or neurosis
Secondary headaches			
Sinusitis	Over involved sinus (referred frontal or vertex in sphenoid sinusitis)	Occurrence increased in allergy seasons and with infection	Associated upper respiratory tract infection, sinus tenderness, postnasal drip
Posttraumatic	Unilateral or bilateral, frontal or occipital	Temporally linked with trauma; may persist for ≥ 2 yr	Associated dizziness, occasional syncope, mild thought disorder, sleep disturbance, anxiety/depression
Pseudotumor cerebri	Variable, often generalized or retroorbital	Weekly to daily; often worse in AM	Visual obscurations, 6th nerve palsy, papilledema, normal CT/MRI

Temporal arteritis	Unilateral pain in temporal or occipital scalp	Onset usually > age 45	Visual symptoms, polymalgia rheumatica, jaw claudication, tender palpable scalp artery, increased sedimentation rate
Costen's syndrome (TMJ syndrome)	Temporomandibular joint (TMJ), temporal scalp, ear, midface, neck	Daily; worse with chewing, talking, bruxism	Anxiety, occlusal problems, "blocked" sensation in ear, joint crepitus, restricted mouth opening
Gradenigo's syndrome	Eye or frontotemporal pain	Constant; occasional throbbing	Lesion of apex of petrous bone, 6th nerve palsy, 5th nerve dysfunction
Raeder's syndrome	5th cranial nerve distribution, usually forehead	Constant; throbbing	Horner's syndrome, 5th and 6th nerve palsies, internal carotid artery or middle fossa lesion
Cervical spondylosis	Occipital-temporal	Constant; worse in AM	Neck pain, history of neck trauma, arthritis
Eye disease	Orbital, periorbital, temporal	Often daily	Glaucoma, refraction errors
Meningitis	Generalized	Acute or subacute onset; increasing pain over hours to days	Fever, lethargy, variable neurologic signs, stiff neck
Subdural hematoma	Generalized with focality depending on location of hematoma	Subacute onset; constant pain	Dulling of sensorium, focal neurologic signs, focal skull percussion tenderness
Tumor	Variable	Increasing in frequency, and intensity; constant in late stages; AM prominence	Worse in supine position and improved upright, focal signs, projectile vomiting
Hypertensive	Generalized, throbbing	Often acute onset; early AM	Need to rule out hemorrhage
Subarachnoid hemorrhage	Generalized; worst headache of life	Acute onset	Family history, loss of consciousness, meningeal signs, focal neurologic signs, 3rd nerve palsy, back pain

Acute, new-onset head pain can be associated with life-threatening disease as in the case of subarachnoid hemorrhage. Pain from subarachnoid hemorrhage usually peaks within 1 to 5 minutes, while pain from vascular head pain syndromes such as migraine usually builds up less rapidly. Many patients who initially state that their headache was sudden in onset will, with more careful questioning, indicate that the pain builds up over a 30- to 60-minute period. In subarachnoid hemorrhage, 30 to 50% of patients lost consciousness briefly at onset, a rare pattern in recurrent vascular headaches. Acute severe headache can also be a manifestation of cluster or trigeminal neuralgia.

LOCATION OF PAIN. Vasodilation and traction or inflammation of vessels and nerves in the anterior and middle cranial fossae may cause pain referred to the anterior portions of the head including the temporofrontal region of the scalp, the periorbital areas, and the face. Pain from lesions arising in the posterior fossa is referred to the back of the head behind the vertex and in the upper part of the neck. Some investigators believe that disorders involving the upper cervical spine can result in occipital head pain radiating forward to the temporal regions. Pain at the vertex is an important symptom that may herald disease in the pituitary fosa or the underlying sphenoid sinus.

PAIN QUALITY. Tension headaches are usually generalized and are often described as squeezing or feeling "like a band around my head." The pain is usually nonthrobbing and may be associated with the significant muscle tension in the neck and proximal areas of the shoulders. Unilateral pain is seen in migraine, trigeminal neuralgia, and cluster headache. In migraine, the pain is experienced in the temporal and frontal regions of the scalp in contrast to the periorbital or retro-orbital pain of cluster headache. In over half of patients with migraine, the pain takes on a throbbing quality, corresponding to the pulse, at some point during the headache. In trigeminal neuralgia, the sharp, repetitive, lancinating pain follows one of the three major divisions of the fifth cranial nerve. Cluster headache may be throbbing but more often has a constant boring quality to it.

TIME OF DAY. Tension headaches characteristically build up slowly throughout the day, and may improve as evening comes on; they seldom interfere with sleep. They may be present on awakening in patients who have daily headaches. Migraine headaches occur at any time of the day, frequently in the early morning, being present on awakening or sometimes waking the patient from sleep. They also occur following periods of stress. Because a supine posture tends to increase the intracranial pressure, an early morning occurrence of head pain suggests increased intracranial pressure, particularly if the pain remits shortly after rising. Other conditions associated with early morning headache include sinus congestion, glaucoma, new-onset high blood pressure, hypoglycemia, and cervical spondylosis. Conversely, "low-pressure" headache occurring either spontaneously or following lumbar puncture is worsened by the upright posture and relieved by lying down.

ASSOCIATED SYMPTOMS AND PRECIPITATING FACTORS. Nausea and vomiting are characteristic of migraine, cluster headache, and advanced cases of increased intracranial pressure. Photophobia, motion sickness, and scalp tenderness are also characteristic of migraine. In temporal arteritis there may be muscle pain consistent with polymyalgia rheumatica, tenderness of the scalp or scalp arteries, jaw claudication, and visual blurring or frank visual loss.

Certain foods, such as packaged meats containing nitrates, or withdrawal from alcohol or coffee can precipitate vascular headaches. Some medications, such as nitroglycerin, characteristically cause headaches, and birth control pills often increase the severity and frequency of migraine. Daily use of ergotamines or compound medications containing barbiturates can result in "rebound" headaches, which subside on gradual withdrawal from those medications.

Vascular headaches associated with menses typically occur just prior to the onset of bleeding and often last 1 to 3 days. Although a well-established headache pattern may commonly change dramatically just prior to or during menopause, a thorough reevaluation of the patient is indicated when this occurs, just as it would be if a major change in headache pattern occurred at any other time in the patient's life.

Other possible precipitating factors include head trauma, emotional stress, fatigue, and infection.

Physical Examination
Certain aspects of the general examination require particular attention. Eyes should be examined for impaired vision, disconjugate gaze, glaucoma, optic atrophy, pupillary asymmetry, subhyaloid hemorrhage, and signs of papilledema. The head and neck should be examined for bruits over the eyes and carotid arteries, and palpated for painful areas, masses, or evidence of trauma. The scalp, sinuses, temporal arteries, and temporomandibular joints should be palpated for tenderness. Lateralized percussion tenderness over the cranial vault can be a sign of subdural hematoma, subdural empyema, or subarachnoid cyst. In 35 to 77% of patients with temporal arteritis (giant cell arteritis), firm, tender, enlarged arteries may be found in the scalp. Giant cell arteritis need not be located in the temporal vessels. Cases exhibiting involvement of the posterior scalp arteries with occipital head pain have been described. The neck should be examined for unusual proportions (suggesting abnormalities at the craniocervical junction), masses, range of motion, and nuchal rigidity.

Abnormalities found on the neurologic examination should lower the threshold for neurologic consultation and/or further evaluation.

Laboratory Evaluation
If the history suggests a primary headache syndrome and both general and neurologic findings are normal, extensive laboratory evaluation is not needed. A number of studies have shown that few CT-detected abnormalities, leading to a change in therapeutic approach, are found in such patients. Routine screening for unsuspected medical conditions (e.g., uremia) may be helpful, and erythrocyte sedimentation rate (ESR) should be measured in patients over 50 years old, to rule out temporal arteritis. Cervical spine or sinus radiographs may be useful when the patient localizes pain to these areas specifically. Cervical spine pathology, most commonly spondylosis, can result in pain over the occiput, with bilateral spread to the temporal areas. Cervical spine films are most important in patients with coexisting rheumatoid arthritis, where occipital head pain may signal odontoid erosion and significant craniocervical instability. Sinus films, either radiographs or CT, should be ordered when the patient has pain over the frontal or maxillary sinuses, or over the vertex (sphenoid sinus pain referral pattern).

CT is necessary when secondary headache is suspected, but may give confounding results in primary headache syndromes. As many as 20% of patients with classic migraine have transient, focal, low-density parenchymal lesions, maximal at 3 to 4 days following attacks. There have been reports of an increased incidence of cortical atrophy in patients with severe migraine, but the significance of these changes is unclear.

Nonspecific abnormal findings on CT may lead to further unnecessary diagnostic testing. Conversely, normal results may lead to a false sense of security. Headache from chronic meningitis, nasopharyngeal tumor, or craniocervical junction abnormalities, for instance, is compatible with a normal-appearing, routine CT scan. Testing must therefore be individualized using clinical judgment. CT scans are clearly indicated in five circumstances: (1) when the history suggests a specific diagnosis other than a primary headache; (2) when the examination is abnormal; (3) when a patient with a chronic headache syndrome develops new features; (4) when there are atypical features, for example, new onset of migraine in an elderly patient; and (5) when the patient is HIV-positive or otherwise immunocompromised. When these indications for further workup do not exist, it is reasonable to follow the patient's clinical course.

MRI of the head and neck further defines abnormalities found on CT, and is the best initial imaging study when the history and physical examination suggest lesions involving the posterior fossa, the craniocervical junction and upper spine, the pituitary, or the meninges. It is more sensitive than CT in patients with HIV infection and headache.

Lumbar puncture, in most cases preceded by CT or MRI to rule out a mass, is indicated in patients with fever or other evidence of active infection, malignancy, HIV infection or other immunocompromised states, delirium, dementia, seizures, or progressive neurologic deterioration not otherwise defined.

Treatment
Patient education and a sympathetic physician-patient relationship must be at the core of therapy for all primary headache syndromes. Patients should be reassured that the headaches do not represent a life-threatening disorder and encouraged to participate actively in their own treatment. Because finding the best therapy may require several trials, patients should not be led to expect instant results.

The first step is to attempt to modify the triggering factors and stressors that contribute to the headache. Medicines, dietary factors (e.g., chocolate, processed meats, caffeine withdrawal), and personal habits (e.g., smoking, alcohol, sleep deprivation) that may worsen the condition should be explored with the patient and appropriate changes or modifications discussed. Birth control pills should be discontinued in patients with migraine. Work and domestic stresses should be discussed and ameliorated if possible. Sometimes psychotherapy is useful.

Relaxation and biofeedback training have been shown to be effective for both migraine and muscle contraction headaches. Various techniques are available and include progressive relaxation using guided imagery, or biofeedback using temperature or electromyographic end points on the hand or scalp. Simple relaxation techniques that require no special equipment should be attempted before more elaborate and expensive alternatives are instituted. Instructing friends or relatives in how to massage the affected painful area may also be helpful.

Often psychological support, attention to precipitating factors, and some form of relaxation therapy are all that is required, especially for simple tension headache or for headaches related to acute stress. The question should not be *which* medication to start but *whether* to start any medication at all. If headaches are disrupting the patient's life or if the pain is perceived as quite severe, and if simple measures have failed, pharmacologic treatment should be considered.

Medication for headaches can be given in three different ways: (1) for symptomatic relief of acute painful episodes, (2) for prevention of headache after warning signs have appeared (abortive therapy), and (3) as prophylactic therapy to reduce the frequency of headaches. For vascular headaches without aura, abortive therapy can be tried if begun early in the course of an attack. The decision to attempt prophylactic therapy should be made only after symptomatic therapy has failed. The patient must clearly understand the purpose of prophylaxis and must not take the medicine to relieve acute pain.

Symptomatic Treatment for Tension or Migraine Headache
Headaches frequently respond well to simple measures, such as aspirin, acetaminophen, or nonsteroidal anti-inflammatory drugs (NSAIDs). These drugs are best given singly, although a combination of acetaminophen with aspirin or an NSAID can sometimes provide enhanced pain relief over a single agent. Proprietary combinations of aspirin, caffeine, and a small amount of barbiturate may provide effective analgesia for moderate head pain, particularly when there is a significant muscle contraction component. However, daily use of such medication can result in persisting "chronic daily headache" or recurrent rebound headache. Because of their addictive potential, narcotic medications should be used in a limited fashion in treating headaches of a benign nature. Intramuscular or rectal opiates are commonly used to treat very severe attacks of migraine. It should be remembered that no medication, no matter how it is given, is likely to completely relieve the pain of severe migraine. The goal is to make the patient as comfortable as possible while the headache runs its course. Antiemetics and fluid supplementation are indicated in some cases. Morphine suppositories can be used when repeated injections are impractical. However, the continued use of narcotics, even over a short period of days, may result in a mild withdrawal syndrome when they are discontinued, with recrudescence of the headache. Many patients with severe migraine report that opiates do not relieve the pain but merely allow them to sleep and that sleep provides them the best relief. Hence, a sedative such as chloral hydrate or a barbiturate, which allows the patient to sleep until the pain subsides, may be more effective than narcotics.

Recently, some investigators used intravenous dihydroergotamine, 1 mg every 8 hours, as adjunctive therapy for migraine. They reported excellent results both acutely and in patients who had had the headache for several days. Intravenous prochlorperazine (Compazine), 10 mg given over 3 minutes, has also been reported to be effective acutely.

Abortive Treatment
Tension headache can occasionally be aborted by escaping from the precipitating situation. Learned biofeedback and relaxation techniques, massage, and over-the-counter nonsteroidal medications are also effective. Muscle relaxant medications are sometimes effective but are too sedating for frequent use.

In classic migraine, abortive therapy can be used if an aura is clearly identifiable. Various preparations of ergotamine are available, and include Cafergot and Bellergal for oral use, Ergomar for sublingual use, Medihaler Ergotamine for inhalational therapy, and suppositories. Patients may have nausea and vomiting at the onset of an attack, making oral administration difficult. Any of the sublingual, inhalant and suppository forms may help to circumvent this difficulty, but the individual patient response, including side effects, is highly variable. Systemic absorption is most rapid and complete with the inhalational and rectal forms. Intensification of nausea and vomiting as well as paresthesias and numbness of the extremities are side effects of the ergotamines. It is best to give the maximum nonnauseating dose of ergotamines at the beginning of a headache rather than relying on multiple smaller doses given over a longer period of time. Daily use of ergots can result in "rebound" headache. If this is suspected, complete withdrawal over a 4- to 6-day period is indicated. Ergots are contraindicated in patients with hypertensive cardiovascular disease, hepatitis, renal failure, and pregnancy. Oral isometheptene is effective for abortive therapy and had fewer side effects than the ergots. Because of its overall lower efficacy, it is usually prescribed as a second-line drug when ergots cannot be used or are ineffective.

For cluster headaches, abortive therapy is more difficult because of the relatively rapid buildup and short duration of head pain. However, ergotamine compounds have been effective in aborting some attacks and should be tried. Sublingual or inhalant medications are more likely to be effective because of their more rapid onset of action and their availability despite vomiting. Oxygen inhalation at 4 to 8 L per minute is effective in some patients and can be used at home. In one study it was as effective as ergotamine. Intranasal lidocaine has also been reported to be effective in some patients with cluster headache.

Prophylactic Treatment
Tension, migraine, and cluster headaches can all be treated prophylactically. General guidelines for the use of prophylaxis include headaches occurring more than 3 times a month or incapacitating headache for more than 2 days per month. Prophylaxis should only be used after other modes of therapy have failed. Trials of prophylactic medications should be made for periods of at least 2 months each and, if effective, carried to as long as 6 months. If the headaches remit, the drug should be tapered intermittently to prevent chronic side effects and to take advantage of naturally occurring remissions.

For vascular headaches associated with menses, prophylactic treatment should begin 5 days before the anticipated period, with a nonsteroidal agent, a long-acting ergotamine-containing compound, isometheptene, or cyproheptadine, continued through the menses. Diuretics are not very effective, even when significant perimenstrual swelling is present.

For migraine, a number of medications have efficacy. These include the tricyclic antidepressants, particularly amitriptyline; beta-blockers (propranolol, nadolol, timolol, atenolol, and metoprolol); some of the calcium channel blockers (nifedipine); and some of the NSAIDs (ibuprofen, aspirin). Methysergide can be effective but has dose-related side effects that preclude its routine use. Daily low-dose ergotamine (sustained-release Bellergal) can be effective for short periods of time. Monoamine oxidase inhibitors are sometimes used in patients refractory to other modes of therapy.

Combination therapy is sometimes used when it is not specifically contraindicated by the drug combination itself. Two-drug therapy can include a beta-blocker with a tricyclic, or either class of medication with low-dose ergotamine on a daily basis. While both amitriptyline and propranolol are effective in a wide range of patients, treating depressed patients with amitriptyline and hypertensive patients with propranolol reduces the number of medicines needed to manage both conditions. A useful approach in refractory migraine is to rotate through a series of medications or combinations for a trial period of 2 to 3 months each until the most effective treatment is found. The patient's cooperation will be improved if it is explained that an empirical approach must be taken.

The method of trying a series of prophylactic medications for 2- to 3-month periods is

Table 100-2. Medications for prophylaxis of headache

Medication	Indication	Dosage	Effects and advantages	Adverse effects
Propranolol (Inderal) (nadolol, timolol, atenolol also effective)	Migraine	20 mg bid to start Up to 240 mg/day (propranolol)	Side effects relatively rare; effective β-adrenergic blocker; long-acting forms now available	Bradycardia; contraindicated in chronic renal failure, congestive heart failure, asthma; rebound cardiac effects; depression
Amitriptyline (Elavil)	Migraine, tension	10–25 mg hs to start Up to 100–150 mg/day (hs)	Antidepressant action separate from antiheadache action; once-daily dosing; blocks serotonin reuptake at nerve terminal	Sedation, dry mouth, orthostatic hypotension, rare urinary retention, weight gain
Methysergide (Sansert)	Migraine, cluster	2–12 mg/day divided doses	Very effective prophylaxis for migraine and cluster; serotonin antagonist, antihistaminic	Abdominal discomfort, peripheral vasoconstriction, angina, muscle cramps, and retroperitoneal, endocardial, and pleural fibrosis
Cyproheptadine	Migraine	12–24 mg/day	Physiologic effects similar to methysergide; side effects uncommon	Sedation, dizziness, pedal edema, dry mouth, occasional diarrhea, weight gain
Bellergal (contains ergotamine, belladonna, and phenobarbital)	Migraine, tension	1 bid, sustained release	Few side effects; somewhat effective for tension headaches	Sedation, ergot side effects

Drug	Indication	Dose	Comments	Side effects/Contraindications
Midrin (contains isometheptene, dichloralphenazone, and acetaminophen)	Migraine, tension	For acute attack 2 PO at onset; 1/hr up to 5 capsules in 12 hr	Effective for aborting migraines; useful in low doses prophylactically; little nausea	Contraindicated with glaucoma, hypertension, and heart and liver disease
Diazepam (Valium)	Tension	2–10 mg/day	Muscle relaxant; long-acting	May induce dependency, withdrawal syndrome, depression
Aspirin (ibuprofen also effective)	Migraine, tension	325 mg qid	Effective in some patients as prophylaxis; inexpensive, simple	GI side effects, antiplatelet activity
Lithium	Cluster	Start at 300 mg tid and adjust according to serum levels	Especially effective in chronic cluster	Nephrogenic diabetes insipidus, tremor, GI symptoms, confusion, hypothyroidism
Indomethacin (Indocin)	Chronic paroxysmal hemicrania, ice pick–like headaches	25–50 mg tid	Mechanism unknown but effective	GI side effects, may induce headache
Corticosteroids (prednisone)	Cluster, migraine	60 mg/day for 7–10 days with rapid taper	Effective in cases of severe acute exacerbation	Cataracts, diabetes, osteoporosis, Cushing's syndrome, mood changes
Nifedipine (Procardia)	Migraine, cluster	10 mg bid–20 tid	Relatively rapid onset (a calcium channel blocker)	Nonvascular headache, flushing, edema; cannot be used with β-blockers

also effective for preventing tension headache, although the range of medications is more limited. NSAIDs, nonsedating muscle relaxants, and massage and biofeedback techniques are the most effective. When depression is clearly a component of the clinical syndrome, tricyclic antidepressants can be very effective. They may also be extremely useful in patients with both migraine and tension headaches.

Cluster headaches can be effectively prevented by a variety of medications, as outlined in Table 100-2. Lithium and methysergide are both quite effective, but both require close follow-up by a physician familiar with their use. Calcium channel blockers have also been reported to be effective in patients with cluster headaches. A 10-day course of histamine desensitization is effective in producing prolonged remissions in some patients refractory to other therapy. The daily headaches of chronic paroxysmal hemicrania, a recently described form of cluster headache, can be effectively prevented by relatively low doses of indomethacin.

When treatment with medications is unavoidable, the simplest and safest should be tried first. When medications fail or when there is a question about the diagnosis, early referral to a neurologist or neurosurgeon is indicated. One study of the effect of such referrals found that in more than two-thirds of patients, a timely evaluation by a specialist reduced the overall frequency of physician visits for headache.

Aronoff GM, ed. Special issue on headache. Clin J Pain 1989; 5:1–127.
A single issue devoted to multiple aspects of headache diagnosis and management. Includes 20 well-referenced articles on migraine, cluster, tension headache, headache in children, inpatient treatment, and the pharmacologic management of pain, among other clinically useful topics. An excellent resource.

Blau JN, Thavapalan M. Preventing migraine: a study of precipitating factors. Headache 1988; 28:481–3.
Careful review of factors that may be important in nondrug therapy for migraine.

Clouch C. Non-migranous headaches: classification and management. Br Med J 1989; 299:70–2.
A good way of organizing treatment regimens for patients with nonvascular headaches.

Couch JR, Diamond S. Status migrainosus: causative and therapeutic aspects. Headache 1983; 23:94–101.
Common approaches used by practitioners faced with this difficult problem.

Dalessio DJ, ed. Wolff's headache and other head pain. 4th ed. New York: Oxford University Press, 1987.
This classic text includes data on the mechanisms of many head pain syndromes.

Diamond S, Dalessio DJ, eds. The practicing physicians approach to headache. 4th ed. Baltimore: Williams & Wilkins, 1986.
Very useful guide for designing diagnostic and treatment strategies, particularly for patients refractory to many modes of therapy.

Edmeads, J. The worst headache ever. 2. Innocuous causes. Postgrad Med 1989; 86:107–10.
Sensible approach to a difficult clinical problem.

Hollander H, Stringari S. HIV associated meningitis: clinical course and correlations. Am J Med 1987; 83:813–6.
Headache presentation and course in HIV infection.

Jones J. Randomized double-blind trial of intravenous perchlorperazine for the treatment of acute headache. JAMA 1989; 261:1174–6.
A fast, safe, non–opiate-based treatment for acute vascular headache.

Kudrow L. Paradoxical effects of frequent analgesic use. Arch Neurol 1982; 33:335–41.
Highlights the problem of chronic daily headache and rebound headache with overuse of analgesics.

Lance JW. Mechanism and management of headache. 4th ed. Boston: Butterworth, 1982.
Reviews a large clinical experience and provides discussion of the mechanisms of headache as well as detailed suggestions for treatment.

Lovshin LL, ed. Proceedings of the International Headache Colloquium. Headache 1988; 28:652–88.
Journal issue devoted to diagnosis and treatment of migraine, cluster, analgesic rebound headaches, and the emergency management of headache, among many other topics.

Raskin NH. Headache. 2nd ed. New York: Churchill Livingstone, 1988.
Excellent, up-to-date reference reviewing current treatment approaches and hypotheses of headache. Well referenced.

Headache. In: Vinken PJ, et al, eds. Handbook of clinical neurology 4. Amsterdam: Elsevier, 1986.
Comprehensive treatment of head pain from multiple clinical experts in the field.

101. SEIZURES: EVALUATION
John A. Messenheimer

Seizures are paroxysmal disturbances of behavior and/or consciousness that result when abnormally active neurons fire together in a sustained burst. *Epilepsy* is a term used to describe chronic recurrent seizures; the equivalent term *seizure disorder* may be preferable to patients because the lay public often erroneously associates the term epilepsy with inherited degenerative neurologic disease.

Seizures and seizure disorders are classified according to their clinical manifestations and their electroencephalographic (EEG) characteristics. A major distinction is made between partial seizures, involving a limited area of the brain, and generalized seizures, in which the activity of both cerebral hemispheres is affected. Partial seizures may spread to become secondarily generalized seizures. The International Classification of Seizures and the Epilepsies is summarized, in an abbreviated form, as follows:

I. Partial seizures
   A. *Simple partial seizures* involve a focal region of the brain, with motor, sensory, autonomic, or psychic symptoms reflecting the area from which the seizure originates. They do not produce an alteration of consciousness.
   B. *Complex partial seizures,* formerly known as "temporal lobe epilepsy" and "psychomotor epilepsy," are characterized by a transient confusional state in which consciousness is either lost or impaired. In contrast to partial simple seizures, they involve brain structures associated with maintaining normal consciousness; these foci are usually in or near the limbic cortex, most often the structures of the mesial temporal lobe (*hippocampus and amygdala*).
II. Primary generalized seizures
   A. *Generalized tonic-clonic seizures,* formerly called "grand mal," result from abnormal discharges in widespread areas of the brain, with loss of consciousness and tonic-clonic motor activity. This is the most frequently encountered form of primary generalized seizure.
   B. *Absence seizures,* formerly called "petit mal," are characterized by brief (< 30 seconds) episodes of staring and unresponsiveness, and are primarily encountered in children. Juvenile myoclonic epilepsy, a type of absence seizure that usually begins in adolescence, is characterized by associated myoclonic activity and may also be accompanied by generalized tonic-clonic seizures.
III. Partial seizures evolving to secondarily generalized seizures
   These seizures begin as partial seizures and progress to generalized tonic-clonic seizures. Most adult-onset generalized seizures are actually secondarily generalized from focal brain areas.

Establishing the Diagnosis
The first, yet often the most difficult, question to answer is whether the patient has had a seizure or not. Distinguishing a seizure from other forms of paroxysmal behavioral

disturbances, as well as identifying the type of seizure activity, can often be done from the clinical history. Details of the event should be obtained both from the patient and from witnesses. The classic features of the three most common types of seizure activity should be sought.

Generalized tonic-clonic seizures begin with the tonic contraction of all extremities. They may be associated with a loud vocalization, tongue biting, and incontinence, but the absence of any of these events should not be used as an argument that a seizure has not occurred. Cyanosis is a common feature and its presence should be determined in the history. Following the tonic phase, the clonic phase is associated with repetitive clonic motor activity involving all extremities. The motor activity usually lasts from 1 to 5 minutes, and is followed by a longer postictal period in which the patient progresses from unresponsiveness, to stupor or confusion, to full alertness. Patients are amnestic for the generalized motor portion of the seizure and for some of the postictal period. If, however, the generalized seizure began as a partial seizure or with very brief generalized seizure activity, the patient may report symptoms prior to the loss of consciousness. A feeling of exhaustion is common in the postictal period. Muscle soreness within 1 to 2 days after the seizure may occur in patients who have experienced violent motor activity. The type of motor activity (clonus versus tremor) and the lack of responsiveness during the event help to distinguish this type of seizure from nonepileptic events. Partial seizures that secondarily generalize often produce generalized tonic-clonic seizures with asymmetric motor activities and/or postictal deficits. The clinical entities most often confused with generalized tonic-clonic seizures are pseudoseizures and syncopal episodes, which are discussed further below.

Complex partial seizures are the most prevalent seizure disorder in adults and vary considerably in presentation. Most of these seizures begin with a motionless stare, which is preceded in many cases by a warning or aura. The aura may be difficult for the patient to describe, but is recognized as a familiar, often unpleasant sensation. Other manifestations of the aura, which is actually a simple partial seizure, may include vague epigastric discomfort, feelings of déjà vu, or olfactory hallucinations. The stare lasts for several seconds and is often associated with automatisms (lip smacking, swallowing, or chewing movements), which then may be followed by automatic behaviors such as fumbling with clothing or other items. These automatisms are characteristic of complex partial seizures, and help to distinguish them from absence seizures. The degree of impairment of consciousness during the seizure is quite variable. Witnesses usually describe the patient as staring and unresponsive to them during the seizure, although some patients may talk and respond partially, even assuring those around them that they are all right. Patients' reactions may range from complete amnesia for the event and denial that anything has happened to memories of hearing people talk to them but being unable to answer. The seizure ends gradually in a transition to a postictal confusional state, often making it difficult to determine precisely when the seizure has ended. The total seizure duration is usually from 1 to 4 minutes. The severity of the postictal confusional state is often proportional to the duration of the seizure. Patients consistently underestimate the duration of these events, probably because memory function is suspended during all or a part of the seizure. The clinical entities most commonly confused with complex partial seizures are absence seizures and anxiety or panic attacks.

Absence seizures are primarily a disorder of children, characterized by brief episodes of staring and unresponsiveness, or sometimes merely slowed response times. Episodes last only seconds, are often accompanied by rhythmic eye blinking, and terminate without any postictal confusion or disorientation. They may occur many times a day. Patients usually describe a brief gap in their awareness of their environment. Usually these seizures can be precipitated by hyperventilation. Other types of seizure activity, such as myoclonic jerking, may complicate absence seizures, and some patients go on to develop generalized tonic-clonic seizures. A syndrome of mycoclonus, absence seizures, and generalized tonic-clonic seizures characterizes juvenile myoclonic epilepsy, which is further distinguished by four to six per second spike and wave discharges on EEG. Absence seizures usually cease by age 20; their appearance after puberty or persistence into young adulthood should lead to consideration of complex partial seizures.

Ictal stupor is a form of status epilepticus characterized by a prolonged confusional state. This unusual presentation typically occurs in older patients (> 50 years old) with no history of seizures or psychiatric difficulty. The clinical presentation is quite varied and may include an acute psychotic reaction. While some patients exhibit recurrent absence-like attacks amidst their confusion and some eventually have a generalized tonic-clonic seizure, many patients never exhibit any clear sign of seizure activity and can only be diagnosed by identifying the characteristic continuous discharge of spike and wave activity on EEG. The diagnosis should be suspected in any patient with sudden behavioral change and no prior psychiatric history.

Distinguishing Seizures from Other Conditions

A variety of other conditions have symptoms in common with and may be confused with seizures.

Syncope is most likely to be erroneously identified as a seizure when it is accompanied by either tonic (posturing or stiffening) or clonic motor activity. It is estimated that motor activity is associated with syncope in 50 to 60% of cases. This may occur as a result of cerebral ischemia when the syncopal episode is severe or prolonged, particularly when the patient is prevented from falling to a horizontal position. Despite the resemblance to a seizure, these motor phenomena are not associated with EEG evidence of seizure activity. Syncopal episodes are often preceded by light-headedness, a dimming of vision, diaphoresis, and pallor, whereas the onset of a seizure is usually abrupt. Recovery from syncope is rapid (within 30 seconds), with an almost immediate clearing of mentation, while more prolonged confusion is often seen following a seizure. Syncope is not associated with the automatisms (e.g., lip smacking) seen in complex partial seizures.

Vascular events such as transient ischemic attacks and migraine headaches may resemble seizures. Localized ischemia may produce paroxysmal episodes of tingling that mimic a partial simple somatosensory seizure, or transient aphasia similar to a partial complex seizure. An ischemic etiology is also suggested by transient weakness or other neurologic signs and symptoms characterized by the loss of function. Todd's paralysis, a transient asymmetric postictal weakness following a partial or secondarily generalized seizure, may be extremely difficult to distinguish from an ischemic cerebrovascular event. Vertebrobasilar insufficiency may result in drop attacks, without a loss of consciousness. Such episodes are usually accompanied by other symptoms referable to the brain stem, such as dizziness, diplopia or other visual deficits, and dysarthria.

Hyperventilation and anxiety attacks may be confused with partial complex seizures. Symptoms may include dizziness, paresthesias, carpopedal spasm, and syncope. However, attacks typically last much longer and are more variable than true seizures; patients are not usually amnestic for the event, and usually describe intense anxiety throughout the episode. Symptoms can often be reproduced by having the patient hyperventilate voluntarily, but this should be done with caution since partial and primary generalized absence seizures may also be precipitated by hyperventilation.

Transient global amnesia is a prolonged episode of memory impairment, usually lasting from 4 to 8 hours and occurring without language problems, automatisms, or other neurologic accompaniments. The cause is undetermined. Although the abrupt onset and associated confusion may suggest complex partial seizure acitivity, episodes are much longer (hours versus minutes) and patients are, other than being amnestic, quite capable of complex interactions during attacks. Recurrences are infrequent.

Pseudoseizures are a poorly understood phenomenon in which paroxysms, most often resembling generalized tonic-clonic seizure activity, occur without any EEG evidence of seizure activity. Most of these patients are not malingering, but are experiencing emotional or psychogenic behavioral alterations. There are no absolute criteria for distinguishing pseudoseizures from true epileptic events; the diagnosis is further complicated by the fact that many patients with pseudoseizures also have a genuine seizure disorder. Pseudoseizures should be suspected when seizures fail to respond to standard therapy, when the behavioral manifestations are not stereotyped from one seizure to another, and when the motor activities are not of the typical tonic-clonic type. The correct recognition of pseudoseizures often requires the use of video monitoring and EEG telemetry and should never depend only on the observation of behavioral events. In many cases, very complex bizarre motor and behavior patterns have been shown to be epileptic by the use of such monitoring.

Diagnostic Evaluation

A seizure is a symptom of brain dysfunction. The workup should attempt to identify an etiology. The likely causes vary with the age of the patient at the onset of the first seizure, but the single largest diagnostic group in all ages includes those without a clear etiology. The most commonly identified causes in young adults (18–45 years) are drugs and drug withdrawal (especially alcohol), tumor, and trauma; in older adults, tumor, trauma, and cerebrovascular events are more likely to be identified. The evaluation may have to be repeated in the future; low-grade gliomas, for instance, can easily be missed on computed tomography (CT). The likelihood of determining the etiology is increased when the seizure has a focal component.

History should include a description of the attack from both the patient and observers. A family history of seizures and any previous central nervous system insults should be identified. The frequency, duration, and variability of events should be determined. Is there an aura? Can precipitants such as alcohol, sleep deprivation, or menstruation be identified? Chronic alcohol users are at risk of developing a seizure disorder, apart from the classic context of alcohol withdrawal due to trauma and infections associated with this condition. The ability to abort an attack is described by patients with some forms of partial seizures and should not contradict the diagnosis of epilepsy. Episodes occurring at night, rather than other times of the day, suggest real seizures rather than pseudoseizures.

Physical examination should include a careful search for focal neurologic signs or deficits, as well as indications of other underlying diseases.

Routine laboratory tests should include a complete blood count and serum chemistries to detect possible metabolic abnormalities such as hypoglycemia, hyponatremia, hypocalcemia, uremia, and hepatic insufficiency. A marked metabolic acidosis may be noted in blood drawn in the immediate postictal period. This is a transient nonspecific abnormality that is a result of the seizure and not the cause.

EEG is an essential part of the seizure workup. It can provide important information to aid in classifying the seizure and the presence of abnormalities can suggest metabolic or structural disorders that may not be evident by imaging or routine laboratory studies. However, the EEG cannot by itself either establish or eliminate the diagnosis of a seizure. Depending on the type of disorder and the conditions of the study, the EEG may be normal between seizures in 10% of patients with seizure disorders, even when repeated studies are performed after adequate sleep deprivation. In addition, approximately 2% of the normal population have epileptiform abnormalities in their EEGs but no clinical history of seizures.

The yield of the EEG in identifying the type of seizure varies considerably. Absence seizures have a characteristic 3-per-second spike and wave pattern found in the period of time between seizures (interictal period) in 80% of patients with this disorder. Juvenile myoclonic epilepsy is associated with 4-per-second spike and wave discharges. In patients with complex partial seizures, only about 50% have abnormal findings on a single EEG done during an awake state; the likelihood of positive results may be increased to 80 to 90% by repeating the study during sleep or after sleep deprivation. In generalized tonic-clonic seizures, the initial EEG is normal in up to 20% of patients, and nonspecifically abnormal in another 40%.

The EEG should be performed in a reputable laboratory with appropriately trained technologists and physicians; an improperly recorded or interpreted study may lead to a missed or mistaken diagnosis. Use of telephone transmission EEG services is discouraged, as this may introduce artifact into the record and often omits the historical and behavioral observations by the technologist that are essential to the clinical interpretation. If epileptiform activity is not found on the first tracing, a repeat study should be obtained after the patient has been sleep deprived. In some cases, further information may be obtained by referring the patient for a more intensive study. Various types of EEG monitoring, with or without simultaneous videotape recording of behavior, are available. If the seizure frequency is sufficiently high, these techniques may permit EEG recording during a seizure, which is almost always conclusive in determining a correct diagnosis and classification of the seizures.

CT or *magnetic resonance imaging* (MRI) is required in any adult with a new onset of seizures. Although the yield is low in young people (< age 30) with generalized seizures and normal findings on examination, the availability and noninvasiveness of imaging studies has led to their routine use, even when the likelihood of detecting a structural or vascular lesion is small.

MRI is more sensitive in detecting most lesions that cause seizures. CT may fail to detect lesions that have the same density as the surrounding brain, or are near bone (as are many areas of the brain with the lowest seizure thresholds).

Lumbar puncture (LP) may reveal elevation of cerebrospinal fluid (CSF) protein or CSF pleocytosis, suggesting infection, vasculitis, or occult central nervous system (CNS) malignancy. LP is contraindicated in the presence of any structural lesion, increased intracranial pressure, or a bleeding disorder, and should never be performed in any seizure patient without first obtaining an imaging study. LP is mandatory if there is suspicion of CNS infection; in other patients its yield is very low. In the absence of contraindications, most neurologists recommend LP in patients with seizures of recent onset, because it may detect low-grade infection, neoplasia, or vasculitis that may not be evident on other studies.

Follow-up

When the initial evaluation is normal, the search for etiology should be repeated in 6 to 12 months. This is particularly important in the newly diagnosed patient with recurrent seizures, but should also be considered in patients who are seizure-free on anticonvulsant drug therapy, because normal imaging studies do not completely eliminate the possibility of a structural lesion. If the patient has been seizure-free without anticonvulsant medications, repeat evaluation is probably not necessary. If there is any question regarding the diagnosis, the patient should be referred to a neurologist who specializes in seizure disorders.

Engel J. Seizures and epilepsy. Contemporary neurology series. Vol. 31. Philadelphia: FA Davis, 1989.
An excellent and thorough review of the basic science, clinical, and psychosocial issues pertaining to epilepsy.

Scheuer ML, Pedley TA. The evaluation and treatment of seizures. N Engl J Med 1990; 323:1468–74.
An excellent brief review.

Penry JK, ed. Epilepsy. Diagnosis, management, quality of life. New York: Raven Press, 1986.
A short, excellent overview of the diagnosis and treatment of epilepsy from a primary care perspective.

Hauser WA, Hesdorffer DC, eds. Epilepsy, frequency, causes, and consequences. New York: Demos, 1990.
An outstanding and detailed review of the literature regarding various risk factors for epilepsy, including prognostic factors, potential genetic risks, and others.

Aminoff MJ, et al. Electrocerebral accompaniments of syncope associated with malignant ventricular arrhythmias. Ann Intern Med 1988; 108:791–6.

DeMaria AA, et al. EEG in cough syncope. Neurology 1984; 34:371–4.
Two articles illustrating the high frequency of nonepileptic, convulsive-like movements during syncope.

Delgado-Escueta AV, Enrile-Bacsal FE. Juvenile myoclonic epilepsy of Janz. Neurology 1984; 34:285–94.
An excellent description of the various presentations of this treatable form of epilepsy.

Miller JW, et al. Transient global amnesia: clinical characteristics and prognosis. Neurology 1982; 37:733–7.
Reviews the clinical characteristics of transient global amnesia in 277 patients. Although 23.8% of the patients had recurrent episodes, they were not at increased risk for subsequent stroke.

Ellis JM, Lee SI. Acute prolonged confusion in later life as an ictal state. Epilepsia 1978; 19:119–28.

Guberman A, et al. Nonconvulsive generalized status epilepticus: clinical features, neuropsychological testing, and long term followup. Neurology 1986; 36:1284–91.
Two articles illustrating the many variations in clinical presentation of this not uncommon presentation of epilepsy.

Hauser WA, Ng SKC, Brust JCM. Alcohol, seizures, and epilepsy. Epilepsia 1988;29:Suppl. 2:S66–S78.

Ng SKC, et al. Alcohol consumption and withdrawal in new-onset seizures. N Engl J Med 1988; 319:666–73.
Two thorough presentations of old and important new information regarding the relationship between alcohol and seizures.

Scott DF. Recognition and diagnostic aspects of nonepileptic seizures. In: Riley TL, Roy A, eds. Pseudoseizures. Baltimore: Williams & Wilkins, 1982.
Clear, concise presentation of the literature dealing with pseudoseizures.

Sperling MR, et al. Prolactin in partial epilepsy: an indicator of limbic seizures. Ann Neurol 1986; 20:716–22.
An excellent discussion of hormonal changes associated with seizures.

Williamson PD, Wieser HG, Delagado-Escueta AV. Clinical characteristics of partial seizures. In: Engel J, ed. Surgical treatment of the epilepsies. New York: Raven Press, 1987:465–75.
An excellent description of the variable clinical features of complex partial seizures.

102. TREATMENT OF SEIZURES
John A. Messenheimer

Who Needs Treatment?
Not every patient who has had a single seizure will require treatment with anticonvulsant medication. Those who have had a single seizure provoked by a known precipitant, such as an underlying metabolic disorder or toxic effect, may have no further recurrences. The recurrence rate for patients who present with a first unprovoked seizure, with a normal neurologic examination, imaging studies (computed tomography or magnetic resonance imaging), and electroencephalography (EEG), and with no previous history of brain injury is approximately 25% over 5 years. Once a second seizure has occurred, however, 90% of patients continue to have seizures. The 5-year recurrence rate of patients with a remote history of brain injury or evidence of focal neurologic deficits is 50 to 70%. Other factors that can significantly influence recurrence rates include specific EEG findings and a family history of epilepsy. The decision to initiate or not initiate anticonvulsant therapy must take into account many variables, including the patient's work situation and willingness to experience a seizure recurrence. This decision is best made in consultation with a qualified neurologist, because it may rest on the interpretation of subtle clinical, historical, or laboratory findings.

Drug Therapy
The ultimate goal of treatment is the complete control of seizures and restoration of normal activities, with no significant side effects and preferably with a single agent. This goal is achievable in approximately 60% of patients. A small proportion of patients, perhaps 20%, will require two or more drugs, and 15 to 20% will be intractable to medical therapy, continuing to have at least occasional seizures despite optimal anticonvulsant therapy. Anticonvulsant drugs are symptomatic therapy, and a complete response to treatment does not mean that the patient does not have a progressive process at work.

Principles of Drug Therapy
Treatment is initiated with a single drug. The usual initial doses, as well as other parameters, for primary anticonvulsants are listed in Table 102-1. In general, the dose is increased

Table 102-1. Pharmacologic parameters for anticonvulsant drugs

Drug	Half-life (hr)	Days to steady state	Bound fraction (% of total)	Initial dose	Maintenance dose range	Therapeutic optimal range (µg/ml)
Carbamazepine (Tegretol)	14–27	3–4	70–90	100 mg bid	400–1600 mg qd	4–12
Ethosuximide (Zarontin)	20–60	7–10	0	250 mg bid	500–1500 mg qd	40–100
Phenobarbital (various)	50–150	14–21	40–60	60 mg qhs	60–240 mg qhs	15–40
Phenytoin (Dilantin)	10–30	7–10	90	300 mg qd	300–500 mg qd	10–20
Valproic acid* (Depakene)	8–15	1–2	90	15 mg/kg/day	500–4000 mg qd	50–150

*Also available in enteric-coated tablets as the closely related drug divalproex sodium (Depakote).

until either the seizures are controlled or toxic symptoms are encountered. Blood levels of anticonvulsant drugs are used initially to determine whether the "therapeutic range" has been reached, and later to document compliance and to define the individual patient's blood level correlates of seizure control or toxicity. The "therapeutic range" for each drug is a statistically defined optimal range, representing the range of levels for which the majority of patients have a reduction in seizures without toxic side effects. Individual patients, however, may have seizure control established or exhibit toxic symptoms with levels well outside of this range.

Drug levels should be measured when the patient is at steady state for a particular dosage, which usually occurs after the patient has been on that dosage for five half-lives of the drug (see Table 102-1). Variations in half-life are the norm. Shorter half-lives are seen in cases of comedication with enzyme-inducing drugs (with the exception of valproic acid, all anticonvulsants induce enzymes), whereas longer half-lives are associated with single-drug therapy. If trough levels cannot be obtained, the time of the last dose of medication should be noted when blood samples are drawn, and correlated with the results. An effort should be made to always obtain blood samples from the patient at approximately the same time of day, preferably at trough. Blood levels of anticonvulsants represent a total of both the protein-bound and unbound or "free" fractions. Although only the free drug is available to the brain for anticonvulsant effect, in general the fractions are proportional and the total correlates with the levels in the brain. For phenytoin, which is highly protein-bound, this proportion may be upset by a reduction in serum protein, such as occurs in renal or hepatic insufficiency or hypoalbuminemia, or when another drug, such as aspirin or another anticonvulsant, competes for serum protein-binding sites. The result is a marked increase in the free drug fraction, so that patients may be toxic with total drug levels well within or even below the "therapeutic range." This phenomenon may also occur with other protein-bound drugs, such as valproic acid, and to a lesser extent, carbamazepine, but is generally of little practical significance.

If the original anticonvulsant chosen is ineffective, a second drug should be started while the initial drug is continued at the maintenance dosage. Once the blood level of the second drug reaches the therapeutic range, the first drug should be slowly tapered. Blood levels should be checked first after the new drug has been at a maintenance dosage sufficiently long to reach steady state, or sooner if toxic symptoms appear. Emerging toxic symptoms are not necessarily due to the new drug but may reflect secondary elevations of the first drug induced by the second or may be due to drug interactions. Patients should be warned of this lest they lose confidence in the second drug before it has been given a fair trial. Seizure recurrence during the tapering of the first drug should be dealt with by increasing the dosage of the second drug rather than aborting the withdrawal of the first drug. The goal is to maintain single-drug therapy. The rate of tapering of a drug is controversial, but in general it should not exceed a one-third dosage reduction for every five half-lives of the drug. Once the first drug is tapered and eliminated, the blood level should again be checked so that any interaction of the first with the second will be detected and dosage adjustments made before a seizure occurs.

Most patients do not require more than one drug for adequate seizure control. Occasionally, in the process of making the adjustments described above, the need for two drugs will be objectively documented. Although it may be necessary for the control of seizures, the combination of two or more anticonvulsants often leads to increased toxicity, which may be more debilitating than the seizures. When a patient appears to require more than one drug, a neurologist should be consulted.

Selection of a Drug
The choice of an agent for initial therapy depends on the type of seizure.

PRIMARY GENERALIZED TONIC-CLONIC SEIZURES. Carbamazepine, phenytoin, and valproic acid are all effective, but one or the other may be better tolerated. Phenobarbital may also be effective and has the advantages of a low cost and a long half-life (which improves compliance); it causes sedation in some patients but many tolerate it well.

ABSENCE SEIZURES. The drugs of choice for classic absence seizures are ethosuximide and valproic acid. Ethosuximide is only effective for absence seizures, while valproic acid has a much broader spectrum. Valproic acid is the drug of choice if absence seizures are associated with either myoclonus or generalized tonic-clonic seizures, particularly in juvenile myoclonic epilepsy.

PARTIAL SEIZURES. Carbamazepine or phenytoin are the initial drugs of choice. Some patients respond to valproic acid, phenobarbital, or primidone as secondary drugs.

Commonly Used Anticonvulsants
Because of concerns regarding the use of generic anticonvulsants in the treatment of epilepsy, the following discussion of specific drugs assumes that brand name preparations are being used. While some patients may be able to maintain seizure control using generic anticonvulsants, the use of generic compounds tends to introduce a greater degree of fluctuation in blood levels than would be expected with the brand name preparations. This may or may not be acceptable to the individual patient. For patients in whom the therapeutic window in drug levels is narrow, consistency in the dosing and availability of medication may be critical.

Phenytoin (Dilantin) is an excellent first-line drug for partial seizures as well as for primary or secondary generalized tonic-clonic seizures. It may exacerbate absence seizures, and should be avoided if these are present.

Phenytoin can usually be started at a typical maintenance dose of 300 mg/day. A loading dose of 15 mg/kg results in therapeutic drug levels within a day; without a loading dose, therapeutic drug levels are reached in five half-lives, or about 1 week. Maintenance therapy is often given as a single bedtime dose of Dilantin capsules, which are manufactured in slow-release form. Other formulations require divided dosing. If daily doses of greater than 300 mg are required, it is best to divide the dose, to avoid large fluctuations in blood levels, over a 24-hour period. Unlike other anticonvulsants, phenytoin's kinetics are nonlinear; the enzyme system metabolizing phenytoin may be saturated within the therapeutic range, and once this occurs, an increase in the dose, or the addition of another drug that displaces phenytoin from its binding sites, can result in very high blood levels. For example, an increase in the daily dose of phenytoin from 300 to 400 mg may result in a marked increase in blood levels, raising them from the subtherapeutic to the toxic range. To avoid toxicity, adjustments in phenytoin doses above 300 to 400 mg should be made in increments of 50 or 30 mg. Phenytoin is metabolized in the liver and is highly protein-bound. The presence of hepatic disease or renal disease with hypoproteinemia may result in an increase in the free fraction of the drug, with toxic symptoms at lower total levels than normal. This effect may also be seen with the concurrent administration of certain medications, typically aspirin and valproic acid. Other drugs may affect phenytoin metabolism, with a resulting decrease in phenytoin levels. Because of considerable interindividual variation in drug metabolism, the addition of any new medication should cause anticipation of possible drug interactions. If toxic symptoms appear, blood levels, including a free phenytoin level, should be measured. Further information about phenytoin drug interactions is contained in the volume by Engel, listed in the references.

The most common side effect (3–5%) of phenytoin is rash due to an allergic reaction, within the first 2 weeks of treatment; patients with rashes should be seen and evaluated immediately, and phenytoin discontinued if the rash is suspected to be drug-related. Other common side effects include gingival hyperplasia, which may be controlled somewhat by vigilant mouth care, and hirsutism, which is seen more commonly in young women. Coarsening of the facial features resulting from thickening of the subcutaneous tissue around the nose and eyes also occurs, usually in children. While these side effects are cosmetic, they may be distressing to patients and necessitate choosing an alternative drug. Prolonged therapy with phenytoin has been associated with megaloblastic anemia, which responds to folate, osteomalacia from inactivation of vitamin D, and peripheral neuropathy. Competitive binding of phenytoin to thyroid-binding globulin results in artifactually lowered thyroxine (T_4) levels. Toxic side effects include ataxia, nystagmus, drowsiness, slurred speech, confusion, and possible exacerbation of seizures. Prolonged exposure to toxic levels of phenytoin may result in cerebellar atrophy and ataxia, which is not reversible on withdrawal of the drug. Very rarely, a syndrome of lymphadenopathy with high spiking fevers, arthralgias, a Stevens-Johnson–type exfoliative dermatitis, or bone marrow suppression may occur.

Carbamazepine (Tegretol) is an excellent first-line drug for generalized tonic-clonic seizures as well as partial seizures. It is not effective for absence seizures and may exacerbate seizure activity in some cases of mixed or atypical absence seizures.

Treatment with carbamazepine is initiated slowly, with daily doses of 100 to 200 mg, in order to avoid transient, usually visual side effects, such as blurred or double vision, and/or dizziness. The dosage can be increased every 5 to 7 days to a total daily dose of 600 mg/day. Further dosage changes should be made on the basis of the blood level. Carbamazepine may, over a period of weeks, induce the enzymes necessary for its own metabolism; this results in lower drug levels and/or a shorter half-life at the same drug dosage. During the initial 1 to 3 months of treatment, it may be necessary to increase the dosage to maintain stable drug levels. Levels should be checked several weeks after therapy is initiated, to determine whether this has been a significant factor. Because of its variable half-life, divided dosing of carbamazepine is necessary; twice-a-day administration is often possible, although some patients experience transient side effects 1 to 2 hours after a dose, which usually responds to increasing the dose frequency to three or four times a day. Carbamazepine is better absorbed with food and should be consistently taken with meals.

Carbamazepine is usually well tolerated. Visual disturbances are the most common side effect. Symptoms of toxicity include nystagmus and diplopia, often associated with ataxia; these symptoms may also occur at the initiation of treatment if dosages are increased too rapidly. Inappropriate secretion of antidiuretic hormone is occasionally seen; abnormal results on liver function tests are unusual. Reversible leukopenia and thrombocytopenia are occasionally seen; generally white blood cell counts of less than 3000 per cubic millimeter (or absolute neutrophil counts $< 1000/mm^3$) or platelet counts of less than 100,000 per cubic millimeter indicate a need to reduce the dosage. Aplastic anemia has occurred, but appears to be very rare. Baseline and periodic follow-up blood counts should be obtained every few weeks until the dosage is stable, and at longer intervals thereafter.

Phenobarbital is effective for either partial or generalized tonic-clonic seizures, but not for absence seizures. Its low toxicity, long half-life, and low cost are tremendous advantages over other anticonvulsant medications. Adults usually require 60 to 120 mg/day, which, because of the long half-life, may be given as a single bedtime dose.

Drowsiness is the major side effect of phenobarbital, and the major limitation to its usefulness. Tolerance to the sedation rapidly develops in many patients, but elderly patients may experience confusion or other subtle mental status changes.

Primidone (Mysoline) is a barbiturate that is metabolized to phenobarbital and to phenylethylmalomide (PEMA). Both of these metabolites as well as primidone itself have anticonvulsant activity. It is used as a second-line drug for treating tonic-clonic seizures and partial seizures. Because administration of primidone actually involves three active substances, side effects occur more frequently, and supervision by a neurologist is advisable.

Valproic acid (Depakene, Depakote) is indicated as a first-line drug for absence seizures or for generalized tonic-clonic seizures and as a second choice in partial seizures refractory to phenytoin and carbamazepine. Initial doses should be low (250 mg), increasing every 5 to 7 days to a total dose of 15 mg/kg. Subsequent adjustments should be based on blood levels and the patient's response. Common side effects, affecting about 10% of patients, include gastrointestinal irritability and transient hair loss. Less common central nervous side effects include tremor, diplopia, and ataxia. Thrombocytopenia and coagulation defects have been reported. Hepatic toxicity is a potential problem and occurs in both a mild form characterized by asymptomatic, dose-dependent elevations of liver enzymes, and a much less common but potentially fatal form, heralded by the typical prodromal symptoms of hepatic dysfunction. The risk of the latter is age-dependent (the greatest at under 2 years) and is strongly related to polypharmacy with other anticonvulsants. The risk of this complication in all patients using valproic acid as monotherapy has been estimated as 1 per 37,000; there are no reports of hepatic fatalities in patients over the age of 10 using valproic acid as monotherapy.

Ethosuximide (Zarontin) is indicated only for absence seizures, primarily seen in children. Treatment is initiated at 250 mg/day (15–40 mg/kg/day in children and increased to 750–1500 mg/day in adults). Side effects include gastrointestinal disturbance, agitation, and rarely, thrombocytopenia.

General Treatment Measures

Activity Limitations
Advice to patients regarding activity limitations should be individualized, with a goal of avoiding injury without undue restrictions. Activities will obviously be more limited for patients with frequent or poorly controlled seizures than for those whose seizures are rare, consistently preceded by an aura, or occur only during sleep. In general, activities during which even a momentary loss of consciousness could be fatal, such as scuba diving, rock climbing, or airplane piloting, cannot be permitted. Depending on the characteristics of the seizures, other potentially dangerous activities, such as swimming, bathing, and working with machinery, fire, or electricity, can sometimes be undertaken if proper supervision is available. For instance, patients with seizure disorders may swim safely in the presence of someone who knows they are epileptic and is capable of rescuing them if a seizure occurs. When a seizure disorder interferes with work activity, patients may be eligible for vocational rehabilitation programs. Information about such programs and other social aspects of epilepsy may be obtained from The Epilepsy Foundation of America (1828 L Street, N.W., Washington DC 20036) or from local and state epilepsy associations. Many regional epilepsy groups are active and represent a major resource for these patients.

Driving
Regulations on driving a motor vehicle vary from state to state, but in most the newly diagnosed seizure patient is not permitted to drive for some period of time, and a seizure-free interval is required before driving may be resumed. Patients whose seizures do not involve a loss of consciousness, such as those with simple partial seizures, may have fewer restrictions. State requirements regarding notification of the Department of Motor Vehicles about the patient's condition also vary, and treating physicians must become familiar with the laws in their state.

Avoiding Seizure Precipitants
A number of factors tend to precipitate seizures in some patients and should be avoided. These may include sleep deprivation, fever, strobe lights, psychological stress, and certain drugs that lower the seizure threshold, including some antidepressants and antipsychotics. Excessive alcohol intake can also lower the seizure threshold, especially during the withdrawal phase, but nonalcoholic patients with seizure disorders can usually tolerate occasional alcohol intake without a resulting increase in seizure frequency.

Common Clinical Problems

Recurrent Seizures
Unless medical intractability has been established and documented, each seizure recurrence should prompt an evaluation (blood level and review of the record) and a change in treatment (either a dosage increase or a switch to a new drug). If seizures continue despite optimal therapy with anticonvulsants, the patient should be referred to a neurologist specializing in seizure disorders. Medically intractable patients may be candidates for treatment with experimental drugs or for surgical procedures. A patient who experiences a seizure recurrence after being seizure-free for a long interval (> 1 year) or a patient in whom the pattern (frequency or characteristics) of the seizures changes should be re-evaluated as a newly diagnosed seizure patient, including a search for a structural etiology for the seizures.

Discontinuing Anticonvulsant Medication
Patients who have been seizure-free for more than 2 years may be candidates for withdrawal of the medication. The overall recurrence rate in such patients is approximately 40%, usually occurring in the first year after medication is discontinued. An EEG should be obtained prior to drug withdrawal; the presence of generalized spike and wave activity is associated with an increased risk of recurrence. While there is little consensus on other factors that predict the likelihood of seizure recurrence after anticonvulsant withdrawal, focal seizures are more likely to reappear than are generalized ones, and single seizures have a low recurrence rate (25%) if they are not associated with clinical, radiographic, or electrophysiologic evidence of a focal neurologic abnormality.

Withdrawal of medication must be undertaken only after careful consideration of the risks involved. The patient must fully understand and be willing to accept the risks and potential consequences of a seizure recurrence, and be willing to endure restrictions such as not driving for a period of time, usually at least 6 months, during and after the withdrawal period. No amount of seizure-free time can absolutely guarantee that seizures will not recur during or after withdrawal of the medication.

Pregnancy and Anticonvulsants

Seizure frequency remains unchanged during pregnancy in about half of epileptic patients, but both increased and decreased seizure frequency may also occur. Seizure frequency increases are often due to decreases in the serum levels of the medication, resulting from pregnancy-related alterations in metabolism, volume of distribution, and protein binding of anticonvulsants.

Although low, the risk of birth defects is approximately 2 to 3 times normal, with an overall frequency estimated at 4 to 6% in babies born to epileptic mothers. The most commonly associated anomalies include cleft lip and palate, and cardiac septal defects. The role of anticonvulsant drugs in this process is unclear; congenital anomalies occur with increased frequency even in untreated epileptic patients, and while the risk is higher in treated patients, these patients are also more likely to have additional contributing genetic or biochemical factors. All anticonvulsants have been implicated in this process and none is considered totally safe. Neural tube defects have been associated with valproic acid (1% risk). Trimethadione, an anticonvulsant rarely used today, is contraindicated in pregnancy due to the presence of birth defects in over 50% of the fetuses exposed to it. No medication is assumed to be entirely safe.

At the present time, the following guidelines are suggested:

1. Females of childbearing potential who are taking anticonvulsants must be informed, prior to pregnancy, of the potential risks of these medications. Many of the more serious defects occur in the first trimester, so waiting until the pregnancy is recognized is often too late.
2. All anticonvulsants, with the exception of valproic acid, are enzyme inducers and may cause increased metabolism of steroid hormones, consequently reducing the effectiveness of birth control pills. Women taking anticonvulsants should therefore be warned that birth control pills containing low concentrations of hormones may be ineffective in preventing pregnancy.
3. Consultation with a neurologist specializing in the treatment of epilepsy is recommended prior to pregnancy, to be certain that anticonvulsant medication is indicated and to consider alteration of the current regimen to one that may have a lower risk to the fetus. While generalized tonic-clonic convulsions themselves may pose risks to the fetus from hypoxia, acidosis, or trauma, patients with partial or absence seizures may, in some cases, be able to discontinue drugs during pregnancy.
4. Continued follow-up throughout the pregnancy at monthly intervals is required, to monitor side effects and blood levels.
5. Supplements of vitamin K, at least during the last month of gestation, must be given to reduce the risk of neonatal hemorrhage. Folic acid supplements during the pregnancy may reduce the risk of defects.
6. It should be emphasized that despite these concerns, approximately 95% of infants born to mothers who are taking anticonvulsant medication are normal. A diagnosis of epilepsy and treatment with anticonvulsant medication are not, by themselves, sufficient reason to discourage pregnancy, particularly in women in whom the seizures are well controlled with a single drug at relatively low serum levels.

Engel J. Seizures and epilepsy. Contemporary neurology series. Vol. 32. Philadelphia: FA Davis, 1989.
An excellent and very thorough review of the basic science, clinical, and psychosocial issues pertaining to epilepsy.

Scheuer ML, Pedley TA. Current concepts: the evaluation and treatment of seizures. N Engl J Med 1990; 323:1468–74.
A brief review of the issues discussed here.

Penry JK, ed. Epilepsy. Diagnosis, management, quality of life. New York: Raven Press, 1986.
A short but excellent overview of epilepsy from the primary care perspective.

Nuwer MR, et al. Generic substitutions for antiepileptic drugs. Neurology 1990; 40:1647–51.
Excellent discussion of the issue of generic anticonvulsant medication.

Mattson RH, et al. Use of oral contraceptives by women with epilepsy. JAMA 1982; 45:55–9.
Guidelines for the use of anticonvulsants in women using birth control pills.

Andermann F. Identification of candidates for surgical treatment of epilepsy. In: Engel J Jr, ed. Surgical treatment of the epilepsies. New York: Raven Press, 1987:51–70.
Discussion of the criteria used to select patients likely to benefit from surgical treatment.

Hauser WA, et al. Seizure recurrence after a first unprovoked seizure: an extended follow-up. Neurology 1990; 40:1163–70.
Recent update of an important previous study dealing with the risks of recurrence after an initial seizure, which also included a discussion of previous reports and important methodologic issues in studies of this type.

Callaghan N, Garrett A, Goggin T. Withdrawal of anticonvulsant drugs in patients free of seizures for two years: a prospective study. N Engl J Med 1988; 318:942–6.
A recent discussion on withdrawal of anticonvulsants in an adult population.

Dreifuss FE, et al. Valproic acid hepatic fatalities: a retrospective review. Neurology 1987; 37:379–85.
A comprehensive review of hepatotoxicity of valproic acid. Clear guidelines for safe use.

Janz D, et al, eds. Epilepsy, pregnancy and the child. New York: Raven Press, 1982.
Dalessio DJ. Current concepts: seizure disorders and pregnancy. N Engl J Med 1985; 312:559–63.
Yerby MS. Problems in the management of the pregnant woman with epilepsy. Epilepsia 1987; 3:Suppl:529–36.
Reviews that discuss treatment of the mother and risks to the child.

103. TRANSIENT ISCHEMIC ATTACKS AND CAROTID BRUITS
John S. Kizer

Transient Ischemic Attacks

Transient ischemic attacks (TIAs) are focal neurologic deficits that spontaneously resolve within 24 hours. They are the initial manifestation of only 15 to 20% of arteriosclerotic cerebrovascular events.

Prognosis
The onset of TIAs indicates an increased risk for future cerebral infarctions. Estimates based on prospective follow-up of patients with TIAs indicate a 3-year risk of stroke of any severity of about 20% and a 5-year risk of 30 to 40%, with the majority of new strokes occurring within the first 6 to 12 months after the onset of TIAs. Over the same period, the risk for a disabling or fatal stroke is about 10 to 11%. The same studies suggest that over a 5-year period, about 80% of the patients presenting with TIAs will improve or become asymptomatic if they do not suffer a stroke or heart attack within the first year. No more than 25 to 30% of patients with cerebral infarctions will have antecedent TIAs. Thus, if one assumes that cerebral infarctions account for two-thirds of all strokes (with hemorrhagic and embolic strokes constituting the majority of the other third), more than 80% of all major cerebrovascular events occur without warning.

Pathogenesis

The pathogenesis of TIAs is not understood. It is clear that transient cardiac arrhythmias and episodic hypotension are unlikely causes. Possible mechanisms include the transient formation of platelet microaggregates at local stenoses, subintimal hemorrhage into existing atheromas, localized vasospasm at atherosclerotic plaques, waxing and waning of the size of in situ thromboses, and fibrin and platelet microemboli from ulcerations or stenoses of intra- and extracranial vessels (including the thoracic aorta).

It should be emphasized that not all TIAs are accompanied by large-vessel atherosclerotic disease, and in fact fewer than 10% of all ischemic strokes derive from the tributaries of such a stenosis. Moreover, it is also not certain that lacunar TIAs and infarcts are pathophysiologically related to cortical TIAs and infarcts.

While the immediate cause of TIAs is uncertain, it is quite clear that the presence of TIAs implies diffuse cerebrovascular disease, which in turn is part of a diffuse systemic vasculopathy. Thus, TIAs mark not only a risk for future stroke but also an increased risk for death from other cardiovascular diseases. In fact, death from myocardial infarction occurs 2 to 4 times more frequently than death from stroke. Therefore, therapeutic interventions to prevent the development of stroke in patients with TIAs must take into account that the onset of TIAs represents a late stage in the development of progressive systemic vascular disease.

Evaluation

Differential Diagnosis

In the majority of patients, TIAs are associated with arteriosclerotic cerebrovascular disease. Before the diagnosis of ischemic TIAs can be certain, other illnesses that can present as transient focal neurologic deficits must be considered in the differential diagnosis. These include hypercoagulable states such as polycythemia, thrombocytosis, clotting factor deficiencies, or Trousseau's syndrome. Migraine, focal seizures, syncope, cranial arteritis, intracranial bleeding, hypoglycemia, vasculitis, hyperviscosity syndromes, aneurysms, tumors, emboli, multiple sclerosis, Sneddon's syndrome, hemoglobinopathies, and disorders of the labyrinthian systems producing vertigo may also initially present with transient neurologic dysfunction.

Although the presence of the lupus anticoagulant or antiphospholipid antibodies has been suspected to increase the risk of stroke, their significance outside the setting of a rheumatologic disease is highly controversial.

Laboratory Diagnosis

The diagnosis of obstructive cerebrovascular disease may be supported by the presence of cranial or carotid bruits and confirmed by a variety of noninvasive studies: ocular–ear lobe plethysmography, ultrasound imaging of the extracranial vessels, dynamic brain scans, and spectral analysis of Doppler ultrasound scans of extracranial vessels. The sensitivity and specificity of these noninvasive diagnostic procedures are quite variable when compared to standard arteriography. For example, the sensitivity and specificity of a carotid bruit indicating obstructive disease of the carotids may each be only 50 to 65%. Moreover, oculoplethysmography may give false-negative results in as many as 50% of patients in the presence of bilateral carotid stenoses, because this procedure depends on a comparison of pulse delays between the right and left sides. Duplex ultrasonography (B-mode anatomic imaging coupled with pulsed Doppler ultrasound to assess blood flow) is the most sensitive and specific of the noninvasive tests (sensitivity 85%, specificity 90%). Doppler ultrasonography of the carotids (sensitivity 70%, specificity 90%) and periorbital Doppler ultrasonography (sensitivity 70%, specificity 75%) are alternative investigative tools that give the best information when used in combination (sensitivity 90%, specificity 90%). Transthoracic echocardiography has a low diagnostic yield in patients presenting with TIAs and is not recommended for routine screening. On the other hand, when used appropriately, transesophageal ultrasonography is a highly sensitive and specific test for delineating ulcerative disease of the thoracic aorta or intracardiac sources of emboli.

Arteriography remains the most accurate procedure for delineating disease of the cranial vessels. Arteriography, however, is associated with a significant morbidity—between 1 and 5% depending on the patients studied. Visualizing the carotid circulation by means of computerized digital subtraction angiography is safe, with little or no morbidity and few contraindications; however, this test yields less precise images than does classic arteriography and is not recommended.

Noninvasive tests such as ultrasound are inferior to arteriography in the diagnosis of ulcerative plaques of the carotids. Since there is uncertainty about the relationship between ulcerative disease, its treatment, and the prevention of future strokes, the importance of this deficiency is difficult to assess.

Approach to the Patient

In the patient presenting with TIAs, imaging of the central nervous system (CNS) with either computed tomography (CT) or magnetic resonance imaging (MRI) may not be absolutely necessary in every case, but is advised for those patients in whom some factor other than obstructive cerebrovascular disease is a possible cause of the transient neurologic dysfunction. Diagnostic evaluation of the cranial vasculature using ultrasound to localize extracranial obstructions is advised for patients presenting with hemispheral TIAs or nondisabling stroke who would be candidates for surgery if an ipsilateral obstructive carotid lesion were to be found (see Surgical Therapy). Arteriography should be reserved for the clarification of difficult diagnoses or the preoperative evaluation of vascular anatomy.

Treatment

Therapy includes modifications of risk factors such as alcohol consumption, diabetes, smoking, and hypertension, and attempts to alter the consequences of established cerebrovascular disease.

Modification of Risk Factors

The risk of stroke is generally proportional to the degree and duration of hypertension, and there is solid evidence that treatment of hypertension will prevent the initial occurrence of strokes. Whether such treatment will prevent the occurrence of a second or third stroke is disputed. Currently, there is no evidence that improved control of diabetes by generally available means lessens the risk of future stroke. Carotid disease may diminish in those who discontinue smoking, and heavy consumption of alcohol is a risk factor for both hemorrhagic and ischemic stroke.

Anticoagulant and Antiplatelet Drugs

Attempts to modify the progression and sequelae of ischemic cerebrovascular disease with either anticoagulants or platelet antiaggregants are based on the rationale that platelets and the coagulation cascade are likely to be involved in atherogenesis and cerebral infarction. Implicit in this rationale, however, is the untested assumption that similar mechanisms underlie the pathogenesis of TIAs and cerebral infarction.

ANTICOAGULANTS. Over the past 20 years, numerous controlled and uncontrolled studies investigated the hypothesis that chronic oral anticoagulation of patients presenting with TIAs prevents the occurrence of strokes. These studies did not show any significant protection from the future development of stroke, although the overall cardiovascular mortality may have been slightly reduced. In patients chronically anticoagulated following a myocardial infarction, there may be a 10 to 20% reduction in the risk of stroke, an observation that suggests a higher proportion of embolic strokes in this setting (perhaps from mural thrombi).

ANTIPLATELET THERAPY. There have been 13 controlled trials of the efficacy of aspirin for the treatment of TIAs and ischemic cerebrovascular disease. Meta-analysis of these trials suggests a 20% reduction in the risk of *nonfatal* stroke and a 30% reduction in *nonfatal* myocardial infarction, with no definable difference between high- and low-dose aspirin therapy. No evidence can be adduced that this protective effect extends to women, possibly because fewer women than men were enrolled in these trials. A similar analysis of 10 controlled trials of aspirin in the secondary prevention of myocardial infarction suggests odds reductions of nearly 40% in the rate of *nonfatal* stroke, again reflecting a possible reduction in embolic disease. Overall, there is a small, but significant 15% reduction in overall vascular *mortality*. Most studies suggest that both low- and high-dose aspirin regimens are equally effective. Dipyridamole and sulfinpyrazone have not been shown to add to the therapeutic efficacy of aspirin.

In controlled trials of aspirin in the primary prevention of cardiovascular disease, however, treatment does not reduce overall mortality and an increase in hemorrhagic strokes offsets any reduction in infarctive strokes. Therefore, aspirin is not recommended for the primary prevention of cerebrovascular disease in patients at low risk. Interestingly, evidence from one clinical trial suggested a beneficial effect of aspirin in preventing the progression of multi-infarct dementia. On the other hand, there is no evidence available to determine the therapeutic efficacy of aspirin in Binswanger's encephalopathy (subcortical periventricular myelopathy).

No convincing data support the use of omega-3 fatty acids (fish oil) in the primary or secondary prevention of cerebrovascular disease.

One small controlled study (60 patients) suggested that pentoxifylline (400 mg tid) is twice as effective as aspirin in preventing recurrent TIAs and is equally effective in preventing permanent stroke. Without more substantial evidence, however, pentoxifylline cannot be recommended at this time as a substitute for aspirin.

Two recent studies examined the potential value of the antiplatelet drug ticlopidine in the prevention of ischemic cerebrovascular disease. In patients with a recent stroke, 500 mg daily resulted in a 20% relative risk reduction of stroke and stroke-related death and a 23% relative risk reduction of stroke, myocardial infarction, and vascular death. The overall rate of death was unchanged. When compared to aspirin in patients with TIAs, reversible ischemic neurologic deficits (RINDs), or minor strokes, ticlopidine reduced the 3-year relative risk of stroke and stroke death by 21% and overall vascular death by 12%. The rate of side effects with ticlopidine is approximately 50% higher than that observed with aspirin. Men and women benefit equally. The implications of the observed increase in cholesterol levels (9%) are unknown since recent secondary prevention studies suggested that ticlopidine may acutely reduce the frequency of myocardial infarction.

Thrombolysis
There is growing interest in the use of enzymatic thrombolysis (streptokinase, tissue-type plasminogen activator) in the treatment of threatened or incipient thrombotic or embolic stroke. At present, there is no convincing evidence that such an approach is either safe or effective and its use must be considered experimental.

Vasodilator Therapy
There is no evidence to support the use of vasodilators in cerebrovascular disease, except as they are indicated in the control of systemic hypertension.

Surgical Therapy
The surgical approach to the treatment of TIAs is based on the belief that extracranial vascular disease is a cause of TIAs and a harbinger of cerebral infarction.

The most common surgical approach to the treatment of TIAs is carotid endarterectomy. Surgery of the vertebrobasilar system is rarely performed because this area is relatively inaccessible and because of the disputed belief that TIAs in the distribution of vertebrobasilar arteries have a better long-term prognosis than do TIAs occurring in the distribution of the internal carotid arteries. Anastomosis of the superficial temporal artery to the internal carotid artery, to bypass obstructive lesions, is a third surgical approach.

Two randomized, prospective studies that evaluated the role of extracranial carotid surgery in the management of TIAs were completed prior to 1984. The first study (the Joint Texas Study) was unable to demonstrate that carotid endarterectomy improves survival rate or decreases the risk of stroke in patients presenting with TIAs. In the second study (by Shaw et al.), randomization was halted after the first 41 patients were assigned, because of the statistically higher rate of early stroke and death in the group randomized to undergo surgery.

Contrasting with these earlier studies, the European Carotid Surgery Trial presented an interim report on a randomized trial of carotid endarterectomy for 2518 symptomatic patients with hemispheral TIAs or nondisabling stroke and an ipsilateral carotid stenosis. The medically treated group usually received aspirin, treatment of definite hypertension, and advice to stop smoking. The trialists reported a highly significant, 84% relative reduction in the risk of fatal or disabling *ipsilateral* ischemic stroke following surgery (8.4% absolute risk to 1.1% at 3 years) for patients with high-grade stenosis (> 70%). If, however, the risk of death or disabling stroke within 30 days of surgery (3.7%) is added to the surgical tally, the absolute risk for fatal or disabling ipsilateral stroke is reduced from 8.4% to 4.8% (a relative risk reduction of 40%). Following endarterectomy, for *all* disabling or fatal strokes at 3 years of follow-up, the risk is reduced from 11% to 6%, a reduction just reaching statistical significance. For any stroke lasting more than 7 days, the risk is reduced from 22% to 13% (with a 30-day surgical risk of 7.5%), a highly significant reduction. Because most of the risk of stroke in the control subjects diminished after the first year following the onset of TIAs, the trial suggests that delayed surgery may not generate the same benefits. Importantly, there was no reduction in the frequency of strokes in other tributaries. In patients with low-grade stenosis (< 30%), surgery appeared to be contraindicated. For those with moderate stenosis (30–69%), no recommendations could be made from the study.

Coincident with the published report of the European trial, the North American Symptomatic Carotid Endarterectomy Trial published results of a randomized trial of 1000 patients that appear to parallel the results of the European trial. A recent multicenter study also evaluated the efficacy of anastomosing the superficial temporal artery to the middle cerebral artery for the treatment of occlusive or obstructive atherosclerotic disease of the internal carotid artery. Surgery was not shown to be more effective than medical therapy in the prevention of stroke or recurrent TIA. More importantly, the early complications of stroke and death were 2.5 times higher in the surgical group.

Therapeutic Approach to the Patient
At present, the best available evidence suggests that extracranial carotid surgery prevents many of the fatal or disabling ischemic strokes ipsilateral to a high-grade carotid stenosis (> 70%) in patients presenting with TIAs or a nondisabling stroke when the symptoms are appropriate to the stenosis. Placed into an epidemiologic perspective, 100 such patients would require treatment to prevent five fatal or disabling strokes. Thus, advice as to the value of surgery for a given patient with TIAs obviously requires a careful assessment of the risks and benefits, and the potential therapeutic efficacy of newer medical treatments such as ticlopidine. Moreover, fewer than 10% of patients who have developed a cerebral infarction have an appropriately placed large-vessel lesion, data indicating that the vast majority of patients destined to develop symptomatic, ischemic cerebrovascular disease must be offered supportive care.

For all patients, both those offered surgery and those for whom surgery is not indicated, therapy for TIAs should include the cessation of smoking and excessive alcohol consumption, control of hypertension, and reduction of other risk factors for ischemic heart disease. In addition, daily aspirin therapy is also recommended until more experience is gained with other antiplatelet drugs such as ticlopidine and pentoxifylline.

Asymptomatic Carotid Bruits

Asymptomatic carotid bruits are found in approximately 5 to 7% of adults; their distribution in men and women is nearly equal, and their frequency increases with age. Patients presenting with a carotid bruit have an increased risk of overall cardiovascular mortality, with the frequency of death from myocardial infarction being 2 to 4 times greater than that of death from stroke. In patients with asymptomatic carotid bruits, the 8-year incidence of stroke is between 4 and 12%, a risk 2 to 4 times greater than the risk in patients who do not have a carotid bruit.

Carotid bruits are a marker of cerebrovascular disease, rather than the direct cause of future strokes. Only two-thirds of subsequent strokes in people with carotid bruits are secondary to cerebral infarction; subarachnoid and intracerebral hemorrhage and embolic strokes account for the majority of the remaining third. Also, a majority of cerebral infarctions that occur in patients with asymptomatic carotid bruits are located in vascular territories unrelated to the carotid bruit. Moreover, prospective follow-up of patients with carotid stenosis suggests that fewer than 35% will have progressive disease and that of the few that proceed to complete occlusion, 40% will do so without symptoms. Only about 10% of all cerebral infarctions (all distributions) have an antecedent carotid bruit. Of considerable importance is the observation that a carotid bruit may have a sensitivity and specificity of only 50 to 65% for carotid disease.

Many clinicians have advocated carotid endarterectomy for patients presenting with asymptomatic carotid bruits, arguing from the results of trials for symptomatic patients that surgery reduces the long-term risk of stroke and death. There is little evidence to support this approach. Because the risk of stroke in patients with TIAs and an ipsilateral high-grade stenosis appears to diminish after the first year, there is reason to believe that a stenosis accompanied by TIAs is pathologically more "active" than is a silent stenosis. This suggestion is also supported by the more frequent occurrence of a stroke ipsilateral to an "active" stenosis (a stenosis accompanied by ipsilateral TIAs) than ipsilateral to a silent stenosis. Current trials of endarterectomy for asymptomatic disease are underway.

At the present time, care of the patient presenting with an asymptomatic carotid bruit includes modification of the risk factors for stroke (hypertension, smoking, and diabetes) and other risk factors for total cardiovascular mortality. There are no data on which to recommend the use of aspirin although there is reason to believe that aspirin may slightly reduce overall vascular mortality.

Prophylactic Endarterectomy in Patients Undergoing Surgery

The rate of stroke is about 0.5% in general surgical patients and about 1 to 3% in patients undergoing coronary artery bypass grafting (CABG). Many clinicians have advocated prophylactic carotid endarterectomy in asymptomatic patients with carotid bruits before surgery, especially CABG, in the belief that endarterectomy will prevent surgically related strokes. This approach cannot be recommended for several reasons: (1) The risk of stroke in patients with carotid bruits during CABG is elevated only minimally, if at all, compared to patients without bruits. (2) The majority of strokes are either embolic or perioperative, implying that hypercoagulability or some anomaly of postoperative physiology other than the carotid stenosis is causative. (3) The risk of complications from endarterectomy is double the risk of perioperative stroke. (4) The incidence of neurologic deficit following coronary artery bypass surgery is not significantly greater among patients with angiographically documented carotid artery disease than in those without carotid disease. (5) Limited direct evidence suggests that prophylactic endarterectomy is not effective.

Veterans Administration Co-operative Study Group on Antihypertensive Medications. Effect of treatment on morbidity in hypertension. JAMA 1970; 213:1143–52.
Clinical trial of antihypertensives in reducing cardiovascular morbidity.

Bauer RB, et al. Joint study of extracranial arterial occlusions. JAMA 1969; 208:501–18.
Randomized prospective study of carotid endarterectomy in the patient presenting with TIAs.

Shaw PA, et al. Carotid endarterectomy in patients with transient cerebral ischemia. J Neurol Sci 1984; 64:45–53.
Randomized prospective study of carotid endarterectomy in the patient presenting with TIAs. The ethics committee halted the study when it became clear that early morbidity and mortality of the surgical group were unacceptably higher than in the medical group.

Joint Committee for Stroke Resources. XIV. Cerebral ischemia: the role of thrombosis and of antithrombotic therapy. Stroke 1977; 8:147–75.
Comprehensive review of studies relating to the use of anticoagulants for preventing stroke in the patient with TIAs.

Heyman A, et al. Risk of stroke in asymptomatic persons with cervical arterial bruits. N Engl J Med 1980; 302:838–41.

Wolf PA, et al. Asymptomatic carotid bruit and the risk of stroke—the Framingham Study. JAMA 1981; 245:1442–5.
In this and the preceding study, the risk of stroke is shown to be small. The distribution and type of stroke were not predicted by the location of carotid stenosis.

Antiplatelet Trialist's Collaboration. Secondary prevention of vascular disease by prolonged antiplatelet treatment. Br Med J 1988; 296:320–31.

Meta-analysis of the trials of aspirin in the secondary prevention of vascular disease in patients with myocardial infarction and cerebrovascular disease.

Ropper AH, et al. Carotid bruit and the risk of stroke in elective surgery. N Engl J Med 1982; 307:1388–90.
Prospective study suggests that the risk of operative stroke does not differ between patients with and those without carotid bruit.

Hennerici M, et al. Natural history of asymptomatic extracranial arterial disease: results of a long-term prospective study. Brain 1987; 110:777–91.
Low rate of strokes (0.4%/year), and progression of disease over a median follow-up of 29 months were observed in only 36%.

Chambers BR, Norris JW. Outcome in patients with asymptomatic neck bruits. N Engl J Med 1986; 315:860–5.
Those with high degrees of stenosis have a greater stroke rate. Strokes occur in the tributary of the diseased vessel, however, no more frequently than by chance alone. Eighteen patients went on to total unilateral stenosis, but only 10 had any symptoms.

Health and Public Policy Committee, American College of Physicians. Position paper; diagnostic evaluation of the carotid arteries. Ann Intern Med 1988; 109:835–7.
Discussion of the laboratory methods used to diagnose carotid artery disease.

Yutsu F, Hart R. Asymptomatic carotid bruit and stenosis: a "reappraisal." Stroke 1983; 14:301–4.
Discusses clinical significance of carotid bruit.

Faught E, Trader SD, Hanna GR. Cerebral complications of angiography for transient ischemia and stroke: prediction of risk. Neurology (NY) 1979; 29:4.
Eighteen (12.2%) of 147 patients had cerebral complications; in 8 (5.4%), they were present at discharge from the hospital.

Harrison MJG, et al. Cerebrovascular disease and functional outcome after coronary bypass surgery. Stroke 1989; 20:235–7.
Postoperative neuropsychological deficits are not higher among patients with angiographically visible carotid artery disease.

Hass WK, et al. A randomized trial comparing ticlopidine hydrochloride with aspirin for the prevention of stroke in high risk patients. N Engl J Med 1989; 321:501–7.
Suggests efficacy of ticlopidine in preventing strokes greater than with ASA.

Gent M, et al. The Canadian American Ticlopidine Study (CATS) in thromboembolic stroke. Lancet 1989; 2:1215–20.
Argues for the efficacy in patients with treated stroke. The severity of strokes that occurred, however, was not lessened.

EC/IC study group. Failure of extracranial/intracranial arterial bypass to reduce the risk of ischemic stroke. N Engl J Med 1985; 315:860–5.
Results of an international randomized trial show no benefit, and in fact surgical patients fared worse than medical patients. The surgical complication rate was 2.9%, and 80% of TIAs improved over 5 years.

European Carotid Surgery trialists collaborative group. MRC European Carotid Surgery Trial: interim results for symptomatic patients with severe (70–90%) or with mild (0–29%) carotid stenosis. Lancet 1991; 337:1235–43.
Largest randomized trial of carotid endarterectomy.

North American Symptomatic Carotid Endarterectomy Trial collaborators. Beneficial effect of carotid endarterectomy in symptomatic patients with high-grade carotid stenosis. N Engl J Med 1991; 325:445–53.
Results similar to those of the European study.

Sacco RL, et al. Infarcts of undetermined cause: the NINCDS stroke data bank. Ann Neurol 1989; 25:382–90.
Describes the pathologic findings for 1805 cases of stroke.

104. PARKINSONISM
Axalla J. Hoole and Colin D. Hall

Parkinsonism is not a single disease but a clinical syndrome characterized by a resting tremor, a slowing of voluntary movements, muscle rigidity, and gait abnormalities. It may appear as the predominant problem or as an incidental finding in patients with other diseases.

The prevalence of parkinsonism is estimated to be 1 case per 100 people over 50 years old. Before the advent of levodopa (L-dopa), parkinsonism was associated with an increase in the death rate. Since then, studies of patients taking L-dopa have shown a decrease in the number of deaths attributable to parkinsonism.

Causes
Most patients with parkinsonism have idiopathic Parkinson's disease (paralysis agitans). This disease usually develops in patients over 50 years old and affects men and women equally and whites slightly more frequently than blacks. Von Economo's encephalitis lethargica was recognized as a cause of parkinsonism after the pandemic of 1918 to 1920. Other viruses have occasionally been associated with sequelae that have parkinsonian features, but infection has not been established as a major cause of parkinsonism.

Drugs such as phenothiazines (especially chlorpromazine), butyrophenones (especially haloperidol), and less commonly methyldopa, metoclopramide, and reserpine have been associated with a dose-dependent form of parkinsonism. Symptoms have been reported within days following high dosages, but the usual course is for symptoms to develop after weeks of therapy. Parkinsonism usually disappears within weeks after stopping the drug but may persist longer, particularly following depot injection. Recently, the illicit street drug MPTP was recognized as causing permanent symptoms of parkinsonism.

Manifestations
The major features of established parkinsonism are tremor, bradykinesia, and muscle rigidity. The presentation of Parkinson's disease varies considerably from one patient to another in both the presence and the severity of these symptoms. Early symptoms of parkinsonism may include muscle aches and fatigue; early signs include decreased strength of speech, decreased spontaneous blinking, and unilateral gait disturbance with decreased arm swinging.

The characteristic resting "pill-rolling" tremor of the thumb and forefinger is seen in approximately two-thirds of patients. The tremor worsens with anxiety or tension, usually diminishes with movement of the limb, and disappears with sleep. Starting in the hand, the tremor may remain relatively restricted or eventually involve the arm and leg on the same side and then the opposite extremities.

Bradykinesia is an inability to initiate movement. This is often the most disabling aspect of the disease. Because patients have trouble adjusting position, maintaining balance is difficult and falls are frequent.

Rigidity is bilateral and affects both extensor and flexor muscles; however, there is no loss of strength. Resistance to passive motion is continuous ("plastic rigidity"), unless a superimposed tremor imparts a "cogwheel" effect to the rigidity.

The gait of patients with parkinsonism is characteristic. Early in the course of disease, there is a unilateral loss of arm swinging; later both arms are involved. Starting to walk becomes more difficult, and the patient eventually develops a gait pattern in which the upper part of the body is thrust forward to initiate walking and the patient goes forward with small rigid steps chasing his or her center of gravity (festinating gait). The patient is often more unsteady when turning. Eventually, even stopping becomes a problem.

Characteristic changes in voice, facial features, and handwriting also occur. Hoarseness is an early sign and may be followed by a loss of vocal strength. Ultimately, there is little face or lip movement, and speech becomes blurred and hard to understand. Facial expression is characteristic and referred to as "mask-like." Changes are bilateral, as opposed to the usual unilateral changes in patients with seventh nerve lesions. The glabellar response is positive: When the patient is asked not to blink and then tapped on the bridge of the nose, he or she will blink with each tap and not have the usual spontaneous suppression of response to the tap. Handwriting becomes smaller and may show the regular movements of the tremor.

Other clinical findings include blepharospasm (fluttering of the eyelids after they are shut) and sialorrhea (production of a greasy, thick sebum) accompanied by a scaly dermatitis over the forehead and face.

Evaluation

Diagnosis is almost entirely based on clinical findings. Laboratory tests are not usually performed unless the evaluation suggests that the course is unusual, there is a focal neurologic deficit, or the parkinsonism is associated with an underlying disease that requires further testing. When the differential diagnosis includes multiple cerebral infarcts, normal-pressure hydrocephalus, or progressive supranuclear palsy, computed tomography (CT) or magnetic resonance imaging (MRI) may be helpful.

Differential Diagnosis

When only one feature of the disease is present, diagnosis may be difficult. In some patients, the tremor is minimal or absent, and rigidity and postural problems are the predominant complaints. In these patients, parkinsonism may be difficult to distinguish from depression, or in younger patients, from early Huntington's disease or Wilson's disease. Rarely, patients in whom only the muscles controlling phonation are involved present with a speech disorder.

The tremor of parkinsonism should not be confused with postural tremors and cerebellar intention tremor. Postural tremor is worsened by positioning (as when the arms are outstretched), is diminished by rest, and is not accompanied by rigidity or bradykinesia. Postural tremors are found in patients with benign essential tremor, a disorder that may be sporadic or may be inherited, and in patients with metabolic problems such as thyrotoxicosis, hypomagnesemia, or alcoholism.

Benign essential tremor can frequently be identified in first- and second-degree relatives of patients with postural tremors. It may diminish or disappear with alcohol consumption, a finding reliable enough to be considered a clinical test by some neurologists. Patients with benign essential tremor may respond to propranolol, 60 to 180 mg/day in divided doses, but not to L-dopa or anticholinergics.

The intention tremor of cerebellar dysfunction worsens with purposeful use of the hands. A confusing factor may be that up to 10% of patients with parkinsonism also have an intention component of their tremor.

Other conditions in which some manifestations of parkinsonism are often present include multiple cerebral infarcts and Alzheimer's disease as well as less common problems such as progressive supranuclear palsy and Shy-Drager syndrome. In these conditions, the triad of tremor, rigidity, and bradykinesia is generally a less significant part of the overall picture. Occasionally, cerebral atherosclerotic disease may be indistinguishable from Parkinson's disease, but in atherosclerosis, parkinsonism usually appears as part of a stepwise progression of little strokes, other local neurologic deficits are identifiable, and tremor is frequently absent. In Alzheimer's disease, dementia is the principal finding; the dementia associated with idiopathic parkinsonism is less profound and is not an early finding. However, as intellectual function is being more thoroughly evaluated, dementia is emerging as a more important finding.

Parkinsonism may also be associated with or be a sequela of brain damage resulting from severe metabolic disorders, such as hypoglycemia, hyponatremia, anoxia, and renal or hepatic failure. Normal-pressure hydrocephalus, which presents as a gait disturbance as well as incontinence and deteriorating intellectual ability, may also be confused with parkinsonism. Frontal lobe neoplasms, such as meningioma, may closely mimic the features of parkinsonism and should be considered when there is a rapid onset of symptoms.

Parkinsonism may also be confused with problems associated with diminished facial movement and flat expression, including hypothyroidism and psychiatric disorders such as depression.

Treatment

Principles of Drug Therapy
Drug treatment of parkinsonism is based on manipulating the brain neurotransmitter system with either dopaminergic or anticholinergic agents, or both. In parkinsonism there is a decrease in levels of the neurotransmitter dopamine in the substantia nigra. Since dopamine suppresses striatal systems that are stimulated by acetylcholine, decreased levels of dopamine or blockage of its effects by such drugs as phenothiazines lead to uncontrolled effects of acetylcholine. The most frequently used drug is L-dopa, which crosses the blood-brain barrier and is decarboxylated to dopamine. Other drugs sometimes employed are bromocriptine and pergolide mesylate, which are dopaminergic agonists, and amantadine, whose mode of action is unclear but is believed to stimulate release of dopamine from neurons. The two most frequently used anticholinergic drugs are trihexyphenidyl (Artane) and benztropine mesylate (Cogentin).

A recent and very exciting development has been the use of a monoamine oxidase inhibitor, selegiline (formerly known as deprenyl), which not only has proved to be of benefit in relieving mild symptoms but also may prevent progression of the disease process. There is controversy as to whether the optimal time to start treatment with L-dopa or carbidopa–L-dopa (Sinemet) is earlier or later in the course of the disease. Because long-term studies indicate a decline in the benefit of L-dopa after the first 5 years of treatment, there is concern that starting early will result in side effects occurring sooner and the medication losing its effectiveness. On the other hand, withholding treatment until later in the course does not allow the patient to benefit at the time the medication may be most effective and most helpful. The following is a reasonable approach:

Medications are begun only after all drugs that can cause parkinsonism have been withdrawn for 4 weeks.

If the patient has parkinsonian features but is functioning relatively normally, the physician may observe without treatment. Alternatively, patients who have convincing evidence of parkinsonism may be offered treatment with selegiline (Eldepryl), with the hope of delaying the progression of symptoms. The cost of this drug ($4/day in 1990) may be prohibitive for many patients.

If significant symptoms develop, or remain after treatment with selegiline, then further medications, such as amantidine, anticholinergics, or carbidopa–L-dopa should be added.

If symptoms are mild but still troublesome, anticholinergics or amantidine may be prescribed as described below. Amantadine may be a preferable first step in elderly patients because of their lower tolerance to anticholinergic side effects.

If tremor is the paramount feature, and the patient is functioning well, a trial of anticholinergics is worthwhile.

If the patient still is unable to function satisfactorily either in the home or at work, carbidopa–L-dopa should be started. If the patient is already taking anticholinergics or amantidine, withdrawal of these medications should be tried after satisfactory therapeutic results are achieved with carbidopa–L-dopa or L-dopa. Selegiline may be continued.

If the patient has failed to respond satisfactorily to a maximum dose of L-dopa or carbidopa–L-dopa or if the optimal effect declines as the disease progresses, amantidine, anticholinergics, and bromocriptine should be added, in that order, and evaluated. If any one of these is unhelpful, it should be withdrawn. However, there is a cumulative effect from these agents, and some patients will benefit from taking all of them.

Specific Drugs
Selegilene (formerly deprenyl, marketed as Eldepryl) is a monoamine oxidase B inhibitor that was recently suggested to have a role in preventing the progression of parkinsonism. It may also have a mild effect in improving clinical symptoms. The dosage is 5 mg twice a day. Side effects are infrequent, but when added to carbidopa–L-dopa, the L-dopa side effects may be increased. The medication is very expensive.

Amantadine, 100 mg 2 times a day, may improve the symptoms of parkinsonism. Its effects are usually short-lived (weeks or months) but occasional patients experience long-term benefits. It is used primarily in mild cases or as an adjunct to L-dopa, but may be employed as initial therapy, particularly in elderly patients as an alternative to anticholinergics. Side effects are fewer than with alternative agents, but include hallucinations, psychosis, and a harmless livedo reticularis.

Anticholinergics are used in mild cases and to relieve tremors. Frequently used agents are trihexyphenidyl (Artane), 2 to 5 mg 2 to 3 times a day, and benztropine mesylate (Cogentin), 1 to 2 mg 2 to 3 times a day. Neither of these agents has an established benefit over the other, and patients who do not respond to one may respond to the other. Other anticholinergics used occasionally include procyclidine (Kemadrin), biperiden (Akineton), and diphenhydramine (Benadryl). Common side effects that are usually well tolerated include dry mouth, blurred vision, and dizziness. Constipation may require the use of a mild laxative. More serious side effects that may limit the use of anticholinergics in elderly patients include acute confusion and urinary retention.

L-*Dopa (usually given as Sinemet)* has its greatest effect on bradykinesia, but also may be useful for treating all the clinical features of parkinsonism except intellectual dysfunction. In order to reduce its peripheral side effects, nausea, vomiting, postural hypotension, and cardiac arrhythmias, L-dopa is usually given with carbidopa. The latter is a decarboxylase inhibitor that prevents the conversion of dopa to dopamine outside the brain. If nausea and vomiting occur, it happens generally early in the course of treatment. The dosage may be reduced and then increased more gradually. Taking carbidopa–L-dopa with food may also prevent gastric disturbance. Hypotension, which is usually a late effect, may be helped by wearing support hose.

A carbidopa–L-dopa combination (Sinemet) is available in several strengths: Scored tablets contain 10 mg of carbidopa with 100 mg of L-dopa, or 25 mg of carbidopa with either 100 or 250 mg of L-dopa. This combination should be started slowly and titrated up to effective levels. A typical starting dosage is one 25/100-mg tablet given twice a day. After 2 days, this can be increased to one tablet 3 times a day, and then after a few days, increased to one tablet 4 times a day. This must be individualized for each patient, but most do not require or tolerate more than a maximum of 700 mg of L-dopa per day at a dosage schedule of 4 times per day; some clinicians add another drug, such as bromocriptine, to the regimen when levels reach only 400 mg of L-dopa per day.

The major side effects of carbidopa–L-dopa develop after months or years of therapy. They are due to the effects of the medication on the central nervous system. The most common are dyskinetic movement disorders; orofacial dyskinesia is most frequent, followed by athetoid movements and dystonic posturing, which can mimic Huntington's disease, tardive dyskinesia, or other degenerative neurologic disorders.

Psychiatric disturbances resulting from long-term therapy range from depression to acute psychosis with mania and frightening hallucinations. Vivid nightmares are a clue that a psychosis may be developing. If these symptoms appear, the dosage must be abruptly reduced or terminated. With improvement, the dosage may again be titrated upward, but a reappearance of symptoms may prevent optimal therapeutic levels from being reached. Other antiparkinsonian medications may also cause psychosis, and if the patient is receiving combination therapy, it may be necessary to withdraw all medications and restart them one at a time to verify which is causing the difficulty. As this will lead to a rapid increase in parkinsonian symptoms, it may be necessary to have the patient hospitalized.

After months or years of therapy, often with a dosage that has been previously well tolerated, the "on-off" phenomenon may develop. During the day, the medication may quite suddenly lose its effectiveness and the patient may become markedly bradykinetic. These spells may last minutes to hours. At times, they can be helped by increasing the doses or rearranging the dosage schedules to give smaller doses of carbidopa–L-dopa more frequently. Other patients may find that reducing dietary protein enhances the effect of carbidopa–L-dopa. The addition of ancillary medications such as bromocriptine may also be helpful. A sustained-release form of L-dopa/carbidopa has recently become available and may be effective in reducing some of the difficulties associated with fluctuations in serum levels. A conversion table is available with the product literature.

Other specific but uncommon effects of L-dopa or carbidopa–L-dopa include cardiac arrhythmias. Rarely, darkening of urine and sweat and a change of taste may occur, but these do not require modification of therapy.

Treatment must be individualized, both the amount and frequency of carbidopa–L-dopa and the use of other drugs. Most significantly affected patients find an effective dosage is one that gives reasonable but not complete relief from parkinsonian features. At the onset of therapy, it should be explained to the patient that completely alleviating symptoms and signs often leads to unacceptable side effects. Patients who remain intellectually intact can be given significant latitude to change the timing and amount of medication taken throughout the day.

Bromocriptine (Parlodel) is a dopaminic agonist that is less likely to cause dyskinesias, but is significantly less effective than L-dopa. It may be most effective when added to L-dopa or carbidopa–L-dopa in a dosage of 2.5 mg twice a day, increasing by 2.5 mg/day each week to a usual maximum of 15 mg; some patients tolerate up to 30 mg. Nausea, vomiting, and postural hypotension are milder than with an L-dopa preparation. More serious are visual hallucinations, nightmares, and acute confusional states.

Pergolide mesylate (Permax) is an alternative dopamine agonist that can be used in conjunction with carbidopa–L-dopa if bromocriptine is ineffective. It is given as 0.05 mg/day for 2 days, and then increased by 0.1 mg/day every third day until it is therapeutically effective to a total of 5 mg/day, given in two to four doses. The side effects include hallucinations, hypotension, gastrointestinal disturbance, and cardiac ectopy in patients with heart disease. Increasing dyskinesia may require a reduction of the carbidopa–L-dopa dosage.

Drug Holidays

In some patients, drugs may eventually lose their efficacy. "Drug holidays," in which the patient is hospitalized and all drugs are stopped for about a week and then reinstituted, are sometimes used for this situation. In some patients there may be significant improvement, and lower maintenance dosages may be required. This procedure may also be helpful when, after lengthy treatment, the physician and patient cannot clearly identify whether minor increases and decreases in L-dopa dosages are proving helpful or deleterious. Because of the risks associated with the immobility that results when medications are withdrawn, drug holidays should not be undertaken without consultation with a neurology specialist.

Surgery

Stereotactic thalamotomy has limited usefulness in patients with disabling tremor that is unresponsive to drugs. Attempts at surgically inserting dopamine-producing tissues into the brain remain primarily experimental.

Reynolds NC. The tremor syndrome: is it Parkinson's disease? Wis Med J 1981; 80:29–30.
A short review of the differential diagnosis of tremors.

Mental symptoms and parkinsonism (editorial). Br Med J 1973; 2:67–8.
A discussion of the causes of these problems.

Clinical therapeutic rounds: individualization of drug therapy for the parkinsonian patients. JAMA 1975; 233:1198–201.
Stresses the need for adapting therapy to individual patients.

Duvoisin RC. Parkinson's disease: a guide for patients and family. 3rd ed. New York: Raven Press, 1990.
A good guide for both family and physicians.

Klawans HL, Glantz RH. Ten years of L-dopa in parkinsonism. Guidelines Neurosci 1980; 4:1.
A review of persistent therapeutic dilemmas.

Hachinski V. Timing of levodopa therapy. Arch Neurol 1986; 43:407.
An editorial discussion of two articles in this issue, which compare early versus late initiation of treatment with L-dopa.

Liberman AN. Treatment of Parkinson's disease. Mayo Clin Proc 1988; 63:1046–9.
An editorial that discusses the use of dopamine agonists in conjunction with L-dopa.

Ahlskog JE, Muenter M. Treatment of Parkinson's disease with pergolide: a double blind study. Mayo Clin Proc 1988; 63:969–78.

Jankovic J. Long-term study of pergolide in Parkinson's disease. Neurology 1985; 35:296–9.
Kurlan R, et al. Long-term experience with pergolide therapy of advanced parkinsonism. Neurology 1985; 35:738–42.
Three well-designed studies that document the effectiveness of pergolide.

Golbe L. Deprenyl as symptomatic therapy in Parkinson's disease. Clin Neuropharmacol 1988; 11:381–400.
A good review of this drug and its use in Parkinson's disease.

The Parkinson Study Group. Effect of deprenyl on the progression of disability in early Parkinson's disease. N Engl J Med 1989; 321:1364–71.
A report from an ongoing study that describes the beneficial effects of deprenyl.

105. BELL'S PALSY
Robert S. Dittus

Bell's palsy (idiopathic facial paralysis) is an acute peripheral paresis or paralysis of the seventh cranial (facial) nerve for which a specific etiology cannot be determined. It has an annual incidence of about 20 per 100,000 population.

Although the cause of Bell's palsy is unknown, the most widely accepted theory is that it results from a postviral inflammatory lesion of the peripheral nerve; hereditary and vascular factors may also be contributory. In some cases, the facial nerve is the only clinically symptomatic nerve in a more diffuse polyneuropathy.

Risk Factors
Bell's palsy occurs with a fairly uniform distribution worldwide. It can occur at any age. The median age of onset is 40 years old; it is less common below the age of 15. Men and women are equally affected. The incidence appears to be increased in pregnancy, especially during the third trimester. Ten percent of patients with Bell's palsy have had a previous episode. Eight percent give a positive family history for the condition, although a true familial predisposition has not been established. Hypertension and diabetes mellitus appear to be more prevalent among patients with Bell's palsy.

Clinical Manifestations
Prodromal symptoms and their relative frequencies include upper respiratory tract infection (20%), headache (10%), fatigue (3%), and fever (2%). Facial numbness (32%) and spasm (22%) have also been observed in the prodrome. Weakness in the distribution of the facial nerve occurs acutely and unilaterally and can range from a mild paresis to complete paralysis. There is no predilection for either side of the face. Other presenting signs and symptoms include epiphora (tears collecting in and flowing over the lower eyelid, 68%), pain (62%), ageusia (57%), hyperacusis (29%), and diminished tears (17%). The pain is usually in or behind the ear, may be moderate to severe, and does not usually persist beyond 7 to 10 days. Retroauricular tenderness or edema may occur, and the chorda tympani may be erythematous. Hypoesthesia involving the distribution of cranial nerves V and IX is not uncommon.

Paralysis of the facial musculature produces a loss of all voluntary, associated, and emotional movements of the affected side of the face. Although sparing of the forehead musculature is often claimed to be an absolute discriminant in separating central from peripheral etiologies of facial nerve paresis, in one large series 5% of patients with Bell's palsy had sparing of the forehead musculature. As a result of the weakness, the affected side is expressionless, with a smoothing of the forehead wrinkles, a widening of the palpebral fissure, and a loss of the nasolabial fold. The corner of the mouth sags on the affected side, and the mouth is drawn to the unaffected side. The ipsilateral eyebrow may be lowered or elevated. The patient loses the ability to wink, but Bell's phenomenon is preserved (attempted eye closure results in an upward rotation of the eye).

Natural History

Approximately 50% of patients with Bell's palsy suffer only a partial loss of strength in the distribution of the facial nerve. Untreated, almost all will recover with normal function; nearly 90% of patients will recover within 3 to 6 weeks and the remainder within 3 to 6 months. Those few whose recovery is not complete will still have a result that is functionally and cosmetically satisfactory.

The other half of patients develop a complete paralysis, usually within a few days but occasionally evolving over the first week following the onset of symptoms. Of patients having complete paralysis, 50 to 60% will have a normal full recovery, 20 to 30% will have a satisfactory result, and 10 to 20% will be left with a severe palsy. Disfiguring contractures and synkinesis may occur. The symptoms resolve over several months.

There is no way of giving an accurate prognosis early in the course of the disease. A younger age and earlier onset of recovery are associated with a better ultimate degree of recovery. Diminished lacrimation occurs in 40% of patients whose recovery is ultimately incomplete; its presence increases the likelihood of an abnormal recovery from 25 to 50%. Diminished salivary flow also occurs in less than half of the patients whose recovery will be abnormal; its presence increases the likelihood of an abnormal recovery about twofold. A variety of electrical tests have been used to follow the course of nerve degeneration in hopes that this information will have early prognostic value. None has met with universal acceptance but facial nerve conduction studies may help establish a prognosis when they are performed 5 days or later after the onset. A normal or near-normal evoked muscle response indicates a demyelinating lesion, which should have a good prognosis. A low-amplitude response indicates axonal injury and carries a poorer prognosis. Since the prognostic information from these tests is not provided until about day 5, these tests cannot guide decisions on initial therapy; however, the provision of more accurate prognostic information may reduce patient anxiety over the subsequent weeks.

Diagnosis

Bell's palsy is by definition a diagnosis of exclusion. Five groups of disorders account for 98% of all cases of isolated facial nerve paralysis: Bell's palsy (60–70%), trauma (15–20%), otitis media (5–10%), herpes zoster oticus (4–6%), and tumors (3–5%). In the remaining 2%, the paralysis occurs in the presence of a variety of other disorders including infectious diseases (chickenpox, coxsackievirus, encephalitis, mastoiditis, infectious mononucleosis, influenza, meningitis, rubella, syphilis), metabolic abnormalities (diabetes mellitus, hyperthyroidism), and neurologic syndromes (cerebrovascular disease, Guillain-Barré syndrome, multiple sclerosis, myasthenia gravis).

When a patient presents with an acute unilateral facial weakness, the history and physical examination, including otologic and neurologic examination, are the most helpful guides in establishing a diagnosis. The following findings suggest a diagnosis other than Bell's palsy: simultaneous bilateral facial palsies, unilateral facial weakness that slowly progresses over 3 weeks with or without facial hyperkinesis, and failure of facial function to return within 6 months after an acute onset. Tumors are found in 30% of patients with recurrent unilateral facial palsy.

Many additional tests have been used to screen for primary causes and to attempt to locate the site of the lesion. An audiogram can detect hearing loss (which is not consistent with the diagnosis of Bell's palsy). Schirmer's test, to assess the adequacy of lacrimation, can be used for management; if tearing is diminished, patients should be treated with eye lubricants. Additional tests should be considered on an individual basis. Tests that are sometimes performed but have been shown not to be routinely helpful include sedimentation rate, glucose, VDRL, fluorescent treponemal antibody absorption (FTA-ABS), heterophil test, serum viral titers, cerebrospinal fluid analysis, mastoid radiographs, and temporal bone computed tomography (CT) scans.

Treatment

Therapy for Bell's palsy is controversial. There is no evidence that vasodilatation or electrotherapy alters the course of the disease. Because it is currently believed that inflammation and edema of the facial nerve play a role, both steroids and surgery have been advocated in order to decompress the nerve physically in its potentially confining pathway through the fallopian canal. Several studies both claim and refute the efficacy of both steroid therapy and surgical intervention. However, because of flaws in the study designs, none of the published series offers conclusive evidence for or against the use of either therapy. Both continue to be offered and investigated. In patients with no contraindications, the usual steroid therapy has consisted of oral prednisone (approximately 1 mg/kg/day) in two or more divided doses daily initially and for several days, with subsequent dosage reduction to a completion of therapy in 2 weeks.

Because the eyelids may not close completely, attention should be given to supportive care of the eye by providing adequate lubrication (in the form of artificial tears) and protection (by an eye patch) if necessary. If a patient has suffered permanent severe dysfunction, a variety of rehabilitative surgical procedures may be considered to improve facial appearance and function.

Adour KK, et al. The true nature of Bell's palsy: analysis of 1,000 consecutive patients. Laryngoscope 1978; 88:787–801.
Review of epidemiologic, clinical, and laboratory data.

May M, Hardin WB. Facial palsy—interpretation of neurologic findings. Laryngoscope 1978; 88:1352–62.
Detailed discussion of otoneurologic findings in 400 patients with Bell's palsy.

Huizing EH, et al. Treatment of Bell's palsy. Acta Otolaryngol (Stockh) 1981; 92:115–21.
Analysis of the literature on therapy.

Adour KK. Diagnosis and management of facial paralysis. N Engl J Med 1982; 307: 348–51.
Review of facial paralysis including Bell's palsy.

May M. Facial nerve disorders. Am J Otol 1982; 4:77–88.
Review article with special attention to rehabilitative surgery.

Peitersen E. The natural history of Bell's palsy. Am J Otol 1982; 4:107–11.
Description of the natural history of Bell's palsy in 1011 untreated patients.

Katusic SK, et al. Incidence, clinical features, and prognosis in Bell's palsy, Rochester, Minnesota, 1968–1982. Ann Neurol 1986; 20:622–7.
Population-based study of 206 incident cases of Bell's palsy.

May M, Hughes GB. Facial nerve disorders: update 1987. Am J Otol 1987; 8:167–80.
Review of facial nerve disorders including Bell's palsy.

Stankiewicz J. A review of the published data on steroids and idiopathic facial paralysis. Otolaryngol Head Neck Surg 1987; 97:481–5.
A catalog and summary of the effectiveness of steroids in Bell's palsy.

May M, Croxson GR, Klein SR. Bell's palsy: management of sequelae using EMG rehabilitation, botulinum toxin, and surgery. Am J Otol 1989; 10:220–9.
Discussion of therapy for patients having debilitating facial dysfunction as a result of Bell's palsy.

106. DEMENTIA IN THE ELDERLY
Alan K. Halperin and Mary K. Goldstein

Altered mental status is a common finding in the elderly. Approximately 5 to 10% of people older than 65 years and 20% of those older than 80 years have clinically important intellectual impairment. As many as 50% of the patients in nursing homes and mental hospitals may have such impairment.

Dementia is an impairment of memory, judgment, and other higher cortical functions, which characteristically presents with an insidious onset. It has an organic etiology, although the cause may not always be identified clinically. Dementia must be distinguished from delirium, an acute confusional state that is common in acutely ill elderly patients and may be superimposed on an underlying dementia. Delirium is usually reversible when its precipitating cause (e.g., medication, electrolyte imbalance, infection, cardiovascular event) is resolved. Since delirium may be the only sign of illness in an elderly patient, the danger is that an altered mental status resulting from delirium will be ascribed to dementia, and the underlying condition will not be sought or treated.

Causes of Dementia

Irreversible Causes
The major irreversible causes of dementia in the elderly (and their relative frequencies, as a percent of all dementias) include Alzheimer's disease (54%), multi-infarct dementia (13%), and Huntington's disease (5%). Pathologic examination of the brain of patients with Alzheimer's disease reveals a degenerative process involving cortical neurons, without significant ischemic lesions. This process is characterized clinically by a gradual and progressive decline of intellectual function. In contrast, patients with dementia secondary to multiple cerebral infarctions frequently have a stepwise decline in intellectual functioning. A form of vascular dementia that is being increasingly identified with sensitive imaging techniques is known as Binswanger's disease (multifocal leukoencephalopathy), and is characterized by multiple, small periventricular white matter lesions.

Potentially Reversible Causes
Recent estimates are that 11% of dementias are reversible (8% partial reversibility and 3% total). The most common causes (and frequencies) include drugs (28%), depression (26%), various metabolic factors (16%), and normal-pressure hydrocephalus (11%).

Normal-pressure hydrocephalus results in progressive dementia, gait disturbances, and urinary incontinence. In most patients, the cause is unknown, although it may be secondary to a blockage of cerebrospinal fluid reabsorption. In some patients, it is secondary to other central nervous system diseases such as previous subarachnoid hemorrhage, meningitis, and tumors.

A variety of disorders, none by itself very common, account for a significant number of apparent dementias. A partial list includes metabolic problems such as hyperthyroidism, hypothyroidism, Addison's disease, Cushing's disease, steroid treatment, hypoglycemia, hypercalcemia, and hypopituitarism; metabolic and electrolyte disturbances such as hepatic encephalopathy, hyponatremia, and uremia; nutritional deficiencies such as Wernicke-Korsakoff syndrome found in alcoholics, anemias associated with vitamin B_{12} or folic acid deficiency, and pellagra; and cerebral infections such as tuberculous and fungal meningitis, brain abscess, and neurosyphilis.

Diagnostic Strategy

It should never be assumed that dementia is irreversible until a careful evaluation has been completed. However, familiarity with the reversible causes of dementia, a thorough history and physical examination, and a few laboratory and radiologic tests are frequently all that are needed.

History
The history should first establish that the presentation is consistent with a dementia syndrome, differentiating it from delirium. While both are characterized by global cognitive impairment, delirium is acute in onset, lasts days or weeks, and has a fluctuating course. A dementia progresses over months to years. The delirious patient manifests rapid changes in level of consciousness, while the demented patient has impaired cognition in the presence of a clear sensorium. Dementia must also be differentiated from depression presenting with a loss of cognitive abilities, an uncommon but important phenomenon termed pseudodementia. Depression is likely to have a more rapid and recent onset and to be accompanied by a history of depression and by pervasive affective change, including

distress over the cognitive loss. The history should then be directed at characterizing the nature and progression of the dementia and uncovering clues to causal or contributing factors. When a patient's reliability as a historian is at issue, it is important to obtain additional history from external sources. Close family members can be helpful in assessing the severity and progression of impairment and behavioral or intellectual changes. Past medical records should be reviewed.

The dementia associated with Alzheimer's disease begins with subtle memory loss and errors of judgment. Later, impairments in judgment, orientation, intellect, and memory become more prominent. The ability to comprehend, assimilate, and integrate new information is impaired and attention to usual social amenities is decreased. In the late phase, the patient's personality and identity can be totally lost. Mood disturbances frequently occur and range from apathy and listlessness to suspiciousness and anger. The factors influencing the progression of disease are unknown, and the rate of progression is variable. In cases of multi-infarct dementia, patients or their families may be able to remember a specific time when intellectual and cognitive function began to deteriorate. A family history of Huntington's disease suggests that as the cause.

An accurate drug and alcohol history is important because many widely used drugs can cause or exacerbate brain dysfunction. The most commonly implicated are alcohol, tranquilizers, sedatives, hypnotics, antidepressants, antihypertensives including sympatholytics and diuretics, anticonvulsants such as phenytoin and barbiturates, anticholinergics, and miscellaneous other drugs such as levodopa, corticosteroids, and cimetidine.

Patients should also be asked about prior treatment for syphilis, focal neurologic symptoms, and brain trauma. Chronic subdural hematomas and subarachnoid hemorrhages can cause reversible dementia. Acute intellectual changes may be superimposed on a chronic low level of function, so assessment of change from baseline is important. The review of systems may rule out coexisting systemic diseases contributing to the dementia.

Physical Examination

A thorough physical examination is necessary to rule out systemic diseases that can cause reversible dementia. Special attention should be given to possible causes of poor cerebral perfusion, such as congestive heart failure. Neurologic examination begins with a screen of mental status to confirm the presence of cognitive impairment and to distinguish dementia, delirium, and depression. All three can involve disturbances in memory, intellectual function, and orientation. Delirium is characterized by a fluctuating level of consciousness, increased or reduced psychomotor activity, attentional deficits, distractibility, and a disturbed sleep-wake cycle. Depression is said to manifest itself with more "don't know" than "near-miss" answers; however, this may not always be the case. Administration of a depression screening questionnaire validated for use in early dementia (e.g., the Geriatric Depression Scale) may identify a depressed patient. Impairment of memory can be detected by digit or object recall (short-term memory) and questions about historical events that are compatible with the patient's educational background. Intellectual function can be tested by simple calculations or interpretation of proverbs. Visual-spatial function, often impaired relatively early in the course of Alzheimer's disease, may be evaluated by asking the patient to draw a clock face or copy a simple figure. The office examination can also include simple screening tests, such as the Mini-Mental State Examination (Folstein), which evaluates memory, orientation, language, constructional ability, and attention.

Neurologic examination should include a funduscopic examination for papilledema, an indication of increased intracranial pressure. Cranial nerve examination should look for visual field defects (lesions of the optic pathway), disturbances of extraocular movements (dysfunction of cranial nerves III, IV, and VI), and pupillary reactivity (tertiary syphilis). Abnormal movements such as tremors (Parkinson's disease) and tardive dyskinesia should be observed. A sensory examination should be performed to rule out the dorsal and lateral column disease of vitamin B_{12} deficiency. Sensorimotor findings are not expected in Alzheimer's disease until quite late in the course. Frontal lobe signs such as the grasp reflex, oral responses, palmar-mental reflex, and glabella tap reflex are nonspecific indications of diffuse cerebral dysfunction and are frequently present in the later stages of dementia.

The presence of gait disturbances may also aid in diagnosis. Focal gait abnormalities may be secondary to stroke or tumor; small shuffling steps and unstable gait may result from normal-pressure hydrocephalus, ataxia, or cerebellar disease secondary to alcoholism, tumors, strokes, or hypothyroidism. A shuffling and rigid gait is characteristic of Parkinson's disease, and a slapping, wide-based ataxic gait suggests tabes dorsalis or subacute combined degeneration.

Laboratory Tests
Considerable controversy concerning the appropriate testing strategy exists. There is general agreement on the usefulness of a complete blood count (CBC) and glucose, electrolyte, calcium, creatinine, and thyroid-stimulating hormone levels. Neurologic disorders may be caused by a cobalamin deficiency in the absence of anemia or macrocytosis, so some experts recommend the routine use of cobalamin (vitamin B_{12}) levels, and serum methylmalonic acid or total homocysteine if the cobalamin level is in the low-normal range. Other experts, citing evidence that the principal cerebral symptoms of cobalamin deficiency do not constitute a classic dementia syndrome, recommend this testing only if a confusing clinical picture requires it. Other tests (e.g., serologic studies, human immunodeficiency virus (HIV) assay, and heavy-metal screening) may be ordered selectively as suggested by clinical findings.

Computed tomography (CT) scans of the head can detect subdural hematomas, intracranial tumors, normal-pressure hydrocephalus, multi-infarct dementia, and atrophy consistent with Alzheimer's disease, that is, atrophy out of proportion to that expected by age alone. Magnetic resonance imaging (MRI) is superior to CT in detecting multiple focal cerebral lesions, and may help distinguish vascular dementia from Alzheimer's disease. Results must be interpreted with recognition that two forms may coexist. This is of diagnostic significance but unfortunately does not often provide therapeutically useful information. Positron emission tomography (PET) and single-positron emission computed tomography (SPECT) can show a pattern of changes in cerebral blood flow and metabolism. They are promising research tools that may allow specific diagnosis of Alzheimer's disease in the future. An electroencephalogram (EEG) is generally not helpful except for demonstrating the typical findings of Creutzfeldt-Jakob disease. A normal EEG, however, does provide evidence against a metabolic disorder. A lumbar puncture should not be performed routinely, but should be done when tertiary syphilis or another central nervous system infection is suspected (e.g., when headache, fever, focal neurologic signs, or rapid course are part of the presentation). Because the diagnostic tests used to confirm the presence of normal-pressure hydrocephalus are controversial, a neurologist and neurosurgeon should be consulted when this diagnosis is suspected. The evaluation of dementia is best done on an outpatient basis because changes in environment, such as hospitalization, can exacerbate symptoms.

Treatment

Specific Therapy
Specific therapy of potentially reversible dementias is directed at the underlying cause. If depression is present, either as a primary cause or coexisting with dementia, antidepressants should be used cautiously. Nortriptyline and desipramine tend to have a lower frequency of anticholinergic side effects, which makes them preferable in elderly patients. These agents should be started at very low dosages (10–25 mg/day), and titrated up slowly. Monoamine oxidase (MAO) inhibitors and electroconvulsive therapy may, in selected patients, be more appropriate; a psychiatrist experienced in the care of geriatric patients should be consulted if initial therapy with tricyclics is unsuccessful.

The effectiveness of therapy for normal-pressure hydrocephalus is controversial. Improvement with shunt therapy is more likely if the condition is secondary to a prior cerebral insult and in patients in whom the gait disturbance preceded the dementia.

It is controversial whether drugs improve cognitive function in demented patients. Ergoloid mesylates (Hydergine), 1 to 2 mg 3 times a day for 3 to 6 months, may help improve mobility or self-care, or even improve cognitive function in an occasional patient, but are no better than placebo for most patients. There is no evidence that the use of vasodilators, psychostimulants, dopaminergics, neuropeptides, cholinergic substances, or precursors of psychotropic agents improve cognitive function. Tetrahydroaminoacridine is currently under investigation, but is highly controversial.

Management

Supportive measures are directed at maintaining functional capacity and assisting the patient and family in planning for the future. General principles include the following:

1. Coexistent medical conditions should be aggressively treated. Maximal medical therapy of conditions such as congestive heart failure and pulmonary disease may keep the patient more comfortable and more functional, thus improving the quality of life and relieving the caregiver's stress.
2. Changes in the environment should be minimized because they frequently result in mental deterioration. Hospitalization and admission to a nursing home therefore should be avoided if possible.
3. Behavioral management should be the first approach to aggressive behavior. Tasks should be broken down to manageable steps, environmental noise levels reduced, and daily exercise provided. Any sudden change in behavior should prompt a search for a physical (e.g., a dental abscess or other painful condition) or an environmental cause.
4. When other methods of treatment fail, drugs may be targeted specifically to symptoms. If severe agitation with psychotic thinking is present, haloperidol (Haldol) in low dosages of 0.5 to 1.0 mg daily may be helpful. If nocturnal wandering or sleep disturbance is a problem, chloral hydrate or a short-acting benzodiazepine, such as lorazepam or triazolam, may be useful for intermittent treatment. As for other elderly patients, drugs with anticholinergic effects should be avoided.
5. Sensory impairments, such as visual and hearing deficits, should be corrected.
6. Support groups for families of patients with Alzheimer's disease may help them to have more realistic expectations and fewer feelings of guilt and anger. Such groups may also offer practical suggestions for managing problems related to daily activities such as driving, bathing, and toileting. For information about patient care and educational programs, contact Alzheimer's Association, 919 N. Michigan Ave., Suite 1000, Chicago, IL 60611, (312) 335-8700 or (800) 272-3900 (for family members).
7. Social services such as visiting health nurses, homemaker aides, home-delivered meals, physical therapy, respite care, senior citizen centers, and day care centers for the elderly can be invaluable resources to patients and family.

It is appropriate for the primary care physician to discuss with the patient, early in the course of a dementia, preferences regarding future medical care, including code status, treatment of acute illness, chronic enteral feeding, and designation of a surrogate decision maker. Every attempt should be made to honor the patient's wishes and to involve even the more severely demented patient, to the extent possible, in decision-making.

Katzman R. Alzheimer's disease. N Engl J Med 1986; 314:964–73.
A review of diagnoses, theories of causation, and treatments.

Van Horn G. Dementia. Am J Med 1987; 83:101–10.
An extensively referenced discussion of different types of dementia, and the major representative syndromes.

Roman G. Senile dementia of the Binswanger type. JAMA 1987; 258:1782–8.
Reports the increased identification of small subcortical lesions with MRI and CT scans. Discusses risk factors and implications for treatment.

Lipowski Z. Delirium in the elderly patient. N Engl J Med 1989; 320:578–82.
A review of the significance, presentation, diagnosis, and management of delirium, summarizing the features that help to distinguish it from dementia and psychosis.

Francis JF, Kapoor WN. Delirium in hospitalized elderly. J Gen Intern Med 1990; 5:65–79.
Thoroughly reviews the terminology, diagnostic criterion, differential diagnosis, prognosis, and management of delirium.

Clarfield AM. The reversible dementias: do they reverse? Ann Intern Med 1988; 109: 476–86.
A critical, comprehensive review of 32 reported studies. Finds that the frequency of reversible dementia may be overstated.

Barry PP. The diagnosis of reversible dementia in the elderly: a critical review. Arch Intern Med 1988; 148:1914–8.
Another excellent review of the causes of reversible dementia, including a discussion of the methodologic flaws of previous studies.

Lindenbaum J, et al. Neuropsychiatric disorders caused by cobalamin deficiency in the absence of anemia or macrocytosis. N Engl J Med 1988; 318:1720–8.
In a consecutive study of 141 patients with neuropsychiatric abnormalities due to cobalamin (vitamin B_{12}) deficiency, 40 (28%) were found to have no anemia or macrocytosis; of the 14 patients with mental or psychiatric abnormalities, all had accompanying sensory deficits.

Larson EB, et al. Diagnostic tests in the evaluation of dementia: a prospective study of 200 elderly outpatients. Arch Intern Med 1986; 164:1917–22.
Recommends a small number of screening tests; other tests should be ordered selectively.

Applegate WB Jr, Blass JP, Williams TF. Current concepts in geriatrics: instruments for the functional assessment of older patients. N Engl J Med 1990; 322:1207–14.
A guide to the screening tools available to assess cognitive function, physical function, and emotional state in elderly patients.

Council on Scientific Affairs. Magnetic resonance imaging of the central nervous system. JAMA 1988; 259:1211–22.
Discusses MRI findings in dementia. Reports that MRI has demonstrated that Binswanger's disease may be a common cause of dementia, and MRI shows patterns not seen by CT in normal-pressure hydrocephalus. Otherwise, MRI has not exceeded CT in its ability to evaluate dementia.

Winograd CH, Jarvik L. Physician management of the demented patient. J Am Geriatr Soc 1986; 34:295–308.
A practical review designed to assist clinicians in managing the symptoms and problems that confront demented patients and their caregivers. Also includes the Mini-Mental State Examination (Folstein).

Katz I, Curlik S, Lesher E. Use of antidepressants in the frail elderly. Clin Geriatr Med 1988; 4:203–22.
A review of depression in the elderly, including differential diagnoses, with special attention to nortriptyline.

Mace NL, Rabins PV. The 36-hour day: a family guide to caring for persons with Alzheimer's disease, related dementing illnesses, and memory lost in later life. Baltimore: Johns Hopkins University Press, 1991.
A practical and detailed reference book designed for families of demented patients, but an excellent resource as well for clinicians who advise them. Most appropriate for moderate or severe degrees of dementia.

Cohen D, Eisdorfer C. The loss of self: a family resource for the care of Alzheimer's disease and related disorders. New York: WW Norton, 1986. (paperback edition—New York: New American Library, 1987.)
A sensitive guide for families of demented patients, using patient examples and the patients' own words. Includes material appropriate to the early stages of dementia.

Yamkner BA, Mesculam M-M. β-amyloid and the pathogenesis of Alzheimer's disease. N Engl J Med 1991; 325:1849–57.
Reviews evidence for a major role of β-amyloid protein in causing Alzheimer's disease and hypothetical prospects for treatment.

XV. PSYCHIATRIC PROBLEMS

107. ANXIETY
John J. Haggerty, Jr.

Patients with a problem of "nerves" account for about 10 to 30% of encounters in a general medical practice. They may complain of being "shaky," "tense," "irritable," or "uptight," or the diagnosis may be made in the course of evaluating a somatic complaint. The major dilemmas facing the clinician are deciding which patients require special treatment and choosing between pharmacologic and nonpharmacologic treatment approaches.

Evaluation
The information required for initial treatment should include a full description of the symptoms and the life circumstances surrounding their onset; this can be obtained in about 30 minutes of uninterrupted interviewing. The following specific questions should also be asked:

1. *What has been the overall course of the symptoms?* Generalized anxiety disorder typically begins in early adult life and recurs intermittently. Anxiety arising for the first time in middle or late life often indicates another disorder such as depression or occult somatic disease.
2. *How disabling is the anxiety?* Has the patient experienced panic attacks or developed a fearfulness about driving or being in public places (agoraphobia)?
3. *Does the patient have a chaotic or stable life pattern?* Frequent moves, shifting relationships, or physician switching, for example, suggest a personality disorder and diminish the possibility that antianxiety medication can be used successfully.
4. *Does the patient's drinking pattern suggest alcoholism?* The most sensitive indicators are the need for a morning eye-opener and annoyance over criticism about drinking.
5. *Has there been chronic sedative use?* If so, the anxiety may be caused by drug withdrawal.
6. *Does the patient use stimulants such as cocaine or amphetamines? What is his or her caffeine consumption?*
7. *Are there vegetative symptoms of depression?* These include a loss of appetite, weight loss, early morning awakening, a loss of energy, decreased libido, and diurnal mood variation (feeling worse in the morning).
8. *Is the patient being abused or exposed to other real life threats?*

Differential Diagnosis

Generalized Anxiety Disorder
Among patients presenting with symptoms of anxiety, 10 to 30% will fall into one of the specific categories listed below. The remaining majority of patients are likely to suffer from generalized anxiety disorder. This is a chronic, recurrent condition that typically has its onset in young adulthood. The symptoms are nonspecific and include excessive worry, muscular tension, fatigue, autonomic hyperactivity (palpitations, dry mouth, dizziness, and diarrhea), and increased vigilance. Its cause is unknown.

Panic Disorder/Agoraphobia
Sudden, recurrent panic attacks (choking, palpitations, dyspnea, and extreme apprehension) characterize this dramatic subgroup of anxiety disorders. This disorder is not uncommon, but is frequently underreported due to the perceived bizarreness of the complaints. Patients with panic anxiety disorder often develop agoraphobia, a fear of being in public areas. Panic anxiety disorder is frequently mistreated with sedatives but often responds quickly to a combination of antidepressant medication and behavior modification. Psychiatric referral is usually indicated.

Depression
Depressive illness is the most common psychiatric disorder seen in general medical practice, often appearing in the guise of nonspecific nervousness, rather than as the "classic" retarded depression described in psychiatric textbooks. It is important to recognize affected

patients, since primary depression is specifically responsive to antidepressant medication. The diagnosis can usually be made by inquiring into the usual symptoms of depression such as sadness, anhedonia, appetite change, anergia, and poor concentration. Persistence of two or more of these symptoms beyond 1 to 2 weeks generally implies the presence of a medication-responsive depression (see Chap. 108). Anxiety that appears for the first time after the age of 40 should probably be considered evidence of depression until proved otherwise.

Alcohol and Drug Abuse
Alcoholism, the most frequently encountered form of drug abuse, is the underlying factor in at least 5% of cases of chronic anxiety seen in general clinic settings. Anxiety may be a part of either intoxication or withdrawal states. Problem drinking can usually be uncovered by straightforward questioning about drinking patterns. It is usually unproductive to attempt to treat anxiety while drinking continues. Other drugs, when abused, may be associated with anxiety syndromes. These include amphetamines and caffeine, over-the-counter sympathomimetics, hallucinogens, cocaine, and sedative-hypnotics.

Personality Disorder
Identifying features of a significant personality disorder include familiarity with multiple sedatives, a history of repeated suicide gestures, a demanding presentation, and angry, disparaging attitudes toward clinical providers. Sedatives offer no real benefit for the kind of anxiety experienced by these patients and should be avoided. The best approach is to offer a firm, consistent physician-patient relationship, a task requiring no small degree of skill and tolerance.

Hidden Violence and Other "Unmentionable" Traumas
Unrecognized spouse abuse was found to be the main underlying factor in half of the female mental health referrals from a rural primary care clinic. These patients usually presented with nonspecific manifestations of anxiety. The history of traumatic beating, easily elicited on questioning, was largely overlooked by the primary providers, who simply prescribed sedatives for their patients' symptoms. Women who have been raped and members of stigmatized minorities are additional examples of individuals who may feel inhibited about disclosing the real traumas underlying their anxiety.

Undiagnosed Physical Illness
Undiagnosed physical illness underlies anxiety in about 4% of patients. Common causes include hyperthyroidism, cardiovascular disease, and medication (e.g., steroids, aminophylline, anticholinergics, sympathomimetics, and occasionally sedatives).

Acute Psychotic Decompensation
Although generally self-evident, acute psychoses may occasionally be hidden under vague anxiety complaints and superficially intact thinking. Bizarre bodily concerns or fears of bodily "disintegration" are tip-offs to the presence of psychosis, which nearly always requires a major tranquilizer (e.g., chlorpromazine, thioridazine, haloperidol) along with expeditious psychiatric referral.

Prognosis
A number of well-constructed follow-up studies have shown that most patients with untreated generalized anxiety disorder have no more than mild disability 20 years after the initial diagnosis, although symptoms usually return intermittently throughout life. Despite the proliferation of therapeutic techniques and agents, treatment has not been shown to alter the life course of this condition.

Treatment
These findings argue for an approach that emphasizes long-term management over short-term cure. At present there are four basic options to consider for the patient with generalized anxiety disorder: (1) reassurance in the context of an ongoing physician-patient relationship, (2) medication, (3) psychotherapy, and (4) relaxation and stress management techniques. Flexibility is recommended, with the major emphasis determined by the clini-

cian's working style and the availability of treatment resources. The psychological makeup of individual patients, cost, and possible adverse effects should all be considered.

Reassurance
Reassurance alone is indicated when daily functioning is relatively unimpaired, when there are identifiable and understandable stressors, when the patient fears dependence on medication, or when the interview itself has an observable calming effect on the patient. The relationship with the physician is the active ingredient, and reassurance is more likely to be successful when supplemented by regular visits, adequate listening, and the skillful use of suggestion.

Medication
Despite recent controversies, the bulk of evidence seems to support the utility of antianxiety agents in properly selected patients. Benzodiazepines (Table 107-1) remain the treatment of first choice, with clinical studies reporting their overall effectiveness in relieving subjective anxiety as 70 to 75%, compared to 35% for placebo. These drugs blunt hyperarousal regardless of the cause and reduce symptoms in both idiopathic and reality-based anxiety states. The benzodiazepines have relatively few major adverse effects. Dependence and withdrawal have now been well documented but are relatively rare. Psychological dependence is estimated in 1% of patients treated. Withdrawal symptoms usually require the equivalent of at least 40 mg of diazepam (Valium) per day for more than 20 weeks. Unlike most of the other sedative-hypnotics, these drugs have amazingly little effect on respiration and other basic life-support functions; death due to deliberate or accidental overdose is extremely unusual.

Most authorities recommend intermittent use with treatment intervals limited to 1 to 4 months. A useful strategy is to inform the patient of the time-limited nature of the symptoms and then to explain that medication will prove most effective when it is limited to periods of undue stress. This often provides the stimulus for a previously avoided review of the patient's life circumstances and identification of mutually agreed-on "red flag" situations that will signal the need for future courses of medication.

All the benzodiazepines are roughly similar in efficacy for generalized anxiety disorder, and in side effects. Choosing between different benzodiazepines for this purpose is largely a matter of choosing between drug half-lives. The long half-lives of the most commonly used drugs (50 hours for diazepam and 30 hours for chlordiazepoxide) are generally considered an advantage in young, physically healthy patients. In patients with impaired metabolism (particularly the elderly), a long half-life can lead to toxic drug accumulations; in such patients, drugs with a short half-life, such as lorazepam (Ativan) and oxazepam (Serax), are preferable.

Regular doses of benzodiazepines designed to achieve and maintain stable and adequate serum levels are generally more effective for generalized anxiety disorder than are "as needed" doses. Standard practice is to start a patient on a low-to-moderate standing dose, and then to increase the dose or frequency of administration every 2 to 7 days until anxiety symptoms are under reasonable control. Patients are then maintained on this dosage for a period ranging from several weeks to several months. Typical starting dosages are 10 to 20 mg/day of diazepam, 25 to 50 mg/day of chlordiazepoxide, 30 to 60 mg/day of oxazepam, 0.5 to 1.5 mg/day of alprazolam, or 0.5 to 1.5 mg of clonazepam. In elderly patients, short-acting preparations are preferred (see Table 107-1), and doses should be lower. A strategy of using "as needed" doses only might be more appropriate for anxiety symptoms that are limited to clearly identifiable situations. Medications used in this fashion are more effective when given in anticipation of stressful periods rather than after anxiety has appeared. The frequency of administration is determined by the half-life of the specific agent being used. A single daily dose may be sufficient to maintain a pharmacologic steady state when long-acting drugs like diazepam or chlordiazepoxide are used. Clonazepam is given twice a day, and alprazolam 3 to 4 times a day. Because medication half-life may vary from patient to patient, it is best to be flexible with regard to dosage schedule. Intangible factors also play a role. For example, the subjective efficacy of the long-acting drugs diazepam and chlordiazepoxide is increased by giving them 3 times a day, probably because of the "boost" that occurs during the 4- to 6-hour period of rising blood levels following oral ingestion. An alternative pharmacologic approach is to use the nonbenzodi-

Table 107-1. Benzodiazepines used in the treatment of anxiety

	Available dose (mg)	Dose range (mg/day)	Approximate equivalent dose (mg)	Frequency of administration	Relative rapidity of effect after oral administration	Half-life (hr)
Long-acting						
Diazepam (Valium, others)	2, 5, 10	5–40	5	qd–tid	Rapid	20–70
Chlordiazepoxide (Librium, others)	5, 10, 25	25–100	10	qd–tid	Rapid	5–30
Clorazepate (Tranxene, others)	3.75, 7.5, 15	11.25–60.00	7.5	qd–tid	Rapid	30–200
Clonazepam (Klonopin)	0.5, 1, 2	0.5–3.0	0.5	bid	Intermediate	18–50
Short-acting						
Lorazepam (Ativan, others)	0.5, 1, 2	2–8	1	tid–qid	Intermediate	10–20
Alprazolam (Xanax)	0.25, 0.5, 1	0.5–4.0	0.25	tid–qid	Rapid	6–20
Oxazepam (Serax, others)	10, 15, 30	15–60	15	tid–qid	Intermediate–slow	5–15

azepine antianxiety agent buspirone. It has the advantage of being nonsedating and having little if any potential for dependence or abuse. While the response to buspirone is often gratifying, it usually takes about 2 weeks to develop. For this reason, buspirone is only suitable for the long-term management of generalized anxiety disorder. Unlike the benzodiazepines, it will not help acute stress-related symptoms. High-potency benzodiazepines, such as alprazolam and clonazepam, and/or antidepressants (either tricyclic or monoamine oxidase inhibitors) are the most appropriate treatment for patients with panic attacks. Beta-blockers are not a good treatment for generalized anxiety disorder, but may occasionally be useful for the individual with performance-related anxiety ("stage fright") who wishes to reduce sympathetically mediated anxiety symptoms (palpitations, tremulousness) without risking sedation.

Psychotherapy
Psychotherapy requires a relatively large investment of effort by both patient and therapist, making it the most costly alternative in the treatment of anxiety. The indication for psychotherapy lies less in the anxiety symptoms themselves, which are time-limited, than in the potential benefit of resolving persistent underlying problems affecting human relations, achievement, or self-concept. Controlled studies give no edge to any particular school of psychotherapy but do indicate that patients in therapy improve at a greater rate than do control subjects; up to twice as many patients improve, depending on the outcome criteria used. Patients who preferentially respond to psychotherapy generally (1) can identify, or be helped to identify, a specific source of emotional turmoil, usually interpersonal; (2) are willing to accept partial responsibility for difficulties, as well as motivation to changes; and (3) are able to tolerate expression of anxiety-producing emotions.

Relaxation and Stress Management Techniques
Relaxation techniques are thought to work by breaking an anxiety feedback loop maintained by overly responsive voluntary muscle contraction. Modalities include meditation, systematic desensitization, and biofeedback. Teaching the patient to achieve deep muscle relaxation is the basic component of all three. In stress management training, the patient is taught new cognitive strategies for identifying and dealing with common types of stressors. Programs combining these approaches can be found in many university medical centers, Veterans Administration (VA) medical centers, or freestanding stress treatment units. Reported success rates as high as 90% may reflect self-selection and may not necessarily generalize to clinic or practice populations. Attempts have been made to make some of this technology available to physicians in the form of commercially marketed relaxation tapes that can be given to patients for self-instruction. Although these may prove useful in relatively mild cases, experience indicates that relaxation is insufficient in itself and must be combined with individualized behavioral interventions in the hands of an experienced trainer to exert full benefit. Treatment can often be completed in a matter of months. Overall, these techniques work best for people who are somewhat compulsive and task-oriented or who have identifiable anxiety cues and a predominance of symptoms related to motor tension.

Wheeler EO, et al. Neurocirculatory asthenia (anxiety, neurosis, effort syndrome, neurasthenia). JAMA 1950; 142:878–89.
This classic and still relevant article describes the long-term course of anxiety disorder in a cohort of 167 cardiology patients with "anxiety neurosis" (generalized anxiety disorder or panic anxiety disorder) who were followed up 20 years after the initial diagnosis. Twelve percent were fully recovered; 15%, disabled; and the rest, intermittently symptomatic with minimal disability.

Roth M. Anxiety disorders and the use and abuse of drugs. J Clin Psychiatry 1989; 50: Suppl:30–5.
A review of the worldwide use of benzodiazepines, prepared by a key figure in the development of the modern pharmacotherapy of anxiety. The prevalence of occasional benzodiazepine use in the United States is 11 to 12%. Chronic use occurs in 1 to 2% of adults. Chronic users tend to be older and have chronic medical illness. Accepted practice is to discontinue benzodiazepine treatment after several months, taking 6 to 8 weeks to do so.

With some overlap, one-third of long-term users have major depression. One-third have panic disorder. One-half have chronic anxiety disorder.

Lydiard RB, Roy-Byrne PP, Ballenger JC. Recent advances in the psychopharmacological treatment of anxiety disorders. Hosp Community Psychiatry 1988; 38:1157–65.
Summarizes new data regarding pharmacologic approaches for generalized anxiety disorder, panic anxiety disorder, phobias, and obsessive compulsive disorder.

Tyrer P. Current status of B-blocking agents in the treatment of anxiety disorders. Drugs 1988; 36:773–83.
Reviews the advantages and limitations of beta-blockers for anxiety. They are most effective for prominent but not extreme somatic and autonomic symptoms such as palpitation and tremor, but do not relieve anxiety itself. Their main advantage is the lack of abuse potential.

Sheehan DV. Panic attacks and phobias. N Engl J Med 1982; 307:156–8.
Describes the appearance and treatment of panic/agoraphobic syndromes.

Liebowitz MR. Antidepressants in panic disorders. Br J Psychiatry 1990; 155:Suppl 6:46–52.
Discusses the practical aspects of treatment. Sensitivity to side effects requires slow titration in panic disorder patients.

Kutash IL, et al. Handbook on stress and anxiety. San Francisco: Jossey-Bass, 1980.
An in-depth presentation of theory and practice. Chapters on behavior therapy and biofeedback training provide useful descriptions of stress management and relaxation-based procedures.

Greist JH, Jefferson JW, Marks IM. Anxiety and its treatment. Washington, DC: APA Press, 1986.
A comprehensive and well-balanced review for patients. Describes syndromes, medication, behavior therapy, and self-help strategies.

108. DEPRESSION
John J. Haggerty, Jr.

Depressed feelings affect an estimated 12 to 40% of patients encountered in primary care practices. The main task of evaluation is to identify the 5% of these patients who have the specific psychobiologic disorder, major depression, that is known to respond to medication.

Diagnosis
The clinical differentiation between the medication-responsive disorder and the nonspecific symptom is not always simple. Superficial attributes of the presenting complaint, such as the intensity of emotional distress, or the presence or absence of exogenous stressors, are no longer thought to be helpful in making this distinction.

At present, the most frequently used approach is to determine the extent to which depressive mood is accompanied by signs and symptoms that have been shown to be markers of the medication-responsive disorder. These are thought to reflect underlying hypothalamic dysfunction and include the following:

1. Decreased or increased appetite, weight change
2. Insomnia or increased sleeping
3. Observable change in psychomotor activity, either agitation or retardation
4. Persistent inability to enjoy usually pleasurable activities, including sex
5. Fatigue
6. Feelings of worthlessness or guilt
7. Slowed thinking or decreased concentration
8. Recurrent thoughts of death or suicide

The daily presence of four or more of these, along with sadness or apathy, for at least 2 weeks is generally taken as unequivocal evidence for a depressive disorder. A history of depressive episodes increases the likelihood that the current condition is indeed depression. If the patient is experiencing a depressive syndrome for the first time, it is usually possible only to make the general diagnosis of major depressive episode. The subsequent clinical course may lead to a more specific diagnosis of a unipolar or bipolar disorder (see below). Although several biologic markers for depression (nonsuppression of cortisol following dexamethasone administration, blunted thyrotropin [TSH] response to thyrotropin-releasing hormone [TRH] infusion, rapid eye movement [REM] latency on polysomnography) have been identified, none as yet has sufficient sensitivity or specificity to be of use to primary care physicians.

In primary care settings, many depressed patients do not entirely fulfill the criteria listed above. The issue of whether or not to give antidepressant medications to patients with only two or three criteria was addressed in a 3-year follow-up of 100 patients who felt depressed but did not fully meet the diagnostic criteria for a major depressive episode. Forty percent eventually developed the full-blown syndrome and so might have been helped by medications. Family history of depression and abrupt onset of dysfunction helped in identifying potentially treatment-responsive patients.

Depression is particularly likely to escape attention in elderly patients, where it may present with impaired cognitive function. Cultural expectations that the elderly are naturally either sad or confused add to the oversight. Since it is not uncommon for first episodes of depression to occur in old age, clinicians should be certain to inquire about telltale changes in mood, sleeping, eating, and activity whenever they evaluate generalized decline in elderly patients.

Contributing Causes
Undiagnosed medical illness often presents as depression; it should be considered in the evaluation of any depressed patient, particularly those with endocrine dysfunction, infectious disease, or neoplasm, notably pancreatic cancer. Depression may be mimicked by these conditions or be an independent condition requiring treatment in its own right. Commonly used medications that can cause depression include propranolol, methyldopa, reserpine, antianxiety drugs, and corticosteroids.

Unipolar Versus Bipolar Disorder
It is helpful to determine whether the underlying pattern of illness fits best with a diagnosis of unipolar or bipolar (manic-depressive) disorder. These are now thought to represent distinct illnesses with different modes of inheritance and response to treatment. Since the depressive symptoms are indistinguishable, it is usually necessary to rely on the patient's history to decide in which category he or she belongs. In unipolar disorder, there are one or more episodes of depression alone, whereas in bipolar disorder manic episodes are also observed at some point in the patient's lifetime. Manic states are typified by extended periods of elevated mood, ability to get by with minimal sleep, or buying sprees. A history of manic-depressive illness in family members should also be elicited. If any of these findings is present, the patient may have bipolar disorder, and psychiatric consultation is advisable. Unipolar disorder occurs at least 20 times more frequently than bipolar disorder. Therefore, it is usually safe to assume a unipolar disorder for nearly all first episodes of depression. It is useful, however, to make the distinction when possible because of the exquisite responsiveness of bipolar disorder to lithium and other mood stabilizers, and the risk of precipitating mania by using antidepressants alone in susceptible individuals.

Course and Prognosis
Regardless of the type of depressive disorder, dysfunction is usually episodic. Recurrence is the rule, and 75% of patients can expect to have more than one episode during their lifetime. Approximately 15% of patients have chronic symptoms. These individuals tend to be treatment-resistant. When untreated, symptomatic intervals average 4 to 8 months. Intervening asymptomatic periods vary in length from months to decades but as a rule are longer than symptomatic intervals. The first episode of unipolar depression generally occurs in early to mid adulthood. However, onset can occur as early as infancy.

Patients with depressive disorder typically function well when not depressed. The prognosis for return to premorbid function is fairly good, particularly if treatment is prompt and complete. However, up to 15% of patients with depressive disorder attempt suicide. This is about 30 times the population average. Also, patients' actions during symptomatic intervals may have lasting consequences.

Suicide Assessment

Active or passive wishes to be dead are a common and expectable part of the symptom complex of depression. Suicidal fantasies do not in themselves contraindicate primary care management. The main task is to identify patients who have specific or persistent self-harm urges in addition to fantasies. The best approach is to be direct. All patients with depression, regardless of severity, should be asked in a matter-of-fact fashion whether they have lost their desire to be alive. Next, the frequency of suicidal thoughts should be ascertained, as well as whether a specific method of self-harm has been envisioned. Does the patient struggle greatly with the thoughts, or can they be dismissed with relative ease? The patient should be rapidly referred to a trained psychiatric clinician if any of the following are found: (1) The patient is not certain that he or she can avoid enacting suicidal fantasies; (2) the frequency or intensity of suicidal thoughts is accelerating; (3) there is a history of suicide attempts; or (4) factors that might seriously compromise judgment, including psychosis, severe emotional perturbation, or substance abuse, have been identified.

Drug Therapy

Non–Monoamine Oxidase Inhibitor Antidepressants
Non–monoamine oxidase (MAO) inhibitor antidepressants are the treatment of choice for most patients suffering a major depressive episode. This category of drugs includes the tricyclics, tetracyclics, and trazodone (now collectively designated "heterocyclic"), as well as several newer, chemically distinct agents (fluoxetine, bupropion) (Table 108-1).

All drugs in this class demonstrate a similar overall effectiveness in placebo-controlled studies, that is, improved mood and vegetative functioning in around 60 to 70% of patients with clear-cut depressive syndrome. A given patient, on the other hand, may respond to one drug but not another. Although the biochemical reasons for this are partially understood, this has not led to clinically useful predictions of which drug to start. Since the individual patient's response patterns to drugs do not change and are often familial, it is useful to ask which drugs have proved effective in the past, either for the patient or for family members.

If this information is not available, the next best approach is to select an antidepressant on the basis of its side effects. Sedative, anticholinergic, and hypotensive effects of each drug appear in different proportions. The heterocyclic agents all slow cardiac conduction, whereas the newer agents have little or no adverse cardiac effects. As a general rule, "secondary" (demethylated) antidepressants such as desipramine and nortriptyline have fewer cholinergic and hypotensive effects than do their "tertiary" (nondemethylated) counterparts such as amitriptyline and imipramine. These differing side effect profiles can frequently be used to the patient's advantage. For example, amitriptyline will fit a patient with insomnia; imipramine or desipramine, someone who fears oversedation; and trazodone, a man with benign prostatic hypertrophy. The demethylated agents nortriptyline and desipramine are good choices for elderly patients who have increased sensitivity to anticholinergic and hypotensive effects. Protriptyline, maprotiline, and amoxapine have additional side effects that should limit their use by primary care physicians.

Fluoxetine and bupropion have unique side effect profiles. Fluoxetine lacks anticholinergic, orthostatic, and cardiotoxic effects and has a very minimal potential for lethal overdose. This makes it an attractive, although expensive, first-choice alternative, particularly for patients with cardiac illness. Unlike most other antidepressants, it does not cause inappropriate weight gain; indeed its anorectic effect may limit its use in some patients. Its lack of sedative-hypnotic properties is a boon for some, but not all patients. On the negative side, fluoxetine can cause intolerable restlessness, nausea, anorexia, and headaches. Because some active metabolites have an extremely long half-life, rapid dosage escalation (< every 2 weeks) is not possible, and a relatively long washout period may be necessary when switching to another antidepressant. Five weeks of washout is necessary

Table 108-1. Commonly used antidepressants

	Doses available (mg)	Dose range (mg)[a]	Anticholinergic	Orthostasis	Sedation
Heterocyclic agents					
Tertiary amines					
Amitriptyline (Elavil, others)	25, 50, 100, 150	50–300	High	Moderate	High
Doxepin (Sinequan, others)	25, 50, 100, 150 10 mg/ml of liquid	50–300	High	Moderate	High
Imipramine (Tofranil, others)	10, 25, 50	50–200	Moderate	High	Moderate
Secondary amines					
Desipramine (Norpramin, others)	20, 25, 50, 100, 150	50–300	Low	Moderate	Low
Nortriptyline (Aventyl, others)	10, 25, 50, 75 10 mg/5 ml of liquid	50–250	Moderate	Low	Moderate
Protriptyline[b] (Vivactil)	5, 10	15–40	Low	Low	Very low
Other amines					
Amoxapine[c] (Asendin)	25, 50, 100, 150	50–400	Moderate	Low	Low
Maprotiline[d] (Ludiomil)	25, 50, 75	50–225	Moderate	Moderate	Moderate
Newer agents					
Fluoxetine (Prozac)	20	20–80	None	Very low	Very low
Trazodone (Desyrel)	50, 100, 150, 300	100–600	None	High	High
Bupropion (Wellbutrin)	75, 100	100–450	None	Very low	Very low

[a] In elderly patients, both the initial dose and the limits of the dose range are lowered.
[b] Protriptyline has a very long half-life, and therefore carries a risk of prolonged toxicity; note that doses are much lower than for the other heterocyclic agents.
[c] Amoxapine is metabolized to loxapine, a neuroleptic drug that carries the potential of tardive dyskinesia.
[d] Maprotiline is associated with an increased risk of seizures.

when switching from fluoxetine to an MAO inhibitor. Bupropion also lacks cholinergic and cardiotoxic effects, but has some bothersome adverse effects such as agitation and seizures that diminish its utility as a first-choice treatment.

Drug dosage is quite variable, mainly due to large individual differences in drug metabolism. Primary care physicians often prescribe insufficient amounts. Usually a healthy middle-aged adult will require 150 to 250 mg/day of a tricyclic antidepressant. The long half-life of all drugs in this class allows lumping as much of the daily total as possible in a single bedtime dose.

When a tricyclic antidepressant is used, the typical practice is to start with an initial 25- or 50-mg nighttime dose and then increase into the therapeutic range in stepwise fashion over the next 5 to 10 days. Lower starting doses (10 or 25 mg at bedtime) are appropriate in older patients and those with a history of sensitivity to medications. The patient should be advised to expect dry mouth, constipation, dizziness on standing, and sedation. Some will also experience tremulousness and increased anxiety, particularly with imipramine. If any of these symptoms become excessive, the dosage should be held at tolerable levels for 1 to 2 weeks. Since patients tend to develop tolerance to side effects, it is often possible to resume increasing the dosage toward therapeutic levels after such a wait. If adverse effects are still excessive, a different antidepressant should be tried. Dosage changes should be approached more cautiously in the elderly, who are more likely to develop side effects of all types. A pretreatment electrocardiogram is generally advisable in patients over the age of 45, as well as a brief review of medicines, both prescription and over-the-counter, that might potentiate anticholinergic effects.

Symptoms respond to medication at different rates. Sleeping often responds quickly, particularly if a tricyclic is used. Mood, appetite, and energy, however, may take 4 to 6 weeks to improve. If a patient has not responded to a presumably adequate dosage (up to 250 mg/day of most tricyclic antidepressants) by this time, a blood sample should be obtained to determine whether nonresponse represents wrong dosage, noncompliance, or wrong treatment. If the antidepressant concentration is below the therapeutic range, then the medication dosage should be increased. If it is within accepted limits, then the medication should be changed or the diagnosis reconsidered. Therapeutic ranges for older antidepressants such as the tricyclics have been well validated. Those available for newer agents such as trazodone, fluoxetine, and bupropion cannot yet be interpreted with the same degree of precision, but are nevertheless useful for "ball park" determinations of under- or overdosing. Patients who fail to respond to trials of at least two different drugs probably warrant psychiatric referral.

Once response occurs, medication should be continued for the 6 to 8 months that the depressive syndrome would normally run. When the drug is discontinued, it should be weaned over several weeks. Overly rapid discontinuation of tricyclics, in particular, may cause a cholinergic rebound syndrome consisting of insomnia, abdominal pain, and anxiety. Individuals with frequently recurring depressive episodes may benefit from long-term maintenance on antidepressants.

All antidepressants are potentially toxic. Single doses of tricyclics exceeding 2 g are frequently fatal. In normal doses, the main areas of concern for heterocyclics are central nervous system toxicity in the elderly (who often respond to one-third to one-half the usual amount) and potential cardiotoxicity in patients with preexisting heart disease. Because most heterocyclic antidepressants have quinidine-like and hypotensive effects, they should be used with considerable caution in patients with serious conduction abnormalities, specifically including first- and second-degree heart block and left bundle-branch block, and during recuperation from myocardial infarction. Fluoxetine and bupropion are the only drugs with unequivocal safety in these situations and in patients with serious arrhythmias. All the medications discussed here are relatively safe in mild-to-moderate congestive heart failure.

Lithium

Lithium clearly blunts acute manic attacks and, when taken chronically, will prevent both manic and depressive episodes in patients with bipolar disorder. It may also help some patients with treatment-resistant depression, particularly when it is given in combination with an antidepressant.

Monoamine Oxidase Inhibitors
MAO inhibitors are receiving increased attention in the treatment of depressive episodes that do not respond to the tricyclic antidepressants. They seem particularly useful for patients with a marked degree of anxiety. They are not, however, drugs of first choice for most primary care physicians.

Thyroid Hormone
Thyroid hormone (T_3) has been reported to potentiate the antidepressant drug response and to decrease the side effects in some treatment-resistant depressions. This has important research implications but is not yet an approved indication.

Neuroleptic-Antidepressant Combinations
Neuroleptic-antidepressant combinations are rational treatments only for patients with psychotic depressions or during the first days of an agitated depression. The neuroleptic adds an unwarranted risk for tardive dyskinesia that is otherwise best avoided.

Nondrug Therapy

Electroconvulsive Therapy
Recent public sentiment has obscured the fact that electroconvulsive therapy has a higher overall efficacy than does any drug presently available for the treatment of depression, and is no more dangerous. Present indications include psychotic depression and drug failure. Complications are rare with modern techniques. Transient and circumscribed memory loss may occur; however, controlled studies have not documented other significant alterations in mental functioning.

Psychotherapy
Depression is one of the few illnesses for which it has been clearly demonstrated that medication and talking have an additive effect. Antidepressants, for example, are less effective than psychotherapy for improving self-esteem and social functioning and diminishing suicidal feelings. It is generally recommended, therefore, that depressive patients receive both treatments concurrently.

The literature favors an active, encouraging approach that focuses on current interpersonal functioning and downplays the exploration of deep-seated psychodynamics. Fortunately, the recommended technique for accomplishing these aims is generally within the abilities of most nonpsychiatrists.

A typical course of psychotherapy might involve weekly 30- to 45-minute sessions over 2 to 3 months. The initial aim is to help the patient diminish feelings of guilt and to relax excessive self-demands. This is accomplished by explaining that diminished functioning is the result of a treatable and nonvolitional illness, by legitimizing slowing down as necessary for recovery from any illness, and by being willing to tolerate the patient's temporarily increased dependency. A deep exploration of feelings in the early stages of treatment is likely to increase guilt and is best avoided at this point.

As the patient starts to improve (3–4 weeks), the focus should move to the exploration of the patient's current interpersonal milieu. The goals now are to allow catharsis, to identify current precipitants, and to facilitate the repair of relationships that have been damaged by the depressive syndrome. In the final stages of therapy, the clinician and patient work together on a cognitive level to identify distorted self-views involved in the depression and to characterize situations that might lead to future depressions. Not all patients are capable of reaching this last stage, and in many cases, the provider will have to be content with simple symptom reduction and catharsis. Individuals who unearth difficulties with emotional adjustment that persist beyond resolution of the depressive syndrome, and who are sufficiently verbal, should be considered for referral to more intensive psychotherapy.

Keller MB. Unipolar depression. In: Frances AJ, Hales RE, eds. Annual review of psychiatry. Vol. 7. Washington, DC: American Psychiatric Press, 1988:147–275.
This comprehensive update covers all aspects of depression.

Nielsen AC, Williams TA. Depression in ambulatory medical patients. Arch Gen Psychiatry 1980; 37:99–1004.
In a group of 500 medical group practice patients evaluated for depression, 12% were at least mildly depressed, and 4 to 5% had moderate depression of the type that would probably respond to medication. Physicians identified only one-fourth of the latter group. The merits of routine screening for depression are discussed.

Keller MB, et al. Treatment received by depressed patients. JAMA 1982; 248:1848–55.
Even when recognized, depression is still grossly undertreated. Only 3% of subjects referred to a large collaborative depression study had previously received a standard antidepressant trial. Most had been inappropriately treated with anxiolytics.

Cohen-Cole SA, Harpe C. Diagnostic assessment of depression in the medically ill. In: Stoudemire A, Fogel BS, eds. Principles of medical psychiatry. Orlando: Grune & Stratton, 1987:23–36.
The fact that depression often coexists with other illnesses may contribute to its underdiagnosis in medical settings. This chapter provides a concise orientation to the interaction between depression and medical illness.

Akiskal HS, et al. Differentiation of primary affective illness from situational, symptomatic and secondary depression. Arch Gen Psychiatry 1979; 36:635–43.
Patients who only partially met criteria for major depression were followed longitudinally. Forty percent subsequently developed clear-cut evidence for unipolar or bipolar disorder. The remaining 60% comprised a heterogeneous mix of personality disorder, adjustment reaction, and other miscellaneous problems. Strong family history was the best predictor of "true" depressive disorder.

Blazer DG. Affective disorders in late life. In: Busse EW, Blazer DG, eds. Geriatric psychiatry. Washington, DC: American Psychiatric Press, 1989: 369–402.
This review focuses on the epidemiology, diagnosis, and management of late life depression.

McGreevey JF Jr, Franco K. Depression in the elderly: the role of the primary care physician in management. J Gen Intern Med 1988; 3:498–507.

Fitten LJ, et al. Depression: UCLA geriatric grand rounds. J Am Geriatr Soc 1989; 37:459–72.
Two complementary articles reviewing the diagnosis and treatment of depression in elderly patients.

Amsterdam J, Brunswick D, Mendels J. The clinical application of tricyclic antidepressant pharmacokinetics and plasma levels. Am J Psychiatry 1980; 137:653–62.
This article summarizes the probable therapeutic ranges for various tricyclic antidepressants and discusses how to use drug level measurements in clinical decision-making.

Glassman AH, et al. Cardiovascular effects of tricyclic antidepressants. In: Meltzer HY, ed. Psychopharmacology: the third generation of progress. New York: Raven Press, 1987:1437–42.
The cardiotoxicity of tricyclic antidepressants tends to be overestimated. This reference provides a detailed description of the differential effects of tricyclic antidepressants on blood pressure and cardiac conduction, rhythm, and mechanical function.

Roose SP, Glassman AH. Cardiovascular effects of tricyclic antidepressants in depressed patients with and without heart disease. J Clin Psychiatry Monogr 1989; 7(2):1–18.
This article reviews the effect of tricyclics on pulse, blood pressure, rhythm, left ventricular function, and conduction, with data on the newer nontricyclic agents.

Jefferson JW, et al. Lithium encyclopedia for clinical practice. 2nd ed. Washington, DC: APA Press, 1983.
This book is an excellent source of basic information on this increasingly useful drug. It is available in paperback.

Dimascio A, et al. Differential symptom reduction by drugs and psychotherapy in acute depression. Arch Gen Psychiatry 1979; 36:1450–6.
In a randomized treatment study, ambulatory patients receiving a combination of antide-

pressants and short-term weekly psychotherapy did better than those receiving either treatment alone. Treatments affected different symptom clusters and had an additive effect when used together.

Beck AT, et al. Cognitive therapy of depression. New York: Guilford Press, 1979.
This book specifically deals with the psychotherapy of depression. It describes an active, time-limited approach that can be used with some modification in primary medical practices, and contains case vignettes and a useful chapter on how to combine psychotherapy with medication.

109. INSOMNIA
Jeffery J. Fahs

Sleep requirements vary considerably from one individual to another. Insomnia can be defined as the subjective perception of inadequate sleep, accompanied by disturbed daytime functioning, with complaints such as irritability, difficulty concentrating, somnolence, or fatigue. Approximately one-third of the adult population has insomnia in a given year, and 15 to 20% of these people consult a clinician for the problem. This complaint is more common among the elderly. Appropriate treatment depends on establishing the cause of the sleep disorder.

Transient Insomnia
Transient insomnia, brought on by environmental events, affects most people at some time in their lives. It generally lasts less than 3 to 4 weeks and remits with resolution of the precipitating circumstances. Phase-shift insomnias, such as are caused by "jet lag" or changing work shifts, result from a dyssynchrony between the individual's sleep-wake pattern and external demands. This insomnia resolves when the sleep schedule becomes resynchronized with the prevailing clock time or work demands. Transient insomnia can be treated with the short-term use of a hypnotic agent.

Persistent Insomnia
This heterogeneous group of disorders is generally defined as more than 4 weeks of difficulty sleeping.

Psychophysiologic Insomnia
Psychophysiologic insomnia usually results from a combination of factors leading to a conditioned arousal at bedtime. During a period of particular stress, individuals who are predisposed to sleeping poorly may begin to develop negative learned associations with the usual nightly routine and setting. This results in a vicious cycle of overconcern, apprehension, and frustration about not being able to fall asleep. Often there is improvement in sleep when this cycle is disrupted, such as by a vacation. This type of insomnia may be difficult to treat and may be confounded by the appearance of secondary psychological difficulties (e.g., decreased self-esteem, social withdrawal) as well as a dependence on hypnotic medications. The basic treatment is guided by principles of sleep hygiene, as described under Sleep Hygiene Measures. The chronic use of hypnotic agents should be avoided, though intermittent, short-term use may be warranted. Success has been reported with relaxation, cognitive, and other behavioral therapies.

Psychiatric Disorders
Patients with an affective disorder may present with a primary complaint of insomnia. There are often coexisting disturbances of other vegetative functions (e.g., appetite, weight change, sexual interest and/or activity), a change in the general level of activity and interests, feelings of sadness or elation, and suicidal thoughts, and the patient may have had previous psychiatric treatment. If depression is believed to be the cause of the insomnia, and if pharmacologic therapy is indicated, a bedtime dose of one of the sedating

tricyclic antidepressants (e.g., amitriptyline or doxepin) is a logical choice. Insomnia associated with a psychotic condition is suggested by the presence of a thought disorder, hallucinations, or delusions; for these, referral to a psychiatrist is usually appropriate.

Drugs
Chronic use of hypnotics usually exacerbates insomnia. As tolerance to a previously effective agent develops, patients may increase the dose, only to find that sleep continues to worsen. In these cases, it must be assumed that the agent is no longer beneficial, and gradual withdrawal from the hypnotic is necessary. Sleep usually worsens temporarily while the drug is being discontinued, and the patient should be reassured that this effect is transient; another drug should generally not be substituted. Alcohol use causes fragmented sleep, and chronic alcoholism is associated with serious sleep disruption. Of course, stimulating agents such as sympathomimetic agents (e.g., coffee/caffeine) may cause insomnia.

Nocturnal Myoclonus and Restless Legs Syndrome
Nocturnal myoclonus and restless legs syndrome are especially common among the elderly. Nocturnal myoclonus is a sleep-related movement disorder marked by rhythmic, periodic contractions of the leg muscles that lead to partial or full arousals, often without the patient remembering the leg movements or even the repeated arousals. Restless legs syndrome, which usually coexists with nocturnal myoclonus, is a dysesthesia of the legs that is relieved only with movement, and thus interferes with the onset of sleep.

Sleep-Wake Schedule Disorders
Delayed sleep phase syndrome is defined by a sleep onset and a wake time that are both later than desired, whereas advanced sleep phase syndrome, which is more common among the elderly and often accompanied by a decreased total sleep time, indicates a sleep onset and arousal that are too early. In extreme forms, these may result in a complete reversal of the normal sleep-wake pattern. Like jet lag and shift work, these disorders represent a dyssynchrony between an individual's circadian rhythm and external demands or expectations. These patients may present with insomnia; treatment usually revolves around attention to sleep hygiene, measures to readjust the circadian rhythm such as exposure to bright light or other "time-givers" (e.g., regular mealtimes, activity schedules), and chronotherapy which involves a gradual readjustment of bedtime.

Other Conditions
Many medical problems, especially those accompanied by pain or other discomforts, are associated with insomnia. *Sleep apnea syndrome* can cause either insomnia or excessive daytime sleepiness. Sleep is punctuated by repetitive apneic episodes with arousals marked by gasping for air, choking, or even cacophonous snoring, of which the patient may be unaware.

Diagnostic Strategy
The "sleep history" is the most important source of information for determining the etiology of a sleeping difficulty. Transient insomnias are differentiated from persistent insomnias by the duration of the problem. Other data should include the following.

Nature of the Complaint
Is the problem falling asleep, staying asleep, or waking too early? Difficulty initiating sleep may point to a psychophysiologic insomnia or a schedule disorder, while early awakening may be a clue to depression. If there are multiple awakenings, the cause of the arousals should be determined (e.g., nocturia or pain). Excessive daytime sleepiness associated with insomnia may indicate the sleep apnea syndrome, in which case the presence of auxiliary symptoms must be clarified.

What are the initiating, aggravating, and alleviating factors? The presence of a clear environmental stressor suggests a psychophysiologic or psychiatric insomnia. Drugs may be implicated. A change in work schedule may point to a schedule disorder. The position of the bed or number of pillows may alter the insomnia associated with gastroesophageal reflux or pulmonary disease, while a change in setting may alleviate persistent psychophysiologic insomnia. The clinician should also attempt to quantitate the patient's perception of the problem (e.g., how long it takes to fall asleep) in order to gauge the response to treatment.

Sleep Patterns

What are the activities and rituals before bedtime? Physically or mentally stimulating activities in the evening contribute to insomnia, while relaxing activities and a regular ritual may pave the way for sleep. When does the patient sleep, and are there daytime naps? Answers to these questions may point to a schedule disorder or fragmented sleep. A 24-hour sleep-wake diary may help to diagnose and quantitate the problem. What is the sleep environment? For example, is the bed comfortable? Is the room too hot or cold? Are there noises, lights, or other distractions?

Sleep-Related Phenomena

Are there repeated leg movements, suggesting nocturnal myoclonus, or loud snoring and choking, which may indicate periods of apnea? Questioning the bed partner may be invaluable in detecting these problems.

Drug History

A drug history must include all current and recently discontinued prescription medications, as well as illicit drugs, over-the-counter preparations, alcohol, caffeine, and nicotine. The insomnia due to stimulants and withdrawal from sedatives is well recognized, but other commonly prescribed medications, such as propranolol, can also cause insomnia. In addition, the tricyclic antidepressants and lithium may worsen nocturnal myoclonus and its associated insomnia.

General Health

Any medical condition, such as rheumatoid arthritis, in which pain is a problem may cause insomnia. In other medical conditions, such as hyperthyroidism and congestive heart failure, insomnia may be a prominent symptom.

Emotional Status

Is a primary psychiatric disorder present? The history should particularly note any signs and symptoms of depression.

Further Evaluation

In most cases, an accurate diagnosis of insomnia can be made in the clinician's office on the basis of the history, physical and mental status examinations, and additional laboratory studies and consultations as indicated. Some patients may require referral to a sleep disorders center for further evaluation and treatment planning. The specific criteria for when to make such referrals remain rather unclear or controversial, and one must rely largely on clinical judgment and common sense. However, those patients in whom sleep apnea is suspected and those in whom insomnia is persistent and refractory to appropriate and adequate treatment probably warrant such a comprehensive evaluation, including polysomnography.

Treatment Strategies

Treatment should be directed toward the cause of the insomnia whenever this is possible. However, certain general treatment strategies are helpful.

Reassurance, Education, and Counseling

Explaining the general nature of sleep, the varying individual needs for sleep, the age-related changes in sleep, and the lack of long-term detrimental effects from short-term sleep loss may reassure the patient, elicit cooperation, and help to avoid the inappropriate and excessive use of sleeping medications.

Sleep Hygiene Measures

Sleep hygiene measures are based on common sense, clinical experience, and sleep research. They are the backbone of treatment for a variety of sleep disorders, though they must be individualized to properly guide this treatment.

Table 109-1. Benzodiazepines used as hypnotics

Drug	Doses available	Usual adult dose (mg)	Onset of action	Half-life
Flurazepam (Dalmane, others)	15-, 30-mg capsules	15–30	Rapid	Long (50–100 hr)
Temazepam (Restoril, others)	15-, 30-mg capsules	15–30	Slow	Intermediate (10–17 hr)
Triazolam (Halcion)	0.125-, 0.25-mg tablets	0.125–0.5	Rapid to intermediate	Short (1.5–5.5 hr)
Quazepam (Doral)	7.5-, 15-mg capsules	7.5–15.0	Intermediate to slow	Intermediate to long (25–40 hr)

1. Establish regular retiring and arising times.
2. Avoid daytime naps.
3. Make the environment comfortable for sleep (e.g., quiet)
4. Use the bed only for sleep, not for eating, watching television, or lying awake.
5. Avoid evening stimulation. Daily physical exercise may contribute to an improvement in sleep, but physical exercise late in the day will lead to physiologic arousal. Mental stimulation before sleep will, likewise, contribute to arousal.
6. Engage in relaxing activities before sleep, possibly including structured relaxation training.
7. Avoid the use of stimulants (e.g., caffeine and nicotine) and alcohol in the late afternoon and evening.

Hypnotic Drugs

The clearest indication for sleeping medications is the short-term treatment of transient insomnia; they may be taken prophylactically when the patient knows that he or she will suffer from insomnia. In addition, there is a role for the intermittent and short-term use of hypnotics in some cases of persistent insomnia, including nocturnal myoclonus, psychophysiologic insomnia, and selected psychiatric disorders. However, chronic use should generally be avoided, and hypnotics are contraindicated in sleep apnea, pregnancy, alcoholism, and situations requiring nighttime alertness. Hypnotics play a relatively minor role in the rational treatment of persistent insomnia.

The benzodiazepines are presently the drugs of choice. Any of them may be used, although only four—flurazepam (Dalmane), temazepam (Restoril), triazolam (Halcion), and quazepam (Doral)—are currently approved specifically for use as hypnotics. These drugs, their typical doses, and pharmacokinetic properties are described in Table 109-1. If a patient is already taking a benzodiazepine during the day, that same benzodiazepine may be used at bedtime for sleep to avoid polypharmacy. (See Table 107-1, describing the benzodiazepines used as anxiolytic agents.) If a patient is not taking a sedative-hypnotic drug, treatment may be initiated with one of the hypnotic benzodiazepines at the lower therapeutic dosage; these are typically taken about 30 minutes before retiring, but temazepam, which has a delayed onset of action, may need to be taken up to 2 hours before bedtime. The choice of a particular benzodiazepine usually depends on the pharmacokinetic profile (especially the absorption rate and half-life) and the resulting clinical effects; those with a long half-life are associated with an impairment of daytime functioning (i.e., "hangover") of which the patient may be unaware, while those with a short half-life are associated with rebound insomnia on discontinuation and anterograde amnesia. These drugs must be prescribed judiciously, for only short periods (usually no more than 2 weeks), and monitored carefully lest the patient's difficulty be exacerbated.

In rare situations, the benzodiazepine hypnotics may not be appropriate, because of sensitivity or a lack of efficacy. In those situations, several alternative pharmacologic treatments are available. Despite being one of the oldest sedative-hypnotic agents, chloral hydrate remains a safe and effective agent, especially when used in its lower dosages. L-Tryptophan has been suggested as a "natural" alternative and may be effective for some individuals; however, its recent association with the eosinophilia-myalgia syndrome demands that it be avoided until its safety is established. Over-the-counter preparations typically contain antihistamines, with the potential for anticholinergic side effects; for this reason, as well as a general lack of established efficacy, they cannot be enthusiastically recommended, and should be avoided in elderly people. The tricyclic antidepressant agents (e.g., nortriptyline or amitriptyline) may have a role in the treatment of insomnia when they are used at low dosages (10–25 mg). While antipsychotic agents (e.g., thioridazine) have been recommended for the treatment of insomnia, their use is probably best limited to those psychiatric conditions with symptomatic insomnia (e.g., psychosis, delirium, or dementia).

Erman MK. Insomnia. *Psychiatr Clin North Am* 1987; 10:525–39.
   The title is somewhat misleading because this article reviews a range of sleep-related subjects, including sleep physiology, functions of sleep, and the whole range of sleep disorders.

Gillin JC, et al. The diagnosis and management of insomnia. *N Engl J Med* 1990; 322:239–48.
A superb article that briefly reviews the diagnostic considerations and nonpharmacologic treatment approaches for insomnia, but is particularly useful for its review of pharmacologic treatments.

Gottlieb GL. Sleep disorders and their management: special considerations in the elderly. *Am J Med* 1990; 88:29S–33S.
An excellent review of the differential diagnostic and therapeutic considerations for insomnia in the geriatric population; a nicely balanced presentation of the role for hypnotic medications. (This article is part of a supplement issue of the American Journal of Medicine which includes a number of additional very good reviews of insomnia and its treatment.)

Greenblatt DJ, et al. Pharmacokinetic determinants of dynamic differences among three benzodiazepine hypnotics: flurazepam, temazepam, and triazolam. *Arch Gen Psychiatry* 1989; 46:326–32.
A careful comparative evaluation of three of the benzodiazepine hypnotics, with particular attention to sedation and memory impairments.

Hauri PJ. Primary insomnia. In: Karasu TB, ed. *Treatments of psychiatric disorders*. A task force report of the American Psychiatric Association. Section 23, Vol. 3. Washington, DC: American Psychiatric Press, 1989; 2424–33.
An excellent review of this group of insomnias, which is defined as not being secondary to another medical or psychiatric condition. This chapter contains a particularly good section on nonpharmacologic treatment.

Jacobs EA, et al. The role of polysomnography in the differential diagnosis of chronic insomnia. *Am J Psychiatry* 1988; 145:346–9.
While probably overstating the therapeutic difference that the revised diagnoses make, this article does point out that polysomnographic evaluation may alter the diagnosis in a substantial number of insomniac patients.

Mendelson WB. Pharmacotherapy of insomnia. *Psychiatr Clin North Am* 1987; 10:555–63.
Concentrating exclusively on the use of benzodiazepines, this short article quickly reviews their pharmacology, indications, efficacy, and concerns regarding their use.

Mendelson WB. Insomnia related to medical conditions: sleep apnea and nocturnal myoclonus. In: Karasu TB, ed. *Treatments of psychiatric disorders*. A task force report of the American Psychiatric Association. Section 23, Vol. 3. Washington, DC: American Psychiatric Press, 1989: 2433–38.
These two conditions, which may not make themselves known until the patient is comprehensively evaluated, are not infrequent causes of insomnia, with particular treatment implications.

Moran MG, et al. Sleep disorders in the elderly. *Am J Psychiatry* 1988; 145:1369–78.
A particularly helpful review, with emphasis on the differential diagnosis and pharmacologic treatment, in this growing segment of our population who are particularly prone to insomnia.

National Institute of Mental Health. Consensus conference report: drugs and insomnia: the use of medications to promote sleep. *JAMA* 1984; 251:2410–14.
An excellent short overview, without references, of insomnia, with particular attention to the cautions to be employed with pharmacologic treatment.

Prinz PN, et al. Geriatrics: sleep disorders and aging. *N Engl J Med* 1990; 323:520–6.
Reviews normal age-related changes in sleep, the variety of sleep disorders most of which present as insomnia, and the use of sedative-hypnotic drugs.

Schmidt PJ. Evaluation and treatment of sleep disorders in the medical setting. *Gen Hosp Psychiatry* 1988; 10:10–15.
A helpful guide to remind one of the various medical illnesses and medical treatments that may lead to a complaint of disturbed sleep.

110. PROBLEM PATIENTS
Douglas A. Drossman

Within every clinical practice, physicians can identify patients they designate as "problem" patients. These patients comprise a heterogeneous group who may have no specific medical or psychiatric diagnosis but are characterized by the behavior they exhibit within the health care system and the reactions they elicit in the physicians caring for them. Consider a typical case history:

A patient presents with long-standing physical complaints that are difficult to characterize. Review of past workups is unrevealing. With each new physician visited, more invasive procedures were done to exclude "organic disease." Treatment has been empirical, unsuccessful, and sometimes harmful. The patient states that others have concluded "nothing is wrong," or "it is in my head," but he knows it is real. He hopes you will find the answer and help where others have failed. By the end of the visit, additional studies seem unnecessary, yet with no specific diagnosis, you wonder if something has been overlooked. The patient strongly states that there are no emotional problems. He demands that something be done *now* for these unbearable symptoms.

Although psychosocial factors play a part in the illnesses of many medical patients, problem patients are typically unwilling or unable to acknowledge an asssociation between stress or emotional factors and their illness. As a result, the physician finds it difficult to obtain relevant data for diagnosis or treatment. Such patients may see each new problem within a long history of chronic or recurrent symptoms as another acute episode that requires immediate relief. Their demands for the physician to "do something" tend to heighten the physician's sense of uncertainty and may also produce feelings of ineffectiveness. This may result in any of several inappropriate physician behaviors: pursuit of unneeded diagnostic studies in an attempt to ameliorate the sense of uncertainty ("furor medicus"), anger toward the patient in whom "nothing is wrong," or dismissal with a statement that the problems are emotional, sometimes accompanied by an undesired referral to a psychiatrist. Since the "problem" with "problem patients" exists to a great degree within the physician-patient interaction, the physician who recognizes these maladaptive behavior patterns early may forestall unneeded studies and treatments and make more effective plans of patient care.

Recognition
Although problem patients do not fall into any specific diagnostic categories, they commonly exhibit a number of identifiable behavior patterns. These include the following:

1. Personalized or bizarre description of the symptoms (e.g., pain "as if seared by hot coals")
2. Persistent complaints with demands for the physician to "do something"
3. Symptoms determined in whole or part from a meaningful fantasy or experience (e.g., chest pain developing after the death of a parent from cardiac disease)
4. Temporal association of the symptoms to stress events
5. Long history of nonspecific complaints and poorly documented illnesses
6. Reluctance to accept the role of psychosocial factors in the illness
7. Resistance to improvement due to the presence of benefits derived from illness (e.g., family attention, disability, expiation of guilt feelings through suffering)

Evaluation
Evaluation should include an initial history and physical examination, which should be repeated as needed when new or different symptoms develop. The story of the illness should be obtained in as unbiased a fashion as possible and in relation to the events that may have contributed to its onset and presentation. The approach should communicate the physician's willingness to hear all aspects of the illness, whether biologic or psychological. The interview should encourage the spontaneous reporting of information through the

patient's own associations. Leading questions or those that elicit "yes" or "no" answers should be avoided at first. More direct and specific questions can be asked later to characterize the illness better and to help confirm the diagnostic possibilities.

Specific Disorders

Patients with certain psychiatric disorders or personality patterns also commonly present with physical complaints and may interact with their physician in ways that result in their being labeled as problem patients. However, early recognition of these specific disorders can lead to more directed and appropriate plans of patient care. These entities include the following.

Psychophysiologic Reaction

Psychophysiologic reaction is an exaggerated physiologic response to anxiety-producing situations, with symptoms such as palpitations, diarrhea, or the hyperventilation syndrome. Many individuals may develop these reactions at one time or another. However, some patients may present with frequent episodes as part of an underlying chronic anxiety disorder. The physician should try to determine possible stressors and, if not possible to remove them, encourage patient adaptation through support, counseling, or appropriate referral.

Conversion Reaction

Conversion reaction is an unconscious adaptive process whereby mental distress is ameliorated through its symbolic representation as a physical symptom. Conversion reactions can occur in any individual as a response to stress (e.g., development of chest pains in the grieving spouse of a heart attack victim). More frequently they develop in patients with the propensity to focus on somatic concerns. Disorders may manifest as loss of bodily function, such as paralysis, or symptoms of pain. Treatment will vary depending on the nature of the stress, the patient's personality and coping style, and the degree of impairment in daily function. When the condition is disabling, psychiatric consultation is usually needed.

Hypochondriasis

Hypochondriasis is a personality variant in which patients maintain a chronic preoccupation with bodily function. They display an unrealistic interpretation of physical sensations as being abnormal, maintain a persistent fear of harboring serious disease, and are preoccupied with a variety of vague and shifting complaints. Many of these patients have limited social relationships outside of the health care system, and their complaints serve to maintain self-esteem and to provide a means of social communication. Treatment often includes accepting them without challenging the illness and maintaining a commitment to regular brief office visits without a need to respond to every complaint.

Pain-Prone Personality

Individuals with this disorder report a long-standing history of numerous dramatic events, operations, and pain episodes. They also seem to display an intolerance of success manifested by a difficulty in holding jobs, a proclivity to submit to demeaning experiences, and the development of symptoms during relatively good periods of life. Patients with this personality pattern often come from an early environment of violence, deprivation, and physical or sexual abuse, with parents who displayed inconsistent behavior or rigid discipline. Alcoholism and broken marriages in the family are common. It is believed that the pain and suffering serve as a means of atonement for early established feelings of self-devaluation and guilt. The physician should recognize that these patients often succumb to a variety of iatrogenic procedures and have a high potential for drug abuse.

"Depressive Equivalent"

The "depressive equivalent" disorder has been called a "masked depression," for the patient attributes sadness, sleep disturbance, and loss of weight and appetite to bodily complaints rather than to an emotional disorder. This misinterpretation can also be made by the physician who fails to explore the circumstances preceding the onset of illness. These patients may respond to supportive psychotherapy or antidepressant medications.

Somatic Delusion
Patients with somatic delusions describe bizarre beliefs about their symptoms (e.g., a headache is caused by the brain being split into pieces). The symptoms are not described metaphorically; the patients truly believe it is happening. These patients have significant psychic disorganization (e.g., schizophrenia) and require psychiatric referral.

Treatment
The therapeutic approach to problem patients must be individualized. The following guidelines are useful.

Establish a Therapeutic Relationship
Establish a therapeutic relationship with a mutual sense of trust and understanding of both physician and patient needs and expectations. The physician's goals should be the following: (1) Accept the adaptive value of the illness, and do not attempt to achieve premature resolution. Often the illness has existed for many years and has resulted in secondary benefits (e.g., increased attention from family, privilege of the "sick role"). (2) Make no promises that cannot be met (e.g., for quick symptom relief). (3) Involve the patient in the treatment plans. This frees the physician from the implied obligation to be the one responsible for the patient's well-being and fosters a greater sense of patient independence and emotional maturity. (4) Accept a commitment for possibly long-term treatment. Initially one to three appointments per month for 15 to 30 minutes are recommended. During these sessions, continued efforts should be made to elicit the patient's own associations and affective state. When symptoms are reported, the physician should not always feel compelled to treat them. When the patient recounts the misfortunes of continued pain and suffering, the physician should communicate an understanding of how difficult it must be to go on with such distress. When the patient focuses on significant thoughts and feelings, the physician should gently encourage them without forcing their disclosure. As symptoms improve, the visits can be decreased in frequency. It is probable that a commitment to continued care through regular though infrequent visits (twice per year when the patient is well) will reinforce the physician's interest and minimize late-night calls and "emergency" visits.

Do Not State That the Problem Is "Emotional"
Problem patients are unable to accept the significance of emotional factors in their illnesses. For this reason, it is best to reassure those with unwarranted fears and volunteer nothing more than they are prepared to accept. To state that the problem is "emotional" may set some patients up as adversaries. If asked by a patient whether or not the problem is "all in my head," the physician should state that it is important to consider the role of all factors in the illness, be they psychological or otherwise. The physician needs to communicate a desire to work with the patient, not to diagnose a disease to treat.

The patient's awareness of an association between emotional factors and illness is not necessary for improvement and should not be a goal of treatment.

Resist the Impulse to Order Unnecessary Diagnostic Studies
The decision for diagnostic studies should be based on careful evaluation of the objective clinical data, not solely on the patient's demands. When a reasonable assessment of the problem has developed from the history and physical examination, the physician must have the confidence *not* to order unnecessary diagnostic studies just to "rule out organic disease." If the complaints are not readily understood, it is wiser to temporize than to commit oneself to a treatment plan with uncertain effectiveness. In time, as the issues become clarified, better diagnostic and treatment choices can be made.

Accept Illness as the Interaction of Biologic and Psychological Determinants
The identification of psychological factors does not exclude a concurrent somatic illness. The physician must also be alert to the development of new disease in patients who "cry wolf."

Reset Goals for Clinical Improvement
To derive satisfaction from the care of these patients requires that the physician set realistic treatment goals. Often improvement should be gauged by the patient's level of

daily function (e.g., work, church, social activities) *despite* the illness rather than by resolution of the symptoms.

Be Aware of Personal Attitudes
The patient's maintenance of the sick role is not necessarily countertherapeutic, but it can be frustrating to the physician whose goal is to make the patient symptom-free. Labels such as "crock" or "turkey" applied to such patients signal the physician's frustration and sense of helplessness. Medicine is not an exact science, and physicians must tolerate uncertainty; however, recognition of the psychosocial dimensions of these patients' illnesses can often lead to greater physician security as their patients' problems are put into clear perspective.

Drossman DA. The problem patient: evaluation and care of medical patients with psychosocial disturbances. Ann Intern Med 1978; 88:366–72.
Presents in more detail the characteristics of problem patients and offers a treatment approach.

De Vaul RA, Faillace LA. Persistent pain and illness insistence: a medical profile to proneness to surgery. Am J Surg 1978; 135:828–33.
Identifies the "polysurgery" patient and reports behavioral patterns that lead to physician errors in clinical judgment.

Somatoform disorders. In: Diagnostic and statistical manual of mental disorders. Revised 3rd ed. Washington, DC: American Psychiatric Association, 1987: 255–67.
The current standardized psychiatric nomenclature for patients who somatize.

Altman N. Hypochondriasis. In: Strain JJ, Grossman S, eds. Psychological care of the medically ill: a Primer in liaison psychiatry. New York: Appleton-Century-Crofts, 1975:76–92.
A discussion of hypochondriasis from a psychodynamic perspective.

Engel GL. "Psychogenic" pain and the pain-prone patient. Am J Med 1959; 26:899–918.
A classic presentation of the adaptive value of pain and suffering for a subgroup of patients with chronic pain.

Kaplan C, Lipkin M Jr, Gordon GH. Somatization in primary care: patients with unexplained and vexing medical complaints. J Gen Intern Med 1988; 3:177–90.
A well-referenced review, discussing theories of somatization, differential diagnosis, and management.

Smith GR, Mansons RA, Ray DC. Patients with multiple unexplained symptoms. Arch Intern Med 1986; 149:69–72.
A study of a group of 41 patients with somatization disorder; subjects had multiple medical complaints with negative medical evaluations, functional disability, and average medical charges of $4700 annually.

Brown HN, Vaillant GE. Hypochondriasis. Arch Intern Med 1981; 141:723–6.
Discusses five troublesome medical responses to hypochondriasis and presents suggestions for management.

111. GRIEF
Eric W. Jensen

Grief, the reaction to loss, is a defined syndrome with predictable psychological and somatic symptoms, occurring in response to various types of losses, such as the loss of a loved one, a body part, or self-esteem. It involves a process of realization that helps an individual accept inwardly the reality of an event that has already occurred in the external world. The term *bereavement,* often used interchangeably with *grief,* usually refers to the normal reactions and behaviors following the death of an important person in one's life.

Clinical research indicates that a loss can contribute to the development of a wide range of somatic and psychological disorders. While the relationship between bereavement and ill health is not necessarily a causal one, the altered emotional state seems to contribute to the development of disease. The bereaved state is associated with a measurable abnormality in immune function and higher mortality and morbidity during the first year of bereavement.

Although most people regard the feelings of grief as "normal" and do not seek professional help, others may turn to physicians for relief of grief-related symptoms, such as anxiety, insomnia, anorexia, or depression, particularly in the 12 to 18 months after a loss. An inquiry about recent losses during the initial evaluation of patients presenting with perplexing physical and psychological problems may help identify unresolved grief reactions, thereby circumventing the need for extensive laboratory studies and procedures.

Timely recognition and treatment of abnormal grief reactions may help prevent their prolongation, as well as the physical and psychological complications that can result from failure to grieve completely.

Phases of the Normal Grief Process

The phases of the grief process, as well as the mental and physical vulnerabilities that may arise, have been identified in many studies. Although death of a loved one is used here as an example of a grief reaction, similar reactions may occur in response to other losses.

Because there is marked variability in the expression of uncomplicated grief, and in the sequence, duration, and intensity of the phases of the grief process, it is important that the clinician recognize unusually severe or chronic symptoms. Uncomplicated grief reactions usually proceed through several phases. Prolonged somatic manifestations and/or a loss of self-esteem may indicate a depressive disorder that requires psychiatric evaluation and treatment.

Initially, the impact of the loss is manifested as shock and disbelief. There may be a marked dichotomy between the intellectual awareness of the loss and the apparent emotional response. Individuals often describe this as a feeling of "numbness." This denial is a normal defensive response, protecting the individual from overwhelming stress until other defenses and support are available. This initial period of shock and denial is brief, typically lasting 2 weeks or less.

The developing awareness of the loss that follows is marked by sadness, guilt, regrets, and feelings of helplessness and emptiness. Persons in this phase often cry easily and suffer from anorexia, sleep disturbances, and other somatic complaints. They may have difficulty concentrating, and performance at work and other activities may be impaired. The emotional pain leads to an intellectual understanding of the extensive ramifications of the loss. There may be anger over the loss and resultant hurt, guilt, and numerous regrets, for example, over unexpressed affection, lack of interaction with the deceased person, or unresolved conflicts. Ordinarily, this stage lasts several weeks, but may persist for up to 6 months.

Resolution consists of an evolving reestablishment of emotional, physical, and mental equilibrium. While this process is rarely final, the bereaved individual is able to place the loss in a larger context and begin to seek new social relationships and interests. In deaths resulting from chronic illness, the survivors often experience relief that the pain and suffering of a protracted illness are over.

Estimates of the length of time for "completion" of the uncomplicated grief process range from 6 weeks to 18 months, but the duration and intensity of the grief process vary markedly. Individuals vary in their inherent ability to adjust to loss and change. Other factors that may contribute to individual variation include: age, duration and extent of illness prior to death, circumstances of death (such as sudden death, suicide, or murder), level of dependence on or emotional closeness with the deceased, unresolved conflicts, cultural aspects of mourning, and acceptance or denial of death.

Social supports and institutionalized rituals tend to facilitate the grief process, while societal or cultural values that discount the impact of loss and minimize the expression of grief may tend to slow it. Losses in childhood have been implicated in difficult and prolonged grief later in life.

Symptoms of Uncomplicated Grief Reactions
Uncomplicated grief reactions progressing as described above may be accompanied by acute symptoms. These symptoms, which usually occur after the initial phase of shock and denial, have been characterized as follows:

1. Somatic distress, including feelings of tightness ("lump") in the throat or chest ("heartache"), crying, shortness of breath and sighing respirations, an empty feeling in the stomach ("butterflies"), choking sensation, sensation of muscular weakness and fatigue, and intense subjective distress with agitation and depression, may occur in waves lasting 20 minutes to 1 hour. These symptoms are usually transitory.
2. Preoccupation with the image of the deceased may include transient auditory and visual hallucinations. These may be vivid enough to frighten the bereaved person, who fears they indicate a loss of contact with reality.
3. Feelings of guilt may take several forms, including blaming oneself for betrayal or neglect of the deceased person, guilt over responsibility for the death or loss, and guilt at surviving.
4. Hostile reactions may be directed, sometimes inexplicably, at family, friends, or physicians who attempt to comfort. The bereaved person may be irritable or withdrawn. Anger may also be focused on the deceased.
5. Daily patterns of functioning may be disrupted. The bereaved person may lose interest in usual activities, have difficulty attending to tasks, and feel restless and distracted.

In recent years, a number of studies have documented the immune and neuroendocrine changes that accompany bereavement. These studies have shown a correlation of grief with lowered T-lymphocyte production, and increased production of adrenocorticoids and catecholamines. It is possible that these alterations account for the increased morbidity and mortality associated with bereavement. However, the complex relationships between grief, physical and emotional reactions to loss, immune and endocrine status changes, and illness remain unexplained.

Incomplete or Pathologic Grief

Failure to Grieve
When grief is excessive, prolonged, delayed, or inhibited, failure to resolve the grief process may occur. Social factors that contribute to the failure to grieve include population mobility, which may separate the bereaved person from family and other traditional forms of support; societal expectations to be "strong," which may make it difficult for individuals, especially males, to express their sorrow; and a loss that is unrecognized or even denied, such as after an abortion or when a loved one dies while committing a crime.

Arrested Grief
Psychological factors may prolong the usual emotional denial of the loss, even if it is recognized intellectually. In fact, bereaved persons can become arrested in any phase of the grief process. Factors that may contribute to arrested grief include excessive dependence on the deceased, marked ambivalence, or the reawakening of an old loss that was never resolved. Multiple losses often place the bereaved at a greater risk for prolonged or arrested grief.

Manifestations of Pathologic Grief
Pathologic grief results in distortions of the normal grief phases. Affected patients can present to the primary care physician with a number of different manifestations including depression, hypochondriasis, conversion disorder, development of medical illness or exacerbation of a preexisting somatic condition, and exacerbation of underlying organic brain syndromes or psychotic states. Other manifestations of pathologic grief include perpetual mourning, loss of social interactions, altered relationships, reclusive behavior or hostility, and self-destructive behavior.

The diagnosis of pathologic grief should be strongly considered when a person has failed to grieve following a significant loss, becomes arrested in one of the phases of grief, or presents with a somatic complaint without a physiologic basis that does not resolve in a short period of time. The individual may have refrained from crying, avoided participation in the funeral, and sought to put thoughts of the deceased out of his or her mind. Symptoms that occur on or around the anniversary of a loss may indicate unresolved grief and may be accompanied by an inability to talk about someone who has died some time ago without becoming emotionally distraught. Interviews characterized by themes of loss suggest unresolved grief, particularly if the patient has physical symptoms similar to those of the dead person.

Treatment

While patients with the many physical and psychological symptoms of grief are often encountered, active intervention may not be necessary if the grief process is proceeding as expected. Clinicians should remain alert for signs of pathologic grief and underlying physical illness. Patients may fear that their physical and psychological symptoms are abnormal or indicate the onset of more serious mental illness. Reassurance that such symptoms are to be expected, and encouragement to continue the process of grieving can help patients avoid delayed or unduly prolonged grief. Some patients may benefit from supportive weekly or biweekly meetings, allowing the opportunity to discuss previous experiences with the deceased, and the grieving process.

In addition, research has shown that a high percentage of patients with uncomplicated grief benefit from participating in grief support groups. The group setting allows patients to recognize the symptoms of grief in other people, and it provides a forum for expressing emotion that may be difficult to express elsewhere. A number of organizations have been found by bereaved parents, spouses, friends, and others. For example, The Compassionate Friends, a national organization with local chapters, provides support for bereaved parents and siblings coping with the death of a child of any age; they may be contacted through their national office (P.O. Box 3696, Oak Brook, IL 60522-3696; telephone (708) 990-0010). Groups may also be located through local departments of social services, schools of social work, mental health centers, or grief counselors.

Pathologic grief can be treated in many cases by encouraging the individual to recognize the loss. Because denial of the loss or the resultant feelings is a common trait of this disorder, treatment of pathologic grief by the primary care physician involves helping the patient to recognize and verbalize the thoughts and feelings that have been avoided. Patients who are complex or unremitting should be referred for psychiatric evaluation and treatment.

The grief process is marked by tremendous individual variation; patients with similar losses may have very different expressions of grief. Familial and social supports, the social context, and the values of the patient's culture and family influence the acceptance or denial of loss. Understanding these relationships makes it possible to use the following general principles to make an individual treatment plan:

1. *Listen carefully, and allow emotional expression.* Encourage a discussion of the thoughts and feelings about the loss, and offer support.
2. *Reassure and educate.* After a careful evaluation, patients benefit from the assurance that they are undergoing a normal and necessary process and are not medically or mentally ill.
3. *Facilitate the expression of feelings.* Reconstruction of memories helps the patient express the feelings of loss necessary for grief. Specific questions about the appearance or character of the deceased, or activities prior to death may be useful.
4. *Allow negative feelings.* Ambivalence about the loss is common, but can inhibit grieving. Encourage the expression of both positive and negative feelings. The balance of contrasting feelings helps the patient place the loss in perspective.
5. *Deal with multiple losses one at a time.*
6. *Do not overmedicate.* Sedative-hypnotics may be requested by patients and used effectively during the acute stages of bereavement, but their prolonged use may interfere with the natural course of uncomplicated grief and should be avoided.

7. *Remain objective.* The expression of personal feelings can be helpful, but the physician should guide and facilitate, not interfere, with the expression of grief.

Brown JT, Stoudemire GA. Normal and pathological grief. JAMA 1983; 250:378–82.
This article describes the three phases of normal grief and the problems that arise when the grieving process becomes pathologically delayed or distorted. Guidelines are provided for physician recognition and management of grief.

Swenson JR, Dunsdale JE. Hidden grief reactions on a psychiatric consultation service. Psychosomatics 1989; 30:300–6.
This study found that a significant number of medical and surgical patients referred for consultation suffered from acute or unresolved grief. Cases are presented and management implications discussed.

Calabrese JR, Kling MA, Gold PW. Alterations in immunocompetence during stress, bereavement, and depression: focus on neuroendocrine regulations. Am J Psychiatry 1987; 144:1123–34.
This article provides an overview of the immune system and reviews clinical studies of the impact of bereavement and other stressors on immunologic and neuroendocrine functions.

Irwin M, Daniels M, Weiner H. Immune and neuroendocrine changes during bereavement. Psychiatr Clin North Am 1987; 10:449–65.
This article summarizes recent studies that showed an association between bereavement and changes in immune and neuroendocrine status. Possible relationships between hormonal function and immunity are explored.

Lieberman PB, Jacobs SC. Bereavement and its complication in medical patients: a guide for consultation liaison psychiatrists. Int J Psychiatry Med 1987; 17:23–39.
This article provides a diagnostic and therapeutic framework for recognizing normal and pathologic grief in its various manifestations. This information can be of help to all physicians who deal with primary care.

Middleton W, Raphael B. Bereavement: state of the art and state of the science. Psychiatr Clin North Am 1987; 10:329—43.
The authors review the origins of our current knowledge about the grief process. They point to the need for major new research initiatives to advance our scientific understanding of this process and guide our therapeutic interventions.

112. ALCOHOLISM
JudyAnn Bigby

Between 20 and 40% of patients in general medical hospitals and 10 and 20% of patients in a typical ambulatory practice have alcoholism, defined as any use of alcohol that has adverse effects on health and/or impairs social, occupational, and family functioning. Primary care clinicians are in a unique position to identify patients at risk for alcoholism, patients with early alcoholism, and patients whose use of alcohol places them at risk for diseases such as hypertension, cerebrovascular disease, and cancer. Steps to intervention in patients with alcoholism may be summarized as follows:

1. Screen for alcoholism and be aware of early signs and symptoms.
2. Gather information about alcohol use, concentrating on evidence of loss of control, adverse consequences, evidence of tolerance or addiction, and quantity and frequency.
3. Present concerns about alcohol use to the patient in a concrete, nonjudgmental fashion.
4. Devise a treatment plan and offer to continue to follow the patient.

Categories of Alcohol Abuse

Patients at Risk for Alcoholism
Patients particularly at risk for alcoholism include those with a family history of alcoholism in a first-degree relative; those who started drinking at an early age; those with a history of other drug abuse; those with behavioral problems early in life; and those in certain occupational circumstances, such as unsupervised night shift jobs, jobs with high accessibility to alcohol during working hours, and where there is social pressure from colleagues to drink.

Patients with Alcoholism
In practice, it is not always easy to distinguish patients who have alcoholism from patients who are problem drinkers or those who may be characterized as heavy drinkers. In general, *alcoholics* have evidence of at least one of the following four manifestations of alcoholism: (1) loss of control of drinking, (2) adverse consequences as a result of alcohol use, (3) evidence of tolerance or addiction to alcohol, and (4) drinking in quantities and at a frequency that are excessive. Alcoholism is a chronic problem and according to the *Diagnostic and Statistical Manual of Mental Disorders* (DSM-IIIR) criteria, must be present for at least 1 month.

Problem Drinkers
Problem drinkers may have one or more of the features of alcoholism but may be in social situations where their drinking is viewed as normal and the problematic drinking behavior may not be chronic. The classic example of the problem drinker is the person who binges on weekends, at parties or other social gatherings, and may suffer adverse consequences such as fighting or being stopped for driving under the influence, but who may not in fact be an alcoholic. The drinking problem is related to the social circumstances, such as for a college student living on campus or with a group of other students where heavy drinking on weekends is not unusual. Once the individual is removed from that setting or realizes an adverse consequence has occurred, the drinking problem ceases.

Heavy Drinkers
Heavy drinkers are those who drink on a daily basis and consume more than the equivalent of three glasses of alcohol (12 oz. of beer, 6 oz. of wine, 1 oz. of whiskey, and 4 oz. of sherry are equivalent to one glass of alcohol) per day. Heavy drinkers may not experience any social or immediate medical consequences of drinking. However, epidemiologic studies demonstrate that heavy drinkers have excess mortality due to accidents, cardiovascular disease, and cancer.

Patients with Medical Risks from Drinking
Patients who do not have clear evidence of alcoholism are at risk for certain adverse consequences of chronic daily drinking, such as hypertension and recurring trauma. Hypertension may be easier to control when alcohol intake is limited to less than two drinks per day.

Screening for Alcohol Use
All patients should be screened for the amount of alcohol consumed. In many instances, it may take several visits before enough information can be gathered to characterize the patient's drinking as normal or abnormal, and to categorize the type of consumption.

For patients who are currently drinking, the screening process should center around the patient's relationship to alcohol and any loss of control of drinking, evidence of tolerance or addiction, and adverse consequences of drinking.

Screening Questions
The CAGE questionnaire is an inexpensive, brief interview that can be used in the process of taking a routine medical history. It includes the following four questions:

1. Have you ever felt the need to *cut down* on your drinking?
2. Have you ever been *annoyed* by criticism of your drinking?

3. Have you ever felt *guilty* about your drinking?
4. Have you ever had a morning *eye-opener* after a night of drinking?

Patients who answer yes to two or more of the questions have a high risk for having alcoholism. The positive predictive value of two affirmative responses has been reported to be 80 to 100%. Affirmative answers on the CAGE questionnaire should be followed up. For example, patients who indicate that they have felt a need to cut down on drinking should be asked to explain what prompted the concern, whether there was success in previous attempts to cut down, and why drinking resumed, and to describe the feeling after cutting down or discovering the inability to cut down. Pursuing positive responses in this way is helpful to distinguish patients with problem drinking from those with alcoholism.

Other screening tools include the Michigan Alcoholism Screening Test (MAST), the Self-Administered Alcoholism Screening Test (SSAST), and the Short MAST. The MAST is the most extensively validated instrument and is reported to have a sensitivity and specificity of approximately 85% but is too long to be used during routine history taking. The SSAST and the Short MAST have not been used extensively in an ambulatory population, nor have they been tested for reliability.

Simple questions such as "Have you ever had a drinking problem?" and "When was your last drink?" have also been shown to be helpful screening questions in the ambulatory setting.

Laboratory Tests

The traditional laboratory tests used to screen individuals for alcoholism, such as liver function tests, mean corpuscular volume (MCV), and blood alcohol level, are less sensitive and specific than standardized screening questionnaires and questions. For example, the MCV is elevated in less than 30% of patients with alcoholism and in one study had a negative predictive value of 40%.

Early Signs and Symptoms of Alcoholism

Patients may complain of insomnia, depression, nightmares, poor memory, and nervousness, which are general complaints that may stem from the depressive effects of alcohol or may represent mild withdrawal. Nonspecific abdominal complaints, sexual dysfunction, and evidence of repeated trauma may also be clues to alcoholism. Epidemiologic studies demonstrate that hypertension increases with the quantity of alcohol consumed.

Physical signs of alcoholism appear in late-stage alcoholism and their presence is not useful in confirming a suspicion of alcoholism. Patients in the early or mid stages of alcoholism will be missed if evidence of liver disease, pancreatitis, cognitive impairment, and other secondary effects of alcohol on organ systems are relied on to confirm the diagnosis.

Confirmatory Data

If routine screening, other information from the history, laboratory test results, or evidence on physical examination suggests a diagnosis of alcoholism, efforts should be made to confirm the diagnosis by obtaining concrete evidence of the adverse consequences of alcohol. Information about job performance or absenteeism from work, legal difficulties such as being accused of driving under the influence, or other social problems can be obtained from the spouse and other family members. An individual with difficulty at work should be asked whether he or she has ever been approached by a supervisor or colleague about alcohol on their breath while on the job. Individuals with family-related problems should be offered the opportunity to have family members come in to discuss problems.

If a patient has a history of alcoholism and is currently abstinent, the length of abstinence should be established, as well as how abstinence was achieved, and how the patient currently feels about drinking. Referral for individual or family counseling may be needed depending on the answers to these questions and the length of abstinence.

Presenting the Diagnosis

The problem of alcohol abuse should be discussed with the patient at whatever level of certainty the data support. Specific data from the history, physical examination, and laboratory tests that support the diagnosis are more useful than a generalized concern about drinking, and the problem should be expressed as explicitly as possible. The clinician can acknowledge the possibility that a patient may feel uncomfortable on hearing the diagnosis and should describe all the reasons why alcohol is a problem for the patient: "I'm concerned that alcohol may be your major problem. Your hypertension, the difficulty you are having with your wife, your recent demotion at work, and your laboratory tests all point to alcohol as the major problem." At the time that the diagnosis is presented, the patient should be given information regarding alcoholism as a disease and the natural history of alcoholism, and most importantly, it should be made clear that treatment exists. A patient is more likely to respond to a nonjudgmental assessment of the problem than to simply being told he or she should stop or cut down on the drinking. However, some patients will find it difficult to hear what the clinician has to say about the diagnosis, and may respond angrily or with denial. This can be frustrating, but clinicians should recognize that the impact of their intervention sometimes is not apparent for several months.

Controlled trials have demonstrated the efficacy of counseling alone to decrease the adverse consequences of heavy drinking. In one study, heavy drinkers identified by questions and by abnormal gamma glutamyl transaminase (GGT) results were randomized to two groups. One group received counseling about the effects of alcohol on their GGT and another group did not receive counseling. The group who received counseling had a lower rate of absences from work, hospitalizations, and mortality related to alcohol abuse. In another trial, patients with evidence of problem drinking identified during a hospitalization were counseled by a nurse. Twelve months later, they had a lower rate of alcohol consumption, compared to controls.

Patients with a family history of alcoholism can be educated about the implications of a positive family history and the risk for substance abuse in other family members. Male offspring of alcoholics carry 4 times the risk of developing alcoholism compared to the general population; females, twice the risk.

Treatment

The physician and patient should together establish goals for treatment. Although accepting the diagnosis, patients may still resist any formal type of intervention such as counseling or attendance at Alcoholics Anonymous (AA) meetings. The physician can then enter into contracts with patients about what they would be willing to do to stop drinking and how long it would take for them to stop. Patients who agree to a specific time of follow-up with a specific plan in mind may be more likely to engage in formal treatment than others would. If a patient refuses to accept alcoholism as the diagnosis, the physician can continue care but should emphasize alcoholism as the primary diagnosis and continue to educate the patient about the need for treatment. In most cases, individuals will not follow up with specific alcoholism treatment unless they are willing to acknowledge a problem. Individuals with crises such as threatened job loss or divorce are an exception.

In addition to helping patients identify a specific treatment plan, clinicians can follow them during the early stages of recovery. Caregivers should be aware of evidence of the prolonged abstinence syndrome (anxiety, difficulty sleeping, continued urge to drink), the tremendous sense of loss, and the vulnerability for relapse in the first weeks to months of abstinence. Patients should be educated about the temporary nature of these problems and the need for treatment to help deal with them should they occur. A relapse should be used as an opportunity for education (a demonstration of loss of control), congratulations for the period of abstinence achieved, and a re-evaluation of the treatment plan.

Referral

Referral to treatment resources will depend on availability in the community. Treatment options include outpatient therapy, inpatient treatment, self-help groups such as AA, and private counseling. Employee assistance programs are also valuable resources for devising treatment plans.

While no particular treatment for alcoholism has proven effectiveness compared to other treatments, treatment in both the outpatient and the inpatient setting does increase the number of days of abstinence, decreases the number of days lost from work, and decreases the amount of health care utilization. Outpatient treatment includes group therapy, family therapy and education, and individual counseling, with or without the use of self-help groups. It may be most appropriate in individuals with social supports, with steady jobs, and minimal denial. Inpatient treatment may be necessary for those who have failed outpatient treatment, have few social supports, or have an impending crisis (job loss, divorce, legal difficulty). Without treatment, about one-third of alcoholics will continue to drink, about one-third will die, and the remaining third will become abstinent or improve.

AA and other self-help groups have not been assessed as formal treatment for alcoholism. AA offers individuals the opportunity to join a fellowship of people with a common goal: the desire to stop drinking. Meetings function as self-help groups without a determined leader. Persons initially beginning an AA program are welcomed, but not forced to participate in meetings, an approach billed as "attraction, not coercion." By the use of short phrases and slogans, individuals are given guidance about ways to achieve and maintain sobriety. The principles for recovery are presented in the "Twelve Steps" and focus on restructuring the alcoholic's life-style. The Twelve Steps have a religious overtone to them but there are specific AA meetings where religiosity is tempered, just as there are meetings for all types of people with alcoholism (such as nonsmokers, women, gays, Spanish-speaking). In order to make an effective referral to AA, physicians can describe what patients might expect at meetings and help to identify a meeting at which the patient will feel comfortable by calling a central office telephone number, available in most communities.

Disulfiram

Disulfiram (Antabuse) has been used as an *adjunct* to the treatment of alcoholism since 1948. It has been shown to be effective in decreasing the number of days that alcohol is consumed and decreasing the frequency of hospitalizations due to complications from alcohol. Disulfiram produces a highly unpleasant reaction, including nausea, vomiting, flushing, sweating, headaches, chest pain, and other symptoms, when even small amounts of alcohol are ingested; it serves as a deterrent to alcohol consumption because patients know that they will become ill if they drink while taking it, and for up to two weeks after it is stopped.

Indications for disulfiram include patients willing to participate in treatment, patients who are prone to relapse (e.g., have failed less structured approaches), and patients who require extra support in crisis situations. It is contraindicated in patients who have drunk while taking disulfiram, and those with cardiovascular disease, advanced liver disease, or chronic renal failure. The usual dosage is 250 to 500 mg daily for a week and then 250 to 500 mg 3 times weekly. Patients should abstain completely from alcohol for 72 hours prior to beginning disulfiram.

Barnes HN, Aronson M, Delbanco TL, eds. Alcoholism: a guide for the primary care physician. New York: Springer, 1987.
  A practical approach to the early diagnosis and management of alcoholism, with emphasis on outpatient treatment, withdrawal, and care of special populations.

Kristensen H, et al. Identification and intervention of heavy drinkers in middle-aged men: results and follow-up of 24–60 months of long-term study with randomized controls. J Alcohol Clin Exp Res 1983; 20:203–9.
  Identification of heavy drinkers, followed by counseling and repeated feedback of GGT results, resulted in lower rates of absenteeism, hospitalization, and mortality from alcohol use.

Chick J, Lloyd G, Crombie E. Counseling problem drinkers in medical wards: a controlled trial. Br Med J 1985; 290:965–7.
  Patients counseled by a nurse had lower rates of alcohol consumption after 12 months of follow-up.

Bush B, et al. Screening for alcohol abuse using the CAGE questionnaire. Am J Med 1987; 82:231–5.
  The CAGE questionnaire had a positive predictive value of 62 to 100% and performed better than liver function tests or the MCV in identifying problem drinkers.

Cyr M. Wartman S. The effectiveness of routine screening questions in the detection of alcoholism. JAMA 1988; 259:51–4.

There was a high prevalence of alcoholism in an outpatient population. Simple questions about drinking were useful in identifying alcoholics.

Klatsky AL, et al. Alcohol consumption and blood pressure: Kaiser-Permanente multiphasic health examination data. N Engl J Med 1977; 296:1194–2000.
Daily consumption of three or more drinks was associated with significantly increased blood pressure.

Fuller RK, et al. Disulfiram treatment of alcoholism: a Veterans Administration cooperative study. JAMA 1986; 256:1449–55.
Disulfiram treatment did not improve rates of abstinence, time to relapse, or employment status but did result in significantly fewer drinking days and reduced medical complications.

Beresford TP, et al. Comparison of CAGE questionnaire and computer-assisted laboratory profiles in screening for covert alcoholism. Lancet 1990; 336:482–5.
The CAGE questionnaire was more sensitive (76%) and specific (94%) for recognition of alcohol dependence than computer-assisted laboratory data profiles, which did perform better than chance alone.

XVI. INFECTIOUS DISEASES

113. SEXUALLY TRANSMITTED DISEASES
Eliseo J. Pérez-Stable

Many communicable diseases have been shown to be transmitted during sexual contact. Gonorrhea, syphilis, chancroid, lymphogranuloma venereum (LGV), and granuloma inguinale (donovanosis) have been considered to be the five classic sexually transmitted diseases (STDs). The newer sexually transmitted microorganisms include *Chlamydia trachomatis; Ureaplasma urealyticum;* herpes simplex viruses (HSVs); the hepatitis viruses; cytomegaloviruses (CMVs); papilloma virus; traditional enteric pathogens such as *Entamoeba histolytica, Giardia lamblia,* and *Shigella* species; and the human immunodeficiency virus (HIV).

Regardless of sexual orientation, the risk of STDs is directly proportional to the number of different lifetime sexual partners a person has. STDs are generally more common in younger persons and in those of less advantaged socioeconomic background, and are less common in women who have sex only with other women. Women taking oral contraceptives have been reported to have a greater incidence of chlamydial infections, possibly because of an increased incidence of cervical ectopy, which in turn facilitates the growth of endocervical organisms. Clinical manifestations of STDs are more subtle in women than in men, and complications, in particular pelvic inflammatory disease (PID) and its sequelae, are far more serious.

This chapter is divided into two sections: the first deals with common pathogens and the second describes the management of common clinical syndromes.

COMMON PATHOGENS

Gonococcal Infections
Neisseria gonorrhoeae causes urethritis, epididymitis, prostatitis, pharyngitis, cervicitis, salpingitis, and disseminated gonococcal infections (DGIs). Men have approximately a 25% risk of acquiring gonorrhea by contact with an infected female, while transmission from an infected male to a woman (or to another man) occurs about twice as often. The greatest economic and social consequence of gonococcal infections is PID, which results in an increased risk of ectopic pregnancy and infertility. Complications of gonorrhea can be minimized by accurate diagnosis and effective treatment of the early clinical syndromes (urethritis and cervicitis).

Clinical Presentations
Urethritis, prostatitis, epididymitis, proctitis, and cervicitis are discussed in the section on common clinical syndromes.

Gonococcal pharyngitis usually results from orogenital sexual contact, more often from fellatio than cunnilingus. Most gonococcal pharyngeal infections are asymptomatic, although sore throat and cervical adenitis may be caused by gonorrhea. Diagnosis depends on culture, since the presence of other *Neisseria* species within the pharynx renders Gram's stain nonspecific.

DGI is seen in 1 to 3% of all patients presenting with genital gonococcal infections, with 75% of all cases occurring in women. Early in its course, DGI presents with polyarthralgias, small joint tenosynovitis, and up to 20 peripherally located pustular skin lesions with a broad erythematous base. A later phase of DGI, more commonly encountered in practice, presents as tenosynovitis and/or a monoarticular arthritis. Gram's stain and culture of the skin lesions and inflamed joints have a low yield. Cultures of the urethra, pharynx, and rectum give a higher yield despite a lack of local symptoms. The isolation of *N. gonorrhoeae* from one of these sites is sufficient for diagnosis in patients with a typical clinical presentation.

Patients with DGI should be hospitalized for initial intravenous therapy until clinical improvement occurs. Penicillinase-producing *N. gonorrhoeae* (PPNG) as a cause of DGI is unusual. Patients with recurrent DGI should be evaluated for complement deficiencies.

Table 113-1. Treatment guidelines for gonococcal infections

UNCOMPLICATED URETHRAL, ENDOCERVICAL, OR RECTAL INFECTIONS
Preferred regimen:
  Ceftriaxone, 250 mg IM once, *plus* doxycycline,* 100 mg PO bid × 7 days
Alternative regimens:
  Any of the following alternatives should be given with doxycycline,* 100 mg PO bid × 7 days
    Spectinomycin, 2 g IM once (recommended in penicillin allergy)
    Ciprofloxacin, 500 mg PO once (contraindicated in pregnancy)
    Norfloxacin, 800 mg PO once (contraindicated in pregnancy)
    Cefuroxime axetil, 1 g PO once, with probenecid, 1 g PO
    Cefotaxime, 1 g IM once
    Ceftizoxime, 500 mg IM once
  The following are to be used only if infection was acquired from a source proved not to have penicillinase-producing *Neisseria gonorrhoeae* (PPNG)
    Amoxicillin, 3 g PO once, with probenecid 1 g PO
    Ampicillin, 3.5 g once, with probenecid, 1 g PO
    Procaine penicillin G, 4.8 million U IM once, with probenecid, 1 g PO

PHARYNGEAL INFECTION
Ceftriaxone, 250 mg IM once, *or* ciprofloxacin, 500 mg PO once
Plus doxycycline, 100 mg PO bid × 7 days

*During pregnancy, erythromycin, 500 mg qid × 7 days, should be substituted for doxycycline.

Antibiotic Resistance
While the incidence of reported gonococcal infections has declined recently, representing the first significant downward trend in over 30 years, the spread of infection due to antibiotic-resistant *N. gonorrhoeae* is a rapidly growing problem. There are two major types of antibiotic resistance: a chromosomally mediated relative resistance and absolute resistance from plasmid-mediated PPNG. Beginning in 1985, epidemic outbreaks of PPNG have been reported throughout the United States, and in some areas PPNG infections constitute 25% of all gonococcal infections. PPNG-infected patients have been predominantly inner-city residents, members of ethnic minority groups, and heterosexuals.

Because of the increasing proportion of gonorrhea caused by antibiotic-resistant strains (especially PPNG), treatment regimens effective against PPNG are highly preferable. Test-of-cure cultures should be performed on all patients treated with a regimen not effective against PPNG (Table 113-1) 3 to 5 days after antimicrobial therapy is completed.

Treatment
The current Centers for Disease Control (CDC) recommendations for the treatment of gonococcal infections are summarized in Table 113-1. Single-dose therapy is highly preferable for treating uncomplicated gonococcal infections. Because coexisting chlamydial infection has been documented in up to 45% of patients with gonorrhea, all patients treated for gonorrhea should also receive an antibiotic effective against chlamydia, such as *doxycycline* (100 mg PO twice a day) or *tetracycline* (500 mg 4 times a day) for 7 days. The daily cost of generic doxycycline is now equivalent to the daily cost of tetracycline, and the less frequent dosing results in better compliance. The cost is $1 to $2 per treatment course. For patients who cannot take a tetracycline (e.g, pregnant women), erythromycin base (500 mg orally 4 times daily) may be substituted. While dual therapy of gonococcal infections with a tetracycline is recommended to eradicate possible coexisting chlamydial infections, sole therapy with tetracycline should be strongly discouraged because plasmid-mediated resistance to tetracycline in gonococcal isolates has been reported in 23 states. Monotherapy with tetracycline has also been found to fail in up to 10% of women treated for gonococcal cervicitis in the absence of resistant strains.

Further advantages and disadvantages of alternative regimens for uncomplicated gonorrhea are as follows:

Ceftriaxone, 250 mg intramuscularly once, is effective against PPNG, works at all sites of gonococcal infection, and is safe during pregnancy. It is also probably effective against incubating syphilis, but ineffective against coexisting chlamydial infection. Official CDC dose recommendations are for 250 mg but a therapeutic success rate of higher than 98% has been reported with 125 mg of ceftriaxone. The smaller dose may be preferred because it is less expensive and can be administered in a volume (0.5 ml) small enough to be administered in the deltoid muscle. The cost is about $8 per 250-mg dose. Test-of-cure cultures after treatment with ceftriaxone are not essential.

Spectinomycin, 2 g intramuscularly once, is the preferred alternative for patients who cannot take ceftriaxone. Spectinomycin is not adequate for pharyngeal gonorrhea and does not treat coexisting chlamydial infection or incubating syphilis. The cost is $10 per dose.

Ciprofloxacin, 500 mg orally as a single dose, is the recommended alternative to ceftriaxone in patients with uncomplicated pharyngeal gonorrhea. Ciprofloxacin is also an alternative for gonococcal infections at other sites.

Other single-dose antibiotic alternatives for urethral, endocervical, rectal, or pharyngeal infections include *norfloxacin,* 800 mg orally; *cefuroxime axetil,* 1 g orally, with probenecid, 1 g; *cefotaxime,* 1 g intramuscularly; and *ceftizoxime,* 500 mg intramuscularly. There is less extensive experience with these regimens and their costs are generally higher than those of comparable regimens. The quinolones (ciprofloxacin and norfloxacin) are contraindicated during pregnancy and in children 16 years or younger.

Ampicillin (3.5 g), *amoxicillin* (3 g), and *procaine penicillin G* (4.8 million U), each with probenecid (1 g), are adequate for treatment of gonorrhea if the infection was acquired from a source proved not to have PPNG. The procaine penicillin G regimen is effective for gonococcal infections at each mucosal site, but ampicillin and amoxicillin are not effective for pharyngitis or proctitis. Routine susceptibility testing and comprehensive test-of-cure evaluations are required for patients treated with these regimens. The cost is less than $1 for oral regimens and about $8 for procaine penicillin G; lower drug costs may be offset by the cost of the additional follow-up needed.

Management of Contacts

Sex partners within the preceding 30 days of patients with documented gonococcal infections should be examined, cultured, and treated presumptively with an antibiotic regimen effective against both gonorrhea and chlamydia. Treatment of contacts should not await the results of cultures or the onset of symptoms. Positive findings in cultured material from sex contacts of a patient known to have gonorrhea necessitate clinical follow-up and contact tracing of sex partners for examination and treatment.

Chlamydial Infections

C. trachomatis is the most common sexually transmitted pathogen in the United States today and causes clinical syndromes quite similar to mucosal gonococcal infections (urethritis in men and cervicitis in women). However, the prevalence of asymptomatic infections is substantially higher, and persons with chlamydial infections may remain asymptomatic for extended periods of time. *C. trachomatis* coexists in 45% of women and 25% of heterosexual men with gonorrhea. Homosexual men with gonorrhea are reported to have less frequent coinfections with *C. trachomatis.* Sexually active adolescent boys evaluated in teen clinics have been found to harbor urethral chlamydia 8 to 9% of the time.

Diagnostic Tests

Tissue culture of *C. trachomatis* is the best test for laboratory diagnosis. Although cultures have close to 100% specificity, it is estimated that 10 to 20% of organisms fail to grow on culture, so that the sensitivity is about 80 to 90%. Charges for chlamydial cultures are usually $35 or higher, although proponents of widespread use insist that the cost can be substantially lowered. Adequate specimen collection and transport to the laboratory are important variables in the successful isolation of chlamydia. Endocervical specimens should be collected after first swabbing the cervix to remove exudate and mucus; in order to obtain adequate cells for culture, the os should then be swabbed for 10 seconds, preferably using a cytobrush. Similarly, rectal cultures should be collected by swabbing the rectal mucosa. Culture of male urethras is rarely indicated.

Nonculture diagnostic methods that are available commercially detect chlamydial antigen and provide a faster diagnosis than does tissue culture. Because specificity and sensitivity of antigen detection tests are compared to the "gold standard" of tissue culture, the test characteristics are inferior. Thus, antigen detection tests should be reserved for routine use in populations with a prevalence of infection of at least 6 to 10% and where standard tissue culture evaluations are not available. Newer antigen detection tests provide results in 15 minutes with a specificity approaching 100%, but the sensitivity continues to be about 90% when compared to culture tests. However, these test characteristics were established in protocol settings with experienced technicians and results may not be as good in an office setting where tests are performed only occasionally.

Enzyme-linked immunosorbent assay (ELISA) performed in clinical laboratories requires a spectrophotometer and takes approximately 4 hours; kits using this method designed for office use do not require special equipment and take 10 to 30 minutes. The sensitivity of this test varies from 67 to 90% and specificity, from 92 to 97% when compared to culture tests. The positive predictive value of the ELISA can range from 32 to 87% depending on the population studied. The advantages of the ELISA are easy transport of specimens, the lack of dependence on a specially trained observer, and the ability to test large numbers of specimens at a time. The *direct-smear fluorescent antibody test* using monoclonal antibodies takes 30 to 40 minutes and requires precise specimen collection, a high-quality fluorescence microscope, and an experienced microscopist for interpretation. The test stains infectious chlamydia particles in epithelial cell scrapings from infected sites. The sensitivity is better than 90% and the specificity is better than 98% when compared to tissue culture. Positive predictive values of this test have ranged from 80 to 95% in populations with a prevalence of chlamydial infections between 10 and 30%.

Clinical Strategies
Empiric therapy may be used in the absence of any laboratory diagnosis if the clinical presentation and epidemiologic risk profile suggest the presence of chlamydia. Adolescents, young pregnant women, and patients at STD and family planning clinics are all at higher risk for chlamydia. Screening of asymptomatic patients at greatest risk for chlamydia infection may be warranted when the prevalence exceeds 6 to 10%. Pregnant women with multiple partners should undergo screening cultures.

Treatment
The treatment of chlamydial infections is summarized in Table 113-2. Doxycycline or tetracycline is the drug of choice; treatment with erythromycin or sulfisoxazole is an acceptable alternative regimen.

Table 113-2. Treatment of chlamydial infections*

Indication	Therapy
Regimens of choice	Doxycycline, 100 mg PO bid for a minimum of 7 days, *or*
	Tetracycline, 0.5 g PO qid for a minimum of 7 days
Alternative regimens	Erythromycin, 0.5 g PO qid for a minimum of 7 days, *or*
	Sulfamethoxazole, 1.0 g PO bid for 10 days
Treatment failure or relapse	Switch to erythromycin if tetracycline was used initially and vice versa
Recurrent treatment failure or relapse	Doxycycline or erythromycin as above for 3–4 wk
Lymphogranuloma venereum	Above regimens continued for a minimum of 2–3 wk

*Nongonococcal urethritis (chlamydial and nonchlamydial), mucopurulent cervicitis, and related syndromes.

Lymphogranuloma Venereum
Specific serotypes of *C. trachomatis* also cause a separate STD syndrome known as lymphogranuloma venereum (LGV). LGV most frequently presents as a painful inguinal lymphadenopathy without clinically evident genital lesions. The initial papule or ulcer of LGV is noticed by less than one-third of infected men and an even lower proportion of women. Clinical diagnosis can be confirmed by culturing aspirate from an enlarged inguinal node. Sinus tract formation with subsequent chronic drainage was common prior to the availability of antimicrobials, but is rarely seen today. Treatment is with doxycycline or other antimicrobials effective against chlamydia for a minimum of 2 to 3 weeks. LGV can also cause proctocolitis.

Syphilis
Reported cases of infectious (primary and secondary) syphilis, caused by the spirochete *Treponema pallidum*, have been increasing in the United States since 1987. Rates are currently the highest since 1950, and some authorities estimate that the number of actual cases is approximately 10 times that reported. During the late 1970s, 70% of infectious syphilis occurred among homosexual or bisexual men but the number of cases among these groups appears to be decreasing in some areas. In contrast, increasing rates have been noted among urban black and Latina women and heterosexual men of all racial and ethnic groups.

Clinical Presentation
Primary syphilis presents as a nontender ulcer or chancre. The average incubation period is 21 days, but can vary from 3 to 90 days. The chancre begins as a papule and develops into a painless ulcer with an indurated border and clean base. Multiple chancres occur in about 25% of patients, and tender ulcers are present in 10%. Painless regional lymphadenopathy is present in 50 to 70% of patients. Although usually located in the genital areas, syphilitic chancres may appear on any affected site.

The secondary stage of syphilis usually develops about 6 weeks after the chancre has healed, but may overlap with primary syphilis. Clinical manifestations of secondary syphilis may involve any organ system; cutaneous and mucosal lesions are the most frequent. The typical maculopapular rash is symmetric, nonpruritic, usually present over the palms and soles, but more pronounced over the trunk than the extremities. Scaling and necrosis may produce psoriatic-appearing or pustular lesions. Two other classic lesions of secondary syphilis include hypertrophic coalesced papules that form in moist intertriginous areas (condylomata lata), and raised painless gray plaques on an erythematous base occurring in the mucous membranes of the oral cavity. Constitutional symptoms and generalized lymphadenopathy are frequent. Epitrochlear adenopathy in particular is an important clue to the diagnosis. Hepatitis occurs in about 10% and acute meningitis in about 1%, and less commonly, renal involvement, splenomegaly, eighth nerve deafness, optic neuritis, iritis, osteitis, and gastropathy are observed.

Abnormalities of the cerebrospinal fluid (CSF) occur in 25 to 40% of patients with early syphilis. Lumbar puncture is not recommended for the routine evaluation of primary or secondary syphilis unless clinical signs and symptoms of neurologic involvement exist, since findings do not affect therapy.

Diagnosis
The diagnosis of syphilis rests on direct microscopy and/or serologic studies. Darkfield microscopic examination of a suspicious lesion provides a prompt and accurate diagnosis in experienced hands, but is not available in most clinical settings. Direct fluorescent antibody tests for syphilis are available from many public health laboratories and can provide a rapid diagnosis for patients with suspicious ulcers.

The Venereal Disease Research Laboratories (VDRL) slide flocculation test and the rapid plasma reagin (RPR) agglutination test detect the nonspecific antibodies produced in response to infection by *T. pallidum* and are the most commonly used tests for diagnosing syphilis. Antibodies are first detected in the patient's serum 4 to 6 weeks following infection, or up to 3 weeks after the primary chancre develops. In primary syphilis, the VDRL or RPR is reactive in 70 to 80% of patients, while in secondary syphilis, tests are reactive in nearly 100%. Specific treponemal tests are required to confirm the reactive

VDRL or RPR. Sequential serologic tests should be done with either VDRL or RPR each time by the same laboratory. Although both tests are equally valid, RPR titers tend to be slightly higher and the two are therefore not comparable.

The fluorescent treponemal antibody absorption test (FTA-ABS) and the *T. pallidum* hemagglutination assay (TPHA-TP) are the most widely used specific treponemal tests. Tremponemal tests are more sensitive and specific than either the VDRL or RPR test but should not be used as the initial screening test in diagnosing syphilis. Once the treponemal test becomes reactive, it usually remains positive even after appropriate antibiotic therapy.

Treatment and Follow-up
Therapy for syphilis is summarized in Table 113-3. One intramuscular injection of benzathine penicillin G is sufficient treatment for primary or secondary syphilis. In patients with penicillin allergies, skin testing is recommended to confirm the allergy, with desensitization if necessary. Procedures for skin testing and desensitization are included in the *1989 Sexually Transmitted Disease Treatment Guidelines* published by the CDC. Doxycycline or tetracycline for 2 weeks is an effective alternative that requires careful follow-up to ensure adherence to therapy. Erythromycin, 500 mg orally 4 times a day for 2 weeks, can be used if desensitization to penicillin is not possible and if patients cannot tolerate doxycycline or tetracycline. However, preliminary reports suggest that erythromycin is inadequate in pregnant women with syphilis and in patients coinfected with HIV. Thus, whenever possible benzathine penicillin should be used in all patients with early syphilis. Preliminary data suggest that ceftriaxone, 250 mg intramuscularly daily for 10 days, is also effective. Caution must be used in treating a penicillin-allergic patient with a cephalosporin. Careful follow-up is mandatory when alternative regimens are used.

Following appropriate therapy, quantitative titers of VDRL at 3, 6, 12, and 24 months after treatment are recommended to monitor the response. Patients with adequately treated primary syphilis should have either very low titers (< 1:8) or nonreactive nontreponemal antibody tests (VDRL or RPR) by 12 months. Similar results should be observed in treated patients with secondary syphilis by 24 months. Patients with HIV infection should have more frequent follow-up, with serologic testing at 1, 2, 3, 6, 9, 12, and 24 months. A fourfold increase in titer at any time may represent treatment failure or reinfection. If reinfection is ruled out, CSF examination and treatment with a regimen effective against neurosyphilis is recommended.

HIV and Syphilis
Coinfection with HIV may alter the natural history of syphilis and lead to earlier manifestations of neurosyphilis that are more difficult to treat. In an HIV-infected person with clinical findings suggesting that syphilis is present but with negative serologic findings, alternative methods of diagnosis such as biopsy of lesions should be used. Penicillin regimens should be used whenever possible in all HIV-infected patients with syphilis. Some authorities advise that the CSF be examined and/or treatment appropriate for neurosyphilis be given for all patients coinfected with syphilis and HIV. Further study is needed to address the need for lumbar punctures in evaluating early syphilis, the efficacy of currently recommended therapy, and the possible effect of HIV infection on the progression of syphilis and its response to therapy. (See Chap. 114 for further discussion).

Contacts
Persons exposed to a patient with infectious syphilis within the previous 90 days should be examined clinically, tested serologically, and treated presumptively for early syphilis.

Herpes Simplex Viruses
Infections with HSVs are the most common cause of genital ulcers in sexually active adults (Table 113-4). The continued upward trend in the number of patient consultations for genital herpes infections may reflect both the intense media attention and the availability of acyclovir. HSVs are characterized by latent infection following an acute episode despite vigorous host response, symptomatic or asymptomatic reactivation that may occur at any time, and oncogenic potential. Latent infection with HSV occurs within neurons and thus recurrent episodes manifest over a smaller area of skin than the initial episode.

Table 113-3. Treatment for syphilis*

Indication	Penicillin therapy	Therapy for patients with penicillin allergy	Comments
Early syphilis: primary, secondary, latent of < 1 yr	Penicillin G benzathine, 2.4 million U total IM at a single session	Doxycycline, 100 mg PO bid for 15 days *or* Erythromycin, 500 mg PO qid for 15 days *or* Ceftriaxone, 250 mg IM qd for 10 days	Consider CSF examination in patients with HIV infection.
Syphilis of > 1 yr: latent, cardiovascular, late benign	Penicillin G benzathine, 2.4 million U IM once a wk for 3 successive wk (7.2 million U total)	Doxycycline, 100 mg PO bid for 30 days *or* Erythromycin, 500 mg PO qid for 30 days	Before using nonpenicillin therapy, in treatment failure patients, or if neurologic signs or symptoms are present, CSF examination should be performed to rule out asymptomatic neurosyphilis. Some authorities advise doing this before penicillin therapy also. All patients with coexisting HIV infection should have a CSF examination.
Neurosyphilis	Aqueous penicillin G, 12–24 million U/day IV, divided into q4h doses, for 10–14 days; follow with penicillin G benzathine, 2.4 million U IM weekly for 3 doses	Confirm allergy and obtain expert consultation to determine optimal therapy	Alternative regimen if outpatient compliance can be ensured. Procaine penicillin G, 2.4 million U IM daily, plus probenecid, 500 mg PO qid, both for 10–14 days. Follow with penicillin G benzathine, 2.4 million U IM weekly for 3 doses.

*Based on Centers for Disease Control recommendations.

Table 113-4. Genital ulcers: differential diagnosis

Causes	No./size	Pain/tenderness	Appearance	Inguinal nodes	Diagnostic tests	Treatment
Herpes simplex viruses	Groups of multiple ulcers of uniform size—2–10 mm	Uniformly present	Erythematous border surrounds lesions; many stages present (papules, vesicles, ulcers, crusting)	Present in primary infection; tender; variable in recurrences (40–80%)	Viral cultures; scraping base for Giemsa or Wright's stain	Local care; analgesics; acyclovir, 200 mg PO 5 ×/day
Primary syphilis	Classically a single lesion; >1 in nearly half of series; size may vary; when mutiple—4 mm–2 cm	Usually painless, pain if superinfected	Base is relatively clean; edge indurated	Present and painless	Darkfield examination; RPR or VDRL, FTA-ABS confirmatory	Penicillin benzathine or doxycycline (see Table 113-3)
Chancroid	Usually single lesions with much variation in size; multiple lesions	Uniformly present	Base is necrotic; edge ragged, not indurated	Present in ½; painful and unilateral	Gram's stain of exudative borders; culture	Erythromycin or ceftriaxone (see text)
LGV	Single 1–2-mm lesion of short duration	Present only occasionally	Shallow ulceration with clean base	Usually appear after ulcer resolves; painful; bilateral in ⅓	Chlamydial cultures of an involved node; serologic titers ≥ 1:512	Doxycycline (see Table 113-2)
Granuloma inguinale (donovanosis)	Single or multiple	Not tender even when massive lesions	Granulation tissue with beefy red lesions; edge often stark white	Rare	Crushed tissue stained with Wright's or Giemsa preparations	Gentamicin; chloramphenicol; ampicillin; tetracycline

Both HSV-1 and HSV-2 can be sexually transmitted. HSV-1 typically infects the oral mucosa and HSV-2 usually infects the genital area. However, about 10 to 20% of the time the opposite is seen. Genital infections with HSV-1 are less likely to recur (14–25%) than those caused by HSV-2 (60–88%). Other than usual location, no distinguishing clinical findings differentiate HSV-1 from HSV-2.

Clinical Presentation
Primary infection with HSV usually presents with systemic symptoms of fever, malaise, and anorexia, shortly followed by the appearance of a characteristic painful vesicular rash. Tender bilateral inguinal lymphadenopathy frequently accompanies the primary infection, but is variable in recurrent infections. The initial vesicles may persist for several days before progressing through the well-defined ulcer, crust, and healed stages in 1 to 3 weeks. Ulcers in the oral mucosa may be so painful that patients are unable to eat and genital lesions may cause dysuria. HSV proctitis presents with frequent urgent bowel movements producing small amounts of liquid stool with occasional blood. Local complications include a neurogenic bladder with urinary retention and bowel dysfunction secondary to sacral radiculomyelitis. The duration of illness is 2 to 4 weeks.

In recurrent episodes, patients typically report a 1- to 2-day prodrome of localized paresthesias, pruritus, or burning at the site of subsequent vesicular lesions. Systemic symptoms are milder, viral shedding lasts a mean of only 2 days, and the local involvement is usually less extensive. Illness lasts only 5 to 10 days but there is wide variability as to the frequency and duration of recurrences.

Diagnosis
A typical clinical presentation of primary or recurrent HSV is sufficient for diagnosis by an experienced clinician. If viral cultures are not available, treatment decisions and counseling may be based on clinical impressions alone. Tissue culture for HSV takes 24 to 96 hours, but is the most sensitive and specific test. Techniques are simple and the cost can be limited to less than $20 per specimen. Immunofluorescent assays of scrapings from lesions, using monoclonal antibodies and some DNA hybridization procedures, have approached the sensitivity of viral cultures and provide a faster diagnosis for half the cost. Although the antigen detection tests may substitute for tissue culture in the clinical management of acute HSV infections, the indications for using these diagnostic tests may be limited. A definitive diagnostic test for a patient who desires that level of certainty requires HSV culture. In addition, cultures differentiate HSV-1 and HSV-2, which has prognostic implications for recurrences.

A Tzanck smear of a vesicular lesion can confirm a diagnosis of herpes virus if multinucleated giant cells are present. However, false-negative rates approach 25% and the test is nonspecific since it cannot differentiate HSV from varicella zoster virus (VZV) when evaluating nongenital lesions. The sensitivity of all laboratory methods for detecting HSV is higher in vesicular than in ulcerative lesions. Serologic assays have little value in diagnosing acute HSV infections, cannot distinguish HSV-1 and HSV-2, and are best used in epidemiologic studies to identify patients with past infections.

Treatment
Chemotherapy with acyclovir for HSV infections has been a pioneering step in the treatment of viral infections. Topical acyclovir is not recommended for the treatment of HSV, as studies have shown minimal therapeutic benefit in primary infections and no demonstrable benefit over placebo in recurrent infections.

Treatment of the first clinical episodes of HSV with oral acyclovir, 200 mg by mouth 5 times a day for 7 to 10 days, has been shown to significantly decrease viral shedding, speed resolution of symptoms, and shorten the time to crusting and healing from about 14 to about 7 days when compared to placebo. In patients with primary HSV proctitis, acyclovir is given in the higher dosage of 400 mg orally 5 times a day for 10 days. Acyclovir therapy for the first clinical episodes may be continued until clinical resolution occurs. In patients with severe systemic disease or complications necessitating hospitalization, intravenous acyclovir (5 mg/kg of body weight) is indicated.

The benefit of oral acyclovir in the treatment of recurrent HSV is considerably less than that in primary infections. Shortening the duration of symptoms and viral shedding by 1 to 2 days was the most significant impact shown in placebo-controlled trials. Self-initiated acyclovir therapy, 200 mg orally 5 times a day or 800 mg orally twice a day, at the very beginning of the prodrome may provide the most benefit in selected patients with recurrent HSV. The time to subsequent recurrence is not changed by acute treatment with oral acyclovir.

Patients with genital HSV infection should be informed about the potential for recurrences. Frequent or severe recurrences of genital HSV may have a substantial impact on a patient's social function, and suppressive therapy (see below) may be indicated for some. Professional counseling and herpes support groups may also be helpful.

Management of Pregnant Patients

Pregnant women without life-threatening HSV infection should not be treated with systemic acyclovir for recurrent genital herpes because its safety has not been established. The risk of neonatal transmission of HSV from an infected mother is highest among women with primary infection near the time of delivery and it is low among women with recurrent herpes. Viral cultures during pregnancy are not routinely indicated because the results do not predict viral shedding at the time of delivery. At the onset of labor, women without symptoms (including prodrome) or signs of genital herpes may have vaginal deliveries. Cultures of the birth canal at delivery may be helpful for making decisions about neonatal management.

HIV Coinfection

Patients with immunodeficiency have more severe clinical manifestations of HSV infection and are at greater risk for dissemination and systemic complications. Some health care providers recommend therapy with acyclovir in higher than standard doses for all patients with HIV infection, but neither the need nor the proper increased dosage has been conclusively established. Immunocompetent as well as immunocompromised patients who fail initial treatment may benefit from an increased dosage of acyclovir. Patients with acyclovir-resistant strains of HSV and HIV have been successfully treated with foscarnet. In these situations, the primary provider should consult an expert in infectious diseases.

Suppressive Therapy

Long-term daily suppressive therapy may reduce the frequency of reactivation among patients with a minimum of more than 6 episodes per year and/or disabling herpes recurrences. Virologic documentation of HSV infection should be completed before long-term therapy is started. Treatment for 4 months resulted in fewer recurrences (25 versus 100%) and a prolongation in the time to the first episode (120 versus 18 days) when compared to placebo. All patients had recurrences within 3 months after completing acyclovir treatment. The recommended regimen for suppressive therapy is 200 mg 2 to 5 times a day or 400 mg 2 times a day, but some studies have used 800 mg once a day. Long-term experience with daily chemosuppression for up to 3 years indicates that the effectiveness persists as long as acyclovir is continued and the toxicity appears to be minimal. Because acyclovir-resistant strains of HSV have been isolated from patients treated with daily suppressive therapy, use of this regimen must be selective. The CDC recommends that after 1 year of continuous suppressive therapy, acyclovir be discontinued and the recurrence rate reassessed.

Management of Contacts

Patients should be advised to abstain from sexual activity while lesions are present. Because sexual transmission of HSV has been documented in the absence of recognized clinical lesions, and daily suppressive therapy decreases but does not eliminate viral shedding, condoms should be used during all sexual exposures to persons with known HSV infection. Sex partners of patients with HSV infection who have genital lesions may benefit from evaluation, but there is little value in evaluating asymptomatic partners.

Chancroid

Chancroid is caused by *Hemophilus ducreyi*, a gram-negative coccobacillus. In 1986, 3418 cases, the largest number since 1952, were reported. Chancroid is now established as an endemic disease in selected areas of the United States. In a CDC analysis of 9 outbreaks of chancroid in 1981 to 1987, involving 5409 cases, the male-female ratio averaged 10:1, and men patronizing prostitutes were involved in 6 of the outbreaks. Blacks and/or Latinos were the principal ethnic groups involved in all of the outbreaks.

Clinical Presentation and Diagnosis
The incubation period from the time of exposure varies from 1 to 14 days, with an average of 7 days. Lesions are generally confined to the genitalia and are characterized by extensive local necrosis. Genital ulcers are usually single and uniformly tender, with a characteristic necrotic base and a nonindurated ragged edge. Ulcers vary in size from 1 to 22 mm and unilateral tender lymphadenopathy is present in 50% of patients. Fluctuant bubos may occur in up to one-third of patients even after appropriate antibiotic therapy has started, and aspiration through adjacent healthy skin is the treatment of choice. Complications of untreated chancroid include fistula formations to the skin, bladder, or intestine.

Clinical suspicion is essential to the diagnosis. Although a low incidence in the past has led most U.S. practitioners not to suspect it, chancroid must be considered a possibility in any patient with a painful genital ulcer. Gram's stain of a genital ulcer scraping showing typical gram-negative coccobacillary bacterium is specific, but at best the sensitivity is only 50%. Since there are no serologic markers for *H. ducreyi*, culture is the best method of diagnosing chancroid. Cultures should be obtained from the perimeter of the ulcer and not from the necrotic base. Special culture media must be used for this fastidious organism and many suspected cases are not confirmed. The microbiology laboratory must be advised that the clinician suspects *H. ducreyi*, since isolation requires incubators set at a lower temperature than usually used.

Treatment and Follow-up
The susceptibility of *H. ducreyi* to various antimicrobials varies throughout the world. The recommended treatment of chancroid in the United States is oral erythromycin, 500 mg 4 times a day for 10 days, or ceftriaxone, 250 mg intramuscularly in a single dose. Acceptable alternative regimens include trimethoprim-sulfamethoxazole, one double-strength tablet (160 mg/800 mg) twice a day for 7 days or four double-strength tablets in a single dose; amoxicillin, 500 mg, plus clavulanic acid, 125 mg, 3 times a day for 7 days; and ciprofloxacin, 500 mg orally twice a day for 3 days. Empiric treatment for the other common causes of genital ulcers, syphilis or herpes, is inadequate for chancroid.

Successful treatment of chancroid results in symptomatic improvement within 3 days and a resolution of lesions and clearing of exudate within 7 days after therapy has started. Patients should be followed until all lesions are completely healed. Lymphadenopathy resolves more slowly and may on occasion require needle aspiration even if an effective antimicrobial is used.

Treatment failures are defined by a lack of clinical improvement by 7 days after therapy was initiated. In this setting, the clinician should consider an alternative diagnosis or coinfection with another STD. Patients with poor adherence to multiple-dose oral regimens may be retreated with single-dose or supervised regimens. However, resistant *H. ducreyi* may also explain treatment failures and susceptibility testing should be performed on isolates from patients who show no clinical improvement with recommended therapies. Patients with HIV infection also do not respond as well to recommended antimicrobial regimens, especially to single-dose treatment.

Management of Contacts
Sex partners of patients with *H. ducreyi* from within the 10 days preceding the onset of symptoms should be examined and treated with a recommended regimen, whether symptomatic or not.

Common Clinical Syndromes

Urethritis
Urethritis is an inflammatory process of the anterior urethra presenting with a urethral discharge and/or dysuria. It is the most common clinical syndrome caused by sexually transmitted pathogens in men. Although a subset of women with acute urethral syndrome

have an STD, most frequently caused by *C. trachomatis,* the parallel clinical syndrome in women is cervicitis.

The three established infectious causes of urethritis are *N. gonorrhoeae, C. trachomatis,* and *U. urealyticum.* Gonococcal urethritis accounts for 30 to 50% of all cases, with higher rates among persons of less privileged socioeconomic status. *C. trachomatis* causes 30 to 50% of cases and *U. urealyticum* an estimated 10 to 25%. As many as 15% of cases occur without an identifiable cause. Since nongonococcal urethritis (NGU) became reportable only recently, its true incidence can only be estimated. Community-based studies, however, indicate that NGU is 2 to 3 times as common as gonococcal urethritis.

Differential Diagnosis

Although most clinicians suspect urethritis in sexually active men complaining of a urethral discharge, dysuria is the only complaint in up to one-third of patients. Gonococcal urethritis typically presents with a spontaneous or expressible, purulent discharge ("drip") and dysuria within 5 days of exposure. In patients with NGU, symptoms are generally milder and the incubation period can be as long as 5 weeks. Discharge usually must be expressed in patients with NGU and may be absent completely. Because of the considerable clinical overlap between gonococcal and nongonococcal urethritis, Gram's stain should be performed for every patient.

Gram's stain of a urethral discharge is a simple, inexpensive, and rapid method of diagnosis and is highly reliable in experienced hands. Urethral specimens for Gram's stain can be obtained from a spontaneous discharge or from a discharge expressed by stripping the anterior urethra. In patients in whom a discharge is not spontaneous or expressible, a calcium alginate swab is inserted at least 2 cm into the anterior urethra and a smear is made. To maximize the yield, a urethral smear should be obtained at least 2 hours after urination. Calcium alginate swabs are preferred over cotton swabs for obtaining culture specimens because cotton inhibits certain strains of *N. gonorrhoeae.*

The presence of four polymorphonuclear leukocytes (PMNs) per high-power field on Gram's stain of a urethral discharge is abnormal. Typical gram-negative diplococci located in the cytoplasm of PMNs are seen in 90% of men with gonococcal urethritis. This microscopic finding results in a positive gonococcal culture 98% of the time in men with urethritis. Routine culture of the urethra for *N. gonorrhoeae* is not necessary with definitive findings on Gram-stain smear. However, the presence of atypical gram-negative diplococci or extracellular gram-negative diplococci only does not reliably predict or exclude the diagnosis of gonorrhea and a culture is then necessary.

Gram's stains showing PMNs but no gram-negative diplococci exclude gonorrhea as the cause of urethritis in 98% of patients and is diagnostic of NGU without further tests. A negative gonococcal culture in the presence of urethritis is also sufficient to confirm a diagnosis of NGU. Cultures or direct antigen detection methods for *C. trachomatis* in men with urethritis are rarely if ever indicated.

Asymptomatic gonococcal urethritis in men is so infrequent (< 1%), even in STD clinics, that screening cultures are not recommended. Asymptomatic infections should be sought in male contacts of women with PID, DGI, or positive screening cultures for gonorrhea. Up to 40% of these men may have a positive culture for *N. gonorrhoeae.*

Treatment and Follow-up

Treatment of men with uncomplicated gonococcal urethritis is summarized in Table 113-1. All patients with suspected or confirmed gonococcal infections should receive simultaneous treatment with a regimen effective against *C. trachomatis.* If Gram's stain shows PMNs without gram-negative diplococci, then treatment for NGU with doxycycline, tetracycline, or erythromycin as outlined in Table 113-2 is sufficient. Sexual abstinence is strongly advised during the treatment period.

A follow-up visit is recommended 1 week after the completion of treatment in order to document clinical resolution and complete contact tracing. Patients with suspected gonorrhea treated with a regimen ineffective against PPNG should have a test-of-cure culture. Men treated for NGU do not need further laboratory tests; those who fail to respond clinically to doxycycline should be treated empirically with erythromycin, since 5 to 10% of *U. urealyticum* is resistant to doxycycline. Up to one-third of men with NGU have recurrences within 6 weeks of therapy. Although reinfection should always be considered,

NGU without culturable *C. trachomatis* or *U. urealyticum* has been shown to be the most likely to recur. Although the reasons for these observations are not known, some experts believe that unidentified etiologic agents or noninfectious causes (e.g., trauma) may be responsible. Sex contacts of men with NGU should be examined and treated with antimicrobials independent of symptoms.

Complications
Epididymitis and prostatitis occur as local complications of gonococcal urethritis in no more than 2 to 3% of patients, whereas the rate was about 15% before antimicrobials were available. *N. gonorrhoeae* causes up to one-third of acute epididymitis in men under 35 years old, but *C. trachomatis* is a more prevalent pathogen in this clinical syndrome. These complications are frequently but not always accompanied by symptomatic urethritis. Sexually transmitted pathogens are less frequent in men older than 35 years, when enteric bacteria become important etiologic agents. Treatment regimens effective against both gonorrhea and chlamydia (see Table 113-1) are recommended for epididymitis suspected to be caused by a sexually transmitted pathogen.

Genital Ulcers
HSVs are the most common cause of sexually transmitted genital ulcers, with syphilis and chancroid the next most prevalent causes in the United States. Because the presence of ulcerated genital lesions probably has facilitated the transmission of HIV among heterosexuals in Africa, the increasing incidence of syphilis and chancroid in the United States is of particular concern. The transient ulcers of LGV are infrequently noticed by the patient; patients with LGV usually present with the subsequent inguinal adenopathy. Granuloma inguinale (also known as donovanosis or granuloma venereum) is caused by the gram-negative bacterium *Calymmatobacterium granulomatis*. It presents with single or multiple nontender ulcers that gradually enlarge and may cause extensive tissue destruction. Donovanosis is rare in the United States but common in developing countries and should be suspected in patients presenting with genital ulcers after contacts overseas.

Differential Diagnosis
The differential diagnosis of genital ulcers is summarized in Table 113-4. The etiology of genital ulcers can usually be determined by a combination of clinical signs and simple laboratory tests.

The presence of the typical prodrome preceding the appearance of a cluster of painful vesicles that ulcerate and crust is sufficient to make a clinical diagnosis of genital herpes. Viral culture or an antigen detection test can confirm the diagnosis; culture is necessary before considering chronic treatment with acyclovir.

The first clinical sign of primary syphilis is the appearance of a solitary papule that subsequently ulcerates in its central portion and is often covered by a crust. The chancre is almost always painless, and ranges from a few millimeters to 2 cm in size, with induration of the surrounding tissue. It usually heals in 1 to 5 weeks regardless of therapy and rarely leaves a noticeable scar. The diagnosis of primary syphilis is confirmed by serologic studies at the time of presentation, repeated 6 weeks later if the results are initially negative.

Genital ulcers caused by *H. ducreyi* are distinguished from syphilitic chancres by the presence of pain and irregular borders, and the absence of indurated edges. Gram's stain confirms the diagnosis in about 50% of patients; cultures are more sensitive but must be carefully done (see the section on chancroid above). Clinical follow-up after empiric therapy may be necessary to confirm the diagnosis.

LGV causes transient small ulcers that typically resolve by the time the patient presents with painful inguinal adenopathy; when these ulcers are seen, syphilis should be ruled out and clinical follow-up will determine the presence of LGV.

Granuloma inguinale is diagnosed by the finding of typical intracellular bacilli (Donovan bodies) in histiocytes of tissue from lesions; smears are prepared by crushing the tissue between two glass slides and staining it with Wright's or Giemsa stain.

Treatment
The treatment of specific causes of genital ulcers is summarized in Table 113-4 and in the preceding sections on specific pathogens. Sex contacts of any patient with a genital ulcer

due to syphilis, chancroid, LGV, or donovanosis should be treated whether symptomatic or not. Symptomatic contacts of patients with HSV infection may benefit from evaluation and counseling.

Vaginitis and Cervicitis
Trichomoniasis is almost always an STD; male partners of women with trichomoniasis are usually asymptomatic but should be treated with metronidazole. The role of sexual transmission in bacterial vaginosis is uncertain. Vulvovaginal candidiasis is usually not an STD but transmission to men can occur and manifest as candidal balanitis; unless this occurs, treatment of sex partners is not necessary. (See Chap. 74 for further information on diagnosis and treatment.)

Cervicitis is the female clinical counterpart to urethritis in men; the clinical syndrome can be caused by *N. gonorrhoeae, C. trachomatis,* and HSV. The clinical presentation is characterized by vaginal discharge with associated lower abdominal or pelvic pain, and an inflamed and tender cervix with visible discharge from the os. HSV can be diagnosed by the visualization of multiple vesicular lesions and ulcers but may require confirmation with a culture or antigen detection test. Culture for gonorrhea is mandatory in all women with cervicitis. Gram's stain of cervical discharge cannot be relied on to make the diagnosis, since typical gram-negative diplococci inside PMNs are seen in only about half of patients with cervicitis due to *N. gonorrhoeae.* Mucopurulent cervicitis, however, is most frequently caused by *C. trachomatis* and treatment for both etiologies is recommended. Maintaining a high clinical suspicion of and providing early intensive therapy for cervicitis, pending the culture results, may help prevent the consequences of PID.

Proctitis, Colitis, and Enteritis
Sexually active persons with diarrhea, tenesmus, and abdominal cramps may have proctitis, colitis, or enteritis caused by an organism transmitted by sexual contact. Transmission is facilitated by receptive anal intercourse or oral-anal sexual activity. With the exception of rectal gonococcal infection, these syndromes occur predominantly in homosexual men.

Proctitis is an inflammation limited to the rectum (distal 10–12 cm) and presents with anorectal pain, tenesmus, urgency, and frequent bathroom visits with small amounts of mucus or blood. Gonococcal, chlamydial, and herpetic etiologies are the most common sexually transmitted causes of proctitis. Differentiation among the causes of proctitis is not possible on clinical presentation alone. Anoscopy should be performed to confirm the presence of inflammation and to obtain specimens for Gram's stain and cultures. In order to obtain adequate specimens for gonococcal, chlamydial, and HSV cultures, a swab should be pressed onto the rectal mucosal surface via an anoscope for about 30 seconds. Gram's stain of anal discharge may show the typical intracytoplasmic gram-negative diplococci characteristic of *N. gonorrhoeae,* but the absence of this finding does not rule out a gonococcal etiology. In the absence of a diagnostic Gram's stain showing gonorrhea or typical vesicles of HSV infection, cultures should be obtained for the three etiologic agents. Empiric treatment of sexually transmitted gonococcal and chlamydial proctitis is with ceftriaxone, 250 mg intramuscularly, plus doxycycline, 100 mg orally 2 times a day, for 7 days and should be initiated pending the culture results. Alternative regimens are listed in Table 113-1. HSV proctitis occasionally causes neurologic involvement, including paresthesias, erectile difficulties, urinary bladder dysfunction, and gluteal pain, and should be treated with systemic acyclovir. Among patients coinfected with HIV, herpes proctitis may be especially severe.

Colitis presents with the clinical symptoms of proctitis plus diarrhea and/or abdominal cramps, and the colonic mucosa is inflamed proximal to 12 cm. Etiologic organisms include *Shigella* species, *Campylobacter jejuni, E. histolytica* (amebiasis), and rarely, *T. pallidum* or *C. trachomatis* (LGV).

Enteritis transmitted sexually presents as diarrhea without signs of proctitis. In homosexual men at risk, it is usually caused by *G. lamblia.*

Shigella and *Campylobacter* infections present as an acute onset of diarrhea, with blood and mucus frequently appearing after the first 2 days. The most important initial diagnostic test is examination of the stool for leukocytes, which are absent in viral gastroenteritis. Definitive etiologic diagnosis depends on stool cultures, but fecal leukocytes are found in 90% of patients with shigellosis and in at least 75% of those with *Campylobacter* infections.

The drug of choice in treating *Shigella* infections has been trimethoprim-sulfamethoxazole, one double-strength tablet (160/800 mg) by mouth 2 times per day for 7 days. Treatment of *Campylobacter* infections with erythromycin, 500 mg 4 times per day, is also recommended. Ciprofloxacin, 500 mg orally 2 times a day for 7 days, is effective for both *Shigella* and *Campylobacter* infections.

Amebiasis has varied presentations, ranging from vague abdominal pains associated with a nonspecific change in bowel habits, to frequent and bloody stools associated with severe pain, tenesmus, fever, and dehydration. Giardiasis is usually a mild illness characterized by loose stools interspersed by constipation, belching, flatulence, and nonspecific epigastric complaints. Blood and mucus in the stool are rare findings in giardiasis. Diagnosis of amebiasis or giardiasis depends on an examination of stool specimens for ova and parasites by experienced staff in a parasitology laboratory. Symptomatic amebiasis should be treated with metronidazole, 750 mg by mouth 3 times per day for 10 days, plus either iodoquinol, 650 mg by mouth 3 times per day for 20 days, or diloxanide furorate, 500 mg by mouth 3 times per day for 10 days. The drug of choice for giardiasis is quinacrine, 100 mg by mouth 3 times daily for 7 days, and metronidazole, 250 mg by mouth 3 times daily for 7 days, is an alternative regimen.

Venereal Warts

Condylomata acuminata are warts involving the genitalia, the anus, or oral pharyngeal surfaces, resulting from infection with the human papilloma virus (HPV). An estimated 1 million consultations for condyloma acuminatum occurred in the United States during 1981, with the majority of cases being in young adults. Transmission of HPV occurs in 65% of sex partners of persons with active condylomata, with an incubation period of 2 to 3 months. Certain types of HPV have been strongly associated with genital dysplasia, and all women with anogenital warts should have an annual Pap smear.

Diagnosis of condyloma acuminatum is based on its typical appearance and presentation; the warts begin as tiny papules, which as they grow may merge to form large verrucous lesions. The most common sites are the posterior vaginal introitus and the labia, but warts may also be found in the perianal area, urethra, vagina, cervix, and mouth. Intravaginal warts may be difficult to visualize without magnification. Women with cervical warts or with evidence of papilloma virus on Pap smear (suggested by the mention of koilocytosis on the report) should be referred for colposcopic examination. Atypical, pigmented, or persistent warts should be biopsied.

Treatment of condyloma acuminatum is directed at removal of the exophytic warts and amelioration of any accompanying symptoms. HPV is not eradicated by any of the therapeutic options, and recurrences are common. Cryotherapy with liquid nitrogen or a cryoprobe is the treatment of choice in most clinical situations. Podophyllin, 10 to 25% in a compound tincture of benzoin, may be used as an alternative treatment of external genital, perianal, or urethral meatus warts; with the surrounding skin protected by talc or petroleum jelly, it is applied to a limited area per session, and washed off in 1 to 2 hours. Treatments may be repeated at weekly intervals. Podophyllin is teratogenic and therefore its use is contraindicated during pregnancy. An alternative agent that may be used in pregnancy is trichloroacetic acid (80–90%); it is applied to external genital, perianal, or anal warts in a manner similar to podophyllin, with talc or baking soda used to remove the unreacted acid. Electrodesiccation/electrocautery is an option for external genital, perianal, or oral warts. Surgical removal of oral or anal lesions is sometimes done but may lead to scarring. Management of all cervical warts or of extensive or refractory warts in other areas should be carried out by an expert.

Patients with known active condyloma acuminatum should abstain from intercourse until the lesions have resolved. Use of condoms after active lesions have resolved is encouraged to minimize possible transmission.

Prevention of Transmission

Most STDs are transmitted solely from person to person. Abstinence or sexual intercourse with one mutually faithful uninfected partner is the best method of preventing the transmission of STDs. Persons who are known or suspected to have an active STD should refrain from sexual activity until they are no longer capable of transmitting the etiologic agent.

Proper use of condoms with each act of sexual intercourse can reduce, but not eliminate, the risk of STDs. Laboratory tests have shown latex condoms to be effective mechanical barriers to HIV, HSV, cytomegalovirus, hepatitis B virus, *C. trachomatis,* and *N. gonorrhoeae.* Natural membrane condoms, which contain small pores, do not prevent the passage of HIV or hepatitis B virus. Condom use has increased among homosexual and bisexual men but much education is needed to target high-risk heterosexual men and women.

The data on other barrier methods are more limited. A randomized comparative study among high-risk women in Bangkok showed that users of the nonoxynol 9–impregnated contraceptive sponge had partial protection against chlamydia and gonorrhea, but an increased risk of candidiasis.

All health care providers share responsibility for the control of STDs in their community. Local health departments should be notified of all cases of gonorrhea, primary and secondary syphilis, chancroid, enteric pathogens, and other STDs as required by law. (Chlamydia is now reportable in a few states, including California, but not yet in most others.) All named contacts should be treated whenever a regimen effective against clinical infections is available. This is especially important for female contacts, because infection is more frequently silent and disease potentially more severe. The identity of the index case need not be revealed to the contact; confidentiality must be maintained as strictly as possible during contact investigations.

Centers for Disease Control. 1989 sexually transmitted disease treatment guidelines. MMWR 1989; 38(S-8):1–43.
The most recent revision of STD treatment recommendations from the CDC belongs in every practitioner's office. This is not updated annually, but "when necessary," usually every 4 to 5 years. In addition to being published in MMWR as referenced above, it is also available in booklet form from Technical Information Services (E-06), Center for Prevention Services, Centers for Disease Control, Atlanta, GA 30333.

Boslego JW, et al. Effect of spectinomycin on the prevalence of spectinomycin-resistant and of penicillinase-producing *Neisseria gonorrhoeae.* N Engl J Med 1987; 317:272–8.
Experience in treating U.S. servicemen in Korea showing that 8 of 97 patients treated with spectinomycin alone had unsuccessful treatment because of resistant strains.

Braff EH, Wibbelsman CJ. Asymptomatic gonococcal urethritis in selected males. Am J Public Health 1978; 68:779–80.
Urethral cultures of men presenting to an STD clinic for symptoms unrelated to urethritis, showing a prevalence of asymptomatic infection of 0.9%.

Brunham RC, et al. Mucopurulent cervicitis—the ignored counterpart in women of urethritis in men. N Engl J Med 1984; 311:1–6.
Visualization of yellow mucopurulent endocervical secretions and the presence of 10 or more PMNs correlate with cervical C. trachomatis infection.

Centers for Disease Control. Condoms for prevention of sexually transmitted diseases. MMWR 1988; 37:133–8.
Reviews the evidence supporting the use of condoms and the rationale for promoting their use in preventing STDs.

Centers for Disease Control. Antibiotic-resistant strains of *Neisseria gonorrhoeae.* Policy guidelines for detection, management and control. MMWR 1987; 36: Suppl 5S:1S–18S.
Summary of the problem and recommendations for control.

Centers for Disease Control. *Chlamydia trachomatis* infections—policy guidelines for prevention and control. MMWR 1985; 34: Suppl 3S:53S–74S.
Summary of CDC policy guidelines.

Corey L, Spear PG. Infections with herpes simplex viruses. N Engl J Med 1986; 314: 686–91, 749–58.
Excellent review of the clinical and biologic aspects of HSV.

Douglas JM, et al. A double-blind study of oral acyclovir for suppression of recurrences of genital herpes simplex virus infection. N Engl J Med 1984; 310:1551–6.
Randomized trial showing the benefit of acyclovir in suppressing or decreasing recurrences in patients on continuous therapy.

Handsfield HH, et al. Asymptomatic gonorrhea in men. N Engl J Med 1974; 290:117–23.
Report showing that 40% of male contacts of women with PID had positive urethral cultures for gonorrhea despite the absence of symptoms.

Holmes KK, et al, eds. Sexually transmitted diseases. New York: McGraw-Hill, 1988.
Superb reference on all aspects of STDs.

Hook EW, Holmes KK. Gonococcal infections. Ann Intern Med 1985; 102:229–43.
Excellent review of the clinical and laboratory aspects of infection.

Judson FN. Management of antibiotic-resistant *Neisseria gonorrhoeae*. Ann Intern Med 1989; 110:5–7.
Discusses strategies for treatment of PPNG and others.

Lafferty WE, et al. Recurrences after oral and genital herpes simplex virus infection—influence of site of infection and viral type. N Engl J Med 1987; 316:1444–9.
HSV-1 genital infections recur less frequently than do HSV-2 infections.

Reichman RC, et al. Treatment of recurrent genital herpes simplex infections with oral acyclovir. JAMA 1984; 251:2103–7.
Clinical trial showing the marginal benefit of treatment of recurrent HSV with acyclovir—about 1 day less of symptoms and viral shedding in the treated group.

Rosenberg MJ, et al. Effect of the contraceptive sponge on chlamydia infection, gonorrhea, and candidiasis. JAMA 1987; 257:2308–12.
Study in Bangkok among high-risk women showing the relative efficacy of barrier contraceptives in preventing chlamydia and gonorrhea.

Schmid GP, et al. Chancroid in the United States: reestablishment of an old disease. JAMA 1987; 258:3265–8.
Report from the CDC documenting the increased incidence, established endemic foci, and frequent misdiagnosis by clinicians.

Stamm WE. Diagnosis of *Chlamydia trachomatis* genitourinary infections. Ann Intern Med 1988; 108:710–17.
Review of the clinical and laboratory aspects of chlamydial infections, with practical recommendations for the use of rapid antigen detection tests. A strong case is made for the wider use of tissue culture in making the diagnosis.

Stamm WE, et al. Effect of treatment regimens for *Neisseria gonorrhoeae* on simultaneous infection with chlamydia trachomatis. N Engl J Med 1984; 310:545–9.
Documents the high prevalence of coexisting chlamydial and gonococcal infections and the 10% failure rate of tetracycline alone for gonococcal cervicitis.

Strauss SE, et al. Suppression of frequently recurring genital herpes. N Engl J Med 1984; 310:1545–50.
Documented in a placebo-controlled trial that chronic suppressive therapy with acyclovir is safe and effective in decreasing HSV episodes while treated. Recurrences resumed after acyclovir was stopped, with a trend toward less frequent and less severe episodes.

114. MANAGEMENT OF HIV-INFECTED PATIENTS
Mitchell H. Katz

An estimated 1 million persons in the United States are infected with the human immunodeficiency virus (HIV). Over 95% of these persons belong to one of four major risk groups: gay or bisexual men; injection drug users; recipients of blood products prior to 1985, including hemophiliacs; and sex partners of people in these risk groups. The ultimate proportion of infected patients who will develop acquired immunodeficiency syndrome (AIDS) is unknown. However, there is increasing evidence that appropriate treatment and prophylaxis prevent opportunistic infections and prolong survival early in the course of infection.

Primary care physicians have an important role to play in the care of HIV-infected people. Given the large number of HIV-infected individuals, it would be impossible for specialists to provide care for all infected individuals. More importantly, primary care physicians bring special skills to the care of HIV-infected patients, including a familiarity with treating multisystem illness and in dealing with difficult psychosocial issues.

Diagnosing HIV Infection

HIV infection is identified by the presence of HIV antibodies. The two widely available antibody tests are the enzyme-linked immunosorbent assay (ELISA) and Western blot tests. The ELISA is the usual screening test; it is less expensive than and equally sensitive to the Western blot, but is less specific (more false-positive results). Therefore patients who have a persistently positive result on ELISA (> 2 tests) should have a confirmatory Western blot test, and only those with positive results on both tests should be considered HIV-positive. These tests have a combined sensitivity and specificity of 99.9%. In low-risk populations, where the true prevalence of HIV seropositivity is less than 1 in 1000, a positive result may be more likely to be a false-positive than a true-positive result. Patients with indeterminate Western blot results may subsequently convert to a positive result, and should have a repeat Western blot or an alternative confirmatory test.

Antibody testing should always be accompanied by pre- and posttest counseling. Pretest counseling should explain the difference between an anonymous and a confidential test. In anonymous testing the person tested need not reveal his or her name. This is provided through a nationwide network of alternative test sites. Patients who choose to have confidential testing outside of these sites need to be informed that their test result will be part of their medical record, and billing such tests to insurance companies may prejudice coverage. Posttest counseling for HIV-positive individuals should include emotional support, referral to agencies that provide supportive services, and plans for medical treatment. Because of the emotional impact of HIV antibody tests, results should not be disclosed over the telephone or by mail; instead patients should plan a second visit to receive their results in person.

Physicians should urge seropositive persons to notify their partners who are at risk. When seropositive persons are reluctant to disclose their result to their partners, clinicians should discuss the importance of disclosure in a supportive manner. If the patient refuses, many state laws allow, but do not require, physicians to disclose the antibody test result to at-risk partners.

Regardless of the test result, all patients tested should be educated about the transmission of the disease. It should be emphasized that the virus cannot be transmitted through casual contact, but only through sexual relations, injection drug use, or blood products, and that transmission can be prevented by avoiding an exchange of fluids (sperm, vaginal fluids, blood) during sexual relations and by using clean needles for injection drug use. Barrier methods such as condoms decrease the risk of transmission but do not eliminate it. There are no well-documented cases of transmission of disease through open-mouth kissing, but there remains a theoretic risk of transmission.

Individuals who test antibody-negative need to be alerted that seroconversion usually occurs within 6 months of exposure. Individuals with a more recent exposure should return for repeat testing. There are reports of high-risk individuals who tested negative for HIV antibodies but had evidence of HIV infection on DNA amplification techniques (polymerase chain reactions) or viral culture. Such cases are uncommon.

Definition of AIDS and AIDS-Related Complex

The Centers for Disease Control (CDC) surveillance definition of AIDS specifies the presence of an opportunistic infection (e.g., *Pneumocystis carinii* pneumonia [PCP], cryptococcal meningitis) or an HIV-related neoplasm (e.g., Kaposi's sarcoma). For these diagnoses, serologic evidence of HIV antibody is not necessary to fulfill AIDS criteria. In 1987, the CDC added to the list of AIDS-defining illnesses documented diarrhea for longer than 1 month, significant weight loss, and dementia, in patients with HIV antibodies.

The CDC has proposed expanding the AIDS definition to also include all HIV-infected adults with a positive HIV serology and a CD4 lymphocyte count less than or equal to

200 cells μ/L. It is hoped that the new definition will improve surveillance efforts of HIV-disease and enable HIV-infected patients to qualify earlier for needed social service benefits.

The term *AIDS-related complex* (ARC) has been used to denote patients who are HIV-positive and symptomatic, but do not fulfill the CDC criteria for an AIDS diagnosis. In general, this group of patients is very heterogeneous, ranging from patients with generalized lymphadenopathy to those with debilitating weakness and chronic fevers. Many clinicians therefore avoid the term *ARC*.

Medical Evaluation and Monitoring

History

Progression to AIDS is rare in the 2 years following seroconversion; it occurs in 20% of patients 6 years after infection, and in 50% of patients 10 years after infection. Birthplace and travel history provide clues to the diagnosis of endemic infections, such as histoplasmosis and coccidioidomycosis.

Symptoms and Signs

Because many of the symptoms associated with early HIV infection are subtle, patients may not mention them. Of particular concern are systemic symptoms: fever, night sweats, weight loss, and decreased energy. The early physical signs of infection tend to manifest themselves in organs (especially the mouth and the skin) that usually receive only a cursory examination in asymptomatic patients. Hairy leukoplakia, oral candidiasis, and Kaposi's sarcoma are of particular importance because when they occur in otherwise healthy people, they are almost pathognomonic for HIV infection.

Hairy leukoplakia appears as white hair-like projections, usually on the side of the tongue. Unlike candidiasis, hairy leukoplakia cannot be removed by swabbing. While the lesions of hairy leukoplakia and candidiasis themselves are generally not problematic, both are associated with an increase in the rate of progression of HIV disease.

Kaposi's sarcoma can be flat or raised, red, pink, or purple lesions that generally do not blanch. Although they can appear anywhere on the body, they tend to have an acral distribution: the tip of the nose, the ear, the penis, and the lower extremities. They also are commonly seen on mucosal surfaces such as the hard palate.

Laboratory Studies

Recommended baseline studies include a complete blood cell count with differential cell and platelet counts, sedimentation rate, lactate dehydrogenase (LDH) level, serum rapid plasma reagin (RPR) or VDRL test, a purified protein derivative (PPD) skin test with a control skin test (such as *Candida albicans* antigen), a chest radiograph, and an absolute helper T-cell (CD4) count.

HELPER T-CELL (CD4) MEASUREMENT. The CD4 count is the most widely accepted prognostic marker and a criterion for the administration of zidovudine (AZT) and PCP prophylaxis. The risk of developing AIDS is linearly related to the CD4 count. Patients with CD4 counts under 200 cells μ/L have a poor prognosis, with over 80% developing AIDS within 3 years. In contrast, patients with counts above 400 cells μ/L have only about a 15% risk of developing an AIDS-defining illness within 3 years. As expected, the 3-year risk of developing AIDS for patients with counts between 200 and 400 cells is intermediate; about 45% develop AIDS.

The CD4 count has several limitations: It is dependent on laboratory techniques; varies in an individual person by time of day (lower in the morning); decreases with concurrent viral infections; and represents a quantitative, rather than qualitative, assay of immune function. The variation in CD4 counts by laboratory and by time of day may be 50 to 75 cells, with even larger variations occurring with intercurrent illness. Because the trend in CD4 counts is more reliable than any individual value, counts should be checked every 3 to 6 months, depending on the stage of illness. Other prognostic tests, including the beta-2-microglobulin and p24 antigen, may be requested by patients. These tests are generally less useful than CD4 counts in planning therapy.

OTHER LABORATORY PARAMETERS. Hematologic abnormalities associated with HIV infection include anemia, leukopenia (especially lymphopenia), and thrombocytopenia. Although the sedimentation rate is a nonspecific test, it tends to increase gradually with the duration of HIV infection. An abrupt increase is consistent with a new opportunistic infection or malignancy. A baseline LDH level is useful for future diagnostic evaluations because abrupt increases in LDH values are consistent with PCP or B-cell lymphoma.

Serologic tests for syphilis in HIV-infected patients must be interpreted with caution, since antibody tests may not be accurate in patients with disordered antibody production. Falsely negative RPR or VDRL tests in secondary syphilis and falsely negative confirmatory tests (fluorescent treponemal antibody absorption test [FTA-ABS]) have been reported. Moreover, treatment failures with standard therapy have occurred in HIV-infected patients. The CDC currently recommends a very aggressive diagnostic and therapeutic approach. All HIV-infected patients with a positive RPR or VDRL test for longer than 1 year, or for an unknown duration, should receive a lumbar puncture with a cerebrospinal fluid (CSF) cell count and a CSF VDRL test. Patients with normal results on CSF evaluation should be treated for late latent syphilis with penicillin G benzathine, 2.4 million U given intramuscularly weekly for 3 weeks, and have titers measured at follow-up. Patients with pleocytosis or positive CSF VDRL test should be treated for neurosyphilis with penicillin G potassium, 2 to 4 million U given intravenously every 4 hours for 10 days, or penicillin G procaine suspension, 2.4 million U given intramuscularly daily, with probenicid, 500 mg 4 times a day for 10 days. Current treatment recommendations for primary and secondary syphilis are the same as in HIV-negative individuals, but because of treatment failures, greater vigilance should be given to follow-up titers and neurologic examinations.

The *PPD skin test* is most sensitive for exposure to *Mycobacterium tuberculosis* (*M. tuberculosis*) when it is performed early in the course of HIV infection because anergy generally occurs later. For example, one study showed that all patients with active *M. tuberculosis* 2 or more years prior to an AIDS diagnosis have a positive PPD, while only 30% of those with active *M. tuberculosis* after or concurrent with an AIDS diagnosis have a positive PPD.

Because some patients are anergic, a baseline chest radiograph is necessary to rule out active tuberculosis. Patients whose chest film shows an infiltrate, especially when associated with hilar or mediastinal adenopathy, should be evaluated by sputum smears and cultures for mycobacteria. Patients with acid-fast bacilli on sputum smear should be treated with a minimum of three drugs for *M. tuberculosis* until a definitive diagnosis is made. HIV-infected patients with a positive PPD (> 5 mm of induration) and a normal-appearing chest film should receive isoniazid for a year regardless of their age.

Antiviral and Prophylactic Treatment Measures

Zidovudine (AZT), Formerly Azothymidine
AZT has been shown to slow the course of HIV infection. A randomized, multicenter trial showed that AZT, compared to placebo, decreased opportunistic infections, decreased the incidence of HIV encephalopathy, and increased survival in patients with prior PCP and those with severe ARC. More recent studies demonstrated that AZT, compared to placebo, decreases the rate of development of severe ARC and AIDS in patients with mild ARC (e.g., thrush or hairy leukoplakia) and in patients who are asymptomatic but with CD4 counts below 500 cells µ/L.

AZT dosing remains controversial but recent studies indicated that lower dosages are equally efficacious with fewer side effects. For asymptomatic patients, 100 mg 5 times a day is recommended; because of the difficulties of complying with such frequent administration, some clinicians recommend 3-times-a-day dosing, using 200 mg in the morning and evening and 100 mg at midday. For individuals with later stages of infection, 200 mg 3 times a day is recommended. AIDS patients with neurologic disease may benefit from higher dosages.

The toxicity of AZT can occur early or in the long term. Early side effects include headaches, malaise, nausea, vomiting, bloating, constipation, and disordered sleep. These effects occur in varying intensity in about 40% of patients, but almost always remit spontaneously within 6 weeks. Long-term side effects include macrocytic anemia and neutropenia, which are unresponsive to vitamin supplementation but do respond to drug reductions and drug "holidays." Less common side effects include hepatitis and myositis.

Complete blood cell counts with platelet and differential counts should be checked every 2 weeks for the first month of therapy, and then every 1 to 3 months if counts are stable. Liver function and a creatine phosphokinase (CPK) level should be checked every 3 months. AZT can be given concomitantly with most drugs except probenecid, which decreases the elimination of AZT. Initial studies found that patients who took acetaminophen with AZT were more likely to become neutropenic. Most clinicians believe this association was confounded; that is, patients who used acetaminophen had more febrile illnesses causing the neutropenia. Therefore, acetaminophen need not be avoided. Although not absolutely contraindicated, it is prudent to interrupt AZT therapy during initial treatment of serious opportunistic infections (e.g., PCP, toxoplasmosis, cryptococcal meningitis) because of the combined bone marrow toxicity of multiple drugs.

In vitro resistance to AZT has been demonstrated in patients who have been taking AZT for longer than 6 months. While the finding of in vitro resistance is consistent with the clinical observation that AZT is not as effective for the majority of AIDS patients after 18 months, this should be interpreted cautiously. The patients in whom resistance was demonstrated were clinically doing well and the isolates were not resistant to other related dideoxynucleosides (e.g., didanosine [ddI]). Whether resistance will develop in patients treated with AZT who have less advanced disease, in whom there is a lower body reservoir of virus, is unknown.

Didanosine (ddI) and Dideoxycytidine (ddC)
Both ddI and ddC have been shown to increase CD4 counts in HIV-infected patients. ddI has been approved for patients who are intolerant to AZT or who are deteriorating despite AZT therapy. The most serious side effect of ddI is pancreatitis, which occurs in about 9% of patients and has resulted in about 10 deaths among the initial 14,000 patients who have taken the drug. Other side effects include peripheral neuropathy, dry mouth, and agitation. The drug must be taken on an empty stomach (1 hour before or 2 to 3 hours after meals), and two tablets must be taken at the same time to provide an adequate amount of buffering agent. Dosage is by weight with patients between 50 and 74 kg receiving two 100-mg tablets twice a day. Administration of ddI can interfere with absorption of other drugs, such as dapsone, which require an acid medium for absorption.

ddC is available through the drug company as an investigational agent for patients who are intolerant to AZT or who are deteriorating despite AZT therapy (1-800-ddC-21HIV). Two common side effects seen with ddC are peripheral neuropathy and aphthous ulcers.

Pneumocystis carinii *Pneumonia Prophylaxis*
Prior to the advent of prophylaxis, PCP occurred in 80% of AIDS patients and was the index diagnosis in 60%. Two types of prophylaxis can be distinguished: secondary and primary. Secondary prophylaxis should be given to all patients after an episode of PCP, even if they are on antiviral therapy. Bronchoscopies done long after the resolution of PCP have revealed a persistence of *P. carinii* cysts. Primary prophylaxis is based on natural history studies demonstrating that 18% of patients with CD4 counts below 200 cells μ/L will develop PCP within a year. Since there is a linear increase in PCP risk as counts decrease from 500 cells μ/L, the exact cutoff for starting prophylaxis is controversial. PCP prophylaxis is not usually offered to patients with CD4 counts above 300. In questionable cases, other prognostic indicators such as persistent fevers, thrush, and hairy leukoplakia should be considered.

There are three commonly used methods of prophylaxis: aerosolized pentamidine, oral trimethoprim-sulfamethoxasole, and oral dapsone. Aerosolized pentamidine, 300 mg monthly, has been shown to decrease the incidence of PCP in patients at risk, compared to both historical control subjects and patients randomized to receive lower dosages of aerosolized pentamidine. Bronchospasm sometimes occurs with treatment, but can be prevented with inhaled bronchodilators. Occurrences of PCP during inhaled pentamidine therapy are generally mild and typically occur in the apical regions where less of the inhaled drug is deposited. Several cases of disseminated *Pneumocystis* in people receiving aerosolized pentamidine have been reported but are rare. Patients with a history of PCP who are given aerosolized pentamidine are at increased risk of pneumothorax. Aerosolized pentamidine is costly, not widely available, and may be less effective than the two oral regimens. Therefore, most patients should be given one of the two oral regimens, with aerosolized pentamidine reserved for patients who do not tolerate the oral regimens.

Trimethoprim-sulfamethoxazole, one double-strength tablet 3 times a week, has been shown to decrease the occurrence of PCP. Side effects at this low dose are uncommon, but include anemia, neutropenia, fever, and rash with a small risk of Stevens-Johnson reaction.

Dapsone (100 mg twice a week) is inexpensive and appears to be well tolerated and effective as a method of prophylaxis. Side effects include anemia and rash. Glucose-6-phosphate dehydrogenase (G-6-PD) levels should be checked prior to the administration of dapsone.

Immunizations

HIV-infected patients should receive pneumococcal and influenza vaccines. Patients who are negative for hepatitis B surface antigen and at continued risk for exposure (e.g., homosexual men, injection drug users) should receive hepatitis B vaccine. Antibody responses to vaccines are suboptimal in HIV-infected patients, but the earlier vaccines are given in the course of HIV infection, the greater the likelihood of achieving protective antibody titers. Live vaccines, such as oral poliovirus and yellow fever vaccines, should be avoided.

Herpes Simplex Prophylaxis

Some clinicians treat all patients with a history of herpes simplex attacks with chronic suppressive acyclovir therapy (200 mg tid). The rationale is that HIV-infected patients tend to get more severe herpes attacks than do immunocompetent hosts, and that active herpes simplex infections may stimulate the HIV virus. Acyclovir is generally well tolerated, even with the concurrent administration of AZT, although acyclovir resistance has been reported.

Approach to Common Symptoms and Problems

Fever

Fever is the most common symptom reported by HIV-infected individuals. Because of the myriad of possible etiologies, the evaluation depends on the stage of HIV infection, the acuity of the symptoms, and the presence of localizing symptoms.

At the time of seroconversion, many patients have an acute illness characterized by several weeks of high fevers, pharyngitis, lymphadenopathy, rash, and neurologic symptoms. The illness typically occurs 6 weeks after exposure. Treatment is symptomatic, with HIV antibody testing performed, if the patient consents, after all symptoms have resolved.

Many HIV-infected patients will have nightly fevers with sweats prior to any AIDS diagnosis. Generally such patients feel well and the fevers are due to the primary effects of the virus. Such patients should have PPD testing and a chest radiograph to rule out tuberculosis.

In patients who present with new fevers, the evaluation proceeds according to the organ system affected (see below). If the patient has no symptoms other than fever, and the temperature is higher than 101.5°F (38.6°C), then blood cultures for bacteria and mycobacterium and a serum cryptococcal antigen test should be performed. Patients with PCP almost always have at least minor respiratory symptoms, but cases of PCP in patients presenting with fever alone have been reported. Therefore, patients with fever in whom no other cause is found should be evaluated for PCP with a chest radiograph and a serum LDH level, with further evaluation depending on the patient's clinical condition. For unclear reasons, AIDS patients are more likely to have allergic reactions from antibiotics, especially sulfa drugs, and drug-related fever should be considered. AZT also has been associated with fever.

Aggressive treatment of fever can help prevent dehydration. Nonsteroidal anti-inflammatory agents are generally more effective in reducing fever in AIDS patients than are aspirin or acetaminophen. Patients with fever and long-standing neutropenia due to their underlying disease do not generally require hospitalization unless they appear septic (e.g., hypotensive), are using injection drugs, or are neutropenic due to chemotherapy for an AIDS-related malignancy.

Respiratory Symptoms
Respiratory symptoms—cough, shortness of breath, chest congestion, or chest tightness—pose a diagnostic dilemma. Respiratory symptoms are common in the general population and the majority of episodes even among HIV-positive individuals will be self-limited viral infections. On the other hand, HIV-infected patients are at risk for PCP, a life-threatening pneumonia requiring prompt treatment.

Evaluation of patients with HIV risk factors and respiratory symptoms includes a chest radiograph and determinations of the sedimentation rate and LDH level. Patients with a normal-appearing chest film, sedimentation rate less than 50 mm/hr, and an LDH less than 220 U/L have a very low risk of PCP and can be followed clinically. In a continuity care setting, where a patient may have had a CD4 count done in the 6-month period prior to the occurrence of respiratory symptoms, a CD4 count greater than 250 cells μ/L makes a diagnosis of PCP very unlikely.

Patients with a unilateral infiltrate on chest film should be treated for community-acquired pneumonia, as both pneumococcal and *Hemophilus influenzae* pneumonia occur more commonly in HIV-infected individuals than in the general population. Further evaluation for PCP should be performed if the patient does not improve in 3 to 5 days because between 10 and 15% of patients with PCP have a focal infiltrate. Patients with an elevated sedimentation rate or LDH level need to be followed closely for PCP, even if the chest film appears normal, because between 15 and 20% of ambulatory patients with PCP will have a normal-appearing chest film. If such patients do not improve rapidly, they should be evaluated further with a sputum induction for PCP. Sputum inductions are performed by having patients inhale a mist of 3% saline solution from an ultrasonic nebulizer. In institutions with experience performing sputum inductions, the sensitivity is between 50 and 80%. Even with inductions performed under the best of conditions, however, patients with negative sputum stains may have PCP. Patients whose clinical presentation is consistent with PCP, or who are seen at institutions without the capability of performing sputum induction, should have bronchoscopy with lavage. Nonspecific indicators of PCP include decreased carbon monoxide diffusing capacity and an abnormal-appearing gallium scan. These tests can be helpful in excluding the diagnosis of PCP (when the results are completely normal) or in providing additional evidence of the need for bronchial lavage.

Patients whose chest films show the classic radiographic appearance of PCP—diffuse interstitial or perihilar infiltrates—should be aggressively evaluated for PCP, with sputum induction and bronchoscopy if sputum stains are negative. Because of the enormous psychological significance of an AIDS diagnosis, and the morbidity of treatment for PCP, empiric therapy for PCP should be avoided, except while awaiting results from sputum induction or bronchial lavage.

Patients receiving PCP prophylaxis tend to have atypical presentations of PCP, with very subtle respiratory symptoms. Diagnosis of PCP in patients on prophylaxis requires a high index of suspicion. Arterial blood gases are generally not helpful in the diagnosis of PCP, because patients with PCP may have near-normal resting blood gases while patients with other types of pneumonia may have marked hypoxia. However, arterial blood gas results have therapeutic significance in determining whether patients with pneumonia who are short of breath can be treated as outpatients or whether they require hospitalization.

Patients who are not severely hypoxic (arterial oxygen tension [pO_2] > 60–70 mm Hg) may be treated for PCP as outpatients. The two most common oral regimens are trimethoprim-sulfamethoxazole (15 mg/kg in 3 to 4 doses/day) and trimethoprim (300 mg 3 times a day) with dapsone (100 mg/day). Patients frequently develop a pruritic erythematous maculopapular rash after 7 to 10 days of trimethoprim-sulfamethoxazole. If there is no involvement of the mucous membranes and no desquamation of skin, treatment can be cautiously continued with the use of diphenhydramine (25–50 mg 4 times a day). Other common side effects with trimethoprim-sulfamethoxazole include drug-related fever, neutropenia, anemia, and hepatitis. Patients who have such reactions can be switched to trimethoprim-dapsone. Patients should have a normal G6PD level prior to the start of dapsone. In addition to rash, anemia, neutropenia, and hepatitis, patients on trimethoprim-dapsone can develop methemoglobinemia, and should have methemoglobin levels checked every 7 days. Patients with moderate to severe PCP (O_2 saturation < 90%) should be treated with steroids along with specific treatment. PCP treatment should be for a minimum of 14 days, and ideally 21 days, with secondary prophylaxis of PCP starting as soon as possible after treatment of the acute illness.

Mouth Lesions
Oral candidiasis typically appears as removable white plaques. It can also appear as erythematous plaques, usually on the palate. Treatment of these lesions should begin with topical agents such as clotrimazole troches (3–5 times a day), which are more effective and easier to use than swishes. Recalcitrant cases can be treated with ketoconazole (200 mg once or twice a day) or fluconazole (50–100 mg once a day). Candidiasis should be treated until there are no plaques left in the mouth. After this occurs, use of one troche per day will frequently prevent recurrences. Angular cheilitis (fissures at the corners of the mouth) are usually also caused by *Candida,* and can be treated with ketoconazole cream.

Hairy leukoplakia does not generally require treatment. Spontaneous remissions with acyclovir and AZT are reported. HIV-infected patients are prone to gingivitis probably because of an overgrowth of mouth flora. Chlorhexidine rinses, along with dental cleaning, are helpful for this problem. Ulcerations of the gums (necrotizing ulcerative gingivitis) and severe periodontal disease may require antibiotics (metronidazole, 250 mg 4 times daily for 4–5 days); such patients should be referred to an oral surgeon with experience in treating HIV-infected patients.

Headache
Headache, particularly when accompanied by fever, can portend serious infection in an HIV-infected patient. If the headache is new and serious (not relieved by nonopiate pain relievers), the patient should undergo emergency brain imaging. The choice of computed tomography (CT) with contrast media or magnetic resonance imaging (MRI) depends on the local resources. In general, MRI is more sensitive for diagnosing brain lesions, especially toxoplasmosis, in AIDS patients.

Toxoplasmosis is the most common neurologic opportunistic infection, typically appearing as multiple ring-enhancing lesions on CT scan. Patients with a brain scan consistent with toxoplasmosis can be treated as outpatients if mental status changes do not prevent them from complying with an outpatient regimen. Therapy should be initiated with pyrimethamine, 100 to 200 mg loading dose and 50 to 75 mg daily, with sulfadiazine, 4 to 6 g daily in 4 divided doses, and folinic acid, 10 to 50 mg daily. A follow-up scan should be performed 2 weeks after toxoplasmosis therapy is started. Solitary brain lesions on MRI are consistent with non-Hodgkin's lymphoma. Therefore, for patients with a solitary lesion, stereotactic brain biopsy should be considered.

If the brain scan of a patient with headache and fever appears normal and the patient has a nonfocal neurologic examination, one of two strategies should be employed, depending on the severity of symptoms, availability of tests, and patient preferences. Patients should have either a serum cryptococcal antigen and a serum RPR (or VDRL) performed, with watchful waiting, or a lumbar puncture. The most common meningitis in HIV-infected patients is cryptococcal. The serum cryptococcal antigen (CRAG) is 80 to 95% sensitive for cryptococcal meningitis. If the test is negative, the likelihood of cryptococcal meningitis is low. A patient with a positive antigen, at any titer, should have a lumbar puncture. A lumbar puncture should also be performed if the neurologic examination is abnormal or if symptoms persist. A lumbar puncture is done to rule out bacterial meningitis (rare), cryptococcal meningitis with a false-negative serum CRAG, neurosyphilis with a false-negative serum VDRL, and lymphomatous meningitis. Elevated CSF cell counts, which are primarily lymphocytic and accompanied by negative cultures, are consistent with primary HIV or other viral meningitides and usually remit spontaneously. Headache without fever has a similar differential diagnosis, but is less likely to represent a serious opportunistic infection. If the neurologic examination is normal, then the evaluation should include a careful history of both therapeutic drug use (AZT is a major cause of headache) and recreational drug use, a discussion of psychosocial stresses, a serum CRAG and an RPR test, and a therapeutic trial of a pain reliever. If the headache persists, a CT or MRI should be performed, along with a lumbar puncture.

Mental Status Changes
Mental status changes are quite common in HIV-infected patients, especially patients who have already had an AIDS-defining opportunistic infection. All the neurologic syndromes that cause headache, including toxoplasmosis, cryptococcal meningitis, neurosyphilis, and lymphomatous and viral meningitis, can present exclusively as mental status changes. HIV encephalopathy is a dementing illness that presents as a gradual change in mental status, impairing short-term memory and other cognitive skills. Diagnosis is by exclusion: a CT scan or MRI showing no masses (but atrophy greater than usual for the patient's age) and nondiagnostic CSF findings. Neuropsychiatric testing may quantitate deficits and help distinguish HIV encephalopathy from depression (pseudodementia). Other common treatable causes of changes in mental status include electrolyte disturbances and overuse of benzodiazepines and opiate pain relievers.

Seizures
First seizures should be evaluated by CT or MRI and a lumbar puncture. HIV encephalitis is the most common cause of seizures, but is a diagnosis of exclusion based on negative findings on imaging studies and a CSF evaluation. Patients with a single seizure should be treated with phenytoin, as seizures have a high rate of recurrence in this population. Because treatment with an antiseizure medicine is recommended regardless of electroencephalography (EEG) results, the EEG has an unclear role in the evaluation of an HIV-infected patient with seizure.

Visual Disturbances
Complaints of visual changes must be taken very seriously in HIV-infected individuals. Cytomegalovirus (CMV) retinitis, which tends to occur late in the course of HIV disease, is rapidly progressive without treatment. Patients typically complain of decreased visual acuity. Funduscopic examination shows fluffy white or yellow exudates with perivascular hemorrhages. These lesions need to be distinguished from cotton-wool spots, which are common benign lesions in HIV-infected patients. Cotton-wool spots appear as small, white, indistinct spots without hemorrhage. Because the distinction between these lesions can be difficult for the nonspecialist, and because CMV retinitis usually begins peripherally where it can be missed with indirect ophthalmoscopy, patients with acute visual changes should be seen immediately by an ophthalmologist.

Diarrhea
Diarrhea in HIV-infected patients is usually infectious in origin. The gamut of organisms is considerable, ranging from bacteria (e.g., *Campylobacter, Salmonella, Shigella*) to viruses (CMV, adenovirus) and protozoans (*Cryptosporidium, Entamoeba histolytica, Giardia*). While many of the agents that cause diarrhea in HIV-infected patients also cause diarrhea in immunocompetent patients, the major differences are that in HIV-positive patients the symptoms tend to be more severe; bacteremia and concomitant infection occur more often in other abdominal organs, especially the biliary system; and relapses of diarrhea with the same organism occur more frequently.

The diagnostic evaluation should include a stain for fecal white blood cells, stool culture, and three specimens for ova and parasites (including modified acid-fast staining for *Cryptosporidium*). If stool examination does not yield an etiology and symptoms continue, patients should be evaluated by sigmoidoscopy and biopsy. HIV-infected patients who have diarrhea for longer than 1 month, and in whom no etiologic factor is found, are considered to have a presumptive diagnosis of AIDS. In many such cases, a primary effect of the HIV virus on the colonic epithelium is the underlying cause and patients may improve with AZT therapy. Patients with severe diarrhea, unresponsive to standard symptomatic treatment with agents such as bismuth subsalicylate or diphenoxylate hydrochloride with atropine sulfate, may benefit from paregoric or tincture of opium.

Weight Loss
Weight loss in HIV-infected patients is generally multifactorial including a hypermetabolic effect of opportunistic infections or the HIV itself (HIV cachexia), chronic anorexia, chronic nausea and vomiting due to drugs (e.g., AZT, sulfa drugs) or to infections of the

hepatobiliary tree, and chronic diarrhea. Screening for opportunistic infections proceeds through an evaluation of the organ systems for which there are localizing complaints (e.g., cough, headache). Liver function tests are helpful for diagnosing the presence of hepatitis, but are not usually therapeutically helpful, except in the cases of drug-induced hepatitis. Some patients given an appetite stimulator such as megestrol acetate (80 mg 4 times a day) will gain weight. Diarrhea is best treated as outlined above. Many patients require enteral dietary supplementation to increase calorie consumption (e.g., Ensure), and a few patients who have disabling vomiting or unrelenting diarrhea, and otherwise good functional status, may benefit from total parenteral nutrition.

Skin Problems

Skin problems are common in HIV-infected individuals, and include bacterial, fungal, viral, neoplastic, and other dermatitides.

Staphyloccocal infections usually present as folliculitis or superficial abscesses. Folliculitis is best treated with topical clindamycin. Use of an antibacterial soap such as chlorhexidine gluconate (Hibiclens) may prevent relapses. Abscesses often require incision and drainage, along with systemic antibiotics (dicloxacillin, 500 mg 4 times a day).

Fungal rashes can occur on any part of the body, and respond well to topical antifungal creams (e.g., ketoconazole 2% daily). Herpes simplex virus outbreaks should be treated with acyclovir (200 mg PO 5 times a day) to speed recovery and prevent progressive local disease. HIV-infected patients who develop herpes zoster infection should be treated with acyclovir to prevent dissemination (800 mg PO 5 times a day). Steroids should not be used. Patients with disseminated herpes or zoster infection with ophthalmic involvement should be hospitalized for intravenous acyclovir therapy.

Warts are common among HIV-infected individuals. Molluscum contagiosum (warts with cratered centers), in particular, have a propensity for spread and should be treated with liquid nitrogen. Kaposi's sarcoma lesions, which are cosmetically bothersome to patients, can be treated with intralesional vinblastine sulfate (Velban) with good results. When Kaposi's lesions occur on the lower extremities, they are frequently associated with lymph edema, and patients may benefit from electron-beam therapy. Systemic chemotherapy is reserved for patients with aggressive skin Kaposi's sarcoma or visceral disease (e.g., gastrointestinal, pulmonary).

Seborrheic dermatitis occurs with increased incidence in HIV-infected individuals. It responds well to topical hydrocortisone and antifungal creams. The latter is used because scrapings of seborrheic dermatitis in HIV-infected individuals have shown the fungus *Pityrosporon ovale*.

Xerosis, with persistent itching, can be a perplexing problem for HIV-infected patients. Emollients and antipruritic lotions provide relief.

Supportive Care

Many HIV-infected patients are understandably depressed or anxious. Primary care physicians can counter feelings of helplessness by offering patients a promise of ongoing care, supportive counseling, and referral to local support groups and, when appropriate, mental health professionals. Depression that becomes disabling may be treated with antidepressants. Benzodiazepines should be used cautiously in the treatment of anxiety, especially in patients with HIV encephalopathy.

Patients should be counseled about the adverse effect of job changes on their health insurance coverage. Those without health insurance should be informed of benefits they are entitled to through state Medicaid programs. Federal programs administered locally may provide costly drugs such as AZT for patients whose insurance coverage does not include them. Physicians should encourage patients to discuss their feelings about the future use of medical interventions, such as respirators, feeding tubes, and hospitalization, and to execute a durable power for health care. The latter is especially important when the patient would prefer someone other than a family member, such as a close friend or partner, to make decisions about their care should they become incapacitated.

Patients can be taught to monitor and report signs of opportunistic infections, such as high fevers, shortness of breath, severe headache, and visual changes. By emphasizing the treatable nature of most opportunistic infections, particularly when detected early, clinicians can enlist patients to participate aggressively in their own health care.

The serious nature of HIV infection, coupled with the limits of medical therapy, lead some patients to use "alternative treatments"—vitamins, herbs, or drugs with untested efficacy. Because some alternative therapies have side effects or interact with standard therapy, clinicians should ask patients in a nonjudgmental fashion whether they are using alternative therapies. Often it is impossible to assess whether these alternative therapies are beneficial. Therefore, it is best to openly discuss these issues with patients, and encourage them to bring in articles from the popular press or relay experiences that friends using similar treatments have had.

The explosion of information about HIV treatment can overwhelm generalists. While it is impossible to keep abreast of all developments in the field, it is possible to research questions by using local resources such as HIV specialists, state medical associations, or AIDS newsletters such as *AIDS Clinical Care* or *AIDSFILE* (see references). Patients with unusual manifestations of disease may be referred to HIV specialists while the generalist maintains primary responsibility for the patients' care. Physicians should identify local specialists interested in caring for HIV-infected patients, especially ophthalmologists, otolaryngologists, dentists, and psychiatrists. Home health nursing agencies can provide hospice and other supportive home services.

Centers for Disease Control. Recommendations for diagnosing and treating syphilis in HIV-infected patients. MMWR 1988; 37:600–2, 607–8.
A concise summary of treatment guidelines.

Dismukes WE. Cryptococcal meningitis in patients with AIDS. J Infect Dis 1988; 157: 624–8.
Discussion of the clinical manifestations, diagnostic tests, and therapy of cryptococcal meningitis.

Faulstich ME. Psychiatric aspects of AIDS. Am J Psychiatry 1987; 144:551–6.
Review of neuropsychiatric syndromes in AIDS patients, as well as the psychosocial issues of healthy HIV-infected individuals.

Glatt AE, Chirgwin K. *Pneumocystis carinii* pneumonia in human immunodeficiency virus-infected patients. Arch Intern Med 1990; 150:271–9.
A review of the diagnosis, treatment, and prophylaxis of PCP.

Levy RM, Bredesen DE, Rosenblum ML. Neurologic complications of HIV Infection. Am Fam Physician 1990; 41:517–36.
A thorough review of the neurologic manifestations of HIV infection, along with photographs of CT scans of patients with HIV encephalitis, toxoplasmosis, and CNS lymphoma.

Moss AR, et al. Seropositivity for HIV and the development of AIDS or AIDS related condition: three year follow-up of the San Francisco General cohort. Br Med J 1988; 296:745–50.
Data on the association between CD4 counts, as well as other prognostic markers, and progression to AIDS.

Poland GA, Love KR, Hughes CE. Routine immunization of the HIV-positive asymptomatic patient. J Gen Intern Med 1990; 5:147–52.
Discussion of the use of the hepatitis B, pneumococcal, influenza, and tetanus-diphtheria vaccines in HIV-infected people.

Sande MA, Volberding PA, eds. The medical management of AIDS. 2nd ed. Philadelphia: WB Saunders, 1990.
A useful reference for diagnosis and treatment of HIV-related illnesses.

Volberding PA, et al. Zidovudine in asymptomatic human immunodeficiency virus infection. N Engl J Med 1990; 322:941–9.
Multicenter, randomized, double-blind trial of AZT versus placebo in HIV-infected patients with CD4 counts below 500 cells/mm^3. The trial demonstrated a significantly decreased rate of progression to advanced ARC and AIDS in those patients who received AZT.

Yarchoan R, Mitsya H, Broder S. Clinical and basic advances in the antiretroviral therapy of human immunodeficiency virus infection. Am J Med 1989; 87:191–200.
A detailed review of the pharmacologic approaches to anti-HIV therapy, including AZT, ddI, ddC, and CD4, along with a discussion of resistance to AZT, AZT use in pregnant women, and combination therapy.

AIDS Newsletters
AIDS Clinical Care. Useful summaries of common infections in HIV-infected individuals, along with diagnostic algorithms, a question and answer column, and reviews of current research. Published monthly, $68.00/year. AIDS Clinical Care, P.O. Box 9085, Waltham, MA 02254-9085.

AIDSFILE. Discussions of common manifestations of AIDS, along with interviews with AIDS experts, and selected annotated references. Published quarterly. Available free. AIDSFILE, San Francisco General Hospital, Ward 84, 995 Potrero Avenue, San Francisco, CA 94110.

115. HERPES ZOSTER
Terrie Mendelson

Herpes zoster, or "shingles," is a reactivation of latent varicella (chickenpox) infection characterized by pain, paresthesias, and vesicular cutaneous eruptions along single or adjacent dermatomes. It demonstrates no seasonal, ethnic, or gender preference and may occur in persons of any age, though it is uncommon in healthy children and young adults. The attack rate is doubled in persons over the age of 50; it has been estimated that half the population will have been afflicted by age 85. The disease is more common in patients with impaired cellular immunity, particularly those undergoing chronic immunosuppressive therapy for organ transplantation or with a history of Hodgkin's or other lymphomas. Its incidence appears to be increased among those infected with the human immunodeficiency virus (HIV), but it does not currently constitute a diagnostic criterion for symptomatic HIV disease. There is no evidence to support the notion that herpes zoster is a marker for occult malignancy in apparently healthy persons.

Because an episode of herpes zoster does not confer immunity against further attacks, zoster may recur; no particular predilection has been demonstrated for recurrence within the same dermatome. Multiple recurrences of herpes zoster have been documented, but are distinctly uncommon, and cultures of characteristic lesions will usually yield a diagnosis of herpes simplex virus infection.

Pathogenesis
Varicella zoster virus is thought to penetrate cutaneous endings of sensory nerves at the time of primary infection and ascend to sensory dorsal root ganglia, remaining latent within those neurons. A variety of conditions may subsequently result in reactivation and include an age-associated loss of cell-mediated immunity for varicella zoster virus, generalized immunosuppression, and local irradiation or trauma. Under such conditions, the virus is hypothesized to replicate in the ganglia and their associated sensory nerves, producing an active ganglionitis as well as the classic vesicular cutaneous lesions. Transient viremia may follow, but dissemination and spread to the viscera rarely occur in immunocompetent persons.

Clinical Manifestations
Herpes zoster characteristically presents with burning pain or paresthesia in a dermatomal or segmental distribution, accompanied by an erythematous maculopapular rash which progresses over several days to easily recognizable clusters of vesicles, pustules, and crusts. Low-grade fever, malaise, and regional lymphadenopathy commonly accompany the cutaneous manifestations. New crops of lesions may continue to erupt for 3 to 5

days; complete healing of crusted lesions and resolution of pain occur over 3 to 4 weeks in most cases. The vesicular lesions remain infective until crusted over.

The lesions of herpes zoster typically appear in a unilateral, dermatomal distribution, with occasional spread to adjacent dermatomes. Distribution is most commonly thoracic, particularly in the T-5 dermatome, followed by cranial, cervical, and then lumbar segments. Involvement of the ophthalmic division of the fifth cranial nerve may present with extraocular muscle dysfunction, mydriasis, ptosis, and keratoconjunctivitis. The ophthalmic nerve's nasociliary branch innervates the nasal tip as well as the cornea and iris; thus, lesions on the tip of the nose mandate ophthalmologic consultation even in the absence of obvious ocular involvement. Zoster oticus, resulting from the involvement of cranial nerves VII, VIII, IX, and X, may manifest with pain, vesicular lesions in the auditory canal, a loss of taste sensation in the anterior two-thirds of the tongue, and ipsilateral facial paralysis (Ramsay Hunt syndrome).

Characteristic prodromal sensory symptoms may infrequently occur without the subsequent development of cutaneous lesions (*zoster sine herpete*), resulting in mistaken diagnoses and extensive evaluation for thoracic or abdominal pain of unknown etiology.

Infectivity

Persons lacking immunity to varicella may become infected acutely via contact with the vesicle fluid from a patient with herpes zoster, although the attack rate is much lower than that following exposure to a primary case of varicella. The greatest risk exists for young children who have not yet been infected with "chickenpox" and who come in contact with a relative or caretaker with herpes zoster. Similarly, immunocompromised patients lacking protective antibody to varicella may develop a primary varicella infection following exposure to vesicle fluid from a person with zoster. Because herpes zoster always represents reactivation of varicella virus, only chickenpox, and not herpes zoster, can result from exposure to a patient with zoster.

Diagnosis

The diagnosis is usually made on the basis of a characteristic clinical syndrome; in most cases, the typical dermatomal distribution of vesicular or crusted lesions will allow accurate differentiation from impetigo, pustular psoriasis, or herpes simplex. Clinical diagnosis may be supported by the demonstration of intranuclear inclusions and multinucleated giant cells in Wright-stained scrapings of a vesicle base (Tzanck smear), though this technique cannot differentiate between herpes simplex and zoster viruses. When such differentiation is desirable, as in the case of an immunocompromised patient with diffuse vesicular eruptions, cultures of vesicle fluid are indicated. Viral culture and fluorescent monoclonal antibody staining of vesicle fluid are highly sensitive and specific, though not yet available at all medical centers. Serologic techniques to measure viral antibody titers are less useful, as zoster demonstrates some cross-reactivity with herpes simplex.

Complications

The most common complication of herpes zoster is postherpetic neuralgia, characterized by neuropathic pain along involved segments that may persist for months or years after the cutaneous lesions heal. Its incidence is low in children and young adults, but increases with age to approach 50% by age 60. There has been some suggestion that this complication may occur more frequently in diabetic patients, but this has not been well documented in any study to date.

Since the primary site of infection with herpes zoster is within the nervous system, asymptomatic abnormalities of the cerebrospinal fluid (CSF) are common and should not cause concern; the majority of patients will demonstrate transient CSF lymphocytic pleocytosis and elevated protein levels. Involvement of the ophthalmic division of the trigeminal nerve may result in a severe keratoconjunctivitis, and all patients with zoster in this distribution should therefore be referred promptly for ophthalmologic evaluation. Infection along sacral dermatomes frequently results in acute urinary retention. True meningoencephalitis, cerebellar ataxia, and transverse myelitis occur rarely.

Transient motor paralysis may occur if motor nerves originating in the same spinal segment with the affected cutaneous nerve are involved; onset typically occurs within a few weeks of the rash, and complete recovery is seen in more than 75% of affected patients within several weeks.

Cutaneous dissemination of herpes zoster occurs in less than 2% of patients, primarily in the immunocompromised. The prognosis in these patients is much poorer due to a greater likelihood of visceral involvement.

Treatment

Analgesia
The treatment of uncomplicated acute herpes zoster should focus on analgesia and symptomatic relief. Salicylates, codeine, and the local application of topical ethyl chloride or lidocaine sprays are often sufficient to provide adequate analgesia. Although there are few clinical data documenting its efficacy, topical capsaicin (Zostrix; a naturally-occurring substance P depleter) is newly available, and it is anecdotally reported to be beneficial for pain relief. Antihistamines and drying lotions provide effective relief for pruritus. Oral steroids do not decrease the severity or duration of acute zoster pain to a significant degree.

Antiviral Agents
Specific antiviral therapy is indicated for acute herpes zoster in immunocompromised patients (including those with HIV infection) in order to decrease the risk of dissemination. Because of the potential for more serious complications in diabetics, the elderly, and those with involvement of the ophthalmic branch of the fifth cranial nerve, antiviral agents are recommended for use in these patients as well. Their relatively high cost does not warrant use in the younger, immunocompetent patient population.

Since the demonstration of its greater efficacy and minimal toxicity, acyclovir has largely replaced vidarabine for the treatment of herpes virus infections. Because the sensitivity of varicella zoster virus to acyclovir is 10-fold less than that of herpes simplex, much higher dosages (800 mg PO 5 times qd or 1500 mg IV qd for 7 days) are required for the treatment of herpes zoster. Clinical investigations to date have demonstrated that treatment with acyclovir within 72 hours of symptom onset results in a statistically faster resolution of pain and healing of lesions, though the differences may not be clinically significant.

Prevention of Postherpetic Neuralgia
Antiviral therapy does not affect the incidence or duration of postherpetic neuralgia. Oral steroids (prednisone, 60 mg qd for 6 days with rapid taper) have been investigated for this use, but their efficacy remains controversial. Steroids should not be used in immunocompromised persons due to the potential for reducing their resistance to opportunistic infection. Concerns about an increased risk for disseminated zoster have not been supported by clinical studies.

Treatment of Postherpetic Neuralgia
Treatment of this debilitating and sometimes chronic disorder may prove frustrating for patients and physicians alike. Usual analgesic agents are typically ineffective unless used in combination with a tricyclic antidepressant such as amitriptyline (50–75 mg qhs). Transcutaneous electrical nerve stimulators may provide temporary local analgesia. Phenothiazines and anticonvulsants have been recommended by some, but there are no definitive data to support their use. Patients who have this complication may be reassured to learn that the majority will have complete resolution of pain within a year; for those few with a prolonged course of severe pain, sympathetic blockade or dorsal root entry zone surgical lesions may be required.

Prevention

The only effective prevention for herpes zoster is prevention of primary varicella infection; there is no effective means for clearing latent varicella virus from the sensory ganglia. A varicella vaccine is being developed to prevent primary chickenpox in children, and this might logically be expected to decrease the incidence of herpes zoster if it comes into widespread use. Zoster immune globulin, obtained from the sera of convalescing zoster patients, can be used to prevent chickenpox in exposed susceptible patients, but has no role in the prevention of herpes zoster.

Esmann V, et al. Therapy of acute herpes zoster with acyclovir in the non-immunocompromised host. Am J Med 1982; 73(1A):320–5.
Early treatment with acyclovir increased the rate of lesion healing and hastened the resolution of acute pain by several days, but had no effect on the incidence of postherpetic neuralgia.

Loeser JD. Herpes zoster and post-herpetic neuralgia. Pain 1986; 25:149–64.
An excellent, readable review with an extensive list of references.

McKendrick MW, et al. Oral acyclovir in acute herpes zoster. Br Med J 1986; 293:1529–32.
In a group of elderly, immunocompetent patients, treatment with oral acyclovir initiated within 48 hours of symptom onset resulted in slightly faster healing and diminished pain.

Melbye M, et al. Risks of AIDS after herpes zoster. Lancet 1987; 1:728–31.
Homosexual men with herpes zoster demonstrated a high rate of progression to AIDS over a 6-year period in this retrospective chart review study. Comparable rates were not determined for homosexual men without zoster; zoster may simply be a marker for HIV infection in this population.

Portenoy RK, et al. Acute herpetic and post-herpetic neuralgia: clinical review and current management. Ann Neurol 1986; 20:651–64.
A succinct review of the pathology, clinical features, and therapeutic management of herpes zoster and its complications.

Shepp DH, et al. Treatment of varicella zoster virus infection in severely immunocompromised patients: a randomized comparison of acyclovir and vidarabine. N Engl J Med 1986; 314:208–12.
A prospective, randomized trial demonstrating that intravenous acyclovir is more efficacious than vidarabine for the treatment of varicella zoster infection in immunocompromised hosts.

Schmader SE, Studenski S. Are current therapies useful for the prevention of postherpetic neuralgia? A critical analysis of the literature. J Gen Intern Med 1989; 4:83–9.
A critical review of the data concerning the effectiveness of steroids and antiviral therapy in reducing the incidence of postherpetic neuralgia.

Straus SE, et al. NIH conference. Varicella zoster virus infections: biology, natural history, treatment and prevention. Ann Intern Med 1988; 108:221–37.
A lucid review summarizing current concepts and treatment recommendations.

Watson PN, Evans RJ. Post-herpetic neuralgia: a review. Arch Neurol 1986; 43:836–40.
A review of the literature concerning pharmacologic prophylaxis and treatment for postherpetic neuralgia.

116. INFECTIOUS MONONUCLEOSIS
Jack D. McCue

Infectious mononucleosis (IM) results from infection with Epstein-Barr virus (EBV). Most EBV infections are asymptomatic; symptomatic illness rarely occurs in children under 5 years old, and even adolescents have a less than 50% chance of developing typical IM as a result of EBV infection. Clinically apparent infections seem to occur most frequently in populations in whom primary exposure to EBV is delayed until the second decade of life, and perhaps because of this, IM is most often diagnosed in adolescents from higher socioeconomic groups. Symptomatic IM appears to be caused primarily by the host response to antigenic changes in B lymphocytes, the primary host cells for EBV. A vigorous T-lymphocyte proliferative response to EBV-infected B lymphocytes is largely responsible for the adenopathy and atypical lymphocytosis. The inflammatory response and killing of EBV-infected lymphocytes may also be the cause of fever, pharyngitis, and hepatitis characteristic of IM.

Clinical Manifestations
Patients with typical IM are nearly always in their teens or 20s. After a 30- to 50-day incubation period, there may be a brief nonspecific prodrome followed by the triad of pharyngitis, fever, and adenopathy. Malaise and fatigue may be disproportionately severe.

Pharyngitis is present in over 80% of patients, and about 50% have exudate. In some cases (so-called anginose pharyngitis), the signs and symptoms are much more severe than in streptococcal pharyngitis. Palatal petechiae occurring at the junction of the hard and soft palates are seen in 25% of patients; while not diagnostic of IM, they suggest the diagnosis. The degree of fever correlates with the overall severity of the illness. Temperatures commonly reach 39°C (102.2°F) and many exceed 40°C (104.0°F) in acutely ill young adults. Significant adenopathy is nearly universally noted, and its absence should make one doubt the diagnosis of IM. In acute disease, the nodes may be massively enlarged and tender. IM is one of the few diseases of healthy persons that cause significant posterior cervical adenopathy. About half of patients have a mild to moderately enlarged spleen, which may be slightly tender. The enlargement usually peaks in the second week of illness.

Palpable hepatomegaly occurs in about one-fourth of patients, although jaundice is unusual. Mild right-upper-quadrant tenderness on percussion is very common. In a few instances, IM may present as hepatitis.

Rashes

Rashes are not helpful in making the diagnosis because they are infrequent and of variable appearance. Up to 100% of patients receiving ampicillin develop an extensive maculopapular rash, presumably due to immune complexes from cross-reacting antibodies; a similar reaction occurs less often with other drugs and antibiotics.

Although present in only 10 to 20% of patients, facial, particularly eyelid, edema is rarely encountered in other illnesses of young adults and may, therefore, suggest IM.

Atypical Infectious Mononucleosis

Up to 25% of patients present with atypical illness, especially those under 10 or over 50 years old. The common atypical representations include fever of unknown origin, leukemia or lymphoma, arthralgia-myalgia syndromes, aseptic meningitis and encephalitis, pneumonia, fever and rash of unknown cause, nonspecific gastrointestinal complaints, and mild jaundice.

Clinical Course
In the typical case of IM, sore throat and fever last about a week and adenopathy regresses in less than a month. Fatigue resolves more slowly; usually daily tasks can be resumed after 2 to 4 weeks. Rapid onset of symptoms and severe sore throat and fever seem to be associated with a prolonged recovery. Most cases of prolonged fatigue probably represent post-IM depression or psychological problems unrelated to EBV infection. An inability to study and perform at pre-illness levels may cause students to become further depressed when they fall behind in studies.

The chronic fatigue syndrome is not caused by EBV infection, although viruses are included among its hypothesized etiologies. Chronic EBV infections have been documented, but are rare and severe and usually occur in immunocompromised patients. The attribution of fatigue to "chronic mono" impedes the elucidation of its real causes and may divert attention from psychosocial problems.

Complications and Sequelae
Although very few patients experience complications from IM, awareness of the possibility can prevent their occurrence. This is particularly true for splenic rupture, which is usually due to trauma before the third week of illness, but which may also occur spontaneously or after apparent recovery. All patients with IM should be instructed to seek medical attention promptly for abdominal pain. The duration of the risk for splenic rupture after IM infection is not known, but it is recommended that strenuous activity or participation

in contact sports not be resumed for at least 1 to 2 months after the resolution of splenomegaly; since the latter may not be clinically detectable in a large proportion of patients, some recommend that all patients with IM avoid vigorous exercise for 1 to 2 months.

Airway obstruction from pharyngeal edema and massive tonsillar enlargement is also rare but potentially life-threatening; patients in whom impending obstruction is suspected should be hospitalized because tracheostomy or intubation may become necessary. Interstitial pneumonitis has been noted in 3 to 5% of patients, and it usually resolves without complication. Pleural effusions have also been reported.

Hematologic complications include hemolytic anemia, which is usually mild and asymptomatic and is estimated to occur in up to 3% of patients. Mild thrombocytopenia is not uncommon, but severe thrombocytopenia and other hemorrhagic phenomena may also occur. Neutropenia, sometimes severe, has been reported.

Neurologic complaints probably occur in less than 1% of patients, and include meningoencephalitis, aseptic meningitis, Guillain-Barré syndrome, transverse myelitis, facial nerve palsy, seizures, optic neuritis, peripheral neuropathies, and psychoses.

Cardiac complications include myocarditis, which is usually asymptomatic and recognized by nonspecific electrocardiographic changes, and pericarditis, which is very rare.

Renal involvement may be reflected by transient minor abnormalities on urinalysis (microscopic hematuria, pyuria, and proteinuria) in up to 15% of patients. These findings are usually self-limited, and there is controversy as to whether nephritis due to IM actually occurs.

Diagnosis

Clinical Presentation

The triad of fever, adenopathy, and pharyngitis is usually due to a common viral or streptococcal pharyngitis, not IM. Streptococcal pharyngitis may coexist with IM but is probably not any more prevalent in IM patients than in healthy persons. Posterior cervical adenopathy and the presence of splenomegaly help distinguish an IM pharyngitis from a streptococcal one.

Of the possible causes of atypical lymphocytosis, only infection with cytomegalovirus (CMV) is commonly confused clinically with atypical IM in older adults. The diagnosis of CMV mononucleosis and the less common toxoplasmosis mononucleosis is made serologically. The syndrome of heterophile-negative persistent fatigue and pharyngitis without atypical lymphocytosis usually has another viral or psychiatric cause.

Heterophil Antibodies

The "spot" tests for heterophil antibodies are about 95% specific and about 90% sensitive. False-positive results are nearly always trace or 1+ and may occur in patients recovering from asymptomatic IM, since the spot test result can remain positive for several months. False-negative results are usually encountered in atypical IM in young children and older adults. The degree of positivity of the antibody test does not reliably correlate with the severity of clinical illness. A false-negative spot test result will usually turn positive in 1 to 2 weeks after the onset of symptoms. Rarely is a third spot test justified after two tests, done a week apart, show negative results. It is rarely necessary to confirm a spot test result with a classic Paul-Bunnell heterophil titer.

The white blood count is usually elevated in acute IM. Nearly all patients have an absolute lymphocytosis with more than 4500 mononuclear cells/mm^3 and a relative lymphocytosis of greater than 50%. While atypical lymphocytosis occurs in many illnesses, it ordinarily exceeds 10% of white blood cells only in IM. Atypical lymphocytes are usually T cells that are larger than normal lymphocytes, with irregular "folded" cytoplasmic borders, an increased amount of cytoplasm with vacuoles, and an irregular nucleus.

Specific Anti-EBV Antibodies

The commonly available anti-viral capsid antigen (VCA) IgG assay has limited diagnostic value when positive because a fourfold rise in IgG titer is seen in only about 10% of patients and the anti-VCA IgG titer remains elevated at about 1:40 for life after EBV infection. A negative test, however, virtually rules out IM, since titers peak near the time of onset of symptoms. The presence of anti-VCA IgM antibody, on the other hand, is highly diagnostic, since it acutely rises to 1:5 or higher and returns to 0 within a few months. Assays for anti-VCA IgM are more difficult to perform than IgG assays but are now more commonly available. Additional antigen and antibody assays are also performed in special laboratories, but like anti-VCA assays are difficult to interpret and should be ordered only for serious diagnostic dilemmas.

Other Laboratory Abnormalities
Hemolytic anemia is rare. Mild thrombocytopenia is common. Liver enzymes are nearly always mildly elevated. Low-grade hyperbilirubinemia is common, but elevations above 5 mg/dl or enzyme elevations over 10 times normal should suggest some other diagnosis. Nonspecific electrocardiographic changes, false-positive serologic tests for syphilis, and positive rheumatoid factor assays occur rarely.

Treatment

Most patients with IM require nothing more than symptomatic therapy, such as aspirin or acetaminophen for fever and anesthetic throat lozenges or gargles for pharyngitis. Aspirin and other nonsteroidal anti-inflammatory agents, like indomethacin, in high dosages (150 mg/day for adults) are said to relieve some symptoms of IM, but this assertion has not been tested by controlled trials. Acyclovir is ineffective, even in very high dosages.

Isolating patients with IM is unnecessary. Although the presumed mode of transmission is contact with EBV-containing oropharyngeal secretions, and the illness is sometimes popularly called the "kissing disease," there is little epidemiologic evidence of a space-time clustering of IM or of prior exposure of IM patients to others with IM. Therefore, patients need not be restricted from close contact with others.

The use of corticosteroids for IM is controversial. In controlled studies, they have been proved to be superior to placebo in ameliorating fever and pharyngitis; they may also result in an improved sense of well-being and a shortened duration of illness. The use of corticosteroids is universally recommended in patients with potential airway obstruction and favored for patients with neurologic, hematologic, or cardiac complications. The usual dosage is 1 mg/kg of prednisone daily for 3 days, then tapered over 7 to 10 days. Some proponents recommend that corticosteroids also be used in most patients with severely symptomatic but uncomplicated IM, to help them return to normal functioning more quickly and possibly to prevent post-IM depression or a loss of significant time from schoolwork. Other authorities are reluctant to administer potent anti-inflammatory agents during an infection, although one study of their effects on lymphocytes in IM showed no deleterious responses.

Antibiotics are indicated only for the treatment of group A beta-hemolytic streptococcal pharyngitis and possibly for anginose pharyngitis. Foul (anaerobic) breath and massively swollen and painful oropharyngeal tissues may indicate the presence of a polymicrobial bacterial pharyngitis that may respond to treatment with penicillin or metronidazole. Antibiotics in general and ampicillin in particular should be avoided because of the very high incidence of associated rash.

Chang RS. Infectious mononucleosis. Boston: Hall, 1980.
Extensively referenced book covering nearly all aspects of EBV infection and IM.

Hoagland RS. Infectious mononucleosis. New York: Grune & Stratton, 1976.
Classic account of clinical IM.

Schooley RT, Dolin R. Epstein-Barr virus (infectious mononucleosis). In: Mandell GL, Douglas RG, Bennett JE, eds. Principles and practice of infectious diseases. 3rd ed New York: Wiley, 1990:1172–1185.

Cheeseman SH. Infectious mononucleosis. Semin Hematol 1988; 25:261–8.
Comprehensive reviews of clinical and laboratory aspects of IM.

Halery J, Ash S. Infectious mononucleosis in hospitalized patients over forty years of age. Am J Sci 1988; 295:122–4.
A cause of fever of unknown origin and abnormal findings on liver function tests.

Straus SE. The chronic mononucleosis syndrome. J Infect Dis 1988; 157:405–12.

Manu P, Lane TJ, Matthew DA. The frequency of the chronic fatigue syndrome in patients with symptoms of persistent fatigue. Ann Intern Med 1988; 109:554–6.

Kroenke K, et al. Chronic fatigue in primary care: prevalence, patient characteristics, and outcome. JAMA 1988; 260:929–34.
Differing opinions on the chronic fatigue syndrome: You decide!

Gold DG, et al. Chronic fatigue. A prospective clinical and virologic study. JAMA 1990; 264:48–53.
No evidence of ongoing EBV infection was demonstrated in a population of 26 patients with chronic fatigue.

Andersson J, et al. Effect of acyclovir on infectious mononucleosis: a double-blind, placebo-controlled study. J Infect Dis 1986; 153:283–90.
High-dose intravenous acyclovir had little effect on the course of symptoms of IM.

Brandfonbrener A, et al. Corticosteroid therapy in Epstein-Barr virus infection. Effect on lymphocyte class, subset, and response to early antigen. Arch Intern Med 1986; 146:337–9.

Bender CE. The value of corticosteroids in the treatment of infectious mononucleosis. JAMA 1967; 199:97–9.

Pront C, Dalrymple W. A double-blind study of 82 cases of infectious mononucleosis. J Coll Health Assoc 1966; 15:62–6.
Three controlled studies showing the beneficial effects of corticosteroids in reducing fever and adenopathy.

Rutkow IM. Rupture of the spleen in infectious mononucleosis: a critical review. Arch Surg 1978; 113:718–20.
An excellent review of this serious complication, with very conservative recommendations not necessarily supported by the data.

117. INTESTINAL PARASITES
Richard A. Davidson and Terrie Mendelson

Parasitic disease is not rare in the United States. Over 20% of inhabitants in the southeast and south central states are infected with intestinal nematodes. The most common pathogenic enteric parasitic infections of immunocompetent adults include the protozoal infections giardiasis and amebiasis; and the helminth infections ascariasis, trichuriasis, enterobiasis, strongyloidiasis, and hookworm. Among immunocompromised persons, particularly those infected with the human immunodeficiency virus (HIV), infections with the coccidian protozoan parasites *Cryptosporidium* and *Isospora belli* are recognized as a common source of chronic and often severe diarrheal illness.

Parasitic infections cause a variety of symptoms and signs, most of which are nonspecific. Infection may be suspected in the presence of the clinical presentations summarized in Table 117-1.

Laboratory Diagnosis
Ordinarily an enteric parasitic infection is confirmed when the diagnostic stage of the parasite is demonstrated in stool or duodenal contents. Diarrheal stools, which are likely to contain trophozoites as well as cyst forms, should be examined by a well-trained laboratory technician within 30 minutes of passage; if a delay is necessary, the stools should be preserved in polyvinyl alcohol or refrigerated to promote the survival of trophozoites. Formed stools most frequently contain cyst, egg, or larval forms, and prompt examination is therefore less crucial. A concentration technique is often employed to improve the chances of detecting eggs and cysts when they are present in small numbers. At least 50% of infections with intestinal parasites can be demonstrated in one stool specimen; three specimens will detect 80 to 90% of all recognized infections.

Infections with *Giardia* and *Strongyloides* are occasionally not detectable by stool examination alone; when these organisms are suspected and stool examinations are negative,

Table 117-1. Clinical settings in which parasitic infections should be considered.

Clinical setting	Potential parasitic infection
Eosinophilia	Hookworm, strongyloidiasis, ascariasis
Unexplained anemia	Hookworm
Malabsorption	Giardiasis, strongyloidiasis, cryptosporidiosis
Gastrointestinal bleeding	Amebiasis, trichuriasis, hookworm
Wheezing	Ascariasis, trichuriasis, hookworm, strongyloidiasis
Pruritic, urticarial, and maculopapular skin rashes	Hookworm, ascariasis, strongyloidiasis
Dysentery	Amebiasis, giardiasis, trichuriasis, cryptosporidiosis, isosporiasis
Rectal itching	Enterobiasis
Unexplained gastrointestinal symptoms	All
Recent immigration from endemic area	All
Human immunodeficiency virus infection	Cryptosporidiosis, amebiasis, giardiasis, isosporiasis, strongyloidiasis

an evaluation of duodenal contents obtained by endoscopy or string test (Enterotest) may be necessary. To perform the string test, an encapsulated length of braided cotton string is swallowed; the proximal end is taped to the cheek, and the distal end is carried into the duodenum. The string is removed after 3 to 4 hours and the bile-stained segment is examined microscopically for parasites.

Enterobiasis (pinworm), in contrast to infections with other intestinal parasites, is infrequently diagnosed by stool examination; the "Scotch-Tape test" may be performed by touching clear cellophane tape to the perineum, preferably before the morning bowel movement, and examining the tape for eggs under a microscope.

Eosinophilia occurs in infections with most parasites that have an extraluminal stage, including *Ascaris, Strongyloides,* and hookworm. Eosinophilia is not typically seen in amoebic dysentery, giardiasis, and enterobiasis. Approximately 90% of patients diagnosed with strongyloidiasis have peripheral eosinophilia, making this a reasonably effective screening test for this infection. However, eosinophilia may be absent in patients who are taking corticosteroids or have chronic infections. There is no clear association between the degree of eosinophilia and the burden of infection.

Giardiasis

Giardia lamblia is a water-borne protozoan with widespread distribution. Infection occurs when *Giardia* in the cyst stage, which is resistant to water chlorination, is ingested. Excystation occurs in the upper gastrointestinal tract, and motile trophozoites reproduce and live in the duodenum. Infection is usually contracted from a contaminated water supply and can occur epidemically or sporadically, depending on the source of exposure. The organism is endemic in some western areas of the United States, where it may contaminate mountain stream water and thereby infect campers. There is an increased incidence of *Giardia* infection in homosexual men, apparently because of person-to-person spread; outbreaks have also been reported in day-care centers.

Symptoms of giardiasis vary widely, from none at all to explosive, watery, malodorous diarrhea. In extreme cases, alterations in small-bowel mucosa lead to malnutrition, which is reversible with treatment of the infection. Eosinophilia is rarely seen. When stools are examined, cysts are found more frequently than are trophozoites. As noted, a single Enterotest examination may be more sensitive than three stool examinations.

Quinacrine is the drug of choice for treating all stages of giardiasis, and is usually effective in a dosage of 100 mg 3 times daily for 5 days. Metronidazole is a commonly prescribed alternative therapy that is equally efficacious but is not approved by the Food and Drug Administration for this use. Furazolidone is an effective alternative, but is less readily available and carries a higher incidence of side effects. Careful follow-up 10 to 14 days after treatment is recommended in order to demonstrate eradication of the organism. When there is a strong clinical suspicion of giardiasis, a therapeutic trial of quinacrine is a reasonable approach if stool examinations fail to reveal evidence of parasitic infection.

Amebiasis

Amebiasis results from the ingestion of cysts of *Entamoeba histolytica*. The mode of transmission is fecal-oral, resulting from either inadequate hand-washing or anal sexual intercourse. Infection is frequently asymptomatic, and may be detected only by identifying the characteristic cysts in formed stool. Clinically apparent intestinal amebiasis presents as diarrhea of variable severity, ranging from mild, intermittently loose stools to profuse, explosive, and bloody dysentery. Extraintestinal infection typically presents as an expanding mass lesion, most commonly in the right hepatic lobe where it may mimic a pyogenic liver abscess. Less commonly, amoebic abscesses may form in the pericardium, pleural space, lung, or central nervous system.

Diagnosis is based on the demonstration of either cysts or trophozoites of *E. histolytica*. As many as seven types of nonpathogenic amoebae that can be confused with *E. histolytica* may colonize the gastrointestinal tract; therefore, final identification is best left to a well-trained laboratory technician. Ordinarily, trophozoites are found only in loose stools examined soon after passage; cysts may be found in formed or loose stools and remain recognizable for a longer period of time.

Eosinophilia is typically absent in all forms of amebiasis. The most frequently used serologic test is the amoebic indirect hemagglutination titer (AIH); it is most useful for extraintestinal disease, where it is 95% sensitive in detecting infection. The sensitivity of this test falls to 85% for active intestinal infection, and it is not able to identify asymptomatic cyst passers.

The need for treatment of asymptomatic infection has been a subject of debate for some time. Although studies carried out both in the United States and in Third World countries have demonstrated that only 10% of asymptomatic infections will progress to clinically apparent disease, the importance of asymptomatic carriers as a reservoir of infection has led to the current recommendation to treat all patients with documented infection.

All forms of amebiasis usually respond to treatment with metronidazole, 750 mg 3 times daily for 10 days. For dysenteric or extraintestinal infection, this should be followed with iodoquinol, 650 mg 3 times daily for 20 days. Paromomycin, 25 to 35 mg/kg/day in three divided doses for 7 days, is an alternative to iodoquinol for mildly symptomatic intestinal infection. The treatment of choice for asymptomatic cyst passers is diloxanide furoate, 500 mg 3 times daily for 10 days; unfortunately, this drug is currently available only through the Centers for Disease Control (CDC). Effective alternative treatments for asymptomatic infection are paromomycin or iodoquinol.

Ascariasis

Ascaris lumbricoides is a common nematodal infection in the United States and is present throughout North America. The infection is contracted by ingesting eggs, which are usually found in fecally contaminated soil. Thus, the infection is most prevalent in children, though it may also occur in adults. The worm is large (up to 35 cm in length), and the typical infection consists of 8 to 10 worms.

Eosinophilia is present during larval migration, but is often absent in adults with chronic infections. Symptoms are typically limited to intermittent mild abdominal pain, and diarrhea is uncommon. The most serious sequelae of infection are host sensitization, which may cause an allergic reaction indistinguishable from bronchial asthma, and complications due to the migration of adult worms: bile duct obstruction, acute hemorrhagic pancreatitis, peritonitis, and intestinal obstruction in cases of heavy infestation.

Eggs are readily demonstrable in stool. No serologic tests are yet available. When a patient or parent reports passage of a worm that is over 1 cm in length, it should be considered an *Ascaris*.

Therapy is with mebendazole, 100 mg twice daily for 3 days. An equally effective alternative therapy consists of pyrantel pamoate, 11 mg/kg once. Both drugs act by paralyzing the worm, thus allowing its excretion in the stool. In mixed parasitic infections, *Ascaris* should be treated first, as other antihelminthic agents will cause it to migrate.

Trichuriasis
Trichuris, also known as whipworm, is extremely common; for example, 46% of the population surveyed in 1974 at Hilton Head Island, South Carolina, were infected. Eggs are ingested most frequently by children in fecally contaminated soil. The eggs mature in the jejunum and embed into the colonic mucosa at maturity. Infections in adults are typically asymptomatic, but children and heavily infested adults may develop anemia, blood-streaked diarrhea, nausea, vomiting, and rectal prolapse. The eggs, which are quite distinctive, can be found in the stool. Eosinophilia may occur with acute infection. The treatment of choice is mebendazole, 100 mg twice daily for 3 days.

Enterobiasis
As many as 200 million people worldwide may be infected with pinworm, including 18 million in the United States and Canada. The infection is spread by a hand-to-mouth transmission of eggs, and is usually acquired by scratching the perianal region. Other household members are frequently infected, presumably because eggs may be inhaled with house dust. In one study of houses with several infected children, 222 of 241 house dust samples were found to contain pinworm eggs.

The worm matures in the upper gastrointestinal tract and lives in the cecum; the gravid female migrates to the perineum to lay her eggs, resulting in the common symptoms of perianal and vaginal pruritus. Eosinophilia is distinctly unusual. Diagnosis is most effectively establishing by using the Scotch-Tape test (described under Laboratory Diagnosis), though three serial daily examinations may detect only 90% of cases.

The treatment of choice is pyrantel pamoate, 11 mg/kg in a single dose. A repeat dose 2 weeks later is strongly recommended. This medication may cause nausea and vomiting. Alternative therapies include mebendazole, 100 mg in a single dose and repeated in 2 weeks, or piperazine, 65 mg/kg daily for 7 days. It is advisable to thoroughly wash bedclothing and linens following treatment in order to prevent recurrence. Hand-washing is the most effective means of reducing infection of household contacts, and efforts to minimize house dust may also provide benefit.

Hookworm
Necator americanus, the New World hookworm, is found throughout the United States. Its life cycle includes penetration through the skin and a molting stage in the lung, which typically produces a pronounced eosinophilia. Acute infection causes few symptoms; the characteristic lassitude, exertional dyspnea, weakness, and dizziness develop insidiously as the result of a progressive hypochromic, microcytic anemia. The adult worm attaches and reattaches to the intestinal mucosa many times daily, and secretes an anticoagulant that causes persistent bleeding from prior attachment points. Each worm may cause 0.03 to 0.15 ml of blood loss per day.

Diagnosis is usually made by identifying the egg stage in stool; in milder cases, concentration techniques may improve the diagnostic yield. The eggs may be confused with those of *Trichostrongylus,* a prevalent nonpathogen. The treatment of choice is mebendazole, 100 mg twice daily daily for 3 days; pyrantel pamoate may be used as an alternative therapy.

Strongyloidiasis
Strongyloidiasis, while somewhat less common than the previously described infections, has a higher rate of mortality. Like hookworm, the larvae penetrate the skin, and adults live in the upper gastrointestinal tract. Typical symptoms are crampy abdominal pain, intermittent diarrhea, and nausea; unlike hookworm, *Strongyloides* do not cause profound anemia.

Most infections cause eosinophilia and can be diagnosed by finding one of the larval stages, a 2-mm worm, in the stool; eggs are usually not passed. Under certain conditions, particularly in patients with deficient cell-mediated immunity due to chronic corticosteroid use, organ transplantation, or acquired immunodeficiency syndrome (AIDS), the worm undergoes a metamorphosis to a different larval stage. It then penetrates the intestinal wall and enters the bloodstream in large numbers, resulting in sepsis and multiorgan failure. Approximately 50% of such cases of "hyperinfection" are fatal.

Therapy for strongyloidiasis is thiabendazole, 25 mg/kg twice a day for 2 days; a repeat course 1 week later is recommended, particularly if the patient is immunocompromised. Two courses of therapy are 96% effective.

Cryptosporidiosis and Isosporiasis

Homosexual men are at risk for intestinal infection with a variety of enteric organisms, which result in what has been termed the "gay bowel syndrome." Organisms commonly identified in stool samples from patients with this chronic and recurrent diarrheal syndrome include *G. lamblia, E. histolytica,* a variety of nonpathogenic *entamoebae, Cryptosporidium,* and *I. belli.* The latter two are animal pathogens that cause only brief, self-limited diarrhea in immunocompetent persons, but often lead to severe, chronic dysentery in those infected with HIV. *Cryptosporidium* may also infect the biliary tract and lead to inflammation of the papilla of Vater, papillary stenosis, and sclerosing cholangitis.

The incidence of chronic cryptosporidiosis among AIDS patients in this country is 3 to 4%; as many as 15% of Haitians with AIDS are infected with isosporiasis. Both infections may result in profound dehydration, weight loss, malnutrition, and electrolyte depletion due to the large volume and prolonged duration of diarrhea. The diagnosis is made by identifying the characteristic oocysts in stool samples treated with a modified acid-fast stain; most clinical laboratories do not perform this analysis unless it is specifically requested.

At present, there is no effective therapy for the treatment of cryptosporidiosis; spiramycin has been studied, but has yielded disappointing results to date. Therefore, the mainstays of therapy for this disorder are careful attention to fluid and electrolyte repletion and the administration of antidiarrheal agents such as loperamide (Imodium) or codeine. Recent data suggest a possible role for the use of sandostatin in some patients. Health care workers should exercise scrupulous infection precautions when attending to infected patients in order to avoid spreading this untreatable infection to other susceptible individuals.

Isosporiasis, which occurs less commonly, responds readily to treatment with trimethoprim-sulfamethoxazole, one double-strength tablet 4 times daily for 10 days, then twice daily for 3 weeks. Recurrent infection is common, but responds to repeated therapy.

Fanning M, et al. Pilot study of sandostatin therapy of refractory HIV-associated diarrhea. Dig Dis Sci 1991; 36:476–80.
Early investigation of a promising new therapy.

Birkhead G, Vogt RL. Epidemiologic surveillance for endemic *Giardia lamblia* infection in Vermont. The roles of waterborne and person-to-person transmission. Am J Epidemiol 1989; 129:762–8.
Giardiasis was the most common reportable disease in Vermont and resulted in significant morbidity. Both water-borne and person-to-person transmissions were found to be important factors in causing nonoutbreak-related cases.

Davidson RA. Amebiasis. Conn's current therapy. Philadelphia: WB Saunders, 1989: 38–40.
A recent review of the diagnosis and treatment of amebiasis.

Davidson RA. Issues in clinical parasitology: I. The treatment of giardiasis. Am J Gastroenterol 1984; 79:256–61.
A review of the major controlled trials of medications used in the treatment of this common infection. A discussion about possible risks of carcinogenesis with the use of metronidazole is included.

Davidson RA, Fletcher RH, Chapman LE. Risk factors for strongyloidiasis A case-control study. Arch Intern Med 1984; 144:321–4.
The risk of strongyloidiasis was increased in whites, males, patients taking corticosteroids, and patients with gastric surgery or hematologic malignancy.

Gathiram V, Jackson TF. A long study of asymptomatic carriers of pathogenic zymodemes of *Entamoeba histolytica*. S Afr Med J 1987; 72:669–72.
This study reports a 10% incidence of amoebic colitis among a large cohort of asymptomatic cyst passers over 1 year of observation. The authors recommend treatment of asymptomatic infection based on documentation of its spread to previously uninfected household members.

Genta RM. Predictive value of an enzyme-linked immunosorbent assay (ELISA) for the serodiagnosis of strongyloidiasis. Am J Clin Pathol 1988; 89:391–4.
The availability of a relatively accurate ELISA will tremendously simplify the diagnosis of Strongyloides *infection. This test has a positive predictive value of 97% and a negative predictive value of 95% in a selected population.*

Schneiderman DJ, Cello JP, Laing FC. Papillary stenosis and sclerosing cholangitis in the acquired immunodeficiency syndrome. Ann Intern Med 1987; 106:546–9.
This report describes biliary tract involvement with cryptosporidiosis in AIDS patients.

Scowden EB, Schaffner W, Stone WJ. Overwhelming strongyloidiasis. Medicine 1978; 57:537–44.
The authors clearly describe how hazardous this infection may be when it occurs in patients with altered immune status.

Smith JW, Wolfe MS. Giardiasis. Annu Rev Med 1980; 31:373–83.
This is an excellent, thorough review of this common infection.

Smith PD, Janoff EN. Infectious diarrhea in human immunodeficiency virus infection. Gastroenterol Clin North Am 1988; 17:587–98.
The authors provide a thorough review of the protozoan, fungal, bacterial, and viral enteric infections commonly encountered in this population.

Soave R. Cryptosporidiosis and isosporiasis in patients with AIDS. Infect Dis Clin North Am 1988; 2:485–93.
This is an excellent review of the epidemiology, pathogenicity, clinical profile, and therapy of these protozoan enteric infections in AIDS patients.

118. TUBERCULOSIS
Eliseo J. Pérez-Stable

Tuberculosis in the United States has become a disease of the elderly, foreign-born, nonwhite minorities, and persons with human immunodeficiency virus (HIV) infection. In 1987, the elderly comprised 27.3% and foreign-born individuals, 22.6% of newly reported cases. Case rates are more than 4 times higher in nonwhite compared to white elderly patients; nursing home residents are particularly susceptible to new infection. Foreign-born individuals with newly reported tuberculosis originated from Mexico (23.3%), the Indochinese countries (13.4%), the Philippines (12.5%), Haiti (6.3%), Korea (5.8%), and China (4.3%). Finally, HIV infection markedly increases the risk of tuberculosis. The seroprevalence of HIV in patients with newly diagnosed tuberculosis has been reported to be 20 to 30% in areas with high rates of acquired immunodeficiency syndrome (AIDS), and 4 to 11% of patients with AIDS also have tuberculosis.

Screening for Tuberculosis
Persons with asymptomatic tuberculosis infection can be identified through tuberculin skin testing; of the reactors, between 5 and 15% will develop active tuberculosis during their lifetime. An effective preventive strategy is to perform tuberculin skin testing in

groups at high risk for tuberculosis and to treat tuberculin reactors who are at greatest risk for reactivation with isoniazid preventive therapy.

Screening with skin testing is strongly recommended in high-risk populations, such as persons infected with HIV; close contacts of persons known to have pulmonary tuberculosis; persons with medical risk factors; foreign-born persons from high-prevalence countries; medically underserved low-income populations including minorities, alcoholics, and injection drug users; residents of long-term care facilities and correctional institutions; and persons employed in hospitals, clinics, day-care centers, schools, and correctional institutions.

The Tuberculin Skin Test

Tuberculin skin testing is the only available method to screen for tuberculosis infection (chest radiographs identify only current pulmonary infections), and it is essential that it be performed and interpreted appropriately. The 5–tuberculin unit (TU) (intermediate-strength) tuberculin test should always be used, applied intradermally by the Mantoux technique. The 250-TU (second-strength) tuberculin test has an unacceptably high proportion of reactions due to nontuberculous mycobacteria. The belief that patients with a history of tuberculosis have more severe necrotic reactions to tuberculin tests is not supported by the data, and should not be used as a reason to use the 1-TU (first-strength) tuberculin in adults.

Reading tuberculin tests is based on palpating the skin for induration borders and measuring the induration diameter transverse to the long axis of the forearm. Accurate measurement may be facilitated by applying a ballpoint pen to help define induration borders; the reading in millimeters should then be recorded in the chart. Erythema should be disregarded.

The definition of a positive tuberculin test result was recently revised by the American Thoracic Society and Centers for Disease Control, using three cutoff values for positive tests:

1. Household or close contacts of an active case, persons with a clinical suspicion of tuberculosis, and anyone with HIV infection should be considered positive when 5 mm of induration or more is present.
2. A reaction of 10 mm of induration or more is considered positive in other persons with additional risk factors for tuberculosis not in the above-mentioned risk groups. These include foreign-born persons from high-prevalence countries, injection drug users, homeless persons, residents of nursing homes and correctional institutions, and persons with other medical conditions associated with a risk of tuberculosis (discussed below under Isoniazid Preventive Therapy).
3. In the remainder of the population, a positive reaction is defined as 15 mm of induration or more, minimizing false-positive results.

Conversion from a negative to positive result signifies a high risk of developing active disease. Tuberculin conversion is defined for persons younger than 35 years as an increase in induration of at least 10 mm to a reading of 10 mm or more within a 2-year period. In persons older than 35 years, a 15-mm increase to a reading of 15 mm of induration or more within a 2-year period defines a tuberculin converter.

Because of the *booster phenomenon,* a two-step tuberculin skin testing protocol is recommended for persons who will undergo serial tuberculin skin tests. This phenomenon reflects the recall of waned immunity, and is defined operationally as a positive reaction to a second skin test given after an initial test was negative. Boosting occurs in all age groups but increases substantially in persons older than 55 years. In persons undergoing serial tuberculin tests, the increase in the size of the reactive induration with repeat testing may be interpreted as a conversion and lead to unnecessary preventive therapy with isoniazid (INH); establishing true reactivity with two-step testing can prevent this. In the two-step protocol, the first test is read 7 days after application; a second test is applied on day 7 if there is less than 10 mm of induration, and the second test is then read at 2 to 3 days. This strategy maximizes the proportion of positive tests on initial evaluation. A comparison of day 2 and day 7 readings of tuberculin tests showed that the yield of positive tests was similar for each reading, with over 80% of positive tests on day 2 remaining positive on day 7. Thus, there is no need to have a tuberculin test read in an emergency room because of weekends or holidays.

Ambulatory patients with clinical tuberculosis have a positive tuberculin skin test at least 95% of the time at diagnosis, but false-negative results can occur. Any person with a recent infection with *Myobacterium tuberculosis* may have a negative result at the initial evaluation; a repeat test is indicated 6 to 12 weeks later. Between 17 and 24% of hospitalized patients with clinical tuberculosis will have negative tuberculin tests. In most cases, positive skin tests occur 2 weeks after the patients start antituberculosis therapy and improve their nutritional status. False-negative tuberculin tests may also occur up to 6 weeks after the administration of live viral vaccines, and with immunosuppressive therapy or diseases affecting the lymphoid tissue. The rate of false-negative results among persons infected with HIV depends on the severity of immunosuppression. Most persons with asymptomatic HIV infection and tuberculosis will have a positive tuberculin test.

A history of *bacille Calmette-Guérin* (BCG) vaccination should be ignored in interpreting skin test results. After BCG vaccination, tuberculin reactivity wanes at a rate of about 10% per year, unless repeated doses of BCG (or tuberculin) are administered. Most patients in the United States with a history of BCG vaccination are from areas of the world with a high prevalence of tuberculosis. Hence, a positive tuberculin test is more likely to be due to *M. tuberculosis* infection than to BCG.

Isoniazid Preventive Therapy

The American Thoracic Society and the Centers for Disease Control recommend INH preventive therapy (IPT) in the following categories of individuals, in order of priority:

Persons with positive (≥ 5 mm) on the purified protein derivative (PPD) test and HIV infection regardless of age. The lifetime risk of developing tuberculosis disease among HIV-infected persons with positive PPD results is estimated to be at least 30%.

Household and other close contacts of potentially infectious cases of pulmonary tuberculosis regardless of age or tuberculin status. Household contacts of an active case have a 2 to 5% likelihood of developing active tuberculosis in the first year.

Newly infected persons or documented converters on the tuberculin skin test regardless of age. Such persons have a 3 to 5% risk of active tuberculosis in the first year.

Persons with positive PPD (≥ 5 mm) and an abnormal chest radiograph without active tuberculosis. They have a 1 to 4.5% risk of active tuberculosis in the first year. Isolated calcified granulomas do not increase the risk of reactivation.

Persons with a positive PPD (≥ 10 mm) and medical conditions reported to increase the risk of tuberculosis. These include silicosis, prolonged therapy with corticosteroids (equivalent of ≥ 20 mg of prednisone for at least 1 month), immunosuppressive therapy of other types, malignancies, chronic renal failure, weight of 10% or more below ideal body weight, insulin-requiring diabetes mellitus, jejunoileal bypass, gastrectomy, and pregnancy (wait until after delivery to administer INH).

Tuberculin reactors (≥ 15 mm) younger than 35 years with no other risk factors. Adults with a positive PPD but normal chest radiographs have a risk of 0.1% per year of developing active tuberculosis. This risk is cumulative over the person's lifetime. The cutoff point of 35 years old for preventive treatment is based on the negligible risk of hepatitis from INH under this age.

Effectiveness

Strong evidence supports the use of IPT in high-risk settings. Randomized, placebo-controlled, blinded clinical trials consistently indicate a 70% reduction in the number of cases of tuberculosis over 3 to 5 years of follow-up. Subjects included household contacts, schoolchildren, institutionalized persons, and poor populations. A randomized controlled trial in 28,000 participants with inactive pulmonary tuberculosis confirmed the benefit of IPT in preventing active tuberculosis over a follow-up of 5 years. Patients were randomized to one of four treatment regimens with the following results:

	TUBERCULOSIS CASES (NO.)	REDUCTION (%)
Placebo	97	0
3 months of INH	76	21
6 months of INH	34	65
12 months of INH	24	75

Persons with any radiographic abnormalities less than 2 cm^2 did equally well with 6 or 12 months of IPT.

Cost-benefit analyses demonstrate that 6 months of IPT is the optimal strategy for individuals with a normal chest film and no other risk factors. Thus, in persons with normal chest films or in household contacts of an index patient receiving 6- or 9-month chemotherapy regimens, a 6- or 9-month duration of IPT is recommended. Patients with abnormal chest films or with HIV infection should receive a full 12 months of IPT to maximize benefit.

Risks of Isoniazid
Elevations of serum aminotransferases (transaminases), aspartate aminotransferase (AST; SGOT) or alanine aminotransferase (ALT; SGPT), occur in 10 to 20% of persons taking INH. Clinical hepatitis is infrequent and is directly related to an increase in age:

AGE (YR)	HEPATITIS RISK
< 20	Rare
20–34	Up to 0.3%
35–49	Up to 1.2%
50–64	Up to 2.3%
≥ 65	Up to 5.0%

The risk of hepatitis was also related to alcohol intake, occurring in 0.64% of nondrinkers, 1.08% of occasional drinkers, and 2.65% of daily drinkers. However, persons who abuse alcohol are also at an increased risk of tuberculosis, and this should not be used as a reason not to recommend INH. The presence of chronic liver disease probably increases the risk of INH-related hepatitis as well.

Peripheral neuropathy occurs in less than 1% and is preventable with pyridoxine (vitamin B$_6$) supplements of 10 to 25 mg/day. Pyridoxine should be given to persons older than 65 years, pregnant women, diabetics, alcoholics, patients with chronic renal failure, poorly nourished persons, and anyone with any other predisposition to peripheral neuropathy.

Other side effects from INH include vague and minor difficulties with concentration that can almost always be avoided by administering the dose at night. Dizziness and occasional gastrointestinal upset are reported. INH interferes with the metabolism of phenytoin and disulfiram, leading to an increase in the serum levels of these drugs; their doses should be appropriately adjusted.

Managing the Patient on Isoniazid Prophylaxis
Before beginning IPT in a person with a reactive tuberculin test, active tuberculosis should be ruled out by a chest radiograph. If radiographic abnormalities more extensive than granulomas are present, active disease should be ruled out with sputum cultures. Chest films that do not change for at least 1 year would also be evidence for inactive disease, but, if in doubt, sputum specimens should be obtained.

INH is administered in a daily dose of 300 mg. Symptoms should be monitored in person or by telephone at *monthly* intervals. Baseline liver function tests are not recommended for individuals younger than 35 years unless there is a history of excessive alcohol use or liver disease. Baseline and periodic testing of AST (SGOT) levels during the course of IPT should be done in older persons. Asymptomatic persons with an AST level above 250 IU (approximately 5 times the upper limits of normal) or with a threefold increase over an elevated baseline should discontinue INH. In addition, any symptom compatible with hepatitis that is not readily explained by a transient illness mandates a temporary cessation of INH. If the AST level is normal, then INH can be restarted. If the AST is elevated in the presence of symptoms, INH should be stopped. Most reported deaths from INH-related hepatitis have occurred when the patients were continued on the drug through the jaundice stage.

Standard Therapy

Pulmonary tuberculosis usually presents with productive cough of more than 3 weeks' duration, fatigue, loss of appetite and weight, fever, and occasionally hemoptysis. Up to 20% of ambulatory patients with tuberculosis are asymptomatic. Persons with HIV infec-

Table 118-1. Drugs used for the treatment of tuberculosis

Drug	Daily dose	Activity	Adverse effects
First-line antituberculosis drugs			
Isoniazid (INH)	5 mg/kg up to 300 mg	Bactericidal; penetrates all body fluids and cavities	Hepatitis, neuropathy, hypersensitivity, CNS, acne
Rifampin (RIF)	10 mg/kg up to 600 mg	Bactericidal	GI upset, induces microsomal enzymes, orange body fluids, fever, purpura, hepatitis
Pyrazinamide (PZA)	15–30 mg/kg	Bactericidal in acid environment	Hepatitis, gout, GI upset, rash
Ethambutol (EMB)	15 mg/kg	Bacteriostatic	Retrobulbar neuritis, rash, gout
Streptomycin	15 mg/kg IM	Bactericidal	Vertigo, hearing loss, renal toxicity
Ciprofloxacin	500 mg PO bid	Bactericidal	GI upset, rash, contraindicated in pregnancy
Second-line antituberculosis drugs			
Para-aminosalicylic acid (PAS)	150 mg/kg	Bacteriostatic	Hypersensitivity, GI upset
Ethionamide	15–20 mg/kg	Bactericidal	Hepatitis, GI upset
Cycloserine	15–20 mg/kg	Bacteriostatic	Headache, depression, psychosis, seizures
Kanamycin	15–30 mg/kg IM	Bactericidal	Renal toxicity
Capreomycin	15–30 mg/kg IM	Bactericidal	Renal toxicity

tion are more likely to present with extrapulmonary tuberculosis (40% compared to 15%) with unusual manifestations.

Principles of Therapy
Multiple drugs (Table 118-1) must be included in the regimen from the start.
Organisms must be susceptible to the drugs used.
Bacteriologic response should occur within the expected time.
A single drug should never be added to a failing regimen.
Drug treatment must continue for a sufficient period of time.
The promotion and monitoring of compliance are essential.

Short-Course Chemotherapy Regimens
Short-course chemotherapy regimens using INH and rifampin for 6 to 9 months are as effective as longer courses of treatment. The choice of drugs to use in short-course chemotherapy for tuberculosis is based on treating distinct subpopulations of tubercle bacilli. First, the rapidly dividing subpopulation of extracellular organisms is readily killed by INH, rifampin, and streptomycin, when given in bactericidal doses. A second subpopulation of organisms is thought to exist in solid caseous material, generally growing slowly, but with spurts of metabolic activity. Rifampin seems to be the most effective drug in

killing these intermittently growing organisms. The third group of organisms is postulated to exist within the acidic environment of macrophages. It is assumed that the efficacy of pyrazinamide, which is active in an acid environment, results from its ability to kill these intracellular organisms.

The use of combinations of antituberculosis drugs in short-course chemotherapy should be guided by the following generalizations: A minimum duration of 6 months of therapy is necessary to achieve low relapse and failure rates. INH should be used for the full duration of any treatment regimen unless there are specific reasons, such as adverse effects or bacterial resistance, to exclude it. Rifampin is an essential drug for any regimen of less than 12 months. Pyrazinamide given in the initial 2 months improves the efficacy of 6-month regimens. There are no additional benefits to continuing pyrazinamide beyond the initial 2 months in regimens containing both INH and rifampin. Ethambutol, in doses usually given, is not as effective as pyrazinamide when given in the initial phase. After an initial daily phase of treatment, twice-weekly administration of appropriately adjusted doses of drugs is as effective as daily administration and may increase adherence. Directly observed outpatient treatment also improves adherence. Hospitalization is not necessary unless indicated for other reasons.

Current American Thoracic Society and Centers for Disease Control recommendations for standard therapy of tuberculosis offer two major alternatives:

9 months of INH and rifampin (with or without ethambutol). The bacteriologic relapse rate after 12 to 120 months of follow-up is only 1.9%.

6 months of INH and rifampin, supplemented by pyrazinamide (with or without ethambutol or streptomycin) for the first 2 months. This is as equally effective as the 9-month regimen, but the rate of adherence is higher. The bacteriologic relapse rate after 12 to 48 months of follow-up is only 1.6%.

In both regimens, the intermittent administration (after 2–4 weeks of daily therapy) of appropriate doses has comparable results to daily treatment throughout.

Treatment of tuberculosis in HIV-infected patients should be continued for a minimum of 9 months and for at least 6 months beyond the time of documented culture conversion as evidenced by three negative cultures.

Drug resistance leads to much lower success rates. If drug resistance is suspected, at least three drugs should be used in the initial phase of treatment. The percentage of *M. tuberculosis* cultures with primary drug resistance has decreased over the past decade to between 3 and 5% for INH and streptomycin; it is much lower for other agents. Drug resistance is more prevalent in certain situations. In the United States, primary drug resistance rates vary by ethnic group: Asians, 14.8%; Latinos, 11.8%; blacks, 6.1%; whites, 4.9%; and Native American, 4.1%. Moreover, in the developing world the reported rates of resistance to INH or streptomycin are often above 20% and occasionally in excess of 50%. Thus, immigrants from a developing country should be assumed to have INH-resistant disease until proved otherwise.

If patients with INH-resistant organisms are treated with INH and rifampin alone, they are likely to develop resistance to rifampin within several weeks after therapy was started. If the prevalence of INH resistance is more than 5% (or perhaps under any circumstances), treatment should be started with three or four drugs (including INH). Previously treated individuals should be assumed to have drug resistance until proved otherwise. Persons treated previously with regimens that did not contain both INH and rifampin are much more likely to have drug-resistant organisms on recurrence. Individual regimens for patients with drug-resistant tuberculosis should contain at least two agents that the patient has not received previously. For such patients, consultation should be obtained from the local or state health department or from a physician experienced in treating drug-resistant tuberculosis. In contrast, persons who relapse after apparently successful treatment with an INH-rifampin regimen generally have fully sensitive organisms and can be re-treated with the same regimen.

Evaluation After Starting Antituberculosis Chemotherapy
Considerable improvement or a resolution of symptoms is expected within the first month of effective chemotherapy. In patients who presented with positive sputum cultures, repeat cultures should be obtained at *monthly* intervals until sputum conversion is documented.

Patients are considered noninfectious after 2 weeks of therapy. After 3 months of treatment, more than 90% of such patients should convert to negative cultures. Failure to convert the sputum generally means either the organisms are resistant to the agents being used or the patient is not taking the drugs. Long-term follow-up sputum cultures are not needed if bacteriologic conversion is demonstrated and the patient has had a favorable clinical outcome. A chest radiograph at 3 months is optional and one at the completion of treatment is desirable (assuming there are no clinical changes necessitating a new film).

Rieder HL, et al. Tuberculosis in the United States. JAMA 1989; 262:385–9.
A state-of-the-art review of tuberculosis epidemiology from the Centers for Disease Control. Develops the concept that tuberculosis is a disease limited to high-risk groups and amenable to targeted treatment efforts.

American Thoracic Society/Centers for Disease Control. Diagnostic standards and classification of tuberculosis. Am Rev Respir Dis 1990; 142:725–35.
Revision of these groups' statement summarizing the data and expert opinion on the transmission and pathogenesis of tuberculosis, diagnostic mycobacteriology, and use of the tuberculin skin test.

Centers for Disease Control. Screening for tuberculosis and tuberculous infection in high-risk populations; and the use of preventive therapy for tuberculous infection in the United States: recommendations of the Advisory Committee for the Elimination of Tuberculosis. MMWR 1990; 39:1–12.
Report outlining strategies that will lead to the elimination of tuberculosis. Primary care clinicians should emphasize screening and recommend preventive therapy in high-risk/ prevalence groups.

Slutkin G, Pérez-Stable EJ, Hopewell PC. Time course and boosting of tuberculin reactions in nursing home residents. Am Rev Respir Dis 1986; 134:1048–51.
Evaluation of the two-step strategy for placing and reading tuberculin skin tests, showing that there were similar proportions of positive readings on day 2 and day 7. PPD test results can be read up to 7 days after placement.

Thompson NJ, et al. The booster phenomenon in serial tuberculin testing. Am Rev Respir Dis 1979; 119:587–97.
Study conducted by the Centers for Disease Control to help define the booster phenomenon; it occurred at all ages studied but increased with age.

Ferebee SH. Controlled chemoprophylaxis trials in tuberculosis: a general review. Adv Tuberc Res 1970; 17:28–106.
A scholarly and comprehensive review of INH trials conducted during the first two decades of tuberculosis chemotherapy. A classic.

IUAT Committee on Prophylaxis. Efficacy of various durations of isoniazid prevention therapy for tuberculosis: five years of follow-up in the IUAT trial. Bull WHO 1982; 60:555–64.
Placebo-controlled trial evaluating the efficacy of INH in preventing pulmonary tuberculosis in patients with abnormal chest films. Compared to placebo, 12 months of INH resulted in a 75% reduction in the number of cases at 5 years.

Kopanoff DE, Snider DE, Caras GJ. Isoniazid-related hepatitis: a US Public Health Service cooperative surveillance study. Am Rev Respir Dis 1978; 117:991–1001.
Study quantifying the risk of INH-related hepatitis in asymptomatic adults, with increasing age and daily alcohol use as major risk factors.

Stead WW, et al. Benefit-risk considerations in preventive treatment for tuberculosis in elderly persons. Ann Intern Med 1987; 107:843–5.
Review of the usefulness of tuberculin skin testing and benefits of INH preventive therapy in elderly persons. If the indications are appropriate, age should not be used as a reason not to administer INH in elderly persons.

American Thoracic Society/Centers for Disease Control. Treatment of tuberculosis and tuberculosis infection in adults and children. Am Rev Respir Dis 1986; 134:355–63.
These groups' official statement on standard therapy.

Centers for Disease Control. Tuberculosis and human immunodeficiency virus infection: recommendations of the Advisory Committee for the Elimination of Tuberculosis (ACET). MMWR 1989; 38:236–50.
Emphasis on the high risk of active tuberculosis with coincident HIV infection makes identification and early INH therapy a public health priority.

Combs DL, O'Brien RJ, Geiter LJ. USPHS tuberculosis short-course chemotherapy trial 21: effectiveness, toxicity, and acceptability: the report of final results. Ann Intern Med 1990; 112:397–406.
Clinical trial comparing 9 months of INH and rifampin to 6 months of INH and rifampin supplemented by 2 months of pyrizinamide at the start. Confirms that both regimens have equal efficacy, but there are fewer adverse reactions and there is better adherence with the 6-month regimen.

Dutt AK, Moers D, Stead WW. Smear-negative, culture-positive pulmonary tuberculosis: six-month chemotherapy with isoniazid and rifampin. Am Rev Respir Dis 1990; 141:1232–5.
Patients with radiographic abnormalities consistent with pulmonary tuberculosis and negative smears and cultures for tuberculosis had excellent results with 6 months of INH and rifampin alone.

119. VIRAL HEPATITIS
Terrie Mendelson and Bernard Lo

It is important to distinguish among the several viruses that cause acute viral hepatitis because of the differences in prognosis for patients and indications for prophylactic treatment of contacts.

Hepatitis A, formerly called infectious hepatitis, is spread by fecal-oral transmission. Fecal excretion of the virus starts about 2 weeks before the onset of jaundice and usually ceases by the second week of illness. Hepatitis A is not spread by blood or other body secretions. Transmission is usually person to person and sporadic; however, common-source outbreaks that are traceable to contaminated water or food and to day-care centers caring for children in diapers can occur. Sexually active male homosexuals are at increased risk. The illness is self-limited and there is no resulting carrier state or chronic liver disease. In the United States, approximately 50% of middle-aged people from a middle-class background have serologic evidence of prior hepatitis A infection.

Hepatitis B, formerly called serum hepatitis, is transmitted by blood, other secretions, and contaminated needles and from mother to infant. It is additionally distinguished from hepatitis A by an asymptomatic carrier state and potential sequelae, including chronic persistent or chronic active hepatitis, cirrhosis, and hepatocellular carcinoma. Groups at increased risk for hepatitis B are shown in Table 119-1.

Hepatitis C, caused by a recently discovered RNA virus, is responsible for many cases of what was formerly termed *non-A, non-B hepatitis*. This virus is now recognized to account for up to 90% of cases of posttransfusion hepatitis and approximately 40% of sporadic non-A, non-B hepatitis. Hepatitis C also appears to be responsible for a large proportion of cases of nonalcoholic chronic liver disease; anti–hepatitis C antibodies (anti-HCV) have been found in the serum of 82% of patients with cryptogenic cirrhosis and 27% of patients in Los Angeles with hepatocellular carcinoma. Antibody to the virus has been demonstrated in 42% of injection drug users, making this population an important reservoir of infection. Unlike hepatitis A and B, the incubation period for hepatitis C is not dose-related; symptoms similar to those of hepatitis B may occur 4 days to 8 weeks follow-

Table 119-1. Groups at risk for hepatitis B virus (HBV) infection

	Prevalence of serologic markers of HBV infection	
	HB_sAg (%)	All markers (%)
High risk		
Immigrants/refugees from areas of high HBV endemicity	13	70–85
Users of parenteral drugs	7	60–80
Homosexually active males	6	35–80
Household contacts of HBV carriers	3–6	30–60
Patients in hemodialysis units	3–10	20–80
Intermediate risk		
Prisoners (male)	1–8	10–80
Health care workers with frequent blood contact	1–2	15–30
Low risk		
Health care workers without frequent blood contact	0.3	3–10
Healthy adults (first-time volunteer blood donors)	0.1	3–5

ing infection. Transmission of this disease, as for hepatitis B, is person to person via intimate or sexual contact or an exchange of blood.

Hepatitis D, or delta hepatitis, is caused by a defective RNA virus that occurs only in association with hepatitis B. Though it may produce typical viral hepatitis, which is clinically indistinguishable from acute hepatitis A, B, or C, it is frequently responsible for the cases of fulminant hepatitis among persons who are chronically or acutely infected with hepatitis B. Mortality rates in such patients approach 75%, and a failure of supportive medical therapy may necessitate emergent liver transplantation. The prevalence of antibody to hepatitis D shows no relation to gender, race, or geographic location within the United States, but is increased in injection drug users and in those homosexually active men with large numbers of sex partners. Its mode of transmission appears to parallel that of hepatitis B. Hepatitis D is principally important for its role in exacerbating hepatitis B infection.

Hepatitis E virus, which has been demonstrated but not yet isolated, appears to cause a sporadic, rapidly resolving, enterically transmitted form of *non-A, non-B hepatitis*.

Diagnosis

Clinical Evaluation
The history and physical examination help establish the cause and severity of the illness. The classic presentation of acute viral hepatitis is malaise, followed by anorexia, nausea, and right-upper-quadrant discomfort. Jaundice and dark urine are findings in icteric patients. The spectrum of disease ranges from asymptomatic and anicteric infections to fulminant hepatitis with coma and death.

History should include drug use (prescribed, illicit, over-the-counter, and injection) as well as transfusions and contact with hepatitis patients. Hepatitis A tends to have a more acute, influenza-like onset and a milder clinical course. Prodromal symptoms of serum sickness (fever, rash, and arthritis) preceding jaundice suggest hepatitis B. The finding of elevated hepatic transaminase levels following transfusion is characteristic of hepatitis C. Development of acute or fulminant hepatitis in a carrier of hepatitis B suggests hepatitis D.

Nonviral causes of acute hepatitis must be considered in the differential diagnosis: alcohol, drugs (aspirin, acetaminophen, isoniazid, rifampin, methyldopa, phenytoin, and halothane), toxins (paraquat, *Amanita* mushrooms), and infectious (syphilis, bacterial sepsis, leptospirosis, and Q fever).

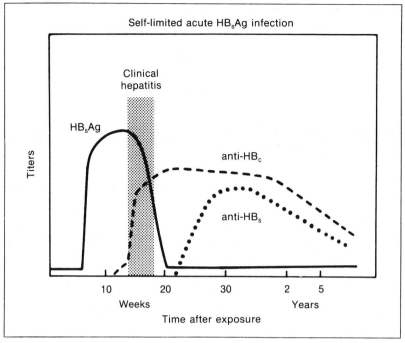

Fig. 119-1. Time course for the appearance of hepatitis B abnormalities.

Laboratory Evaluation

Liver function tests show 20- to 50-fold elevations of aminotransferases (transaminases) but only moderate increases in alkaline phosphatase levels. The elevations of bilirubin are variable; many patients are anicteric, with a bilirubin below 2.5 mg/dl. The degree of elevation of these liver enzymes is not indicative of disease severity. A better indicator is an abnormal prothrombin time that is not corrected by vitamin K; this finding reflects an impaired hepatic synthesis of clotting factors. The hemoglobin and leukocyte count are usually normal.

Serologic tests are necessary to establish the specific agent responsible for viral hepatitis. IgM anti–hepatitis A virus antibody (anti-HAV) is detectable at the time of clinical illness and is specific for acute hepatitis A. However, IgG anti-HAV is not helpful in the diagnosis of acute infection because it persists for years and may be present from a previous infection.

Serologic tests for hepatitis B include hepatitis B surface antigen (HB_sAg), hepatitis B surface antibody (anti-HB_s), hepatitis B core antibody (anti-HB_c), and e antigen (HB_eAg). The time course of appearance of these abnormalities is illustrated in Figure 119-1.

HB_sAg is the earliest and most useful marker. In 10% of instances, however, it is never detectable, and in others, it disappears before the patient visits the physician. Moreover, HB_sAg is not specific for acute hepatitis and may denote chronic rather than acute infection.

Anti-HB_c is found in patients with acute, chronic, or previous infection. IgM anti-HB_c may become a reliable test that is specific for acute infection. Unlike anti-HB_s, anti-HB_c does not confer immunity.

The presence of HB_sAb indicates immunity to infection from hepatitis B, although a few cases of infection in patients with HB_sAb have been reported. Such rare patients may have very low titers of HB_sAb, a falsely positive test for HB_sAb, or infection with a different subtype of HB_sAg.

HB_eAg is found only in patients who are positive for HB_sAg. In chronic carriers, patients

Table 119-2. Serologic tests for acute viral hepatitis

HB$_s$Ag	IgM anti-HAV	Etiology
−	+	Acute hepatitis A
+	+	Acute hepatitis A in chronic hepatitis B carrier
+	−	Acute hepatitis B or acute non-A, non-B hepatitis in chronic hepatitis B carrier[a]
−	−	Acute hepatitis B or acute non-A, non-B hepatitis[b]

[a] Anti-HB$_c$ would not be useful in distinguishing these possibilities.
[b] Anti-HB$_c$ would distinguish these possibilities; it is positive in acute hepatitis B when HB$_s$Ag is negative, and it is negative in non-A, non-B hepatitis.

with chronic HB$_s$Ag hepatitis, and HB$_s$Ag-positive "needlestick donors," its presence indicates greater infectivity.

An enzyme-linked immunosorbent assay (ELISA) for anti-HCV was released in May of 1990. This serologic test has already gained widespread use in blood banks, where it is expected to identify the approximately 1.2% of asymptomatic donors who are infected with hepatitis C. "Surrogate markers" for non-A, non-B hepatitis that were previously used included anti-HB$_c$Ab and elevated alanine aminotransferase (ALT; SGPT) levels; these detected only 50% of infected donors. It has been estimated that 64.7% of chronic, post-transfusion non-A, non-B hepatitis could be prevented through the widespread screening of blood donors for hepatitis C. The newly-developed anti-HCV assay has limited usefulness in diagnosing acute hepatitis C infection, as the average time required for the development of detectable antibody is 22 weeks.

A serologic test is also available for detecting antibody to the hepatitis D virus. Indications for its use are primarily epidemiologic, as it occurs only in association with HB$_s$Ag and its detection does not change either the treatment or the prognosis of the illness.

No serologic test is yet available for the putative hepatitis E virus.

Routinely ordering a complete panel of serologic tests for diagnosing acute hepatitis is costly and unnecessary. In most instances, IgM anti-HAV and HB$_s$Ag tests are sufficient (Table 119-2). In a few cases, serologic tests do not distinguish acute from chronic hepatitis B infection.

Management of Acute Hepatitis

The treatment of all forms of acute hepatitis involves supportive care and avoidance of potential hepatotoxins. For most patients, the disease is self-limited and can be managed on an outpatient basis. Indications for hospitalization are an inability to maintain adequate oral intake, insufficient care at home, and fulminant hepatitis (often manifested by encephalopathy, hypoglycemia, and coagulopathy). Activities should be limited primarily by patient symptoms; enforced bed rest in young, otherwise healthy patients has been shown not to be helpful. Alcohol and drugs that are not essential are usually discontinued because of the fear of additional, drug-induced hepatic damage. However, there is no definitive evidence establishing such comorbidity. Similarly, there is no evidence that special diets alter the course of the disease.

No medications have been shown to alter the course of acute viral hepatitis. Controlled trials have shown corticosteroids to be of no benefit; they may indeed be detrimental in patients who are Hb$_s$Ag-positive. Vitamin K may correct a prolonged prothrombin time. Sedatives are contraindicated, especially in a patient with agitation or an altered mental status, because they can mask or precipitate fulminant hepatitis. If an antiemetic is considered, phenothiazines should be avoided because of the risk of cholestasis as an idiosyncratic reaction.

Fulminant hepatitis is treated with supportive intensive care, focusing on the management of hypoglycemia, electrolyte and acid-base disorders, encephalopathy, and antibiotic treatment of accompanying bacterial sepsis. Liver transplantation may be indicated for intractable cases without involvement of other major organ systems.

Liver biopsy is rarely indicated for patients with acute hepatitis. Occasionally it may be used to distinguish viral from alcoholic or drug-related hepatitis. Biopsy results do not alter the treatment, however, and histologic findings early in the course of acute viral hepatitis do not establish prognosis.

Serial evaluation of the patient is necessary to confirm clinical and biochemical resolution of the infection. In hepatitis B, 5 to 10% of patients remain positive for HB_sAg for longer than 6 months. In non-A, non-B hepatitis not related to transfusions, chronic liver disease is rare. Fluctuations in or worsening of the liver function test results are common during acute hepatitis C and do not necessarily signify chronic hepatitis. In some patients with chronic infection, liver biopsy may be indicated to provide prognostic information or to guide therapeutic decisions.

Management of Contacts

Household contacts of patients with hepatitis A are at risk; virus shedding has been documented for as long as 2 weeks after the appearance of jaundice, although in most instances it ceases at about 1 week. This risk can be reduced by careful hand-washing by the patient after defecation and by administering immune serum globulin (ISG) to household contacts. For adults, 2 ml of ISG administered intramuscularly reduces the incidence of hepatitis in contacts by 70%. Although many adults already have immunity to hepatitis A, screening is not recommended. ISG is inexpensive and safe; concerns about the potential for transmitting human immunodeficiency virus (HIV) or other viral infections through ISG have not been borne out in clinical or research experience.

ISG prophylaxis is not required after casual contact at school or work. It should, however, be considered in two special situations. In day-care centers, staff and children exposed to a child in diapers with hepatitis A may be given ISG. Also, because a food handler with hepatitis A may cause a common-source outbreak, ISG should be considered for patrons and other employees of a restaurant.

Because hepatitis B is spread by blood, saliva, and semen, intimate and sex contacts of the patient are at risk; casual contacts, however, such as colleagues at work, are not at risk. Kissing, sexual intercourse, and sharing eating utensils, razors, toothbrushes, and intravenous needles should be discontinued until the patient no longer has HB_sAg. In most patients, HB_sAg disappears by a few weeks after the resolution of clinical illness.

Hepatitis B immune globulin (HBIG), which contains high titers of anti-HB_s, may be effective prophylaxis for sex contacts. In one study, sex partners of HB_sAg-positive individuals were screened for the presence of anti-HB_s; those without detectable antibody titers were randomized to receive either ISG or HBIG. The incidence of clinical hepatitis in the partners who received HBIG was 4%, whereas 27% of partners treated with ISG developed clinical hepatitis. The same study found no benefit for household contacts treated with HBIG. Based on these limited data, the Centers for Disease Control (CDC) now recommends one 5-ml dose of HBIG for sex contacts of hepatitis B-infected individuals. HBIG is probaby ineffective if it is given later than 14 days after the last contact. Screening the contact for susceptibility by assaying for anti-HB_s is reasonable if the contact has a high likelihood for prior hepatitis B infection and if it will not delay the administration of HBIG. Homosexual male contacts should receive hepatitis B vaccine with HBIG. Heterosexual contacts should receive a second dose of HBIG if the index patient is still positive for HB_sAg 3 months later.

There is no effective prophylaxis against hepatitis C or D.

Management of HB_sAg Carriers

HB_sAg carriers comprise about 0.2% of the general population and up to 10% of the high-risk groups outlined in Table 119-1. The evaluation of carriers should include a careful history, physical examination, and liver function tests. Symptoms of liver disease (jaundice, malaise, anorexia, and weight loss) and a history of injection drug use or exposure to blood should be sought. If the findings of this evaluation are negative, liver biopsy is not indicated because it shows serious disease (chronic active hepatitis, cirrhosis, or hepatocellular carcinoma) in fewer than 5% of patients. Although a liver biopsy may give diagnostic or prognostic information, it unfortunately does not lead to effective therapy.

Sex and household contacts of HB_sAg carriers are at risk for developing hepatitis B. Carriers positive for HB_eAg are especially contagious; serologic evidence of infection develops in 78% of their sex contacts, compared to only 25% of contacts of patients who are

HB_eAg-negative. However, testing for HB_eAg is not clinically useful because patients who test negative may still be contagious. The presence of HB_eAg does not increase the risk for nonsexual household contacts.

HBIG is not effective prophylaxis for contacts of carriers because of its short-term effect. However, hepatitis B vaccine probably will prove effective.

Management of Chronic Hepatitis

The prognosis in patients with chronic active hepatitis B and C is poor: of patients with chronic hepatitis B who tested positive for antibody to the e antigen, 54% developed cirrhosis within 5 years in one large study. The demonstration that loss of hepatitis B viral replication is associated with remission from chronic disease has led to the search for immunomodulatory and other classes of drugs that might impair viral replication. Although corticosteroids have been used with moderate effect on active hepatic inflammation, they do not induce remission in the majority of patients. The best evidence to date for effective chemotherapy is for the use of interferon alfa; in several recent studies of chronic hepatitis B and non-A, non-B, approximately one-third of treated patients achieved clearance of detectable viral DNA at 3 to 6 months after treatment. The long-term benefit and risk for this still-investigational therapy are not yet known.

Prevention of Hepatitis B

Vaccine

Recombinant hepatitis B vaccine is over 90% effective in reducing subsequent hepatitis B in male homosexuals and in dialysis patients and staff. It will probably be shown to be effective for other high-risk groups: household contacts of chronic HB_sAg carriers, cancer patients, drug addicts, patients and staff in institutions for the mentally retarded, health care workers with frequent blood contact, and children of HB_sAg-positive mothers. Adults who are not in these high-risk groups do not require vaccination.

Vaccination is unnecessary in people who are immune (positive for anti-HB_s) or who are carriers of HB_sAg. Screening is cost-effective before vaccination when the expected prevalence of serologic markers and the attack rate are high, as in male homosexuals. The best screening test before vaccination is anti-HB_c, which identifies HB_sAg carriers as well as most previously infected persons.

Immunization requires three doses, with the second and third doses given after 1 and 6 months. Immediate side effects are no greater than with placebo. The long-term risks are unknown, but none have been detected in up to 10 years. Anti-HB_s is induced in over 90% of healthy recipients and persists for at least 5 years. Administration of the vaccine to unscreened patients appears safe, even when such patients are found to have been HB_sAg- or anti-HB_s-positive prior to vaccination.

Indications for vaccination and guidelines for screening undoubtedly will change as more information is available and as costs are reduced. The indications for hepatitis B vaccine are discussed further in Chapter 124.

Passive-Active Immunization

Giving both HBIG and vaccine induces both immediate and long-term protection against infection. The simultaneous administration of HBIG does not reduce the effectiveness of the vaccine. Studies on infants of mothers positive for HB_sAg have shown that passive-active immunization is 90% effective. Generalizing from these neonatal data, the CDC now recommends combined passive-active immunization for needlestick, ocular, or mucous-membrane exposure to HB_sAg-positive blood, even though no clinical studies of passive-active immunization have been carried out in these settings.

Needlestick Exposure

Accidental inoculation with the blood of hepatitis patients is a hazard for some health care workers. Because of cost, prophylaxis with HBIG or vaccine is given only when "donor" blood is proved to be positive for HB_sAg. Donors who have acute hepatitis or who are in the high-risk groups (see Table 119-1) should be tested for HB_sAg. A single dose of ISG may be given while waiting for the results. If the donor is positive for HB_sAg, one dose of HBIG and the first dose of vaccine are given to the recipient as soon as possible after exposure. The remaining two doses of vaccine are given as usual 1 and 6 months later. A second dose of HBIG is not necessary.

Alternatively, HBIG alone without vaccine can be given after exposure. The first dose of HBIG is given as soon as possible; a second dose is given 1 month later. In one study, HBIG reduced the incidence of abnormal serum aminotransferase levels from 5.9% to 1.4% in this setting.

If the "donor" is unlikely to be positive for HB_sAg (e.g., a hospitalized patient without liver disease), testing for HB_sAg and administering HBIG are not cost-effective and are not recommended. In such low-risk situations and in situations in which the "donor" cannot be identified, ISG is often given as prophylaxis, although there is no evidence that it is effective.

After needlestick exposures, health care workers should be counseled as well about the risk of human immunodeficiency virus (HIV).

Alexander GH, Williams R. Natural history and therapy of chronic hepatitis B virus infection. *Am J Med* 1988; 85:143–6.
Remission from chronic hepatitis B infection is associated with the loss of viral replication. Review of the available agents reveals that only interferon alfa has demonstrable benefit in up to one-third of treated patients.

Alter HJ, et al. Detection of antibody to hepatitis C virus in prospectively followed transfusion recipients with acute and chronic non-A, non-B hepatitis. *N Engl J Med* 1989; 321:1494–1500.
Assays were performed for antibody to hepatitis C virus in a group of patients with posttransfusion non-A, non-B hepatitis and in their blood donors. Hepatitis C virus was clearly established as the predominant agent for transfusion-associated non-A, non-B hepatitis. "Surrogate" assays for ALT and anti-HB_c would have detected only half the anti-HCV–positive donors identified in the transmission of hepatitis among this group.

Dienstag JL, et al. Hepatitis A virus infection: new insights from seroepidemiologic studies. *J Infect Dis* 1978; 137:328–40.
The article presents an epidemiologic and clinical review of hepatitis A.

Fattovich G, et al. Long-term follow-up of anti-HB_e-positive chronic active hepatitis B. *Hepatology* 1988; 8:1651–4.
Fifty-four percent of anti-HB_e–positive patients with chronic hepatitis B developed cirrhosis during a mean histologic follow-up period of 4.5 years, mainly in association with continuing hepatitis B virus replication or hepatitis D infection.

Hoofnagle JH. Serologic markers of hepatitis B virus infection. *Annu Rev Med* 1981; 32:1–11.
This is a concise review of hepatitis B serology.

Immune globulins for protection against viral hepatitis. *Ann Intern Med* 1982; 96:193–7.
Recommendations of the CDC for ISG are presented.

Lange WR, Cone EJ, Snyder FR. The association of hepatitis delta virus and hepatitis B virus in parenteral drug abusers. 1971 to 1972 and 1986 to 1987. *Arch Intern Med* 1990; 150:365–8.
Anti–hepatitis D seropositivity was widespread in parenteral drug abusers as early as 1971. Antibody prevalence was unrelated to gender, ethnicity, or geographic location but was positively associated with HB_sAg seropositivity.

Mulley AG, Silverstein MD, Dienstag JL. Indications for use of hepatitis B vaccine, based on cost-effectiveness analysis. *N Engl J Med* 1982; 307:644–52.
A decision analysis of different strategies for screening and vaccination for hepatitis B is presented.

Postexposure prophylaxis of hepatitis B. *Ann Intern Med* 1984; 101:351–4.
New recommendations for passive-active immunization after needlestick exposure and for HBIG in sex contacts of patients with acute hepatitis B are given.

Sanchez-Tapias JM, et al. Hepatitis C virus infection in patients with nonalcoholic liver disease. *Ann Intern Med* 1990; 112:921–4.
The prevalence of anti-HCV in 1495 asymptomatic blood donors was 1.2%. Anti-HCV was found in the serum of 82% of patients with cryptogenic liver disease, and was not present in patients with high-titer antinuclear antibodies.

Saracco G, et al. Serologic markers with fulminant hepatitis in persons positive for hepatitis B surface antigen. A worldwide epidemiologic and clinical survey. *Ann Intern Med* 1988; 108:380–3.
Among patients positive for HB_sAg with fulminant hepatitis, only 52% were attributed to hepatitis B infection alone in this worldwide study. Thirty percent of cases were caused by coinfection or superinfection with hepatitis D virus, and in 18.5% of cases, no obvious superimposed factor was found.

Seeff LB, Koff RS. Passive and active immunoprophylaxis of hepatitis B. *Gastroenterology* 1984; 86:958–81.
The authors present a recent, comprehensive, thoughtful review.

Yu MC, et al. Prevalence of hepatitis B and C viral markers in black and white patients with hepatocellular carcinoma in the United States. *J Natl Cancer Inst* 1990; 82: 1038–41.
In a Los Angeles study of patients with hepatocellular carcinoma, serologic markers for hepatitis B and C were obtained and compared with their prevalence in matched controls. The relative risk for hepatocellular carcinoma in patients testing positive for anti-HCV was 10.5; for patients with one or more markers for hepatitis B, 7.0; and a synergistic effect on risk was demonstrated.

XVII. ALLERGIC CONDITIONS

120. URTICARIA
Rebecca A. Silliman

Urticaria (hives) is an eruption of transient erythematous papules or wheals resulting from dilatation of small capillaries within the dermis and extravasation of fluid into the interstitium. The lesions are pruritic and worsened by scratching. Angioedema is a related condition in which the lesions are nonpruritic and involve deeper tissues, sometimes resulting in asymmetric swelling of a body region.

About 20% of the population experiences urticaria and/or angioedema at some time during life. The severity ranges from a single fleeting episode to a chronic recurring problem. There is overlap between the syndromes of acute and chronic urticaria, and the duration of the acute illness is variably defined between 6 weeks and 6 months depending on the source quoted. Urticaria and angioedema can occur together or separately, but since they are similar in treatment and prognosis, they are usually considered to be part of the same process.

Two syndromes can be confused with urticaria/angioedema but they have different mechanisms and clinical course. Hereditary angioneurotic edema is a rare entity characterized by recurrent episodes of angioedema, laryngeal edema, and colicky abdominal pain, frequently accompanied by a family history of sudden respiratory death. Urticarial vasculitis is an uncommon and incompletely understood syndrome with features of both urticaria and vasculitis, which should be considered in patients with atypical or chronic urticaria. It differs from urticaria in being nonpruritic, although it may cause a burning sensation. It usually persists for over 24 hours and may be associated with blisters, purpura, and pigmentary changes. Other features of immune complex disease may be present to a variable extent, including arthritis or arthralgias, hypocomplementemia, and glomerulonephritis.

Causes
Many different factors can cause urticaria or angioedema (Table 120-1). Hives are often due to an allergic reaction, but a variety of nonimmunologic factors can also induce them, including chemicals and drugs, bacteria, animal substances, physical agents, and stress. Cholinergic urticaria and dermatographism are common types of nonimmunologic urticaria. Cholinergic urticaria is triggered by emotion, heat, exercise, or temperature change and induced by acetylcholine. Dermatographism is an exaggerated response to cutaneous stimuli, in which hives result from relatively mild skin trauma such as scratching or pressure from tight clothing. With both immunologic and nonimmunologic mechanisms, mast cells and basophils are stimulated, resulting in the release of a variety of mediators. Regardless of mechanism, re-exposure may cause recurrence.

Urticaria usually appears within minutes of exposure to the offending agent, but its appearance may be delayed for more than 24 hours. Lesions should disappear within 24 hours of initial appearance; a longer duration suggests another pathogenetic mechanism.

Urticaria is enhanced by heat, fever, exercise, emotional stress, alcohol, hyperthyroidism, and menstrual/menopausal status. It may be worsened by aspirin as well as by drugs that cause degranulation of mast cells (e.g., morphine, codeine, guanidine, reserpine).

Diagnostic Approach
Evaluation of the patient with urticaria is guided by the following principles: (1) A successful search for etiology is most likely in the acute syndrome, (2) a history and physical examination will provide the most valuable information in this search, (3) symptomatic treatment will be virtually the same in all cases, and (4) the identification of an etiologic agent or an underlying disease can aid therapy.

Although in more than 90% of cases the cause for urticaria is never found, the causative agents most likely to be identified are new drug and food exposures. Penicillin is the major drug offender, but almost any drug can be implicated. Aspirin can both cause and exacerbate urticaria, particularly the chronic type, and is included in many combination drugs. A careful drug history should include over-the-counter medications. Remember also that penicillin may be present in trace amounts in a wide variety of dairy products. Nuts,

Table 120-1 Causes of urticaria and angioedema

Cause	Examples
Drugs	Penicillin, morphine, aspirin
Foods	Nuts, berries, shellfish, chocolate, tomatoes, cheese
Infections	*Streptococcus,* coxsackievirus, *Candida*
Inhalants	Pollens, dust
Penetrants	Cosmetics, animal dander and saliva
Insect bites and stings	Fleas, mites
Internal disease	Rheumatic fever, lymphoma, hypothyroidism
Genetic abnormalities	Vibratory angioedema, familial cold urticaria, hereditary angioneurotic edema
Complement activation	Henoch-Schönlein purpura, systemic lupus erythematosus
Psychological factors	Stress
Physical agents	Cholinergic urticaria, cold urticaria, pressure urticaria

fish, berries, eggs, shellfish, chocolate, tomatoes, and cheese are frequent food product offenders, as are additives such as dyes or benzoic acid and naturally occurring salicylates.

Several features of the urticarial lesions themselves can suggest the etiology. One- to 3-mm wheals, occasionally with satellite wheals and surrounding erythematous flares, are characteristics of cholinergic urticaria. Papular urticaria on the lower extremities of children frequently results from insect bites. Pruritic linear wheals suggest dermatographism. When the lesions are limited to exposed areas, light or cold may be to blame.

Often the etiology is not obvious from either historical data or the characteristics of the lesions. In an otherwise healthy patient, symptomatic therapy may be prescribed, and the search need not be pursued. When urticaria persists or recurs, the less frequent causes should be considered. These causes may not be obvious; for instance, inapparent infections such as tinea pedis or asymptomatic vaginal trichomoniasis have been implicated. In addition, the drug and food history should be reviewed again, since these are still the most likely etiologic agents.

With chronic symptoms, a more aggressive evaluation of diet is justified. Patients should be instructed to write down all foods eaten during the 24 hours prior to each attack. While ingestion often results in the development of lesions within minutes, attacks can occur as late as 24 hours after ingestion of the offending agents; exposure more remote than 24 hours is unlikely to be related. When symptoms are frequent or continuous, a short-term trial of a rigid elimination diet is warranted.

Laboratory evaluation should be based on clues elicited from the history and physical findings. When no such clues are found, tests may be employed to screen for common asymptomatic disease and as an aid in reassuring the patient. These tests might include a complete blood cell count to identify anemia, eosinophilia, or white cell count abnormalities and a urinalysis to look for cells or proteins. Other tests should be ordered to follow up clues elicited from the history, physical examination, or screening laboratory tests (e.g., stool examination for ova and parasites or cryofibrinogen levels). However, without evidence of a particular agent, further testing, including skin testing, is not useful. If urticarial vasculitis is suspected, suspicious lesions should be biopsied.

In some patients, urticaria will recur for more than 6 months and persist for as long as 10 years. Because of the annoying symptoms and the frequency of inadequate response to therapy, the physician may be tempted to undertake further laboratory investigation. However, the search for a cause in chronic urticaria is usually unsuccessful. A review of 236 patients at the Mayo Clinic found that the primary etiologic factor was either psychogenic (22%) or undetermined (70%) in 92% of patients.

Treatment

In those situations in which a specific etiologic agent is identified, avoidance is the most important intervention. Antihistamines and sympathomimetic drugs are the mainstay of therapy in both acute and chronic urticaria. Recurrences may be decreased by minimizing triggering or modifying factors such as psychological stress. Elimination of aspirin or aspirin-containing drugs may also help. Modulators of cutaneous vasodilation, such as alcohol, heat, or exertion, should be decreased when possible.

Sympathomimetic Drugs

Sympathomimetic drugs such as epinephrine and ephedrine are most useful in the treatment of acute or severe urticaria, particularly if it is associated with anaphylaxis. A recommended approach to the patient with acute urticaria is to administer subcutaneous epinephrine (0.2–0.5 ml of 1:1000 aqueous epinephrine) in conjunction with an oral antihistamine. This initial treatment should be followed by a long-acting subcutaneous epinephrine preparation (Sus-Phrine) or oral preparation (ephedrine) and an antihistamine for the ensuing 24 to 48 hours.

Antihistamines

Antihistamines are believed to benefit about 80% of patients. A wide variety of agents is available, but the choice of drug must be based on the duration of action, side effects, and costs, since controlled trials comparing efficacy are few. Hydroxyzine (Atarax or Vistaril) in dosages of 10 to 25 mg 4 times a day may have a more powerful antipruritic effect and more prolonged inhibition of the wheal flare response than other antihistamines. It has been reported to be superior in the treatment of dermatographism and, like cyproheptadine (Periactin), is especially effective in cholinergic urticaria. Other antihistamines commonly used include chlorpheniramine, 4 mg 4 times a day, and diphenhydramine (Benadryl), 25 to 50 mg 4 times a day. A new generation of antihistamines (e.g., terfenadine) with less central nervous system penetration has recently been introduced. These drugs hold considerable promise because of a demonstrated efficacy and a better side effect profile.

When faced with side effects or no response, it is advisable to switch from one class of antihistamines to another. Alternative antihistamines are listed by class in Table 20-1; note that cyproheptadine, a piperazine appropriate for use in urticaria, is not included in the table because it is used primarily for pruritus, and not in the treatment of rhinitis.

Corticosteroids

Corticosteroids are rarely indicated but may be helpful to control severe attacks and in the therapy of serum sickness, pressure urticaria, and complement-mediated urticaria with vasculitis. There are no controlled trials to support the use of steroids, and it is generally believed that they have no place in the treatment of other types of acute and chronic urticaria.

Mathews KP. Urticaria and angioedema. J Allergy Clin Immunol 1983; 72:1014.
A comprehensive review of pathophysiology, evaluation, and treatment.

Garmon WR. Urticarial vasculitis: report of a case and review of the literature. Arch Dermatol 1979; 115:76–80.
Case report and an extensive literature review, which place this entity in the continuum of immune complex disease.

Champion RH. Drug therapy of urticaria. Br Med J 1973; 4:730–2.
A succinct approach to drug therapy.

Guin JD. Treatment of urticaria. Med Clin North Am 1982; 66:831–49.
Reviews pathogenesis and patient evaluation as well as treatment.

Rhoades RB, et al. Suppression of histamine-induced pruritus by three antihistaminic drugs. J Allerg Clin Immunol 1975; 55:180–5.
A double-blind crossover study of diphenhydramine, cyproheptadine, and hydroxyzine. Hydroxyzine was superior in suppressing pruritus.

Burrall BA, Halpern GM, Huntly AC. Chronic urticaria. West J Med 1990; 152:268–76.
Discusses causes and control of chronic urticaria; notes that the cause is not identified in more than 75% of cases.

Grant JA, et al. Double-blind comparison of terfenadine, chlorpheniramine, and placebo in the treatment of chronic idiopathic urticaria. J Allergy Clin Immunol 1988; 81:574–9.
This randomized trial comparing terfenadine, chlorpheniramine, and placebo demonstrates the superiority of terfenadine in controlling symptoms, with fewer side effects.

121. "BEE" STINGS
Rebecca A. Silliman

Stings by members of the *Hymenoptera* order (honeybees, yellow jackets, wasps, hornets, and fire ants, to be referred to as "bees" throughout this chapter) are common, but fatal reactions to these stings are not. Forty to fifty such deaths are reported annually, although experts believe that the actual number is greater. These deaths, which follow systemic reactions to stings, are characterized by urticaria and/or angioedema, respiratory distress from laryngeal edema or bronchospasm, or anaphylaxis with shock. Abdominal pain and/or nausea may also be experienced. While the majority of systemic reactions occur in children, most deaths are in adults and often have been attributed to underlying cardiovascular disease.

Bee venoms contain a wide variety of pharmacologically active peptides and amines. Although the various venoms are similar in composition, there is no antigenic cross-reactivity between honeybee and vespid (yellow jacket, hornet, wasp) venoms. Individuals sensitive to honeybees are often not sensitive to the vespids, and vice versa. Within the vespid group there does appear to be some antigenic cross-reactivity, but the role of this in clinical sensitivity is not well documented.

Local Reactions

Nonallergic local reactions are characterized by pain, itching, and swelling at the sting site. The typical appearance is a central red sting site surrounded by a clear wheal, which extends into a red flare. Edema formation is variable.

Therapy is symptomatic. If the stinger is still in the skin, it should be carefully flicked away with a fingernail or removed with tweezers. Local application of cold compresses and calamine lotion may be soothing. An aspirin tablet rubbed on a moistened sting site will also provide pain relief, which will persist with repeated moistening. Meat tenderizer, if placed on the sting site early, may also lessen pain and itching through enzymatic degradation of the venom. A mild topical corticosteroid cream (e.g., 1% hydrocortisone) and/or oral antihistamines (e.g., diphenhydramine, 25–50 mg qid) help relieve itching. Patients should be reassured that they are not at increased risk for developing the more serious systemic reactions.

Predicting Systemic Reactions

The natural history of systemic reactions is variable and unpredictable. Patients with a history of a systemic reaction, therefore, pose diagnostic and therapeutic problems. The history of a previous systemic reaction does not predict future reactions, nor does the absence of such a history mean that one is less likely to have anaphylaxis in the future. Laboratory testing can also be misleading. In one study of patients with a history of systemic reaction to sting, only 40% of those with positive tests to venom had a systemic reaction when subsequently stung. Likewise, immunoglobulin E (IgE) antibody determinations (RAST testing) are associated with both 20% false-positive and 20% false-negative rates. Experience with the combination of these two tests (skin testing and IgE measurements) has been limited, although anaphylaxis has been observed in skin test–positive and IgE-negative patients. In vitro determination of human leukocyte histamine release is even less helpful. The test requires sophisticated equipment, and cells from 15% of insect-allergic patients will fail to release histamine when challenged with anti-IgE.

Thus the clinician cannot predict accurately who is at risk for future systemic reactions, either by history or by laboratory tests. In general, however, children who have had a systemic reaction tend to experience progressively less severe reactions and lose their sensitivity altogether, while adults are more likely to retain their sensitivity.

Preventing Systemic Reactions

Since systemic reactions of any degree can be quite terrifying, patients need education about the probability of future episodes, preventive strategies, and treatment.

Avoiding Stings

Avoiding stings is an important preventive measure and can be accomplished without significant restriction of activities. Yellow jackets cause most accidental stings because of their wide geographic distribution and because they build their nests in the ground. Wearing shoes helps protect against stings on the feet. Close-fitting clothing should be worn so that the insects cannot get to the skin. Dark-colored clothing attracts insects, but gray, white, or red materials do not. Also, shiny jewelry and scented perfume, soaps, and lotions should be avoided. Keeping garbage in containers with tight-fitting lids will deter bees. If a nest or hive is built in the vicinity of a patient's home, it should be removed, preferably by a professional exterminator. Lastly, an insect-sensitive person should drive with the car windows closed. If a bee becomes trapped in the car, the driver should stop and help the insect out using a cloth or handkerchief.

Treatment of Reactions

In addition to receiving these instructions, a sensitive person should be taught what to do if stung. The honeybee is the only member of the *Hymenoptera* order that leaves its stinger behind in the victim. A person stung by a honeybee should remove the stinger carefully because there still may be venom remaining in the venom sac. Squeezing the sac or leaving the stinger in place will force any residual venom into the skin.

Sting-sensitive patients (those who have experienced a systemic reaction) should receive a prescription for an emergency treatment kit (e.g., Ana-Kit, Hollister-Stier Laboratories). These kits contain a preloaded syringe of epinephrine and a chewable antihistamine. The kit insert should be carefully reviewed with patients to make sure that they understand how to administer the epinephrine. They also must recognize when the solution has become inactivated (it turns pink-brown) and needs replacement. Patients not on immunotherapy should be instructed to administer the epinephrine and seek immediate medical attention. Those on immunotherapy need not be seen by medical personnel unless the epinephrine fails to relieve bronchospasm, laryngeal edema, or hypotension. This will allow for more intensive therapy, including fluid replacement, additional epinephrine, and bronchodilators as necessary.

Immunotherapy

While the prevention of stings and the treatment of reactions is straightforward, the prevention of systemic reactions in a sting-sensitive person is not. The first decision is whom to treat. A general, though perhaps controversial, recommendation is that any patient who has had generalized urticaria, angioedema, bronchospasm, or anaphylactic shock should be skin-tested and treated with the appropriate immunotherapy. Initial testing and immunotherapy should be performed by an allergist, although continued therapy can easily by supervised by a generalist in collaboration with an allergist.

Skin-testing should be performed at least 4 to 6 weeks after a sting to avoid false-negative results. The aim is to determine specifically which hymenopteran caused a reaction. Whole-body extracts became widely used in the 1950s, and their efficacy was reported to be 90 to 95%. However, these studies were neither well designed nor well controlled. The occurrence of treatment failures plus in vitro evidence of an immunologic response to venom but not to whole-body extract led investigators at Johns Hopkins to conduct a small controlled trial comparing venom to whole-body extract and placebo. Venom therapy was found to be superior to both placebo and whole-body extract. The study has been criticized and results questioned because of methodologic weaknesses. However, it provides the best evidence to date. The Food and Drug Administration approved the use of venom immunotherapy in 1979, and it is now considered the treatment of choice. The Johns Hopkins group reports a 98% protection rate for sting-sensitive adults. Patients should be treated with the venom of the insects to which they are sensitive. As noted previously, patients sensitive to honeybees are usually not sensitive to the vespids. Within the vespid group, there may be some cross-reactivity resulting in multiple positive skin test results. Only those patients with both positive skin tests and a history of systemic reactions to different vespids (e.g., hornet and yellow jacket) should receive more than a single venom. For example, sensitivity to both hornets (yellow and white-faced) and yellow jackets is known to occur, and a mixed venom preparation that contains these three is commercially available.

Different dosing regimens have been advocated, with varying incidences of both local and systemic reactions. These rates are comparable to those experienced in other forms of immunotherapy (e.g., ragweed hay fever). Because an average sting contains about 50 µg of proteinaceous material, 100 µg has been empirically chosen as a maintenance dose. This should fully protect patients against at least two stings. Whether a smaller maintenance dose is as effective is not known. A recent study compared three different dosing frequencies and found no difference in rates of either local or systemic reactions. However, since the immunologic response was greater and the number of injections fewer with the more rapid regimen, the authors recommend a program of seven bimonthly injections beginning with 15 µg divided into two doses separated by 30 minutes. Every 2 weeks the dose is doubled until maintenance (100 µg) has been reached. A more conservative approach begins with 0.01 µg and increases to 100 µg over 6 to 8 weeks with two to three injections per weekly visit. In either case, dose increases are adjusted in response to reactions. After the maintenance level has been attained, hyposensitivity is maintained by injections every 1 to 2 months.

The optimal duration of therapy is unknown. However, the risks of chronic therapy appear to be minimal, based on findings in a study of beekeepers and their families who have long-term and repeated exposure to honeybee venom. Therapy has been discontinued in patients whose IgE levels have become undetectable, with untoward effects observed from future stings. Further investigations, however, are clearly necessary.

McLean DC. Insect sting allergy. Prim Care 1987; 14:513–21.
A practical approach for the primary care physician.

Golden DK, Schwartz HJ. Guidelines for venum immunotherapy. J Allergy Clin Immunol 1986; 77:727–8.
Guidelines for clinicians developed by the Committee on Insects of the American Academy of Allergy and Immunology.

Valentine MD. Insect venom allergy: diagnosis and treatment. J Allergy Clin Immunol 1984; 73:299–304.
An up-to-date review of the state of the art from the allergist's viewpoint.

Lichtenstein LM, Valentine MD, Sobotka AK. Insect allergy: the state of the art. J Allergy Clin Immunol 1979; 164:5–12.
An excellent treatment of the subject.

Reisman RE. Stinging insect allergy. J Allergy Clin Immunol 1979; 64:3–4.
A companion article to Lichtenstein (above), which stresses areas where important information is still lacking.

Rubenstein HS. Bee-sting diseases: Who is at risk? What is the treatment? Lancet 1982; 1:496–9.
A critical appraisal of systemic reaction risk and the evidence of immunotherapy efficacy. Many questions are raised but no solutions offered. Rubenstein does not feel that immunotherapy is justified.

Yunginger JW, et al. Immunological and biochemical studies in beekeepers and their families. J Allergy Clin Immunol 1978; 61:93–101.
A report of two cross-sectional studies of beekeepers and their families. Compared to controls, both beekeepers and family members had higher IgE antibody levels. However, no clinically significant hematologic, renal function, or blood chemistry abnormalities were found.

XVIII. HEALTH MAINTENANCE

122. PREVENTIVE CARE
Russell Harris

Preventive care may be more effective than intervening after disease is established. While current evidence does not support a preventive approach for all health problems, it is clear that attention to a limited prevention agenda could have a substantial effect on death and suffering from several conditions. Health problems may be prevented by four basic methods: screening tests to find disease at an early, treatable stage; modification of risk factors, usually by counseling and patient education; immunizations for infectious disease; and specific prophylaxis for some infectious and other diseases. The list of diseases that can be prevented in one of these ways is not long, but growing.

This chapter concludes with a table presenting a limited preventive agenda of screening tests, counseling, and immunizations. More detailed tables by age group are available in the guide prepared by the U.S. Preventive Services Task Force, which is listed in the references and also includes extensive discussions of preventive interventions for 60 different illnesses and conditions.

Screening

Although screening has been advocated for a number of conditions, only a few satisfy the three criteria for screening: (1) that the condition be an important cause of suffering or death, (2) that there be an effective treatment that has proved to be more effective for early than late disease, and (3) that the screening test be accurate (i.e., sensitive and specific) and acceptable to patients. Screening for conditions that meet these criteria, followed by appropriate intervention, is therefore a major priority of preventive care.

Cardiovascular Disease
Mortality from cardiovascular disease has fallen 40% since the late 1960s, simultaneous with a reduction of three risk factors: cigarette smoking, hypertension, and high blood cholesterol.

SMOKING. All patients should be screened regularly for cigarette smoking; reduction in the risk for cardiovascular disease occurs almost immediately after smoking cessation. Additional benefits and intervention techniques are discussed below, under counseling, and in Chapter 130.

HYPERTENSION. This should be screened for routinely at office visits, using a well-calibrated sphygmomanometer. Mild hypertension (diastolic pressure of 90–104 mm Hg) should not be diagnosed until at least three elevated pressures have been obtained over several weeks. A large benefit of treatment has been demonstrated for patients with moderate or severe hypertension (diastolic pressure $\geq$ 104 mm Hg), and all such patients should receive pharmacotherapy. The magnitude of the benefit of treating mild hypertension is smaller (primarily in reducing stroke) and must be weighed against the side effects of medications. These issues are discussed further in Chapter 25.

CHOLESTEROL. Reducing cholesterol levels can reduce the incidence and mortality of cardiovascular disease in asymptomatic middle-aged men (aged 30–64 years) with initial serum cholesterol levels above 250 to 260 mg/dl. Data are lacking for women, and for younger and older patients. However, since the incidence of coronary disease increases in postmenopausal women, approaching that of men about 10 years older, it seems reasonable, until new studies are reported, to extrapolate the findings in men to women in their 40s and 50s.

Thus, asymptomatic men 30 years or older, and women 40 years or older, should be screened every 5 years for high blood cholesterol. The presence of a strong family history of coronary disease or other cardiac risk factors (e.g., smoking, hypertension, diabetes) should prompt consideration of earlier screening. Dietary treatment should be instituted in patients with a serum cholesterol level of 260 mg/dl or higher on several determinations, or in patients with other risk factors who have a cholesterol level of at least 240 mg/dl. If after 6 months, dietary therapy has not succeeded in lowering cholesterol below these treatment thresholds, drug therapy should be considered. Some may wish to base therapy on further characterization of lipids into high-density lipoprotein (HDL) and low-density lipoprotein (LDL) (see Chap. 126).

The question of whether there should be an upper age limit for cholesterol screening is difficult to answer. Since large studies of cholesterol treatment have required 6 to 8 years of therapy before a benefit is realized, patients unlikely to live longer than 6 to 8 years, or for whom diet or drug therapy would present a significant burden, may not benefit from screening. (See Chap. 126.)

Cancer Screening

CERVICAL CANCER. Screening appropriate women with the Pap smear to find early, treatable lesions is effective in reducing mortality from cervical cancer. Although the death rate from cervical cancer has been declining for some years, an estimated 6000 women still died of this disease in 1990. Most deaths occur in women who have not had previous screening, and these women tend to be older, low income, and minority.

All sexually active women with an intact cervix should be screened with a Pap smear, except for women over the age of 65 years who have had multiple negative results. Priority should be given to women without previous negative results. Women who have had a hysterectomy that removed the cervix (for reasons other than previous cervical cancer) cannot get cervical cancer and need not be screened. Women who have not engaged in sexual intercourse at all, or who are not currently sexually active and have had several negative results on Pap smears, are also at essentially no risk. Women over 65 years old who have had consistently negative Pap smear results rarely develop invasive cervical cancer, so screening these women is not mandatory.

The optimal frequency of Pap smears has been debated. Screening every 3 years reduces the risk of invasive cervical cancer by more than 90%; there is only minimal additional benefit to more frequent screening. Some argue that the number of false-negative results (variously estimated at 0–20% of women with cervical pathology) dictates that Pap smears be done more frequently. Most false-negative results, however, are likely due to poor collection rather than interpretive errors. Thus, adequate training of physicians and nurses in Pap smear technique, and use of the cytobrush (which has been shown to obtain endocervical cells at a higher rate than the spatula), are better approaches to the problem of false-negative results than is increasing the frequency of testing.

BREAST CANCER. About 75% of all cases of breast cancer occur in women 50 years or older. There is good evidence that screening women aged 50 to 74 years with regular mammography and clinical breast examination (CBE) can decrease mortality from breast cancer by 30%. All women in this age group should be screened with mammography and CBE every 1 to 2 years. Women 75 years or older are at high risk for breast cancer and thus should also be considered for screening with CBE and mammography. Since the benefit begins to occur about 5 years after screening begins, women who are unlikely to live longer than 5 years need not be screened. Physiologically younger women, however, may benefit. (See also Chapter 131, for technique of clinical breast examination and other information.)

Although cancer occasionally occurs in women younger than 40 years, the overall risk in asymptomatic women is very low: Routine screening would likely do more harm than good in these women. Women in their 40s are in an intermediate-risk group: higher than women in their 30s but lower than women older than 50. Mammography is not as good a test in premenopausal women and has never been shown to save lives in women under 50 years old: Screening mammography need not be done routinely for women in their 40s, but may be reserved for those with a history of breast cancer in a mother, sister, or daughter. It is reasonable to carry out screening with CBE beginning at age 40.

A common error is to use mammography to determine whether women with breast lumps should be referred for biopsy. As the CBE often detects breast cancer invisible by mammography, a woman with a dominant lump should be referred, regardless of mammographic findings. (See Chap. 80.)

COLORECTAL CANCER. Colorectal cancer causes more deaths in the United States than any other cancer except lung cancer, and is curable if found early. The digital rectal examination can detect palpable lesions in the rectum, probably less than 10% of colorectal cancers. The two primary screening tests for colorectal cancer are, therefore, fecal occult blood testing and sigmoidoscopy. Unfortunately, at present it is not clear whether either of these tests is sensitive and specific enough to save lives from this disease. A reasonable policy to determine whether to screen for colorectal cancer should be based on individual risk and patient preferences. Major risk factors are increasing age (colorectal cancer is rare before age 40), a positive family history for colorectal cancer in a first-degree relative (increases risk by a factor of two to three), ulcerative colitis (which increases risk after 10 years of disease duration), and certain uncommon familial syndromes. For patients in one of these high-risk categories who are interested in screening, sigmoidoscopy every 3 to 5 years with or without annual fecal occult blood testing may be of benefit. Further information about screening for colon cancer is included in Chapter 51.

PROSTATE CANCER. Prostate cancer is common (> 100,000 cases annually, recently overtaking lung cancer as the most common nonskin cancer in men) and potentially fatal (> 28,000 deaths each year). Unfortunately, screening tests, such as the digital rectal examination and serum tumor markers (e.g., prostatic acid phosphatase and prostate-specific antigen), are inaccurate, missing many cases and incorrectly labeling normal patients as being positive for the disease. In addition, there is evidence that while nearly half of older men have prostate cancer, only about 1 in 380 men with the disease actually die from it. Successful screening for prostate cancer could, thus, subject many to unnecessary procedures and therapy. Thus screening for this disease is not currently recommended, but research should be a high priority.

Screening for Other Health Problems

VISUAL ACUITY SCREENING. The prevalence of undetected problems of visual acuity increases dramatically with age. Over 45% of people more than 75 years old have visual problems from cataracts alone; interventions, including cataract surgery in appropriately selected patients, can improve physical and subjective functioning. Thus, patients 65 years or older should be screened annually. Techniques include simple questioning (e.g., Has your vision changed recently? Do you have difficulty reading the newspaper? Do you have difficulty identifying someone across the room?) and Snellen chart testing. As visual acuity of at least 20/40 is required for moderate activity, patients with worse acuity, or with changing vision, should be referred to an ophthalmologist.

GLAUCOMA SCREENING. Primary open-angle glaucoma is an important cause of visual problems. The prevalence of this condition increases with age, to about 4% in people aged 75 years or older; it is higher in African-Americans and people with diabetes. Unfortunately there is not presently an acceptable way for primary physicians to detect early glaucoma. Tonometry, the traditional screening test, detects intraocular hypertension, a condition that is a risk factor for, but not synonymous with, glaucoma. Even in trained hands, tonometry detects only about 50% of people with glaucoma, and only about 1% per year of patients with ocular hypertension develop the visual field defects typical of glaucoma. In the absence of a glaucoma screening test suitable for use in primary practice, clinicians should have a low threshold for referring older and African-American patients to ophthalmologists for visual symptoms. Patients with diabetes for over 10 years should have an annual ophthalmology visit to check for retinopathy as well as glaucoma. (See Chap. 10, for further discussion of diagnosis and treatment.)

HEARING SCREENING. The prevalence of hearing impairment increases with age, with about 25% of people over 65 years old reporting a significant problem. A recent study found that over half of screened, hearing-impaired patients continued to wear prescribed hearing aids 8 hours or more each day, with improved social and emotional functioning. Patients 65 years or older should be screened every 5 years, with either simple screening questions such as the Hearing Handicap for the Elderly—Screening Version (HHIE-S, a

10-item self-administered questionnaire) or a hand-held audiometer. These two methods have been tested and found to be reliable and accurate; testing using a whisper and a watch tick is sometimes also used for screening. Assuming the physical examination does not reveal impacted cerumen, patients who report difficulty, or those with a 40-dB or greater hearing loss at 1000 or 2000 Hz in either ear, should be referred to an otolaryngologist.

THYROID SCREENING. Depending on the diagnostic criteria used, as many as 10% of women 40 years or older can be found to have "abnormal" results on thyroid function tests indicative of previously unknown hypo- or hyperthyroidism. The prevalence of such abnormal results is considerably less in men and younger women. However, many "abnormal" patients never develop symptoms or signs of thyroid disease, and even in those who do, there is no good evidence that treating these conditions at a presymptomatic stage is better than starting therapy at the onset of symptoms. Thus, screening asymptomatic patients for thyroid disease is unwarranted, but having a low threshold for testing patients with vague and nonspecific symptoms is a good idea.

TUBERCULOSIS SCREENING AND PROPHYLAXIS. More than 90% of current cases of active tuberculosis in the United States come from a pool of between 10 and 15 million people with asymptomatic infection. The great majority of people in this asymptomatic pool can be identified by tuberculin testing of high-risk groups, using the 5 TU Mantoux test.

The Centers for Disease Control (CDC) Advisory Committee for the Elimination of Tuberculosis (ACET) recommends screening persons in the following high-risk groups who have not previously been treated or had a positive result on the Mantoux test:

Persons with human immunodeficiency virus (HIV) infection, or other medical conditions that have been reported to increase the risk of tuberculosis (e.g., diabetes mellitus, gastrectomy, chronic renal failure, high-dose corticosteroid therapy, malignancies)
Close contacts of persons with newly diagnosed infectious tuberculosis
Injection drug users known to be HIV-seronegative
Persons with possible old tuberculosis on chest films
People who come to the United States from high-prevalence countries
Medically underserved low-income groups
Residents of nursing homes
Residents of correctional institutions
Children and adolescents
Health care workers

Repeat testing at 6- to 24-month intervals should be carried out in those persons at continued risk of exposure to active tuberculosis. The appropriate use of isoniazid prophylaxis is discussed in Chapter 118.

HIV TESTING. Voluntary screening for HIV is recommended for persons with possible exposure. Such individuals include homosexual and bisexual men, individuals with sexually transmitted diseases (STDs), prostitutes, injection drug users, recipients of blood transfusions from 1978 to 1985, persons infected with tuberculosis, and the sex partners of all such persons. Seropositive persons, even if asymptomatic, benefit from a monitoring of CD4 lymphocyte counts and appropriate treatment with prophylactic zidovudine and aerosol pentamidine. (See Chap. 114 for further information.) Such treatment has been shown to improve survival of HIV-infected persons. Furthermore, the treatment for syphilis and tuberculosis might be altered for seropositive persons. HIV screening also has public health benefits, since persons identified as seropositive may alter behaviors that transmit the virus.

Clinicians can maximize the benefits of screening and minimize the harms by educating and counseling patients before HIV testing, discussing the confidentiality of HIV results, urging patients to disclose positive results to sex partners, and advising patients on how to reduce high-risk behaviors. In patients without high-risk behaviors who desire HIV testing, the positive predictive value of HIV testing may be substantially increased if tests are performed in reference laboratories and if further confirmatory tests are run on a second blood specimen. Screening low-risk individuals for HIV infection is not useful either for the individual or for public health, because in this situation most positive tests would be false-positive, providing misinformation with all of its unfortunate consequences.

Counseling and Patient Education

Physician counseling and patient education concerning the reduction of risk factors can have a substantial impact on several health problems.

Smoking Cessation

An estimated 390,000 Americans die each year from smoking-related diseases, including cardiovascular disease, cancers (lung, larynx, oral cavity, esophagus, pancreas, urinary bladder), chronic lung disease, and others. Smoking cessation, even after many years, markedly decreases the toll of these diseases: almost immediately for cardiovascular disease, and gradually over about 10 years for lung cancer and chronic lung disease. A 1990 report by the Surgeon General noted that persons who quit smoking have one-half the risk of dying over the next 15 years as those who continue to smoke. And smoking cessation is possible: More than 38 million Americans have stopped smoking.

Despite the acknowledged benefits of smoking cessation, many physicians do not undertake such counseling, and report feeling ill-prepared and ineffective at getting patients to stop smoking. A review of studies on smoking cessation interventions, however, found that success depended not on novel or unusual techniques but was the product of individualized advice and assistance, repeated over time in different forms by several sources. Physicians who patiently offer their patients strong, ongoing, personalized support, including follow-up visits and the involvement of nonphysician staff, will eventually have the greatest success.

Further information about counseling efforts, use of nicotine gum, and nationally available educational materials and programs is discussed in Chapter 130.

Prevention of Injuries

Injuries are the leading cause of death in people under the age of 45 years. About half of these deaths are due to motor vehicle injuries, which may be prevented through counseling about the most important modifiable risk factors: (1) drinking alcohol before driving, and (2) not using occupant protection systems such as seat belts and air bags.

About 40% of persons killed in automobile crashes are intoxicated with alcohol. Physicians are often not aware of patients who have alcohol problems, but there are indirect methods, such as the CAGE questions, that allow identification of at least some of these people. (See Chap. 112.) Physician identification and counseling of such persons could well contribute to a reduction in alcohol-related motor vehicle injuries.

The use of occupant protection systems has been shown to reduce moderate and serious motor vehicle injury by 50%, yet less than half of Americans wear seat belts. Even if physician counseling were only successful for a small percentage of patients, motor vehicle injuries are so frequent that many lives would likely be saved.

Dietary Fat Consumption

Our understanding of the effect of diet on health and disease is incomplete. There is an increasing amount of research in this area. However, we do know that diet is one of the determinants of serum cholesterol, an important risk factor for coronary heart disease (CHD), and that reducing dietary cholesterol, total fats, and saturated fats can reduce cholesterol levels and the risk of CHD. There is also increasing evidence that high levels of animal fat in the diet may be a risk factor for colon cancer. Thus, all patients should be counseled about dietary fat intake, including possible fat substitutes and low-fat ways of preparing food. (See Chap. 145.)

Exercise

There are many theoretic ways that regular exercise might improve health. Some of these (such as reduced risk of CHD and improved insulin sensitivity in diabetics) are better supported by research evidence than others (such as improved mental health). Overall, there is sufficient evidence of a benefit to recommend regular exercise to all patients without a contraindication (such as congestive heart failure, increasing angina pectoris, dissecting aneurysm, thrombophlebitis, serious cardiac arrhythmia, moderate or severe

Table 122-1. A preventive care agenda

I. SCREENING

Problem	Test	Frequency	Target Group
Smoking	Ask about tobacco use	Regularly	All patients
Hypertension	Blood pressure	Every 1–2 yr	All patients
High blood cholesterol	Serum cholesterol	Every 5 yr	Men: age ≥ 30 yr Women: age ≥ 40 yr
Cervical cancer	Pap test	Every 3 yr	Sexually active women
Breast cancer	Mammography and clinical breast exam (CBE)	Every 1–2 yr	CBE: women aged ≥ 40 yr Mammography: women aged ≥ 50 yr
Colorectal cancer	Sigmoidoscopy	Every 3–5 yr	High-risk patients (e.g., patients over 40 with a positive family history)
Cataracts	Ask about vision, do Snellen chart testing	Annually	Patients aged ≥ 65 yr
Hearing impairment	Ask about hearing, use handheld audiometer	Every 5 yr	Patients aged ≥ 65 yr

II. COUNSELING

Message	Target Group
Tobacco cessation	Patients using tobacco
Injury prevention (alcohol use, seat belts)	All patients
Decreased dietary fat consumption	All adult patients
Regular exercise	All patients
Information about birth control	Women of childbearing age, adult men
Safe sex	Sexually active patients
Advanced directives	Older patients, patients with chronic disease likely to shorten life

Table 122-1 (continued)

III. IMMUNIZATIONS
See Chapter 124, for more detailed discussion of indications for immunization and schedules for administration.

Type	Frequency	Target Group
Influenza vaccination	Annually	Patients with chronic disease, all patients aged ≥ 65 yr
Pneumococcal vaccination	Once, repeat every 6 yr in some high-risk groups	Patients with chronic disease, all patients ≥ 65 yr
Hepatitis B vaccination (preexposure)	One series of 3 injections	Health care workers, hemodialysis and hemophiliac patients, homosexual men, heterosexual patients with multiple partners, IV drug users, patients with STDs
Measles vaccination	Initial, with revaccination for students entering college, and for health care workers without evidence of immunity	All adults without contraindications born after 1956 who lack documentation of immunization with live vaccine on or after the first birthday, physician-diagnosed measles, or laboratory evidence of immunity
Rubella vaccination	Once	Adults without contraindications who lack documentation of immunization on or after first birthday, physician-diagnosed rubella, or laboratory evidence of immunity
Tetanus toxoid	Every 10 yr	All patients

aortic stenosis, severe anemia, marked obesity, severe arthritis). The exercise prescription must be tailored to the individual, but several general principles can be followed.

First, the best type of exercise appears to involve using the major muscle groups in repetitive movement over a period of 20 to 30 minutes. Gardening, cycling, swimming, jogging, or walking briskly are ideal activities. Second, to minimize injury any exercise program should be started slowly, gradually working into the desired intensity, duration, and frequency. High intensity is not required for health benefits; some of the greatest benefits have been found in previously sedentary people beginning a moderate exercise program. To be effective, a program must be carried out regularly, ideally 3 or more times each week. Seasonal programs have only seasonal benefits. Exercise electrocardiography for asymptomatic, generally healthy people planning on adopting a new exercise program is not necessary. See Chapter 127.

Birth Control
Counseling about birth control (and STD prevention) may be among the most useful ways for physicians to spend office visits with teens and young adults. It is estimated that 30% of unmarried teens 15 to 19 years old have sexual intercourse without using contraception. Although the overall frequency of unintended pregnancy is uncertain, unplanned adolescent pregnancy often has severe negative consequences for both baby and mother. Effective birth control techniques are discussed in Chapter 75. The effectiveness of physician coun-

seling to encourage these techniques is likely to be optimized by using a nonjudgmental approach and respecting confidentiality.

Prevention of Sexually Transmitted Diseases
There has recently been a large increase in the frequency of STDs in the United States. Those at highest risk are teenagers and young adults, people with multiple sex partners, and homosexual and bisexual men. Effective techniques to decrease the risk of STDs include monogamous sexual relationships, use of condoms, refraining from anal intercourse, and not having sex with partners whose infection status is uncertain. The effectiveness of physician counseling in changing sexual behavior is uncertain, but physicians do come in frequent contact with persons at risk and thus have an opportunity to counsel. The first step is a nonjudgmental approach to taking a sexual history and understanding the patient's knowledge of and attitudes toward prevention practices. The physician should then provide clear information, preferably both oral and written, with periodic reinforcement. (See Chap. 113.)

Advance Directives
Patient preferences regarding life-sustaining treatment and care at the end of life should be respected. Since patients may become incompetent to make medical decisions through either accident or illness, physicians should encourage advance discussion of such preferences, rather than waiting for the most terminal, intensive-care stage of a disease. Such prior discussions can prevent the anguish that often occurs when decisions must be made for incompetent patients whose wishes are unknown. Studies of patients with chronic illnesses have shown that most welcome such discussions, that most appreciate the physician taking the initiative in raising the issues, and that important information has been learned. Often, an ongoing dialogue that involves other family members can be established and can make eventual decision-making much easier.

While establishing this dialogue is the most important reason for physicians raising the issue, many patients are also interested in information about advance directives such as the Living Will and Durable Power of Attorney. Neither document is legally complex. The Living Will is a statement signed by the patient that provides guidelines for treatment should the patient be unable to participate in decision-making, but is usually restricted to use during a terminal illness. The Durable Power of Attorney applies to a wider range of medical circumstances, and allows the patient to designate a surrogate decision-maker, preferably someone with whom he or she has discussed preferences for terminal care, to make decisions for the patient. In either case, the patient retains the right to participate in decision-making if he or she is able to do so, and may make changes or revoke either document at any time. Advance directives should be discussed with at least older and chronically ill patients, and earlier documents should be reviewed periodically. The patient should also be encouraged to share these discussions with other important persons who might be concerned in decision-making at the end of life. The Patient Self-Determination Act, which took effect in December 1991, mandates wider discussion of advance directives as a condition of receiving Medicare funding. Hospitals, nursing homes, and health maintenance organizations are required to give patients written information on advance directives when they are admitted or enrolled.

Immunizations
The three most important adult immunizations to target for prevention efforts are influenza vaccination, pneumococcal vaccination, and hepatitis B vaccination. All are aimed at important causes of suffering and death in large groups of patients. Tetanus immunization status should be assessed in all patients; tetanus toxoid is indicated for those inadequately immunized, and in particular for older adults, who are less likely to have ever received a primary series. Vaccination for rubella is recommended for susceptible women of childbearing age and for health care workers. Vaccination for measles is recommended for adults born after 1956, particularly those working in medical settings, who do not have documentation of immunization with live vaccine after age 1 year, a history of measles *diagnosed by a physician*, or serologic evidence of immunity. Indications and schedules for these and other immunizations are discussed in detail in Chapter 124.

Prophylactic Interventions

Effective postexposure prophylaxis regimens are available for a number of infectious diseases, including tuberculosis, hepatitis A and B, *Hemophilus influenzae* type b, meningococcal infection, and rabies. These interventions apply to specific clinical situations and are not part of routine health maintenance.

Prophylactic interventions for other conditions include postmenopausal estrogen for the prevention of osteoporotic fractures (discussed in Chap. 66) and aspirin for those at high risk of myocardial infarction (see Chap. 29).

Implementing a Preventive Policy

Although the "prevention agenda" outlined above is not a lengthy one, it may still be difficult to ensure that it is accomplished for most patients. As most patient visits involve a complaint or a chronic problem, finding time to talk about preventive care can be a challenge. While some patients make routine preventive care visits, this approach has become less popular as the prevention agenda has moved away from the "complete physical" to targeting a limited number of issues relevant to a patient's age and sex group. Many physicians have found that an efficient model is to integrate prevention into usual illness-related care. This might include such steps as:

1. Deciding on a "prevention policy," indicating which prevention services the physician wants to make sure are delivered to a high percentage of eligible patients
2. Developing a computerized or manual "prompting system" to remind the practice which patients are targeted for which services
3. Working with nonphysician staff to efficiently respond to the "prompt" (e.g., by having the secretarial staff complete mammogram order forms or the nurses gather information about cigarette smoking and exercise) and to develop procedures for services such as influenza vaccinations to be delivered without occupying a formal physician visit
4. Assigning a place in the medical record to record the date of the preventive service and the results
5. Developing a "call back" system, similar to those in many dentists' offices, to remind patients about follow-up or repeat prevention services

Such efficient office "systems" should allow physicians to accomplish a larger share of the limited, but extremely important, prevention agenda.

Hayward RSA, et al. Preventive Care Guidelines: 1991. Ann Intern Med 1991; 114:758–83.
A very useful summary of the recommendations of major expert groups, documenting the broad areas of agreement and the reasons for areas of disagreement.

Ransohoff DF, Lang CA. Screening for colorectal cancer. N Engl J Med 1991; 325:37–41.
An excellent, brief review of fecal occult blood test and endoscopy screening for colorectal cancer, concluding that "screening of asymptomatic persons without known risk factors is not justified at this time."

U.S. Preventive Services Task Force. Guide to clinical preventive services. Baltimore: Williams & Wilkins, 1989.
Succinct reviews of the effectiveness of 169 preventive interventions, with practical recommendations. This best single reference to the entire field of preventive care should be on every physician's desk.

Goldbloom RB, Lawrence RS. Preventing disease: beyond the rhetoric. New York: Springer, 1990.
Another publication from the U.S. Preventive Services Task Force, including background papers on many topics. There are especially good chapters on physical activity, smoking cessation, STDs, breast cancer screening, and colorectal cancer screening.

Ford DE, Whelton PK, Gordis L. Frontiers in disease prevention. J Gen Intern Med 1990; 5: Suppl.
Proceedings of a conference exploring the U.S. Preventive Services Task Force report. There are especially useful articles on the adverse effects of screening, the costs of prevention, and computerized reminder systems for preventive care.

Oboler SK, LaForce FM. The periodic physical examination in asymptomatic adults. Ann Intern Med 1989; 110:214–26.
Reviews the evidence for performing components of the physical examination in asymptomatic nonpregnant adults. In addition to screening procedures for which the efficacy has been established (blood pressure determination, breast examination, and Pap test), the authors recommend several other maneuvers at varying frequency (measurement of weight, visual acuity, hearing, examination of skin, cardiac auscultation, and abdominal palpation aneurysm in men older than 60). Contains 140 references.

Garber AM, Sox HC, Littenberg B. Screening asymptomatic adults for cardiac risk factors: the serum cholesterol level. Ann Intern Med 1989; 110:622–39.
The most balanced and objective review of a controversial area.

International Agency for Research on Cancer Working Group on Evaluation of Cervical Cancer Screening Programmes. Screening for squamous cervical cancer: duration of low risk after negative results of cervical cytology and its implications for screening policies. Br Med J 1986; 293:659–64.
An international collaborative study, with data from 10 large screening programs throughout the world, finding that screening more often than every 3 years adds little reduction to invasive cervical cancer rates.

Eddy DM. Screening for cervical cancer. Ann Intern Med 1990; 113:214–26.
A cost-effectiveness analysis of the important issues in cervical cancer screening.

Lichtenstein MJ, Bess FH, Logan SA. Validation of screening tools for identifying hearing-impaired elderly in primary care. JAMA 1988; 259:2875–8.
An evaluation of several methods to screen for hearing impairment.

Anda RF, Williamson DF, Remington PL. Alcohol and fatal injuries among US adults. JAMA 1988; 260:2529–32.
A prospective study finding a dose-response relationship between self-reported alcohol use and subsequent fatal injury.

Council on Scientific Affairs, American Medical Association. Alcohol and the driver. JAMA 1986; 255:522–7.
A review of the evidence about alcohol consumption and motor vehicle injuries, and a statement of the American Medical Association policy.

Centers for Disease Control. Progress toward achieving the national 1990 objectives for injury prevention and control. MMWR 1988; 37:138–40, 145–9.
A surveillance report, showing some progress toward reducing the motor vehicle fatality rate, at least partly attributable to a decrease in fatalities associated with high blood alcohol levels and an increasing use of seat belts.

Lo B, et al. Voluntary HIV screening: weighing the benefits and risks. Ann Intern Med 1989; 110:727–733.
Analyzes the scientific and ethical considerations in HIV testing.

Rhame FS, Maki DG. The case for wider use of testing for HIV infection. N Engl J Med 1990; 320:1248–54.
Advocates wider use of HIV testing than is currently practiced.

Coates TJ, Lo B. Counseling patients seropositive for human immunodeficiency virus. West J Med 1990; 153:629–34.
A practical discussion of what to say when the test result is positive.

Shmerling RH, et al. Discussing cardiopulmonary resuscitation: a study of elderly outpatients. J Gen Intern Med 1988; 3:317–21.
Finucane TE, et al. Planning with elderly outpatients for contingencies of severe illness: a survey and clinical trial. J Gen Intern Med 1988; 3:322–25.
Two articles discussing the issues and patient preferences regarding advance directives.

Lo B, Steinbrook RL. Beyond the Cruzan case. Ann Intern Med 1991; 114(10):895–901.
Compelling reasons for physicians to encourage patients to give explicit advance directives, with advice on how to get information on laws in individual states.

123. ATHLETIC PHYSICALS
Desmond K. Runyan and Sally S. Harris

Although much has been written about preparticipation athletic physicals, there is little agreement about the objectives, frequency, and content of the ideal examination. Current recommendations are based on epidemiologic knowledge gained from observational studies. However, in the absence of a formal evaluation of many of the recommended diagnostic maneuvers, one must still rely largely on clinical experience and "expert" opinion. This chapter summarizes those recommendations that have the strongest support and presents a rational outline for the athletic physical.

Objectives
Most experts in sports medicine would limit the preparticipation examination to a search for conditions that put the athlete at risk for adverse effects (injury, illness, or death) due to participation in sports. But because the athletic examination is frequently used as a substitute for routine health care for young adults who may have no other contact with the health care system, some advocate a complete evaluation of general health status and physical fitness. However, there is no evidence that a more extensive examination is advantageous. The limited, focused athletic physical identifies relevant problems economically and fulfills legal or regular requirements for athletic program participation by school-age children, adolescents, and young adults.

Format
Examination by the personal physician has the advantage of accessible records, patient rapport, opportunity for personal follow-up, and often a more comfortable setting. Group examinations involving serial organ system examinations by different examiners have the advantages of special equipment and expertise, with higher identification rates of abnormalities as well as lower costs. Single-file "lineup" examinations by a solo examiner provide inadequate conditions for physical diagnosis and patient privacy and have been condemned by experts in sports medicine.

The frequency of examination is controversial. The traditional practice of examinations done yearly or even for every sports season is inefficient and inappropriate. In healthy young athletes, the yield of disqualifying conditions on initial examination is low (0.2–1.2%) and will be even lower on repeat examination. Since most unsuitable candidates are disqualified on the initial examination, a comprehensive first physical with a subsequent evaluation limited to a review of the medical history will be adequate for the vast majority of athletes. Other examinations will be needed only to evaluate the rehabilitation status of acquired conditions.

Components of the Athletic Physical

Medical History
The majority of disqualifications of athletes will be based on history alone. With a specific goal of identifying those conditions that proscribe athletic participation, a brief and focused history should include (1) general health status; (2) past injuries or hospitalizations; (3) drug and alcohol use; (4) limitations of function; and (5) review of cardiac, pulmonary, and musculoskeletal systems.

It has been suggested that athletes with the potential for sudden death may be identified in advance by asking about syncope during exercise and about a family history of sudden death, because sudden death in young athletes has been associated primarily with hypertrophic cardiomyopathy, for which the presence of syncope as well as a positive family history is common. However, in a review of 29 athletes who died suddenly, most did not have evidence of risk on either prior histories or physical examinations. One study suggested that the risk of sudden death for an individual with a history of syncope is increased only in those patients for whom a cardiac etiology can be determined, usually based on history or physical examination alone.

General Physical Examination
The yield from physical examination is low, reflecting the low prevalence of disqualifying conditions among young athletes. The findings that most commonly triggered referral in several recent series were musculoskeletal conditions in need of rehabilitation and heart murmurs, most of which subsequently proved to be benign. The majority of athletes with conditions warranting referral can be identified on the basis of history alone and are subsequently cleared for sports participation. The routine physical examination is therefore a relatively small component of the preparticipation screening assessment of athletes.

Otoscopy, ophthalmoscopy, and the traditional hernia examination have not been found to be important or useful in the absence of a relevant history. Assessment of pubertal maturity by examination of the genitalia in prepubertal boys has not been shown to be useful in identifying individuals at risk of injuries in school contact sports; differences in muscle strength correlate better with the risk of injury.

Cardiopulmonary Examination
Despite the paucity of data demonstrating real benefits, it is standard practice that each athlete receive a cardiopulmonary examination early in his or her athletic career. This should include blood pressure measurement, palpation of peripheral pulses, and auscultation of the heart. Soft pulmonic murmurs are common and of little or no clinical importance. The murmur of valvular aortic stenosis, when heard, is usually found in the second right intercostal space as a crescendo-decrescendo ejection murmur, radiating to the carotids. It may be preceded by a systolic ejection click. In contrast, the murmur of hypertrophic subaortic stenosis is described as intermittent in character and may be heard best at the left sternal border without an accompanying click. The murmur is intensified by exercise or the Valsalva maneuver.

Several authorities recommend that each athlete be required to run and/or walk for 12 minutes and then be examined immediately afterward for evidence of hemodynamic abnormality or exercise-induced asthma. Exercise-induced asthma and hypertension are the most frequent occult conditions found during preparticipation examinations, but are not usually grounds for disqualification. Unfortunately, screening has not proved to be effective for identifying individuals at risk for sports-related sudden death. In particular, there is no demonstrated role for the routine use of electrocardiography or echocardiography for screening in the absence of a suggestive history.

Orthopedic Examination
The orthopedic examination is perhaps the part of the examination that is most useful in identifying problems that may lead to injury. A history of previous injury is the principal determinant of the risk for future injury, and the examination should determine whether there are residual deficits. The knee and ankle are the joints at greatest risk, but the examination can be tailored to include other previously injured joints, or those involved in specific sports.

Evaluation of knee strength should be part of a routine examination. A study of West Point cadets in athletic competition suggested that the majority of leg and knee injuries are actually re-injuries. Cadets found to have a difference of as little as 10 lb. in strength between legs on extensive knee strength testing were referred to a program to rehabilitate the weaker leg, and the subsequent rate of knee injuries fell precipitously. Similar reductions in the rate of knee injuries have been noted in high school athletes who underwent general voluntary preconditioning programs.

Knee strength is most accurately determined using a weight-lifting apparatus. Measuring and comparing the midthigh muscle bulk of each leg, along with clinically testing the muscle strength, may prove a reasonable proxy for more elaborate measurement, but the diagnostic accuracy of this approach has not been established.

Flexibility and ligamentous laxity have not been found to correlate with the risk of sports injuries. Although one early study found such a correlation in regard to ligamentous injuries of the knee in professional football players, these findings have not been found to hold true in subsequent studies of varying age groups in several different sports.

Down Syndrome
Evaluation of the athlete with Down syndrome is of particular concern because of the widespread participation of these individuals in Special Olympic sports programs. Atlan-

toaxial instability is associated with Down syndrome (10–20%), is usually asymptomatic, and is believed to progress gradually with age. Whether such individuals are at increased risk of subluxation is not known. Individuals with Down syndrome in whom subluxation has occurred generally have a history of preceding neurologic signs and symptoms for several months. Evidence of atlantoaxial instability on cervical spine radiographs (atlantoaxial interval > 5 mm) has not been found to be predictive of subluxation. However, current recommendations based on prudent judgment suggest obtaining cervical spine radiographs for all athletes with Down syndrome and excluding those with atlantoaxial instability from participating in contact sports and sports that cause maximal neck flexion.

Laboratory Testing
There is no evidence from six large studies of athletic physicals that routine testing of the blood or urine identifies individuals who should be excluded from athletic participation. In the absence of a positive history, hemoglobin analysis is unlikely to reveal an anemia that will have an adverse impact on performance. Urinalysis is also unproductive. One study noted that 40 of 701 children had abnormal urine protein concentrations on screening, but none was found to have any urinary tract abnormality on more extensive evaluation. Other screening tests are only indicated in populations where the prevalence of some disqualifying condition (e.g., tuberculosis) is sufficiently high to warrant screening in the absence of symptoms.

Disqualifying Conditions
The most recent guidelines for disqualification from sports participation are the 1988 recommendations of the American Academy of Pediatrics, shown in Table 123-1. Disqualification from nonstrenuous noncontact sports is rarely necessary, but disqualification from strenuous or contact sports may be necessary either during an acute illness or because of chronic disease. The final decision should be based on individual patient assessment, the physician's clinical judgment, and the patient's understanding and acceptance of the inherent risk associated with sports participation in the presence of preexisting medical conditions.

Fields K, Delaney M. Focusing the pre-participation sports examination. J Fam Pract 1990; 30:304–12.
A recent summary, concurring with the approach described in this chapter.

Goldberg B, et al. Pre-participation sports assessment—an objective evaluation. Pediatrics 1980; 66:736–44.
An analytic report on more than 700 screening physicals, examining the utility of the process. In this study, the positive findings were not related to subsequent problems during participation.

Runyan D. The pre-participation examination of the young athlete. Defining the essentials. Clin Pediatr 1983; 22:674–9.
Discusses the athletic physical and contraindications to participation in sports, expanding on the material in this chapter.

Maron BJ, et al. Results of screening a large group of intercollegiate competitive athletes for cardiovascular disease. J Am Coll Cardiol 1987; 10:1214–21.
An examination of the risk of sudden death in athletes. Based on a prospective screening evaluation of 501 intercollegiate student athletes, the authors suggest that a systematic preparticipation screening program is not an efficient means of detecting clinically important cardiovascular disease in young athletes.

Riser WL, et al. A cost-benefit analysis of preparticipation sports examinations of adolescent athletes. J School Health 1985; 55:270–3.
A cost-benefit analysis of preparticipation sports examinations of 763 adolescents, with suggestions on ways to improve the generally unfavorable cost-benefit ratio. In addition, findings from four previous studies on preparticipation sports examinations are reviewed.

Durant RH, et al. The preparticipation examination of athletes: comparison of single and multiple examiners. Am J Dis Child 1985; 139:657–61.

Table 123-1. Recommendations for participation in competitive sports

	Contact/ Collision	Limited Contact/ Impact	Noncontact		
			Strenuous	Moderately Strenuous	Nonstrenuous
Atlantoaxial instability	No	No	Yes*	Yes	Yes
*Swimming; no butterfly, breast stroke, or diving starts					
Acute illnesses	*	*	*	*	*
*Needs individual assessment, e.g., contagiousness to others, risk of worsening illness					
Cardiovascular					
Carditis	No	No	No	No	No
Hypertension					
Mild	Yes	Yes	Yes	Yes	Yes
Moderate	*	*	*	*	*
Severe	*	*	*	*	*
Congenital heart disease	†	†	†	†	†
*Needs individual assessment					
†Patients with mild forms can be allowed a full range of physical activities; patients with moderate or severe forms, or who are postoperative, should be evaluated by a cardiologist before athletic participation.					
Eyes					
Absence or loss of function of one eye	*	*	*	*	*
Detached retina	†	†	†	†	†
*Availability of American Society for Testing and Materials (ASTM)–approved eye guards may allow competitor to participate in most sports, but this must be judged on an individual basis.					
†Consult ophthalmologist					

Inguinal hernia	Yes	Yes	Yes	Yes	Yes
Kidney: absence of one	No	Yes	Yes	Yes	Yes
Liver: enlarged	No	No	Yes	Yes	Yes
Musculoskeletal disorders	*	*	*	*	*
*Needs individual assessment					
Neurologic					
History of serious head or spine trauma, repeated concussions, or craniotomy	*	*	Yes	Yes	Yes
Convulsive disorder					
Well controlled	Yes	Yes	Yes	Yes	Yes
Poorly controlled	No	No	Yes†	Yes	Yes‡
*Needs individual assessment					
†No swimming or weight lifting					
‡No archery or riflery					
Ovary: absence of one	Yes	Yes	Yes	Yes	Yes
Respiratory					
Pulmonary insufficiency	*	*	*	*	*
Asthma	Yes	Yes	Yes	Yes	Yes
*May be allowed to compete if oxygenation remains satisfactory during a graded stress test					
Sickle cell trait	Yes	Yes	Yes	Yes	Yes
Skin: boils, herpes, impetigo, scabies	*	*	Yes	Yes	Yes
*No gymnastics with mats, martial arts, wrestling, or contact sports until not contagious					
Spleen: enlarged	No	No	No	Yes	Yes
Testicle: absence or undescended	Yes*	Yes*	Yes	Yes	Yes
*Certain sports may require protective cup.					

Source: Committee on Sports Medicine. Recommendations for participation in competitive sports. Pediatrics 1988; 81:737–9. Reprinted with permission.

A study comparing the effectiveness and findings of group examination with the individual evaluation in the physician's office: The station-type examination identifies more conditions than the individual examination does.

Davidson RG. Atlantoaxial instability in individuals with Down syndrome: a fresh look at the evidence. Pediatrics 1988; 81:857–65.
An examination of the conventional wisdom of radiographic screening of athletes with Down syndrome.

124. IMMUNIZATIONS
Eliseo J. Pérez-Stable

Immunizations are probably the most cost-effective tool in preventive medicine. In active immunization, antibody or antitoxin is produced in response to the administration of a vaccine or toxoid. In passive immunization, temporary immunity is provided by the administration of preformed antibodies or antitoxin. Specific vaccine indications in adults will vary by factors such as life-style, occupation, medical conditions, and travel plans. A detailed history of immunization should be recorded in all medical charts.

Tetanus Toxoid
Tetanus is a rare disease in the United States with only 101 cases reported in 1987 and 1988. About 75% of cases follow acute injuries such as puncture wounds, lacerations, and abrasions, but tetanus can also result from chronic skin lesions (such as stasis or decubitus ulcers and abscesses) and injection drug use. Almost all reported cases occur in adults, with 67% occurring in persons over 50 years old. Only about 50% of older adults have protective levels of circulating antitoxin, compared to 90% of younger adults. In a health care maintenance setting, elderly patients are less likely to get tetanus toxoid even though they are at greater risk for clinical tetanus.

Tetanus-diphtheria toxoid (Td) is recommended for routine use in adults. Three intramuscular doses comprise a primary series. The second dose is given 4 to 8 weeks after the first dose and the third dose is given 6 to 12 months after the second. Clinical tetanus may occur in persons reporting a completed primary series. Thus, boosters are recommended every 10 years as a part of routine health maintenance, unless the patient sustains a tetanus-prone wound. The cost of Td is about 60¢ per dose.

Although minor side effects, such as a sore arm (40%), swelling at the site (20%), and itching (10%), are common, these can be more severe when the interval is inappropriately decreased. A history of neurologic or severe hypersensitivity reaction following a previous dose is a contraindication to Td. Pregnant women should receive Td if eligible, but waiting until the second trimester is a reasonable precaution.

For clean, minor wounds, Td should be administered only to update the primary series. For other wounds, tetanus prophylaxis depends on the immunization history. Td should be given if more than 5 years has passed since the last booster. Tetanus immune globulin is recommended in other than clean, minor wounds when the individual has received no more than one Td dose in the past. If the immunization history is uncertain, it should be assumed that no doses of Td have been given. A primary Td series and tetanus immune globulin should be administered.

Measles Vaccine
The incidence of measles has been greatly reduced by effective vaccines and widespread immunization campaigns. But because 5 to 20% of young adults remain susceptible, up to 20 to 30% of cases now occur among adolescents and young adults, and outbreaks of measles on college campuses have increased. Encephalitis or death occurs in approximately 1 per 1000 measles cases; the risk is greater in adults than in children.

The live attenuated virus used to prevent measles produces a mild or unapparent, noncommunicable infection. Antibodies develop in 90 to 95% of individuals after a single, subcutaneous 0.5-ml dose. Pregnancy and altered immune states are contraindications to live viral vaccines. Persons with a history of anaphylactic hypersensitivity to neomycin or with anaphylactic reactions to eating eggs should not be immunized with measles vaccine. The side effects include fever, which occurs in 5 to 15% of vaccinees beginning 5 to 12 days after vaccination and lasting 1 to 2 days. Transient rashes have been reported in 5%. The incidence of encephalitis after measles vaccination is lower than the observed background incidence of encephalitis of unknown cause. The frequency of side effects is not related to age.

Measles vaccine is indicated for all adults born after 1956 who do not have documentation of immunity. A history of immunization without medical record documentation was of no benefit in predicting immunity to measles.

Persons vaccinated with the inactivated measles virus vaccine (available from 1963 to 1967) are at risk of developing atypical measles when they are exposed to the natural virus. They should be revaccinated with the current attenuated live vaccine. Forty to 55% of persons who previously received killed measles vaccine develop reactions, usually fever, malaise, and myalgias, after live vaccination.

Because many measles cases reported in 1989 and 1990 outbreaks occurred in previously immunized children and young adults, the Centers for Disease Control (CDC) revised its recommendations for measles prevention. Adults born after 1956 who received only one dose of measles vaccine should be revaccinated, particularly during an outbreak, on entering college, or starting employment. Adults working in medical settings should be targeted for measles vaccination. Documentation of two doses of measles vaccine or other evidence of measles immunity should be reported. Evidence of measles immunity can be provided by proper physician-diagnosed measles disease, serologic evidence of measles immunity, or birth before 1957.

Rubella Vaccine

Prevention of congenital rubella syndrome is the goal of rubella immunization programs. As with measles, the incidence of rubella has been greatly reduced by the widespread use of the vaccine in children. In 1988, only 221 cases of rubella were reported in the United States, with 58% of cases occurring in persons 15 years or older. In addition, there was only one case of congenital rubella syndrome reported to the CDC. However, an estimated 10 to 15% of young adults remain susceptible to rubella and limited outbreaks continue to be reported from universities and places of employment, especially hospitals.

Rubella vaccine is indicated for all susceptible adults, particularly women of childbearing age, college students, and health care workers. Health care workers who might be exposed to patients infected with rubella or who might have contact with pregnant patients should have documentation of immunity or vaccination. Serologic testing of all women of childbearing age is an expensive strategy that has been questioned, because follow-up rates of immunization are low. Thus, rubella vaccination of women who are not pregnant and have no history of vaccination is justifiable without serologic testing.

The live attenuated rubella virus vaccine is prepared in human diploid cells and is administered subcutaneously in a single 0.5-ml dose. Lifetime immunity is provided to over 90% of vaccine recipients. Side effects to rubella vaccine include arthralgias of the peripheral joints in up to 40% of vaccine recipients; frank arthritis occurs infrequently. Symptoms begin 3 to 25 days after immunization and last from 1 to 11 days. Persistent or chronic arthritis is uncommon. Adult women have a greater incidence of arthralgias and arthritis than do children. Rubella vaccine should not be given to persons who are immunocompromised or to persons with anaphylactic reactions to neomycin. While pregnancy is considered a contraindication to rubella vaccination, there seems to be little (if any) increased risk of congenital rubella. In a prospective registry, no cases of congenital rubella syndrome have been reported for 267 infants whose mothers were vaccinated during pregnancy.

Mumps Vaccine

The incidence of mumps, like other childhood diseases, has been greatly reduced since the introduction of live virus vaccine, but outbreaks among adolescents and young adults in educational and occupational settings have increased in recent years. In adults, mumps can cause orchitis in up to 20% of men and oophoritis in 5% of women. Although worrisome, this complication is usually unilateral and rarely causes sterility. Nerve deafness occurs in 1 per 15,000 patients.

A single 0.5-ml dose of live attenuated mumps vaccine administered subcutaneously results in protective antibodies in 90% of recipients. Parotitis and central nervous system dysfunction from mumps vaccine have been reported rarely. Rashes, pruritus, and purpura have been temporally associated with mumps vaccine, but these are uncommon. Persons with a history of anaphylactic reactions after egg ingestion or neomycin administration should not be immunized.

Mumps vaccine is indicated for adults born after 1956 without documented evidence for physician-diagnosed mumps, prior vaccination, or laboratory evidence of immunity. Pregnant women and immunodeficient persons should not receive the mumps vaccine.

Polio Vaccine

There have been no indigenous cases of wild-type poliovirus–caused disease reported in the United States since 1979, but paralytic poliomyelitis could reappear if the current high levels of immunity are not maintained by routinely immunizing children.

The newly licensed, enhanced-potency poliovirus vaccine is preferred for adults requiring immunization because the risk of oral polio vaccine–associated paralysis is greater in adults than in children. A primary series consists of three 0.5-ml doses given subcutaneously—two doses given 4 to 8 weeks apart and a third dose given 6 to 12 months after the second. The inactivated polio vaccine contains trace amounts of neomycin and streptomycin; although hypersensitivity reactions are possible, no serious adverse reactions have been documented. Oral polio vaccines are associated with paralysis in vaccine recipients with a risk of 1 case per 520,000 doses distributed.

Routine polio vaccination of adults who have not had a primary series is not recommended, except in persons who are at increased risk of exposure to the wild polioviruses. Travelers to developing countries who have not previously been immunized should receive a full primary series or, if previously immunized, a single booster dose. Health care personnel in close contact with patients who may excrete polioviruses should have a complete primary series.

Influenza Vaccine

Influenza epidemics have been associated with 10,000 to 50,000 excess deaths annually during 1957 to 1986, with 80 to 90% occurring in persons over age 64. Deaths result not only from the influenza infection itself but also from an associated increase in cardiopulmonary deaths. In addition to excess deaths, influenza epidemics cause an excess of 172,000 hospitalizations per epidemic at an estimated cost of $600 million. At least 40% of these hospitalizations occur in adults younger than 65 years who have no explicit indications for being vaccinated. The vaccine is up to 90% effective in preventing clinical illness among young healthy adults, but only 40 to 70% effective in the elderly. However, nursing home residents vaccinated against influenza have a two- to fivefold reduction in radiographic evidence of pneumonia, hospitalization, and death when compared to nonvaccinated residents.

Influenza A viruses are most commonly associated with epidemics. These viruses undergo almost yearly antigenic drifts; a major change in virus antigens is known as an antigenic shift. These antigenic drifts and shifts require new vaccines to be formulated each year in anticipation of new antigens. Antigenic variation also occurs with influenza B viruses, although less frequently. Disease from influenza B viruses tends to be less severe than that caused by influenza A viruses.

Influenza vaccine is an inactivated virus administered as a single intramuscular 0.5-ml dose during the fall each year. The vaccine should be administered by early November to achieve the maximal duration of protection throughout the winter months, but vaccination as late as January protects recipients. Annual vaccination is required because influenza virus vaccines have a short duration of immunogenicity. Minor side effects are common and include a sore arm and swelling in up to 40% of recipients. A flu-like illness of malaise and low-grade fevers persisting for 1 to 2 days occurs in no more than 5% of the vaccine recipients. Severe immediate hypersensitivity reactions are extremely rare and are most likely caused by the tiny amounts of residual egg protein in vaccines given to persons with a history of anaphylactic reactions to eggs. Patients should be asked whether they have trouble breathing after eating eggs. Hives, swelling of the lips or tongue, cardiovascular collapse, and acute respiratory distress after eating eggs are absolute contraindications to influenza vaccine. In patients receiving intermittent immunosuppressive therapy, vaccine should be given during a drug-free interval to improve immunogenicity. There is no association between the current vaccines and the Guillain-Barré syndrome.

Influenza vaccine programs should target the groups at greatest risk from complications of influenza infection. In a decreasing order of priority, these include:

Adults with chronic disorders of cardiovascular or pulmonary systems that are severe enough to have required regular medical follow-ups or hospitalization during the preceding year

Residents of nursing homes and other chronic care facilities housing patients of any age

Otherwise healthy individuals 65 years or older

Adults with chronic metabolic diseases (including diabetes mellitus), renal dysfunction, hemoglobinopathies, or immunosuppression (including human immunodeficiency virus [HIV] infection) severe enough to require regular medical follow-up or hospitalization during the preceding year

Young adults requiring chronic aspirin therapy, and thus at high risk of Reye's syndrome

Persons capable of transmitting influenza viruses to high-risk persons should also be vaccinated. Examples are health care workers who have contact with high-risk patients, providers of home care, and household contacts of high-risk persons. Individuals providing essential community services may consider vaccination in order to minimize disruption of the services during an outbreak. Pregnant women have not had excess mortality from influenza except during the two great pandemics of this century. The vaccine has no known teratogenicity and should not be withheld from pregnant women, especially those at high risk from influenza complications. Persons at risk who travel should be protected, and while the risk of influenza in the tropics is present throughout the year, the season of greatest activity in the Southern Hemisphere is April through September.

Only 55 to 60% of nursing home residents, 22 to 32% of noninstitutionalized elderly persons, and 10% of high-risk younger adults receive influenza vaccine each year. More effective vaccination programs should be developed for ambulatory care and patients discharged from hospitals during the fall. The involvement of nonphysician staff to offer the vaccine or to provide information to patients significantly increases the use of influenza vaccination. Postcard, personal, and telephone reminders by physicians and nurses have also been effective. Medicare has covered flu shots for the elderly since 1988.

Pneumococcal Polysaccharide Vaccine

Pneumococcal infections cause an estimated 40,000 deaths annually, and antibiotics and intensive care units have not changed the mortality from pneumococcal bacteremia during the first 5 days of hospitalization. Elderly persons are particularly at risk. The effectiveness of pneumococcal vaccine has been estimated to be between 64 and 70%, although an efficacy in immunodeficient patients has not been shown.

A 23-valent polysaccharide vaccine against pneumococcal disease was licensed in 1983, replacing the 14-valent vaccine. The 23 capsular types in the vaccine cause 88% of cases of pneumococcal bacteremia. In most patients, pneumococcal vaccine is administered only once, 0.5 ml intramuscularly. Mild local reactions such as erythema, pain, and induration occur in 50%; severe allergic reactions, fever, rash, or myalgias occur in less than 1% of vaccine recipients. Anaphylactoid reactions are estimated at 5 per million doses administered.

An emerging consensus is that pneumococcal vaccine should be given to all healthy elderly persons before they develop immunodebilitating chronic diseases. As with influenza vaccine, more effective immunization programs need to be developed. In addition to the elderly, it is recommended that the following adults receive pneumococcal vaccine:

Immunocompetent adults who are at increased risk of pneumococcal disease or its complications, including persons with cardiovascular disease, pulmonary disease, cirrhosis, alcoholism, cerebrospinal fluid (CSF) leaks, and diabetes mellitus, and those 65 years or older

Immunocompromised adults with an increased risk for pneumococcal disease or its complications, including patients with sickle cell anemia, splenic dysfunction or asplenia, Hodgkin's disease, lymphoma, multiple myeloma, chronic renal failure, nephrotic syndrome, and conditions associated with immunosuppression such as organ transplantation and HIV infection

Pneumococcal vaccine should be given at least 2 weeks prior to elective splenectomy or the initiation of immunosuppressive therapy. Patients with multiple myeloma have an adequate antibody response only 30% of the time.

Persons who receive the 14-valent pneumococcal vaccine should not be revaccinated with the 23-valent vaccine since the increased coverage is modest.

Revaccination every 6 years should be considered for persons who are at highest risk of fatal pneumococcal infection such as asplenia. Rapidly declining antibody levels have been confirmed in persons with nephrotic syndrome, renal failure, and organ transplants, and they should also be revaccinated. Elderly persons and patients with HIV infection should also be considered for revaccination. Local adverse reactions are not increased with revaccination at 6 years. Recommendations for the timing of revaccination in other groups are not clear at this time.

Hepatitis B Vaccine

Vaccination can prevent acute hepatitis B virus (HBV) infection and the sequelae of fulminant hepatitis, chronic active hepatitis, cirrhosis, hepatocellular carcinoma, and neonatal transmission. Genetically engineered HBV vaccine is now generally used. Plasma-derived vaccine must be used in persons with a known allergy to yeast, which is used in preparing the genetically engineered vaccine; because of its greater immunogenicity, plasma-derived vaccine is also administered to hemodialysis and other immunocompromised patients.

HBV vaccine is administered intramuscularly in the deltoid in three 1-ml (10-µg or 20-µg) doses; the initial dose is repeated at 1 and 6 months. Protective antibodies are produced in over 90% of healthy adults completing a series. The side effects have been mostly limited to soreness and erythema at the injection site in 15 to 20% of patients, lasting 1 to 2 days. For hemodialysis patients or other immunocompromised persons, the recommended dose of HBV vaccine is 40 µg for each of the three doses, whether the plasma-derived or genetically engineered vaccine is used. The HBV vaccination series costs at least $100 plus administrative costs. (Manufacturers in Asia produce HBV vaccine for $5–$21 per series.)

Prevaccination serologic screening is cost-effective when the expected prevalence of immune individuals is high and the cost of screening is reasonable. Using the total antibody (anti-HB_c) to hepatitis B core antigen (HB_cAg) (both IgG and IgM) for serologic screening identifies carriers and almost all previously infected persons. Neither group requires vaccination. The test using the antibody (anti-HB_s) to hepatitis B surface antigen (HB_sAg), on the other hand, does not identify carriers. If the radioimmunoassay (RIA) anti-HB_s test is used for screening, a minimum of 10 RIA sample ratio units should be used to designate immunity, even though 2.1 is the usual designation of a positive test.

Preexposure HBV vaccination is recommended for:

1. Newborns whose mother is HB_sAg-positive. All pregnant women should be screened for HB_sAg. Selective screening programs identify only 35 to 65% of HB_sAg-positive mothers.
2. Sex partners and household contacts of HBV carriers.
3. Homosexually active men.
4. Clients and staff of institutions for the developmentally disabled. Staff of nonresidential day-care programs attended by known HBV carriers should also be vaccinated.
5. Hemodialysis patients. Vaccination of patients early in the course of renal disease results in higher seroconversion rates and antibody levels.
6. Users of illicit injectable drugs.
7. Recipients of clotting-factor concentrates.
8. Health care and public safety workers with frequent blood contact who are at risk of trauma that may result in the percutaneous or permucosal introduction of HBV, or who may potentially transmit HBV to patients or persons attended. The risk among health care professionals is highest during the professional training period and, when possible, vaccination should be completed during training. Despite the presence of

HBV vaccine programs in selected hospitals, only 36% of persons at high risk had actually received vaccine. In the past, some persons were mistakenly concerned that plasma-derived HBV vaccine could be contaminated with HIV virus, despite the use of preparation procedures that inactivate similar viruses and a lack of evidence of higher rates of acquired immunodeficiency syndrome (AIDS) or seroconversion in recipients. The availability of the genetically engineered vaccine should alleviate any residual concerns. Management after a needlestick, scalpel wound, or mucous-membrane exposure is discussed in Chapter 119.

9. Families adopting children from countries of high HBV endemicity should have the children screened for HB_sAg. If adoptees are HB_sAg-positive, family members should be vaccinated.
10. Other contacts of HBV carriers in special situations, such as those caring for children with aggressive behavior or with skin diseases.
11. Special high-risk populations with high endemicity of HBV infection. These include Alaskan natives, Pacific Islanders, and immigrants from eastern Asia and sub-Saharan Africa.
12. Inmates of long-term correctional facilities.
13. Heterosexually active persons with multiple partners.
14. International travelers to endemic areas who plan to stay for more than 6 months.

Targeting high-risk groups for HBV vaccination has not had a substantial impact on the incidence of disease, and an alternative strategy is universal vaccination of all persons.

HBV vaccine–induced antibody levels decline steadily with time and up to 50% of adult vaccine recipients have low or undetectable antibody levels by 7 years. However, clinical (or viremic) HBV infections in persons with a decrease in antibody levels are rare. Booster doses of vaccine and routine serologic tests to assess antibody levels are not recommended in vaccine recipients with a normal immune status. The possible need for booster doses after longer intervals has yet to be established. For hemodialysis patients, booster doses should be given when the antibody levels decline to less than 10 mIU/ml, as determined by annual serologic testing.

Rabies Vaccine

Human rabies is a rare disease in the United States, accounting for zero to two deaths per year since 1980. Possible rabies exposure, on the other hand, is common: About 20,000 persons are vaccinated yearly, and 100 to 200 persons are bitten by animals subsequently proved to be rabid. Rabies prophylaxis for bite wounds is discussed in Chapter 138.

Preexposure immunization for rabies may be considered for individuals with unusual risk, such as veterinarians, zoo keepers, and speelunkers. A series of three intramuscular injections or intradermal injections of human diploid cell rabies vaccine produces excellent antibody levels; the series consists of an initial dose, repeated at 7 and 28 days. If a continuous or frequent risk of exposure is likely, boosters every 6 months to 2 years are advisable.

HIV Infection and Immunizations

There is no convincing evidence that immunizations accelerate the clinical course of HIV infections. Caution should be used in administering live viral vaccines to patients with symptomatic HIV infection. For adults, pneumococcal vaccine is recommended and vaccines against influenza and HBV should be considered. *H. influenzae* type B conjugate vaccine should also be considered because HIV-infected patients are at greater risk for severe infection by this encapsulated bacterium.

Patients with asymptomatic HIV infection may not develop adequate antibody responses to vaccination. For example, only about one-half of HIV-infected men develop protective antibodies after HBV vaccine. While such patients still should be immunized, concerns regarding follow-up HB_sAb levels have been raised. Antibody responses to influenza and pneumococcal vaccines are near-normal in asymptomatic HIV-positive persons. On average, less than 50% of patients with symptomatic HIV infection have an adequate antibody response to these vaccines.

Committee on Immunization. American College of Physicians. Guide for adult immunization. 2nd ed. Philadelphia: American College of Physicians, 1990.

A practical, well-organized, easy to use guide that summarizes current issues in adult immunization. It belongs in every practitioner's office.

Williams W, et al. Immunization policies and vaccine coverage among adults. Ann Intern Med 1988; 108:616–25.
A scholarly review of the public health approach to immunizations for adults, with policy recommendations. The sections on influenza and pneumococcal vaccines provide persuasive arguments for a more proactive office- or hospital-based immunization program.

Immunization Practices Advisory Committee (ACIP). Diphtheria, tetanus, and pertussis: recommendations for vaccine use and other preventive measures. MMWR 1991; 40(RR-10):1–28.
Summary recommendations for primary tetanus prevention and management in wound care.

Centers for Disease Control. Measles prevention: recommendations of the Immunization Practices Advisory Committee (ACIP). MMWR 1989; 38(No. S-9):1–18.
Discusses in detail the morbidity of measles infection, epidemiology of preventable cases, and rationale for revised recommendations for measles vaccine.

Centers for Disease Control. Rubella vaccination during pregnancy—United States, 1971–1986. MMWR 1987; 36:457–61.
A prospective registry of 267 infants born to mothers who received rubella vaccine during pregnancy, showing no cases of congenital rubella. One-third of mothers received vaccine during the first 8 weeks of pregnancy.

Kaplan KM, et al. Mumps in the workplace: further evidence of the changing epidemiology of a childhood vaccine-preventable disease. JAMA 1988; 260:1434–8.
Describes the workplace epidemic including clinical morbidity in adults and discusses the importance of immunizing susceptible adults.

Robertson SE, et al. Clinical efficacy of a new, enhanced-potency, inactivated poliovirus vaccine. Lancet 1988; 1:897–9.
Increased efficacy of inactivated vaccine demonstrated.

Immunization Practices Advisory Committee. Prevention and Control of Influenza. MMWR 1991; 40(RR-6).
Statement from the CDC published annually in the MMWR, summarizing epidemiology, public health importance, and clinical issues regarding the prevention of influenza. Vaccine content and recommendations for immunization are discussed in detail.

Douglas RG. Prophylaxis and treatment of influenza. N Engl J Med 1990; 322:443–50.
A review of the influenza vaccine and antiviral therapy for the prevention and treatment of influenza.

Patriarca PA, et al. Efficacy of influenza vaccine in nursing homes. JAMA 1985; 253:1136–9.
A retrospective cohort study of nursing home residents, showing that patients who did not receive influenza vaccine had an increased risk of respiratory illness (by 2.6), hospitalization (by 2.4), infiltrate on chest radiograph (by 2.9), and death (by 5.6). Influenza vaccine reduces the severity, morbidity, and mortality of influenza infections.

Margolis KL, et al. Frequency of adverse reactions to influenza vaccine in the elderly. JAMA 1990; 264:1139–41.
A double-blind, crossover study of either influenza vaccine or saline placebo, followed 2 weeks later by the alternative agent. This study of over 330 U.S. veterans found that mild and limited soreness (20% after vaccine vs 5% after placebo) of the arm was the only significant symptom associated with the vaccine.

Immunization Practices Advisory Committee. Pneumococcal polysaccharide vaccine. MMWR 1989; 38:64–8, 73–6.
CDC recommendations on target groups for pneumococcal vaccine and a summary of epidemiology, public health rationale, and clinical issues.

Bolan G, et al. Pneumococcal vaccine efficacy in selected populations in the United States. Ann Intern Med 1986; 104:1–6.
Epidemiologic approach to demonstrating the efficacy of pneumococcal vaccine by comparing serotypes in vaccine recipients and nonrecipients with positive blood cultures. The authors conclude that among vaccine recipients there was a 64% reduction in the expected cases caused by vaccine serotypes.

LaForce FM, Eickhoff TC. Pneumococcal vaccine: an emerging consensus. Ann Intern Med 1988; 108:757–9.
Editorial summarizing data that support the use of pneumococcal vaccine and proposing that universal immunization of elderly adults may be the most effective public health strategy.

Sims RV, et al. The clinical effectiveness of pneumococcal vaccine in the elderly. Ann Intern Med 1988; 108:653–7.
A case-control study of 122 patients, aged 55 years or older, with Pneumococcus cultured in usually sterile fluids, excluding the severely immunocompromised. The estimated efficacy was 70% (95% confidence intervals, 37–86%).

Centers for Disease Control. Protection against viral hepatitis: recommendations of the Immunization Practices Advisory Committee (ACIP). MMWR 1990; 39(No. RR-2):1–26.
Summary of public health and clinical issues in the prevention of hepatitis. The section on HBV includes rationale for each of the high-risk groups.

Hadler SC. Are booster doses of hepatitis B vaccine necessary? Ann Intern Med 1988; 108:457–8.
Editorial commenting on the concerns raised about the possible need for booster doses of vaccine. The data are not persuasive.

Miriam JA, et al. The changing epidemiology of hepatitis B in the United States: need for alternative vaccination strategies. JAMA 1990; 263:1218–22.
No risk factors were identified in 30 to 40% of cases of acute HBV infection in four sentinel counties from 1981 to 1988. The overall incidence remained constant and consideration should be given to universal immunization.

Mulley AG, Silverstein MD, Dienstag JL. Indications for use of hepatitis B vaccine, based on cost-effectiveness analysis. N Engl J Med 1982; 307:644–52.
Detailed analysis of the cost-effectiveness of using an HBV vaccine and of screening prior to vaccination.

Szmuness W, et al. Hepatitis B vaccine—demonstration of efficacy in a controlled clinical trial in a high-risk population in the United States. N Engl J Med 1980; 303:833–41.
Randomized clinical trial showing the effectiveness of HBV vaccine in a high-risk population, with equal adverse effects in vaccine and placebo recipients.

Practices Advisory Committee: Rabies prevention—United States. MMWR 1984; 33(28):393–408.
Recommendations for pre- and postexposure prophylaxis, and information on the adverse effects and contraindications.

Collier AC, et al. Antibody to human immunodeficiency virus (HIV) and suboptimal response to hepatitis B vaccination. Ann Intern Med 1988; 109:101–5.
No antibody response to HBV vaccine in 7 of 16 HIV-positive patients, compared to 6 of 68 HIV-negative patients.

Huang KL, et al. Antibody responses after influenza and pneumococcal immunization in HIV-infected homosexual men. JAMA 1987; 257:2047–50.
Antibody responses to influenza virus and pneumococcal vaccines were comparable in asymptomatic HIV-infected men and non–HIV-infected men. A subsequent study showed that less than 50% of patients with symptomatic HIV infection had adequate antibody response.

125. CARDIAC RISK FACTOR MODIFICATION
Mark A. Hlatky and Stephen B. Hulley

Coronary heart disease (CHD) is the leading cause of death in the United States today, as well as a major cause of suffering, disability, and expense. This chapter focuses on four aspects of risk for CHD: (1) What are the independent risk factors? (2) How strong is the relationship between the risk factor and disease? (3) Is an efficacious and feasible intervention available? (4) Does reduction in the risk factor reduce risk?

Risk factors for CHD most consistently observed in prospective studies include high blood pressure, cigarette smoking, high blood cholesterol, low levels of high-density lipoprotein (HDL) cholesterol, obesity, glucose intolerance, and sedentary life-style. Each of these factors independently increases an individual's risk of CHD by two- to threefold. Moreover, risk factors interact so that CHD risk may be over 10 times higher in individuals who have several risk factors than in those who have only one. In general, there is an increasing risk of CHD with increasing level of the risk factor, with no clearly apparent breakpoint or threshold.

Age, sex, and a family history of premature CHD are also important factors that predict CHD. Although the risk attributable to them cannot be modified, they are important because they increase the absolute risk for the individual, thereby increasing the cost-effectiveness of interventions directed at the modifiable risk factors.

Effect of Risk Factor Reduction on CHD

Hypertension
A diastolic pressure of 90 mm Hg is conventionally used to diagnose mild hypertension. Patients with high levels on several visits should reduce salt intake and, if obese, lose weight. Drug treatment should be considered in those patients whose diastolic pressure remains above 95 after a few months of nonpharmacologic treatment, particularly in older patients and those with other risk factors. Randomized, controlled trials of treating patients with hypertension have demonstrated a substantial reduction in total mortality, due primarily to a lower incidence of stroke and other complications of hypertension.

The controversy over treatment of isolated systolic hypertension in the elderly has been recently addressed by the Systolic Hypertension in the Elderly Program. A stepped-care approach significantly reduced the incidence of stroke and coronary heart disease in that study. Systolic hypertension merits treatment, starting with dietary intervention and adding drug therapy if needed.

Smoking
The CHD risk associated with cigarette smoking rises steadily with increasing cigarette consumption and is not appreciably diminished by the use of filtered, as opposed to unfiltered, cigarettes. Cigarette smoking also increases the CHD risk in nonsmokers who live with a person who smokes.

Several observations strongly suggest that cessation of cigarette smoking reduces the risk of CHD. In the Framingham Study, the CHD incidence, after adjusting for other risk factors, was more than 50% lower in persons who quit smoking as compared with those who continued to smoke. Other cohort studies that controlled for potential confounding by other CHD risk factors found that the risk of CHD among those who had quit smoking for at least 1 year was similar to the risk of lifelong nonsmokers. The evidence regarding smoking and CHD, combined with the studies linking cigarette smoking with cancer and chronic lung disease, supports vigorous efforts at smoking cessation (see Chap. 130).

Total Cholesterol and HDL Cholesterol
The potential efficacy of interventions aimed at changing the levels of these lipids is discussed in Chapter 126.

Glucose Intolerance
Diabetes is a strong, independent risk factor for the development of CHD, but the efficacy of therapy on risk reduction is not known. Insulin injections and oral hypoglycemic agents

reduce hyperglycemia, but neither eliminates the underlying metabolic disorder. While treatment of diabetes can control symptoms due to hyperglycemia and may forestall microvascular diabetic complications, its value for the prevention of CHD is not established.

Type A Behavior
The popular view that aggressive, competitive, chronically rushed individuals are more likely to die of heart disease has not been confirmed by recent epidemiologic studies. While it seems reasonable to advise patients to reduce the stress in their lives, in order to be more comfortable if nothing else, more extensive interventions on "coronary-prone behavior" are of uncertain benefit.

Sedentary Life-style
Many nonexperimental studies have demonstrated that vigorous, active people develop heart disease less often than sedentary individuals. There has been controversy about whether exercise is actually protective or whether people who choose to exercise are at lower risk for other reasons. The balance of current evidence favors protection (see Chapter 127). Experimental studies of exercise in CHD prevention have been inconclusive, chiefly due to the small numbers of individuals studied and the unwillingness of many sedentary people to increase their habitual level of physical activity. Although the direct effect of exercise on CHD risk remains uncertain, beneficial effects on other risk factors, such as serum HDL cholesterol and obesity, are established. Thus, an exercise program is an important adjunct to CHD prevention.

Obesity
Obese individuals have a high incidence of CHD, even when other risk factors are taken into account. Obesity also affects CHD risk by increasing other risk factors. Weight loss reduces blood pressure, improves glucose tolerance, increases HDL cholesterol, and lowers total (or low-density lipoprotein) cholesterol. Thus, interventions aimed at obesity are a valuable component of any CHD risk reduction program.

Aspirin Therapy
Aspirin therapy has received attention as a preventive measure. Coronary thrombosis appears to be the precipitating factor for the serious acute manifestations of CHD: sudden cardiac death, acute myocardial infarction, and unstable angina pectoris. Aspirin in the dose of 325 mg every other day was shown in the Physician Health Study to reduce significantly the risk of coronary events, but also slightly increased the risk of hemorrhagic stroke. The potential benefits of aspirin therapy are greater in subjects at high risk for coronary artery disease as a result of being older (> 50 years) or having multiple cardiac risk factors. The optimal dose and timing of aspirin therapy for the purpose of primary prevention remain unsettled.

Practical Implications
With the exception of aspirin and treatment of hypertension and high blood cholesterol, the interventions discussed have not been unequivocally shown by randomized clinical trials to be effective in preventing CHD. However, the evidence for quitting smoking, becoming physically fit, and avoiding obesity is persuasive. Moreover, the recent decline in heart disease mortality, which may be related to improved control of risk factors, provides additional encouragement for preventive efforts. On this basis, the objectives in Table 125-1 are offered as guidelines for physicians and patients interested in taking steps to prevent CHD. On the other hand, it is undeniable that CHD does develop in individuals without risk factors, and that some individuals with multiple risk factors remain free of CHD. These facts should caution us from being judgmental or overly dogmatic in dealing with healthy asymptomatic individuals, for there is still much to learn about coronary disease and its prevention.

The first step in any intervention program is an assessment of modifiable risk factors, including the patient's smoking and exercise history, and measurements of weight, blood pressure, and serum cholesterol. After this assessment, the physician can discuss the overall risk of the patient's developing CHD, explore patient attitudes, and formulate specific, individualized recommendations. Since no single factor causes CHD, preventive

Table 125-1. Modifiable risk factors and their potential for CHD prevention

Risk factor	Treatment goal	Appropriate target for intervention	Comment
Cigarette smoking	Nonsmoker	Yes	Top priority
Hypertension	Diastolic BP < 90 mm Hg	Yes	Use of drugs for mild hypertension is controversial
Total cholesterol > 240 mg/dl	> 10% decrease	Yes	Avoid using drugs except in those at very high risk
Obesity	Ideal weight	Probably	Both direct and indirect effects
Sedentary life-style	Physical fitness	Probably	Direct, indirect effects likely
HDL cholesterol	?	Rarely	Increased by exercise
Type A behavior	?	No	Risk factor status uncertain
Glucose intolerance	Good control	No	Evidence for CHD reduction discouraging

measures should be based on an integrated approach to multiple risk factors. Intervention seems particularly likely to benefit those individuals who have several risk factors, because the risk associated with any one factor is greater in the presence of other risk factors.

Many measures directed at CHD prevention can be initiated in the physician's office, such as treating hypertension and high blood cholesterol, and encouraging smoking cessation and dietary modification. The latter efforts may be aided by referral to special intervention programs and professional dietitians. (See also Chaps. 130 and 145.)

Compliance with a preventive program is often difficult for asymptomatic patients, since the disease may not strike until many years in the future. The physician should transmit conviction of the value of the recommendations wholeheartedly and consider the life-style and family setting of the patient in developing advice. For some measures, such as smoking cessation, weight loss, and exercise, the immediate benefits in well-being, improved body image, and social interactions may prove more of a motivation than the potential long-term benefits in CHD prevention. Educational pamphlets, posters, and other materials (available from the American Heart Association and other organizations) can reemphasize the consequences of risk factors and outline skills helpful in achieving life-style changes.

The 1988 report of the Joint National Committee on detection, evaluation and treatment of high blood pressure. Arch Intern Med 1988; 148:1023–38.
Summarizes recommendations for the treatment of hypertension.

SHEP Cooperative Research Group. Prevention of stroke by antihypertensive drug treatment in older persons with isolated systolic hypertension. Final results of the systolic hypertension in the elderly program (SHEP). JAMA 1991; 265:3255–64.
Demonstrates the value of treating isolated systolic hypertension.

Svendson KH, et al. Effects of passive smoking in the MRFIT. Am J Epidemiol 1987; 126:783–95.
Demonstrates an increased relative risk in the nonsmoking spouses of smokers.

Rosenberg L, et al. The risk of myocardial infarction after quitting smoking in men under 55 years of age. N Engl J Med 1985; 313:1511–4.

A case-control study suggesting that the risk of myocardial infarction in former cigarette smokers decreases within a few years of quitting, to a level similar to that in men who have never smoked.

Toronto Working Group. Asymptomatic hypercholesterolemia: a clinical policy review. J Clin Epidemiol 1990; 43:1021–117.
A comprehensive and critical evaluation of cholesterol intervention.

The Expert Panel. Report of the National Cholesterol Education Program Expert Panel on detection, evaluation and treatment of high blood cholesterol in adults. Arch Intern Med 1988; 148:36–69.
Provides guidelines for the treatment of cholesterol, including a description of dietary and pharmacologic therapy.

Working Group on Management of Patients with Hypertension and High Blood Cholesterol. National Education Program Working Group report on the management of patients with hypertension and high blood cholesterol. Ann Intern Med 1991; 114:227–37.
Addresses the management of patients with multiple cardiac risk factors, with an emphasis on hypertension and high blood cholesterol. Both nonpharmacologic therapy and drug treatment are discussed.

University Group Diabetes Program. Effects of hypoglycemic agents on vascular complications in patients with adult-onset diabetes: VII. Mortality and selected nonfatal events with insulin treatment. JAMA 1978; 240:37–42.
A late report from this well-known study, which failed to demonstrate a beneficial effect of treatment on vascular complications.

Obermen A. Exercise and the primary prevention of cardiovascular disease. Am J Cardiol 1985; 55:10D–20D.
An overview of the data on exercise.

National Institutes of Health Consensus Development Conference. Health implications of obesity. Ann Intern Med 1985; 103:981–1077.
A series of background papers and a consensus statement on obesity.

The Steering Committee of Physicians Health Study Research Group. Findings from the aspirin component of the ongoing Physicians Health Study. N Engl J Med 1988; 318:262–4.
Reports a reduction by almost half in the incidence of myocardial infarction in physicians taking aspirin 325 mg every other day.

126. HIGH BLOOD CHOLESTEROL: SCREENING AND INTERVENTIONS
Robert B. Baron

Increased levels of blood cholesterol are associated with an increased risk of coronary heart disease (CHD), and lowering blood cholesterol will reduce the incidence of CHD. The primary tasks of office management of high blood cholesterol are the appropriate detection and evaluation of those patients at greatest risk, and the rational use of diet and drug therapy.

Rationale for Reducing Cholesterol to Prevent CHD
Considerable evidence from epidemiologic, genetic, physiologic, and animal studies has long suggested a strong, causal link between elevated levels of blood cholesterol and CHD. Five recent studies, however, have added sufficient additional evidence to justify an aggressive detection and treatment approach to high blood cholesterol.

The long-term follow-up of the men screened for the Multiple Risk Factor Intervention Trial demonstrated that levels of 240 mg/dl doubled the risk of death from CHD in 6 years, when compared to blood cholesterol levels of 200 mg/dl. Levels of 300 mg/dl doubled the risk again. This study also clearly demonstrated that the relationship between elevated blood cholesterol, CHD mortality, and total mortality was virtually identical to the relationship between hypertension and the same end points.

The Lipid Research Clinic Coronary Primary Prevention Trial (LRC-CPPT), a randomized study of cholestyramine in middle-aged men with high blood cholesterol clearly demonstrated that lowering total and low-density lipoprotein (LDL) cholesterol resulted in a decrease in CHD. The Helsinki Heart Study, a randomized study of gemfibrozil in middle-aged men, confirmed that lowering LDL cholesterol decreased the risk of CHD and demonstrated that raising high-density lipoprotein (HDL) cholesterol also resulted in a decrease in cardiac events. The changes in LDL and HDL cholesterol each accounted for approximately 50% of the benefit.

The Coronary Drug Project, which studied middle-aged men with a history of myocardial infarction (MI), showed that after 11 years, men who took niacin for 5 years as part of the initial Coronary Drug Project had an 11% decrease in total mortality. This finding was particularly important because neither the LRC-CPPT nor the Helsinki Heart Study resulted in a decrease in total mortality with drug treatment.

The Cholesterol-Lowering Atherosclerosis Study, a randomized trial of cholesterol-lowering drugs in men who recently had coronary artery bypass graft surgery, reviewed coronary arteriograms before and after drug treatment. Drug-treated subjects developed fewer new atherosclerotic lesions in both native and graft vessels and had regression of preexisting lesions not seen in the control group.

Patient Evaluation
The National Cholesterol Education Project (NCEP) guidelines for the management of high blood cholesterol are as follows:

Initial Classification by Total Cholesterol
Adult patients aged 20 to 70 years should have total cholesterol measured at least once every 5 years. These initial measurements can be nonfasting. Levels below 200 mg/dl are classified as "desirable" and can be rechecked in 5 years. Levels above 200 mg/dl should be remeasured, and if, on average, they remain above 200 mg/dl, further evaluation is required.

Patients with an initial total cholesterol above 200 mg/dl should be categorized as either at high or low risk for CHD on the basis of history and physical findings and a blood HDL cholesterol level. Those patients at high risk of CHD are more likely to benefit from cholesterol reduction. Patients are considered to be "high risk" if they have a history of CHD, including a definite MI or angina, or at least two of eight other risk factors for CHD. These include male sex, a family history of premature CHD (definite MI or sudden death of a parent or sibling before age 55), cigarette smoking (>10 cigarettes/d), hypertension (treated or not treated), low HDL cholesterol (< 35 mg/dl in men, < 45 mg/dl in women), diabetes mellitus, history of definite cerebrovascular or occlusive peripheral vascular disease, or obesity (> 30% over "desirable weight").

High-risk patients with total cholesterol averaging 200 mg/dl or higher and low-risk patients with total cholesterol levels at 240 mg/dl or higher should have the LDL cholesterol level estimated as described below. Low-risk patients with average total cholesterol levels of 200 to 239 mg/dl should be given dietary advice and re-evaluated in 1 year.

Classification by LDL Cholesterol
LDL cholesterol is estimated from fasting measurements of other serum lipids using the following equation:

LDL cholesterol = Total cholesterol − HDL cholesterol − (Triglycerides/5)

In patients with triglyceride levels above 400 mg/dl, this equation is less accurate and LDL cholesterol must be measured by ultracentrifugation. Patients are further classified based on their LDL cholesterol. The LDL cholesterol is emphasized diagnostically to eliminate those patients with elevated HDL cholesterol and/or elevated triglyceride levels who despite elevated levels of total cholesterol are not at increased risk of CHD.

Patients with high LDL cholesterol (> 160 mg/dl) or borderline LDL cholesterol (130–159 mg/dl) should be clinically evaluated for secondary causes of high blood cholesterol,

Table 126-1. Treatment guidelines

	Initiation LDL level	Minimal LDL goal
Dietary treatment		
Without CHD or with < 2 other risk factors*	≥ 160 mg/dl	< 160 mg/dl
With CHD or with ≥ 2 other risk factors*	≥ 130 mg/dl	< 130 mg/dl
Drug treatment		
Without CHD or < 2 other risk factors*	≥ 190 mg/dl	< 160 mg/dl
With CHD or ≥ 2 other risk factors*	≥ 160 mg/dl	< 130 mg/dl

*Risk factors include the following: male sex, definite MI or sudden death of a parent or sibling before age 55, smoking more than 10 cigarettes/d, hypertension, HDL cholesterol < 35 mg/dl, history of definite cerebrovascular or occlusive peripheral vascular disease, or body weight > 30% over desirable weight.

such as hypothyroidism, nephrotic syndrome, diabetes mellitus, obstructive liver disease, and medications that increase LDL levels such as progestins and anabolic steroids. In severe cases, family members should also be assessed to detect familial lipid disorders. Treatment should then be initiated according to the guidelines outlined in Table 126-1.

HDL Cholesterol
HDL cholesterol is a powerful, inverse, independent predictor of CHD in most populations, particularly in women. It should be measured in all patients with initial total cholesterol higher than 200 mg/dl to complete the risk factor profile. A number of studies have shown that individuals with elevated LDL cholesterol may be protected from much of the anticipated increased risk of CHD if the HDL cholesterol is also high (> 85 mg/dl). In such instances, especially in individuals without evidence of CHD, deferring treatment with medications may be reasonable.

HDL cholesterol need not, however, be measured in patients with a total cholesterol level of less than 200 mg/dl, or as a screening test, for several reasons. First, although individuals with a low HDL cholesterol and a low LDL cholesterol level appear to be at increased risk of CHD, individuals with this lipid profile are relatively uncommon. Moreover, no clinical study has yet shown that raising the HDL cholesterol in subjects with normal LDL cholesterol is advantageous. Secondly, the total cost of cholesterol detection would increase significantly if all individuals required measurement of both HDL and total cholesterol. Third, measurement of HDL cholesterol has not yet been fully standardized. One survey of the proficiency of HDL cholesterol measurement in 14 clinical laboratories revealed interlaboratory variations of 9 to 38%. Even in the best laboratories, the standard deviation of HDL cholesterol measurement is 3 mg/dl. Thus, a true HDL cholesterol of 43 mg/dl, for example, could be reported as anywhere between 37 mg/dl and 49 mg/dl 95% of the time. Since small errors can importantly affect the clinical interpretation of HDL levels, the risk of incorrectly classifying patients, particularly those with normal LDL levels, is great. Finally, although a number of nonpharmacologic measures are able to raise HDL cholesterol (weight loss, exercise, smoking cessation), each is sufficiently beneficial that they can be recommended to patients interested in reducing CHD risk without knowledge of the HDL cholesterol.

Triglycerides
There is little evidence to support an independent relationship between blood triglycerides and CHD. Fasting blood triglycerides should, however, be measured in individuals with a total cholesterol level higher than 240 mg/dl and in high-risk patients with cholesterols higher than 200 mg/dl, in order to estimate the LDL cholesterol level. Individuals with

levels above 1000 mg/dl are at increased risk for pancreatitis and should receive diet therapy, including avoidance of alcohol, and, if necessary, medications.

Evaluation of Elderly Patients
Application of these detection and treatment guidelines to the elderly remains controversial. Although cholesterol remains a risk factor for CHD in the elderly, it is a less powerful risk factor. Moreover, virtually all of the cholesterol-lowering trials excluded or contained very small numbers of elderly subjects. The use of cholesterol-lowering medications in the elderly, although not well studied, would be expected to result in a higher rate of side effects and drug interactions. Even diet therapy is of concern, given the already marginal nutritional intakes of many elderly patients.

Arguments in favor of applying these guidelines to older adults are based on their higher prevalence of CHD; although cholesterol is a less potent risk factor in the elderly (a lower relative risk), the absolute number of preventable deaths may actually be greater in the elderly since the prevalence of CHD is so high (a higher absolute risk).

The decision to treat elderly patients must be individualized, considering the patient's physiologic age and functional status, comorbid conditions, usage of other medications, dietary status, life-style issues, and personal preference. The greatest benefit might be expected in elderly patients with multiple risk factors for CHD and those with established CHD. Because of the accelerated rate of progression seen in coronary artery bypass grafts, patients with grafts and concurrent lipid disorders should usually be treated if no contraindications are present.

Recommendations for Women
Although CHD is less common in premenopausal women than in age-matched men, the rate becomes similar approximately 6 to 10 years after menopause. As a result, CHD is the leading cause of death in women, accounting for one-third of all deaths. Unfortunately, none of the clinical trials establishing that lipid modification prevents CHD have included women. Thus, recommendations for female patients are based on observational studies and inferentially from the clinical trials with men.

Observational studies have shown both LDL cholesterol and HDL cholesterol to be important predictors of CHD in women. In older women, HDL cholesterol may be a more potent predictor than LDL cholesterol. Current recommendations are to screen and evaluate women similarly to men. Because male gender is considered one of the factors that determine overall risk status, more women will be categorized as low risk, resulting in the use of the higher cutoffs for treatment as described above. Diet and drug therapy should also be used in the same manner for women as for men.

The lower risk of CHD in premenopausal women is thought to be due to the physiologic effects of estrogen. When given pharmacologically to postmenopausal women, estrogen decreases LDL cholesterol and increases HDL cholesterol by 15 to 20%. Observational studies of postmenopausal women who use estrogen have shown a consistent decrease in CHD. As a result, the use of estrogen as a lipid-modifying agent in high-risk women with lipid disorders is currently under investigation.

Treatment

Diet Therapy
Three common dietary factors account for most of the diet-induced elevations in blood cholesterol: (1) high intake of saturated fatty acids, (2) high intake of dietary cholesterol, and (3) high intake of total calories resulting in obesity. The goal of dietary treatment of high blood cholesterol is reversing these three dietary habits.

Unfortunately, dietary changes are very difficult for many patients. Clinical trials of dietary change have generally resulted in relatively small (approximately 7%) average changes in dietary cholesterol. Physicians commonly have little experience in promoting dietary changes, and most provide only cursory attempts at the dietary treatment of high blood cholesterol. With appropriate guidance, however, many patients are able to change their diets, obviating the need for drug treatment. Reductions in blood cholesterol of greater than 20% can sometimes be achieved. Diet therapy for high blood cholesterol should be tried for 3 to 6 months before drug therapy is begun. A full discussion of diet therapy is found in Chapter 145.

126. High Blood Cholesterol: Screening and Interventions 623

Table 126-2. Lipid-modifying effects of major cholesterol-lowering medications

	LDL cholesterol	HDL cholesterol	Triglycerides
Nicotinic acid	− 15–20%	+ 30–35%	− 25–30%
Resins	− 15–25%	+ 5%	+ 10%
Gemfibrozil	− 15%	+ 15–20%	− 35–50%
Lovastatin	− 20–45%	+ 10%	− 20%

Drug Therapy

Patients with elevated LDL cholesterol who do not respond to 3 to 6 months of intensive dietary therapy should be considered for drug therapy. As noted in Table 126-1, high-risk patients with persistent LDL cholesterol levels of 160 mg/dl or higher and low-risk patients at LDL cholesterol levels of 190 mg/dl or higher are begun on medications. Four classes of medications are currently available for first-line therapy of high blood cholesterol. These are the B-complex vitamin nicotinic acid, the bile acid–binding resins cholestyramine and colestipol, the fibric acid derivative gemfibrozil, and the HMG-CoA reductase inhibitor lovastatin.

The lipid-modifying effects of each agent are summarized in Table 126-2. All of the drugs lower LDL cholesterol effectively, although lovastatin is approximately twice as potent. Nicotinic acid and gemfibrozil are the most efficacious at raising HDL cholesterol. Gemfibrozil, nicotinic acid, and lovastatin all reduce blood triglycerides, while the bile acid–binding resins may increase triglyceride levels.

NICOTINIC ACID. Nicotinic acid has been used to modify serum lipids for many years. Its efficacy and safety are well established by the reduction in recurrent MIs demonstrated in the initial Coronary Drug Project and the decrease in total mortality seen in its long-term follow-up. Although the mechanism of action of nicotinic acid is not fully understood, it decreases very-low-density lipoprotein (VLDL) production in the liver, resulting in a decrease in LDL synthesis.

Nicotinic acid is the least costly of all the lipid-modifying medications but the most difficult to use. Side effects, particularly the cutaneous flushing experienced by almost all patients, limit patient acceptance. The flushing is prostaglandin-mediated and can be significantly inhibited with low doses of aspirin ($1/2$–1 aspirin/day). Beginning with very low doses of nicotinic acid, instructing the patient to take it with food, and carefully informing the patient about flushing can also improve patient acceptance. Sustained-action nicotinic acid preparations, although more expensive and somewhat less effective in raising HDL cholesterol levels, also result in less cutaneous flushing. Other side effects of nicotinic acid include hepatitis, gastrointestinal distress, glucose intolerance, hyperuricemia, and dry eyes. Hepatic toxicity is more likely to occur with sustained-release preparations; in asymptomatic individuals, nicotinic acid can be continued despite mild elevations in liver enzymes. Nicotinic acid should be used with caution in patients with diabetes and liver disease, and avoided in patients with active gout or peptic ulcer disease.

Treatment with nicotinic acid should be initiated with very low doses, typically 100 mg with the evening meal. The dose can be doubled each week until 1.5 g/day is achieved. If the goal LDL cholesterol level is not achieved, the dose can be increased to 3 to 6 g/day in divided doses; such higher doses are frequently necessary.

CHOLESTYRAMINE AND COLESTIPOL. The bile acid sequestrants also have an established record of safety and efficacy as demonstrated by the reduction in CHD in the LRC-CPPT. The sequestrants bind bile acids in the large intestine, resulting in an increase in hepatic bile synthesis from cholesterol. The decrease in hepatic cholesterol results in an increase in LDL receptor activity, stimulating LDL removal from plasma. The sequestrants are not absorbed and have no systemic toxicity, but may interfere with the absorption of other medications and so should be taken either 2 hours before or 1 hour after other drugs.

The use of the sequestrants is limited by their method of administration and side effects.

Administered as a powder mixed with water or juice, the agents commonly cause constipation, nausea, abdominal discomfort, bloating, and dry mouth. Side effects can be decreased by taking the powders with fruit juice instead of water, increasing dietary fiber and fluids to prevent constipation, and taking the medication with meals. A confectionary form and a more pulverized "light" form have recently been marketed to improve patient acceptance.

Treatment is with 4 g of cholestyramine or 5 g of colestipol once or twice daily and is increased to maintenance doses of 16 to 24 g and 20 to 30 g, respectively, in 4 to 6 doses per day. Unfortunately, these medications are quite expensive, especially when purchased in individual packets or in one of the newer formulations.

Because of their lack of systemic toxicity, these medications, when tolerated, may be particularly useful in younger patients and women of childbearing potential. They should be avoided, however, in patients with elevated triglycerides (> 500 mg/dl), because they may further increase triglyceride levels, and in patients with low levels of HDL cholesterol, since other agents are more effective at elevating HDL cholesterol.

GEMFIBROZIL. The safety and efficacy of gemfibrozil have been established by the reduction in CHD demonstrated in the Helsinki Heart Study. Approximately one-half of the demonstrated reduction was thought to be attributed to the reduction in LDL cholesterol achieved by gemfibrozil, and half to the increase in HDL cholesterol.

Gemfibrozil is extremely well tolerated and easier to use than either nicotinic acid or the sequestrants. The most common side effects are gastrointestinal, including dyspepsia, abdominal pain, and cholecystitis. Occasional abnormalities of hematologic parameters, hepatitis, and myositis have been reported. The drug is begun with 300 mg with dinner and advanced as needed to 1200 mg/day in divided doses.

Like niacin, gemfibrozil is particularly useful in patients with an elevated LDL cholesterol and a low HDL cholesterol. It is also used in patients with severe triglyceride elevations (> 1000 mg/dl) to prevent pancreatitis. In some patients with both elevated LDL cholesterol and elevated triglycerides, LDL levels may increase.

LOVASTATIN. Lovastatin competitively inhibits the rate-limiting enzyme in cholesterol synthesis, HMG-CoA reductase, resulting in an increase in LDL receptors and enhanced removal of blood LDL cholesterol. Although the LDL-lowering effect of lovastatin is well known, the effect on CHD incidence and mortality has not been established. Side effects are infrequent, however, and the drug appears to be well tolerated. The most common side effects are gastrointestinal discomfort, headaches, fatigue, and skin rashes. Approximately 2% of patients develop elevations of liver enzyme levels or myalgias and myositis with elevated creatine phosphokinase (CPK) levels requiring discontinuation of the medication. When lovastatin and gemfibrozil are used together, these side effects are approximately 3 times more common. Initial concerns about an increase in lens opacities with lovastatin have not been substantiated.

Lovastatin is begun at 20 mg with the evening meal and can be increased up to 80 mg/day in split doses. Transaminase and CPK levels should be monitored regularly.

OTHER MEDICATIONS. Psyllium seed preparations have been demonstrated in one study to result in a 15% reduction in LDL cholesterol with no effect on HDL cholesterol. The role of psyllium and other soluble fibers is discussed further in Chapter 145.

A number of other drugs are available for modifying lipids, but are not recommended for general use. Probucol lowers LDL cholesterol by 10 to 15% but also decreases HDL cholesterol by 25%. Clofibrate, although approved for triglyceride lowering, has been shown to increase cancers of the biliary tract. Neomycin can lower LDL cholesterol by 20 to 25% but can cause serious nephrotoxicity and ototoxicity and commonly causes diarrhea and abdominal cramps. Dextrothyroxine, an isomer of L-thyroxine, lowers LDL cholesterol levels by making the patient hyperthyroid, resulting in a high incidence of adverse cardiovascular and hypermetabolic effects.

DRUG COMBINATIONS. In patients with inadequate responses to single agents, combinations of the four classes of lipid-modifying drugs can be used. Since each class works by a different mechanism, their effects are synergistic. Drug combinations can also be used to prevent side effects due to high doses of individual drugs. Since nicotinic acid, lovastatin, and gemfibrozil each cause some liver toxicity, monitoring the symptoms of hepatitis and liver enzyme levels is particularly important. Similarly, myositis and CPK elevations are more common in patients taking both lovastatin and gemfibrozil than either drug alone.

REFERRAL. The vast majority of patients with lipid disorders can be successfully managed by primary care physicians. Referral to lipid specialists should be considered for those patients with elevated blood cholesterol who cannot be controlled with the four classes of medications discussed above. Selected patients with severe genetic dyslipidemias, such as homozygous familial high blood cholesterol, should also be referred.

Baron RB. Management of hypercholesterolemia: a primary care perspective. West J Med 1989; 150:562–8.
A clinical review.

Blankenhorn DM, et al. Beneficial effects of combined colestipol-niacin therapy on coronary atherosclerosis and coronary venous bypass grafts. JAMA 1987; 257:3233–40.
The first report of regression of coronary atherosclerosis in subjects intensively treated with lipid-lowering medications.

Canner PL, et al. Fifteen-year mortality in Coronary Drug Project patients: long-term benefit with niacin. J Am Coll Cardiol 1986; 8:1245–55.
The long-term follow-up of the Coronary Drug Project, which showed an 11% reduction in total mortality in subjects who took niacin during the study. This is the first, and only report, of a decrease in total mortality with lipid modification.

Coronary Drug Research Group. Clofibrate and niacin in coronary heart disease. JAMA 1975; 231:360–81.
The initial report of the Coronary Drug Project. This randomized controlled trial of 8341 men aged 34 to 64 with a documented MI showed a decrease in recurrent MIs in men treated with nicotinic acid.

Frick MH, et al. Helsinki Heart Study: primary-prevention trial with gemfibrozil in middle-aged men with dyslipidemia. N Engl J Med 1987; 317:1237–45.
A randomized, double-blinded comparison of gemfibrozil and placebo in 4081 men, aged 40 to 55, with non-HDL cholesterol higher than 200 mg/dl. Gemfibrozil treatment resulted in a 34% decrease in cardiac events.

Garber AM. Where to draw the line against cholesterol. Ann Intern Med 1989; 111:625–6.
A brief comparison of the guidelines for detection, evaluation, and treatment of high blood cholesterol currently recommended in the United States with those recently published in Canada. The Canadian recommendations are significantly less aggressive.

Grundy SM. HMG-CoA reductase inhibitors for treatment of hypercholesterolemia. N Engl J Med 1988; 319:24–33.
An excellent review.

Grundy SM, et al. The place of HDL in cholesterol management: a perspective from the National Cholesterol Education Program. Arch Intern Med 1989; 149:505–10.
An explanation of the decision to keep HDL cholesterol in a somewhat secondary role in the detection, evaluation, and treatment of high blood cholesterol.

Lipid Research Clinics Program. The Lipid Research Clinics Coronary Primary Prevention Trial results: I. Reduction in the incidence of coronary heart disease. JAMA 1984; 251:351–64.

Lipid Research Clinics Program. The Lipid Research Clinics Coronary Primary Prevention Trial results: II. The relationship of reduction in incidence of coronary heart disease to cholesterol lowering. JAMA 1984; 251:365–74.
The two initial reports of the results of the LRC-CPPT, a randomized controlled study of 3806 men, aged 35 to 59, with total cholesterol levels above 265 mg/dl who were given cholestyramine or placebo. Cholestyramine resulted in a 21% decrease in coronary deaths, and the incidence of all coronary end points decreased 17%.

Manninen V, et al. Lipid alterations and decline in the incidence of coronary heart disease in the Helsinki Heart Study. JAMA 1988; 260:641–51.
A follow-up report from the Helsinki Heart Study showing that the benefit from lipid modification with gemfibrozil was approximately equally due to lowering LDL cholesterol and raising HDL cholesterol, but not due to lowering triglycerides.

Martin MJ, et al. Serum cholesterol, blood pressure, and mortality: implications from a cohort of 361,622 men. Lancet 1986; 2:933–6.
Follow-up report on the 361,622 men initially screened for enrollment in the Multiple Risk Factor Intervention Trial. The report showed that compared to average blood cholesterol levels of 200 mg/dl, levels of 240 mg/dl and 300 mg/dl resulted in a two- and fourfold increase in CHD risk, respectively. The report also demonstrated that the relationship between cholesterol, CHD mortality, and total mortality was virtually identical for patients with high blood cholesterol and hypertension.

Choice of cholesterol-lowering drugs. Med Lett Drugs Ther 1988; 30:81–4.
An excellent comparison of medications, including costs.

National Cholesterol Education Program expert panel. Report of the National Cholesterol Education Program expert panel on detection, evaluation and treatment of high blood cholesterol in adults. Arch Intern Med 1988; 148:36–69.
The initial comprehensive report outlining the current recommendations for detection, evaluation, and treatment of high blood cholesterol in the United States.

127. EXERCISE
David S. Siscovick

Clinicians are frequently asked how exercise affects health. Unfortunately, answers are difficult to come by because studies of the potential benefits and risks of exercise appear contradictory.

Benefits
Potential benefits that have been attributed to exercise include (1) reduced risk of coronary heart disease (CHD) morbidity and mortality; (2) reduced levels of cardiovascular risk factors; (3) increased functional capacity, effort tolerance, or work capacity; and (4) improved sense of well-being including less anxiety and depression, better sleep, and better "quality of life."

Coronary Events
Several studies have suggested that asymptomatic persons who do not engage in vigorous exercise have 2 to 3 times the risk of clinical CHD (i.e., angina pectoris, myocardial infarction, sudden cardiac death) compared to vigorous persons. This relationship appears to be independent of other risk factors for CHD. Thus, lack of vigorous exercise is associated with an increase in CHD risk comparable to that for hypertension and cigarette smoking.

It has been suggested that persons with other risk factors, particularly people who are older, are obese, or have a history of hypertension, might benefit the most from vigorous activity. Continued participation in vigorous exercise appears to be necessary to maintain the beneficial effect. However, it is not known whether persons who begin vigorous exercise late in life achieve the same benefit as those who have engaged in exercise throughout life. Although these observations have been based on nonexperimental studies, the U.S. Preventive Services Task Force recently concluded that the available evidence supports the role of exercise in the prevention of clinical CHD.

Cardiovascular Risk Factors
Exercise has been shown to increase high-density lipoprotein cholesterol, fibrinolysis, and insulin sensitivity and to decrease very-low-density and low-density lipoprotein cholesterol

and premature ventricular contractions. Furthermore, associations apparently exist between vigorous exercise and control of hypertension, obesity, glucose intolerance (in maturity-onset diabetes mellitus), and hyperlipidemia. The efficacy of vigorous exercise in either the prevention or long-term treatment of these latter conditions is not established. However, it is generally acknowledged that exercise is favorably associated with factors related to cardiovascular risk.

Functional Capacity
Physiologic studies have repeatedly demonstrated that vigorous exercise increases functional capacity. However, there is disagreement about the time needed for an exercise program to change functional capacity, the magnitude of the increase in functional capacity achievable, and whether older persons differ in their responsiveness to such exercise. Exercise adequate to achieve fitness clearly increases physical work capacity or effort tolerance—a benefit that both patients and physicians consider clinically significant.

General Well-Being
Based on uncontrolled studies of volunteer participants in organized exercise programs, it has been suggested that exercise improves sleep and enhances a person's "sense of well-being." Additionally, exercise has been reported to increase brain endorphin levels. It is a common clinical impression that exercise decreases anxiety and depression; however, proper studies supporting the efficacy of exercise in either the prevention or the treatment of anxiety or depression have not been reported. Despite the absence of controlled evidence, exercise appears to affect the mood of many patients favorably and has been commonly recommended for this purpose.

Risks
Exercise is associated with risks as well as benefits. Two specific exercise-related hazards, sudden cardiac death and musculoskeletal injuries, are of particular importance.

Sudden Cardiac Death
Exercise-related sudden cardiac death is a rare but catastrophic event, occurring in approximately 1 per 20,000 exercisers per year. Epidemiologic studies have demonstrated that the risk of sudden cardiac death is transiently increased sevenfold during vigorous exercise, compared to the risk at other times. The occurrence of sudden cardiac death during exercise is not a random event; vigorous exercise can precipitate sudden cardiac death. The magnitude of the increase in risk during exercise is influenced by the level of habitual activity. The increase in risk during exercise is less for men who are regular exercisers than for men who are more sedentary. Men with prior clinical CHD and sickle cell trait are also at increased risk for exercise-related sudden cardiac death. However, among apparently healthy men and those with prior CHD, there is no evidence that exercising increases the overall risk of sudden cardiac death. In fact, the net effect (the balance between the benefits and risks) of habitual vigorous exercise among apparently healthy persons suggests that habitual exercise reduces the overall risk of sudden cardiac death.

Musculoskeletal Injuries
Few epidemiologic studies have estimated the risks of exercise-related musculoskeletal injuries; they are, however, relatively common but only occasionally require medical attention and result in disability.

Pre-Exercise Evaluation
Medical evaluations before beginning vigorous exercise have been suggested to identify persons for whom exercise might be harmful. Several groups have arbitrarily recommended that all persons over 35 years old and persons less than 35 years old with either a history of cardiovascular disease or CHD risk factors should "see their physician" before increasing their physical activity. In part, this recommendation is based on the conventional wisdom that persons who are at increased risk for CHD are those for whom exercise might be harmful and that unusual activity is particularly likely to be dangerous. Pre-exercise evaluations have also been recommended to identify persons with other cardiac

(e.g., aortic stenosis, congestive heart failure, hypertrophic cardiomyopathy) and noncardiac (e.g., acute infections) contraindications to exercise.

A variety of diagnostic maneuvers have been recommended as part of a pre-exercise evaluation: history, physical examination, chest radiograph, electrocardiogram, exercise tolerance test, complete blood cell count, urinalysis, fasting blood sugar, creatinine, cholesterol, arterial blood gas, pulmonary function tests, echocardiogram, and Holter monitoring. Unfortunately, it is not known whether any of these maneuvers helps identify those otherwise healthy persons for whom exercise increases risk.

Routine exercise testing of all asymptomatic adults before exercise training does not appear to be justified given the low absolute risk of exercise-related death. The likelihood of CHD in an asymptomatic population is low (approximately 5%). As a result, most positive exercise test results in an asymptomatic population would be falsely positive, and a negative result would merely confirm the low likelihood of CHD. Furthermore, the sensitivity of clinically silent ST segment changes on the exercise electrocardiogram for predicting activity-related acute cardiac events appears to be low, approximately 20%. If the results of a screening exercise electrocardiogram were used to target interventions that might reduce the transient increase in risk during activity, it is likely that these efforts would miss approximately 80% of cases of activity-related acute cardiac events among apparently healthy exercisers.

For asymptomatic patients presenting for a pre-exercise evaluation, maneuvers other than a careful history and physical examination should not be performed initially. Those patients with possible cardiac symptoms or a history of heart disease should be more fully evaluated (including an exercise tolerance test) before initiating an exercise program. Many patients and physicians have come to expect that extensive pre-exercise testing be done. The yield from doing so is certainly small, and this practice is not justified by evidence of benefit.

Exercise Prescription

The exact "dose" of exercise needed to achieve specific health benefits is unknown. Guidelines for the quantity and quality of exercise required to develop and maintain "fitness" have been suggested by the American College of Sports Medicine. These recommendations were derived from studies of endurance training programs. Improvement in fitness, measured as maximum oxygen intake, was directly related to the frequency, intensity, and duration of activity. For healthy persons, the usual recommendation is for rhythmic aerobic activity involving large muscle groups—that is, activities like brisk walking, jogging, swimming, tennis, and cross-country skiing that require an intensity of 60 to 90% of maximum heart rate reserve. This amounts to a heart rate of approximately 130 to 135 beats per minute in a young person (50–80% of maximum oxygen intake), of 15 to 60 minutes' duration per occasion, 3 to 5 days per week.

In prescribing exercise, the initial level of fitness is an important consideration. Persons with low levels of fitness (e.g., older persons) can achieve a significant training effect with a sustained heart rate as low as 110 to 120 beats per minute. It is commonly recommended that persons check their pulse during exercise to ensure the proper exercise intensity. However, a rough guide to attaining the necessary intensity is the "perspiration test"; exercise that results in perspiration is usually associated with a pulse above 70% of maximum. Additionally, persons should feel pleasantly fatigued rather than exhausted at the end of a workout. For joggers, a useful guide is the "talk test"; jogging should be at a pace that allows the runner to carry on a conversation with a fellow runner.

When exercise above the minimum threshold of intensity is performed, fitness development is a function of the total kilocalorie energy expenditure in such activities. This training effect appears to be independent of the mode of dynamic exercise. While the minimum level of physical activity necessary to maintain fitness is unknown, there is physiologic evidence to suggest that exercise must be maintained on a "regular" basis to maintain the "training effect." If vigorous exercise is discontinued for several months, fitness levels appear to return to pretraining levels.

When initiating an exercise program, asymptomatic persons should be advised to gradually increase the intensity and duration of their activity over a 1- to 4-week period. If symptoms consistent with cardiovascular disease occur, patients should discontinue exercise and contact their physician. Non–weight-bearing activities, such as swimming as opposed to jogging, appear to be associated with fewer debilitating injuries (e.g., foot, leg, or knee injuries) in beginning exercisers. "Overuse" injuries are common and usually result from engaging in an excessive training load for too long without adequate rest. Performance of stretching exercise and exercises of increasing intensity to "warm up" before engaging in endurance activity and of decreasing intensity to "cool down" after intense exercise is commonly recommended.

Morris JN, et al. Vigorous exercise in leisure-time: protection against coronary heart disease. Lancet 1980; 2:1207–10.
The first clinical episodes of CHD in 17,944 middle-aged male British civil servants prospectively followed for 8½ years are reported in relation to physical activity status during leisure time.

Paffenbarger RS, Wing AL, Hydge RT. Physical activity as an index of heart attack risk in college alumni. Am J Epidemiol 1978; 108:161–75.
Follow-up study of 16,936 Harvard male alumni, aged 35 to 74 years, where risk of the first attack was related inversely to energy expenditure in physical activity.

Powell KE, et al. Physical activity and the incidence of coronary heart disease. Annu Rev Public Health 1987; 8:253–87.
A meta-analysis of over 40 studies that examined the relation between physical activity and CHD.

Siscovick DS, et al. Physical activity and primary cardiac arrest. JAMA 1982; 248:3113–7.
A population-based, case-controlled study supporting the hypothesis that vigorous leisure-time physical activity reduces the risk of primary cardiac arrest.

Cooper KH, et al. Physical fitness levels versus selected coronary risk factors: a cross-sectional study. JAMA 1976; 236:116.
Prevalence study of nearly 3000 men showing an inverse relationship between the level of physical fitness and selected risk factors.

Siscovick DS, et al. The incidence of primary cardiac arrest during vigorous exercise. N Engl J Med 1984; 311:874–7.
An analysis that puts into perspective the risks and benefits of vigorous exercise that relate to sudden cardiac death.

Siscovick DS, et al. Sensitivity of exercise electrocardiography in predicting acute cardiac events during moderate and strenuous physical activity. Arch Intern Med 1991; 151:325–30.
An analysis from the Lipid Research Clinics Coronary Primary Prevention Trial examining the ability of exercise electrocardiography to predict activity-related cardiac events.

American College of Sports Medicine. Position statement on recommended quality and quantity of exercise for developing and maintaining fitness in healthy adults. Med Sci Sports 1978; 10:vii–xi.
Presents guidelines, rationale, and research background for the current recommendations for exercise prescription in healthy adults.

Harris SS, et al. Physical activity counseling for healthy adults as a primary preventive intervention in the clinical setting. Report for the US Preventive Services Task Force. JAMA 1989; 261:3590–8.
Presents an evaluation of the following: (1) the burden of suffering attributable to physical inactivity; (2) the efficacy of physical activity in disease prevention in regard to six medical conditions; and (3) the characteristics of the intervention in terms of simplicity, cost, safety, acceptability, and patient compliance.

Kark JA, et al. Sickle-cell trait as a risk factor for sudden death in physical activity. N Engl J Med 1987; 317:701–2.
An analysis demonstrating a potential interaction between physical activity and sickle cell trait related to the risk of sudden death.

128. MEDICAL ADVICE FOR TRAVELERS
Robert B. Baron

Physicians should be familiar with the health risks of travel and be able to provide advice, immunizations, medications, and follow-up care. Changing patterns of disease and health requirements demand the availability of frequently updated resources such as the Centers for Disease Control's (CDC) annually updated publication *Health Information for International Travel;* the CDC also maintains a telephone information line for international travelers—404-332-4559. In some instances, referral to travel specialists or public health officials is necessary.

Routine Immunizations
All adult patients who travel, regardless of their destination, should be up-to-date with routine immunizations. These are discussed further in Chapter 124.

Tetanus
Adults should have completed a primary series of tetanus-diptheria and receive boosters every 10 years. Some high-risk travelers may benefit from boosters every 5 years since a tetanus-prone wound does not need further treatment with tetanus immune globulin or postexposure booster if the person has been boosted within 5 years.

Measles
Recommendations for the use of the measles vaccine for international travel are currently in flux. Although the incidence of measles remained stable in the United States between 1981 and 1988, a marked increase in cases was observed in 1989. Over 25% of cases in the United States, including several large outbreaks on college campuses, are related to international travel (imported cases and contacts). In adults who travel, revaccination is recommended for individuals born after 1956 who were vaccinated before 1980.

Rubella
Women of childbearing age who are not immune to rubella (and who are not pregnant) should consider immunization prior to travel.

Mumps
Adults without a history of mumps or prior vaccination should be vaccinated prior to travel.

Polio
Although polio is highly endemic in most developing countries, the risk of polio for travelers is very low (approximately 1 case/yr). Adults who received a primary series of polio vaccine as a child should, however, receive a booster when traveling to highly endemic areas (e.g., Amazon basin, India, Nepal). Because of the small, but real risk of vaccine-associated paralytic polio (1/520,000 doses), the enhanced-potency inactivated vaccine is preferred over the oral (live) vaccine for boosting adults.

Pneumococcal Disease
Persons with chronic illnesses and healthy persons over the age of 64 should receive the vaccine prior to travel.

Influenza
Persons with chronic illnesses, particularly of the cardiopulmonary system, the elderly, and health care workers who will be engaged in patient care activities should receive the vaccine prior to travel. Travelers to the tropics should be reminded that while the risk of influenza is present there throughout the year, the season of greatest activity in the Southern Hemisphere is April through September.

Required Vaccinations
Some countries require proof of vaccination against diseases, such as cholera and yellow fever, prior to entry. Smallpox vaccination has not been required or recommended since 1982, due to the apparent eradication of this disease worldwide. An updated list of requirements is published annually and updated biweekly by the CDC. Vaccinations must be documented on the World Health Organization's "International Certificate of Vaccination."

For direct travel from the United States, no country currently requires cholera vaccination but many nations of West and Central Africa require yellow fever vaccination. No vaccinations are required for return to the United States. For travel between developing countries, requirements for vaccination vary. Currently, fewer than 10 nations require cholera vaccination under any circumstances.

Cholera
Unfortunately, the cholera vaccine is only about 50% effective, and is not recommended for travelers to endemic areas unless it is required. Cholera can be largely prevented by following the hygienic suggestions for preventing traveler's diarrhea.

Yellow Fever
Yellow fever vaccine is an effective attenuated live virus vaccine against a disease without specific treatment. Patients who travel to rural areas of countries in the endemic zones should receive this vaccine whether or not it is required by local authorities. Endemic areas include much of equatorial Africa (below 15 degrees latitude North and above 15 degrees South) and jungle regions of South America (Colombia, Brazil, Peru, Bolivia, and Ecuador).

Primary vaccination is with a single dose; boosters are required every 10 years. Yellow fever vaccine requires cold storage and is only viable for 30 minutes after reconstitution. It is only administered at approved centers (identified by calling local health departments).

Vaccinations Recommended in Certain Circumstances
Typhoid
The killed bacterial vaccine, administered as two injections 4 weeks apart, is only about 70% effective and often causes fever, headache, and malaise after each injection. The live attenuated oral vaccine, released in 1990, has comparable efficacy, and fewer side effects (rare incidence of abdominal discomfort, nausea, vomiting, rash, and urticaria). It is administered by enteric-coated capsules, taken on alternate days for a total of four doses.

Since typhoid fever and other *Salmonella* infections can be prevented by hygienic measures and treated with antibiotics, use of either vaccine is optional.

Meningococcal Disease
Although most travelers are at extremely low risk for meningococcal disease, several popular travel destinations have had epidemics warranting vaccination. Travelers to Nepal, the New Delhi region of India, Saudi Arabia, and sub-Saharan Africa should receive the vaccine.

Rabies
Rabies vaccine, an inactivated virus preparation, is only recommended for travelers likely to have contact with potentially rabid animals (veterinarians, animal trainers, spelunkers, etc.) and for travelers spending prolonged periods in countries where rabies is a constant threat (many areas of Latin America, the Far East, and Africa). Preexposure vaccination, however, does not eliminate the need for postexposure prophylaxis (see Chap. 138).

Plague
Plague vaccination is recommended only for travelers to endemic areas likely to have direct contact with wild rodents and rabbits (and their fleas). Plague is found in selected rural, mountainous areas of the Americas, Africa, and Asia and is typically a seasonal disease occurring during warm humid weather.

Japanese B Encephalitis
This mosquito-borne viral illness is prevalent in India and most of Asia. Distribution of the vaccine has been discontinued in the United States since 1987 due to liability concerns. The vaccine is available in Asia and is recommended for those travelers spending prolonged periods in rural Asia.

Hepatitis B
The hepatitis B vaccine is recommended for travelers to highly endemic areas who are likely to have direct contact with blood or secretions of potentially infected people, such as high-risk health workers and travelers likely to have sexual contact with local people. Areas with the highest prevalences of hepatitis B ($\geq 5\%$) include Southeast Asia (including China and Indonesia), South Pacific Islands, sub-Saharan Africa, the interior Amazon basin, and parts of the Caribbean. Three doses are given over a 6-month period. All doses should be given in the deltoid region (rather than the buttock) to enhance absorption. Hepatitis B vaccine will also protect against hepatitis D, also highly prevalent in the developing world.

Hepatitis A
The risk of hepatitis A has been estimated at 1 to 10 per 1000 travelers to the developing world. Travelers staying in the developing world for less than 3 months should receive 2 ml of immune serum globulin (ISG) while those staying 4 to 6 months need 5 ml. Travelers for longer than 6 months need boosters while away. The process used to prepare ISG removes any potential viral particles and no virus has been cultured from ISG. No cases of human immunodeficiency virus (HIV) infection or any other viral illness has ever been documented to result from ISG. Unfortunately, ISG is not effective against enterically transmitted non-A, non-B hepatitis.

Multiple Vaccines
Patients who require multiple vaccines (live and/or inactivated) can receive multiple antigens on the same day at different anatomic sites without an apparent loss of efficacy. Live vaccines, including the oral polio vaccine, measles, mumps, rubella, and yellow fever, should be given at least 14 days prior to or at least 6 weeks after ISG is given. Inactivated vaccines can be given at any time before, with, or after ISG is administered.

Hypersensitivity to Vaccine Components
Vaccines such as yellow fever, produced by growing microorganisms in embryonated chicken eggs may cause hypersensitivity reactions in individuals allergic to eggs and should not be administered to such individuals. Live viruses prepared in cell culture, such as measles, mumps, and influenza, can also lead to anaphylactic hypersensitivity reactions in individuals with known anaphylactic hypersensitivity to eggs.

Vaccination of Individuals with Febrile Illnesses
Individuals with minor illnesses, such as upper respiratory tract infections, can receive vaccinations despite their illness. Individuals with more severe febrile illnesses, however, should postpone vaccinations until they have recovered, to avoid superimposing adverse vaccine effects on their illness or mistaking a manifestation of the illness as an adverse effect of the vaccine.

Traveler's Diarrhea
Unless efforts are made to prevent it, at least one-third of travelers to developing countries will develop "traveler's diarrhea" (emporiatric enteritis, "turista," "Montezuma's revenge," cruise ship cramp, "Delhi belly," the "Aztec two-step"). Careful hygienic measures can prevent most cases. Enterotoxigenic *Escherichia coli* is the most common cause, but many other infectious etiologies are also prevalent, including *Shigella, Salmonella, Campylobacter,* other bacteria (*Vibrios, Aeromonas, Yersinia*), rotaviruses and Norwalk-like viruses, amoeba, *Giardia,* and other enteric parasites.

Characteristically, patients develop a sudden onset of watery diarrhea, usually accompanied by cramps, urgency, nausea, malaise, and low-grade fever. Symptoms usually last 3 to 5 days (longer in children) and resolve spontaneously. Significant fever and purulent or bloody feces should suggest invasive bacteria or parasites; these symptoms are not due to enterotoxigenic *E. coli*.

Traveler's diarrhea can be prevented by careful attention to hygiene, particularly food and water selection. Especially risky foods include tap water and ice, unpeeled fruits and raw vegetables, unpasteurized milk and dairy products, and raw meat and raw seafood. Cooked food exposed to flies can also transmit diarrheal illnesses. Thus, travelers should only eat and drink food and beverages that follow the "Traveler's Rule of P's": peeled, packaged, purified, and piping hot. Tap water can be purified by boiling or by use of iodine tablets. Teeth should also be brushed using purified water.

Numerous studies have shown that traveler's diarrhea can also be prevented by antibiotics and by nonantimicrobial medications. Doxycycline (100 mg/day), trimethoprim-sulfamethoxazole (one double-strength tablet/day), trimethoprim (200 mg/day), and norfloxacin (400 mg/day) have been shown in randomized blinded studies to be consistently effective in reducing the incidence of traveler's diarrhea by 50 to 88%. Antibiotic side effects, however, are common, and prophylactic antibiotics are not indicated in most instances.

Nonantimicrobial medications have also been studied for the prevention of traveler's diarrhea. Bismuth subsalicylate (Pepto-Bismol), taken as a liquid, 60 ml 4 times a day or as a 2 tablets 4 times a day, has been shown to significantly decrease the incidence of traveler's diarrhea. Large doses of bismuth subsalicylate can cause salicylate toxicity in children and in adults taking large doses of salicylates for other illnesses. Difenoxin (the active metabolite of the diphenoxylate Lomotil), loperamide hydrochloride (Imodium), and activated charcoal are ineffective.

A number of measures are available for the effective treatment of traveler's diarrhea. Fluid and electrolyte balance should be maintained by the liberal use of clear liquids (fruit juices, soft drinks, tea, broth). For rapid relief of symptoms, loperamide (4 mg initially, then 2 mg after each loose stool, to a maximum of 16 mg/day) may be taken. Alternatively Pepto-Bismol (30 ml of liquid or 2 tablets every 30 minutes for eight doses and after each bowel movement) can be begun but this regimen takes somewhat longer and is less effective than loperamide. No significant prolongation of infection has been consistently demonstrated with antimotility drugs.

To shorten the duration of the illness from 3 to 5 days to 1 to ½ day, antibiotics can be taken. Three-day regimens of trimethoprim-sulfamethoxazole (one double-strength tablet bid), trimethoprim (200 mg bid), doxycycline (100 mg bid), norfloxacin (400 mg bid), and ciprofloxacin (500 bid) are all effective. A recent study showed the combination of loperamide and trimethoprim-sulfamethoxazole to be more effective than either agent taken alone.

Measures taken to prevent traveler's diarrhea may be individualized according to the plans and preferences of the traveler, and the location of travel. At a minimum, all travelers should be instructed in hygienic precautions and basic treatment measures. Pepto-Bismol or loperamide should be included in the "travel kit" for initial treatment, along with an antibiotic, such as trimethoprim-sulfamethoxazole, for severe cases. Travelers for whom the risk of diarrhea is more threatening than the inconvenience and potential side effects of medications might consider using Pepto-Bismol or one of the effective antibiotics prophylactically.

Malaria

Malaria is one of the world's most common infectious diseases and the most common serious disease of travelers. It is caused by one of four protozoan species of the genus *Plasmodium: P. vivax, P. falciparum, P. ovale,* and *P. malariae*. All are transmitted by the bite of the infected female *Anopheles* mosquito. The disease is characterized by a flu-like illness with fever, headache, malaise, chills, and sweats. It may cause anemia and jaundice; *P. falciparum* infections may cause kidney failure, coma, and death.

Malaria occurs in large portions of the developing world including Central and South America, sub-Saharan Africa, India, Southeast Asia, and Oceania. Although local conditions vary, travelers are primarily at risk when visiting rural areas during the evening and night.

The emergence of chloroquine-resistant *P. falciparum* (CRPF) has made chemoprophylaxis somewhat complicated. Travelers to areas where chloroquine resistance has not been reported (primarily Central America and Haiti) should be given chloroquine phosphate (Aralen), 500 mg weekly, at the same time each week. Chloroquine should be begun 1 to 2 weeks prior to arrival and must be continued for 6 weeks afterward. Travelers with a history of heavy exposure to mosquitoes in malarious areas should also take primaquine phosphate, 26.3 mg/day, during the last 2 weeks of posttravel chloroquine treatment to eradicate the risk of occult, extraerythrocytic (liver) *P. vivax* and *P. ovale*. Screening for glucose-6-phosphate dehydrogenase (G-6-PD) deficiency should be performed in patients at risk prior to prescribing primaquine.

Until recently, travelers to areas with CRPF were advised to take weekly doses of chloroquine and weekly doses of pyrimethamine (25 mg) and sulfadoxine (500 mg) (Fansidar). Since sulfadoxine became available in the United States in 1982, however, severe cutaneous reactions (erythema multiforme, Stevens-Johnson syndrome, and toxic epidermal necrolysis) have been reported, some leading to death. Most reports involved patients simultaneously taking chloroquine.

Recommendations for the prevention of malaria in areas of chloroquine resistance (most of the malarious world) are currently in flux. Mefloquine (Lariam), a new antimalarial similar in structure to quinine, was approved for release in the United States in April 1989. Effective against both chloroquine-resistant and sulfadoxine-resistant strains, mefloquine is now the drug of choice for travelers at risk of infection with CRPF. The currently recommended dose of mefloquine is 250 mg beginning 1 week prior to travel, continuing through the period of exposure and for 4 weeks afterward. At this dose, mefloquine's side effects, gastrointestinal upset and dizziness, are infrequent. Because its quinine-like effects may cause prolongation of the QT interval and sinus bradycardia, it should be used with caution in patients taking beta-blockers, calcium channel antagonists, and other drugs that affect cardiac conduction.

Other regimens that can be used in areas of chloroquine resistance include:

Doxycycline daily (100 mg/day), begun 1 to 2 days before travel to malarious areas, and continued during exposure and for 4 weeks afterward. This is a good regimen for short-term travelers intolerant to mefloquine or for whom the drug is contraindicated. The major side effect is sun-sensitivity reactions.

Chloroquine (weekly) plus proguanil (200 mg/day). Proguanil is also not available commercially in the United States but is available in most international cities. Limited data suggest that the regimen is efficacious in Africa (Kenya) but not in Asia or Oceania (proguanil resistance).

Cloroquine (weekly) and, as needed, sulfadoxine (3 tablets PO as a single dose) during any febrile illness while traveling. This temporary measure should be followed by prompt medical evaluation.

All travelers to malarious areas should be informed on how to prevent exposure to mosquitoes. *Anopheles* mosquitoes feed at night, limiting malaria transmission to the hours between dusk and dawn. Whenever possible, travelers should remain in screened areas, wear clothes that cover most of the body, and liberally use insect repellents with more than 30% *N,N*-diethyl-*m*-toluamide (deet). Additional protection may be afforded by treating clothing with permethrin, a pesticide available as Permanone Tick Repellent. Toxic and allergic reactions to deet have been reported, including anaphylaxis, seizures, and fatal ingestions; preparations should be kept out of reach of children and discontinued if skin eruptions or signs of systemic toxicity are noted. Travelers should also know that malaria can occur despite chemoprophylaxis. Any significant febrile illness occurring during or after travel to endemic areas should be evaluated.

Other Infectious Illnesses

Most travelers are at minimal risk for the development of other tropical illnesses. Nonetheless, travelers to the tropics and providers should be somewhat familiar with the most common serious tropical illnesses and the measures useful in their prevention. The most important of these are additional arthropod-borne diseases, including dengue fever, Japanese encephalitis, filariasis, leishmaniasis, and trypanosomiasis. Measures to protect against mosquitoes, as described above, and other measures to avoid contact with the respective vectors will protect the traveler against these diseases. Schistosomiasis also remains a major global health problem. Transmitted by aqueous contact with infecting cercariae, it can be prevented by avoiding swimming and bathing in slow flowing, snail-infected fresh water.

Patients who travel are also at risk of acquiring the same illnesses for which they are at risk while at home. Most common are respiratory infections, skin infections, and sexually transmitted diseases. Travelers should be advised to carry common remedies for upper respiratory tract infections. Skin infections can be particularly bothersome while traveling in the tropics. Wounds require immediate attention with cleansing and topical antiseptics to prevent cellulitis and abscesses. Erythromycin or other antibiotics with a similar spectrum should be carried in areas where medications are not readily available.

Sexually transmitted diseases may pose a number of difficulties for travelers who are sexually active. Penicillinase-producing *Neisseria gonorrhoeae* (PPNG), for example, is prevalent throughout much of the developing world. All travelers with gonorrhea who have acquired the disease in these areas should be treated with a regimen effective against PPNG, such as ceftriaxone, 250 mg intramuscularly. The spread of HIV infection and acquired immunodeficiency syndrome (AIDS) has increased the urgency of avoiding casual sexual contact while traveling. The use of condoms and the avoidance of sexual practices that involve the exchange of bodily fluids (especially semen and blood) are strongly recommended. Chancroid and granuloma inguinale are also more prevalent in developing countries than in the United States.

Environmental Illnesses

Trauma
The most common cause of death in travelers is trauma, usually due to motor vehicle accidents. Unfortunately seat belts, motorcycle helmets, and other protective devices are not widely available. Travelers must use common sense to avoid particularly high-risk situations such as travel at night and traveling with people who are intoxicated.

Climate
Excessive exposure to extreme temperatures can also cause health problems including heat exhaustion, heatstroke, frostbite, and hypothermia. Careful attention to fluid and electrolyte intake, sun exposure, and adequate clothing can prevent these problems. Sunscreens with sun protection factor (SPF) of 15 or greater effectively protect against sunburn caused by ultraviolet B.

"Jet Lag"
Jet lag can result in disturbed patterns of sleep and wakefulness and can cause fatigue, malaise, and anorexia. Complete adaptation may take as long as 1 week depending on the number of time zones crossed. Although a number of nonpharmacologic measures have been advocated to prevent jet lag, most are either ineffective (diet manipulations) or impractical (light exposure to reset circadian rhythms). General measures such as avoiding alcoholic beverages and maintaining adequate fluid intake during air travel may be helpful. The use of benzodiazepines during air travel is controversial. Instances of transient global amnesia have been reported in air travelers who have taken benzodiazepines and alcohol together. A reasonable approach is to reserve benzodiazepines for inducing sleep after arrival at one's destination.

Motion Sickness
Motion sickness can result from any form of travel, but is most common during travel by boat. Transdermal scopolamine patches are effective for up to 3 days, but must be administered at least 4 hours prior to embarkation. Antihistamines and low doses of benzodiazepines are also effective but may cause sedation.

Altitude Illness
Altitude illness can develop in travelers to altitudes higher than 8000 ft. Most common is acute mountain sickness (AMS). Characterized by headache, nausea, lassitude, and insomnia, it commonly occurs 6 to 48 hours after arrival at a high altitude. Rest and the avoidance of further elevation for 2 to 3 days are recommended. AMS is usually self-limited but in some individuals can progress to high-altitude pulmonary edema and high-altitude cerebral edema.

Altitude illness can be prevented by gradual ascent (no more than 1000 ft/day over 8000 ft or "staging," e.g., spending acclimatization time at intermediate altitudes), adequate hydration, and avoiding overexertion. Acetazolamide (Diamox) can be used to prevent AMS in patients with a known history of previous altitude sickness and for rescuers and others who must ascend rapidly. Acetazolamide is given as 250 mg every 8 hours 1 to 2 days prior to ascent and during the few days at high altitude. Dexamethasone is also effective at preventing AMS at particularly high elevations. Treatment of altitude sickness, particularly in its more severe forms, is immediate descent. Descent of 2000 to 3000 ft will almost always result in improvement of the patient's condition. Acetazolamide can also be used for treatment. Many authorities currently recommend withholding acetazolamide prophylactically, but using it at the first sign of symptoms of AMS.

Designing a Medical Kit

Patients traveling to areas of the developing world where medications are not readily available should bring an adequate supply of selected medications. Any chronic medications and simple first-aid equipment should be included. A basic kit might include: Pepto-Bismol tablets or loperamide (for the initial treatment of traveler's diarrhea), trimethoprim-sulfamethoxazole (for the treatment of severe traveler's diarrhea), antimalarials, a benzodiazepine (for sleep and motion sickness), erythromycin (for skin infections), clotrimazole (for skin and vaginal infection), acetaminophen, a decongestant, hydrocortisone cream (particularly for those inclined toward bad insect bites), insect repellent, and water purification tablets.

Centers for Disease Control. Health information for international travel 1990. Washington, DC: US Department of Health and Human Services. HHS publication no. (CDC) 89-8280.
Published annually (and updated bimonthly), this is the definitive reference for travel advice. Don't leave home without it!

Hill DR, Pearson RD. Health advice for international travel. Ann Intern Med 1988; 108:839–52.
Comprehensive recent review.

Hill DR, Pearson RD. Measles prophylaxis for international travel. Ann Intern Med 1989; 111:699–71.
Summary of the evidence leading to the current recommendation for revaccination.

Advice for travelers. Med Lett Drugs Ther 1990; 32:33–6.
Usual excellent Medical Letter fare. Updated periodically.

Travelers' diarrhea-consensus conference. JAMA 1985; 253:2700–5.
Excellent discussion of epidemiology, etiology, prevention, treatment, and areas of future research. Strong recommendations against prophylactic antibiotics.

Centers for Disease Control. Recommendations for the prevention of malaria in travelers. MMWR 1990; 39(RR-3):1–10, 630.
Mefloquine is now the drug of choice for CRPF. Due to breakthroughs at the dose of 250 mg every other week, the currently recommended dose is 250 mg each week.

Brown KR, Phillips SM. Tropical diseases of importance to the traveler. Adv Intern Med 1984; 59–84.
Comprehensive review including tropical diseases rarely seen by U.S. physicians.

Houston C. Altitude illness: the dangers of heights and how to avoid them. Postgrad Med 1983; 74:231–48.
A practical review of altitude illness and current recommendations for prevention and treatment.

AMA Commission on Emergency Medical Services. Medical aspects of transportation aboard commercial aircraft. JAMA 1982; 247:1007–11.
Reviews the potential effects of high-altitude flight on medical and surgical conditions, with special attention to effects on blood gases and recommended precautions for patients with chronic cardiovascular and pulmonary conditions. Also includes a section advising

physician-passengers on how to respond to common medical problems encountered on commercial flights.

Insect repellents. Med Lett Drugs Ther 1989; 31:45–7.
A concise summary of skin and clothing repellents used against mosquitoes and ticks, reviewing adverse reactions to deet and additional benefits of permethrin clothing spray.

129. OCCUPATIONAL DISEASES AND DISABILITY DETERMINATION
Gary Pasternak and Timothy S. Carey

Primary care physicians often diagnose and treat acute, occupationally related illness or injury and routinely provide ongoing care to patients with chronic diseases that affect their ability to perform in the workplace. Work-related visits fall into one of three categories: preemployment examinations, acute or chronic work-related problems, and disability determination.

The Preemployment Examination
Physicians may be approached by companies to perform preemployment examinations on groups of workers, or asked by an individual patient to perform such an examination. The major purpose of the examination is to determine whether the patient is physically capable of performing the duties or tasks required by the job. The examination must be specifically keyed to the job requirements; physical conditions may well be disqualifying for one job but not for another. Physiologic measurements may be obtained to serve as a baseline against which surveillance for possible future occupational disease may be assessed. An example of such a baseline measurement would be pulmonary function testing in workers who would be exposed to unprocessed cotton dust. The examination also may serve as a periodic health examination and may provide an opportunity for screening for several diseases that may not be related to occupation, but that are important: hypertension, colorectal carcinoma, high blood cholesterol, and others. If the job applicant meets the physical requirements of the job, a clearance is provided. Specific findings from the exam are not routinely sent to the employer. When information that is not germaine to the patient's prospective job is gathered in the course of the examination, as for example the existence of diabetes, the physician should not forward such information to the employer without the express permission of the employee.

Work-Related Injury and Illness
An estimated 20 million work-related injuries and 390,000 work-related illnesses occur each year in the United States. The National Institutes of Occupational Safety and Health (NIOSH) has estimated that annually about 10,000 workers are killed in occupational accidents and 100,000 die from occupational diseases. However, the number of reported illnesses, injuries, and deaths is much lower. Difficulty in estimating the extent of occupational disease is due to several factors: (1) Illness may not be reported because symptoms from occupational diseases are similar to many nonoccupational disorders and not easily recognized or workers may be deterred from reporting a problem because of fear of job loss. (2) Reporting requirements vary from state to state and are not strictly enforced. (3) The long latency between exposure and onset of symptoms (i.e., asbestos exposure and lung cancer) obscures recognition of the work-relatedness of many occupational illnesses.

Evaluation
The occupational history is the critical element in determining the connection between illness and the workplace. What distinguishes this history from the standard medical history is an emphasis on questions aimed at gaining epidemiologic, toxicologic, and industrial hygiene information. Important questions for evaluating an acute or chronic medical problem are:

1. Are the symptoms associated with work? Have these symptoms improved during vacations or weekends?

2. Are other workers experiencing similar symptoms?
3. Does the job involve work with any dusts, fumes, or chemicals or other substances or conditions considered hazardous?
4. Is personal protective equipment (respirator, gloves, special clothing) used and is the ventilation in the workplace adequate?
5. Have levels of toxic substances ever been measured at the worksite?

If exposure to a toxic substance is identified or suspected, the physician should attempt to determine the route (skin absorption, inhalation, ingestion), magnitude, frequency, and duration of exposure. In practice, a reliable estimate of dose often requires specialized evaluation of industrial hygiene in the workplace. However, if the initial history uncovers exposure to a single agent or compound with known toxicity such as lead, then laboratory tests may be indicated.

A more comprehensive occupational history is often needed when the above questions are unrevealing and the physician still suspects occupational disease, or when the medical examination is part of an ongoing medical surveillance of an individual or group with exposure to known hazards such as lead, mercury, asbestos, noise, or respiratory toxins. In particular, illnesses that display a delayed onset from the initial exposure (i.e., asbestosis, berylliosis, silicosis) are often discovered by taking a more detailed history. This additional history should focus on job description and activity rather than job title. For example, a physician may be conducting research on carcinogenic substances or neurotropic viruses; a laborer's main activity may involve cleaning out underground storage tanks containing residual organic solvent compounds; a secretary may be required to sit for prolonged periods entering data at a computer terminal without rest breaks. Detailed histories may be facilitated by use of a standard occupational history form, such as that contained in the *Handbook of Occupational Medicine* (listed in the references).

Many disorders due to either chemical, physical, or biologic agents may go unrecognized because the relationship between the exposure and disease is not generally appreciated by physicians (i.e., carpal tunnel syndrome in clerical workers, Raynaud's phenomenon in workers using vibrating hand tools, neuropsychiatric symptoms in solvent-exposed workers, cancer in workers exposed to ethylene oxide, sleep disturbances in rotating-shift workers). NIOSH has developed a list of leading work-related diseases and injuries aimed at stimulating recognition, surveillance, and prevention of a wide range of occupational diseases. They are listed under the following headings: occupational lung diseases, musculoskeletal injuries, occupational malignancies, severe traumatic injuries, cardiovascular diseases, disorders of reproduction, neurotoxic disorders, noise-induced hearing loss, dermatologic conditions, and psychological disorders. The physician must keep in mind that an occupational illness may be clinically indistinguishable from a similar nonoccupational disease. For example, asthma due to chemical exposure in an auto-body worker may appear indistinguishable from intrinsic asthma or reactive airways due to other environmental stimuli. The ability to establish a link between a disease process and the workplace depends largely on obtaining a thorough occupational history and establishing a source of exposure.

When workplace-related illnesses have substantial overlap with non–workplace-related illness, determining causality may be quite difficult. Association with initiation of the job, relief with weekends and vacations, and trials of changes in job tasks are all useful in identifying the syndrome as work-related. The physician should not be discouraged by a lack of familiarity with job descriptions and potential exposures. Suspicion that a patient may have an occupationally induced illness should prompt the physician to perform diagnostic tests early and seek specialist consultation and treatment when necessary. The following criteria may be helpful in identifying patients needing referral to an occupational medicine specialist: patients with suspected occupational disease whose cases require further investigation such as worksite visits, environmental monitoring, or interaction with public health officials; patients with a disease that may be related to environmental or occupational factors for which the primary care physician is unable to make the etiologic diagnosis; patients who are exposed to a single toxin or hazard that is unfamiliar to the physician; a patient requiring specialized diagnostic testing; a patient requiring expert medical testimony in a legal case.

Resources and Sources of Information
If the hazard is a chemical substance, it is helpful to know its generic ingredients. If the employee does not know this information or is unable to provide a suitable product label or container, then the Material Safety Data Sheet (MSDS) should be requested from the employer. The MSDS is required to list dangerous substances along with the acute health effects. The federal Hazard Communication Standard mandates that employers provide a worker with an MSDS within 72 hours of request. Once the generic compounds are known, then a number of commonly available reference books can be consulted to determine potential acute and chronic health effects. The physician should not be hesitant to contact the employer or supervisor in attempts to obtain more information about exposures.

A worksite evaluation or toxicologic investigation is usually beyond the scope of most practitioners. However, if the situation warrants, more information may be obtained by formally evaluating the worksite, conducting environmental sampling for toxins, or examining other employees. The Occupational Safety and Health Administration (OSHA) can provide assistance concerning legal exposure limits as well as inspect worksites for suspected hazards. The local office of OSHA may be found by calling the federal OSHA office at 202-523-8148. Many states maintain their own OSHA offices, the telephone numbers of which are listed under state government in the phone book. NIOSH also provides information and worksite health evaluations. NIOSH maintains an extensive library and provides assistance in researching occupational health questions. They may be contacted at 513-533-4382. In addition, hospital- or university-based occupational medical centers exist throughout the country. These centers often have multidisciplinary teams staffed by occupational physicians, nurses, industrial hygienists, and specialists with expertise in fields such as occupational dermatology, neurology, and pulmonary disease. The physicians and other specialists in these centers may be consulted by phone.

Disability Determination

Two common sources of income replacement for work incapacity are Workers' Compensation and the Social Security disability programs. Workers' Compensation in the United States is a "no-fault" insurance system for work-related accidents and illness. To qualify as a compensable condition, the worker must demonstrate that the illness or injury arose out of the course of employment. In many instances, such as traumatic accidents, the causal inference is straightforward. However, in instances of occupational illness there may be a long latency period and difficulty establishing a causal link between exposure and disease. If the physician suspects a causal link between a work exposure and a disease, he or she is obliged to so notify the patient and, in some states, directly report the injury or illness to the appropriate state agency.

Social Security disability benefits are available to individuals who meet the following criteria: have not worked for at least 6 months; have income less than approximately $500 per month; meet medical criteria specifying the level of documented disease or impairment needed to qualify for benefits. These criteria are easily obtained by consulting the Social Security Administration publication "Disability Evaluation Under Social Security," available from the U.S. Department of Health and Human Services (see references). If a patient meets the published criteria, granting of disability benefits is likely. Patients who do not meet the published criteria may still qualify for benefits under a number of circumstances. Patients may have a number of moderate impairments that, taken together, are disabling. For example, a patient with moderate obstructive airway disease, angina, and a visual impairment may qualify for benefits even though no single condition meets the medical "listings" of the Social Security Administration. Patients who are illiterate or trained only for manual labor may also qualify for benefits with moderate, rather than severe impairments.

Physicians may take on a variety of roles in interacting with patients in the Social Security disability system, and must be careful to make their role clear to the patient, themselves, and the determining agency. Early on in the disability process, the agency is only interested in comparing clinical information with agency guidelines, and is prohibited from using a disability assessment from a personal physician. In this instance, the primary care physician transfers clinical information to the disability agency. Later on in the disability appeals process, medical opinion provided by the treating physician is welcomed and may be persuasive. Especially useful is physician information describing multiple medical problems and their interactions, which may cause diminished functioning. Physicians may also serve as consultative examiners for the disability determinations agency. In this case they provide information to the agency on specialized conditions (especially psychiatry), or they may attempt to clarify unclear situations. Such examinations are conducted on a fee-for-service basis by a physician other than the applicant's usual physician. Almost never does a practicing physician determine the provision of disability benefits. Provision of clear information to the patient regarding the physician's role can avoid much patient misunderstanding and physician frustration.

McCunney RJ. Handbook of occupational medicine. Boston: Little Brown, 1988.
This recently published, pocket-sized edition summarizes the major areas of occupational medicine, including disorders of all major organ systems, toxicology, medical surveillance, and legal and ethical aspects pertinent to clinical practice.

Gosselin R, et al. Clinical toxicology of commercial products. Baltimore: Williams & Wilkins, 1984.
Provides a list of trade name products and generic ingredients and includes toxicologic information and recommendations for treatment of acute exposures. Excellent first source of information when product name or ingredients are known.

Social Security Administration. Disability evaluation under Social Security. Washington, DC: U.S. Department of Health and Human Services. SSA publication no. 05-10089, 1987.
Contains listings of the impairments necessary to qualify for disability under the Social Security programs.

Cullen MR, Cherniack MG, Rosenstock L. Occupational medicine. N Engl J Med 1990; 322:594–601, 675–83.
Comprehensive review of occupational medicine, concentrating on the primary physician's approach. Includes a discussion of "sick building syndrome," carpal tunnel syndrome, and reproductive consequences of occupational exposures. Contains 265 references.

Carey TS, Hadler NM. The role of the primary physician in disability determination for Social Security and worker's compensation. Ann Intern Med 1986; 104:706–10.
Discusses the process of disability application and award under both the Social Security Disability and Workers' Compensation systems. Emphasizes ways in which the treating physician can assist the patient through an often confusing bureaucratic process.

130. CIGARETTE SMOKING CESSATION
Elizabeth E. Campbell

Despite considerable publicity concerning its negative health effects, cigarette smoking remains the number one cause of preventable mortality in this country. More than 50 million Americans continue to smoke cigarettes and more than 350,000 premature deaths each year are directly attributable to smoking.

Although a steady decline in per-capita cigarette consumption has been reported since 1973, the decline in the prevalence of smoking has occurred primarily among men. Young women and teenage girls are today more likely to smoke than are their male counterparts. The incidence of smoking-related illnesses among women continues to rise, and lung cancer has now replaced breast cancer as the number one cause of cancer mortality among women. Moreover, for both men and women there has been increasing consolidation of the smoking habit among those who continue to smoke. By 1980, the percentage of individuals classified as heavy smokers ($\geq$ 25 cigarettes/day) had reached 35% of male smokers and 24% of female smokers, and this trend continues.

Passive Smoking

Passive smoking, the exposure to smoke emitted from the lit end of a cigarette (sidestream smoke) and to that exhaled by the smoker (mainstream smoke), has received increasing attention as a significant health risk. The 1986 Surgeon General's report stated that the health risks of involuntary smoke exposure to nonsmokers are greater than those associated with a number of federally regulated environmental and occupational toxins. Dose-response curves of urinary and salivary cotinine in heavily smoke-exposed nonsmokers indicate a level of exposure roughly equivalent to smoking one-half to one cigarette a day, a level that has been shown among light active smokers to be associated with an increased risk of lung cancer. In addition, the National Research Council estimated the relative risks of developing lung cancer among nonsmokers married to smokers to be 1.41 to 1.87, compared to subjects not exposed to environmental tobacco smoke. It has been estimated that 21 to 70% of the more than 12,000 lung cancer deaths each year among nonsmokers may be due to environmental tobacco smoke.

Passive smoking has also been linked to a number of nonmalignant respiratory diseases. In a number of studies, adults environmentally exposed to tobacco smoke have been found to have significant reductions in forced expiratory volume in 1 second (FEV_1) and forced midexpiratory flow rates. Moreover, passive smoking has been found to be associated with increased rates of cardiovascular disease among exposed nonsmokers relative to unexposed nonsmokers. Children of smokers have been found to have an increased frequency of both upper and lower respiratory tract infections, asthma, chronic middle-ear effusions, and recurrent and chronic otitis media.

The Role of the Physician

Studies of office-based, smoking cessation counseling have shown that most physicians do not counsel their patients about smoking, even those at particularly high risk from smoking, such as hypertensives and women taking oral contraceptives. Physicians report feeling ill-prepared and ineffective at getting patients to quit smoking, whereas up to 90% of patients say they would like to quit and most indicate they would like their physician's assistance with this process.

Studies of the effectiveness of physician counseling have shown varied results, ranging from essentially no effect of counseling to a 50% cessation rate at 1 year. The highest quit rates have been found in individuals in the perimyocardial infarction period, followed by those with acute smoking-related diseases, and individuals at known high risk for cardiovascular disease. Significant and maintained success rates with otherwise healthy individuals have been more elusive. In a British study of more than 2000 smokers, patients received brief (1–2 minutes) counseling, a quit-smoking pamphlet, and an announcement regarding follow-up during a general medicine encounter. The quit rate at 1 year was 5.1%, compared to 0.3% among patients receiving "usual care." The median quit rate in several other trials in which the patient was simply advised to quit was 6% at 1 year. In other studies in which the physician included more than just simple advice, but incorporated interventions such as "strong advice," warnings, record-keeping, follow-up, compliance contracts, and exhaled carbon dioxide analyses, the median 1-year quit rate was 22.5%. Recent studies suggested that the addition of nicotine replacement therapy for nicotine-addicted individuals may improve success rates. The features shown to be most strongly associated with successful outcomes are multiple motivation methods, involvement of both physicians and nonphysicians in the counseling process, individual encounters between patients and providers, and multiple reinforcement encounters over long periods of time. The National Cancer Institute is currently supporting research into interventions to help patients quit smoking, including physician-based programs, worksite cessation programs, media campaigns, cessation resource task forces, telephone hotlines, and network newsletters for smokers and quitters.

Counseling Patients About Smoking

Successful physician smoking cessation counseling emphasizes: (1) individualized motivation and advice, stressing the positive benefits of quitting; (2) assessing obstacles to quitting and addressing them realistically; (3) pharmacologic treatment of nicotine addiction; (4) contracting for a quit date; and (5) a follow-up program. Benzodiazepines and other tranquilizers, tobacco substitutes (e.g., lobeline or Indian tobacco), and other preparations have not been shown to be effective in helping people to stop smoking, although recent reports suggested a possible role for clonidine in the treatment of nicotine withdrawal.

Motivation
The first step in smoking cessation counseling is to determine the patient's motivation to quit. Motivation may be enhanced by a number of strategies. Smoking should be identified as a problem, and physicians should deliver firm and consistent advice against it. Emphasizing the positive medical, social, psychological, and financial benefits of quitting, however, may provide more effective motivation than warnings about the negative health consequences of continued smoking. Patients should be asked about their own reasons for wanting to quit and expected benefits, so that advice can be personalized. The financial savings from quitting are substantial, ranging from several hundred to several thousand dollars per year. Health benefits include improved vigor and exercise tolerance, fewer upper respiratory tract infections, lowered risk of cardiovascular disease and certain malignancies, and longer life expectancy. Family members no longer exposed to passive smoking may also benefit, with fewer respiratory infections occurring in children, less asthma and atopic disease, lowered risk of chronic obstructive pulmonary disease (COPD), and less risk of lung cancer in the nonsmoking spouse. Social benefits include greater social acceptability, no longer being limited to smoking sections of public places, and providing better role models for children. Psychological benefits include freedom from the dependency on cigarettes and a sense of accomplishment and mastery from having "kicked the habit."

Assessing Obstacles to Quitting
Physicians can help patients assess their own obstacles to quitting, such as nicotine addiction, fear of weight gain, anxiety off of cigarettes, and prior failed attempts at quitting. Questions to determine whether a patient is nicotine-dependent include how soon after awakening the first cigarette is smoked, how many cigarettes are smoked in a day, and what happens in situations in which the patient cannot smoke. Answers that suggest addiction include smoking the first cigarette of the day within 30 to 60 minutes of awakening; a total daily cigarette consumption of more than 20 to 25 cigarettes; and agitation, headaches, nausea, and severe craving in situations in which the patient cannot smoke. Other obstacles should be addressed realistically, acknowledging potential problems and helping the patient to develop plans or strategies by which to deal with them. For example, patients who fear weight gain should be advised that two-thirds of people who quit do not have sustained weight gain 1 year later, and that a 10-lb weight gain is generally not as significant a health risk as a year of smoking 1 to 2 packs per day. Weight gain can also be controlled by dietary changes and physical activity. Anxiety associated with cigarette cessation may be an indication for nicotine replacement therapy. The use of benzodiazepines and other tranquilizers is generally not appropriate. Patients who are discouraged by past failures should be reminded that most exsmokers have quit more than once in the past before successfully quitting cigarettes.

Nicotine Replacement Therapy
Nicotine replacement therapy is the only treatment that has been shown to be effective in the treatment of tobacco dependence, although preliminary data on clonidine are encouraging. Nicotine replacement, in the form of a gum or a transdermal patch, can help treat or prevent the physical withdrawal symptoms associated with smoking cessation while the patient deals with the issues surrounding his or her psychological dependence. Nicotine replacement therapy has no demonstrated role among patients who are not pharmacologically dependent on nicotine. It should not be used by patients continuing to smoke cigarettes. The effectiveness of nicotine gum is based on the systemic absorption of nicotine from the buccal mucosa. Serum levels of nicotine can be maintained at a near-plateau, high enough to suppress the urge to smoke cigarettes, though significantly lower than the peaks induced by cigarette smoking. There is more experience with the gum than with the patches, and some data suggest the patches may be more effective and associated with fewer side effects.

Nicotine gum must be used appropriately in order to be effective, and patients should be carefully instructed in its use. Clinical studies have shown that patients who did not use the gum appropriately or for sufficient duration have uniformly failed to benefit from its use. The gum is available in 2-mg and 4-mg strengths; most patients are begun on the lower-strength preparation. Patients should begin use of the gum when they have actually stopped smoking; at that time they should chew a piece of gum whenever the urge to smoke arises. The gum should be chewed slowly, waiting for the taste or tingle to develop. The gum should then be "parked" in the cheek, along the buccal mucosa, until the taste disappears, or the urge to smoke recurs. This sequence is then repeated over and over, so that a piece of gum should last about 30 minutes. Most patients require 10 to 20 pieces of gum a day when they first stop smoking; patients requiring more may benefit from the 4-mg preparation. Transdermal nicotine patches are available in 21-, 14-, and 7-mg strengths. Most patients are started on 21 mg a day. With both gum and patches, patients are generally maintained on therapy for about 3 months, and subsequently tapered off. Most people have little difficulty giving up replacement therapy. The cost of a 96-piece package of gum is about $24 to $33, translating to a daily cost of $2.50 to $5.10, depending on the number of pieces used. The cost of a month of nicotine patches is about $3 to $4 a day, decreasing below this level as the dose is tapered. This compares to a daily cost of $1.75 to $3.50 for two packs of cigarettes a day. Since nicotine replacement therapy is discontinued within 3 to 4 months, the total cost is under $400 and is substantially less than the annual cost of smoking two packs a day.

While nicotine gum has been a useful adjunct for some patients, others have been unable to use it because of its side effects, which include throat irritation, nausea, dizziness, and abdominal pain. Some of these symptoms may be related to swallowing excess nicotine, and may be controlled by slowing down the rate at which the gum is chewed. Transdermal nicotine patches may be associated with fewer side effects. Nicotine replacement therapy is contraindicated in pregnant patients, and patients with recent myocardial infarctions or life-threatening arrhythmias.

At this time clonidine has not been approved for use in smoking cessation. It might be considered for smokers who are nicotine-addicted and want to quit but cannot use nicotine replacement. Similar to nicotine replacement therapy, clonidine should be used as an adjunct to a smoking cessation program.

Setting a Quit Date

Patients are encouraged to set quit dates within a 2-week period after the decision to quit has been reached. This "lead time" allows them to make psychological and practical preparations for their quit efforts, and to rally support from their family and friends. Smokers should be encouraged to plan other activities for those situations in which they tend to smoke and to dispose of all smoking materials and ash trays the day before their quit date. A holiday, a birthday, or some other special occasion, especially one that removes them from many of their usual smoking cues, can be a particularly effective quit date for some individuals. Conversely, dates that will be predictably more stressful than others should be avoided. A written quit-date prescription or contract may be more effective than a verbal one.

Arranging Follow-up

Follow-up should occur, in person or by phone, within 1 to 2 weeks after the patient's actual quit-date, and on a fairly regular basis thereafter for the first several months. These follow-up visits or phone calls are intended to monitor the patient's progress, to facilitate early intervention with relapses, and to provide additional support and encouragement for the maintenance of abstinence in order to help consolidate the nonsmoking habit. Patients who have successfully quit should be offered the opportunity to discuss difficulties they may be having, such as dealing with high-risk situations around other smokers. Patients who have quit but relapsed should be congratulated for trying and encouraged to learn from the attempt, for example, by questions about what led to the first cigarette and what might help in the next attempt. Patients who have not quit might be asked about the obstacles to trying and should be offered support to try when they are ready.

Table 130-1. Nationally available smoking cessation aids

A. Self-help manuals and kits
  1. The American Lung Association (ALA) offers several manuals, including *Freedom from Smoking in 20 Days* (how to quit), *A Lifetime of Freedom from Smoking* (avoiding relapse), and *Freedom from Smoking for You and Your Baby* (a quit program for pregnant women). A contribution of $7.00 is requested for the manuals, which can be obtained through local ALA chapters, or the American Lung Association, 1740 Broadway, New York, NY 10019. Tel: 212-315-8700.
  2. The American Heart Association offers "In Control," a self-teaching program produced in conjunction with the ALA, which can be used with or without an instructor. Videotapes and the instructor's manual cost $75; the participant program consisting of weekly guides and tables is $25. Free publications including *Calling It Quits*, and *Children and Smoking: A Message to Parents*. Contact a local chapter, or American Heart Association, 7320 Greenville Ave, Dallas, TX 75321. Tel: 214-315-8700.
  3. The American Cancer Society offers a wide variety of materials, including the "I Quit Kit," the *Quitter's Guide—7 Day Plan to Help You Stop Smoking, How to Quit Cigarettes* (targeted to blue-collar workers), and a variety of smoking programs aimed at young people. Also available are several videotapes, including "Death in the West," contrasting the cigarette advertisers' image of the smoker with the realities of smoking-induced illness and death, and "The Feminine Mistake," describing the impact of smoking on women's bodies. Consult a local chapter to obtain these and other materials, or American Cancer Society, 1599 Clifton Road Northeast, Atlanta, GA 30329. Tel: 404-320-3333.
  4. National Cancer Institute offers free publications *Quit for Good* and *Clearing the Air*. Call, toll-free, 800-4-CANCER.
  5. American Academy of Family Physicians (AAFP) offers the "AAFP Stop Smoking Kit" for use in office practice, with audiotapes for physicians and office staff, charting system, and self-help materials for patients. The cost is $50 for AAFP members, $80 for nonmembers. Contact Dr. Herbert Young of the AAFP, toll-free, 800-274-2237.
  6. Shipley RH. *Quit Smart: A Guide to Freedom from Cigarettes*. A clear, supportive and practically oriented, self-help guide. Cost is $6.95, from JB Press, Department B, P.O. Box 4843, Duke Station, Durham, NC 27706.
B. National nonprofit clinics
  1. The American Cancer Society's "FreshStart" program consists of four 1-hr sessions, usually conducted over a 2-wk period. The FreshStart facilitator's guide is a detailed description of how to conduct a "FreshStart" group; the participants' guide is completely self-explanatory, so that it can be used by participants on their own. The frequency of group programs varies by area. The "FreshStart" program is free, although there is some charge for materials and some local organizations charge an incentive fee that is refunded at the end of the sessions.
  2. The ALA's "Freedom from Smoking" program, consisting of seven sessions over a 3-wk period, is held several times a year by most ALA affiliates. The fee is $45.
  3. The Seventh-Day Adventist "Breathe Free Plan to Stop Smoking" consists of eight 1-hr sessions over a 2- to 3-wk period. The program does have a spiritual dimension, which is pursued at the end of each session and which participants are free to skip if they choose. Follow-up phone calls are made to participants at regular intervals over the first year. Several million smokers have been helped by this program and its predecessor, "The Five Day Plan," with reported 1-yr abstinence rates of 14–38%. A $10 charge is sometimes made for educational materials. Contact: General Conference of Seventh Day Adventists, Health and Temperance Department, 6840 Eastern Avenue NW, Washington, DC 20012. Tel: 202-722-6700.
C. Commercial organizations
  1. The "Smokeless" program is a highly structured program including a 1-hr introductory session in which participants commit to quitting, a treatment phase of four 1½-hr meetings on consecutive days, and a maintenance phase consisting

Table 130-1 (continued)

> of three meetings held over a 2-wk period. The program is distributed through the American Institute of Preventative Medicine, and is offered through local hospitals, corporations and health promotion associations in a number of states.
> 2. "Smoke Stoppers" is a 5-wk program that utilizes behavioral modification techniques in a systematic approach to the quitting process. It is conducted locally through hospitals, health organizations, and businesses.

D. Office of smoking and health—The Office of Smoking and Health (OSH) of the US Department of Health and Human Services coordinates programs for research, smoking education, and prevention. It publishes an annual in-depth report on the health effects of smoking and the *Bulletin on Smoking and Health*, a biennial directory of research in the area, and also supplies technical information to researchers. OSH also conducts an extensive public information program, including development of smoking prevention and intervention materials for schools. Contact: Office of Smoking and Health, Department of Health and Human Services, Public Health Service, Centers for Disease Control, Rockville, MD 20857.

Visits or calls can be conducted by the physician or by a nurse trained in smoking cessation counseling.

Smoking Cessation Manuals and Group Programs

Most ex-smokers have quit on their own without help from their physicians and without formal instruction. Table 130-1 lists some of the materials and programs available to physicians and patients who would like help; most of the sources listed have additional pamphlets, posters, videos, and cassette tapes available on request. These can be used alone, or can be valuable additions to a physician counseling program.

Self-help books and kits are generally inexpensive or free of charge. Most emphasize behavior modification techniques and address issues of motivation, obstacles to quitting, techniques for stopping, handling withdrawal symptoms, dealing with relapses, and remaining abstinent. Reported quit rates at 1 year are in the range of 15 to 20%.

Group programs are run by both commercial and nonprofit organizations. The latter programs are significantly less expensive, and rely on group sessions and behavior modification. Commercial programs typically claim higher success rates than those reported by nonprofit groups, but often report quit rates only at the completion of the program, and not 6- or 12-months later. Comparisons between programs are often not appropriate, because the smokers enrolling in each and the type of follow-up studies done may not be comparable.

In addition to nationally run programs, hundreds of local programs exist. Although many use techniques similar to those of more established programs, most have not been thoroughly evaluated. Regional chapters of the American Cancer Society, American Lung Association, and American Heart Association may have information on specific programs available locally.

Fielding JE. Smoking: health effects and control. Parts I and II. N Engl J Med 1985; 313:491–8, 555–61.
Complete review of the health and economic consequences of smoking, including data on the effects of passive smoking and in utero effects of maternal smoking. Measures to control smoking and aid quitters are reviewed.

Fielding JE, Phenow KJ. Health effects of involuntary smoking. N Engl J Med 1988; 319:1452–60.
Comprehensive review of the literature on environmental smoke exposure, and risks to both children and adults.

The Surgeon General's 1990 report on the health benefits of smoking cessation—executive summary. MMWR 1990; 39(RR-12):i–xv, 1–12.
Summarizes the health consequences of smoking cessation, including cardiovascular, respiratory disease, and other nonmalignant disease; malignancies; reproduction; body weight change; and psychological and behavioral changes.

Anda RJ, et al. Are physicians advising smokers to quit? JAMA 1987; 257:1916–9.
Survey data from 5845 smokers showing that less than half had been advised by a physician to quit, even those at significant risk for heart attacks and strokes.

Health and Public Policy Committee, American College of Physicians. Position paper: methods for stopping cigarette smoking. Ann Intern Med 1986; 105:281–91.
Describes available smoking cessation methods and reviews data concerning their effectiveness.

Tonnesen P, Norregaard J, Simonsen K and Sawe U. A double-blind trial of a 16-hour transdermal nicotine patch in smoking cessation. N Engl J Med 1991; 325:311–5.
A double-blind randomized study of nearly 300 smokers comparing transdermal nicotine patches with placebo, showing significantly higher abstinent rates among the treated individuals. There were very few side effects.

Kottke TE, et al. Attributes of successful smoking cessation interventions in medical practice: a meta-analysis of 39 controlled trials. JAMA 1988; 259:2883–9.
Explores the features of smoking cessation trials to determine the program factors most predictive of successful quitting.

Methods used to quit smoking in the United States: do cessation programs help? JAMA 1990; 263:2760–5.
Excellent review describing the characteristics of individuals who have succeeded in quitting smoking and those who have not, and the types of programs followed or efforts made by each group. The accompanying editorial (pp. 2795–6) underscores the messages of this study.

Benowitz NL. Pharmacologic aspects of cigarette smoking and nicotine addiction. N Engl J Med 1988; 319:1318–29.
Describes the physiologic and pharmacologic effects of nicotine and reviews nicotine addiction and replacement therapy.

Cummings SR, et al. Internists and nicotine gum. JAMA 1988; 260:1565–9.
Survey of physicians, revealing incorrect practices in the use of the gum and misunderstanding of its contraindications and side effects.

Glassman AH, et al. Heavy smokers, smoking cessation, and clonidine: results of a double-blind randomized trial. JAMA 1988; 259:2863–6.
Reports on a trial using oral clonidine.

Ornish SA, Zisook S, McAdams LA. Effects of transdermal clonidine treatment of withdrawal symptoms associated with smoking cessation: a randomized controlled trial. Arch Intern Med 1988; 148:2207–31.
Another clonidine study, using patches rather than pills.

131. BREAST CANCER SCREENING
Suzanne W. Fletcher

One in 10 women in the United States will get breast cancer, and of those, one-third will die of it. Frustratingly, treatment advances have not substantially improved the prognosis; once a woman gets breast cancer, her chances of survival are about the same as they were several decades ago. The intent of screening is to find the cancer at an early, curable stage. Presently, less than 50% of breast cancers are found before they have metastasized to axillary nodes.

The incidence of breast cancer rises steadily with age; 70% of cases occur after the age of 50. In order to detect a single case in 20-year-old women, more than 80,000 would have to be examined, whereas about 350 women aged 65 would be have to be examined to find a cancer.

Effectiveness of Screening

The three main breast cancer screening techniques include physical examination of the breasts by a health professional, mammography, and breast self-examination. There is excellent evidence that with the use of physical examination, mammography, or both, breast cancer can be found and treated early enough to prevent one-third of the breast cancer deaths in women aged 50 to 59. This evidence, which includes several randomized clinical trials, is more convincing than the evidence supporting any other type of cancer screening. There is increasing evidence that early treatment after screening also is effective in women aged 60 to 74. No studies have been reported yet for women over the age of 75.

Evidence regarding the effect of physical examination and/or mammography among women aged 40 to 49 has generated a great deal of controversy. Most of the studies reported to date found no protective effect.

Whether physical examination or mammography is the most important screening technique is not yet known. One study, in which over a million examinations were carried out, showed that of the cancers found on screening, mammography detected 89% and physical examination, 58%. Each technique found some cancers that the other missed.

Evidence about breast self-examination is much less conclusive than evidence supporting mammography and/or physical examination. The only study comparing women offered instruction in breast self-examination to women not offered such instruction found no difference in the breast cancer mortality of the two groups after 5 to 7 years of follow-up.

In sum, the evidence suggests that breast cancer is one disease where physicians should increase their efforts in screening by physical examination and mammography, especially in women between the ages of 50 and 75.

Screening Techniques

Physical examination detects over half the cancers found on screening, some of which will have been missed by mammography. In one study performed with silicone models simulating breast tissue, physicians detected 87% of 1.0-cm lumps, 33% of 0.5-cm lumps and 15% of 0.3-cm lumps.

The purpose of screening is to discover breast cancers before they would be visible or easily palpable by the patient. Therefore, some of the recommendations in physical diagnosis textbooks about inspection of the breasts for symmetry, skin dimpling, and visible lumps (all likely to be signs of advanced cancer) are probably not appropriate for a screening examination. Busy clinicians should concentrate on careful palpation of the breasts.

Breast palpation should be done with the patient lying supine. The breast should be made as flat as possible. This is especially important in patients with large breasts. Flattening of the breast can be achieved in two ways: (1) placing the patient's ipsilateral hand on her forehead, or (2) having the patient tilt her hips toward the contralateral side and then rotate her shoulders back toward the side of the breast to be examined. A pillow or folded towel placed under the scapula may help.

Each breast should be palpated carefully, using one hand (whichever is most comfortable for the examiner) and the pads (not tips) of the three middle fingers held together. The fingers should make small circular motions, as if tracing the outer edge of a dime. At each position, three different circles should be made, first with light pressure, then with medium, and finally with deep pressure.

The examination should systematically cover the area bordered by the midaxillary line laterally, the midsternum medially, the clavicle superiorly (in order to include the tail of the breast), and the "bra line" under the breast inferiorly. Many texts recommend a concentric circular pattern, starting at the nipple and making larger and larger circles until the entire breast is covered. However, more thorough coverage of the breast is obtained when a *vertical stripping* pattern is used (Fig. 131-1). With the vertical strip pattern, palpation begins in the patient's axilla. The fingers move down the midaxillary line in a stepwise fashion, making three circles of variable pressure at each new position. When

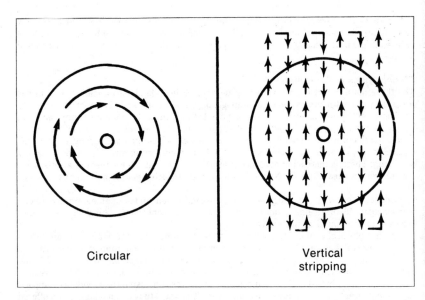

Fig. 131-1. Two commonly recommended patterns for breast physical examination: (1) circular pattern and (2) vertical stripping pattern. Studies of women performing breast self-examination found that women are more thorough and miss fewer areas using the vertical stripping pattern. (From MS O'Malley, SW Fletcher. Clinical breast examination in breast cancer screening. N C Med J 1987; 48:502–4. Courtesy *North Carolina Medical Journal*.)

the fingers have reached the bra line, they move medially slightly (making sure that some overlap occurs), and the examination continues up the chest to the clavicle. The fingers then continue in this fashion to move up and down the chest in vertical strips. The nipple should be examined in the same way as the rest of the breast.

Studies have shown a strong correlation between the duration of breast examination and lump detection. Thorough palpation of a single breast takes at least 2 minutes, much longer than most physicians spend.

It is not always easy to distinguish benign tissue from malignant lesions on physical examination. Normal breast tissue is commonly lumpy, often described as "ropey," "granular," or "pea-like," particularly in the periareolar area and in the upper outer quadrant. Classically, breast cancers are noncystic, hard, nonmoveable, and irregular. However, benign lesions can also have these characteristics, and cancers sometimes do not. Mammography, ultrasound, and/or fine-needle aspiration can help resolve uncertainty. It is important to remember, however, that a negative mammogram does not rule out cancer. Regardless of the result of mammography, highly suspicious findings on physical examination should be pursued further.

Mammography can pick up both single breast masses that clinicians miss on the physical examination (especially small lumps < 1 cm), and areas of microcalcifications associated with cancer, sometimes without any clearly discernible mass. Despite the strong scientific evidence and recommendations for mammography, fewer than half of targeted women have ever had a mammogram, and fewer than one-third get annual mammograms.

A major problem with mammography is its cost. Although the actual cost of mammography has been reported to be as low as $25, most women receiving mammography will be charged $50 to $125. Most women will have to bear this expense themselves because third-party payers usually do not cover charges for screening tests.

Breast self-examination has been recommended by many groups. It is appealing as a method of screening because it is noninvasive and entails no expense. However, it appears that women must be trained, rather than only encouraged, in order to perform adequate examinations for early lump detection. Most recommendations are for monthly self-examinations, which in menstruating women should be performed following the menstrual period. Pamphlets instructing women in the procedure are available from many organizations, including the American Cancer Society and the National Cancer Institute.

As mentioned above, it is not yet clear that breast self-examination decreases breast cancer mortality, especially in women who obtain routine physical examinations and mammography.

Screening Recommendations

The following recommendations reflect those made by a number of expert groups, including the U.S. Preventive Services Task Force, the National Cancer Institute, the American Medical Association, Canadian Task Force on the Periodic Health Examination, the American Cancer Society, and the American Colleges of Physicians, Obstetricians and Gynecologists, and Radiology.

Women Aged 40 to 49

Routine physical examination is generally recommended, although the effectiveness of this procedure *alone* has not been established.

Most of the scientific controversy surrounding breast cancer screening concerns the routine use of mammography in women in this age group. Although breast cancer incidence begins to rise in women aged 40 to 49, studies have yet to show convincing evidence of the benefit from screening. Nevertheless, several national groups recommend routine mammography in this age group every 1 to 2 years.

One problem in screening for breast cancer in young women is the high false-positive rate; most breast lumps found in women in this age group are due to benign breast disease. In one study among women aged 40 to 44, over nine women underwent breast biopsy for every cancer found. The ratio dropped to less than 4:1 in women aged 55 to 59.

Women Aged 50 and Older

Yearly physical examination and mammography are universally recommended for women aged 50 to 74, based on convincing evidence of effectiveness. There are few data available for women over the age of 75.

High-Risk Women

Women under 50 years old are at higher risk for breast cancer if they have a personal history of breast cancer or a mother or sister with a history of breast cancer. Women with first-degree relatives who had bilateral breast cancer before menopause appear to be at extraordinarily high risk for breast cancer (30–50% lifetime incidence), especially if the cancer occurred in both the mother and a sister. These high-risk women should receive both periodic physical examinations and mammography.

Many other possible risk factors for breast cancer have been studied, including history of fibrocystic disease, high socioeconomic status, late age at birth of the first child, and late age of menopause, all having a small but positive correlation with increased incidence of breast cancer. It has not been established that women with any of these risk factors would benefit from aggressive searches for breast cancers before age 50.

O'Malley MS, Fletcher SW, Morrison B. Does screening for breast cancer save lives? Effectiveness of treatment after breast cancer detection following screening by clinical breast examination, mammography, and breast self-examination. In: Lawrence RS, Goldbloom R, eds. Preventing disease. New York: Springer, 1990:251–264.
Summarizes evidence about breast cancer screening.

Shapiro S, et al. Periodic screening for breast cancer. The health insurance plan project and its sequelae, 1963–1986. Baltimore: Johns Hopkins University Press, 1988.
The longest study of breast cancer screening.

Baker LH. Breast cancer detection demonstration project. Five year summary. CA 1982; 32:194–225.
Compares breast cancer detection by physical examination and mammography.

O'Malley MS, Fletcher SW. Screening for breast cancer with breast self-examination. A critical review. JAMA 1987; 257:2196–203.
Suggests that more rigorous research must be done before the effectiveness of breast self-examination can be determined.

UK Trial of Early Detection of Breast Cancer: First results on mortality in the UK Trial of Early Detection of Breast Cancer. Lancet 1988; 1(8608):411–6.
Breast cancer mortality in communities where women were offered training in breast self-examination was the same as that in control communities.

Hill D, et al. Self-examination of the breast. Is it beneficial? Meta-analysis of studies investigating breast self-examination and extent of disease in patients with breast cancer. Br Med J 1988; 297:271–5.
A review, study, and meta-analysis of breast self-examination.

Fletcher SW, O'Malley MS, Bunce LA. Physicians' abilities to detect lumps in silicone breast models. JAMA 1985; 253:2224–8.
Physicians found only 44% of lumps.

Pennypacker HS, Bloom HS, Criswell EL. Towards an effective technology of instruction in breast self-examination. Int J Ment Health 1982; 11:98–116.
A description of the development of a method to teach breast self-examination.

Saunders KJ, Pilgram CA, Pennypacker HS. Increased proficiency of search in breast self-examination. Cancer 1986; 58:2531–7.
A study showing that breast examination is more thorough with the vertical stripping technique than with the circular technique.

O'Malley MS, Fletcher SW. Clinical breast examination in breast cancer screening. NC Med J 1987; 48:502–4.
Describes method for physical examination of the breast.

132. PROSTATE CANCER SCREENING
James L. Fry, Jr.

Adenocarcinoma of the prostate is the most common cancer in males and is second only to lung cancer as the cause of cancer-related death. The National Cancer Institute predicted that there would be approximately 106,000 new cases and 30,000 deaths due to this disease in 1990. The prevalence of this tumor dramatically increases from 9.3 per 100,000 at age 50 years to 937 per 100,000 for those 85 years or older. Only 1% of prostate cancers occur in patients less than 50 years old. Death rates from prostate cancer have increased during the last 60 years, almost entirely because of an increase in mortality of black males, who have the highest incidence of prostate cancer in the world.

Natural History
Cancer of the prostate is thought to arise peripherally, in the outer posterior portion of the gland, and to grow centrally. Most, but not all, prostatic cancers progress through orderly steps, from microscopic disease to nodule, to local extension, to distant metastases. If confined to the prostate gland, prostatic cancer is a curable disease. With all modes of treatment, survival rates are much better for those with localized disease.

The American College of Surgeons survey has estimated that approximately 20% of new patients have clinical extraprostatic disease (stage C), and approximately 25% have metastatic disease (stage D) at the time of diagnosis. These facts are the impetus for the increased interest in screening for prostate cancer. Unfortunately, current screening tests are inaccurate, and rigorous evidence that early detection and treatment improve survival and quality of life is lacking. Approximately 30% of men in the fifth decade and 60% of men in the eighth decade have histologic evidence of prostate cancer at autopsy, but have no clinical symptoms. Only 1 in approximately 400 men with prostate cancer actually dies from the disease. Thus, many individuals have the disease but do not require treatment because the tumor is not clinically apparent throughout their life.

Tests Used for Prostate Cancer Screening

Digital Rectal Examination

Over the years, the standard for prostatic evaluation has been the digital rectal examination (DRE). The hallmarks of prostate cancer on digital examinations are asymmetry, nodularity, and induration.

To differentiate between benign prostatic hypertrophy (BPH) and cancer, imagine a tight fist with the palmar surface facing the examiner. The thenar eminence has a consistency similar to that found with BPH, while the first knuckle of the thumb is similar to the induration of cancer. Once induration is detected, it must be assumed to be cancer of the prostate until proven otherwise. Benign conditions causing hard prostatic nodules include granulomatous prostatitis, prostatic infarct, calcific nodules (stones), and senile atrophy. The most reliable way to differentiate among these lesions is to perform a biopsy. When a nodule or induration is discovered, the patient should be referred to a urologist for evaluation. Ordinarily a needle biopsy is done as an office procedure. Complications, primarily bleeding and prostatitis, occur infrequently and their incidence is further reduced by using transrectal ultrasound to identify the biopsy site.

In five series of over 11,000 patients who were screened for prostate cancer as part of a routine physical examination, the rate of abnormalities on rectal examination ranged from approximately 3 to 10% and the rate of cancer detection from 0.78 to 1.7%. However, the cost of screening all men over 50 years old, if they came solely for the DRE, would exceed $7 billion per year in the United States (including biopsy of those with suspicious lesions). In addition, many patients diagnosed by DRE have advanced-stage disease that may not be treated for cure.

Therefore, DRE, to be cost-effective, should be performed during a routine, complete, yearly physical examination on men over 50 years old, or on men presenting with symptoms of obstructive uropathy.

Serum Tumor Markers

Prostatic acid phosphatase (PAP) has no role in screening for prostate cancer because its sensitivity is low (0–13%) and it usually detects advanced-stage extraprostatic or metastatic disease that is not subject to curative treatment.

Prostate-specific antigen (PSA) is considered a serum tumor marker; small amounts appear in patients with BPH and typically decrease after transurethral resection of the prostate. If the normal limits of serum PSA levels are set in the low range (2–4 ng/ml) the sensitivity is quite high (70–100%), but the specificity is low (47–79%). Many tumors would be detected; however, as many as 50% of all individuals screened would undergo prostate biopsy due to an elevated PSA. The morbidity and cost of such a great number of biopsies are unacceptable. If, however, higher limits of normal are set (< 10 ng/ml), the sensitivity decreases to 30 to 35% but the specificity increases to 96%. In this situation the majority of men with the disease would remain undetected.

While ineffective as a screening test, measurements of serum PSA are of great value in following patients who have undergone radical prostatectomy or definitive radiation therapy for cancer of the prostate. If elevated serum levels of PSA do not drop significantly toward zero 8 to 10 weeks after radical prostatectomy, undetected metastases and a high recurrence rate should be expected in 1 to 4 years. Over 90% of patients who had elevated PSA levels 1 year following radiation therapy were, in one series, found to have positive findings on biopsy. Even moderately elevated levels of PSA in patients with BPH should decrease after transurethral resection of the prostate.

Transrectal Ultrasound

Transrectal ultrasound with ultrasound-guided needle biopsy has become a common office procedure for evaluating the genitourinary system, but is not recommended as a screening test alone.

In five independent series, over 2600 patients were screened for prostate cancer. The sensitivity was high (90–100%), but the specificity was low: Only 20% of suspicious areas that were biopsied were found to contain malignant cells. Furthermore, in a well-controlled study, transrectal ultrasound was not significantly more sensitive than DRE for detecting cancer, but the cost and inconvenience are substantially higher.

Recommendations

No one method has proved to be readily available, cost-effective, and accurate for screening for prostate cancer. However, some combinations of these tests have given greater accuracy in diagnosing cancer. One plan for screening begins with the DRE during a routine physical examination. If the prostate is asymmetric, is indurated, or has nodularity, patients should be evaluated by a urologist. Usually transrectal ultrasonography will be performed; if the results are suspicious, those with an elevated serum PSA will have a needle biopsy of the prostate. Treatment, whether radical surgery, radiation therapy, observation, or hormonal therapy, would then be determined based on the stage and grade of the tumor.

Thompson IM, Ernst JJ. Adenocarcinoma of the prostate: results of routine urologic screening. J Urol 1984; 132:690–2.
This study suggests that screening by rectal examination alone is not sufficient.

Cooner WH, et al. Clinical application of transrectal ultrasonography and PSA in search for prostatic cancer. J Urol 1988; 139:758–61.
Elevated PSA and ultrasonographic results in addition to abnormal findings on digital examination were used to select patients who needed a biopsy.

Hudson MA, Bahnson RR, Catalona WJ. Clinical use of prostate specific antigen in patients with prostate cancer. J Urol 1989; 142:1011–17.
A good discussion of PSA; suggests that the best use may be in monitoring the response to therapy.

Lee F, et al. Prostate cancer: comparison of transrectal ultrasound and digital rectal examination for screening. Radiology 1988; 168:389–394.
Suggests that ultrasound is more sensitive than digital examination in detecting cancer of the prostate.

Chodak GW, Keller P, Schoeberg HV. Assessment of screening for prostate cancer using the digital rectal examination. J Urol 1989; 141:1136–8.
A large study that questions the effectiveness of mass screening for cancer of the prostate.

Chodak GW, Schoenberg HW. Progress and problems in screening for carcinoma of the prostate. World J Surg 1989; 13:60–4.
A good review of the status of screening for prostate cancer.

XIX. MISCELLANEOUS

133. SYNCOPE
M. Andrew Greganti

Syncope is a sudden loss of consciousness that is usually followed by full recovery within minutes. A feeling of "fading" or "blacking out" often precedes the loss of consciousness; however, there is no true prodrome. Because the most frequent underlying pathophysiology is a decrease in cerebral perfusion, syncope usually occurs when the patient is upright. Some causes, particularly cardiac arrhythmias, result in syncope in any position.

The causes of syncope can result in a spectrum of attacks of varying severity. "Near syncope" is at one end of the spectrum and presents as light-headedness, dizziness, or faintness that is not followed by a loss of consciousness. Often its effects may be aborted by lying down. Sudden death, or "irreversible syncope," secondary to cardiac disease is at the opposite end. Classic syncope can be a harbinger of these more serious attacks. Determining where the patient fits in the spectrum is a key goal of clinical evaluation.

Syncope must be distinguished from other syndromes, such as seizures, vertigo, and dizziness, which result in altered consciousness or dysequilibrium. Hypoglycemia, hypoxemia, hypocapnia, and hypercapnia cause altered mental status, but rarely so abruptly that they are confused with syncope. When difficulty is encountered, it is usually in separating true syncope from seizures. Some observations that are helpful in making this distinction are listed in Table 133-1. Of the characteristics listed, the presence or absence of postictal confusion best discriminates between the two. Occasionally, syncope is followed by transient tonic-clonic activity as a result of prolonged cerebral ischemia, produced when a patient is prevented from falling to a horizontal position. Although this raises the question of central nervous system disease, primary neurologic abnormalities are not usually present.

Frequency

The frequency with which the various causes of syncope are encountered varies with the clinical setting and the patient's age. In the community and in first-contact office practice, vasovagal syncope is by far the most common; in fact, many cases are not even brought to a physician's attention. In referral practices, and particularly with older patients, more serious causes are found with greater frequency. In one recent study of patients with syncope who were evaluated in the emergency room, the outpatient clinics, and the inpatient services, 26% of the episodes were due to cardiovascular disease, 26% were noncardiovascular, and 48% were unexplained. This relatively high proportion of unexplained cases has been observed in other studies in a variety of settings. Patients whose syncope remained unexplained had the lowest mortality and those with a cardiovascular cause, the highest. Other studies have documented a 1-year mortality of 20 to 30% for cardiac syncope, up to 10% for unexplained syncope, and 5% for noncardiac causes. Regardless of the frequency, even the relatively uncommon conditions (e.g., complete heart block) must be considered because they are life-threatening and treatable.

Causes of Syncope

Because syncope is by definition transient and self-limited, the physician is rarely called on to treat an attack. Rather, the challenge is to find the underlying cause in order to predict and prevent future attacks and identify the infrequent situations in which syncope is a manifestation of serious, life-threatening disease. Success in defining a specific cause is primarily dependent on methodically taking the patient's history and doing a focused physical examination based on a thorough knowledge of the differential diagnosis.

Vasovagal Syncope

Vasovagal syncope results from a transient decrease in cardiac output because of a combination of peripheral vasodilation and bradycardia. The diagnosis is totally dependent on an accurate history. The episodes typically occur in response to highly stressful settings such as the threat of physical injury, the receipt of bad news, or other anxiety-provoking circumstances. Patients are usually standing at the time of onset, occasionally sitting, and rarely recumbent. Premonitory symptoms include a feeling of warmth, light-headedness,

Table 133-1. Characteristics distinguishing syncope from seizures

Characteristic	Syncope	Seizure
Position	Usually standing	Standing or supine
Onset	Gradual—may be heralded by a "fading" sensation	Abrupt—no prodrome
Skin color	Pale	Normal
Tonic-clonic activity	Occasionally 1 to 2 clonic jerks	Frequent
Personal injury	Occasional	Frequent
Incontinence	Occasional	Frequent
Tongue biting	Occasional	Frequent
Postictal phase	Usually the return to consciousness is prompt; no postepisode confusion	Return to consciousness is slow; postepisode confusion

sweating, epigastric discomfort, and nausea. Associated physiologic changes include a temporary (1–2 minutes) increase in heart rate, blood pressure, total systemic resistance, and cardiac output. This is followed by a reversal of these physiologic changes and increased vagal tone. The result is a pallid, unconscious patient who is hypotensive and bradycardic, but who rapidly recovers when placed in the supine position. A history of other episodes under similar circumstances is especially helpful in making the diagnosis.

Panic Attacks
Stressful circumstances can also be associated with syncope from panic attacks, particularly if the attacks are accompanied by hyperventilation, which reduces cerebrovascular perfusion by lowering blood PCO_2 and, as a result, produces vasoconstriction. It is usually possible, on careful questioning, to elicit one or more of the following characteristics of hyperventilation: stereotyped attacks; onset during times of interpersonal stress or crowding; symptoms of anxiety; heaviness in the chest; paresthesias in the hands, perioral area, and feet; and, in extreme cases, carpopedal spasm and periods of apnea without cyanosis. Having the patient voluntarily hyperventilate during examination may produce the symptoms and provide support for this diagnosis. This can be done unnoticed during the respiratory examination.

Postural Hypotension
A reduction in systemic blood pressure occurs on assuming the upright position, if reflex vasoconstriction is inadequate. The classic history is that of a patient who faints on getting out of bed or up from a chair. Diagnosis is dependent on a careful history of the circumstances surrounding an attack and on the measurement of a standing blood pressure (after the patient has been recumbent for at least 15 minutes). Although a clinically meaningful decrease in orthostatic blood pressure is not strictly defined, a drop of 10 to 20 mm Hg in systolic and diastolic pressure, or a decrease in mean blood pressure of 30 mm Hg or more, increases the likelihood that orthostatic hypotension is the cause of syncope. Any decrease that is associated with symptoms is significant.

When the onset is recent, volume contraction is a common cause, particularly in the elderly. Protracted diarrhea, blood loss, recurrent emesis, poor oral intake, and excessive use of diuretics are the common precipitating factors. Newly prescribed medications that result in autonomic dysfunction have a comparable effect. When syncope is more chronic, autonomic nervous system dysfunction is commonly a problem. This may result from aging, the sympathetic neuropathy of diabetes mellitus, adrenergic blocking drugs, or less common causes—amyloidosis, idiopathic orthostatic hypotension, and Shy-Drager syndrome. Prolonged bed rest predisposes to syncope by deconditioning autonomic reflexes.

Most postural hypotension can be treated by removing the underlying cause(s). When that is not possible (e.g., in the case of autonomic neuropathy), having the patient rise more slowly may help. Alpha-adrenergic agents, 9-alpha fluorohydrocortisone, and monoamine oxidase inhibitors have been used with success in individual cases. Unfortunately, most patients respond suboptimally.

Cough and Micturition
Syncope occurring during severe paroxysms of coughing is probably related to depletion of central blood volume secondary to splanchnic pooling and increased intrathoracic pressure, which, in the standing position, may result in a sudden drop in mean systolic blood pressure. Micturition syncope, which is characteristically seen in young men in their 20s and 30s, is less well understood but probably results from the sudden loss of vascular tone related to the emptying of a full bladder in the standing position. Making either of these diagnoses is totally dependent on an accurate history.

Arrhythmia
A precipitous fall in cardiac output secondary to arrhythmia—either tachycardia or bradycardia—results in syncope. According to one report, syncope was the presenting manifestation of myocardial infarction in 7% of patients over 65 years old. The patient may occasionally experience an "odd sensation," a "fluttering" or "jerking" in the chest, but there are often no symptoms referable to the heart. Abrupt loss of consciousness is followed by a similarly abrupt clearing. The routine ECG may not identify the problem even in cases of myocardial infarction; nevertheless, a cardiogram is warranted. Holter monitoring is more effective, particularly when attacks are frequent (and thus likely to be recorded) and in older patients who are more likely to have arrhythmia as a cause of syncope. Whether the frequency of heart block or tachyarrhythmias is sufficient to support routine 24- or 48-hour monitoring in patients with fainting of uncertain cause remains debatable.

In many patients who have chronic, recurrent syncope and who are suspected of having underlying cardiac disease, the syncopal episodes are so infrequent that routine Holter monitoring is unlikely to be helpful. Early data from studies on loop monitors, which allow more prolonged recording intervals, are encouraging. Cardiology consultation for more invasive diagnostic studies (e.g., intracardiac electrophysiologic techniques) should be considered if life-threatening arrhythmias remain suspect but undocumented. The enthusiasm of some cardiologists for electrophysiologic studies may reflect referral bias, leading to the conclusion that the technique is more effective than it really is. The importance of identifying a treatable cardiac cause has been documented by recent studies showing that patients with a cardiovascular cause of syncope have a three- to fivefold higher incidence of sudden death, than do patients with a noncardiovascular or an unknown cause.

Other Primary Cardiopulmonary Diseases
Careful cardiac examination may provide evidence for entities that commonly produce syncope, including aortic stenosis, hypertrophic subaortic stenosis, mitral stenosis, mitral valve prolapse, pulmonary hypertension, and atrial myxoma. Echocardiography may help to confirm the clinical suspicion of these entities.

Carotid Sinus Syncope
A hypersensitive carotid sinus can cause transiently depressed cardiac output. Episodes are related to activities that stimulate the carotid sinus, such as movement of the neck, shaving, or wearing a tight shirt collar. Unfortunately, questions about these associations and physical examination are usually low in yield. This diagnosis should be considered particularly in the elderly, after other cardiac-related problems have been excluded. The diagnostic test is carotid sinus massage during ECG and hemodynamic monitoring in a setting where resuscitative equipment is readily available. The maneuver should be used with great care in the elderly because of the increased risk of dislodging atheromatous material from carotid plaques. Two abnormal responses are observed: asystole with a significant drop in blood pressure (cardioinhibitory type) and a significant drop in blood pressure without a significant decrease in cardiac rate (vasodepressor type). Treatment of the cardioinhibitory type requires insertion of a pacemaker. There is no effective treatment for the vasodepressor type.

Cerebrovascular Disease
Transient ischemic attacks resulting in hypoperfusion of the vertebrobasilar system may present with a sudden loss of postural muscle tone and consciousness. Although the underlying pathophysiology is usually vertebrobasilar occlusive disease, vertebrobasilar arterial spasm can present similarly during migraine headaches. Commonly there are other symptoms related to structures in the posterior fossa, for example, visual, auditory, or vestibular symptoms. Ischemia secondary to arteriosclerosis of the carotid vessels characteristically does not produce a loss of consciousness except in the setting of bilateral occlusive disease.

Cerebrovascular disease is suspected by history alone. The physical examination is often of little help, although identifying posterior cervical and infraclavicular bruits or a difference in arm blood pressure (vertebral steal syndrome) supports this diagnosis. Definitive diagnosis depends on aortic arch and cerebral angiography; however, these studies do not exclude other causes of syncope even when definitive lesions are found. Unfortunately, practical therapeutic options are very limited in the setting of posterior fossa vascular disease. As a result, the risk-benefit ratio of cerebrovascular evaluation should be carefully considered.

Pulmonary Embolus
Massive pulmonary emboli may obstruct the main pulmonary artery and produce a severe drop in cardiac output with hypotension. Most patients with pulmonary emboli causing syncope (the presenting complaint of 13% of a series of patients with pulmonary embolism) do not live long enough to obtain medical care. On occasion, central obstruction of blood flow is transient because the clot dislodges from central vessels and moves to peripheral pulmonary vessels, allowing more prolonged survival.

Approach to Diagnosis
Successful diagnosis of the cause of syncope, and hence prevention of subsequent attacks, is primarily dependent on methodically taking the patient's history and doing a focused physical examination. A number of studies have confirmed the high yield of the carefully done history and physical examination. In most cases a limited number of studies can be done to substantiate or refute the initial clinical impression. The primary goal is to define the high-risk group of patients with an underlying cardiac cause.

The relatively high mortality of cardiac arrhythmias as causes of syncope warrants hospital admission for cardiac monitoring in patients who present acutely with a history and risk factors highly suspect for underlying cardiac disease. Holter monitoring may be used in patients with less acute presentations when the syncopal episodes are occurring frequently. The development of loop-recorder technology may allow sufficiently long recording intervals (several months) to increase the yield in patients with infrequent episodes. Loop recorders can be activated after a syncopal episode and retrieve information about the cardiac rhythm for the preceding few minutes. The signal-averaged ECG is a relatively new, noninvasive technique that detects low-amplitude, high-frequency signals at the terminal portion of the QRS complex. These signals may serve as the electrophysiologic substrate for ventricular arrhythmias. More specialized testing such as electrophysiologic studies is probably warranted in refractory cases in which the underlying cause remains evasive in the setting of probable cardiac disease. Unfortunately, correlating electrophysiologic findings with a patient's syncopal episodes remains far from clear-cut.

Electroencephalography (EEG) is one of the most commonly used tests. It should be done in those patients in whom a postictal interval or other history makes a seizure disorder highly suspect, keeping in mind that patients with seizures can have normal EEGs. Similarly, abnormal EEGs occur in patients without seizure disorders. CT of the head should also be considered when the findings on history or EEG are highly suggestive of seizures. CT findings are similarly suggestive when the physical examination reveals a focal neurological abnormality.

Other tests such as skull films, lumbar puncture, and cerebral angiography are very low in yield unless the patient's history suggests a new-onset seizure disorder or there is a focal neurologic abnormality on physical examination. Treatment options are often limited even when specific pathology is found on cerebral angiography.

Kapoor WN, et al. A prospective evaluation and follow-up of patients with syncope. N Engl J Med 1983; 309:197–204.
Prospectively evaluates emergency room patients, inpatients, and outpatients and defines specific diagnostic categories with prognostic importance. Concludes that patients with a cardiovascular cause have a strikingly higher incidence of sudden death than do patients with a noncardiovascular or unknown cause.

Eagle KA, et al. Evaluation of prognostic classifications for patients with syncope. Am J Med 1985; 79:455–60.
Prospectively evaluates 176 consecutive patients who presented to an emergency room and concludes that 70% of patients can be placed into either very-high- (cardiac) or very-low- (vasovagal/psychogenic or unknown cause) risk groups.

Kapoor W, et al. Syncope in the elderly. Am J Med 1986; 80:419–28.
Describes the prospective evaluation and prognostic factors in 210 elderly patients as compared with 190 younger patients. Concludes that patients with a cardiovascular cause of syncope are at exceedingly high risk of mortality and sudden death regardless of age. Elderly patients with an unknown or noncardiovascular cause have a higher incidence of sudden death and mortality than do younger patients.

Naccarelli GV. Evaluation of the patient with syncope. Med Clin North Am 1984; 68:1211–30.
Presents a helpful overview of the evaluation of syncope, particularly secondary to cardiac causes.

Lee RT, et al. Long-term survival after transient loss of consciousness. J Gen Intern Med 1988; 3:337–43.
Addresses the factors that influence the long-term outcome of 198 patients who presented to an emergency ward with syncope and concludes that the cause of syncope is significantly correlated with mortality. The long-term mortality was significantly increased in patients with a prior history of coronary or cerebrovascular disease.

Silverstein MD, et al. Patients with syncope admitted to medical intensive care units. JAMA 1982; 248:1185–9.
Reviews the records of 108 patients admitted to a medical intensive care unit and defines the 1-year mortality based on etiology—cardiovascular, noncardiovascular, or unexplained. The cardiovascular group had the highest mortality.

Branch WT. Approach to syncope. J Gen Intern Med 1986; 1:49–58.
Provides a useful overview of the differential diagnosis, available diagnostic tests, the approach to selection of diagnostic tests, and the approach to therapy.

Noble RJ. The patient with syncope. JAMA 1977; 237:1372–6.
An in-depth discussion of the differential diagnosis based on pathogenic mechanisms.

Luxon LM, et al. Controlled study of 24-hour ambulatory electrocardiographic monitoring in patients with transient neurologic symptoms. J Neurol Neurosurg Psychiatry 1980; 43:37.
Presents data that support the value of 24-hour ECG monitoring as a diagnostic tool.

DiMarco JP, et al. Intracardiac electrophysiologic techniques in recurrent syncope of unknown cause. Ann Intern Med 1981; 95:542–8.
Presents data on 25 patients with recurrent, unexplained episodes of syncope. Full electrophysiologic evaluation with programmed stimulation was useful in diagnosis and therapy.

Manolis AS, et al. Syncope: current diagnostic evaluation and management. Ann Intern Med 1990; 112:850–63.
Provides a comprehensive review of the causes, current diagnostic evaluation, and treatment of syncope.

134. EDEMA
William F. Finn

The amount, composition, and distribution of fluid within the body are exquisitely controlled and under normal conditions remain relatively constant. An abnormal accumulation of fluid in the interstitial space is termed edema.

The hallmark of excessive interstitial fluid is transient pitting of the skin or subcutaneous tissue from the brief application of firm pressure. Nonpitting edema is the peculiar bogginess of the skin that occurs in myxedema and the increased thickness of the subcutaneous tissue that occurs as a result of fibrosis induced by chronic inflammation or venous stasis. The specific cause of edema may be suggested by its distribution. Localized edema suggests damage to tissue or mechanical problems; generalized edema suggests abnormalities in the systemic control of salt and water excretion due to heart, liver, or kidney disease.

Localized Edema
Common causes of localized edema include changes in the permeability of capillary walls, an increase in the protein concentration of the interstitial fluid, and/or an increase in venous hydrostatic pressure. Depending on the specific abnormality, the edema may be unilateral or bilateral and, in either case, more prominent in areas below or above the diaphragm.

Loss of Vascular Integrity

Loss of vascular integrity occurs with urticaria and angioneurotic edema. Release of vasoactive substances (histamine, bradykinin, and other polypeptides) alters the permeability of the capillary wall, resulting in leakage of plasma proteins and fluid movement into the interstitial space. Electrothermal injury, excessive radiation, cold exposure, and severe ischemic injury also cause a loss of vascular integrity. In children, idiopathic scrotal edema may occur in response to infections, trauma, or allergies. This condition is self-limiting, is occasionally recurrent, and most often results in unilateral painless swelling of the scrotum. At times, the swelling may extend to the groin, abdomen, and perineum.

Increase in Tissue Oncotic Pressure

An increase in tissue oncotic pressure may result from a reduction in lymph flow, which leads to an increase in interstitial protein concentration. Causes include surgical or traumatic injury, radical mastectomy, radiation therapy, compression or infiltration of the lymphatics with malignant cells, recurrent inflammation (lymphangitis), and Milroy's disease, a form of inherited, congenital lymphedema. The edema associated with lymphatic obstruction often becomes nonpitting and firm because of secondary fibrotic changes in the skin and subcutaneous tissues.

Increase in Hydrostatic Pressure

An increase in hydrostatic pressure, generally due to an increase in venous resistance, favors the movement of fluid into the interstitial space. An increase in the systemic arterial blood pressure does not directly result in edema formation.

Edema above the diaphragm, particularly of the face, is often due to compression of the superior vena cava. The "superior vena cava syndrome" is commonly caused by metastatic carcinoma of the lung, less frequently by tumors or inflammatory lesions of mediastinum, occasionally by aortic aneurysms or traumatic thrombosis, and rarely by endothoracic goiters, mitral stenosis, pericarditis, and mediastinal emphysema.

Unilateral edema of an upper extremity may be due to thrombosis of a subclavian vein, obstruction from neoplasms, or compression from enlarged lymph nodes.

Unilateral leg edema is most commonly the sequela of old fractures, phlebitis, or surgery, which has resulted in abnormalities of the veins or lymphatics. Because these conditions are so common, fluid accumulation from systemic causes may also appear unilaterally. Thus, while unilateral leg edema is usually a result of local problems, cardiac, hepatic, or renal disease cannot be excluded on this basis alone.

Unilateral edema of a lower extremity also frequently results from incompetent valves in the superficial venous system (often accompanied by varicosities), venous thrombosis, or external compression from benign or malignant masses located in inguinal or intra-abdominal areas. A less common cause is tight-fitting clothing.

Bilateral edema below the level of the diaphragm may signify an increased resistance to flow in the right side of the heart or pulmonary vasculature or to obstruction of the inferior vena cava. Conditions such as pulmonary hypertension, pulmonic stenosis, tricuspid insufficiency, and constrictive pericarditis are associated with venous congestion and edema formation. The most common causes of bilateral, lower extremity edema, however, are diseases of the kidney, liver, or heart that result in generalized edema.

Generalized Edema

Except when complicated by hypoalbuminemia, generalized edema indicates an increase not only in the interstitial fluid but also in the sodium content of the extracellular compartment and signifies potentially serious renal, cardiac, or liver disease. In general, edema implies an increase in interstitial fluid of at least 3 L. While this is usually associated with a proportional weight gain, the simultaneous loss of lean body mass may obscure the gradual retention of sodium and water.

Renal Disease

Edema develops as a result of both acute and chronic renal disease. Abnormalities of renal function are usually present, except in the nephrotic syndrome in which edema formation may precede changes in creatinine or urea clearance.

Liver Disease

Liver disease results in ascites when disorganization of the normal architecture of the liver leads to portal venous hypertension. Alone or in combination with other factors, impaired ability to synthesize albumin may result in generalized edema.

Cardiac and Pulmonary Disease

When the classic signs of congestive heart failure are present, the diagnosis is not difficult to establish. However, these abnormalities may be intermittent or associated with other causes of edema. Frequently overlooked is the coexistence of chronic obstructive pulmonary disease.

Nutritional Disease

Kwashiorkor results from a diet high in carbohydrates but insufficient in protein. This condition is frequently associated with hypoalbuminemia, which, along with other factors, results in edema formation. In marasmus due to a low intake of all nutrients, edema is uncommon. When "starvation edema" or "famine edema" occurs, it may be a consequence of the loss of elasticity in tissue structures and the tendency for the extracellular fluid volume to remain at prestarvation levels despite the loss of body weight.

Gastrointestinal Disease

Many diseases are associated with protein-losing enteropathy, including inflammatory diseases, disorders of the mucosal cells, and diseases associated with abnormalities of absorption. In these conditions, edema formation occurs because of an impaired ability to absorb amino acids and subsequent protein depletion and hypoproteinemia.

Other Causes

Idiopathic Edema

Idiopathic edema occurs most commonly in young women in the absence of hepatic, cardiac, or renal disease and without other demonstrable causes. The periodic or cyclical nature of the edema formation and the apparent relation to the menstrual cycle suggests a hormonal basis; however, its pathogenesis remains enigmatic. In overt cases, there is a substantial weight gain during the day, which may range from 1.5 to 2.5 kg. Pitting edema of the lower extremities may occur. The most distressing symptoms include a bloated feeling with abdominal distention, headaches, excessive thirst, and emotional lability.

The weight gain occurs over several days or weeks and often remits with a spontaneous diuresis coincident with or soon after the onset of menses. Signs generally attributable to intravascular volume depletion (a rapid, thready pulse with a narrow pulse pressure along with an orthostatic drop in blood pressure and, in severe cases, syncope) may be present during the early phase of edema formation. In addition, evidence of hemoconcentration with an elevation of the hematocrit can be found in some patients. This constellation of signs and symptoms suggests that women with idiopathic cyclical edema alternate between periods of intravascular volume contraction and edema formation.

Orthostatic Sodium Retention

Some patients are thought to have an abnormal capillary leak of protein resulting in a reduction in blood volume, which is most pronounced in an upright posture. Characteristically, these patients may have no evidence of pitting edema in the morning, but by evening, because of the excessive salt and water retention, the edema is present. In some cases, elevated renin and aldosterone and a significant fall in plasma volume have been found after only 1 hour of standing. There is also a tendency in these patients to retain sodium and water when standing and to be unable to excrete a water load in a normal manner when first given a sodium load.

Diuretic and Laxative Abuse

Diuretic and laxative abuse may paradoxically result in edema formation. Prolonged use of either agent may lead to increased renin and aldosterone levels. When the diuretics are precipitously stopped, rapid salt retention occurs, and may last several days. Unfortunately, the response, particularly in people who are overly concerned with their weight and appearance, is to increase the dose and frequency of the diuretic. It has been claimed that this is the most common cause of idiopathic cyclical edema. If diuretic or laxative abuse is suspected but denied by the patient, the urine can be tested for thiazides or phenolphthalein.

Carbohydrate Loading

Fasting is associated with natriuresis, and conversely, refeeding with antinatriuresis. Patients who alternate between periods of low and high carbohydrate and sodium intake are likely to notice periods of weight gain and even edema formation. Groups of people particularly prone to carbohydrate-induced edema formation include patients who fast during the week but binge on the weekends, travelers forced to alter eating patterns, and some patients with personality traits similar to those with anorexia nervosa. The feeling of bloatedness or the appearance of edema may lead to diuretic use and the possibility of diuretic-induced edema as well.

Heat Edema

Heat exposure is not ordinarily associated with weight gain, but occasionally a transient weight gain of up to 5 kg occurs over several days, accompanied by a decrease in urine volume, edema of the lower extremities, and a feeling of bloatedness. The urine tends to have a high sodium content and the serum sodium concentration is depressed, a series of events that resemble inappropriate antidiuretic hormone secretion. After several days, a spontaneous diuresis usually occurs. The frequency of the occurrence of heat edema is unknown, but it is likely to be more common than generally believed.

Altitude Edema

Life-threatening pulmonary and cerebral edema may develop singly or together during the first week of high-altitude exposure, when acute mountain sickness is most common. Peripheral edema also occurs at high altitudes but may occur in low-altitude hill walkers in the absence of the symptoms of acute mountain sickness. It is possible that the effects of altitude and exercise may be additive in producing the altitude edemas. The specific cause is unknown but may result from an increase in venous pressure.

Drugs

Pharmacologic agents can cause edema formation through a variety of mechanisms. Drugs that promote salt and water retention include potent vasodilators such as hydralazine and minoxidil; nonsteroidal anti-inflammatory drugs; adrenal steroids; estrogens; and phenothiazine tranquilizers such as thioridazine (Mellaril), chlorpromazine (Thorazine), and trifluoperazine (Stelazine) and the thioxanthene derivative thiothixene (Navane). The cancer chemotherapy agent interleukin-2 may cause increased vascular permeability and the vascular leak syndrome, resulting in severe complications such as ascites, hydrothorax, and pulmonary edema within hours of treatment. Insulin therapy of diabetic ketoacidosis may cause peripheral edema as a result of an antinatriuretic effect of insulin on the renal tubules.

Approach to Patients with Edema

The primary consideration in patients with edema is to look for systemic disease. This can usually be accomplished by asking about symptoms of cardiac, pulmonary, hepatic, renal, and gastrointestinal disorders and by a physical examination directed toward possible abnormalities of these organs. In patients with generalized edema, posteroanterior and lateral chest films are indicated to look for congestive heart failure. To look for renal disease, a careful analysis of a freshly voided urine specimen and determination of the serum creatinine or blood urea nitrogen (BUN) levels should be performed. Renal insufficiency may be present without striking abnormalities in the microscopic examination of the urine sediment, and conversely, proteinuria and the nephrotic syndrome may occur without a rise in serum creatinine or BUN levels. Liver function studies are useful because generalized edema may be an early manifestation of liver disease and portal hypertension. The serum albumin concentration should be measured when heavy proteinuria is found, when liver disease is suspected, or when protein-depletion malabsorption is suspected. If the patient has ascites, an abdominal paracentesis should be performed. The fluid should be characterized as a transudate or an exudate, examined for abnormal cells, bacteria, and fungi, and cultured for acid-fast bacilli.

If the chest films, urinalysis, serum creatinine and BUN levels, liver function studies, and serum albumin concentration are all normal and there is no evidence of severe pulmonary or gastrointestinal disease, the cause of the generalized edema formation may be assumed to be idiopathic or cyclical in nature, to be related to drug ingestion, or to be due to changes in climate, diet, or altitude or to one of several endocrinopathies. Further diagnostic efforts are warranted because these situations are not uncommon, are often the source of great anxiety, and may be alleviated by relatively simple changes. A detailed history should be taken about those events that are temporarily related to the onset of the edema; specifically, a chart of daily morning and evening weights through several menstrual cycles should be obtained from female patients. All patients should be asked about drugs that can cause edema, diuretic or laxative abuse, patterns of carbohydrate and salt intake, and sudden changes in climate and altitude. If drug abuse is in question, the urine can be tested for thiazides or phenolphthalein.

In patients with localized edema, a search should be made for evidence of allergic reactions as indicated by the presence of wheals or urticaria. These patients frequently complain of intense itching. The edema from burns or cold exposure is accompanied by inflammatory signs or evidence of tissue damage.

With chronic lymphatic obstruction, reduction of edema may minimize secondary fibrotic changes. Frequent elevation of the involved extremity (to a point above the level of the right atrium), use of support hose, dietary sodium restriction, and diuretics may all be helpful.

When edema is associated with varicose veins, there is usually irreversible deep venous obstruction and incompetent valves. Treatment is designed to reduce the hydrostatic pressure when the patient is erect through the use of fitted stockings and periodic elevation of the legs. Occasionally, it may be necessary to recommend ligation of the perforating veins and removal of the superficial veins (see Chap. 40).

Patients who are believed to have cyclical or idiopathic edema should not be given diuretics, which may eventually worsen the edema. Instead, they should be put on salt restriction and other dietary or drug manipulations.

Anderson RJ, Schrier RW. Renal sodium excretion, edematous disorders, and diuretic use. In: Schrier RW, ed. Renal and electrolyte disorders. 3rd ed. Boston: Little, Brown, 1986:79–139.
An extremely well-presented discussion.

Brenner BM, Stein JH, eds. Body fluid homeostasis. New York: Churchill-Livingstone, 1987.
An in-depth treatise on the major edema-forming states.

McKeown JW. Disorders of total body sodium. In: Kokko JP, Tannen RL, eds. Fluids and electrolytes. Philadelphia: WB Saunders, 1986:63.
Comprehensive presentation combining pathophysiology and clinical medicine.

Baliga R, Lewy JE. Pathogenesis and treatment of edema. Pediatr Clin North Am 1987; 34:639–48.
Excellent review, with particular emphasis on problems in the pediatric population.

135. LYMPHADENOPATHY
Robert H. Fletcher and David J. Weber

Peripheral lymphadenopathy (enlarged lymph nodes) occurring without other findings that point to the cause presents a difficult dilemma for clinicians. On one hand, many of the potential causes are both serious and treatable. On the other hand, the only way to make a definite diagnosis is, in nearly all instances, by a lymph node biopsy. Therefore, a great deal rests on the clinician's judgment as to whether an invasive procedure is necessary.

Causes
The list of possible causes for lymphadenopathy is extensive (Table 135-1). General categories include malignancies, either intrinsic to the node or metastatic; infections of virtually all kinds; antigenic stimulation (e.g., secondary to local injections or systemic, autoimmune diseases); and drugs (specifically phenytoin, but also others if they cause serum sickness). Sarcoidosis is associated with granulomatous adenopathy. For a large proportion of enlarged lymph nodes, no specific cause is determined.

Initial Evaluation
The likelihood of finding an important and treatable cause of lymphadenopathy can be estimated from information available at the time the patient is first seen. Key factors to consider in developing a differential diagnosis of adenopathy are: (1) age of the patient; (2) size, shape, and consistency of the lymph nodes; (3) location of the adenopathy; and (4) duration and rate of change. The judgment to pursue a diagnostic workup or wait is based, in large measure, on these observations.

Likely Causes
Infections are the most common cause of adenopathy; clinical symptoms and signs (i.e., fever, rash tenderness) usually suggest the diagnosis. For nodes that clinicians decide to biopsy, whether at referral centers or community hospitals, a small set of possibilities accounts for nearly all results. About 40% of such nodes are abnormal but without findings from histologic examination or culture that allow a specific diagnosis. Three conditions account for nearly all of the remaining 60% of nodes evaluated: metastatic malignancies (25%), intrinsic malignancy (e.g., lymphoma, 20%), and tuberculosis (10%). The remainder (5%) includes a variety of normal and abnormal tissues. Therefore, the probability that a lymph node will be nonspecifically involved, or reflect one of these three specific conditions, is extremely high even before considering other information.

Age
The likelihood of cancer increases with age. In one series, 25% of biopsied nodes from young people revealed cancer, while 75% of nodes from patients over 75 years old were malignant. Normally, the lymphatic tissue in adolescents and young adults is larger than it is later in life, so that minor degrees of node "enlargement" may not be abnormal in the young.

Table 135-1. Causes of generalized lymphadenopathy in the United States

Infections
  Viral
    Human immunodeficiency virus type 1
    Mononucleosis (Epstein-Barr virus)
    Cytomegalovirus
    Hepatitis B
    Measles
    Rubella
  Bacterial
    Scarlet fever (group A streptococci)
    Brucellosis (*Brucella* species)
    Cat-scratch disease
    Leptospirosis (*Leptospira* species)
    Secondary syphilis (*Treponema pallidum*)
    Glanders (*Pseudomonas mallei*)
  Mycobacterial
    Miliary tuberculosis (*Mycobacterium tuberculosis*)
    Atypical mycobacterial infection
  Protozoal
    Toxoplasmosis (*Toxoplasma gondii*)
  Fungal
    Histoplasmosis (*Histoplasma capsulatum*)
Neoplasms
  Leukemia (chronic lymphocytic, acute, chronic granulocytic)
  Lymphoma (Hodgkin's disease, lymphocytic, histiocytic lymphoma)
  Immunoblastic lymphadenopathy
  Metastases
Collagen vascular disorders
  Systemic lupus erythematosus
  Rheumatoid arthritis
  Juvenile rheumatoid arthritis
Endocrine disorders
  Hyperthyroidism
  Hypoadrenocorticism
  Hypopituitarism
Hypersensitivity states
  Serum sickness
  Drug reactions (especially to phenytoin)
Miscellaneous
  Sarcoidosis
  Lipid storage diseases

Location
The likelihood of finding a specific diagnosis varies with the location from which a node is taken. Abnormal nodes in the neck most often provide a specific diagnosis (70%), followed by those in the axilla (50%) and the groin (40%). This is presumed to be because minor infections in the extremities, particularly the lower ones, increase the prevalence of nonspecifically enlarged ("reactive") nodes in their region. For example, palpable, firm inguinal nodes up to 1 cm in diameter are common in adults. Therefore, one is more inclined to biopsy an enlarged neck node than a groin node. Similarly, if there is a choice of nodes to biopsy (e.g., with generalized lymphadenopathy), it is best to biopsy one in the neck.

Rate of Change
Nodes that enlarge rapidly are more often pathologic than are slowly growing ones. Unfortunately, patients often do not notice when the node first appeared, even in prominent places such as the neck. Also, fear and wishful thinking may color their reports.

Physical Findings
Examination of involved nodes can yield relatively accurate information about the underlying pathophysiologic process. Five observations should be made: size, localization, consistency, inflammation, and fixation. A large size (e.g., > 1 cm) weighs in favor of a specific pathology. Generalized adenopathy is caused by systemic disease, whereas local or regional adenopathy may represent either local (e.g., infection, tumor) or systemic (e.g., human immunodeficiency virus [HIV] infection, tuberculosis) disease. Hard nodes represent metastatic cancer or fibrosis from a previous inflammation (particularly if the nodes are small). Firm or rubbery nodes are associated with lymphomas and leukemia, as well as a variety of infections and antigenic processes. Fluctuant nodes usually represent pyogenic infection, although advanced tuberculosis, and occasionally necrotic tumors, can also result in central liquefaction. Signs of inflammation (e.g., heat, redness) suggest infection or antigenic stimulation. Fixation of nodes to adjacent structures—to each other or to the deep fascia or dermis—represents either neoplasm invading outside the node capsule or organized inflammation.

Diagnostic Tests

Excisional Biopsy
Biopsy of abnormal lymph nodes is the most accurate means of diagnosis. Usually a node is excised in its entirety rather than partially removed, because having as much tissue as possible is useful for histologic diagnosis and because the diagnosis and treatment of some conditions (e.g., mycobacterial adenitis) begin with excision. Most pathologic nodes can be removed under local anesthesia, without admitting the patient to the hospital. The morbidity of the procedure is negligible and is mainly related to infection or damage to local neurovascular structures, especially when the procedure is done in the axilla or groin. Usually it is sufficient to send excised nodes for routine histology and bacterial culture. Occasionally, other tests such as special stains and cultures for mycobacteria, viruses, and fungi are suggested by the clinical situation. When the official pathology report is equivocal (e.g., "atypical hyperplasia"), it may be helpful to talk with the pathologist; so much rests on their interpretation that pathologists are inclined to be conservative for the record.

Needle Biopsy
Needle biopsy, using a thin-bore needle, can be accomplished with negligible morbidity. In published series, about 85% of attempts yield sufficient tissue for diagnosis. Since only a small number of cells are obtained, and tissue architecture is disrupted, it is sometimes not possible to make a firm diagnosis, particularly for intrinsic malignancies. When the biopsy specimen indicates cancer, one can have confidence in the result—that is, there are few false-positive results. However, if the results are negative for malignant cells, one cannot rule out cancer. In one series, 60% of patients whose biopsy specimens were read as negative for cancer subsequently proved to have cancer. Therefore, needle biopsy is most useful when metastatic cancer, as opposed to lymphoma, is suspected and when the results are positive rather than negative.

Aspiration
If a node is fluctuant, it is tempting to aspirate it, since aspiration is a relatively noninvasive procedure. Indeed, aspiration might determine the diagnosis if the cause is infection, either pyogenic or tuberculous, although it is by no means perfectly sensitive for this purpose. However, most of these nodes require either incision and drainage (for pyogenic infection) or excision for diagnosis (e.g., lymphoma) or for cure (e.g., infection with mycobacteria other than *Mycobacterium tuberculosis*). Therefore, aspiration is not, in itself, a particularly useful diagnostic maneuver.

Lymphangiography
Lymphangiography demonstrates the anatomic distribution of abnormal nodes. But lymphangiography cannot determine, with reasonable certainty, the specific process taking place in the nodes.

Strategy for Evaluation

In most situations, the initial management of lymphadenopathy involves a choice between two options: biopsy or waiting. If laboratory tests are done, they should include a complete blood cell count; PPD and control; chest film; and a serologic test for HIV, if the patient is in a group at high risk for HIV infection (see Chap. 114). Occasionally abdominal computed tomography is useful. Beyond these, efforts to find out the cause of isolated peripheral lymphadenopathy indirectly (e.g., by means of elaborate serologic and skin tests) are usually not helpful. Waiting, at least for a short time, is often the preferred course of action. There are virtually no situations in which waiting for up to 2 weeks will result in a lost opportunity for treatment, particularly if the clinical findings do not change appreciably during that time.

When the decision to peform a biopsy is made, one must expect a certain number of nondiagnostic results (in most series about 40%) in order to safely include nearly all pathologic nodes. At times, biopsy is undertaken because of a concern on the part of the patient or physician that cannot be relieved in any other way.

Specific Presentations

Hard Cervical Nodes
A hard cervical node, particularly in the elderly, often represents a metastasis from a cancer arising in the mucosal surfaces of the head or neck. The primary cancer often cannot be visualized without using special instruments to examine relatively inaccessible surfaces (e.g., the nasopharynx) and even then it may not be found. There is evidence that the likelihood of recurrence is less if definitive surgery, often involving radical neck dissection, is done immediately following biopsy, rather than as a second procedure. For this reason when head and neck cancer is suspected, biopsy should be done by a specialist and in the hospital, usually after panendoscopy has been performed, so that if surgery is necessary it can be completed at the same time as the biopsy.

Inflamed Cervical Nodes
Inflamed cervical nodes, particularly in children and young adults, are usually the result of infection with staphylococci, streptococci, or both. Several features of this syndrome are counterintuitive. Usually no primary focus of infection is seen in the mouth or pharynx. Also, patients are often not very febrile or "toxic," although they are usually uncomfortable because of local swelling. If the node is just beginning to become fluctuant, many clinicians first treat the patient with antibiotics chosen to cover staphylococci and streptococci, and then proceed to incision and drainage only if there is no improvement. If the node is frankly fluctuant, it is unlikely that surgery can be avoided.

Tuberculous Adenitis
Tuberculous adenitis presents as an enlarging, mildly symptomatic node of several weeks' to months' duration. The adenitis is usually in the neck and rarely in the axilla or groin. About three-fourths of tuberculous nodes are not fluctuant at diagnosis. Tuberculous adenitis is suspected when the patient has a history of tuberculosis, a positive PPD, or an abnormal-appearing chest film, although only 40 to 90% of patients have these findings. Systemic signs are infrequent, and the disease is usually not active at other sites. The majority of infections in adults are caused by *M. tuberculosis;* in children most cases are caused by atypical mycobacteria. When tuberculous adenitis is suspected, antituberculous drugs are given following node excision until the culture results are available. If culture grows *M. tuberculosis,* antituberculous drugs are continued for 9 to 12 months. If there is evidence of infection elsewhere and the diagnosis can be made without node excision, drugs alone may be curative. For infections with mycobacteria other than *M. tuberculosis,* excision alone is often sufficient, except in persons who are immunocompromised (e.g., with HIV infection).

Genital Ulceration with Regional Adenopathy
Inguinal lymphadenopathy may be associated with a genital ulceration, with the latter usually appearing first. The lymphadenopathy may be unilateral or bilateral. Causes include syphilis, herpes, chancroid, lymphogranuloma venereum, and donovanosis (see Chap. 113).

Cat-Scratch Disease
Chronic tender regional lymphadenopathy, especially of the head and neck, may be due to cat-scratch disease, which usually occurs after the scratch of a kitten or cat, but may also be transmitted by other animals. The disease is caused by an as-yet-unnamed, small, fastidious, pleomorphic, gram-negative bacillus, or its cell wall–deficient variants. Associated malaise and fever each occur in about 30% of patients; less common associated symptoms include splenomegaly, headache, sore throat, rashes, conjunctivitis, and parotid swelling. The disease is usually self-limited and resolves in 4 to 6 weeks. The appropriate role for antibiotics has not been determined. The diagnosis is usually made clinically; node biopsy is not diagnostic, but may show granulomatous inflammation and stellate areas of necrosis.

Lymphadenopathy Associated with HIV Infection
Lymphadenopathy occurs in approximately 50% of persons who develop seroconversion, as the initial manifestation of their HIV infection. This syndrome occurs about 4 to 12 weeks after exposure, and consists of fever, malaise, myalgia, headaches, sore throat, diarrhea, and a maculopapular rash. In the latter stages of HIV infection, many patients develop persistent generalized lymphadenopathy, defined as adenopathy involving two or more extrainguinal sites, of at least 3 months' duration. The nodes are discrete and nontender, and suppuration does not occur. The generalized lymphadenopathy often is one of the manifestations of the AIDS-related complex, which may include fever, weight loss, diarrhea, malaise, and night sweats.

Lymphadenopathy is usually a result of a reaction to HIV proliferation, but may also be caused by cancer (e.g., lymphoma, Kaposi's sarcoma) and infection (e.g., toxoplasmosis, cytomegalovirus, *Mycobacterium avium-intracellulare*). Biopsy should be considered in HIV-positive patients with adenopathy and systemic symptoms or signs, especially if the lymph nodes are increasing in size. However, it is not necessary to subject patients with stable adenopathy to the morbidity of repeated lymph node biopsies.

Libman H. Generalized lymphadenopathy. J Gen Intern Med 1987; 2:48–58.
Concise but thorough review of the causes and clinical approach to generalized lymphadenopathy in the adult.

Swartz MN. Lymphadenitis and lymphangitis. In: Mandell GL, Douglas RB Jr, Bennett JE, eds. Principles and practices of infectious disease. New York: Churchill-Livingstone, 1990:818–25.
Comprehensive review of infectious causes of both regional and generalized lymphadenopathy.

Greenfield S, Jordon MC. The clinical investigation of lymphadenopathy in primary care practice. JAMA 1978; 240:1388–93.
An algorithm for evaluating adults whose initial and most prominent problem is peripheral lymphadenopathy.

Slap GB, Brooks JS, Schwartz JS. When to perform biopsies of enlarged peripheral lymph nodes in young patients. JAMA 1984; 252:1321–6.
Presents a retrospective review of pathology and clinical findings in 123, 9- to 25-year-old patients undergoing lymph node biopsy. Using discriminant analysis, a predictive model was developed to aid in selecting young patients for biopsy.

Lee Y, Terry R, Lukes RJ. Lymph node biopsy for diagnosis. A statistical study. J Surg Oncol 1980; 14:53–60.
The results of 925 consecutive lymph node biopsies for diagnosis, done at Los Angeles County University of Southern California Medical Center between 1973 and 1977.

Betsill WL Jr, Hajdu SI. Percutaneous aspiration biopsy of lymph nodes. Am J Clin Pathol 1980; 73:471–9.
The results of 361 cytologic examinations of specimens aspirated by percutaneous needle biopsy from superficial lymph nodes. Adequate material was obtained from 85%, and 81% of the samples were positive for malignant cells. There were no false-positive results, but over half of the negative results were false-negatives.

Martelli G, et al. Fine needle aspiration cytology in superficial lymph nodes: an analysis of 266 cases. Eur J Surg Oncol 1989; 15:13–16.
Similar to the above study. Analysis of 266 aspirates revealed the sensitivity of cytology for metastatic cancer to be 96.5% and for lymphomas, 67.3%. False-positive results did not occur but false-negative results were common.

Chen J, Wood MH. Tuberculous lymphadenopathy: a collective review with a case report. J Natl Med Assoc 1988; 80:1083–8.
A comprehensive review of clinical manifestations, diagnosis, and therapy of tuberculous adenopathy. Adenopathy in adults is usually due to M. tuberculosis and in children, to other mycobacteria.

Marcy SM. Infections of lymph nodes of the head and neck. *Pediatr Infect Dis* 1983; 2:397–405.
A comprehensive review of infectious causes of lymphadenitis of the head and neck in children and adolescents.

Piot P, Plummer FA. Genital ulcer adenopathy syndrome. In: Holmes KK, et al., eds. Sexually transmitted diseases. 2nd ed. New York: McGraw-Hill, 1990:711–6.

Krockta WP, Barnes RC. Sexually transmitted diseases: Genital ulceration with regional adenopathy. Infect Dis Clin North Am 1987; 1:217–33.
Concise but thorough approaches to diagnosing the syndrome of genital ulceration with regional adenopathy.

Said JW. AIDS-related lymphadenopathies. Semin Diagn Pathol 1988; 5:365–75.
Persistent generalized lymphadenopathy frequently occurs in HIV-infected subjects. Histologic findings are described.

136. HYPOTHERMIA AND COLD INJURY
Alan K. Halperin

Exposure to cold can cause hypothermia or injury in the form of frostbite, trench or immersion foot, or chilblains.

Hypothermia

Hypothermia is defined as a spontaneous drop in core body temperature below 95°F (35°C). It occurs in two very different populations. One group is composed of the elderly sick and derelicts of any age in whom hypothermia accompanies exposure or medical problems. The other group is composed of young, usually healthy people who by bad luck or ignorance have been caught unprepared in severe, cold weather. Approximately 650 deaths per year are attributed to hypothermia; however, this is probably an underestimate because many cases are unrecognized or unreported. Since 1977, the incidence has been increasing.

Risk Factors
In healthy individuals, hypothermia usually occurs in people exposed to prolonged, cold ambient temperatures. However, it can also occur from exposure at higher temperatures (as high as 70°F or 21°C) if thermoregulatory mechanisms are impaired. Most cases of

hypothermia, especially in the elderly or infirm, are a result of exposure to cold plus other factors, such as dampness, alcohol (which causes vasodilation with resultant heat loss and also predisposes to inactivity and trauma), hypoglycemia (which decreases heat production), and infection. Also associated are tranquilizers, sedatives, and hypnotics (which interfere with central hypothalamic regulation); metabolic disturbances (hypoglycemia, hypothyroidism, and hypoadrenalism); miscellaneous diseases, such as sepsis, malnutrition, uremia, and hepatic failure; lesions of the hypothalamus; and spinal cord transection (loss of vasoconstriction). The elderly appear to be particularly susceptible to hypothermia because of an inadequate vasoconstrictive response to cold, a decreased ability to generate heat in response to cold, impaired cold perception, decreased muscle mass, and frequent immobility due to disease or trauma. In a cold environment, any disease, particularly in the elderly, can cause hypothermia.

Evaluation

The initial symptoms of hypothermia—fatigue, weakness, slowness of gait, incoordination, apathy, confusion, decreased judgment, and hallucinations—are nonspecific and can easily be confused with other metabolic disorders. Companions of people developing hypothermia may not recognize the early symptoms, and medical personnel may also overlook this possibility unless there is a high index of suspicion.

If hypothermia is suspected, the patient's temperature should be taken with a low-range rectal thermometer or probe. Errors occur when the thermometer is not shaken down properly or when the patient's temperature is actually below 94°F (34.4°C), the lowest point on the usual rectal thermometer.

The physical findings of hypothermia are also nonspecific. These include decreased blood pressure, heart rate, and respiratory rate; generalized edema of the skin; decreased level of consciousness; dilated and poorly reactive pupils; depressed deep tendon reflexes; and increased muscle tone. Shivering is often absent, particularly in severely hypothermic patients. The remainder of the physical examination should include a thorough search for the associated problems, particularly sepsis and myxedema, that increase the risk for hypothermia. Because of the prominent neurologic findings, signs of head trauma can be obscured, making the evaluation of brain injury difficult.

A continual assessment of cardiovascular findings is important because of the effects of the cold on myocardial irritability and conduction. Atrial fibrillation and sinus bradycardia are the most common arrhythmias. The risk of ventricular fibrillation increases as the core temperature drops below 86°F (30°C) and is greatest below 75°F (24°C). Electrocardiographic changes may include prolonged PR interval, prolonged QRS complex, and the J wave (Osborn wave), which is a small upward deflection or hump early in the ST segment of lateral precordial leads.

In addition to cardiac complications, other important potential metabolic complications include aspiration pneumonia (due to increased secretions and decreased level of consciousness and cough reflex), ileus, pancreatitis, decreased renal function (due to hypovolemia, fluid shift to extravascular space), metabolic acidosis (due to poor tissue perfusion), respiratory acidosis (due to hypoventilation), hyperglycemia (due to an inhibition of insulin release), hypoglycemia, electrolyte disturbances, and rarely disseminated intravascular coagulation. Blood gases must be corrected for temperature, or mistakes in evaluation or treatment can occur. For each 1°C decrease in temperature below 98.6°F (37.5°C), the pH is increased by 0.015, the PCO_2 is decreased by 4.4%, and the PO_2 is decreased by 7.2%.

Treatment

Treatment of hypothermia falls into two categories: first aid in the field and management in a medical facility. In both situations, the approach to rewarming patients is controversial. In mild hypothermia, efforts at rewarming in the field are warranted. But in severe hypothermia, particularly in patients with frozen extremities who have quit shivering and are stuporous, immediate transportation to the nearest hospital is indicated. These patients must be handled gently because jostling may precipitate a cardiac arrhythmia. Wet clothes should be removed and replaced by warm, well-insulated, dry clothing or covering. Both thawing of the extremities and hot liquids taken internally can cause shunting of blood from the extremities into the central circulation, causing a "secondary chill" or "after drop," which can lead to ventricular fibrillation. For patients who are conscious and shivering, tepid sweet drinks are advocated (some recommend warm Jell-O because of the sugar and protein content). In addition to the above, when the patient cannot be removed from the cold environment quickly or when hypothermia is mild, gentle rewarming by direct skin-to-skin contact may be helpful.

Since many patients have hypoglycemia, 50% glucose should be given immediately. If alcoholism is suspected, thiamine should be given with the glucose because a carbohydrate load may precipitate psychosis. Drugs need to be used with extreme caution, as pharmacokinetics are disturbed in hypothermic patients. All drugs are less metabolically active in the hypothermic patient.

All patients with a temperature less than 90°F (32°C) should be admitted to an intensive care unit for continuous monitoring until the temperature is greater than 95°F (35°C). Rewarming can be accomplished by external or internal core warming. External warming can be passive (removing the patient from the cold and wrapping with blankets) or active (immersing the patient in a warm-water bath at 105–133°F [40–45°C] or using a heating blanket). Numerous methods for active core rewarming are available, including warmed intravenous (IV) fluids; inhalation of warmed humidified oxygen through an endotracheal tube or mask; peritoneal dialysis; colonic, gastric, or mediastinal irrigation; and hemodialysis. Of the above, rewarming with warmed IV fluids and warmed humidified oxygen is generally the preferred technique. In cases of severe hypothermia (temperatures below 75°F or 24°C) or refractory arrhythmias (ventricular fibrillation or asystole), peritoneal dialysis should be started.

Prognosis

Because of decreased metabolic requirements, patients may appear dead. However, patients with core temperatures as low as 60.8°F (16°C) have been revived and have fully recovered after as long as 6 hours of cardiopulmonary resuscitation or 90 minutes under water. No conclusions about the reversibility should be made until the patient is rewarmed.

Mortality is more related to the presence of associated diseases than to the degree of hypothermia. When a serious underlying disease is present, such as sepsis, mortality approaches 75%, whereas for accidental hypothermia in healthy individuals, mortality is approximately 6%. The death rate is reduced by prompt recognition, awareness of the potential metabolic complications, and prompt treatment.

Cold Injury

Chilblains

Chilblains come from exposure to nonfreezing cold and thus are most often found on cheeks, hands, and shins. The injury results from the vascular response to cold—vasoconstriction, then vasodilation and edema. After rewarming, the area will appear cyanotic and mildly edematous with burning and pruritus. Re-exposure causes more severe damage in the same areas. These areas may have a heightened response to cold for several years. Treatment is by warming and prevention by wearing protective clothing.

Immersion Foot and Trench Foot

Immersion foot and trench foot are nonfreezing problems caused by exposure to water. In immersion foot, there is direct contact with water; in trench foot, the shod foot is wet. Both are usually associated with more than 12 hours of exposure. The foot appears mottled to waxy, feels cold, and has no pulsations. There is usually no sensation in the foot. On rewarming, there is local swelling, pain, and occasionally blistering. If severe ischemic damage occurs, there may be focal areas of gangrene. This is followed by a phase of recovery that may be associated with weakness, increased sensitivity to cold, and pain with walking. These patients should be evaluated as soon as possible. However, these conditions are often associated with frostbite or hypothermia and frequently should receive inpatient care.

Frostbite

Frostbite is caused by exposure to temperatures below freezing, causing ice crystals to form in tissues. Damage comes from cellular dehydration and ischemia. High-altitude, rapid freezing produces less damage than slow freezing. A combination of high winds and cold is much more dangerous than cold alone. People at risk are those who become wet or immobile, who have compromised arterial circulation to the extremities, who are intoxicated from alcohol, or who have had previous frostbite. The parts of the body most likely to develop frostbite are fingers, toes, nose, and earlobes. The frostbitten extremity appears white, feels firm, has lost sensation, and is usually immobile.

The degree of damage is described as follows:

First degree: Hyperemia and edema on rewarming.
Second degree: Blistering following the above.
Third degree: Necrosis leading to hemorrhagic vesicles and edema.
Fourth degree: The same as above, but there is small-vessel obstruction that leads to ischemic demarcation and loss of tissue.

For "frost nip" (blanching of skin), wrapping the affected part in a dry parka or placing it on the abdomen or axilla of a companion can prevent further injury. In frostbite, the frozen part should not be thawed if there is a chance of refreezing, because refreezing may increase tissue damage. Alcohol, despite giving a temporary feeling of warmth, causes further loss of body heat; tobacco is also contraindicated. The extremity should not be rubbed with snow, immersed in hot or cold water, or covered with salves. Restrictive clothing should be removed and the extremity wrapped in a bulky, loose dressing. Activity should be stopped, and patients should not walk on frostbitten feet. Breaks in the skin, particularly in partially thawed tissue, can lead to infection.

If at all possible patients should be hospitalized for treatment. The accepted rewarming technique is to immerse the frozen part in a water bath at 104°F (40–42°C) until a flush has returned to the most distal part (usually 20–30 minutes). The last steps of thawing can be very painful, and analgesics may be required.

After rewarming, extreme care needs to be taken to avoid infection and trauma. The affected parts should be gently cleaned and cotton placed between the digits. Surgical débridement should be delayed until a sharp line of demarcation between viable and nonviable tissue develops. Blisters should not be broken.

Prevention

Cold injuries can best be prevented by wearing warm, loose, dry clothing in multiple layers on the head, body, and extremities to prevent heat loss. One should keep dry at all costs; materials lose insulation properties when wet. People expecting to be outside for a long time should carry spare dry clothing and food for continuous nibbling (a mixture of nuts, raisins, and candy is ideal).

Edlich RF, et al. Cold injuries. Compr Ther 1989; 15(9):13–21.
Reviews the physiology of temperature homeostasis, and the causes, diagnosis, and treatment of both systemic hypothermia and local cold injuries.

Danzl DF, et al. Multicenter hypothermia survey. Ann Emerg Med 1987; 16:1042–55.
A large multicenter study examining the outcomes of 428 hypothermic patients.

Paton BC. Accidental hypothermia. Pharmacol Ther 1983; 22:331–77.
A comprehensive review of all aspects of hypothermia including the pathophysiology, history, physical examination, and treatment options, and a comprehensive review of the literature.

Ferguson J, Epstein F, Van de Leuv J. Accidental hypothermia. Emerg Med Clin North Am 1983; 1:619–37.
A concise review of major aspects of hypothermia.

Miller JW, Danzl DF, Thomas DM. Urban accidental hypothermia: 135 cases. Ann Emerg Med 1980; 9:456–61.
A comparison of different rewarming methods.

Pa Vee TS, Reineberd EJ. Extreme hypothermia and ventricular fibrillation. Ann Emerg Med 1980; 9:100–1.
Demonstrates the value of prolonged cardiopulmonary resuscitation in hypothermia.

Besdine RW. Accidental hypothermia: the body's energy crisis. Geriatrics 1979; 34:51–9.
A review of hypothermia in the elderly.

Davidson M, Grant E. Accidental hypothermia from a community hospital perspective. Postgrad Med 1981; 70:42–9.
Data on 60 patients.

Fitzgerald FT, Jessop C. Accidental hypothermia: a report of 22 cases and review of the literature. Adv Intern Med 1982; 27:127–43.
An excellent review of practical considerations.

137. HEAT INJURY
Alan K. Halperin

The spectrum of local and systemic reactions to excessive ambient temperature includes heat cramps, heat exhaustion, and heat stroke. Heat cramps are painful tonic contractions of muscles occurring in alert individuals with normal temperatures. Heat exhaustion is characterized by fever greater than 102°F (39°C), sweating, headache, nausea or vomiting, chills, and weakness, with central nervous system changes usually limited to lassitude, mild dizziness, or unsteady gait. Heat stroke is associated with high fever (up to 106°F [41°C]); severe central nervous system disturbances such as confusion, delirium, or coma; absent or diminished sweating; and occasionally hypotension and circulatory collapse. There is no sharp distinction among these three syndromes, and they may occur together.

Heat injury arises under two circumstances. One, called exertional heat injury, occurs in people, often athletes or military recruits, who overexercise in a hot and humid environment. The other, classic heat injury, is principally a disease of the elderly with chronic diseases who are exposed to an elevated ambient temperature. The presentation, metabolic complications, and treatment are similar, but the means of prevention are different.

Risk Factors

Exertional Heat Injury
Exercising in a hot and humid environment is the most common cause of heat injury. Approximately 1% of runners participating in road races develop heat-related injuries, usually heat cramps and heat exhaustion. Risk factors for heat injury include the following:

1. Weather conditions: The incidence of heat injuries increases with ambient temperature, solar radiation, and humidity. An index called the "wet bulb globe temperature index" (WBGT) is a summary of these three conditions; when the WBGT rises above 84.4°F (28°C), the American College of Sports Medicine recommends not running, including races. Running should be done before 9:00 AM or after 4:00 PM during the summer months.
2. Insufficient acclimatization: Exercising in a hot environment produces higher core temperature, higher heart rate, and a marked reduction in exercise capacity. It takes approximately 5 to 10 running sessions in a hot environment for a conditioned athlete to acclimatize. This can be lost after only 2 to 4 weeks.
3. Lack of conditioning: Less-conditioned athletes are less heat tolerant and take longer to acclimatize. Runners who develop heat injury usually have not run for long and have been running few miles, and their training distances have been shorter than race distances.
4. Dehydration: Progressive dehydration commonly occurs during prolonged exercise, even if fluids are supplied. Extreme fluid losses, especially if exercise is begun in a dehydrated state, predispose to heat injury.
5. Age extremes: Both young children and older adults are more susceptible to heat injury because of lower sweating rates and decreased aerobic capacity.
6. Obesity.

7. Prior heat stroke: Runners with a history of heat stroke have higher rates of recurrence. It is not known whether these individuals had preexisting defects in thermoregulation or whether defects developed during the heat stroke episode.

Classic Heat Injury

Heat injury is more common in tropical climates. However, yearly epidemics occur during the summer in temperate climates in places such as the United States. For example, in the summer of 1980, approximately 1265 people died of heat injury; many more were less severely affected and survived. Most reported epidemics occur after more than 48 hours of temperature averaging over 90°F (32.2°C) and relative humidity over 50%. Classic heat injury is predominantly a disease of the elderly exposed to an elevated ambient temperature without air conditioning or adequate shade and at least one of the following risk factors:

1. Chronic disease, such as cardiovascular disease, is the single most important factor in the development of heat injury. Patients with cardiovascular disease have limited cutaneous vasodilatation, do not increase their tolerance to heat with time, have impaired sweat production, and do not increase their cardiac output or heart rate with increasing temperature. Diabetics have some of these same defects.
2. Drugs that can predispose to heat injury include diuretics, which prevent volume expansion and impair vasodilatation; anticholinergics, which inhibit sweating; phenothiazines, which disrupt the hypothalamic thermoregulatory center; and alcohol, which impairs vasomotor control and judgment.
3. Inability to care for self, such as bedridden or demented patients.
4. Obesity.
5. Acute infections.

Metabolic Complications

The primary defense against hyperthermia is evaporative cooling by sweating. If excessive, this can result in disturbances of body water, electrolytes, and renal function. Either hyponatremia or hypernatremia can occur depending on salt water intake. Hypokalemia is frequent and may play a role in cardiovascular instability and rhabdomyolysis. It is hypothesized that brief exposure to elevated temperatures causes hyperventilation and respiratory alkalosis. More prolonged exposure results in lactic acidosis from hypovolemia, hypoxemia, hypotension, and increased metabolic requirements. Arterial blood gases in the presence of hyperthermia must be corrected for body temperature. In general, a rise in 1°C above 98.6°F (37.5°C) will increase the PCO_2 by 4.4% and the PO_2 by 6% and decrease the pH by 0.015. Impaired renal function usually reflects dehydration.

Approximately 10% of patients with severe heat injury develop acute renal failure. Contributing factors include thermal injury, hypotension, dehydration, and rhabdomyolysis. Rhabdomyolysis is associated with dark urine (myoglobinuria), tender muscles, elevated creatine phosphokinase, and commonly hypocalcemia and hypophosphatemia.

Abnormalities of liver function, including elevated serum bilirubin and transaminases, are common but rarely serious. Hypoglycemia or hyperglycemia can occur. Minor abnormalities of coagulation such as prolonged prothrombin time and partial thromboplastin time are common, but disseminated intravascular coagulation is a rare complication. Electrocardiographic changes include nonspecific ST and T wave changes and intraventricular conduction abnormalities. Hemodynamic monitoring has demonstrated that exertional heat injury is usually associated with hyperdynamic circulation with increased heart rate and cardiac output and decreased systemic vascular resistance. In contrast, classic heat stroke usually involves decreased cardiac output and increased peripheral resistance. These distinctions are not absolute; the elderly may not have the cardiovascular reserve to compensate with tachycardia and decreased systemic resistance.

Prevention

Prevention of exertional heat injury follows from the risk factors: not running when the weather is hot, humid, and sunny; ensuring adequate training and acclimatization when beginning exercising or changing locations; liberal intake of fluids; and knowledge of the early symptoms of heat injury. Prompt first aid, followed by appropriate care, can reduce morbidity and mortality.

Individuals at risk during heat waves should be encouraged to wear lightweight, light-colored, and wide-pored clothing of cotton, rather than polyester; change wet clothing; decrease activity; take cool showers; and spend as much time as possible in air-conditioned places. Some cities have established air-conditioning shelters for those at risk.

Treatment

Heat cramps are usually easily treated by giving oral fluids; water is sufficient. Salt tablets and sugar are best avoided because fluid losses are usually hypotonic, and sugar delays gastric emptying. Massaging the affected muscles and rest may also help. Intravenous fluids or muscle relaxants are rarely necessary.

Mild heat exhaustion can be managed where it occurs or in the office. On the other hand, severe heat exhaustion and heat stroke are medical emergencies; usually they require prompt first aid, followed by hospitalization. Treatment is directed toward rapid cooling, support of the cardiovascular system, and increasing renal blood flow. The patient's temperature should be continuously monitored by a rectal probe. Cooling effects should cease when the rectal temperature reaches 102°F (38.8°C), or hypothermia might result. Rapid cooling is best accomplished by the following procedure: Remove the patient's clothing and position the patient in front of a fan. Apply ice packs to the lateral aspect of the trunk, and spray the patient with tepid (40°C or 104°F) water. Massaging the skin, especially the torso and neck, will help to prevent vasoconstriction. Rapid cooling, defined as a reduction of rectal temperature to less than 102 or 103°F (38.9–39.4°C) within an hour from presentation, may increase survival. Rapid fluid administration at room temperature also promotes cooling. Patients should not be immersed in ice baths, because it promotes vasoconstriction, or given chlorpromazine, because it interferes with central thermoregulation.

Fluids are given to correct dehydration. The amount of dehydration is variable, but patients with exertional heat injury tend to have larger fluid deficits. One liter of hypotonic fluid, such as 0.45% saline and 5% dextrose, should be given rapidly and adjusted as volume and electrolytes dictate.

Acute renal failure should be anticipated if hypotension or rhabdomyolysis has occurred. Mannitol, 12.5 g, may be used to promote renal blood flow. If rhabdomyolysis occurs, the urine should be alkalinized.

Antipyretics such as aspirin or acetaminophen are ineffective because their action requires the presence of intact heat-losing mechanisms. Oxygen may be helpful.

Prognosis

Exertional heat injury has an excellent prognosis. In a study of 27 military recruits, there were no deaths and only 1 recruit was not able to return to military duty. In these recruits there were no differences in recovery time or disability between patients with exertional heat exhaustion and heat stroke. The mortality rate reported for classic heat injury using the above-described cooling techniques was 7%. Other studies have reported mortality rates of 40 to 70%. Most of these patients were elderly and were already compromised by having at least two of the following chronic conditions: diabetes mellitus, cardiovascular disease, or mental illness treated with psychotropic drugs. Approximately 50% of those who presented with hypotension died. All those who died failed to regain consciousness and had irreversible brain injury and other complications, such as pneumonia. Most who regained consciousness recovered fully.

Knochel JP. Environmental heat illness: an eclectic review. Arch Intern Med 1974; 133:841–64.
Excellent review of risk factors, pathophysiology, and treatment.

Knochel JP. Heat stroke and related heat stress disorders. Dis Mon 1989; 35:305–77.
An extremely thorough and exhaustively referenced review of the pathogenesis, presentation, and management of heatstroke and other manifestations of environmental heat illness, such as syncope, tetany, cramps, and edema.

Graham BS, et al. Non-exertional heatstroke: physiologic management and cooling in 14 patients. Arch Intern Med 1986; 146:87–90.
Discusses a procedure for lowering core temperature and reports an experience in 14 patients with nonexertional heatstroke.

American College of Sports Medicine position stand on the prevention of thermal injuries during distance running. Med Sci Sports Med 1987; 19:529–33.
Recommendations for preventing exertional heat injury.

Sutton JR, Bar-Or O. Thermal illness in fun running. Am Heart J 1980; 100:778–81.
Review of risk factors for exertional heat injury.

Clark WG, Lipton JM. Drug-related heatstroke. Pharmacol Ther 1984; 26:345–88.
A brief review of the pathophysiology and etiology, with a comprehensive review of drug-related heat stroke.

Olson KR, Benowitz NC. Environmental and drug-induced hyperthermia. Emerg Med Clin North Am 1984; 2:459–75.
A comprehensive review of the pathophysiology, etiology, and management.

Sprung CL. Hemodynamic alterations of heat stroke in the elderly. Chest 1979; 75:364–6.
Hemodynamic findings of eight elderly patients.

Spring CL, et al. The metabolic and respiratory alterations of heat stroke. Arch Intern Med 1980; 140:655–9.
The pathophysiology and metabolic complications in exertional and classic heat injury.

Costrini AM, et al. Cardiovascular and metabolic manifestations of heat stroke and severe heat exhaustion. Am J Med 1979; 66:269–302.
Experience from the Marine Corps at Parris Island, South Carolina.

138. MINOR SOFT TISSUE INJURIES AND INFECTIONS
Sally J. Trued

Many common soft tissue infections and injuries can be well managed in the primary care office setting, provided there is good follow-up and knowledge of the common pitfalls.

Minor Burn Care
Thermal (as opposed to electrical or chemical) burns involving small areas can be managed with careful attention to local wound care techniques. Burns that need referral for specialized care include partial- or full-thickness burns that (1) involve the face, ears, hands, feet, or perineum; (2) are circumferential on extremities where vascular compromise might occur; and (3) involve areas larger than 1% (roughly the area covered by a hand) of the body.

Burns may be classified and characterized as follows:

Superficial (first degree): erythema with minimal edema.
Partial thickness and deep partial thickness (second degree): blistered or moist, red, painful areas in which dermal appendages such as sweat glands or hair follicles are intact; deep partial thickness may be whitened and hypoesthetic.
Full thickness (third degree): charred or whitened anesthetic areas.

Initial care of second- and third-degree burns should begin with gentle cleansing with a mild detergent (such as pHisoHex or Ivory Liquid) and water, followed by débridement of broken blisters or dead skin. Blisters that are initially intact can be left so until they spontaneously rupture or the fluid within becomes cloudy (although some sources advocate early débridement of all second-degree burn blisters, anticipating that they will break on their own from mechanical trauma). The burned area should be covered with a thin layer of silver sulfadiazine cream and a fluffy dressing that will absorb drainage from the burn. Prophylactic antibiotics are not generally indicated. The patient should clean the burn area completely of old cream twice a day (with a gentle soap such as Ivory Liquid and water), dry it well, reapply a thin layer of cream, and reapply the dressing. Follow-up should initially be within 48 hours and at close intervals thereafter until it is clear that healing is established. Tetanus prophylaxis is indicated if the patient has not received either a course of immunizations or a booster within 10 years. First-degree burns such as sunburn may respond to cool compresses and dexamethasone aerosol spray applied topically every 3 hours; this regimen is most effective when it is started within 12 hours of injury.

Burns may be a presentation of child or elder abuse. Injuries that should suggest this possibility include scald burns consistent with "dipping" injuries of the buttocks or extremities, cigarette burns, or iron burns.

Puncture Wounds

Puncture wounds are very common and prone to complications because of the potential for deep inoculation of foreign matter and microorganisms. Some puncture wounds are caused by animal bites (see sections later in this chapter), but many are simple injuries by nails, needles, and so on.

If there is suspicion of bony injury (often the patient suspects this) or foreign body, a radiograph is worthwhile; the radiograph request should specify whether it is for bones or for identification of foreign bodies in soft tissues. It is important to examine for injury to underlying structures, such as tendons or joints. Tetanus immunization status should be determined. The wound area should be cleaned and covered with a dressing, such as clean, dry gauze. Puncture wounds should not be closed with sutures because of the risk of infection. If the wound is on an extremity, elevation facilitates healing.

Puncture wounds that involve the hand are of special concern; entry into the deep spaces of the hand or into the tendon sheaths carries the potential for serious infection. Needle-stick injuries into the distal pulp of the fingers often have a benign course, but occasionally progress to a felon, a tense infection of the distal pulp space that requires drainage by a physician with training in hand care.

Punctures to the plantar aspect of the foot also deserve special attention; if the puncture occurs through a rubber-sole shoe, a piece of rubber or microorganisms may be deeply embedded into the tissues. It is generally recommended that in deep puncture wounds of the plantar foot, a small area of callus be cored out and a careful search for foreign materials be done. The patient should be advised to watch for signs of infection.

Cellulitis

Cellulitis is an infection of the skin and subcutaneous tissue without an actual collection of pus, but with increased warmth, tenderness, redness, and swelling. It is generally preceded by an injury that violates the skin, but may be from infection of hair follicles or sebaceous glands, or of existing superficial ulcers or wounds.

Simple cellulitis of the trunk or extremities of an otherwise healthy patient can be treated with local application of heat, soaks, elevation of an extremity, and oral antibiotics (dicloxacillin, cephalexin) that cover the most common bacteria encountered (group A streptococci, *Staphylococcus aureus*). Close follow-up is warranted, checking for the development of lymphangitis, crepitance, systemic symptoms, or failure to improve over 24 to 48 hours. Anatomic sites of special concern are the head and neck, and in particular the "central triangle" of the face, which drains to the cavernous sinus; infection in this area may warrant hospitalization. Patients with cellulitis of the hands or perineal area likewise should be followed closely, as should debilitated patients in whom the cellulitis may be polymicrobic or include anaerobes.

Hematomas

The accumulation of blood in the subcutaneous tissues after blunt injury is common and sometimes dramatic. After an initial 24 hours of ice packs wrapped in a towel and applied for 20 minutes every 2 to 3 hours, hematomas located in cosmetically or functionally unimportant areas can be managed with local heat and elevation while slow resolution occurs. Although spontaneous resorption may be a long process, attempting hematoma drainage with a needle is generally not recommmended as this may introduce infection into the area. A hematoma that is located on the face or that is disfiguring, an expanding hematoma, or one that develops a bruit deserves referral to a surgical specialist. Hematomas associated with any violation (often very superficial) of the skin can become infected with skin flora and present with erythema, tenderness, or as a fluctuant abscess that requires drainage.

Tetanus Prophylaxis

Although all wounds should be considered tetanus-prone, wounds of special concern are those that are more than 6 hours old; puncture-like; contaminated with dirt, saliva, or feces; contain devitalized or crushed tissue; or already infected. Wound care should always include thorough cleaning, removal of any devitalized tissue or foreign matter, and copious irrigation.

A tetanus immunization history should be obtained from every patient with a recent wound (no matter how superficial), infected ulcer, burn, or animal bite; this should include asking about their primary immunization series and subsequent tetanus toxoid boosters, which should be given every 10 years. Having had the clinical disease does not confer immunity.

The patient who has received inadequate primary immunization but has a "tetanus-prone" wound should receive tetanus immune globulin (TIG) for passive immunity, as well as tetanus toxoid to begin or continue their primary immunization schedule (see Chap. 124 for schedule of primary immunization). There is no contraindication to tetanus immunization for a patient (including a pregnant woman) other than a history of severe hypersensitivity reaction to a previous dose. Local mild or moderate reactions are common and are not a contraindication. Too frequent tetanus toxoid boosters (more often than the guidelines suggest) have been implicated in Arthus-type hypersensitivity reactions characterized by severe local reactions. If there is concern that a systemic reaction represents allergic hypersensitivity, skin testing may be performed. If there is a contraindication to tetanus toxoid administration, an injured patient should be passively immunized. The guidelines for tetanus booster administration in wounds, as established by the Immunization Practices Advisory Committee, are given in Table 138-1.

Ticks

The scalp, neck, axillae, and skinfolds are particularly prone to tick bites. Early discovery and removal decrease the chance of transmission of tick-borne diseases such as Rocky Mountain spotted fever (RMSF), Lyme disease, tick paralysis, Q fever, and tularemia. A tick bites with its mouth parts and attempts to burrow its head under the skin. Some removal techniques may be more harmful than helpful. Putting noxious substances on the tick (such as Vaseline, nail polish, and gasoline) may cause the tick to regurgitate or the mouth parts to break off, thus increasing exposure to infection and impeding removal. Instead, the area should be cleaned with soap and water and tweezers or gloved fingers used to grasp the tick close to the skin; steady traction should be applied without twisting or squeezing, allowing time for the tick to relax its mouth parts. Alternatively, the top of a 25-gauge hypodermic needle or suture needle can be placed between the mouth parts and the skin, and gentle traction applied until the tick releases. If these methods are ineffective, many experienced clinicians recommend lighting and blowing out a match, and holding the warm end near, *but not on,* the body of the tick; the tick will then often climb out itself, to escape the heat. After removal is accomplished, the area should be washed and disinfected with an antiseptic such as alcohol, povidone-iodine (Betadine), or pHisoHex. To avoid contact with ingested blood, never crush the tick with the fingers.

Prophylaxis with antibiotics for RMSF and Lyme disease following tick exposure is ineffective because tetracycline may only prolong the incubation period rather than prevent disease. Patients in endemic areas should be warned to promptly seek medical attention if they develop symptoms suggesting early infection with either of these organisms. For RMSF, the incubation period is 2 to 14 days following exposure, and symptoms of concern are a flu-like febrile illness, with headache, rash, myalgias, nausea, and vomiting. For Lyme disease, the incubation is 3 to 32 days after exposure, and the symptoms include a flu-like febrile illness; the skin lesion of first-stage Lyme disease is erythema chronicum migrans (ECM), an erythematous lesion with a clearing center that may be followed by satellite lesions elsewhere on the body.

Table 138-1. Guidelines for tetanus booster immunization in wounds

Available vaccines:
Td—adsorbed tetanus-diphtheria toxoid, used for most adults, and children ≥ 7 yr; preferable to tetanus toxoid alone.
DPT—adsorbed diptheria-tetanus-pertussis, used for children < 7 yr.
DT—adsorbed diphtheria-tetanus, used for children < 7 if pertussis immunization is contraindicated.
Tetanus toxoid (fluid)—immunizes against tetanus alone; can be given subcutaneously, unlike adsorbed toxoid, which should be given IM; requires 4 rather than 3 doses for primary immunization; ineffective if given simultaneously with TIG; rarely used.
TIG—tetanus immune globulin, for passive immunization; impairs effectiveness of fluid tetanus toxoid if given simultaneously.

Recommended tetanus prophylaxis:

History of tetanus immunization	Clean minor wounds		All other wounds	
	TD*	TIG	TD*	TIG
Unknown status, or inadequate primary immunization	Yes	No	Yes	Yes
< 3 doses of Td, DPT, or DT; or < 4 doses of fluid toxoid				
Adequate primary immunization ≥ 3 doses of Td, DPT, or DT; or ≥ 4 doses of fluid tetanus toxoid	No, if < 10 yr since last dose Yes, if > 10 yr since last dose	No	No, if < 5 yr since last dose Yes, if > 5 yr since last dose	No

*For children < 7 years old, use DPT, or DT if pertussis vaccine is contraindicated.

Spider Bites

Many spiders can bite humans and, with the introduction of microorganisms, cause a local infection. Only two species generally cause significant medical problems. The female black widow spider, a glossy black spider with bright red markings on the ventral abdomen, inflicts a variably painful bite. Local pain or numbness may appear within 30 minutes and systemic symptoms within minutes to 12 hours. The venom of a black widow spider is a neurotoxin that produces central and peripheral nervous excitement with variable clinical manifestations, including anxiety, headache, hypertension, tachycardia, dyspnea, nausea and vomiting, abdominal pain and rigidity, and muscle spasms. The symptoms peak within several hours of the bite and resolve over 48 hours. The treatment is symptomatic, largely aiming to relieve the pain and relax the muscles. Those at risk to develop severe envenomation symptoms, with seizures or uncontrollable muscle spasms, respiratory distress, or shock, are children, the elderly, and those who are debilitated. The available antivenin is equine serum–based and should be used with caution and only in those with severe symptoms; the majority of cases are self-limited and respond to symptomatic treatment.

The brown recluse spider, a small tan or brownish spider with a variably distinct fiddle-shaped design on its dorsal thorax, inflicts a bite that may go unnoticed initially. Within hours to a day or two, the bite site may become ecchymotic and erythematous with a central blanched area; a central vesicle then forms and becomes necrotic, and the necrosis may spread, creating a deep ulcer beneath. The resulting wound often becomes the main issue of management but the systemic symptoms listed below can occur, especially in children, and usually occur within a few hours of the bite (but sometimes taking up to 72 hours). These symptoms include fever, nausea and vomiting, a generalized pruritic rash, and in severe cases, shock and hemolysis. Many bite wounds with minimal local reaction can be treated simply with soaks, dressing, and elevation of the extremity. Severe local reactions with necrosis, or systemic reactions, require referral. All spider bites should receive tetanus prophylaxis.

Mammalian Bite Wounds

Many wounds caused by mammalian bites are relatively superficial, small in size, and not cosmetically or functionally significant; these can be treated with initial care that includes thorough cleansing (using a nontoxic detergent such as Shurclens) and copious irrigation with normal saline, removal of any obviously devitalized tissue, and covering with a clean, dry dressing, and appropriate tetanus prophylaxis. The patient can repeat the cleaning with a gentle soap (e.g., Ivory Liquid) and redress the wound twice a day. Antibiotic prophylaxis, although controversial, in general is indicated for mammalian bites that involve the subcutaneous tissues or below; it should preferably be started within 12 hours of the injury, and continued for 3 to 5 days. If no infection appears by this time, it is safe to stop the antibiotic. Specific coverage for different bites is discussed below.

Bite locations of special concern (and that generally deserve referral) are those on the ears, face, genitalia, hands, and feet. Many bite wounds have some component of crushing or puncture-like injury that leaves partially or fully devitalized tissue as well as deeply inoculated microorganisms. Because of the heavy population of microorganisms in the oral cavities of humans, cats, dogs, and other mammals, infections are, unfortunately, common. Patients especially at risk to develop infection from bite injuries include those with general debilitation, diabetes, and immune disorders; those taking steroids; and those who present with treatment delay of longer than 6 to 12 hours.

Human Bites

The human mouth contains a wide variety of aerobic and anaerobic microorganisms; those that commonly cause infections following bites are aerobic and anaerobic streptococci, *S. aureus*, *Eikenella corrodens*, *Bacteroides*, and *Fusobacterium*. Five-day prophylactic antibiotic regimens (if possible, begun within 12 hours of injury and following the thorough irrigation and débridement described above) include amoxicillin/clavulanate, a broad-spectrum second-generation cephalosporin, or penicillin plus a first-generation cephalosporin. Wounds that present with already established infection should generally be referred for care, except perhaps mild infections of the trunk or extremities (not including the hands).

"Clenched-fist" injuries that occur during fights are of special concern; because the hand is in a flexed position during the contact between the fist and mouth, penetration into the joint can occur with sealing over of the inoculum of microorganisms as the fingers are extended. Patients are often reluctant to discuss the nature of these injuries, so a high level of suspicion is warranted. It is important to examine carefully for tendon injuries and to obtain radiographs for bony injury. Because of the high incidence of infection in these injuries, many hand surgeons recommend hospitalizing all patients with clenched-fist injuries, for elevation of the extremity and parenteral administration of prophylactic antibiotics.

In general, initial closure of bite wounds is not recommended, with the exception of some cosmetically disfiguring wounds of the face or large avulsive injuries of the extremities, both of which require referral for definitive treatment.

A common injury in children (or seizure patients) is that of a tooth penetrating the lower lip during a fall. If a tooth is missing, the lip should be examined carefully to make sure that no tooth is embedded; the wound should then be thoroughly irrigated. In general, closure is not needed if the mucosa only has a small laceration. Penicillin (or erythromycin if the patient has a penicillin allergy) is commonly used for intraoral bite wounds, although most small injuries can simply be watched.

Hepatitis B virus can be transmitted by human bites; the possibility of the biter being in a high-risk group should be ascertained. If so, the guidelines for contaminated needle-stick injuries should be followed, that is, passive prophylaxis with hepatitis B immune globulin (HBIG) and initiation of hepatitis B vaccination three-shot series in high-risk or known positive exposures. The dose for HBIG is 0.06 ml/kg intramuscularly.

The possibility of human immunodeficiency virus (HIV) transmission by human bites is probably a very low but real risk; if the biter is known to be HIV-positive or from a high-risk group, consultation with an infectious disease specialist would be wise.

Dog and Cat Bites

Infection rates for dog bites are generally low, but those for cat bites are quite high. Patients with all but the most superficial cat bites should therefore be treated with prophylactic antibiotics. Streptococci, staphylococci, *Bacteroides, Clostridia,* and *Pasteurella multocida* are among the more commonly cultured organisms in infected bites. Suggested 5-day antibiotic prophylaxis regimens include amoxicillin/clavulanate, penicillin V (excellent coverage against *Pasteurella*), dicloxacillin, erythromycin, or tetracycline. Cat scratches generally contain similar microorganisms (cats lick their paws).

Initial closure of dog and cat bites is not generally recommended, although certain disfiguring or gaping wounds may need referral for consideration of closure on a primary or delayed basis.

Rabies Prophylaxis

Clinical rabies in humans is rare in the United States. Although rabies in domestic animals has nearly been eliminated, rabies in wild animals appears to be increasing in incidence. Animals at high risk for transmitting the rabies virus through bites (or by licking open wounds or mucous membranes) include bats, bobcats, coyote, fox, skunks, and raccoons. Stray dogs and cats, unusual pets such as ferrets, and abnormal-behaving domestic animals are also of concern. The risk from rabbits and rodents is very low.

Because clinical rabies in humans is invariably fatal, primary care physicians must be knowledgeable about postexposure rabies prophylaxis. All bites must be reported to the county animal control office or police, who are responsible for capture and quarantine of suspected rabies cases. If the bite is inflicted by a domestic, rabies-immunized, normal-acting pet, observation of the pet for a few days is adequate. However, if the bite is by a stray or wild animal, that animal should be captured if possible and observed for 10 days; if it becomes ill, it should be killed, the brain examined for the rabies virus, and rabies prophylaxis begun for the victim if necessary. If the animal cannot be identified and observed, and the situation involves a stray, wild, or abnormal-behaving animal, rabies prophylaxis should be undertaken as soon as possible. The rabies virus must travel to the central nervous system to cause disease; thus, a bite on the head or neck should indicate very early prophylaxis, while one on an extremity allows for a short grace period. Many state health departments can give physicians advice about the incidence of rabies in their locale, what animals are likely carriers, and when prophylaxis is warranted.

The Centers for Disease Control (CDC) guidelines for postexposure prophylaxis include local wound care, and both passive and active immunotherapy. Thorough cleansing of the wound with plenty of irrigation to dilute any inoculum is important, followed by débridement of devitalized tissue. For active immunotherapy, human diploid cell rabies vaccine is given intramuscularly at the time of the bite and then subsequently on days 3, 7, 14, and 28; this yields excellent antibody response in virtually all patients. Passive immunotherapy with rabies immune globulin (RIG) at a dose of 20 IU/kg is also necessary and provides immediate protection. It is recommended that one-half of the total dose of RIG be injected into the bite wound site, and the rest given at another site intramuscularly. The CDC recommendations and the listed precautions and contraindications for rabies prophylaxis should be consulted for complete information.

Haynes BW Jr. Emergency department management of minor burns. Top Emerg Med 1981; 3:35–40.
Good discussion of care of common minor burns.

Hess FC, Graff JG. Skin and soft tissue infections. Top Emerg Med 1982; 4:72–81.
A review of the spectrum of infections, abscesses, and cellulitis.

Ginsberg MB. Cellulitis: Analysis of 101 cases and review of the literature. South Med J 1981; 74:530–33.
Discusses organisms involved and appropriate treatment.

Jacobs RJ, Lowe RS, Lanier BQ. Adverse reactions to tetanus toxoid. JAMA 1982; 247:40–2.
A discussion of local reactions, fever, and anaphylactic reactions and their relation to frequent boosters and thimerosal preservative.

Immunization Practices Advisory Committee. Diphtheria, tetanus, and pertussis: guidelines for vaccine prophylaxis and other preventive measures. MMWR 1981; 30:392–408.
The epidemiology of these diseases, available preparations, appropriate immunization schedules, and precautions.

Needham GR. Evaluation of five popular methods for tick removal. Pediatrics 1985; 75:997–1002.
Gentle traction with a gloved finger or tweezers was the recommended method; placing noxious stimuli directly on the tick was not recommended.

Moss HS, Binder LS. A retrospective review of black widow spider envenomation. Ann Emerg Med 1987; 16:188–92.
A practical overview of the clinical presentation and management.

Galloway RE. Mammalian bites. J Emerg Med 1988;6:325–31.
Discussion of risk factors for, and bacteriology of, infections, general wound care, and antibiotic usage.

Callaham M. Controversies in antibiotic choices for bite wounds. Ann Emerg Med 1988; 17:1321–30.
A thorough discussion of the rationale for using or not using antibiotics in bite injuries, with excellent tables and references.

Helmick CG. The epidemiology of human rabies postexposure prophylaxis, 1980–81. JAMA 1983; 250:1990–6.
A study revealing the extent of the unnecessary use of postexposure prophylaxis, and suggestions for improvement.

Practices Advisory Committee. Rabies prevention—United States, 1984. MMWR 1984; 33:398–408.
The complete recommendations of the immunization practices committee for pre- and postexposure prophylaxis, adverse effects, and contraindications.

139. HICCUPS
Raymond F. Bianchi

A singultus, commonly known as a hiccup, is produced by bilateral diaphragmatic and intercostal muscle spasms. The characteristic sound occurs when an inspiratory effort, initiated by the spasm, is aborted by glottic closure.

Causes
The hiccup is a primitive reflex response, involving the phrenic nerve, vagus nerve, and sympathetic chain from T6–12 as the afferent limb, and the phrenic nerve as the efferent limb; it is normally inhibited by descending signals from higher CNS centers. Hiccups can develop either from excitation along the reflex arc, particularly phrenic nerve stimulation, or from suppression of the higher centers, as seen with CNS lesions or metabolic abnormalities. Consequently, treatment can be directed toward either the "hiccup center" in the CNS or the limbs of the reflex arc.

Treatment

Transient Hiccups

Transient hiccups usually result from gastric distention due to overindulgence in food or drink. Because these episodes are brief and self-limited, it is difficult to assess the efficacy of individual treatments. Folk remedies include difficult or distracting tasks like breath-holding, tongue traction, breathing into a paper bag, being frightened, and drinking water from the wrong side of a glass while occluding the ears. Stimulation of the pharyngeal mucosa (e.g., by swallowing 1 tsp of either vinegar or dry granulated sugar) is believed to suppress hiccups by competitive inhibition of afferent fibers.

Intractable Hiccups

Intractable hiccups are empirically defined as persisting for at least 48 hours. The numerous causes are listed in Table 139-1.

The treatment of intractable hiccups remains controversial. In 1932, Mayo stated, "The amount of knowledge on any subject . . . can be considered as being in inverse proportion to the number of different treatments suggested and tried for it. Perhaps one is justified in saying there is no disease which has had more forms of treatment and fewer results from treatment than has had persistent hiccups." The first step in treating intractable hiccups is to identify one of the potentially reversible metabolic or structural etiologies listed in Table 139-1. If none is found, one suggested approach is to insert a nasogastric tube, both to decompress the stomach and to irritate the pharynx. Lack of response indi-

Table 139-1. Causes of intractable hiccups

Psychogenic

Postoperative

Medical

Central nervous system: trauma, vascular insufficiency, tumor, syphilis, encephalitis, sarcoidosis, temporal arteritis, degenerative diseases, syringomyelia, seizure disorder

Neck: goiter, thoracic outlet syndrome

Thorax: diaphragmatic hernia, diaphragmatic tumor, pleurisy, pneumonia, lung abscess, foreign body, aneurysm, asthma, esophageal dysfunction, esophageal cancer, coronary occlusion, pericarditis

Abdomen: duodenal ulcer, cholelithiasis, pancreatic pseudocyst, pancreatic cancer, stomach cancer, colon cancer, metastatic liver cancer, ulcerative colitis, splenomegaly

Urinary tract: hypernephroma, hydronephrosis, prostatism

Toxin/drug: uremia, alcoholism, benzodiazepines

cates the need for drug therapy using an agent that acts either centrally (affecting the hiccup center) or peripherally.

Chlorpromazine has been the most extensively studied of the centrally acting drugs. The recommended dose is 50 mg given as an intravenous bolus; systemic blood pressure must be monitored for hypotension. Success with this therapy is followed by oral chlorpromazine for 10 days. A variety of other drugs are reported to be of value: diphenylhydantoin, haloperidol (5 mg PO tid), orphenadrine (60 mg IM or 100 mg PO), ketamine (0.4 mg/kg IV), and carbamazepine (200 mg PO qid). Evidence that any of these drugs is effective is either anecdotal or difficult to interpret because of the small study sample. Diazepam paradoxically increased the frequency of hiccups in a study of three patients.

Of the peripherally acting drugs, metoclopramide (10 mg PO qid) appears to be the most efficacious. Quinidine sulfate (200 mg PO qid) has been shown to be effective in a small number of patients. Atropine (1 mg IV), edrophonium chloride (10 mg IV), amphetamine (30 mg qd for 1 week), and amyl nitrite have also been recommended. But again, as for the centrally acting drugs, the number of patients tested has been too small to judge efficacy from published studies.

In desperation, unilateral phrenic nerve anesthesia, or crush, has been advocated. The number of patients thus treated has been small, however, and there have been failures—not surprising because hiccups probably result from bilateral hemidiaphragm spasm, and unilateral phrenic nerve trauma would therefore be inadequate therapy.

Samuels LS. Hiccup. Can Med Assoc J 1952; 67:315–22.
Classic review of the subject; the major work favoring the unilateral hemidiaphragm contraction theory of hiccup. Thirty-three etiologies as well as therapy are discussed.

Davis JN. An experimental study of hiccup. Brain 1970; 93:851–72.
The first study to counter the ideas of Samuels. Evidence for bilateral hemidiaphragm and inspiratory muscle involvement is discussed. The author also proposes that hiccups are mediated by a brain stem center separate from the respiratory center.

Nathan MD, Leshner RT, Keller AP. Intractable hiccups (singultus). Laryngoscope 1980; 90:1612–18.
This work adds credence to Davis' theory of an independent hiccup center.

Williamson BWA, MacInture IMC. Management of intractable hiccup. Br Med J 1977; 2:501–3.
Review of all agents that have been advocated in reports in the English language. Protocol for therapy is offered.

140. CHRONIC IDIOPATHIC PAIN
Douglas A. Drossman

Patients with chronic, unexplained, intractable pain present a challenge to clinicians. Such patients may overuse health care resources and experience complications from unneeded diagnostic and therapeutic procedures. Physicians often feel frustrated despite their efforts to help. A behavioral approach to patients with chronic pain is often helpful.

Definition
Chronic idiopathic pain may be defined as frequently recurrent or continuous pain that is poorly related to physiologic events and that lasts longer than 6 months. Chronic pain requires a different approach than acute pain. Acute pain alerts the individuals that damage has occurred within the body; treatment involves removing the damage or providing analgesia while the injury heals. In chronic pain, tissue pathology is less likely to be found. Physical findings and diagnostic studies are negative or any abnormalities found do not explain the symptoms. Furthermore, in chronic pain psychosocial consequences are often profound. Daily functioning (sleep, activities, energy), mood, and interpersonal

interactions are often impaired. Finally, in chronic pain, analgesics (including narcotics) usually are not effective. A multimodal treatment plan for chronic pain includes (1) clarifying the goals of an ongoing relationship with the primary care physician; (2) behavior modification and assistance with coping strategies; (3) pharmacotherapy; and when needed, (4) input from mental health professionals, physical therapists, and anesthesiologists.

Facts and Misconceptions

Chronic pain is often mistakenly assumed to be caused by a specific pathologic process (biomedical model), whereas it is actually a multidetermined disorder (biopsychosocial model). Among patients initially diagnosed to have chronic unexplained pain who are followed prospectively, fewer than 10% are ever given a specific medical diagnosis.

Clinicians may mistakenly assume that patients with chronic pain can be helped only if structural or physiologic abnormalities are identified and specific treatment is instituted. In fact, patients with chronic pain can often improve functioning even though no specific diagnosis is made.

Pathophysiology of Chronic Pain

Pain is a multidimensional phenomenon with sensory, emotional, and cognitive components. Psychological factors can perpetuate the experience of pain after the original stimulus has resolved. According to the gate-control theory, neural mechanisms in the dorsal horn of the spinal cord increase or decrease the conduction of nerve impulses from peripheral nociceptive sites to the spinal cord and brain. Neurotransmitters such as substance P facilitate pain transmission. Conversely, the neurotransmitter enkephalin inhibits substance P release and pain transmission. This system for pain transmission is strongly influenced by serotoninergic areas of the brain that are closely connected with cognitive and emotional centers. Tricyclic antidepressants, which increase serotonin levels, may therefore be useful in the treatment of chronic pain.

The experience of pain may be divided into three dimensions: a sensory-discriminative dimension involving the spinal cord system; a motivational-affective dimension subserved by the reticular and limbic structures; and an evaluative dimension from the cortex, which is influenced by thought and memory. Chronic pain, regardless of etiology, is believed to have more contribution from the motivational-affective and evaluative levels. Thus, regardless of the original etiology, once chronic pain is established, the patient's pain experience and pain behaviors are influenced by the central nervous system and respond to behavioral and psychological therapies.

The perception of chronic pain may persist in the absence of a detectable peripheral source of pain. It has been postulated that prolonged peripheral pain, even of low intensity, may produce self-sustaining or reverberatory neural activity in the central nervous system that leads to chronic pain. Similarly, chronic pain can be ameliorated by relatively brief changes in sensory input that disrupt the central memory-like mechanism (hyperstimulation analgesia). Stimulation of trigger points by needles (e.g., acupuncture), or injection of inert substances can produce prolonged relief of myofascial or visceral pain.

Clinical Presentation

The description of the pain, responses to pain, and associated psychosocial features are often characteristic. The patient's *description of pain* commonly reflects urgency, emotional intensity, and preoccupation with the pain. Multiple other somatic complaints may be present, but symptoms are inconsistent with a somatic process. A history of other types of pain is also common. Symptoms are often described in colorful metaphors, such as "a knife stabbing into my heart."

In response to the pain, patients may focus their efforts and activities on diagnosing and curing the pain. Frequently the patient has seen numerous physicians and has had multiple diagnostic evaluations, including operations. The patient is often frustrated and angry over the failure of previous care. Often there is an implicit or explicit challenge that the current provider will help where the other physicians have failed: "The other doctors haven't understood my problem, but I know that you'll be able to help me." Often the patient gives the physician a double message, such as "I'll do anything to get better, but I can't deal with it any longer." Patients are often very concerned to prove that the pain is real and "not in my head." Patients may be taking high doses of narcotics, and refilling prescriptions may be a major concern. Again, the patient may present a double message: "I don't want to be on all this medicine, but I simply can't go on without them."

Psychosocial features frequently associated with chronic pain include a history of hardship, suffering, and loss, often beginning early in life. Often the patient denies any connection between life events and pain, believing that there is some medical problem that other physicians have missed. The patient may have been independent and stoical until the onset or exacerbation of symptoms. The patient's relationships with other people are often preoccupied with the pain and responses to it. Thus the patient's spouse may be completely dedicated to trying to cure the pain, or alternatively the patient may have become isolated from friends and relatives as the pain has persisted. Feelings of hopelessness, despair, and dependency may be prominent.

Clinical Assessment

1. *What is the patient's life history of illness?* A high frequency of physical complaints, present and past, and of health care visits for these complaints predicts a poorer prognosis. In contrast, patients with a relatively brief history of chronic pain (< 2 years) who do not have an underlying psychiatric disorder, and who are seen in primary care rather than specialty centers, are more likely to improve or recover.

2. *Why is the patient coming now?* Patients with chronic pain often have multiple reasons for seeing the physician. Possible reasons include (a) increased concern about having a serious disease, (b) environmental stressors, (c) worsening of functional status, (d) a "hidden agenda" (e.g., for narcotics, disability, sick role privileges, legitimization of the illness to family or coworkers), (e) exacerbation of psychiatric disturbance, and (f) termination of the previous physician-patient relationship.

3. *What psychosocial factors affect the pain experience and pain behaviors?* Patients with chronic pain frequently report (a) a history of losses (e.g., death of a parent or spouse, or interference with the outcome of a pregnancy) and other traumatic life events that may have begun early in life, (b) a history of physical or sexual abuse, (c) depression and other psychiatric diagnoses, or (d) abnormal illness behaviors and frequent health care utilization. Such other contributing factors should be identified, as they will affect the treatment approach.

4. *What are the patient's perceptions and expectations?* The patient's perceptions and expectations should be addressed from the outset. This permits the physician and patient to agree on realistic treatment goals and minimizes the tendency for physicians to feel "trapped" when the patient holds unrealistic expectations that are not met. Questions to elicit the patient's perceptions and expectations include: "What do you think is causing the pain?", "What are your concerns (or fears) about the pain?", and "What do you hope I will be able to do for you?" In addition, the patient's expectations about diagnostic tests and pain medications need to be ascertained. Patients who bypass these questions by saying "That's why I came to you" or "You're the doctor" are not taking an active role in their health care and are less likely to improve.

5. *What illness behavior is present?* Illness behavior refers to how symptoms are perceived, evaluated, and acted on. Patients with chronic pain often have several "abnormal" illness behaviors: (a) disability disproportionate to detectable disease, (b) a relentless search for validation of an organic disease, (c) placement of control and responsibility for health care with the physician, (d) a sense of entitlement to be cared for by others, or (e) behaviors oriented toward sustaining the "sick role." A major part of treating patients with chronic pain may involve efforts to change such abnormal illness behavior.

6. *How does the pain affect the patient's daily function?* Medical and behavioral intervention will often depend on how much the patient's quality of life is impaired. For example, the patient with chronic pain who begins to decrease activity (e.g., no longer able to work) will require more intervention than the patient with similar reports of pain who can maintain daily activities. Functioning should be assessed in terms of physical activities (e.g., walking, sleeping), psychological well-being (e.g., mood, energy level), social activities (e.g., recreation, relationships with others), and roles (e.g., work).

7. *Is psychiatric illness present?* Patients with coexisting psychiatric disorders have poorer health outcomes. Recognition of a psychiatric disorder can lead to appropriate

treatment with psychotropic medication, psychotherapy, or behavior treatments. Patients with chronic pain, regardless of the cause, are usually depressed. Other diagnoses to consider include anxiety disorder, somatization disorder, alcoholism, drug dependence, and factitious disease.

8. *What are the family or cultural influences on pain behaviors?* Cultural or family explanatory models for pain will affect how the pain is presented to the physician, what the patient expects from the physician, and how the patient responds to treatment. For example, some patients may expect medications to be prescribed and taken in order to legitimize their illness. Other patients may express interpersonal and psychological stress only through physical symptoms and be unwilling to talk explicitly about the underlying psychosocial factors. It is also important to determine how the family has reacted to the patient's illness and what their expectations for care are.

9. *What are the patient's psychosocial resources?* Psychosocial factors that permit the patient to improve daily function *despite* the pain should also be assessed. These include social supports such as family, church, friends, work, and community organizations, and effective coping styles. Good social supports and coping strategies are associated with a better prognosis for patients with chronic pain. Many patients with chronic pain, however, have developed a support system that is centered on dysfunctional illness behaviors. Thus, the spouse may focus his or her own life on taking the patient to the physician or to taking on family roles formerly assumed by the patient.

Treatment Suggestions

A good relationship between the primary care physician and the patient is essential. The expectations for both parties should be explicitly discussed and agreed on. The goal of care should be to help the patient function better despite continuing pain, and not curing the pain or making a definitive diagnosis. Patients need to assume an active role in their care. Physicians should give the patient the option of seeking another caregiver if the patient has expectations for diagnosis or relief of pain that are unacceptable. "I wish I could take away your pain, but I can't. What I can do is to try to help you be more active despite the pain."

Patients should be seen regularly, initially every several weeks, and then less frequently, whether or not they have symptoms. Cutting the link between having symptoms and seeing the physician is crucial. It diminishes the patient's focus on physical symptoms and allows the physician to discuss how the patient is functioning. In addition, it gives the patient confidence that the physician is concerned about him or her. Furthermore, the physician can solve the problem of drop-in visits and long phone calls by making clear that the patient will be seen between scheduled visits only if a new catastrophic illness develops, not if chronic symptoms are exacerbated.

The clinician must accept the patient's pain as real. This does not mean, however, that unwarranted diagnostic or therapeutic maneuvers must be undertaken. The physician should offer to review previous test results, but the expectation should be that previous tests will not be repeated unless they were not adequately done or if new symptoms develop. Because patients with chronic pain often see multiple physicians, there should be an agreement that if the physician agrees to start a therapeutic relationship, all referrals to specialists should be made through the physician, not directly by the patient.

Another topic that needs to be discussed explicitly at the beginning of the relationship is the use of narcotics. The physician should say that his or her style of practice is not to use narcotics on patients with chronic pain and to taper patients who are currently taking narcotics. At times it is difficult to maintain ongoing care without narcotics. In these rare situations, it is best to contract their use to low fixed dosages. Doses as needed are contraindicated: They inappropriately direct the physician-patient interaction toward negotiations over pain medication rather than more long-term adaptive goals.

Behavioral Therapies
Reasonable treatment goals for improving function despite pain can be set jointly by the patient and physician. The key to behavioral treatment is to choose modest goals that can be attained and then to progress to more difficult goals at subsequent visits. By establishing a series of successes, the patient will develop a sense of self-efficacy and become more

involved in his or her own care. Thus, a patient who leaves the house only to see the physician is not ready to embark on a walking program. Instead, the physician and patient should agree to start with something as simple as stretching exercises for a few minutes a day. The important thing is for the patient to do the activities daily and to report back at the next visit. The physician needs to praise the patient for completing the "homework," particularly if the pain is somewhat worse or if it was difficult to carry out. At each visit, the duration or strenuousness of activities can be gradually increased. This approach empowers the patient to take personal responsibility in his or her care and diverts attention away from immediate goals of pain relief through others.

Additional behavioral treatment approaches include *relaxation response, meditation,* and *autogenic training,* all methods associated with reduced sympathetic nervous system activity and muscle relaxation. These processes require both a comfortable environment and the ability of the person to focus on an image, word, or phrase, thereby removing distractions. *Biofeedback* is a technique in which physiologic activity is monitored, and unconscious physiologic information is provided by audio or visual instruments so that the patient can gain control over these functions.

Psychological Consultation and Treatment
Often, psychological consultation and treatment are helpful for patients having chronic pain. When indicated, the referral should be recommended at the outset, as part of an overall plan, rather than when the workup for organic disease reveals negative findings. This minimizes any tendency to view the referral as a rejection by the medical physician. Different approaches include individual psychotherapy, family therapy, group therapy, and cognitive-behavioral therapy. Other behavioral therapies include relaxation exercises, stress management, biofeedback, and self-hypnosis.

Referral is particularly appropriate when a treatable psychiatric disorder is identified, loss of daily functioning or psychosocial impairment is considerable (e.g., total disability, narcotic addiction), the patient identifies stressors that may exacerbate the pain, or the patient is interested in improving coping strategies. In all cases, the referral should be offered as consistent with the goals of adapting to the illness and improving function.

Medications
Nonsteroidal anti-inflammatory drugs, including aspirin, have minimal effectiveness because of their peripheral site of action.

Tricyclic antidepressants are particularly helpful for patients with associated depressive symptoms. Recent study of the serotonin-enhancing tertiary amines (imipramine, amitriptyline, doxepin) also suggested an analgesic effect through action on the descending inhibitory pain control system, and by facilitating endogenous endorphin release. Clinical studies have reported a benefit in many chronic pain disorders (migraine, postherpetic neuralgia, diabetic neuropathy). In one controlled trial of patients with chronic pain, amitriptyline produced a significant decrease in pain intensity and an increase in activity level.

Narcotic analgesics are of no value in chronic pain, and there is great risk for physical and psychological addiction.

Benzodiazepines are of no proven value, and tend to be misused in treating patients with chronic pain syndromes. They may actually increase pain perception, by inhibiting serotonin release.

Multidisciplinary Pain Treatment Centers
Pain treatment centers provide a multidisciplinary team approach toward the rehabilitation of patients with chronic pain. The approach is theoretically rational, and it may be the most efficient method of treating chronic pain. Therapies available at such centers may include transcutaneous electrical nerve stimulation (TENS), nerve blocks, and acupuncture, which may be effective in certain patients. A recent controlled study showed that patients with chronic pelvic pain who underwent an interdisciplinary pain management program had decreased pain scores, decreased anxiety and depression, and improved psychosocial functioning when followed 6 months after the treatment. However, few outcome studies currently exist to determine under what circumstances referral should be made.

Buccini R, Drossman DA. Chronic idiopathic abdominal pain. Curr Concepts Gastroenterol 1988; 12:3–11.
Provides a general overview to the clinical features and diagnostic approach to patients having unexplained chronic abdominal pain.

Melzack R, Wall P. Gate-control and other mechanisms. In: Melzack R, Wall P, eds. The challenge of pain. London: Pelican Books, 1988:165–93.
Reviews the theoretical basis for our understanding of acute and chronic pain.

Klein KB. Chronic intractable abdominal pain. Semin Gastroenterol 1990; 1:43–56.
An excellent and comprehensive review of the epidemiology, pathophysiology, diagnostic approach, and care of patients with chronic intractable abdominal pain. The information provided can be applied to all patients with chronic pain.

Melzack R. Neurophysiological foundations of pain. In: Sternbach RA, ed. The psychology of pain. New York: Raven Press, 1986:1–24.
Reviews the physiologic basis for chronic pain syndromes.

Drossman DA. Psychosocial factors in the care of patients with gastrointestinal diseases. In: Yamada T, ed. Textbook of gastroenterology. Vol. 1. Philadelphia: Lippincott, 1991: 546–61.
A comprehensive approach to understanding the role of psychosocial factors in gastrointestinal illness. The behavioral concepts are applicable to all medical disorders.

Crook J, Weir R, Tunks R. An epidemiological follow-up survey of persistent pain sufferers in a group family practice and specialty pain clinic. Pain. 1989; 36:49–61.
In a study comparing outcomes of patients with chronic pain followed in two clinical settings, pain was no longer reported as a problem in 33% of the patients followed in a family practice clinic, compared to 13% of patients followed at a pain clinic.

Drossman DA. Patients with psychogenic abdominal pain: six years' observation in the medical setting. Am J Psychiatry 1982; 139:1549–57.
Provides 6-year follow-up of 24 patients with chronic abominal pain referred to nonpsychiatric physicians at a medical center. Most patients reported a symptom onset in relation to a major loss, such as death, hysterectomy, or abortion. Only 2 patients had complete relief of pain.

Drossman DA, et al. Sexual and physical abuse among women with functional and organic gastrointestinal disorders. Ann Intern Med 1990; 113:828–33.
Reports on the association of abuse and health outcomes of patients seen at a medical center gastroenterology clinic. A history of abuse was more frequent in patients diagnosed with functional gastrointestinal disorders and, regardless of diagnosis, was associated with more pelvic pain, somatization, physician visits, and surgeries. In only 17% of patients with histories of abuse were these histories known to the patients' physicians.

Pilowsky I, Barrow CG. A controlled study of psychotherapy and amitriptyline used individually and in combination in the treatment of chronic intractable, 'psychogenic' pain. Pain 1990; 40:3–19.
Amitriptyline was effective in increasing patient activity and reducing pain intensity. Psychotherapy improved daily productivity. The roles of these two treatments should be considered complementary.

Miller TW, Kraus RF. An overview of chronic pain. Hosp Community Psychiatry 1990; 41:433–40.
Reviews knowledge about chronic pain and its management, including historical views, assessment, economic factors, and treatment approaches.

Kames LD, et al. Effectiveness of an interdisciplinary pain management program for the treatment of chronic pelvic pain. Pain 1990; 41:41–6.
A randomized controlled study showed a dramatic decrease in pain reporting in the group treated in a multidisciplinary pain control program.

141. MEDICATIONS IN PREGNANCY AND LACTATION
Ronald J. Ruggiero

Health care providers prescribing medications for pregnant patients or counseling pregnant patients about the possible effects of drug exposures must contend with a dilemma: Usually there are only animal and anecdotal human data available about drug exposures during pregnancy. Decisions must be based on the limited amount of information available, as well as on the clinical indication for the drug. While it is best to avoid medications during pregnancy as much as possible, in some cases the risks of untreated illness to both mother and fetus outweigh the risks of exposure to a drug.

The tables included in this chapter are designed to be a quick and concise reference. For further information, readers are directed to the sources named at the end of the chapter; regional poison control centers, local chapters of the March of Dimes, and university drug information services are other good sources of information. For drugs about which few data are available, such as a new drug, it is advisable to contact the manufacturer directly.

Assessing Risks of Drug Exposure
The effects of a drug on a developing fetus depend on the dose and route, concurrent exposure to other drugs, and the time of gestation. During the first 2 fetal weeks, susceptibility to insult may not exist due to a lack of cellular differentiation. The greatest risk of teratogenicity exists during the period of embryonic organogenesis, between about 18 and 60 days after conception, and all drugs should be avoided if possible during this time. Table 141-1 lists the periods of high and low sensitivity of various forming parts. Major morphologic abnormalities occur at highly sensitive times, whereas physiologic defects and minor morphologic abnormalities occur at less sensitive times. In interpreting such charts, it must be remembered that the postconceptual time differs from the weeks of pregnancy, which is traditionally measured from the beginning of the last menses rather than the date of conception. Despite the exponential production of new drugs and chemicals over the last 50 years, the major malformation rate (2.7% of all live births) has remained fairly constant and drug exposure has been thought to be the cause of only 3% of malformations.

Drug Classifications
Since 1980, the Food and Drug Administration (FDA) has required the listing of prescription drugs in categories of teratogenesis, based on available animal and human data. These categories are described in Table 141-2. In general, drugs in categories A through C are considered, with some caveats, safe for use in pregnancy. Drugs in category D can result in adverse effects in pregnant patients, as listed in the "Warnings" section of the drug package insert; they may be needed in a life-threatening situation or serious disease where safer drugs cannot be used or are ineffective. Drugs labeled X are contraindicated

Table 141-1. Timing of human development (postconceptual time in weeks)

Forming part	High sensitivity to teratogens	Low sensitivity to teratogens
Central nervous system	3–6.5	6.5–32 postnatal
Heart	3–6.5	6.5–12
Ears	4–12	12–36
Eyes	4–12	12–36
Arms and fingers	4.5–7.5	7.5–8.5
Legs and toes	4.5–7.5	7.5–8.5
Genitalia	5.5–12	12–38
Teeth	6.5–10	10–36

Table 141-2. FDA Prescription drug-labeling categories for pregnancy

Label as category	Animal studies	Human female control or clinical data
A	Negative	Negative
B	Negative	None
B	Positive	Negative
C	Positive	None
C	None	None
D	None	Positive
X	Positive	Positive

Positive = positive teratogenic results; negative = negative teratogenic results.

Table 141-3. Pregnancy category X and D drugs: probable human teratogens

Azathioprine (D)	Methimazole (D)
Bleomycin (D)	Methotrexate (D)
Barbiturates (D)	Penicillamine (D)
Busulfan (D)	Phencyclidine (X)
Chlorambucil (D)	Phenytoin (D)
Chlordiazepoxide (D)	Primidone (D)
Chlorpropamide (D)	Procarbazine (D)
Coumarin derivatives (D)	Progestins* (D)
Cyclophosphamide (D)	Ribavirin (X)
Dextroamphetamine (D)	Sodim iodine 131 (X)
Diazepam (D)	Tetracyclines (D)
Estrogens* (X)	Thioguanine (D)
Etretinate (X)	Thiotepa (D)
Fluorouracil (D)	Trimethadione (D)
Iodinated glycerol (50% iodine expectorant) (X)	Vaccines, live attenuated (measles, mumps, rubella) (X)
Isotretinoin (X)	Valproic acid (D)
Kanamycin (D)	Vincristine (D)
Lithium (D)	
Menadione** (X)	
Mercaptopurine (D)	

*Low dose combination oral contraceptives currently used have not been shown to be teratogenic when taken during pregnancy.
**If used in third trimester or close to delivery: marked hyperbilirubinemia and kernicterus in the newborn; otherwise, category C by the manufacturer.

in pregnancy, as noted in the "Contraindications" section; safer drugs or other forms of therapy are available.

Several years after the "pregnancy categories" were devised, The Over-The-Counter Drug (OTC) Labeling Warning became required for all OTC medications. It reads as follows: "AS WITH ANY OTHER DRUG, IF YOU ARE PREGNANT OR NURSING A BABY, SEEK THE ADVICE OF A HEALTH CARE PROFESSIONAL BEFORE USING THIS PRODUCT." Patients reading such labels may therefore seek advice from physicians about the use of these products.

Table 141-3 lists category X drugs, those with the greatest teratogenic potential, and category D drugs, which should be avoided if at all possible, although in most instances they have been used without detectable consequences. In some cases, the X category has been designated by the manufacturer, or by an expert body other than the FDA. The details of the liability of these drugs to the fetus are described in the references.

Table 141-4 lists drugs that are considered safe to use during pregnancy, with their ratings and comments about their use.

Table 141-4. Pregnancy category A, B, and C drugs: apparently safe in pregnancy

Drug	Comments
FOR ALLERGIES AND COLDS	
Antihistamines	
Brompheniramine (C)	10 1st-trimester malformations not found with other antihistamines
Chlorpheniramine (B*)	
Cyproheptadine (B)	
Diphenhydramine (C*)	
Hydroxyzine (C*)	
Tripolidine (C)	
Sympathomimetics	
Epinephrine (C*)	
Phenylephrine (C*)	
Phenylpropanolamine (C*)	
Pseudoephedrine (C*)	
Nasal corticosteroids	
Beclomethasone (C*)	Animal teratogen, not human
Flunisolide (C)	Animal teratogen, not human
FOR ANXIETY/DEPRESSION AND INSOMNIA	
Benztropine (C*)	
Chloral hydrate (C)	Possibly the hypnotic of choice
Chlorpromazine (C*)	
Desipramine (C*)	Possible neonatal withdrawal: cyanosis, tachycardia, diaphoresis
Doxepin (C*)	
Fluphenazine (C*)	
Haloperidol (C*)	
Perphenazine (C*)	
FOR CARDIAC ARRHYTHMIAS	
Digoxin (C)	
Disopyramide (C*)	
Isoproterenol (C*)	
Lidocaine (C*)	
Procainamide (C)	
Quinidine (C*)	
FOR ASTHMA	
Albuterol (C)	Transient fetal and maternal hyperglycemia
Aminophylline (C*)	
Beclomethasone (C*)	Animal teratogen, not human
Cromolyn sodium (B)	
Ipratropium bromide (B)	
Isoproterenol (C*)	
Metaproterenol (C)	
Prednisone (B*)	
Terbutaline (B)	
Theophylline (C*)	

Table 141-4. (*Continued*)

Drug	Comments
FOR COUGH	
Codeine (C*)	Risk factor D if high doses for prolonged time: neonatal narcotic withdrawal possible
Dextromethorphan (B*)	
Guaifenesin (C*)	
Terpin hydrate (B*)	
FOR HYPERTENSION	
Atenolol (C)	Observe newborns for 24–48 hr for beta-blockade
Captopril (C)	Embryocidal in animals; possible in utero renal failure
Clonidine (C*)	
Enalapril (C)	See captopril
Hydralazine (C)	
Labetalol (C)	See atenolol
Methyldopa (C*)	
Nadolol (C)	See atenolol
Prazosin (C*)	
Propranolol (C)	See atenolol
Timolol (C)	See atenolol
Verapamil (C)	
FOR INFECTIONS	
Acyclovir (C)	Acyclovir in Pregnancy Registry: 800-722-9292 (call for updates)
Amikacin (C*)	Potential eighth cranial nerve toxicity
Amphotericin B (B*)	
Ampicillin (B*)	
Cephalosporins (B)	
Chloramphenicol (C*)	Gray syndrome in newborns
Clindamycin (B*)	
Clotrimazole (B*)	
Dicloxacillin (B)	
Erythromycin (C)	
Ethambutol (B*)	
Flucytosine (C*)	
Gentamicin (C*)	See amikacin
Isoniazid (C*)	
Lindane (B)	Manufacturer recommends no more than 2 treatments during pregnancy; pyrethins and piperonyl butoxide for lice since they are nontoxic
Mebendazole (C)	Animal teratogen, not human; use only when absolutely needed
Metronidazole (B)	Contraindicated by manufacturer and the CDC in the 1st trimester
Miconazole (C)	
Nafcillin (B*)	
Nitrofurantoin (B*)	Hemolytic anemia if G-6-PD; possibly newborns, whose red blood cells are deficient in glutathione could show hemolysis, although this has never been reported when given at term
Nystatin (B*)	

Table 141-4. (*Continued*)

Drug	Comments
Paromomycin (C*)	Poorly absorbed
Penicillins (B*)	
Piperazine (B*)	
Pyrantel pamoate (C*)	
Pyrazinamide (C*)	
Pyrethins (C*)	
Pyrimethamine (C*)	Folic acid supplementation required
Rifampin (C*)	Possible hemorrhagic disease of the newborn; prophylactic vitamin K_1 is recommended
Spectinomycin (B*)	
Sulfasalazine (B*)	Risk factor D used near term due to possible neonatal kernicterus
Sulfonamides (B*)	See sulfasalazine
Thiabendazole (C)	An animal teratogen only
Trimethoprim (C)	Folate antagonist
Vancomycin (C)	
FOR NAUSEA	
Dimenhydrinate (B)	
Doxylamine (B*)	12.5 mg plus 10 mg of pyridoxine is equivalent to Bendectin, which was never proved to be teratogenic
Metoclopramide (B)	Very effective for hyperemesis
Prochlorperazine (C*)	
Promethazine (C*)	
Pyridoxine (A*)	May be useful for nausea of pregnancy
Trimethobenzamide (C*)	
FOR PAIN	
Acetaminophen (B*)	
Aspirin (C*)	Risk factor D if full dose in 3rd trimester to avoid maternal and fetal hemorrhage
Hydrocodone (B*)	See codeine
Hydromorphone (B*)	See codeine
Ibuprofen (B*)	Risk factor D in 3rd trimester: possible closure of ductus arteriosus in utero; may inhibit labor
Indomethacin (B*)	See ibuprofen
Meperidine (B*)	See codeine
Methadone (B*)	See codeine
Morphine (B*)	See codeine
Naproxen (B)	See ibuprofen
Oxycodone (B*)	See codeine
Pentazocine (B*)	See codeine
Propoxyphene (C*)	See codeine
FOR MISCELLANEOUS USES	
Acetazolamide (C*)	
Betamethasone (C*)	
Caffeine (B*)	High doses associated with increase in spontaneous abortions and in conjunction with smoking may induce lower birth weight than with smoking alone
Cimetidine (B)	
Colchicine (C)	Should be avoided: human lymphocyte cultures show chromosomal damage

Table 141-4. (*Continued*)

Drug	Comments
Cyclamate (C*)	Fetal blood levels are 25%
Cyclosporine (C)	
Dexamethasone (C*)	
Diphenoxylate (C)	
Docusate (C*)	
Glycopyrrolate (B)	
Heparin (C*)	
Levothyroxine (A)	
Nonoxynol 9 (C*)	FDA reports no birth defects (1986)
Paregoric (B*)	See codeine
Phenazopyridine (B)	
Pilocarpine (C*)	
Probenecid (B*)	
Propantheline (C)	
Pyridostigmine (C*)	
Ranitidine (B)	
Ritodrine (B)	
Scopolamine (C*)	At term, fetal tachycardia, decreased heart rate variability, and decreased heart rate deceleration
Senna (C*)	
Simethicone (C*)	
Tetanus toxoid (C*)	Tetanus-diphtheria toxoid recommended if no booster in 10 yr
Tretinoin (B)	If maximal absorption (33%) from 1-g application, this would give only one-seventh of the vitamin A activity from a prenatal vitamin
Vitamin C (A*)	Only intake up to the RDA is recommended
Vitamin E (A*)	

*Those categories marked with an asterisk were not supplied by the manufacturer, but assigned by GG Briggs et al., in *Drugs in Pregnancy and Lactation,* or by the author of this chapter, based on a review of available data.

Medications in Lactation

The basic pharmacokinetics of drug excretion in breast milk have only recently been postulated; the selected references at the end of this chapter give more detail. Not unlike information on the effects of drugs on the fetus, information on the passage of drugs through breast milk and the effects of drugs on the infant is often lacking. Most of the literature citations are single case reports or small series of infants. When data are not found in standard sources, the manufacturer or local drug information centers may be helpful.

To minimize the effect of maternal medications on the nursing infant, (1) the mother should take the drug immediately after breast-feeding; (2) the infant should be observed for unusual signs or symptoms; and (3) drugs that can be safely given directly to the infant, and those known to pass poorly through breast milk, should be used when possible.

Table 141-5 indicates drugs that are contraindicated or that should be given with caution to nursing mothers. Table 141-6 indicates drugs usually compatible with breast-feeding and their unwanted effects on the infant. These are modified from the 1989 recommendations of the American Academy of Pediatrics Committee on Drugs. Finally, Table 141-7 lists commonly used maternal medications that should not affect the breast-feeding infant.

Table 141-5. Drugs that are contraindicated or should be given with caution during breast-feeding

Drug	Possible effect on infant or lactation
Amphetamine	Irritability, poor sleep pattern
Aspartame	Caution if infant has phenylketonuria
Aspirin*	Metabolic acidosis, possible platelet disaggregation, and rash
Bromides	Drowsiness and rash
Bromocriptine	Prevents lactation
Clemastine*	One 10-wk-old reportedly was drowsy, irritable, refused to feed, neck stiffness, and a high-pitched cry
Cocaine	Irritability and tremulousness
Cyclophosphamide	Immune suppression, growth inhibition, and carcinogenesis
Cyclosporine	Immune suppression, neutropenia, growth inhibition, and carcinogenesis
Doxorubicin	Concentrated in milk; immune suppression, neutropenia, growth inhibition, and carcinogenesis
Ergotamine	Vomiting, diarrhea, and convulsions
Heroin	Addiction
Lithium	Infants may average 40% of the maternal serum concentration
Marijuana	THC concentrated in milk
Nicotine	Decreased milk production; shock, vomiting, diarrhea, tachycardia, and restlessness
Methotrexate	Immune suppression, neutropenia, growth retardation, and carcinogenesis
Phencyclidine	Animal studies show milk concentrations to be 10 times that of plasma
Phenobarbital*	Sedation reported in 3 infants, infantile spasms on weaning, and 1 case of methemoglobinemia
Primidone*	Limited conversion to phenobarbital; sedation and feeding problems
Sulfasalazine*	Blood diarrhea in 1 infant whose mother was taking 3 g daily

*The American Academy of Pediatrics recommends that infant blood levels of these drugs be determined.

Table 141-6. Maternal medication usually compatible with breast-feeding

Drug	Reported effect on infant or lactation
Caffeine	Accumulation may occur when mother drinks large moderate-to-heavy amounts causing irritability and poor sleep patterns
Chloramphenicol	Possible bone marrow suppression; milk levels too low to cause gray syndrome
Chlorpromazine	Drowsiness and lethargy reported in 1 infant
Estradiol	Vaginal bleeding on withdrawal

Table 141-6. (*Continued*)

Drug	Reported effect on infant or lactation
Estrogen/progestin	Combination oral contraceptives have decreased milk production only in higher doses no longer used
Ethanol	Drowsiness, diaphoresis, deep sleep, weakness, decrease in linear growth; maternal ingestion of 1 g daily decreases milk ejection reflex; chronic exposure has adverse effects on psychomotor development
Isoniazid	Acetylisoniazid also excreted; periodically examine infant for peripheral neuritis and hepatitis
Methadone	None if mother taking 20 mg in 24 hr
Metoclopramide	Concentrated in breast milk
Metronidazole	After single 2-g dose, discontinue breast-feeding for 12–24 hr to clear the drug
Nalidixic acid	1 case of hemolytic anemia in a G-6-PD infant
Nitrofurantoin	Possible hemolysis if infant has a G-6-PD deficiency
Phenytoin	Methemoglobinemia, drowsiness, and decreased sucking activity in 1 infant
Povidone-iodine	As a vaginal douche, elevated iodine levels in milk
Thiazides	Have been used to suppress lactation (i.e., bendroflumethiazide)

Table 141-7. Maternal medications that should not affect the breast-feeding infant (see also Table 141-6)

Antiinfectives
  Acyclovir   Penicillins
  Aminoglycosides   Pyrimethamine
  Chloroquine   Quinine
  Clindamycin   Rifampin
  Erythromycin   Tetracyclines
  Ethambutol   Trimethoprim
  Isoniazid   Trimethoprim-sulfamethoxazole
Cold remedies (Note: little to no clinical data available)
  Brompheniramine   Guaifenesin with dextromethorphan
  Chlorpheniramine   Phenylpropanolamine
  Diphenhydramine   Tripolidine/pseudoephedrine
  Guaifenesin with codeine
Pain medications
  Acetaminophen
  Aspirin   Methadone (no more than 20 mg/24 hr)
  Codeine   Meperidine
  Ibuprofen   Morphine
  Indomethacin   Naproxen
  Mefenamic acid   Naproxen sodium

Koren G, Pastuszak A. Prevention of unnecessary pregnancy terminations by counselling women on drug, chemical, and radiation exposure during the first trimester. Teratology 1990; 41:657–61.
Discusses the need for better, more effective patient counseling.

Shephard TH. Catalog of teratogenic agents. 6th ed. Baltimore: Johns Hopkins University Press, 1989.
Very comprehensive reference, including chemicals as well as drugs.

Briggs GG, Freeman RK, Yaffe SJ. Drugs in pregnancy and lactation. 3rd ed. Baltimore: Williams & Wilkins, 1990.
The single best reference source for the office. *Drugs in Pregnancy and Lactation: Updates* is a quarterly update to the textbook available by subscription.

Berkowitz RL, Coustan DR, Mochizuki TK. Handbook for prescribing medications during pregnancy. 2nd ed. Boston: Little, Brown, 1986.
Good, small quick reference, but needs revision.

Anderson AJ, Kelley-Buchanan CD. Drugs and pregnancy. In: Knoben JE, Anderson PO, eds. Handbook of clinical drug data. 6th ed. Hamilton, IL: Drug Intelligence Publications, 1988.

Anderson PO. Drugs and Breast Feeding. In: Knoben JE, Anderson PO, eds. Handbook of clinical drug data. 6th ed. Hamilton, IL: Drug Intelligence Publications, 1988.
Two chapters in the clinical drug data handbook.

American Academy of Pediatrics Committee on Drugs. Transfer of drugs and other chemicals into human milk. Pediatrics 1989; 84:924–36.
Recommendations of an expert panel.

Thiels C. Pharmacotherapy of psychiatric disorder in pregnancy and during breastfeeding: a review. Pharmacopsychiatry 1987; 20:133–46.
A rare article in a neglected area.

Buehler BA, et al. Prenatal prediction of risk of the fetal hydantoin syndrome. N Engl J Med 1990; 322:1567–72.
Preliminary results suggest that epoxide hydrolase activity below 30% of the standard will lead to clinical fetal hydantoin syndrome and these fetuses are at risk from other anticonvulsant drugs as well.

142. MOUTH LESIONS
E. Jefferson Burkes, Jr.

Although the clinical appearance of diseases in the mouth is extremely variable, most may be grouped into ulcerative lesions, white lesions, red lesions, and exophytic lesions for descriptive purposes.

Single Ulcers

Trauma
Trauma, as from improperly fitting dentures, is a common cause of oral ulcerations. Healing time is determined by the amount of tissue damage, the location, and in many instances the pathogenic organisms and debris embedded into the tissue. Recognition of the causative agent and its removal, followed by débridement of the ulcer, will usually be sufficient treatment. Trauma on the ventral surface of the tongue in an elderly person may produce a chronic, long-standing ulceration with a central depression and raised margins, resembling cancer. Healing commonly occurs following biopsy. Mouth ulcers should be re-examined within 2 weeks after local factors have been removed; those lesions that have not healed should be further evaluated for the possibility of cancer.

Aphthous Ulcers
Aphthous ulcers (canker sores) are single oval ulcers, 2 to 8 mm in diameter, with regular, broad, red borders, occurring on mobile, nonkeratinized mucosa. From 20 to 50% of people suffer from aphthous ulcers. There is strong evidence that aphthous ulcers result from a cell-mediated or type IV delayed hypersensitivity reaction. These ulcers are painful and last from 1 to 2 weeks. They heal without scar formation but recur at irregular intervals, apparently associated with diverse events such as trauma, psychological stress, gastrointestinal upsets, and menstruation. Recommended treatment is application of a topical anesthetic to the surface, followed by local débridement with hydrogen peroxide on a cotton swab, a rinse of tetracycline, and application of a topical steroid such as triamcinolone acetonide in an oral paste (Kenalog in Orabase) or covered with a gel, such as Zilactin. The tetracycline reduces the number of potentially infective bacteria and has been shown, in controlled studies, to reduce the duration of pain and lesions. Contents of a tetracycline capsule may be applied directly to the ulcer, or dissolved in water and swished in the mouth.

Squamous Cell Carcinoma
Squamous cell carcinoma in the oral cavity is frequently an ulcerative condition in the floor of the mouth and ventral surface of the tongue, more commonly in older individuals and tobacco and alcohol users. Suspicious ulcers lasting longer than 2 weeks should be biopsied.

Other Single Ulcers
Periadenitis mucosa necrotica recurrens produces large long-lasting ulcers that heal with scar formation. Syphilitic lesions may appear as ulcers, as may tuberculosis and fungal infections.

Multiple Ulcers
Multiple ulcers are generally caused by systemic illnesses or viral diseases.

Herpes Simplex Type I
Herpes simplex type I (cold sores) is the most common cause of multiple ulcers. The initial herpesvirus infection, called primary herpetic gingivostomatitis, usually presents during childhood as a febrile illness accompanied by ulcers in the mouth and on the lips. Herpetic ulcers recur almost exclusively on the vermilion border of the lips, gingiva adjacent to the teeth, and hard palate, and are stimulated by trauma, fever, and stress. They begin as small vesicles, which break, enlarge, and coalesce, producing large ulcers with irregular borders. These lesions are painful and last from 1 to 2 weeks. The diagnosis is usually evident from the appearance. Cytology shows a ballooning degeneration of the epithelial cell nuclei and multinucleation. Lysine (500 mg tid) may shorten the course of the acute phase in some patients; maintenance therapy (500 mg qd) may prevent recurrences. Antiviral agents such as acyclovir are appropriate in immunocompromised patients; in immunocompetent patients these costly drugs offer only a minimal shortening in the course of the infection. If steroids are given early, the lesions may spread. Persons examining herpes simplex lesions with an ungloved hand may contract the virus on the fingers (herpes whitlow).

Lichen Planus
Lichen planus is a common condition that can present in the mouth as multiple diffuse ulcers or as white, lacy lines. The ulcerative lesions vary in size and extent and often are bilateral and superficial, with angular margins. Ulcerations may be confined to the gingiva adjacent to the teeth and resemble a severe gingivitis. Lichen planus is characteristically seen in anxious individuals who report irregular exacerbations and remissions. Lichenoid reactions occur with numerous medications. The treatment of choice, topical steroid application in water-soluble or oral paste (Orabase) vehicles, is very effective.

Benign Mucous Membrane Pemphigoid
Benign mucous membrane pemphigoid (BMMP), also a common ulcerative condition, must be differentiated from lichen planus because the eye lesions of BMMP can lead to blind-

ness. BMMP severely affects the gingiva adjacent to the teeth, leaving it red, atrophic, and desquamative. Topical corticosteroids in water-soluble vehicles have been recommended, as well as systemic corticosteroids.

Pemphigus Vulgaris
Pemphigus vulgaris is an uncommon but potentially fatal disease, which may begin with ulcers in the mouth. Diffuse ulceration, rimmed by epithelium that can be easily separated and removed in large sheets, is characteristic. A biopsy showing intraepithelial separation is diagnostic. Topical and systemic steroids are the most effective medications.

Erythema Multiforme
Erythema multiforme (Stevens-Johnson syndrome) presents as an abrupt onset of hemorrhagic ulcers of the lips and oral mucosa. Although it is thought to be an allergic manifestation, in many cases no specific cause is found.

Acute Necrotizing Ulcerative Gingivitis
Acute necrotizing ulcerative gingivitis (trench mouth) is characterized by ulcers occurring only on the gingiva adjacent to and between teeth. It is a fusospirochetal infection, seen in young adults with poor oral hygiene, poor diet, and stress. Patients typically complain about bad breath, bad taste, and pain. Antibiotics like penicillin reduce the acute manifestations; however, thorough cleaning and preventive maintenance (e.g., brushing and flossing, saline rinses, and calculus removal by a dentist) must be accomplished, or recurrence is common and may lead to tooth loss.

White Lesions

Chronic Trauma
Chronic trauma causes oral mucous membranes to become keratinized and therefore white. Removal of the irritant should result in reversal of the lesions. Because white lesions may be premalignant or malignant, especially in patients who use tobacco or alcohol, any lesion that cannot be scraped off or reversed in 2 weeks should be biopsied.

Squamous Cell Carcinoma
Squamous cells carcinoma may be a localized white lesion present in one or more areas in the mouth. Piled up or speckled areas are especially suspicious. Biopsy of suspicious lesions is necessary.

Candidiasis
White plaques that may be rubbed off, leaving an erythematous base, are characteristic of the fungus infection called thrush. The clinical appearance varies from red granular lesions seen commonly under dentures to thick adherent white plaques seen at the corners of the mouth. The plaques contain hyperplastic epithelium invaded by *Candida albicans* hyphae. Hairy leukoplakia is a white lesion seen along the lateral margins of the tongue in immune-deficient patients. There is frequent *Candida* superinfection of this virally induced epithelial lesion, especially in patients with acquired immunodeficiency syndrome (AIDS) (see Chap. 114 for further information).

Oral candidiasis is treated with topical agents such as clotrimazole troches, 3 to 5 times a day, until resolution of all lesions. Troches are more effective than swishes, because contact between the medication and the lesions is more prolonged. Recalcitrant cases can be treated with ketoconazole (200 mg once or twice a day). Hairy leukoplakia alone does not generally require treatment.

Wart-like Lesions
A wart is a localized, rough-surface, usually single, white lesion ranging from 1 to 5 mm in size, caused by a virus. Condyloma accuminatum and papilloma must be considered if multiple, larger wart-like lesions are present. These three lesions are similar in clinical appearance; excisional biopsy is the treatment of choice.

Geographic Tongue
Geographic tongue occurs in 1% of the population; the cause is unknown. It can present as red patches outlined by a white raised border. These lesions change constantly, offer no threat to the patient, and require no treatment.

Nicotine Stomatitis
Nicotine stomatitis occurs in patients who use tobacco heavily. Typically the lesions from snuff occur at the mandibular mucobuccal surface ("snuff dipper's pouch"), while those from cigarettes are mostly on the palate. The oral mucosa may also be diffusely white with areas of white plaque. Because both smoking and dipping snuff are associated with oral cancer, any area of ulceration or focal areas of thickening that persist for 2 weeks should be biopsied to rule out cancer.

Lichen Planus
The most common form of lichen planus is seen as diffuse, interlacing white lines in the buccal mucosa. It may be an incidental finding or may cause the patient extensive irritation. Its relationship to carcinoma is controversial.

Red Lesions

Vascular Lesions
Many localized red lesions are vascular. Hemangiomas in the oral mucosal, when blanched, will often reveal deep feeder vessels. When bleeding or cosmetic appearance is a problem, vascular lesions are treated surgically, or by cryosurgery.

Mucoceles
Mucoceles are red or bluish and are common in the lower lip. They ordinarily persist and cause intermittent swelling and drainage unless they are removed.

Premalignant and Malignant Epithelial Tumors
Premalignant and malignant epithelial tumors may begin as localized or diffuse red patches. A velvety surface with areas of ulceration and small white plaques especially suggests malignant change. A history of tobacco and alcohol use is common when this lesion is found in the floor of the mouth or soft palate.

Other Red Lesions
Shallow, diffuse erosions simulating red lesions may be seen in early or healing vesiculobullous diseases. Candidiasis is commonly a diffuse red granular lesion in the palate under dentures.

Exophytic Lesions

Torus Palatinus and Torus Mandibularis
Torus palatinus and torus mandibularis occur in up to 10% of people. They are lobulated growths of bone in the midline of the palate and on the lingual surface of the mandible, respectively. They grow slowly and seldom cause problems unless the overlying mucosa is injured, exposing bone and causing pain. Removal is unnecessary except in preparation for wearing dentures.

Squamous Cell Carcinoma
Squamous cell carcinoma is the most frequent malignancy of the oral mucosa, accounting for 1 to 3% of all cancers. It occurs in older individuals and especially in those who use tobacco and alcohol. Up to 80% of intraoral carcinomas occur in the floor of the mouth and ventral surface of the tongue. These lesions are hard, with central granular and ulcerated red and white surfaces. Positive differentiation from other lesions is made only by biopsy. Oral cancers spread to regional lymph nodes readily; therefore, examination of the neck as well as the mouth is necessary. Treatment is by surgery or radiation therapy and results in an overall 5-year survival rate of over 50%.

Traumatic Lesions
Soft tumors are generally less likely to be malignant than are firm ones. The most common lesions are responses to injury. Traumatic fibromas are 5- to 15-mm, pink, mobile tumors that occur near the commissure. They enlarge when injured, as in biting.

An abscess from an infected tooth or periodontal disease may drain to the outside through a soft red mass of the gingiva called a parulis (gumboil). They regress when the tooth or periodontal pocket is treated.

Salivary Gland Tumors
Pleomorphic adenoma, the most common benign tumor, occurs in major glands as a firm, well-circumscribed mass that is painless and mobile. Complete surgical removal is the treatment of choice. Significant numbers of malignant salivary gland tumors occur in the minor salivary glands. Ulcerations over masses in the palate, lips, or floor of the mouth, plus pain and/or paresthesia, strongly suggest malignancy.

Referral
When referrals are considered necessary, most should be to dermatologists, since they are familiar with all of the major dangerous diseases of the oral cavity. If cancer is suspected, the referral can be directly to an ear, nose, and throat specialist.

Hooley JR, Whitacre RJ. Principles of biopsy: a self-instruction guide to oral surgery. 2nd ed. Seattle: Stoma, 1980.
Illustrates recommended biopsy principles and techniques for the oral mucosa.

Roitt IM, Lehner T. Immunology of oral diseases. Oxford: Blackwell, 1980.
A textbook incorporating information on immunology as applied to oral lesions and conditions.

Graykowski EA, Kingman A. Double-blind trial of tetracycline in recurrent aphthous ulceration. J Oral Pathol Med 1978; 7:376–83.
A publication stemming from a wide research effort to identify successful treatment for aphthous ulcers.

Decker J, Goldstein JC. Risk factors in head and neck cancer. N Engl J Med 1982; 306:1151–5.
Statistical analysis of factors relating to oral cancer.

Weathers DR, Griffin JW. Intraoral ulcerations of recurrent herpes simplex and recurrent aphthae. JAMA 1970; 82:81–8.
Outlines the clinical differences between herpetic and aphthous lesions.

Cawson RA. Premalignant lesions in the mouth. Br Med Bull 1975; 31:164–8.
Clinical, etiologic, and managerial information about lesions that have a significant risk of becoming squamous cell carcinoma.

Buchner A, Calderson S, Ramon Y. Localized hyperplastic lesions of the gingiva: a clinicopathological study of 302 lesions. J Periodont 1977; 48:101–4.
A review of a biopsy service experience with tumor-like proliferations.

Krutchkoff DJ, Eisenberg E. Lichenoid dysplasia: a distinct histopathologic entity. Oral Surg Oral Med Oral Pathol 1985; 60:308–15.
Histologic evidence of the malignant potential of lichen planus.

Hirsch M, Schooley R. Treatment of herpesvirus infections. N Engl J Med 1983; 309:963–70.
Review of antiviral agents and affected conditions.

Rodu B, Russell CM. Performance of a hydroxypropyl cellulose film former in normal and ulcerated oral mucosa. Oral Surg Oral Med Oral Pathol 1988; 65:699–703.
Describes an adhesive bandage for oral ulcers.

XX. DIETS

143. LOW-SALT DIETS
C. Stewart Rogers

Strict sodium restriction may be required for patients with advanced congestive heart failure (CHF), renal failure, severe hypertension, or cirrhosis with ascites. In the much larger group of patients with mild to moderate hypertension or CHF, modest sodium restriction may allow a reduction in drug therapy to safer or less expensive levels. Dietary sodium restriction may also avoid the need for potassium supplements because potassium loss on diuretics is directly related to sodium intake. A nonpharmacologic approach to sodium reduction is also favored by recent evidence that diuretics raise serum cholesterol levels.

Goals
Salt is 40% sodium (MW = 23) and 60% chloride (MW = 35). Diets may be expressed as milliequivalents of sodium or as milligrams (or grams) of sodium or salt. The usual, unrestricted American diet contains 3 to 5 g of sodium, or 7 to 12 g of salt (130–220 mEq of sodium). Some persons take in more than this; it is unusual for a person with ordinary tastes who satisfies a good appetite to consume much less.

A reasonable goal for patients requiring diuretics for hypertension or CHF would be reduction to 2 g of sodium or 5 g of salt (80 mEq of sodium). This is the level achieved in many studies of salt restriction for hypertension control and has commonly produced a 6– to 8–mm Hg fall in blood pressure. For severe CHF or cirrhosis with ascites, a 1-g sodium diet is often used, and for refractory ascites, temporary diets of 500 mg of sodium are customary. These severely restricted diets are too stringent to be followed by most outpatients.

Implementations
The process of implementing a low-sodium diet includes

1. Choosing a diet prescription.
2. Attracting the serious attention of the patient and family.
3. Communicating principles of diet and providing useful sources of information for shopping, menu planning, and cooking.
4. Adapting diet to food customs of the family.
5. Obtaining accurate data on the composition of available foods.
6. Ensuring access to low-sodium foods (e.g., bread, milk, special preparations).
7. Planning for patients who eat out often.
8. Coordinating low-sodium diet with special prescriptions for potassium, calorie, lipid, and protein contents.
9. Evaluating adherence.

Each of these steps presents obstacles, and rarely are all fulfilled for patients outside of the hospital. It is obvious that ready access to a committed dietitian is essential for full accomplishment of this goal.

The simplest approach, and thus perhaps that most often effective, is to teach the patient/family which foods are to be avoided. Realistically, this method can be expected to reduce grossly excessive sodium intake to 3 g per day and, if sufficiently inclusive, to as low as 2 g per day. The prescription is simple: the use of pickles, salted snack foods, cured meats, canned soups, and table salt must become exceptional rather than routine. Other foods to be curtailed include vegetable juices, salty condiments (catsup, salad dressing, soy sauce), most cheeses, pastas with cheese and tomato sauces, cold (boxed) cereals, and canned vegetables.

Many widely available foods are very low in sodium; all fresh fruits and fruit juices, alcoholic drinks (including beer and wine), hot cereals, fresh meats, and fresh or frozen vegetables, including potatoes. Acceptable levels are found in bread, milk, most desserts, and most seafoods (except for crabmeat and sardines). If patients eat large amounts of margarine or butter, use of unsalted products can save hundreds of milligrams of sodium per day. If severe salt restriction is desired, special bread and milk are available.

Table 143-1. Sodium and calorie content comparison of two meal plans

	Sodium (mg)	Calories
Plan 1		
Breakfast		
Orange juice, 6 oz	4	84
Oatmeal, 1 oz	1	109
Banana	2	68
Eggs (2)	140	160
	147	421
Lunch		
Hamburger, 4 oz	76	249
Lima beans, fresh, ½ cup	1	95
Margarine, unsalted, 1 tsp	1	30
Apple juice, 8 oz	6	110
Ice cream, 1 cup	112	257
	196	741
Supper		
Pork roast, 4 oz	93	292
Applesauce, ½ cup	3	227
Green beans, fresh, ½ cup	3	16
Potatoes, boiled, 5 oz	5	145
Bread, 1 slice	114	76
Margarine, unsalted, 2 tbs	2	200
Beer, 12 oz	18	151
	238	1107
24-hour total	581 mg	2269
Plan 2		
Breakfast		
Tomato juice, 6 oz	659	36
Rice Krispies, 1 cup	340	110
Sausage, two 2-oz patties	520	260
Toast, 1 slice, margarine	150	110
	1669	516
Lunch		
Vegetable soup, 1 cup	823	78
Macaroni and cheese, 1 cup	1086	430
Lima beans, canned, ½ cup	228	82
Dill pickle	1000	10
Buttermilk, 8 oz	257	99
	3394	699
Supper		
Ham, 4 oz	1494	176
Mashed potatoes	632	137
Green beans, canned, ½ cup	319	16
Biscuits, 2	540	208
Margarine, regular, 1 tbs	133	100
Vanilla pudding, ½ cup	200	321
Milk, 8 oz	120	121
	3438	1079
24-hour total	8501 mg	2294

Table 143-1 shows that two representative meal plans, composed of standard and available food, equal in calories and similar in cost, can differ by a factor of 14:1 in sodium content. Plan 1 would satisfy the strictest inpatient approach to refractory ascites, while plan 2 would likely frustrate any routine drug regimen for essential hypertension.

Further information about the sodium and calorie contents of food can be obtained from listings in cookbooks and in pamphlets from the food industry and the American Heart Association. A useful list for physicians and for many patients has been published in *JAMA* (1982; 248:541–3). If specific adjustments of potassium, lipids, or protein are required, it is necessary to consult a dietitian. Likewise, if cost, religious or ethnic customs, or lack of competence are involved, the diet prescription is unachievable without individualization and instruction by a teaching dietitian.

Adherence

Adherence to a diet can be determined by measuring a 24-hour urine for sodium. In the steady state, a person remains in sodium balance, excreting sodium in the urine at approximately the rate of dietary intake. If diuretic therapy has been stable for 2 weeks or more, and if there is no intercurrent illness, a 24-hour urine for sodium (with creatinine to assess completeness of collection) will estimate the sodium intake. Once patients are aware of the purpose of the collection, some may be transiently compliant just before the test, confounding interpretation. In practice, this test is usually reserved for redirecting therapy in refractory hypertension; however, it should be considered before adding a third medication, accepting poor control or adverse drug effects.

The American Dietetic Association. Handbook of clinical dietetics. New Haven: Yale University Press, 1981:G3–16. New edition planned for 1992.
  A concise, practical review of the clinical indications for sodium restriction, including detailed information for menu planning. Includes 62 references to clinical studies, as well as to food lists and cookbooks. The entire handbook would be an excellent resource for a course in clinical nutrition or as an office reference for dietary information.

Hayes A. Sodium and calorie content of common foods (table appended to advances in cardiovascular pharmacology). JAMA 1982; 248:541–3.
  A simple list—quick, clean, and current—of the sodium and caloric content of foods.

Northeast Ohio Affiliate's Low Sodium Cookbook Task Force. Cooking without your salt shaker. American Heart Association in cooperation with the Cleveland Dietetic Association. Dallas: National Center of the National Heart Association, 1978.
  This is an attractive, small cookbook with primary emphasis on recipes with moderately low sodium content. Included are low-sodium ingredients and use of often neglected, alternative flavor enhancers.

Houston MC. Sodium and hypertension: a review. Arch Intern Med 1986; 146:179–85.
  A well-organized review of the pathophysiology, epidemiology, and therapeutics of the relationship of sodium and hypertension.

Australian National Health and Medical Research Council Dietary Salt Study Management Committee. Fall in blood pressure with modest reduction in dietary salt intake in mild hypertension. Lancet 1989; 1:399–402.
  Among the best and most recent of many studies showing that a moderately reduced (80 mEq/d) sodium diet will lower blood pressure an average of 5 mm Hg systolic and 4 mm Hg diastolic, comprising a more useful reduction in a salt-sensitive substrate, and very little in the rest.

144. HIGH-FIBER DIETS
R. Balfour Sartor

High-fiber diets have assumed a major role in the management of constipation, diverticulosis, irritable bowel syndrome, and hemorrhoids. Recent animal and human studies suggest that increased soluble fiber consumption may also improve glucose tolerance in diabetes mellitus and decrease serum cholesterol and triglyceride levels. These benefits are believed to be related to dietary fiber's effects on stool bulk and transit time, glucose absorption, and bacterial fermentation products. Insoluble fiber (wheat bran, psyllium, vegetables) decreases colonic transit time and pressures by increasing fecal bulk (both fecal water

Table 144-1. Dietary fiber in some common foods

Food	Amount	Dietary fiber (g)
Cereals		
All-Bran	1 oz	10.0
Cornflakes	1 oz	0.3
Fruit & Fibre	1 oz	5.0
Raisin Bran	1 oz	3.6
Rice Krispies	1 oz	0.1
Total	1 oz	3.0
Oatmeal (dry)	1 oz	4.5
Shredded wheat	1 oz	2.5
Bread		
White	1 slice	0.6
Brown	1 slice	1.6
Whole wheat	1 slice	2.0
Meats and milk products		
Beef steak	6 oz	0
Whole milk	1 cup	0
Egg	1 large	0
Raw fruits		
Blackberries	½ cup	5.8
Apple	1 small	3.0
Banana	1 medium	1.6
Grapefruit	½	2.6
Orange	1 medium	3.2
Peach	1 medium	1.3
Pear	1 medium	4.1
Raisins	½ cup	5.6
Prunes	5 medium	6.7
Vegetables		
Green beans	½ cup	2.0
Cabbage, cooked	½ cup	2.4
Carrots, raw	1 medium	3.7
Celery, raw	1 stalk	0.7
Corn, canned	½ cup	4.7
Lettuce	1 cup	0.8
Peas, cooked	½ cup	5.4
Potato, baked (without skin)	1 medium	3.1
Rice, white cooked	1 cup	0.4
Summer squash	½ cup	2.2
Tomato	1 medium	3.0

content and dry weight). Nondegradable polysaccharides (cellulose, gums, and lignins) swell in the presence of water to form a gel, which by its sponge-like effect prevents mucosal absorption of water and electrolytes. The water-holding capacity of different types of foods varies widely, depending on their fiber content and individual fiber composition. Wheat bran is the most hydrophilic, holding 4.5 g of water per gram. Soluble fiber (oat bran, beans, citrus fruits) is fermented by colonic bacteria to short-chain fatty acids, which are absorbed and may alter glucose and lipid metabolism. Both soluble and insoluble dietary fibers delay glucose absorption, bind fat and bile acids, and delay gastric emptying, thus promoting satiety with relatively low caloric intake.

The amount of fiber in the diet may be increased both by dietary manipulation (Table 144-1) and the addition of supplemental bran or commercial psyllium preparations. The best source of dietary fiber is from the cereal group: whole-grain breads, bran, whole-grain and oat cereals, and rye crackers. Bran, which is the outer coat of grain that is removed by modern milling, contains the highest known concentration of dietary fiber (44%). Brown bread contains more than twice the fiber content of white bread, while whole-grain bread contains 3 times as much. Legumes (beans and peas) contain more fiber by weight than do root vegetables (carrots and potatoes), and both are higher than leafy green vegetables, which, because of their 90% water content, contain surprisingly little fiber. Fruits contain a moderate amount of fiber, with the best sources being blackberries, dried dates, prunes, raisins, peaches, oranges, and apples. Nuts and popcorn are also good sources of fiber.

Many patients with long-standing symptoms complicated by laxative dependence require supplemental bulk agents to provide at least 10 g of additional fiber per day. This can be accomplished by any of the agents listed in Table 144-2. Of these options, wheat bran is the cheapest ($0.29 per pound in health food stores); it can be mixed with hot cereals or sprinkled on food and in some studies has been found to decrease the colonic transit time more than bulk laxatives do. Bran's beneficial effects are frequently obtained with less supplementation as the colon is gradually "retrained" over a period of months. Commercial psyllium preparations (e.g., Metamucil, Konsyl, Perdiem Plain) can be administered in divided doses (1 tbs bid) and titrated to achieve a beneficial effect (up to 4 tbs/day). It should be noted that sugar-free preparations contain 3 times the psyllium concentrations of flavored formulations.

Potential side effects of a high-fiber diet include calcium, iron, magnesium, and zinc malabsorption by sequestration within the intestines and poor patient acceptance. Nearly all patients experience temporary sensations of gaseousness, abdominal distention, and cramping during the first few weeks of fiber supplementation. Before initiating therapy,

Table 144-2. Representative methods for adding supplemental fiber to the diet

Agent	Average dose/day	Dietary fiber (g)	Cost/day
Cellulose (e.g., Citrucel)	3 tbs	6	0.84
Psyllium powder (e.g., Metamucil, Konsyl, Perdiem)			
Regular	2 tbs	10 (approximate)	0.81
Flavored	6 tbs	10 (approximate)	1.25
Regular, sugar-free	2 tbs	10 (approximate)	0.79
Flavored, sugar-free	2 tbs	10 (approximate)	0.79
Instant mix	6 packets	10 (approximate)	1.35
Fibermed (corn bran, wheat bran, and rolled oats)	2 biscuits	10 (approximate)	0.91
Wheat bran	3 tbs	10	0.02
Oat bran	3 tbs	10	0.07
All-Bran cereal	1 oz (1/3 cup)	10	0.17

the physician must explain these side effects to patients or they will discontinue the diet before beneficial results are obtained. Gradual increases in fiber intake may be better tolerated than sudden radical changes in diet.

Spiller GA, ed. CRC handbook of dietary fiber in human nutrition. Boca Raton, FL: CRC Press, 1986.
Very detailed and well-documented reference giving the definition, methods of analysis, physiologic, and therapeutic effects of dietary fiber.

Anderson JW. Fiber and health: an overview. Am J Gastroenterol 1986; 81:892–7.
A protagonist's view of the beneficial effects of a high-fiber diet in preventing and treating a variety of diseases in Western culture.

Odes HS. Wheat and nonwheat dietary fibers. Is there a choice? J Clin Gastroenterol 1987; 9:131–4.
Sources and effects of therapeutic fiber supplementation.

Cranston D, McWhinnie D, Collin J. Dietary fibre and gastrointestinal disease. Br J Surg 1988; 75:508–12.
A thoughtful review of the epidemiologic and therapeutic relationship of dietary fiber and gastrointestinal diseases.

Kritchevsky D. Dietary fiber. Annu Rev Nutr 1988; 8:310–28.
An extensively referenced discussion of the physiologic effects of fiber.

Vahouny GV. Effects of dietary fiber on digestion and absorption. In: Johnson LR, ed. Physiology of the gastrointestinal tract. 2nd ed. New York: Raven Press, 1987:1623–48.
A thorough review of the effects of dietary fiber on intestinal physiology.

Council on Scientific Affairs. Dietary fiber and health. JAMA 1989; 262:542–6.
A concise review of the data on the physiologic effects of fiber and its role in disease prevention.

Department of Dietetics, Massachusetts General Hospital. Fiber modifications. Diet reference manual. Boston: Little, Brown, 1984:63–9.
Table of dietary fiber in food, by serving size.

Swain JF, et al. Comparison of the effects of oat bran and low fiber wheat on serum lipoprotein levels and blood pressure. N Engl J Med 1990; 322:147–52.
A double-blind, crossover trial demonstrated the lowering of serum cholesterol (by 8%) by oat bran and low-fiber refined wheat. Decreases in cholesterol were a result of diminished dietary fat intake.

145. CHOLESTEROL-LOWERING DIETS
Robert B. Baron

Cholesterol-lowering diets are indicated as first-line therapy for high blood cholesterol. Current recommendations are to initiate diet therapy in low-risk patients with low-density lipoprotein (LDL) cholesterol levels higher than 160 mg/dl and in high-risk patients with LDL cholesterol levels higher than 130 mg/dl (see Chap. 126). All patients with elevated LDL cholesterol should receive 3 to 6 months of diet therapy before treatment with medications. The dietary recommendations for treatment of high blood cholesterol are consistent with the recommendations of the American Heart Association, the National Academy of Sciences, and numerous other panels of experts, for the prevention of coronary heart disease in the public at large.

Dietary Goals
The goal of a cholesterol-lowering diet is to decrease the intake of the three dietary factors that increase blood cholesterol—saturated fatty acids, dietary cholesterol, and excess calo-

ries—and to increase the intake of soluble dietary fiber. The macronutrient composition of cholesterol-lowering diets is shown in Table 145-1. A "step-one" diet is recommended for the first 3 months of therapy; if further reduction in LDL cholesterol is necessary, a "step-two" diet, with further reduction in saturated fatty acids and dietary cholesterol, should be tried.

Total Fat

The typical American diet contains approximately 35 to 40% of total calories as dietary fat. Reduction to 30% of total calories allows for both the required reduction in saturated fatty acids and a decrease in total calories.

Saturated Fat

The reduction of saturated fatty acids is the single most important aspect of cholesterol-lowering diets. In the typical American diet, saturated fatty acids account for approximately 15 to 20% of total calories. In the initial cholesterol-lowering diet, "step one," saturated fatty acids are reduced to less than 10% of calories. A further reduction to less than 7% is indicated in the "step-two" diet. The majority of saturated fatty acids in the US diet are found in meat and meat products, eggs and dairy products, and commercial baked goods that have a high content of tropical oils.

Saturated fatty acids have different effects on blood cholesterol, depending on their carbon chain length. The medium-chain saturates, caprylic (8:0) and caproic (10:0), have little effect on blood cholesterol. The intermediate-chain fatty acid, lauric (12:0), and the long-chain fatty acids, myristic (14:0) and palmitic (16:0), raise the levels of total blood cholesterol and LDL cholesterol. Palmitic acid is the major cholesterol-raising saturate in the U.S. diet. Stearic acid (18:0), however, does not appear to have any significant impact on blood cholesterol. At the present time, these distinctions have little clinical value since foods that are high in short-chain fatty acids, such as butter fat and coconut oil, are also high in intermediate- and long-chain fatty acids, whereas foods high in stearic acid, such as cocoa butter and beef fat, are also high in palmitic acid. These observations, however, may have an important impact on food processing in the future.

Polyunsaturated Fat

When used to replace saturated fatty acids in the diet, polyunsaturated fatty acids result in decreases in blood cholesterol. It is not clear whether the effect is primarily due to the reduction of saturated fat or the addition of polyunsaturates. Since the replacement of saturated fats with monounsaturated fat results in similar reductions of cholesterol, the decrease is most likely due to the reduction in saturated fat. Current U.S. diets contain approximately 7 to 10% of total calories as polyunsaturated fatty acids, predominantly linoleic acid (18:2). Both "step-one" and "step-two" diets contain 10% of total calories as polyunsaturated fatty acids. Previous recommendations to increase the percentage of polyunsaturated fat to even higher levels have been changed because greater quantities of

Table 145-1. Macronutrient composition of cholesterol-lowering diets

Nutrient	Recommended intake	
	"Step-one" diet	"Step-two" diet
Total fat	< 30% of total calories	
Saturated fat	< 10% of calories	< 7% of calories
Polyunsaturated fat	Up to 10% of total calories	
Monounsaturated fat	10–15% of total calories	
Carbohydrates	50–60% of total calories	
Protein	10–20% of total calories	
Cholesterol	< 300 mg/d	< 200 mg/d
Total calories	To achieve desirable weight	

polyunsaturated fats can result in a decrease in high-density lipoprotein (HDL) cholesterol levels. The primary sources of polyunsaturated fats in the diet are vegetable oils such as safflower, sunflower seed, soybean, and corn oil. Although these oils are low in saturated fats and have little inherent LDL-raising potential, they are high in calories (9 kcals/g) and can contribute to increased LDL cholesterol if consumed in quantities that result in weight gain.

Omega-3 Fatty Acids
Also polyunsaturated, omega-3 fatty acids are found predominantly in fish oils, most commonly as eicosapentoic acid (20:5) and docosahexaenoic acid (22:6). The major lipid-modifying effect of these fatty acids is to lower blood triglyceride levels. Little impact on LDL cholesterol is observed, unless omega-3 fatty acids replace saturated fats. Fish oils, however, may prevent coronary heart disease through other mechanisms, including the interference of platelet aggregation or the retardation of fibroblasts and smooth muscle cells in response to arterial wall injury. At the present time, supplements of fish oil are not recommended as part of a cholesterol-lowering regimen, but fish is an excellent dietary substitute for meat.

Monounsaturated Fats
Until recently, monounsaturated fatty acids were thought to have no significant effect on blood cholesterol. Recent evidence, however, suggests that when monounsaturated fatty acids replace saturated fatty acids in the diet, the blood cholesterol decreases to the same degree as with replacement with polyunsaturated fatty acids. The decrease in total cholesterol is due to a reduction of LDL cholesterol; no change is seen in HDL cholesterol or very-low-density lipoprotein (VLDL) cholesterol. The vegetable oils rich in monounsaturated fatty acids include canola oil, olive oil, peanut oil, and some forms of sunflower seed oil, safflower oil, and soybean oil. Peanuts, avacado, olives, hazelnuts, and pecans are also high in monounsaturated oils. Many animal fats also contain significant amounts of monounsaturated oil in addition to large quantities of saturated fats.

Monounsaturated fats occur naturally in the cis configuration. When polyunsaturated fats are hydrogenated, however, transmonounsaturated fatty acids are formed. Transmonounsaturates have recently been found to raise LDL cholesterol and lower HDL cholesterol. Since most margarines are high in transmonounsaturates, they offer no significant advantage over butter; both should be restricted on a cholesterol-lowering diet.

Dietary Cholesterol
Dietary cholesterol has a less important impact on blood cholesterol than saturated fat. Although dietary cholesterol will usually increase blood cholesterol, the effect is more variable and less quantitatively important than the effect of saturated fat. Moreover, the effect of dietary cholesterol is dependent on the saturated fat intake. Individuals on a high-saturated-fat diet will have a significantly greater (two- to threefold) rise in blood cholesterol when fed a diet high in dietary cholesterol than when fed similar quantities while on a low-saturated-fat diet. Dietary cholesterol is found exclusively in animal products including egg yolk, organ meats, some shellfish, and butter fat and in meat, fish, and fowl. Approximately one-third of the daily dietary intake of cholesterol comes from eggs, one-third from dairy products, and one-third from meat. The current average U.S. intake is approximately 450 mg/d. The recommended intake is less than 300 mg/day on a "step-one" diet and less than 200 mg/day on a "step-two" diet.

Total Calories
The ingestion of excess calories resulting in obesity is a major contributor to high blood cholesterol in the United States. Excess calories result in increased blood cholesterol by two complementary mechanisms. The excessive intake of saturated fat and dietary cholesterol that usually occurs with obesity suppresses the activity of LDL receptors. Secondly, excess calories result in the overproduction of VLDL and conversion to LDL. Not all obese individuals, however, have increased blood cholesterol; conversely, weight loss will not always result in a reduction of blood cholesterol. However, weight loss almost always results in decreased blood triglycerides and increased HDL cholesterol. Obesity is also an independent risk factor for coronary heart disease.

Carbohydrates and Dietary Fiber

The replacement of saturated fats in the diet by carbohydrate results in a decreased blood cholesterol level, similar to what occurs with replacement with unsaturated fatty acids. In addition, since carbohydrates contain fewer calories by weight than dietary fats (4 kcal/g versus 9 kcal/g), high-carbohydrate diets may result in less obesity. Diets very high in carbohydrates (> 75% of total calories), however, may result in increased levels of blood triglycerides and decreased HDL cholesterol. Current recommendations are for 55 to 60% of total calories to be derived from carbohydrates, predominantly complex carbohydrates.

Indigestible carbohydrates are called dietary fiber, commonly classified as insoluble and soluble. Insoluble fiber such as the cellulose found in wheat bran adds bulk to the diet and aids in bowel function but has no effect on blood cholesterol. Soluble fibers such as pectins, gums, and psyllium will commonly reduce blood cholesterol. One common soluble fiber, beta-glycan, is found in beans and oat bran. Although large quantities of such foods are necessary to result in significant cholesterol reduction (equivalent to 6 oat bran muffins/day), more moderate intakes of psyllium (1 tsp of sugar-free psyllium 3 times/day) can result in significant reduction (10–15%) in LDL cholesterol.

Alcohol

Alcohol has no significant effect on LDL cholesterol, but does result in increased HDL cholesterol and triglycerides. Most of the increase in HDL is in the HDL_3 subfraction, however, and is thought to offer little protection against coronary heart disease. In general, patients who drink alcohol should limit their intake to two drinks per day for men and one for women. Those who do not drink should not be advised to begin.

Coffee

The effect of coffee on blood cholesterol and cardiovascular mortality remains controversial. Most evidence, including the Framingham Heart Study, suggests that coffee has inconsistent effects on blood cholesterol and no impact on total cardiovascular mortality. Recent evidence suggests that the use of boiled coffee raises blood cholesterol whereas filtered coffee has no effect.

Implementation of Cholesterol-Lowering Diets

In most instances, diet therapy should be initiated by the primary care clinician during a visit especially designated for that purpose. Prior to the visit, patients can be asked to keep a 3- to 5-day record of their food and beverage intake. This record provides a useful screen of patient motivation for dietary change, and provides a data base of food preferences and habits. Although clinical dietitians can provide extremely useful assistance in assessing and designing diets, visits to dietitians should supplement, but not replace, the physician visit.

The "step-one" diet is usually initiated by providing the patient with information about the relation of diet, blood cholesterol, and coronary heart disease; skills to implement dietary change; and support. Patients are provided lists of foods to eat and foods to eat less of (Table 145-2). Specific examples based on the patient's food record are extremely helpful.

Primary care clinicians can help the patient learn behavioral skills that increase adherence to dietary changes. First, they can help the patient set specific goals that are measurable and achievable. Long-term changes are more likely when patients have success in meeting a series of small incremental goals. Recording these goals in the record reinforces the patient's motivation and allows caregivers to provide positive feedback when the goals are met. Second, clinicians can help the patient to analyze the environmental factors that support or impede the desired behavioral changes. For example, what situations or persons or foods will make it difficult for the patient to follow the diet? Once these factors are identified, the patient can actively plan how to counteract them. For example, the patient may need to involve family or friends in the dietary plans. If the patient knows that having certain foods will trigger binges, such foods need to be kept out of the house. Advance meal planning allows for adequate shopping and meal preparation. Third, the clinician can help the patient monitor progress and problems. The goal is to help patients learn to do such monitoring themselves and to take the initiative in addressing problems. Fourth, clinicians can provide positive feedback to reinforce positive behaviors and

Table 145-2. Recommended foods on a cholesterol-lowering diet

Meat, fish, and fowl
Choose
   Fish; poultry without skin; lean cuts of beef, lamb, pork, and veal; shellfish
Decrease
   Fatty cuts of beef, lamb, and pork; spare ribs; organ meats; regular cold cuts; sausage; hot dogs; bacon; sardines; roe

Dairy products
Choose
   Skim or 1% fat milk (liquid, powdered, evaporated), buttermilk
   Nonfat (0% fat) or low-fat yogurt (2%)
   Low-fat cottage cheese (1% or 2% fat)
   Low-fat cheeses, farmer or pot cheeses (all of these should be labeled to have no more than 2–6 g of fat/oz)
   Sherbet, sorbet
Decrease
   Whole milk (4% fat) (regular, evaporated, condensed), cream, half and half, 2% milk, imitation milk products, most nondairy creamers, whipped toppings
   Whole-milk yogurt
   Whole-milk cottage cheese (4% fat)
   All natural cheeses (e.g., blue, roquefort, camembert, cheddar, Swiss), low-fat or "light" cream cheese, low-fat or "light" sour cream, cream cheeses, sour cream
   Ice cream
   Butter and margarine

Eggs and egg substitutes
Choose
   Egg whites (2 whites = 1 whole egg in recipes), cholesterol-free egg substitutes
Decrease
   Egg yolks

Fruits and vegetables
Choose
   Fresh, frozen, canned, or dried fruits and vegetables
Decrease
   Vegetables prepared in butter, cream, or other sauces

Breads and cereals
Choose
   Homemade baked goods using unsaturated oils sparingly, angel food cake, low-fat crackers, low-fat cookies
   Rice, pasta
   Whole-grain breads and cereals (e.g., oatmeal, whole wheat, rye, bran, multigrain)
Decrease
   Commercial baked goods: pies, cakes, doughnuts, croissants, pastries, muffins, biscuits, high-fat crackers, high-fat cookies
   Egg noodles
   Bread in which eggs are a major ingredient

Fats and oils
Choose
   Baking cocoa
   Unsaturated vegetable oils: corn, olive, rapeseed (canola oil), safflower, sesame, soybean, sunflower
   Mayonnaise, salad dressing made with unsaturated oils listed above
   Seeds and nuts
Decrease
   Chocolate
   Butter, margarine, coconut oil, palm oil, palm kernel oil, lard, bacon fat
   Dressings made with egg yolk
   Coconut

Table 145-3. Four steps to a "step-two" diet

1. Determine "desirable weight"
   (weight for height tables)
2. Calculate daily caloric intake
   ($\approx$ 30 kcal/kg)
3. Calculate amount of total calories as saturated fat
   (7% of the value determined in #2)
4. Calculate daily grams of saturated fat intake
   (divide the number derived in #3 by 9)

Example: 45-year-old man, 5 ft 10 in., 175 lb
1. Desirable weight
   154 lb (70 kg)
2. Daily calorie intake
   70 × 30 = 2100 kcal/day
3. Total daily saturated fat calories
   7% of 2100 = 147 kcals
4. Total daily grams of saturated fat
   147 kcals/9 kcals per g = 16.3 g

---

changes in blood cholesterol. In addition to providing such feedback, they can help patients devise ways to reward and reinforce positive changes for themselves.

The further reduction of saturated fat and dietary cholesterol to achieve a "step-two" diet requires a more quantitative approach. By estimating the patient's daily energy requirement, the daily intake of saturated fat (in calories or grams of fat per day) can be calculated. Using food tables, the patient can record daily food intakes and design diets within the guidelines. This process is illustrated in Table 145-3.

Follow-up

Follow-up visits and blood cholesterol measurements should be performed approximately 1 and 3 months after initiation of a "step-one" diet. Patients who achieve the desired response should be seen approximately 2 to 3 times per year to reinforce dietary change. Patients who do not achieve the goal cholesterol level at 3 months can be tried on a "step-two" diet, again with follow-up at 1 and 3 months after initiation. Drug therapy should only be begun if diet therapy for 3 to 6 months fails to achieve the desired result.

Anderson LW, et al. Hypercholesterolemic effects of oat-bran or bean intake for hypercholesterolemic men. Am J Clin Nutr 1984; 40:1146–55.
One of a number of studies demonstrating a significant LDL-lowering effect of soluble fiber.

Bak AAA, Grobee DE. The effect on serum cholesterol levels of coffee brewed by filtering or boiling. N Engl J Med 1989; 321:1432–7.
Boiled coffee raises LDL cholesterol, but filtered coffee does not.

Block G, et al. Nutrient sources in the American diet: quantitative diet from the NHANES II survey: II. Macronutrients and fats. Am J Epidemiol 1985; 122:27–40.
Most saturated fat and dietary cholesterol in the U.S. diet are derived from a relatively short list of common foods.

Bonanome A, Grundy SM. Effect of dietary stearic acid on plasma cholesterol and lipoprotein levels. N Engl J Med 1988; 318:1244–8.
All saturated fats are not created equal. Stearic acid, an 18-chain saturated fatty acid, does not raise LDL cholesterol.

Grundy SM. Monounsaturated fatty acids, plasma cholesterol, and coronary heart disease. Am J Clin Nutr 1987; 45:1168–75.
Monounsaturated fatty acids have the same cholesterol-lowering potential as polyunsaturated fatty acids when used to replace saturated fatty acids in the diet.

Haskell WL, et al. The effect of cessation and resumption of moderate alcohol intake on serum high-density lipoprotein subfractions. A controlled study. N Engl J Med 1984; 43:566–98.
Although moderate alcohol intake raises HDL cholesterol, it occurs in the HDL_3 subfraction, not currently thought to provide significant protection.

Kromhout D, Bosschieter EB, Coulander C. The inverse reaction between fish consumption and 20-year mortality from coronary heart disease. N Engl J Med 1985; 312:1205–9.
Moderate intake of fish (2–3 meals/wk) results in lower mortality from coronary heart disease.

Leaf DA. Cardiovascular effects of omega-3 fatty acids. N Engl J Med 1988; 318:549–57.
Comprehensive review of the effects of omega-3 fatty acids.

Martin AR, Coates TJ. A clinician's guide to helping patients change behavior. West J Med 1987; 146:751–3.
A useful guide emphasizing the skills that primary care clinicians can teach patients to implement dietary change.

Mensick RP, Katan MB. Effect of dietary trans fatty acids on high-density and low-density lipoprotein cholesterol levels in healthy subjects. N Engl J Med 1990; 323:439–44.
Trans–fatty acids, found commonly in margarine, raise LDL cholesterol and lower HDL cholesterol to the same extent as saturated fatty acids (found in butter). Both margarine and butter should be decreased in a cholesterol-lowering diet.

Small DM, Oliva C, Tercyak A. Chemistry in the kitchen: making ground meat more healthful. N Engl J Med 1991; 324:73–7.
A home recipe for lowering the saturated fatty acid and dietary cholesterol content of ground beef.

Wilson PWF, et al. Is coffee consumption a contributor to cardiovascular disease? Insights from the Framingham Study. Arch Intern Med 1989; 149:1169–72.
Coffee consumption has no significant effect on cardiovascular disease.

Wood P, et al. Changes in plasma lipids and lipoproteins in overweight men during weight loss through dieting as compared with exercise. N Engl J Med 1988; 319:1173–9.
Although weight loss is extremely effective at beneficially modifying lipids in overweight men with hyperlipidemia, aerobic exercise is equally effective.

Cookbooks and Patient Resources

Eshelman ER, Winston M. The American Heart Association cookbook. New York: Ballantine, 1985.

Connor SL, Connor W. The new American diet: the lifetime family eating plan for good health. New York: Simon & Schuster, 1986.

Cooper R, Goor N. Eaters choice: a food lovers guide to lower cholesterol. Boston: Houghton Mifflin, 1989.

Griffin GC, Castelli WP. Good fat bad fat: how to lower your cholesterol and beat the odds of a heart attack. Tucson, AZ: Fisher, 1988.

INDEX

Absence seizures, 470
  anticonvulsant drugs for, 476–477
Acetaminophen (Tylenol)
  for headache, 464
  for neck pain, 314
Acetazolamide (Diamox)
  for acute mountain sickness, 636
  for glaucoma, 39
Achalasia
  diagnosis of, 188–189
  with dysphagia, 188–189
  treatment of, 189
Acidosis, metabolic, management of in chronic renal failure, 256
Acoustic neuroma, 47
Acquired immunodeficiency syndrome (AIDS)
  chronic cryptosporidiosis with, 571
  definition of, 550–551
  esophagitis with, 196
  incidence of among HIV-infected population, 549–550
  lower respiratory tract infection with, 103
  newsletters for, 559
  spread of by travelers, 635
  tuberculosis with, 572
Acromegaly
  diabetes with, 393
  and erectile dysfunction, 385
Acromioclavicular joint, 316
Acupuncture, for chronic pain, 686
Acute mountain sickness (AMS), 635–636
  edema with, 660
Acyclovir
  for herpes simplex virus, 541–542
  prophylactic, 554
  for infectious mononucleosis, 566
Adenitis, tuberculous, 665
Adenomas
  autonomously functioning thyroid, 427
  hyperplastic prostatic, 249–251
  thyroid, 417, 419–421
Adenopathy. See Lymphadenopathy
Adenopharyngeal conjunctivitis, 29
Adenosine, for paroxysmal supraventricular tachycardia, 144
Adhesive capsulitis, evaluation for, 318
Adrenal gland, physiology of, 437–438
Adrenal insufficiency
  with corticosteroid administration, 438, 440–441
  and erectile dysfunction, 385
Adrenal steroids, edema with, 660
Adrenergic agents
  decongestant, for allergic rhinitis, 82t
  for glaucoma, 39
Adrenocorticotropic hormone (ACTH), 437
Advance directives, 600
Aerosol bronchodilators, for asthma, 89–91
Afterload reduction, drugs for, 137–138
Aging
  and erectile dysfunction, 384
  and sexual dysfunction in female, 381

Agoraphobia, 501
AIDS. See Acquired immunodeficiency syndrome
AIDS Clinical Care, 559
AIDSFILE, 559
AIDS-related complex (ARC), 551
Albuterol, for asthma, 91
Alcohol
  and cholesterol levels, 709
  and erectile dysfunction, 385
  osteoporosis and, 308
Alcoholics Anonymous (AA), 529–530
Alcoholism, 526
  CAGE questionnaire for, 527–528, 597
  categories of abuse, 527
  confirmatory data for, 528
  determination of, 527
  differential diagnosis of, 502
  drinking pattern suggesting, 501
  early signs and symptoms of, 528
  efficacy of counseling for, 529
  hypertension with, 114
  patients with medical risks from, 527
  presenting diagnosis of, 528–529
  referral for, 529–530
  screening for, 527–528
  steps to intervention in, 526
  treatment of, 529–530
Alginic acid (Gaviscon), for gastroesophageal reflux disease, 193
Alkaline agents, esophageal injury with, 196
Allergen skin testing, 88
Allergens, avoidance of, 89
Allergic conditions, 587–592
Allergic conjunctivitis, 29–30
Allergic rhinitis, 79
  antihistamines for, 81–82, 81t
  diagnosis of, 79–80
  environmental modification for, 80
  immunotherapy for, 83
  sympathomimetic drugs for, 82–83, 82t
  topical corticosteroids for, 83
  treatment of, 80–83
Allopurinol
  for gout, 306–307
  for renal stone disease, 262
Alpha-1-adrenergic receptor inhibitor. See Alpha-1 blockers
Alpha-1-antitrypsin serum levels, for COPD diagnosis, 97–98
Alpha-1 blockers, 122
  for benign prostatic hyperplasia, 251
  for hypertension, 122
Alpha blockers, and erectile dysfunction, 384
Alprazolam, for anxiety, 504t, 505
Altitude edema, 660
Altitude illness, 635–636
Alzheimer's disease, 496–497
Amantadine (Symmetrel)
  for influenza, 63
  for parkinsonism, 490–491
Amaurosis fugax, 43

Amebiasis, 567, 569
  sexually transmitted, 547
  treatment for, 569
Aminoglycosides
  for diverticulitis, 212
  for prostatitis, 246
Amiodarone, to prevent atrial fibrillation, 154
Amitriptyline (Elavil)
  for depression, 508–509t
  for diabetic neuropathy, 407
  for migraine, 465
Amoxicillin
  for chancroid, 543
  for diverticulitis, 211
  for gonococcal infections, 535
  for otitis media, 55
  for sinusitis, 68
Amoxicillin-clavulinic acid, for group A streptococcal pharyngitis, 72
Ampicillin
  for gonococcal infections, 535
  for prostatitis, 246
  for sinusitis, 68
Amputation, for peripheral vascular disease, 181
Anal fissures, 227–228
Analgesics
  for herpes zoster, 562
  for otitis media, 55
Anal skin tags, 225
Anaphylactic shock, with bee stings, 590
Anemia, 443
  detection of, 443
  diagnostic approach to, 443–444
  macrocytic, 446–447
  management of in chronic renal failure, 256
  microcytic reticulocytopenic, 444–446
  normocytic reticulocytopenic, 447
  with reticulocytosis, 447–448
Angina
  clinical evaluation in, 127
  diagnostic strategy in, 130
  laboratory testing for, 128–130
  new-onset, 130
  pathophysiology of, 126
  probability analysis in, 127–128
  progressive, 130
  stable, 127
  stepped-care approach to, 131
  treatment of, 130–132
  unstable, 127, 130
Anginose pharyngitis, treatment of, 566
Angioedema, 587
  causes of, 587, 588t
  diagnostic approach to, 587–588
  treatment of, 589
Angiography
  for angina pectoris, 130
  for peripheral vascular disease, 178
Angioneurotic edema, hereditary, 587
Angiotensin-converting enzyme (ACE) inhibitors
  acute renal failure with, 272
  for afterload reduction, 137, 138
  for chronic renal failure, 254–255
  for congestive heart failure, 137–138
  for diabetic nephropathy, 407
  for hypertension, 120–121
  for proteinuria, 272–273
Angiotensin II, reduced circulating concentrations of, 137–138
Angle-closure glaucoma, 37
  treatment of, 38–39
Angular cheilitis, management of in HIV infection, 556
Ankylosing spondylitis, 321
Anorectal disorders, 225–229
Anorexia nervosa, 16
Anoscopy
  for pruritus ani, 229
  for source of bleeding, 230
Anovulation, 357
  causing abnormal uterine bleeding, 358
  treatment of, 359
Antacids
  for dyspepsia, 199
  for gastroesophageal reflux disease, 193
  interaction of with aspirin, 303
  for peptic ulcer disease, 204
Antianxiety drugs, 503–505, 504t
  and sexual dysfunction in female, 381
Antiarrhythmic drugs, 154
Antibody testing, in HIV infection diagnosis, 550
Anticholinergic drugs
  for asthma, 92–93
  in COPD, 99–100
  for diverticulosis, 211
  for dyspepsia, 199
  and erectile dysfunction, 384–385
  for irritable bowel syndrome, 208
  for parkinsonism, 491
  for peptic ulcer disease, 204
Anticoagulants
  for atrial fibrillation, 154
  for chronic arterial insufficiency, 180
  for thrombophlebitis, 183–185
  for transient ischemic attack, 483
Anticonvulsants
  blood levels of, 476
  commonly used, 477–478
  discontinuing use of, 479–480
  pharmacologic parameters of, 475t
  pregnancy and, 480
  principles of therapy with, 474–476
  problem of, 479–480
  selection of, 476–477
Antidepressants
  commonly used, 509t
  for irritable bowel syndrome, 208
  non-monoamine oxidase inhibitor, 508–510
  and sexual dysfunction in female, 381
  side effects of, 508
  therapeutic range of, 510
Antidiarrheal drugs, 216
AntiDNase titer, for group A streptococcal pharyngitis, 71
Anti-EBV (Epstein-Barr virus) antibodies, 565–566

Antigen tests, for group A streptococcal pharyngitis, 71
Anti-HB$_s$ antibody, 581
Antihistamine-decongestant combinations, 82
Antihistamines
　for allergic rhinitis, 81–82
　avoidance of in COPD, 98
　for bee stings, 590
　classes of, 81t
　elixirs, 74
　for hay fever conjunctivitis, 30
　for nasal symptoms of cold, 61
　for otitis media, 54–55
　for serous otitis, 55–56
　for urticaria, 589
Antihypertensive drugs. *See also* Hypertension
　drugs for hypertension, 117t
　and erectile dysfunction, 384
　impairment of by NSAIDs, 301
Anti-inflammatory drugs. *See* Nonsteroidal anti-inflammatory drugs (NSAIDs)
Antiphospholipid antibodies, 482
Antiplatelet drugs
　for chronic arterial insufficiency, 180
　for transient ischemic attack, 483, 484
Antiprostaglandin drugs. *See* Nonsteroidal anti-inflammatory drugs (NSAIDs)
Antipsychotics, for insomnia, 517
Antipyretics, for heat injury, 673
Antistreptolysin O (ASO) titer, for group A streptococcal pharyngitis, 71
Antithyroid drugs
　for Graves' disease, 420–421
　for hyperthyroidism, 419–420
Antiviral agents
　for herpes simplex, 195, 541–542
　　conjunctivitis, 29
　　keratitis, 24
　for herpes zoster, 562
　for HIV, 552–554
　for influenza, 63
　for prevention of colds, 61
Anti-VCA (viral capsid antigen) IgG assay, 565–566
Anusol-HC, 227
Anxiety, 501
　attacks, 471
　differential diagnosis of, 501–502
　evaluation of, 501
　prognosis of, 502
　treatment of, 502–505
Aortic stenosis
　midsystolic murmur with, 159
　supravalvular, midsystolic murmur with, 159–160
Aphakic spectacles, 36
Aphonia, 76
Aphthous ulcers, 697
ARC (AIDS-related complex), 551
Arrhythmias
　with mitral valve prolapse, 163
　syncope and, 655
Arterial digital subtraction angiography, 178

Arterial disease, of extremities, 177–181
Arterial insufficiency
　acute, 177–179
　chronic, 178–180
　differential diagnosis of, 178
　evaluation of, 178
　skin care in, 179
Arteriography
　for hematochezia, 230–231
　for peripheral vascular disease, 178
　for transient ischemic attacks, 482–483
Arteriovenous shunts, endocarditis risk with, 169
Arthritis, acute gouty, 304–306. *See also* Osteoarthritis; Rheumatoid arthritis
Ascariasis, 567–570
Aspirin
　for angina pectoris, 131
　clinical pharmacology of, 302
　drug interactions of, 303
　for headache, 464
　for neck pain, 314
　for osteoarthritis, 286
　preparations of, 290t
　to prevent deep venous thrombosis, 185
　for rheumatoid arthritis, 288
　and risk of coronary heart disease, 617
　side effects of, 302–303
　toxicities of, 288
Asthma
　acute attack of, 93
　in elderly persons, 94
　evaluation of, 87–88
　exercise-induced, 94
　incidence of, 87
　nocturnal, 93
　occupational, 94
　refractory, 88
　special problems of, 93–94
　treatment for, 89
　　drugs in, 89–93
Asthmatic bronchitis, 95
Athletic physicals, 603–605
　recommendations for participation in, 606–607t
Atrial fibrillation, 151
　diagnosis of, 152
　evaluation of, 152–153
　incidence of, 151
　pathophysiology of, 152
　prevalence of, 151
　prevention of recurrence of, 153–154
　risk factors for, 151
　treatment of, 153
Atrial septal defects, midsystolic murmur with, 159
Atrophic vaginitis, 344–345
　abnormal bleeding with, 359
Atropine
　allergic reaction to, 30
　for intractable hiccups, 682
Audiology referral, 47
Audiometric assessment, 3
Auditory aids, 48
Auditory problems. *See* Hearing, problems with

Auranofin (Ridaura), for rheumatoid arthritis, 289
Austin Flint murmur, 160
Autoimmune thyroiditis, chronic, 428–429
Azathioprine (Imuran), for rheumatoid arthritis, 293
Azotemia, management of in chronic renal failure, 255
AZT. *See* Zidovudine (AZT)

Back pain. *See* Low back pain
Bacterial conjunctivitis, 28–29
Bacterial pharyngitis, group A beta-hemolytic, 566
Bacterial vaginosis, 344
  diagnosis of, 344
  treatment of, 344
Bacteriuria
  with hematuria, 267
  with indwelling catheters, 280–281
  with intermittent catheterization, 279
Baker's cyst, 327
  treatment of, 331
Barium enema, for occult GI bleeding, 232
Barium swallow studies, for dysphagia, 188
Barrett's esophagus, 194–195
Barrier contraceptives, 348–349
  for prevention of STDs, 548
Beclomethasone dipropionate (Beconase, Vancenase), for allergic rhinitis, 83
Bed rest, for low back pain, 323
Bedtime insulin and daytime sulfonylureas (BIDS), 405
Bee stings, 590–592
Behavioral modification therapy
  for chronic pain, 685–686
  for hypertension, 116
  for obesity, 12
Bellergal, for headache, 465
Bell's palsy, 493
  clinical manifestations of, 493–494
  diagnosis of, 494
  natural history of, 494
  risk factors for, 493
  treatment of, 494–495
Benign prostatic hyperplasia, 249
  etiology of, 249–250
  evaluation of, 250–251
  treatment of, 251
Benzalkonium chloride (Zephiran), for cerumen removal, 58
Benzodiazepines
  for anxiety, 503, 504*t*, 505
  for chronic pain, 686
  dosages of, 503–505
  for dyspepsia, 199
  for insomnia, 516*t*
  for irritable bowel syndrome, 208
  for labyrinthitis, 3
  sensitivity to, 517
  used as hypnotics, 516*t*, 517
Benztropine mesylate (Cogentin), for parkinsonism, 491
Bereavement. *See* Grief

Bernard-Soulier syndrome, 450
Bernstein acid perfusion test, 193
Beta-2 selective adrenergic inhaled bronchodilators, 90*t*
Beta-adrenergic bronchodilators, for COPD, 100
Beta-adrenergic drugs, oral, for asthma, 92
Beta-blockers
  for angina pectoris, 131
  for anxiety, 505
  avoidance of in COPD, 98
  for chronic arterial insufficiency, 180
  contraindications for, 120
  and erectile dysfunction, 384
  for hypertension, 119–120
  for glaucoma, 38–39
  for migraine, 465
  for paroxysmal supraventricular tachycardia prevention, 145
  to prevent reinfarction, 141
Bile acid-binding resins, 408
Biliary pain
  with gallstones, 234
  treatment of, 238
Biliary stricture, 239
Binswanger's disease, dementia with, 496
Biofeedback training
  for anxiety, 505
  for chronic idiopathic pain, 686
  for headache, 464
Bipolar mood disorder, 507
Birth control. *See also* Contraception; *specific methods of*
  counseling about, 599–600
  failure rates for, 347*t*
  methods, 347–348
    barrier, 348–349
    intrauterine, 351–356
    oral contraceptive, 349–351
    permanent, 356
  and natural family planning, 348
  use effectiveness of, 346–347
Birth defects, with use of anticonvulsants, 480
Bisphosphonates, for osteoporosis prevention, 310
Black widow spider bite, 678
Bladder
  adrenergic and cholinergic neuroreceptors in, 274
  atonic or neurogenic, 275
  outlet obstruction, with benign prostatic hyperplasia, 249–250
  pressure on, 274
  prolapse of, 274
  stones in with indwelling catheters, 281
  stretch receptors in, 274
  unstable or spastic, 275
Bleeding, abnormal
  causes of, 449–451
  patterns of, 449
  strategy for detecting, 452
  tests for, 451–452
Bleeding time, 452
Blepharitis, 31
Blindness, fleeting, 43

Blood glucose
    goal levels of, 394
    monitoring of in type II diabetes, 405
    self-monitoring of, 399, 405
Blood pressure
    diastolic, 111
    lowering of, 111–112
    systolic, 113
Blood problems, 443–455
B lymphocytes, EBV-infected, 563–564
B mode ultrasonography, in thrombophlebitis
        diagnosis, 183
Body fat, location of, 9–10
Body mass index (BMI), 9
Body weight
    loss of, 15–18
    mortality and, 9–10
    normal fluctuation in, 15
Bone demineralization, 308
Booster phenomenon, 573
Bouchard's nodes
    osteoarthritis in, 283
    x-ray evaluation of, 284
Bougienage, for peptic strictures, 190
Braces, for low back pain, 324
Brain tumor, headache with, 459
Breast
    benign disease of, 370
    biopsy of for breast lumps, 370–371
    clinical examination of, 594
    discharge from, 372
    lumps in, 369–371
    pain in, 371
    physical examination of
        for breast cancer detection, 647–648
        recommended patterns for, 648*f*
Breast cancer
    estrogen effect on, 376
    metastasis of, 646–647
    nipple discharge with, 372
    screening for, 594, 646–649
    women at high risk for, 649
Breast-feeding
    drugs contraindicated during, 694*t*
    drugs used during, 693–694, 695*t*
    maternal medications that should not
        affect infant during, 695*t*
    maternal medication usually compatible
        with, 694–695*t*
Breast self-examination, 647
Bromocriptine (Parlodel)
    for breast pain, 371
    for parkinsonism, 492
Bronchial challenge testing, 88
Bronchiolitis, 95
Bronchitis, 95
    differentiation of from pneumonia, 103
Bronchodilators
    anticholinergic, for COPD, 99–100
    for asthma, 89, 90*t*, 91
    beta-adrenergic, 100
    for cor pulmonale, 102
Bronchoscopy, flexible fiberoptic, 107–108
Brown recluse spider bite, 678
Bumetanide, for congestive heart failure, 136
Bupropion, side effects of, 508–510

Burns, 674–675
Bursitis, 334
    knee, 331
    shoulder, 317
Buspirone, for anxiety, 505

Cafergot, for migraine, 465
CAGE questionnaire, 527–528, 597
Calcific tendinitis
    evaluation for, 318
    treatment of, 320
Calcitonin, for osteoporosis treatment, 310
Calcium
    for osteoporosis prevention, 310
    restriction of for hypercalciuria with renal
        stones, 261
    serum levels of, 432
        lowering of, 434
        measurement of, 431
Calcium channel blockers
    for achalasia, 189
    for angina pectoris, 131
    for cluster headaches, 468
    for dysmenorrhea, 362
    for hypertension, 121–122
    for migraine, 465
    for premature ventricular contractions,
        149–150
Calcium nephrolithiasis
    approaches for prevention and treatment
        of, 263*t*
    treatment of, 262
Calcium oxalate, inhibition of nucleation and
        crystallization of, 262
Calcium stones
    pathogenesis of, 258
    recurrence rate of, 258
Calories
    calculation of requirement of based on
        ideal body weight, 396*t*
    in cholesterol-lowering diet, 708
    consumption with physical activity, 16
Calymmatobacterium granulomatis, 545
Campylobacter infections, sexually trans-
        mitted, 546–547
Campylobacter pylori. See *Heliobacter pylori*
Cancer. See also specific types
    hypercalcemia and, 432–433
    screening for, 594–595
    weight loss with, 15
Candida balanitis, 342
Candida esophagitis, 195
Candida vaginitis, 341
    signs and symptoms of, 341
    treatment of, 341–342
Candidiasis, oral
    with HIV infection, 556
    red lesions and, 699
    white lesions and, 698
Canker sores, 697
Capsaicin (Zostrix), for herpes zoster, 562
Captopril, for hypertension, 120–121
Carbamazepine (Tegretol)
    for seizures, 476–478
    side effects of, 478

Carbidopa-L-dopa (Sinemet)
  for parkinsonism, 490–492
  side effects of, 491
Carbohydrate(s)
  in cholesterol-lowering diet, 709
  diets high in, 13–14
  loading
    edema with, 660
    to prevent exercise-induced hypoglycemia, 411
  restriction diets, 13, 411
Carbonic anhydrase inhibitors, for glaucoma, 39
Cardiac catheterization, endocarditis risk with, 169
Cardiac output, low, 133–134
Cardiac pacing studies, 146
Cardiac rehabilitation programs, post-myocardial infarction, 140
Cardiac risk factor modification, 616
  compliance with programs for, 618
  effects of on coronary heart disease, 616–617
  and potential for coronary heart disease prevention, 618t
  practical implications of, 617–618
Cardiopulmonary diseases, syncope and, 655
Cardiopulmonary examination, in athletic physical, 604
Cardiorespiratory murmur, 158
Cardiovascular system
  disease of
    exercise to reduce risk factors for, 626–627
    screening for, 593–594
  hyperthyroidism effects on, 417
  hypothyroidism effects on, 423
  problems of, 111–171. *See also specific conditions*
  pulsatile tinnitus with anomaly of, 49
Cardioversion, for atrial fibrillation, 153
Carisoprodol (Soma), for nocturnal leg cramps, 338
Carotid bruits, asymptomatic, 485–486
Carotid endarterectomy, 484–485, 486
Carotid sinus massage, 144
Carotid sinus syncope, 655
Carotid surgery, 484–485
Carpal tunnel syndrome, 332–333
  diagnostic studies of, 333
  physical findings in, 333
Cataracts, 32
  clinical findings in, 33
  with diabetes mellitus, 42
  evaluation for, 33–34
  incidence of, 32–33
  optical correction after extraction of, 35–36
  postoperative care for, 35
  treatment of, 34
    complications of, 34–35
    surgical referrals for, 35
    surgical techniques in, 34
Cat bites, 679
Catheterization, urinary, 278–282
  intermittent, 279
  for overflow incontinence, 277

Cat-scratch disease, 666
Cauda equina syndrome, 321–322
CD4 counts
  in HIV infection, 551
  with *Pneumocystis carinii* pneumonia, 553
Cefoxitin, for pelvic inflammatory disease, 368
Cefaclor, for otitis media, 55
Cefizoxime, 535
Cefotaxime, 535
Ceftriaxone
  for chancroid, 543
  for gonococcal infections, 535
  for PID, 368
Cefuroxime axetil
  for gonococcal infections, 535
  for otitis media, 55
Celiac sprue, 219
Cellulitis, 675
Central nervous system
  NSAID effects on, 302
  occult malignancies of, 473
  vertigo with problems of, 2–3
Cephalexin, for diverticulitis, 211
Cephalosporins
  for cystitis, 244
  for diverticulitis, 212
Cerebellar ataxia, vertigo with, 2
Cerebellar function test, 1
Cerebral infarctions, 481
Cerebrospinal fluid, elevated protein in, 473
Cerebrovascular disease, 481–486. *See also specific conditions*
  markers of, 485–486
  syncope and, 656
Cerebrovascular events, risk of, 481
Cerumen. *See* Earwax
Cerumenex Drops, 58
Cervical cancer, screening for, 594
Cervical cap, 348–349
Cervical nodes, 665
Cervical spine
  headache with pathology of, 463
  osteoarthritis of, 284
    pain and, 285
Cervical spondylosis, 312
Cervicitis, infectious, 345
  abnormal bleeding with, 359
  sexually transmitted, 546
Chalazion, 31
  treatment for, 32
Chancroid, 533, 542–543
  clinical presentation and diagnosis of, 543
  management of sexual contacts with, 543
  treatment and follow-up in, 543
Chemotherapeutic agents
  causing esophagitis, 196
  and sexual dysfunction, 381
Chest x-ray
  for acute lower respiratory tract infection, 104
  for COPD diagnosis, 97
  for solitary pulmonary nodule diagnosis, 107
Chickenpox, 561–562
Chilblain, 669

Chlamydia infections
  clinical strategies for, 536
  diagnostic tests for, 535–536
  in PID, 366
  pneumoniae
    differential diagnosis of, 60
    pharyngitis, 73
  psittaci, TWAR strain of, 104
  trachomatis, 533, 535
    infectious cervicitis with, 345
    tissue culture of, 535, 536
    urethritis with, 544
  treatment of, 244, 536
Chloral hydrate, for insomnia, 517
Chlordiazepoxide, for anxiety, 503, 504*t*
Chlorhexidine rinses, 556
Chloroquine
  for malaria prevention
    plus proguanil, 634
    with sulfadoxine, 634
  for nocturnal leg cramps, 338
Chloroquine-resistant *Plasmodium falciparum* (CRPF), 633–634
Chlorpromazine (Thorazine)
  edema with, 661
  for intractable hiccups, 682
Cholecystectomy
  for biliary pain, 238
  for gallstones, 236
  problems following, 239
  prophylactic, 237, 238
  resolution of symptoms with, 236
Cholecystitis, acute, 234
  treatment of, 238
Cholecystography, oral, 235
Cholecystokinin-octapeptide (CCK-OP), 238
Choledocholithiasis, 234
  treatment of, 238
Cholera vaccination, 631
Cholescintigraphy, 235
Cholesteatoma
  with otitis media, 55
  vertigo with, 2
Cholesterol
  dietary, 597, 708
  dietary factors increasing blood levels of, 706–707
  dietary treatment of high levels of, 593–594
  diets lowering, 706–711
  drugs to lower levels of, 408
  high blood levels of
    patient evaluation for, 620–622
    rationale for reducing to prevent CHD, 619–620
    screening and interventions for, 593–594, 619–625
    treatment for, 622–625
  LDL, 112
  and risk of coronary heart disease, 616
  screening for, 593–594
  total, initial classification of CHD risk by, 620
Cholestyramine
  for cholesterol reduction, 623–624

  for dyspepsia, 199
  for lowering cholesterol in diabetics, 408
Cholinergic agents, for glaucoma, 39
Cholinergic urticaria, 587
Chondromalacia patellae, 330
Chronic ambulatory peritoneal dialysis, 407
Chronic fatigue syndrome
  causes of, 7
  definition of, 7
  diagnostic criteria for, 7
  etiology of, 564
  support organizations for, 7–8
Chronic idiopathic pain
  clinical assessment of, 684–685
  clinical presentation of, 683–684
  definition of, 682–683
  facts and misconceptions about, 683
  pathophysiology of, 683
  treatment suggestions for, 685–686
Chronic musculoskeletal pain syndromes, 336–337
Chronic obstructive pulmonary disease (COPD), 95
  clinical course of, 96
  diagnosis of, 96–98
  drug therapy for, 99–101
  incidence of, 95–96
  laboratory evaluation for, 97–98
  oxygen therapy for, 101
  signs of, 96–97
  treatment measures for, 98–99
  treatment of acute infections in, 101
  treatment of cor pulmonale in, 102
Chronic renal failure, 252
  causes of, 252–253
  evaluation of, 253–254
  management of, 254–256
  referral for, 256
  slowing rate of progression of, 254
  treating complications of, 254–256
Chronic venous insufficiency, 173
  clinical presentation of, 173–174
  evaluation for, 174
  treatment of, 174–175
Cigarette smoking. *See* Smoking
Cimetidine (Tagamet)
  and erectile dysfunction, 384–385
  for gastroesophageal reflux disease, 193–194
  for peptic ulcer disease, 203, 204
  and sexual dysfunction, 381
Ciprofloxacin
  for chancroid, 543
  for gonococcal infections, 535
Clavulanic acid, 543
Clenched-fist injuries, 679
Clicking tinnitus, 49
Clindamycin
  for diverticulitis, 212
  plus gentamicin, for PID, 368
Clofibrate
  for cholesterol reduction, 624
  and erectile dysfunction, 385
Clonazepam, for anxiety, 503, 505
Clonidine, for hypertension, 122
Clostridium difficile toxin, diarrhea with, 219

Clotrimazole, 342
Cluster headache, 458
  abortive therapy for, 465
  prophylactic therapy for, 468
Coagulation factor deficiencies, 449–450
Coagulopathies, causing menorrhagia in adolescents, 357
Coarctation of aorta
  continuous murmur with, 160
  hypertension with, 115
Coating agents, for peptic ulcer disease, 204
Cochlear implants, 48
Codeine, 61
Coffee, and cholesterol levels, 709
Coital pain, 380
Colchicine, 306
Cold, exposure to, 667
Cold injury, 669–670
  prevention of, 670
Colds, common, 59–61
Cold sores, 697
Colestipol, for lowering cholesterol, 408, 623–624
Colitis
  diarrhea with, 219
  sexually transmitted, 546
Colon, diverticular disease of, 209–212
Colonoscopy
  for diarrhea, 219
  for occult GI bleeding, 231, 232
  for weight loss evaluation, 17
Color blindness, testing for, 41
Colorectal cancer, screening for, 231, 595
Color vision testing, 41
Common bile duct stones, 234
  removal of, 238
  retained, 239
Complex partial seizures, 469, 470
Compression stockings
  for chronic venous insufficiency, 174
  for varicose veins, 176
Computed tomography (CT)
  for dementia in elderly, 498
  for gallstones, 235
  for headaches, 463
  for hematuria, 268
  for seizures, 472–473
  for solitary pulmonary nodule diagnosis, 107
Computerized digital subtraction angiography, 482–483
Condom external catheter, 281
  complications with, 282
  placement and care of, 281–282
Condoms, 349
  for prevention of STDs, 548
Conductive hearing loss, 45–46
Condyloma acuminatum, 547, 698
Congestive heart failure (CHF), 133
  atrial fibrillation with, 151
  diagnosis of, 134–135
  pathophysiology of, 133–134
  prognosis in, 135
  treatment of, 135–138

Conjunctiva
  foreign bodies in, 21
  evaluation of, 21–22
  treatment for, 22
  inflammation of, 26–30
Conjunctivitis, 26
  acute, 26
  allergic, 29–30
  approach to diagnosis of, 28
  bacterial, 28–29
  causes of, 26
  differential diagnosis of, 26–28
  viral, 29
Constipation
  anal fissures with, 227
  evaluation for, 222–223
  meanings of, 221
  predisposing factors for, 221
  prevention of, 224
  refractory, 224
  signs and symptoms of, 221–222
  treatment of, 223–224, 228
Contact dermatitis, of external ear, 51
Contact lenses
  after cataract extraction, 35–36
  to correct refractive errors, 42
  disposable soft, 42
  gas-permeable, 36
  hard, 35
  soft, 35–36, 42
Continence, urinary, neuroanatomy and physiology of, 274
Contraception. See also Birth control
  barrier methods of, 348–349
  family planning and natural, 348
  oral, 349–351, 352–355t
Contraceptive sponges, 348
Conversion reaction, 520
Cooling
  for hyperthermia, 673
  for rheumatoid arthritis, 293
Cornea
  abrasions of, 24–25
  foreign bodies in, 22–23
  recurrent epithelial erosions of, 25
  rust ring in, 22–23
  trauma of, 26
Coronary artery bypass graft (CABG) surgery
  for angina pectoris, 131–132
  endocarditis risk with, 168
  prophylactic, 486
Coronary atherosclerosis, 127
Coronary Drug Project, myocardial infarction patient study of, 620
Coronary heart disease
  and dietary fat consumption, 597
  with estrogen deficiency, 375
  estrogen therapy and, 378
  evaluation for, 127–128
  evaluation of risk for before exercise program, 627–628
  exercise, 597, 626
    for obesity and, 11
  as leading cause of death, 616

and obesity, 8, 10–11
probability of, 128t
rationale for reducing cholesterol to prevent, 619–620
risk factors for, 616
    effect of reduction of on, 616–617
    reduction of, 617–618
Coronary revascularization, 131–132
Coronary thrombosis, aspirin therapy for, 617
Cor pulmonale, 102
Corsets, for low back pain, 324
Corticosteroid cream, for bee sting, 590
Corticosteroids
    and adrenal physiology, 437–438
    alternate-day, 440
    for COPD, 100
    elevated intraocular pressure with, 39–40
    for gout, 305
    and HPA axis suppression, 438
    for hypercalcemia, 434
    for infectious mononucleosis, 566
    inhaled, for asthma, 91
    intra-articular injections of, rheumatoid arthritis, 293
    for neck pain, 314
    oral, for asthma, 91–92
    for osteoarthritis, 286
    osteoporosis with, 307, 308, 311
    for otitis externa, 51–52
    pharmacology of, 438
    preparations of, 439t
    in prolonged therapy, 438–440
    for rheumatoid arthritis, 293
    short-term, high-dose, 438
    for shoulder pain, 319
    for stress, 441
    therapeutic regimens for, 438–440
    topical
        for allergic rhinitis, 83
        for corneal abrasion, 25
        for urticaria, 589
    withdrawal from, 440–441
Corticotropin
    release of, 437
    stress-induced secretion of, 438
Corynebacterium diphtheriae, 73
Cough, syncope and, 655
Cough suppressants, 105
Counseling
    about smoking cessation, 641–645
    and advance directives, 600
    on birth control, 599–600
    for dietary fat consumption, 597
    exercise, 597–599
    for injury prevention, 597
    for sexually transmitted diseases, 600
    for smoking cessation, 597
C-peptide serum levels, 392
CRAG, in HIV-infected patient, 556
Cranial nerve
    eighth, assessment of function of, 45
    evaluation of, 1
Cricoarytenoid joint arthritis, hoarseness with, 76

Crohn's disease, anal fissures with, 228
Cromolyn sodium (Opticrom)
    for allergic rhinitis, 83
    for asthma, 91
    for vernal conjunctivitis, 30
Cruciate ligament instability, 329f
Crunching tinnitus, 49
Cryptosporidiosis, 571
Cryptosporidium infections, 567
Crystallization inhibitors, for renal stones, 262
Cushing's syndrome
    with corticosteroids, 438
    diabetes with, 393
    and erectile dysfunction, 385
    obesity with, 10
Cyclosporine C, 400
Cyproheptadine (Periactin), for urticaria, 589
Cystine stones, 259
Cystitis
    clinical presentation of, 241–242
    diagnosis of, 243
    management of, 243–244
Cystoscopy
    for benign prostatic hyperplasia, 251
    for hematuria, 268
Cysts, thyroid, 427
Cytologic analysis, 107
Cytomegaloviruses (CMVs), 533
Cytomegalovirus esophagitis, 195
Cytomegalovirus mononucleosis, 565
Cytomegalovirus retinitis, management of in HIV infection, 557

Danazol, for breast pain, 371
Dapsone, for *Pneumocystis carinii* pneumonia, 554
Darkfield microscopy, for syphilis, 537
Dawn phenomenon, 399
Deafness, 45–48
Debrox Drops, 58
Decongestants
    for allergic rhinitis, 82t
    for nasal symptoms of cold, 60–61
    for otitis media, 55
    for serous otitis, 55–56
    for sinusitis, 69
    for vasomotor rhinitis, 84
Deep venous thromboses (DVTs)
    diagnosis of, 182–183
    incidence of, 182
    management of, 183–184
    predisposing conditions of, 185
    prevention of, 185
    treatment of, 184
Degenerative joint disease. *See* Osteoarthritis
Delirium, 497
Dementia
    in elderly, 495–499
    in HIV infection, 557
Dengue fever, 634
Densitometry, for osteoporosis, 309
Dental procedures
    endocarditis risk with, 168
    recommended prophylactic regimen for, 170t

Depression, 506
  antidepressants for, 508–511, 509t
  contributing causes of, 507
  course and prognosis of, 507–508
  diagnosis of, 7, 506–507
    differential, 501–502
    with drug use, 6–7
  fatigue with, 6–7
  management of in HIV infection, 557
  masked, 520
  neuroleptics for, 511
  nondrug therapy for, 511
  suicide assessment with, 508
  unipolar versus bipolar, 507
  weight loss with, 15, 16
Depressive equivalent disorder, 520
De Quervain's disease, 333
Dermatitis
  contact, of external ear, 51
  peripheral venous disease, 174
Dermatographism, 587
Dermatoses, with chronic venous insufficiency, 173–174
Desipramine
  for dementia in elderly, 498
  in elderly patients, 498, 508
  side effects of, 508, 509t
Detrusor instability, 275
  treatment of, 276
Dexamethasone
  for allergic rhinitis, 83
  for altitude sickness, 636
  preparations of, 439t
Dextromethorphan
  for acute lower respiratory tract infection, 105
  for irritable bowel syndrome, 208
Dextrothyroxine, for cholesterol reduction, 624
Diabetes Control and Complications Trial (DCCT), 394
Diabetes (mellitus)
  diagnosis of, 391–393
    criteria for, 391–392
  diarrhea with, 220
  and erectile dysfunction, 385
  gestational, 391, 392
  goals of therapy for, 394
  management of complications of, 406
    macrovascular, 407–408
    microvascular, 406–407
  screening for, 391
  secondary, 393
  type I, 392
    management of, 394–400
  type II, 392
    management of, 401–405
  types of, 391
  ulcer and foot care in, 408
  visual problems with, 42–43
  weight loss with, 15–16
Diabetic nephropathy
  chronic renal failure with, 252
  management of, 406–407
Diabetic neuropathy, management of, 407
Diabetic retinopathy, 406

Diabetic ulcers, care of, 408
Diaphragm, vaginal, 348
Diarrhea
  acute, 212–217
  chronic, 218–220
  management of in HIV infection, 557
  parasitic causes of, 567
  traveler's, 632–633
Diastolic blood pressure
  lowering of, 112
  normal vs. abnormal, 111
Diastolic hypertension
  mild, 112
  moderate-to-severe, 111–112
Diastolic murmurs, 160
Diazepam, 503, 504t
Dicloxacillin, for otitis externa, 52
Dicyclomine (Bentyl)
  for diverticulosis, 211
  for irritable bowel syndrome, 208
Didanosin (ddL), for HIV infection, 553
Dideoxycytidine (ddC), for HIV infection, 553
Diet
  Atkins, 13
  Beverly Hills, 13
  cholesterol-lowering, 622, 706–711
  for constipation, 223
  for diverticulosis, 210
  for dyspepsia, 199
  high-carbohydrate, 13–14
  high-fiber, 704–706
  for insulin-dependent diabetes, 395–396
  for irritable bowel syndrome, 208
  liquid, 18
  low carbohydrate, 13
  low purine, 262
  low-salt, 701–703
  for obesity, 11
  for peptic ulcer disease, 203
  for premenstrual syndrome, 364
  Scarsdale, 13
  single-food, 13
  for type II diabetes, 402–403
  and urticaria, 588
  vegetarian, 13
  very-low-calorie, 12
Diffuse esophageal spasm
  diagnosis of, 189
  dysphagia with, 189
  treatment of, 189
Diflunisal (Dolobid), for rheumatoid arthritis, 288
Digitalis. See also Digoxin
  as cause of death in WPW syndrome patients, 145
  to improve myocardial contractility, 136–137
  premature ventricular contractions with, 147
Digital rectal examination
  for colorectal cancer screening, 595
  for hematochezia, 230
  for prostate cancer, 651
Digoxin. See also Digitalis
  for cor pulmonale, 102
  and erectile dysfunction, 385

for paroxysmal supraventricular tachycardia, 145
Dihydroergotamine, for headache, 464
Diloxanide furoate, for amebiasis, 569
Diltiazem
  for angina pectoris, 131
  for hypertension, 121–122
Diphenhydramine (Benadryl)
  for nocturnal leg cramps, 338
  for parkinsonism, 491
  for rhinitis, 81t
  for sore throat, 61
  for urticaria, 589
Diphenoxylate-atropine (Lomotil), 216
Diphtheria, sore throat with, 73
Dipivefrin, for glaucoma, 39
Direct-smear fluorescent antibody test
  for chlamydial infections, 536
  for syphilis, 537
Disability
  with chronic low back pain, 324–325
  determination of with work-related injury or illness, 639–640
  with rheumatoid arthritis, 294–295
  work-related, 637
Disopyramide
  for premature ventricular contractions, 149
  premature ventricular contractions with, 147
Disseminated gonococcal infections (DGIs), 533
Distal interphalangeal joints, osteoarthritis of, 283
Distance vision testing, 41
Disulfiram (Antabuse), 530
Diuretics
  for afterload reduction, 137
  for congestive heart failure, 135–136
  for cor pulmonale, 102
  edema with abuse of, 660
  and erectile dysfunction, 384
  for headache, 465
  for hypertension, 118–119
  thiazide
    hypercalcemia and, 432, 433
    for osteoporosis prevention, 311
    for renal stone disease, 261
Diverticular disease, 209–212
Diverticulitis, 211–212
Diverticulosis, 209–211
Dix-Hallpike maneuver
  for dizziness, 1
  pathognomonic for paroxysmal positional vertigo, 3
Dizziness, 1–4
Dog bites, 679
Donovanosis. *See* Granuloma inguinale
Dopamine, in parkinsonism, 490
Doppler echocardiography. *See* Echocardiography
Doppler ultrasonography
  for peripheral vascular disease, 178
  for thrombophlebitis diagnosis, 183
  for transient ischemic attack, 482
Down syndrome, evaluation of athlete with, 604–605
Doxazosin, for hypertension, 122

Doxycycline
  for chlamydial infections, 536
  for epididymitis, 248
  for malaria prevention, 634
  for PID, 368
  for prostatitis, 247
  for sinusitis, 68
  for syphilis, 538
  for urethritis, 544
Drug abuse
  differential diagnosis of, 502
  fatigue and, 6
  weight loss with, 16
Drug-induced premature ventricular contractions, 147
Drugs. *See specific agents*
Duodenal ulcer
  complications of, 202
  perforated, 202–203
Durable Power of Attorney, 600
Dysmenorrhea, 360–362
Dyspareunia, 380, 382
Dyspepsia, 197–199
Dysphagia, 187
  causes of, 187
  clinical conditions of, 188–190
  esophageal, 187
  evaluation of, 187–188
  with GERD, 192
  pre-esophageal, 187
  progressive, 187–188
Dysphonia plicae ventricularis, 76
Dsyphoric disorder, late luteal-phase (LLPDD), 362
Dysuria, treatment of in women, 244

Ear problems, 45–58
Ear canal, cleaning of, 52
Ear-nose-throat (ENT) consultation, 46–47
Earwax
  chemical softeners of, 58
  chronic care for, 58
  creation of, 56
  functions of, 56–57
  hearing loss with, 46
  removal of, 57–58
Eating habits, fatigue and, 6
Echocardiography
  for congestive heart failure, 135
  for heart murmur diagnosis, 161
  for mitral valve prolapse, 163–164
  for prosthetic valve evaluation, 166
Echophonocardiography
  for early systolic murmurs, 160
  for heart murmur diagnosis, 161
Echothiophate iodide (Phospholine Iodide), for glaucoma, 39
Ectopic hyperthyroidism, 419
Ectopic pregnancy, 369
Ectropion, 32
Eczematoid dermatoses
  of external ear, 51
  in peripheral venous disease, 174
Edema, 658–661
  with chronic venous insufficiency, 173
  with NSAIDs, 301

Edrophonium
  for intractable hiccups, 682
  for paroxysmal supraventricular tachycardia, 145
Effersyllium, for hemorrhoids, 227
Ehlers-Danlos syndrome, association of with mitral valve prolapse, 162
Elderly
  asthma in, 94
  cataracts in, 33–34
  dementia in, 495–499
  depression in, 507
  dizziness in, 4
  drug selection for hypertension in, 123
  evaluation of cholesterol levels and CHD risk in, 622
  hypothermia in, 668
  ictal stupor in, 470–471
  midsystolic murmurs in, 158–159
  risk of pneumococcal disease in, 611
  systolic hypertension in, 113
  urinary incontinence in, 274–277
Electrical cardioversion
  for atrial fibrillation, 153
  for paroxysmal supraventricular tachycardia, 145
Electrocardiography (ECG)
  for atrial fibrillation diagnosis, 152
  for COPD diagnosis, 97
  in dyspepsia diagnosis, 198
  in mitral valve prolapse management, 164
  for paroxysmal supraventricular tachycardia, 143
  for premature ventricular contraction diagnosis, 148
  resting, 128–129
  signal-averaged, 656
Electroconvulsive therapy (ECT), 498, 511
Electroencephalography (EEG)
  for diagnosis of syncope, 656
  for evaluation of dementia, 498
  for seizures, 472
Electrolyte replacement, for acute diarrhea, 215–216
Electronystagmography (ENG), 3
Electrophysiologic studies
  of rectosigmoid colon, 207
  for syncope diagnosis, 656
Embolectomy, 179
Embolic stroke, 151, 153
Emepronium bromide, causing esophagitis, 196
Emphysema, 95–96
Enalapril, for hypertension, 120–121
Endarterectomy. *See* Carotid endarterectomy
Endocarditis, infective
  with mitral valve prolapse, 163
  patients at risk for, 168
  procedures causing risk of, 168–169
  prophylaxis for, 167–171
  with prosthetic valves, 166–167
  recommended prophylactic regimens for, 169–171
Endocervical polyps, abnormal bleeding with, 359

Endometrial polyps, abnormal bleeding with, 359
Endometriosis, dysmenorrhea with, 361
Endometritis
  causing abnormal uterine bleeding, 358
  treatment of, 359
Endometrium
  atrophic, 359
  biopsy of for abnormal uterine bleeding, 359
  estrogen effect on cancer of, 375–376
Endophthalmitis, fulminant, 34–35
Endoscopic retrograde pancreaticocholangiography, 235
Endoscopic sphincterotomy
  for choledocholithiasis, 238
  for gallstone pancreatitis, 238
Endoscopy, upper GI
  for achalasia diagnosis, 188–189
  for gastroesophageal reflux disease, 192–193
  for peptic ulcer disease, 202
Endovaginal ultrasonography
  for abnormal uterine bleeding, 359
  for PID, 367
End-stage renal disease (ESRD)
  diabetic, 407
  management approaches to, 254
  referral and therapy for, 256
  treatment of, 256
Entamoeba histolytica
  cysts of, 569
  sexually transmitted, 533
Enteritis, sexually transmitted, 546
Enterobiasis, 567, 570
  detection of, 568
Enterotest, for parasitic infections, 568
Entropion, 32
Environmental illnesses, in travelers, 635–636
Environmental modification, for allergic rhinitis, 80
Enzyme-linked immunosorbent assay (ELISA)
  for chlamydial infections, 536
  for hepatitis, 582
  in HIV infection diagnosis, 550
Eosinophilia
  in amebiasis, 569
  in ascariasis, 569
  in parasitic infections, 568
  with strongyloidiasis, 571
Eosinophilia-myalgia syndrome, 517
Eosinophils, with allergic rhinitis, 80
Epicondylitis
  lateral, 333
  medial, 334
Epidemic keratoconjunctivitis, 29
Epidermoid cancer, hoarseness with, 78
Epididymitis, 248
  differential diagnosis of, 248
  treatment of, 248
  with urethritis, 545
Epiglottitis, 73
  hoarseness with, 76

Epilepsy. *See* Seizures
Epinephrine
 for glaucoma, 39
 for systemic reaction to bee sting, 591
 for urticaria, 589
Epithelial tumors, premalignant and malignant, 699
Epstein-Barr virus (EBV)
 antibodies against, 565–566
 in chronic fatigue syndrome, 7
 host cells for, 563–564
 infectious mononucleosis with, 563–566
 sore throat with, 72
Erectile failure, 384–388
Ergotamines
 to abort headache, 465
 rebound headache with, 462
Ergoloid mesylates (Hydergine), for dementia in elderly, 498
Erythema multiforme, 698
Erythrocytosis, 453
Erythromycin
 for chlamydial infections, 536
 for chancroid, 543
 for group A streptococcal pharyngitis, 72
 for *Mycoplasma* infections of ear, 52
 for urethritis, 544
Erythropoietin, 454
 use of in chronic renal failure, 256
Escherichia coli
 fecal, 219
 in traveler's diarrhea, 632–633
 in urinary tract infections in women, 241
Esophageal dysphagia, 187
Esophageal manometry
 for achalasia diagnosis, 188
 for gastroesophageal reflux disease, 193
Esophageal reflux, dysphagia with, 189–190
Esophageal rings, lower, 190
Esophageal sphincter, lower, incompetence of, 191
Esophageal webs, dysphagia with, 190
Esophagitis, 191
 infectious, 195–196
 medication-induced, 196
 physically induced, 196
 reflux, 191–195
Esophagus
 corkscrew, 189
 diffuse spasm of, 189
 dilatation of, 189
 monilial infection of, 190
 physically induced injury of, 196
 pseudodiverticulosis of, 189
 radiation-induced injury of, 196
Estrogens
 for abnormal uterine bleeding, 358
 benefits and risks of, 378
 for benign prostatic hyperplasia, 251
 breast cancer risk with, 376
 for coronary heart disease, 375
 edema with, 660
 endometrial cancer risk with, 375–376
 and erectile dysfunction, 385
 excess of in premenstrual syndrome, 363
 gallbladder disease risk with, 376
 for hot flashes, 373–374
 long-term risks associated with deficiency of, 374–375
 for osteoporosis, 310, 375
 regimens of for postmenopausal therapy, 376–378
 risks and side effects of, 375–376
 starting doses, recommended, in menopause, 377*t*
 uterine bleeding risk with, 376
Ethambutol, for tuberculosis, 577
Ethmoid sinuses, Water's view of, 67*f*
Ethosuximide (Zarontin), for seizures, 476–478, 575*t*
Exercise, 626
 benefits of, 626
 counseling and patient education on, 597–599
 fatigue with inadequate, 6
 for low back pain, 324
 for nocturnal leg cramps, 339
 for obesity, 11
 pre-exercise evaluation for, 627–628
 prescription for, 628–629
 to prevent reinfarction, 141–142
 for rheumatoid arthritis, 293–294
 risk of coronary events with, 626–627
 risk of heat injury with, 671–672
 risks associated with, 627
 for shoulder pain, 318–319
Exercise-induced asthma, 94
Exercise-induced hypoglycemia, 411–412
Exercise testing
 for angina pectoris, 129
 in obesity, 11
Exertional heat injury, 671–673
Exophytic oral lesions, 699–700
Expectorants
 for acute lower respiratory tract infection, 105
 for COPD, 100–101
 for coughs, 61
External urinary catheters, 281–282
Extracorporeal shock wave lithotripsy (ESWL), 237
 for renal stones, 264
Extremities
 arterial diseases of, 177–181
 venous diseases of, 173–177
Eye problems, 21–44. *See also specific conditions*
Eyelid
 disorders of, 31–32
 foreign bodies in, 21

Facial paralysis, idiopathic, 493–495
"False cord hoarseness," 76
Famotidine (Pepcid)
 for gastroesophageal reflux disease, 193–194
 for peptic ulcer disease, 203
Fanconi's anemia, 357
Fasting blood glucose (FBG), 391, 392, 393

Fasting hyperglycemia, 399
Fasting hypoglycemia
  causes of, 410
  diagnosis of, 410–411
  versus postprandial hypoglycemia, 410
Fat. *See also* Cholesterol; Lipoproteins
  dietary consumption of, 597
  monounsaturated, 708
  polyunsaturated, 707–708
  saturated, 707
  total dietary, 707
Fatigue, 5–8
  with infectious mononucleosis, 564
Fatty acids, omega-3, 708
Fecal electrolyte levels, 220
Fecal leukocyte examination, 214–215
Fecal occult blood testing, 231
  for colorectal cancer screening, 595
Female sexual dysfunction, 380
  detection and evaluation of, 380
  intervention for, 382–383
  organic causes of, 381–382
  types of, 380
Fenamates, 298*t*
Fenfluramine, for obesity, 13
Ferrous sulfate therapy, 445–446
Fetus
  assessing risks of drug exposure of, 688
  timing of development of, 688*t*
Fever, with HIV infection, 554
Fiber. *See also* High-fiber diet
  in cholesterol-lowering diet, 709
  dietary, 704*t*, 705
  methods for adding to diet, 705*t*
Fibrillation. *See* Atrial fibrillation; Ventricular fibrillation
Fibroadenomas, breast, 370
Fibrogen degradation product assays, 183
Fibromuscular subaortic stenosis, midsystolic murmur with, 159–160
Fibromyalgia, 336
Fibrositis, 336
Filariasis, 634
Fine-needle aspiration biopsy
  for breast lumps, 369, 370
  for thyroid nodules, 426
Fitz-Hugh-Curtis syndrome, 365
Flavoxate (Urispas), for detrusor instability, 276
Flecainide
  for paroxysmal supraventricular tachycardia prevention, 146
  for premature ventricular contractions, 149
  premature ventricular contractions with, 147
  to prevent atrial fibrillation, 154
Flecainide-like drugs, for premature ventricular contractions, 149
Floaters, in the eye, 43
Fluconazole, for oral candidiasis, 556
Fluid intake
  for acute diarrhea, 215–216
  for heat injury, 673
  for renal stone disease, 261
Fluid retention, in premenstrual syndrome, 363

Flunisolide (Nasalide), for allergic rhinitis, 83
Fluorescein angiogram, intravenous, 42–43
Fluorescein strips, 24
Fluorescent treponemal antibody absorption test (FTA-ABS)
  for HIV infection, 552
  for syphilis, 538
Fluori-Methane, for myofascial pain, 337
Fluoxetine, 509*t*
  for obesity, 13
  side effects of, 508–510
Fluphenazine (Prolixin), for diabetic neuropathy, 407
Flurazepam (Dalmane), for insomnia, 516*t*, 517
Fluttering tinnitus, 49
Folate deficiency, 447
Foley catheter, urine leakage around, 281
Follicular thyroid carcinoma, 427
Food allergy, causing rhinitis, 79
Food intake
  circumstances contributing to decrease in, 17
  decreased, 15
  measures to increase, 18
Foot care, in diabetics, 408
Footwear, for rheumatoid arthritis, 294
Forced expiratory volume in 1 second (FEV1)/forced vital capacity (FVC) ratio
  in asthma, 88
  in COPD, 97
Foreign bodies, ocular, 21–23
Fosinopril, for hypertension, 120–121
Fractures, osteoporosis risk with, 307, 311
Frontal sinuses, Water's view of, 67*f*
Frontal sinusitis, acute, 69
Frostbite, 669–670
Frozen shoulder, evaluation for, 318
Fulminant hepatitis, 582
Functional capacity, exercise to increase, 627
Functional incontinence, 275
  treatment of, 277
Fungal infections
  of external ear, 50–51
  mouth ulcers with, 697
Fungal rashes, with HIV infection, 558
Furazolidone, for giardiasis, 569
Furosemide, for congestive heart failure, 136

Gaisböck's syndrome, 454
Gait analysis, 294
Gait disturbances, in dementia, 497–498
Gallbladder
  estrogen effect on disease of, 376
  gallstones with cancer of, 237
Gallstone ileus, 234
  treatment of, 239
Gallstone pancreatitis, 234
  treatment of, 238
Gallstones
  asymptomatic, 233
  chemical dissolution of, 236–237
  clinical evaluation of, 234–235

clinical syndromes of, 233–234
complications of, 234
diagnostic strategy for, 235–236
incidence of, 233
pathogenesis and epidemiology of, 233
postcholecystectomy problems with, 239
prevention of, 238
silent, 237–238
treatment for, 236–239
Gamma glutamyl transpeptidase (GGT), in diagnosis of alcoholism, 529
Gangrene, with chronic arterial insufficiency, 178
Gardnerella vaginalis, 344
in PID, 366
Gastric bubble, Garren-Edwards, 13
Gastric bypass procedures, for severe obesity, 12–13
Gastric outlet obstruction, 203
Gastric secretory testing, 202
Gastrin, serum levels of, 202
Gastroesophageal reflux disease (GERD), 191
clinical presentation of, 191–192
complications of, 194–195
diagnosis of, 192–193
hoarseness with, 76–77
treatment of, 193–194
Gastrointestinal tract
bleeding of with NSAIDs, 300
edema with disease of, 659
hyperthyroidism effects on, 417
hypothyroidism effects on, 423
NSAID effects on, 300–301
occult bleeding of, 231–232
problems of, 187–240
procedures in
endocarditis risk with, 169
recommended prophylactic regimen for, 171t
Gastroparesis, diabetic, 407
Gastroplasty, 12–13
"Gay bowel syndrome," 571
Gemfibrozil, for cholesterol reduction, 624, 625
Generalized anxiety disorder, 501–503
Genital ulcers
causes of, 545
with chancroid, 543
differential diagnosis of, 539t, 545
with herpes simplex viruses, 538
with regional adenopathy, 666
treatment of, 545–546
Genitourinary tract procedures
endocarditis risk with, 169
recommended prophylactic regimen for, 171t
Gestational diabetes mellitus (GDM), 391, 392
Giant cell arteritis, headache and, 463
Giardia diarrhea, 219
Giardia infections
detection of, 567–568
lamblia, 533, 568
Giardiasis, 568
treatment of, 569
Gingivitis, acute necrotizing ulcerative, 698

Glanzmann's thrombocytopathy, 450
abnormal uterine bleeding with, 357
Glaucoma, 36
acute, differential diagnosis of, 28
classification of, 37
with diabetes mellitus, 42
diagnosis of, 37–38
evaluation for, 37
following cataract surgery, 34–35
ocular side effects of systemic medications for, 39–40
and physiology of intraocular pressure, 36–37
risk factors for, 37
screening for, 39, 595
treatment for, 38
drugs in, 38–39
Glenohumeral joint, 316
Glomerular filtration rate (GFR), reduction of in chronic renal failure, 252
Glomerulonephritis, chronic, 252
Glucocorticoids
pharmacology of, 438
preparations of, 439t
Glucose-6-phosphate dehydrogenase (G6PD) deficiency, 448
Glucose intolerance. See Diabetes (mellitus)
Glucose tolerance
impaired, 393
test, oral (OGTT), 391, 392, 393
Gluten-sensitive enteropathy, diarrhea with, 219
Glycogen storage disease, type I, 435
Glycopyrrolate (Robinul)
for diverticulosis, 211
for irritable bowel syndrome, 208
Goiter, 428
diffuse, 428
multinodular, 428
nontoxic nodular, 430
sporadic diffuse, 429–430
toxic multinodular, 421
toxic nodular, 419
toxic uninodular, 419
treatment of, 421
Goitrous autoimmune thyroiditis, 428–429
Gold sodium thiomalate (Myochrysine), 289
Gold therapy, parenteral, 289
Gold thioglucose (Solganal), 289
Golfer's elbow, 334
Gonococcal infections, 533
antibiotic resistance of, 534
clinical presentations of, 533
management of contacts in, 535
pharyngitis, 533
treatment of, 534–535, 534t
urethritis, 544–545
Gonorrhea, 533
risk of, 533
Gout, 304
acute arthritis and, 304–305
diagnosis of, 305
prophylaxis for, 306
risk of with hyperuricemia, 436
treatment of, 305–307
trophaceous, 305

Gouty nephropathy, risk of with hyperuricemia, 436
Granuloma inguinale, 533
　genital ulcers with, 545
Graves' disease, 418
　extrathyroidal manifestations of, 421
　thyroid enlargement in, 417
　treatment of, 420–421
Grief, 522–523
　pathologic, 524–525
　phases of normal process of, 523–524
　symptoms of, 524
　treatment of, 525–526
Group therapy, for alcoholism, 529
Guaifenesin
　for COPD, 101
　for coughs, 61
Guillain-Barré syndrome
　with influenza, 63
　and influenza vaccine, 611

H2-blockers
　for dyspepsia, 199
　for gastroesophageal reflux, 193–194
　for peptic strictures, 190
　for peptic ulcer disease, 203–204
　side effects of, 203–204
H2-receptor antagonists. *See* H2-blockers
Hairy leukoplakia
　management of in HIV infection, 556
　signs and symptoms of, 551
Hand, osteoarthritis of, 283–286
Hashimoto's disease, 428–429
Hay fever conjunctivitis, 30
HB_sAg
　detection of, 581–582
　hepatitis, chronic, 581–582
　management of carriers of, 583–584
HDL cholesterol
　and CHD risk, 621
　increased levels of, 623, 624
　　and risk of CHD, 620
Headache, 457
　associated symptoms and precipitating factors in, 462–463
　associated with HIV infection, 458–459
　cluster, 458
　evaluation of, 459–463
　incidence of, 457
　location of pain in, 462
　management of in HIV infection, 556
　migraine, 457–458
　posttraumatic, 459
　prophylactic agents for, 466–467t
　prophylactic treatment of, 465–468
　syndromes of, 460–461t
　tension, 457
　time course of, 459–462
　time of day of, 462
　treatment of, 464–468
Health maintenance, 593–652
Hearing
　loss, 45–49
　　with earwax accumulation, 56–57
　　functional, 46

　　sensorineural, 46
　syndromes, 47
　problems with, 45–58
　screening for, 595–596
Hearing aids, 48
Heart murmurs, 157–158
　continuous, 160
　diastolic, 160
　evaluation of, 160–161
　systolic, 158–160
Heart rate, exercise program and, 628
Heat
　for neck pain, 313
　for rheumatoid arthritis, 293
Heat cramps, treatment of, 673
Heat edema, 660
Heat injury (exhaustion/stroke), 671–673
Heberden's nodes
　osteoarthritis in, 283
　x-ray evaluation of, 284
Helicobacter pylori, in peptic ulcer disease, 200, 204–205
Heller's myotomy, for achalasia, 189
Helminth infections, 567, 569–570
Helper T-cell measurement, 551
Helsinki Heart Study, mortality results of, 620
Hemangiomas, oral mucosal, 699
Hematochezia, 230
　evaluation of, 230–231
Hematocrit
　normal, 444t
　in polycythemia, 455
Hematomas, 675–676
Hematopoietic system
　hyperthyroidism effects on, 417
　hypothyroidism effects on, 423
Hematuria, 265
　determination of presence of, 265–266
　diagnostic strategy for, 266
　evaluation for, 266–269
　follow-up for, 269
　referrals for, 269
　screening for, 265
Hemoccult test, 232
Hemodialysis, for diabetic nephropathy, 407
Hemoglobin
　electrophoresis of, 448
　normal, 444t
Hemolysis, with prosthetic valves, 167
Hemophilia A, 450
Hemophilus ducreyi
　chancroid with, 542–543
　genital ulcers with, 545
Hemophilus influenzae
　causing otitis media, 53
　corneal infection with, 28
　epiglottitis with, 73, 76
　type B
　　prophylactic interventions for, 601
　　vaccine for, 613
Hemorrhage. *See also* Bleeding, abnormal
　with duodenal ulcer, 202
　occult gastrointestinal, 231–232
Hemorrhoids, 225
　acute thrombosis and, 226–227

bleeding with, 230
differential diagnosis of, 226
external, 225
  diagnosis of, 226
internal, 225
  diagnosis of, 225–226
pruritus ani with, 228–229
reasons for referral of, 227
treatment of, 227
Hemostasis, normal, 449
Heparin, for acute thrombophlebitis treatment, 184
Hepatitis
nonviral causes of, 580
with NSAIDs, 301
prophylactic interventions for, 601
type A, 579
  vaccination for, 632
type B, 579
  clinical presentation of, 580
  groups at risk for, 580t
  needlestick exposure to, 584–585
  prevention of, 584–585
  serologic tests for, 581
  time course for appearance of abnormalities of, 581f
  transmission by human bites, 679
  vaccine for, 584, 600, 612–613, 632
type C, 579–580, 580
type D, 580
viral, 533
  diagnosis of, 580–582
  fulminant, 582
  management of acute, 582–583
  management of chronic, 584
  management of contacts in, 583
  management of HB$_s$Ag carriers of, 583–584
  non-A, non-B, 579–580
  types of, 579–580
Hepatitis B immune globulin (HBIG)
  as prophylaxis, 583, 584–585
  with vaccine, 584
Herpangina, 74
Herpes simplex conjunctivitis, 29
Herpes simplex keratitis, 24
Herpes simplex viruses, 533, 538–541
  clinical presentation of, 541
  diagnosis of, 541
  esophagitis with, 195
  genital ulcers with, 545
  and HIV coinfection, 542
  infectious cervicitis with, 345
  management of in pregnant patients, 542
  management of sexual contacts in, 542
  pharyngitis with, 74
  prophylaxis for, 554
  suppressive therapy for, 542
  treatment of, 541–542
  type I, 697
Herpes zoster, 560–562
Heterophil antibodies, spot tests for, 565
Hiccups, 681–682
High altitude sickness, 98, 636
High-carbohydrate diets, 13–14

High-density lipoprotein (HDL)
  increase in with estrogen therapy, 375
  and risk of coronary heart disease, 616
High-fiber diets, 704–706
  benefits of, 704–705
  for constipation, 223
  for diverticulosis, 210
  potential side effects of, 705–706
Hip, osteoarthritis of, 284
Hirschsprung's disease, constipation with, 224
Histamine, for headache, 468
HIV. See Human immunodeficiency virus (HIV) infection
Hives. See Urticaria
HMG-CoA reductase inhibitors, for lowering cholesterol in diabetics, 408
Hoarseness, 75–78
"Hollenhorst plaques," 43
Honeymoon cystitis, 241
Hookworm, 567, 570
Hordeolum, 31
  treatment for, 32
Hormones, in premenstrual syndrome, 363
Horner's syndrome, vertigo with, 2
Hot flashes
  incidence of in perimenopausal women, 373
  treatment of, 373–374
Human bites, 678–679
Human chorionic gonadotropin hormone, for obesity, 13
Human immunodeficiency virus (HIV) infection, 533
  antiviral and prophylactic treatment measures for, 552–554
  approach to common symptoms and problems of, 554–558
  diagnosis of, 463, 550
  diarrhea with, 557
  encephalopathy, 557
  fever with, 554
  genital ulcers with, 545
  headache associated with, 458–459, 556
  with herpes simplex virus, 542
  immunizations and, 613
  incidence of, 549–550
  with lymphadenopathy, 664, 666
  management of patient with, 549–559
  medical evaluation and monitoring of, 551–552
  mental status changes in, 557
  mouth lesions in, 556
  parasitic infections in, 567
  respiratory symptoms of, 555–556
  screening for, 596–597
  seizures with, 557
  serologic test for, 665
  skin problems with, 558
  supportive care for, 558–559
  symptoms and signs of, 551
  and syphilis, 538
  transmission by human bites, 679
  tuberculosis with, 572
  visual disturbances in, 557
  weight loss with, 557–558

Huntington's disease, dementia with, 496–497
Hydralazine
  for afterload reduction, 138
  for congestive heart failure, 138
  edema with, 660
  for hypertension, 122–123
Hydration
  for acute diarrhea, 215–216
  for hypercalcemia, 434
Hydrocephalus, normal-pressure, dementia with, 496
Hydrochlorothiazide, for congestive heart failure, 136
Hydrocil Instant, 227
Hydrogen peroxide, for cerumen removal, 58
Hydroxychloroquine (Plaquenil), for rheumatoid arthritis, 292
Hydroxyzine (Atarax, Vistaril), for urticaria, 589
Hyperaldosteronism, hypertension with, 115
Hypercalcemia, 431
  causes of, 432–433
  definition of, 431–432
  drugs causing, 433
  evaluation of, 433–434
  familial, 433
  familial hypercalciuric, 434
  with hyperthyroidism, 418
  management of, 434
  symptoms of, 432
Hypercalciuria, 261
Hyperextension injuries, neck pain with, 312
Hyperglycemia, fasting and, 399
Hyperkalemia
  management of in chronic renal failure, 255
  with NSAIDs, 301
Hyperlipidemia, promoting atherosclerosis, 141
Hypernatremia, with heat injury, 672
Hyperparathyroidism
  hypercalcemia and, 432, 433
  primary, 433
Hyperphosphatemia, management of in chronic renal failure, 255
Hypertension, 111
  atrial fibrillation with, 151
  benefits of treatment for, 111–112
  confirmation of, 114
  detection of secondary, 114–115
  drugs that cause, 114–115
  drug therapy for, 117–123
  general concerns of, 124
  initial evaluation for, 114–116
  isolated systolic, 113
  mild diastolic, 112
  moderate-to-severe diastolic, 111–112
  monotherapy options for, 118t
  nonpharmacologic therapy for, 116–117
  patient education on, 114
  resistant, 123–124
  and risk of coronary heart disease, 616
  risks of, 111
  screening for, 593
  selecting safe and effective therapy for, 115–116
  selective stepped-care for, 124t
  strategies for compliance in therapy for, 116
  strategy for drug selection and initial resistance to, 123
  treatment decisions in, 112–113
Hypertensive nephrosclerosis, 252
Hyperthermia, 671–673
Hyperthyroidism, 416
  causes of, 418–419
  clinical manifestations of, 416–418
  evaluation of suspected, 414–415
  exogenous, 419
  laboratory diagnosis of, 418
  psychological symptoms of, 416
  screening for, 596
  treatment options for, 419–420
Hypertrophic joint disease. See Osteoarthritis
Hyperuricemia, 435–436
Hyperuricosuria
  treatment of, 262
  with uric acid stones, 258
Hyperventilation
  differential diagnosis of, 471
  dizziness with, 1
Hypnotics, 516t
  insomnia and, 514, 517
Hypoalbuminemia, edema with, 659
Hypocalcemia, management of in chronic renal failure, 255–256
Hypochondriasis, 520
Hypocitraturia, 258
Hypoglycemia, 409–412
  with hypothermia, 669
  in premenstrual syndrome, 363
  treatment of, in diabetes, 399–400
Hypoglycemic drugs
  oral, 403, 404t
  for type II diabetes, 403–405
Hypogonadism, and erectile dysfunction, 385
Hypokalemia
  with heat injury, 672
  management of in chronic renal failure, 255
Hyponatremia, with heat injury, 672
Hyposensitization, for allergic rhinitis, 83
Hypotension, postural, 654–655
Hypothalamic dysfunction, 506–507
Hypothalamus-pituitary-adrenal (HPA) axis
  response of to stress, 441
  suppression of, 438
Hypothermia, 667–669
Hypothyroidism, 422
  causes of, 423–424
  causing rhinitis, 85
  clinical features of, 422–423
  evaluation of suspected, 414
  laboratory diagnosis of, 423
  obesity with, 10
  primary, 424
  screening for, 596
  secondary, 424
  subclinical, 422

transient, 424
treatment of, 424–425
Hypothyrotropic hypothyroidism, 424
Hypovolemia, with heat injury, 672
Hysteroscopy, 359

Iatrogenic hypoglycemia, 411
Iatrogenic incontinence, 275
Ibuprofen
  for dysmenorrhea, 361
  NSAIDs, 297t
  for rheumatoid arthritis, 289
Ictal stupor, 470–471
Idiopathic hypertrophic subaortic stenosis (IHSS)
  endocarditis risk with, 168
  midsystolic murmur with, 159
Idoxuridine, allergic reaction to, 30
Imidazole, for candidal vaginitis, 341–342
Imipramine
  for depression, 508–509t
  for detrusor instability, 276
  for sphincter insufficiency, 277
Immersion foot, 669
Immune complex disease, features of, 587
Immune dysfunction. *See* Chronic fatigue syndrome
Immune serum globulin (ISG), 583
Immunizations, 599t, 600, 608–615
  hepatitis B, 584, 600, 612–613
  HIV infection, 554, 613
  influenza, 64, 599t, 600, 610–611
    in COPD patients, 98
  measles, 599t, 600, 608–609
  mumps, 609–610
  passive-active, 584
  plague, 631
  pneumococcal, 599t, 600, 611–612
    in COPD patients, 98
  polio, 610
  rabies, 613
  rubella, 599t, 600, 609
  tetanus, 599, 600, 608, 676, 677t
  for travelers, 630–631
Immunocompromised adults
  parasitic infections in, 567
  risk of pneumococcal disease in, 611–612
Immunoglobulin E antibody determinations, 590
Immunosuppression, infectious diarrhea in, 220
Immunotherapy
  for allergic rhinitis, 83
  for asthma, 93
  for bee stings, 591–592
Impedance plethysmography (IPG), 183
Impedance tympanometry, 54
Indole acetic acids, 297t
Infectious diseases, 533–585
  in travelers, 633–635
Infertility, with PID, 369
Inflammatory bowel disease
  with calcium oxalate and uric acid stones, 258
  signs of, 230
  weight loss with, 16

Inflammatory diarrhea, 219
Influenza, 62–64
  immunization for, 600, 630
  prevention of, 64
  treatment of, 63–64
  vaccine for, 64, 610–611
    and HIV infection, 613
Influenza A vaccine, 610
Influenza B vaccine, 610–611
Inguinal lymphadenopathy, 666
Injury
  cold, 669–670
  heat, 671–673
  minor soft tissue, 674–680
  prevention of, 597
  work-related, 637–639
Inner ear problems, deafness with, 47
Innocent murmurs, 158
Insomnia, 513–517
Insulin-dependent diabetes mellitus, (IDDM), 391, 392
  dietary management of, 395–396
  follow-up for, 400
  insulin therapy for, 396–399
  management of, 394–400
  management of metabolic complications with, 399–400
Insulin
  continuous subcutaneous infusion of, 398
  for insulin-dependent diabetes, 396–397
    initiation of, 398
    monitoring of, 398–399
    regimens for, 397–398
  intermediate, 397
  onset, action, and duration of, 397t
  split-mixed, 397–398
  for type II diabetes, 396–397, 403–405
  ultralente plus regular, 398
Interferon, for cold prevention, 61
Intermittent urinary catheterization, 279
  complications of, 279
Interstitial nephritis
  chronic renal failure with, 252–253
  with NSAIDs, 301
Intestinal tract, parasites of, 567–571
Intraocular lenses, 35
Intraocular pressure
  elevation of with corticosteroids, 39–40
  measurements of, 41
  physiology of, 36–37
Intrauterine devices (IUDs), 351
  dysmenorrhea with, 362
  and risk of PID, 351–356, 366
Intravenous pyelogram (IVP)
  for benign prostatic hyperplasia, 250
  in chronic renal failure, 253
  in discovery of renal stones, 259
  in evaluation of renal colic, 263
  for hematuria, 268
Iodine-induced hyperthyroidism, 419
Iodoquinol, for amebiasis, 569
Iritis, acute, 26–28
Iron deficiency anemia, 444–445
  treatment of, 445–446
Irritable bowel syndrome, 206–208

Ischemic arterial disease, limb-threatening, 177
Ischemic cerebrovascular events, 471
Ischemic ulcers, with chronic arterial insufficiency, 179
Isometheptene, for headaches, 465
Isoniazid
 effectiveness of, 574–575
 patient management with, 575
 resistance to, 577
 risks of, 575
 for tuberculosis, 574–577
Isospora belli infections, 567
Isosporiasis, 571
Isradipine, for hypertension, 121–122

Japanese B encephalitis, 634
 vaccination for, 632
Jejunoileal bypass, 13
Jet lag, 635
Joints, replacement of for osteoarthritis, 286

Kaposi's sarcoma
 with HIV infection, 558
 signs and symptoms of, 551
Keratitis, 26
Keratoconjunctivitis
 epidemic, 29
 vernal, 30
Ketoacidosis, treatment of, 400
Ketoconazole
 for candida esophagitis, 195
 for candidal vaginitis, 342
 for oral candidiasis, 556
Kidney stones. *See* Renal stones
Knee
 acute traumatic events of, 329
 demonstration of effusion of, 327f
 loose bodies in, 330
 mechanical derangements of, 326
 mechanical instability of, 327, 328f
 osteoarthritis of, 284
 physical examination of, 327–328
 recurrent acute painful episodes in, 329–330
 subluxations, recurrent, 330
 torn ligaments of, 329
Knee pain, 326
 chronic aching, treatment of, 330–331
 evaluation for, 326–328
 management of, 328–331
 physical examination of patient with, 327–328
Korotkoff sound, fifth-phase, 111
Kwashiorkor, edema with, 659

Labyrinthitis
 assessment and treatment of, 3
 vertigo with, 3
 viral, 3
Lachman's test, 327, 329f
Lactation, medications in. *See* Breast-feeding
Laparoscopic cholecystectomy, 233
Laparoscopy, 367
Laryngeal mass lesions, 78

Laryngeal nerve damage, hoarseness with, 76
Laryngeal paralysis, 78
Laryngitis
 smoker's, 77
 treatment of, 78
 viral, 76
Late luteal-phase dysphoric disorder (LLPDD), 362
Lateral epicondylitis, 333
Laxatives
 cessation of use of, 223–224
 constipation in conjunction with, 221–222
 edema with abuse of, 660
 noninflammatory diarrhea with use of, 220
LDL cholesterol
 classification of CHD risk by, 620–621
 lowering of and risk of CHD, 620
 removal of from plasma, 623–624
L-dopa, for parkinsonism, 490–491
Left ventricular end-diastolic pressure (LVEDP), elevated, 134
Leg cramps, nocturnal, 337–339
Leiomyomas
 causing abnormal uterine bleeding, 358
 dysphagia with, 190
Leishmaniasis, 634
Lens
 clouding of, 32–36. *See also* Cataracts
 intraocular, 35
LGV. *See* Lymphogranuloma venereum (LGV)
Lichen planus, 697
 white lesions with, 699
Lidocaine, for headache, 465
Lidocaine-like drugs, for premature ventricular contractions, 149
Life-style modification
 for gastroesophageal reflux disease, 193
 post-myocardial infarction, social reinforcement of, 142
Light-headedness
 causes of, 4
 dizziness with, 4
Lipid Research Clinic Coronary Primary Prevention Trial (LRC-CPPT), 620
Lipodermatosclerosis
 with chronic venous insufficiency, 173–174
 treatment of, 174
Lipoproteins. *See also* Cholesterol; High-density lipoprotein; Low-density lipoprotein
 estrogen effect on, 375
Liposuction, 13
Liquid diets, nutritionally complete, 18
Lisinopril, for hypertension, 120–121
Lithium
 for depression, 510
 for headache, 468
 and hypercalcemia, 432
Lithotripsy, 237
Liver
 biopsy of for hepatitis, 582–583
 edema with disease of, 659
 methotrexate effects on, 292

Liver function tests
 abnormal, with heat injury, 672
 carbamazepine effects on, 478
 for hepatitis, 581
 nicotinic acid effects on, 623
 NSAID effects on, 301
 valproic acid effects on, 478
Living Will, 600
Loop diuretics, for congestive heart failure, 136
Loperamide (Imodium), for acute diarrhea, 216
Lorazepam (Ativan), for anxiety, 503
Lovastatin, for cholesterol reduction, 408, 624–625
Low back pain, 320
 bed rest for, 323
 etiology of, 320–321
 evaluation of, 321–322
 physical examination of patient with, 322t
 recurrent and chronic, 324–325
 surgery for, 325
 treatment of acute episodes of, 322–324
Low-calcium diet, 261
Low carbohydrate diets, 13
Low-density lipoprotein (LDL)
 decrease in with estrogen therapy, 375
 in hypertension, 112
Lower esophageal sphincter, 191–192
Lower respiratory tract infections, acute, 103–106
 antibiotic choice for, 106t
 causes of, 103–104
 evaluation for, 104–105
 follow-up for, 105–106
 treatment of, 105
Lower respiratory tract problems, 87–110. *See also specific conditions*
Low-fat diet, 199
Low-flow oxygen therapy
 for COPD, 101
 for cor pulmonale, 102
Low-purine diet, 262
Low-salt diets, 701–703
Low vision, 43–44
Lumbar puncture
 for headache, 463
 for seizures, 473
Lumbar spine
 osteoarthritis of, 284, 285
 x-ray studies of, 322
Lumbosacral spine pain, 285
Lung cancer, and passive smoking, 641
Lupus anticoagulant, 482
Lyme disease, 676
Lymphadenopathy, 662
 associated with HIV infection, 664, 666
 causes of, 662, 663t
 chronic tender regional, 666
 diagnostic tests for, 664–665
 initial evaluation for, 662–664
 location of, 663
 physical findings in, 664
 rate of change of, 664
 specific presentations of, 665–666
 strategy for evaluation of, 665

Lymphangiography, 665
Lymph nodes
 biopsy of, 662, 664
 cervical, 665
 fluctuant, 664
Lymphogranuloma venereum (LGV), 533, 537
 diagnosis of, 537
 genital ulcers with, 545
  differential diagnosis of, 540t
  treatment of, 536t, 537

Macrocytic anemia, 446
 laboratory tests for, 446
 physical examination in, 446
 treatment of, 447
Magnetic resonance imaging
 for headaches, 463
 for seizures, 472–473
Malabsorption
 calorie loss with, 16
 diarrhea with, 217
 laboratory studies for, 17
Malaria, 633–634
Male sexual dysfunction, 384–388
Mammalian bite wounds, 678–680
Mammography, 370–371, 594, 647–649
Manic states, 507
Manipulation, for low back pain, 323
Manometry, for dysphagia, 188
Mantoux test, 596
Marfan's syndrome, association of with mitral valve prolapse, 162
Mastectomy, subcutaneous, 372
Mastoiditis
 hearing loss with, 46
 with otitis media, 55
Maxillary sinuses, Water's view of, 67f
Mazindol, for obesity, 13
Mean corpuscular hemoglobin concentration (MCHC), 444
Mean corpuscular volume (MCV), 443–444
 characterization of, 444t
Measles vaccination, 600, 608–609, 630
Mebendazole
 for ascariasis, 570
 for enterobiasis, 570
 for hookworm, 570
 for trichuriasis, 570
Meclizine, for paroxysmal positional vertigo, 3
Medial epicondylitis, 334
Medullary thyroid carcinoma, 427
 family history of, 426
Mefenamic acid (Ponstel), for dysmenorrhea, 361
Mefloquine (Lariam), for malaria, 634
Meniere's disease
 hearing loss with, 47
 tinnitus with, 48
 treatment of, 3
 vertigo with, 3
Meningitis, headache with, 459
Meningococcal infection
 prophylactic interventions for, 601
 vaccination for, 631

Meningoencephalitis, 63
Meniscal tears, treatment of, 329–330
Menopause, 373
 estrogen therapy for, 375–376
  benefits and risks of, 378
  regimens for, 376–378
 and long-term risks of estrogen deficiency, 374–375
 symptoms of, 373–374
Menorrhagia, 357–358
 definition, 357
 treatment of, 359
Menses, cessation of. *See* Menopause
Menstruation, norms of, 357
Metabolic acidosis, management of in chronic renal failure, 256
Metabolic disorders, 391–441
Metabolism
 hyperthyroidism effects on, 417
 increased rate of with weight loss, 16
Metamucil
 for hemorrhoids, 227
 in high-fiber diet, 705, 705*t*
 for irritable bowel syndrome, 208
Metatarsal phalangeal joints, osteoarthritis of, 283
Metered-dose inhalers (MDIs)
 for asthma, 89–91
 for COPD, 99
 for headache, 465
Methazolamide (Neptazane), for glaucoma, 39
Methimazole (MMI)
 for Graves' disease, 420
 for hyperthyroidism, 419–420
Methocarbamol (Robaxin), for nocturnal leg cramps, 338
Methotrexate, for rheumatoid arthritis, 292–293
Methyldopa, for hypertension, 122
Methylxanthines, breast pain with, 371
Methysergide, for headache, 465, 466*t*, 468
Metoclopramide
 for diabetic neuropathy, 407
 for dyspepsia, 199
 and erectile dysfunction, 385
 for intractable hiccups, 682
Metronidazole (Flagyl, Protostat)
 for amebiasis, 569
 for bacterial vaginosis, 344
 for giardiasis, 569
 for trichomonas vaginitis, 343
Mexiletine, for premature ventricular contractions, 149
Miconazole, for candidal vaginitis, 342
Microcytic reticulocytopenic anemia, 444–445
 evaluation of, 445
 treatment of, 445–446
Micturition, syncope and, 655
Migraine, 457–458
 abortive therapy for, 465
 causes of, 458
 classifications of, 457
 differential diagnosis of, 471
 pain quality in, 462
 precipitating factors of, 458
 prophylactic therapy for, 465
 symptomatic, 464
 time of day of, 462
Milk-alkali syndrome, 433
Minoxidil
 edema with, 660
 for hypertension, 123
Misoprostol (Cytolec)
 NSAIDs, 300–301
 for peptic ulcer disease, 204
Mitral regurgitation
 pansystolic murmur with, 160
 progression of to valve prolapse, 163–164
Mitral valve prolapse, 162
 approach to managing patients with, 164
 complications of, 163–164
 diagnosis of, 162–163
 prevalence of, 162
 silent, 162
Monilial infections, dysphagia with, 190. *See also Candida* esophagitis
Monoamine oxidase inhibitors
 for depression, 498, 511
 for migraine, 465
 for parkinsonism, 490
Mononucleosis, infectious, 563–566
Monounsaturated fats, 708
Morphine suppositories, for headache, 464
Motion sickness, 635
Motor paralysis, with herpes zoster, 561–562
Mouth lesions, 696–700
 exophytic, 699–700
 multiple ulcers, 697–698
 red, 699
 single ulcers, 696–697
 white, 698–699
Mucoceles, 699
Mucokinetic agents, 100–101
Mucormycosis, rhinocerebral, 68
Mucous membrane pemphigoid, benign, 697–698
Multi-infarct dementia, 496
Multinodular goiter, treatment of, 430
Multiple endocrine neoplasia (MEN), type II, 426, 427
Multiple Risk Factor Intervention Trial, long-term follow-up of, 619–620
Multiple sclerosis, vertigo with, 2
Mumps vaccine, 609–610, 630
Murmurs, evaluation of, 157–161
 continuous, 160
 midsystolic (ejection), 158
  causes of, 159–160
  in middle and old age, 158–159
  pathologic, 159–160
 pansystolic (regurgitant), 158, 160
Muscle relaxants, for low back pain, 323
Musculoskeletal system
 exercise-related injuries of, 627
 hypothyroidism effects on, 423
 pain syndromes, chronic, 336–337
 problems of, 283–339
Myasthenia gravis, hoarseness with, 76
Mycobacterial infections, of external ear, 51

Mycobacterium tuberculosis, PPD skin test for, 552
Mycoplasma infections
  of ear, 52
  in PID, 366
  pneumoniae
    differential diagnosis of, 60
    pharyngitis, 73
Myeloproliferative disorder, 454
Myocardial infarction
  atrial fibrillation with, 151
  and mitral regurgitation, 127
  prevention of recurrence and death with, 141–142
  psychological adjustment to, 140
  rehabilitation after, 139–142
  return to physical activity after, 139–140
  return to work after, 141
  sexual activity after, 140
Myofascial disorders, shoulder pain with, 316
Myofascial pain, 337
  management of, 313
  treatment of, 319, 337
Myofascial syndrome, 317
Myofascial trigger points, 337
  neck pain with, 312
Myofascitis, neck pain with, 312
Myotomy, for diffuse esophageal spasm, 189

Naproxen (Naprosyn), for dysmenorrhea, 361
Naproxen sodium (Anaprox), for dysmenorrhea, 361
Narcotics
  avoidance of in COPD, 98
  for chronic pain, 686
  and erectile dysfunction, 385
  for low back pain, 323
Narrow-QRS complex tachycardia, 143
Nasal congestion, drugs associated with, 84
Nasal polyps, 85
Nasopharyngeal cultures, 54
Nasopharyngeoscopy, 84
National Institutes of Occupational Safety and Health (NIOSH)
  information and resources of, 639
  list of work-related disease and injury of, 638
  on occupational accidents, 637
Near vision testing, 41
Necator americanus infection, 570
Neck collar, 313–314
Neck pain, 312–315
Necrotizing ulcerative gingivitis, acute, 698
Needle biopsy
  for lymphadenopathy, 664
  for solitary pulmonary nodule diagnosis, 108
Needle-stick injuries, 675
Neisseria gonorrhoeae, 533–534
  cervicitis with, 345, 546
  pharyngitis, 73
  in PID, 366
  in travelers, 635
  treatment of, 534–535

Neomycin
  cholesterol lowering effects of, 624
  for conjunctivitis, 29
Neosporin, allergic reaction to, 30, 31
Nephritis, interstitial, chronic renal failure with, 252–253
Nephrolithiasis. *See* Renal stones
Nephrolithotomy, percutaneous, 264
Nephropathy
  acute uric acid, 436
  diabetic, 406–407
  gouty, 436
Nephrosclerosis, hypertensive, chronic renal failure with, 252
Nephrotic syndrome
  with NSAIDs, 301
  proteinuria with, 272
Nervous system, problems of, 457–499
Neuralgia, postherpetic, 562
Neural tube defects, with valproic acid, 480
Neurodermatitis, of external ear, 51
Neuroglycopenia, 410
Neuroleptic-antidepressant combinations, 511
Neuropathy, diabetic, 407
Neurosyphilis, 538
Neurotransmitters
  and chronic pain, 683
  and parkinsonism, 490
  in premenstrual syndrome, 363
Nicardipine, for hypertension, 121–122
Nicotine replacement therapy
  gum, 642–643
  transdermal patch, 642–643
Nicotine stomatitis, 699
Nicotinic acid, for cholesterol reduction, 623
Nifedipine
  for angina pectoris, 11
  for dysmenorrhea, 362
  for headache, 465
  for hypertension, 121–122
Nipple, discharge from, 372
Nitrates
  for achalasia, 189
  for afterload reduction, 138
  for angina pectoris, 130–131
  for congestive heart failure, 136
  for diffuse esophageal spasm, 189
Nitroglycerin, sublingual, 131
Nizatidine, for peptic ulcer disease, 203
Nocturia, with benign prostatic hyperplasia, 250
Nocturnal asthma, 93
Nocturnal leg cramps, 337–339
Nocturnal myoclonus, insomnia with, 514
Noise-induced hearing loss, 47
Nonarticular musculoskeletal pain, 335–337
Non-group A beta-hemolytic streptococcal infections, 72–73
Non-insulin-dependent diabetes mellitus (NIDDM), 391, 392, 401–402
  blood glucose monitoring in, 405
  diet for, 402–403
  hypoglycemic drugs for, 403–405
  management of, 402–405

Non-monoamine oxidase inhibitor antidepressants, 508–510
Nonsteroidal anti-inflammatory drugs (NSAIDs), 296
　antihypertensive drug impairment with, 301
　causing esophagitis, 196
　drug interactions of, 302
　for dysmenorrhea, 361–362
　edema with, 600–601
　gastrointestinal side effects of, 300–301
　for gout, 305
　for headache, 464
　　prophylactic, 465–468
　hepatic toxicity with, 301
　in HIV-infected patient, 554
　for infectious mononucleosis, 56
　minimizing risks of, 303
　for neck pain, 314
　for osteoarthritis, 286
　properties of, 297–299t
　renal side effects of, 301
　for rheumatoid arthritis, 288–289
　for shoulder pain, 319
　side effects of, 300–302
Nontoxic nodular goiter, 430
Normocytic reticulocytopenic anemia, 447
Nortriptyline
　for depression, 508, 509t
　in elderly, 498
　for neck pain, 314
Nutcracker esophagus, 189
Nystagmus
　dizziness with, 1
　evaluation for, 1
Nystatin vaginal tablets, 342
　for candida esophagitis, 195
　for candidal vaginitis, 342

Obesity
　and coronary heart disease risk, 617
　definitions of, 9
　degree of, 10
　diets for
　　popular, 13–14
　　very low-calorie, 12
　evaluation for, 10
　failure of treatment for, 9
　health consequences of, 9–10
　history of, 10
　incidence of, 8
　management of severe, 12–13
　motivation for treatment of, 10
　secondary causes of, 10
　treatment of, 11
　　behavior modification and social support in, 12
　　drug, 11
　　exercise, 11
　　medication and devices for, 13
　　for severe case of, 12–13
　　surgical, 12–13
Occult gastrointestinal bleeding, 231
　follow-up of positive tests for, 232
　screening for, 231

Occupational asthma, 94
Occupational disease, and disability, 637–640
Occupational history, 638
　fatigue and, 6
Occupational Safety and Health Administration (OSHA), resources and information of, 639
Occupational therapy, for rheumatoid arthritis, 294
Ocular foreign bodies, 21–23
Odynophagia, 192
Omega-3 fatty acids, 708
Omeprazole (Prilosec)
　for gastroesophageal reflux disease, 194
　for peptic strictures, 190
　for peptic ulcer disease, 204
Open-angle glaucoma, 37
　diagnosis of, 37–38
　screening for, 39
　treatment of, 38–39
Ophthalmopathy, infiltrative, 421
Opiates, for acute diarrhea, 216
Optic disk
　changes in with glaucoma, 38
　glaucomatous cupping of, 37
Oral contraceptives, 349–351
　cancer risk with, 349
　combination pills, 349
　commonly used, 352–355t
　contraindications for, 349–350
　for dysmenorrhea, 361–362
　management of side effects of, 350
　postcoital, 351
　for premenstrual syndrome, 364
　progestogen-only pills, 351
　risk of vascular problems with, 349
　routine follow-up care with, 350–351
　selection of type of, 350
　for hypoglycemia diagnosis, 410
　usefulness of, 411
Oral ulcers, 696–698
Orgasmic function, impairment of in female, 380
Orthopedic examination, athletic, 604
Orthophosphate, for renal stones, 262
Orthostatic proteinuria, 271–272
Orthostatic sodium retention, 660
Osgood-Schlatter disease, 327
　treatment of, 331
Osteoarthritis, 283
　biomechanical factors in, 285
　clinical presentation of, 283
　diagnostic evaluation of, 283–285
　treatment of, 285–286, 330
Osteoarthrosis. *See* Osteoarthritis
Osteogenesis imperfecta, mitral valve prolapse and, 162
Osteomalacia, risk for, 308
Osteophyte formation, 283
Osteoporosis, 307
　causes of, 308
　diagnosis of, 308–309
　with estrogen deficiency, 374–375
　in patients on corticosteroids, 311
　prevention of, 309–311
　treatment for, 309, 375

Otitis externa, 50–53
  malignant, 52
  vertigo with, 2
Otitis media, 53
  clinical features of, 51*t*
  complications of, 55
  diagnosis of, 54
    differential, 50
  hearing loss with, 46
  infectious agents of, 53
  serous, 55–56
  treatment of, 54–55
  vertigo with, 2
Otosclerosis, deafness with, 46
Otoscopy, pneumatic, 45
Overflow incontinence, 275
  treatment of, 276–277
Overuse injuries, 629
Oxicams, 298*t*
Oxybutynin (Ditropan), for detrusor instability, 276
Oxygen therapy
  for COPD, 101
  for cor pulmonale, 102
Oxymetazoline (Afrin), 82*t*
  for nasal symptoms of cold, 60–61
  for rhinitis, 82
Oxypentifylline, for venous ulcers, 175

Pacemakers
  antitachycardia, 146
  capture function in, 155
  complications with, 156
  endocarditis risk with, 169
  failure of, 156
  frequency of use of, 155
  oversensing of, 156
  patient monitoring with, 156–157
  rate responsiveness function in, 155
Paget's disease
  causing hypercalcemia, 432
  evaluation for, 433
Pain
  with anal fissures, 227
  biliary, 234
    treatment of, 238
  breast, 371
  chronic idiopathic, 682–686
    clinical assessment of, 684–685
    clinical presentation of, 683–684
    definition of, 682–683
    facts and misconceptions about, 683
    treatment suggestions for, 685–686
  chronic musculoskeletal, 336–337
  coital, 380
  description of, 683
  ear, 50–51
  knee, 326–331
  low back, 320–325
  lumbosacral spine, 285
  myofascial, 319
  neck, 312–315
  nonarticular musculoskeletal, 335–337
  in peptic ulcer disease, 201
  after removal of corneal foreign body, 23
  with rheumatoid arthritis, 293
  shoulder, 315–320
  with sinusitis, 66
  vision loss with, 43
Pain-prone personality, 520
Palatal myoclonus, tinnitus with, 49
Pancreatic disease, diabetes with, 393
Pancreatic insufficiency, calorie loss with, 16
Pancreaticocholangiography, endoscopic retrograde, 235
Pancreatitis, gallstone, 234, 238
Panic attacks, syncope with, 654
Panic disorder, 501
Papillary necrosis, 301
Papillary thyroid carcinoma, 427
Pap smear, 358
Papular urticaria, 588
Paranasal sinuses, inflammation of, 66–69
Parasites
  intestinal, 567–571
  laboratory diagnosis of, 567–568
Parathyroid hormone (PTH) assay, 433
Paregoric, 216
Parenteral gold therapy, 289
Parkinsonism, 488
  causes of, 488
  drug holidays with, 492
  drugs used for, 490–492
  evaluation of, 489
  manifestations of, 488–489
  treatment of, 490–492
Paromomycin, for amebiasis, 569
Paroxysmal hemicrania, chronic, 468
Paroxysmal positional vertigo
  causes of, 3
  classic findings in, 1–2
  diagnosis of, 3
Paroxysmal supraventricular tachycardia (PSVT), 142–143
  clinical signs of, 143
  diagnosis of, 143–144
  diagnostic cardiac pacing studies of, 146
  ECG of, 143
  electrophysiologic basis for, 143
  prevention of, 145–146
  treatment of, 144–145
Partial seizures, 469
  complex, 470
  drug therapy for, 477
Partial thromboplastin time, activated (aPTT), 450, 451–452
Passive smoking, 641
Patellar dislocation
  acute, 329
  recurrent, 330
Patient education
  on birth control, 599–600
  for dietary fat consumption, 597
  on exercise, 597–599
  for injury prevention, 597
  for smoking cessation, 597
  on STDs, 600
Paul-Bunnell-Davidsohn assay, for EBV infectious mononucleosis, 72
Peak expiratory flow rate (PEFR), in asthma, 88

Pelvic inflammatory disease (PID), 365
　bacteriology of, 366
　causing abnormal uterine bleeding, 358
　clinical findings in, 366–367
　dysmenorrhea with, 361
　evaluation for, 366–367
　with IUDs, 351–356
　prevention of, 369
　risk factors for, 365–366
　sequelae of, 368–369
　treatment of, 359, 367–368
Pemphigus vulgaris, 698
Penicillamine, for rheumatoid arthritis, 289–292
Penicillin, for pelvic inflammatory disease, 368
Penicillinase-producing *Neisseria gonorrhoeae* (PPNG), 533–535
　in travelers, 635
Penile blood pressure, 387
Penile erections
　failure of, 384–388
　physiology of, 384
Penile prostheses, 387–388
Pentamidine, for *Pneumocystis carinii* pneumonia, 553–554
Pentoxifylline (Trental)
　for chronic arterial insufficiency, 180
　for venous ulcers, 175
Peptic strictures, reflux esophagitis with, 189–190
Peptic ulcer disease, 200
　aggressive factors in, 200
　clinical presentation of, 201
　complications of, 202–203
　evaluation of, 201–202
　Helicobacter pylori in, 204–205
　intractability of, 203
　medical therapy for, 203–204
　pathogenesis of, 200–201
　protective factors for, 201
　psychovisceral component of, 204
　risk factors for, 201
　surgery for, 205
Pepto-Bismol, for acute diarrhea, 216
Percutaneous nephrolithotomy, 264
Percutaneous transluminal coronary angioplasty (PTCA), 131–132
Perennial rhinitis, 79
Pergolide mesylate (Permax), for parkinsonism, 492
Periocular foreign bodies, 21
Peripheral vascular disease, 173–186
Peripheral vasodilators, 180
Peritonitis, 365
Peritonsillar abscess, 73–74
Peritonsillitis, 73–74
Periurethral infections, with indwelling catheters, 281
Personality disorder, 502
Peyronie's disease, 385
Pharyngitis
　associated with ulcers, 74
　bacterial causes of, 73
　gonococcal, 533

　group A streptococcal, 70–72
　　antigen testing for, 71
　with infectious mononucleosis, 564
Phenazopyridine (Pyridium), for dysuria, 244
Phenothiazines
　edema with, 600–601
　and erectile dysfunction, 384–385
　premature ventricular contractions with, 147
Phenoxybenzamine, for overflow incontinence, 277
Phentermine, for obesity, 13
Phenylacetic acid, 298*t*
Phenylpropanolamine, for obesity, 13
Phenytoin (Dilantin)
　for nocturnal leg cramps, 338
　for seizures, 475*t*, 476, 477, 478
　side effects of, 477
Pheochromocytomas, diabetes with, 393
Phlebotomy, 102
Phosphate, for renal stones, 262
Phosphorus depletion, causing hypercalcemia, 433
Physical activity, post-myocardial infarction, 139–140
Physical therapy
　for low back pain, 323
　for neck pain, 314
　for rheumatoid arthritis, 293
　for shoulder pain, 318
Pigment gallstones, risk factors for, 233
Pilocarpine, for glaucoma, 39
Pinworm, laboratory diagnosis of, 568
Plague vaccination, 631
Plasma cell dyscrasia syndrome (POEMS), 454
Plasma volume, decreased, 454
Plasmodium species
　chloroquine-resistant *falciparum* (CRPF), 633–634
　and malaria, 633–634
Platelet active agents, 131
Platelet counts, 451
Platelets
　disorders of and abnormal bleeding, 450–451
　drugs affecting, 450*t*
　inhibitors of to prevent deep venous thrombosis, 185
Plica syndrome, 330
Plummer-Vinson web, 190
Pneumococcal vaccine, 599*t*, 600, 611–612
　in COPD, 98
　for travelers, 630
Pneumococcus infections
　causing otitis media, 53
　corneal infection with, 28
　of lower respiratory tract, 103
Pneumocystis carinii pneumonia
　with AIDS, 550
　in HIV-infected patient, 555–556
　prophylaxis for, 553–554
Pneumonia
　differentiation of from acute bronchitis, 103
　with influenza, 63

Polio vaccine, 610
  in travelers, 630
Polyarteritis nodosa, vertigo with cranial nerve involvement in, 2
Polycystic kidney disease, 253
Polycythemia, 453–456
Polycythemia vera
  pathophysiology of, 454
  treatment of, 455
Polymorphonuclear leukocytes, in urethritis diagnosis, 544
Polyunsaturated fat, 707–708
Popliteal cysts, 331
Positional vertigo
  benign, 3
  paroxysmal, 1–2, 3
Positron emission tomography (PET), for dementia in elderly, 498
Postcholecystectomy syndrome, 239
Postcoital contraceptive pills, 351
Postherpetic neuralgia, prevention of, 562
Postmenopausal bleeding, 359
Postprandial hypoglycemia, 411
  diagnosis of, 411
  versus fasting hypoglycemia, 410
  symptoms of, 411
Posttraumatic headache, 459
Postural hypotension, 654–655
Potassium chloride, causing esophagitis, 196
Potassium citrate, for renal stones, 262
Potassium hydroxide (KOH) preparation, in vaginitis diagnosis, 341
Potassium replacement, for congestive heart failure, 136
PPD skin test, in HIV-infected patient, 532
Prazosin
  in BPH, 251
  for hypertension, 122
  for overflow incontinence, 277
Prednisone, for rheumatoid arthritis, 293
Preemployment examination, 637
Pre-esophageal dysphagia, 187
Pregnancy
  anticonvulsants during, 480
  complications of causing abnormal bleeding, 358
  complications of causing menorrhagia in adolescents, 357
  drugs in, 688–693
  ectopic, 369
  management of HSV infection during, 542
  medications in, 688–693
  rhinitis of, 84
  rubella during, 609
  tetanus-diphtheria toxoid in, 608
Preload reduction, drugs for, 135–136
Premature ventricular contractions (PVCs), 147
  diagnosis of, 147–148
  drug-induced, 147
  with mitral valve prolapse, 163
  prevalence of, 147
  and sudden cardiac death, 147
  treatment of, 148–150
Premenstrual syndrome (PMS), 362–364

Presbycusis, 47
Presbyopia, testing for, 41
Preventive care, 593
  agenda for, 598–599t, 601
  counseling and patient education in, 597–600
  immunizations in, 600
  implementation of policy for, 601
  prophylactic interventions in, 601
  screening programs in, 593–597
Primidone (Mysoline), for seizures, 478
Probenecid, for gout, 306
Problem drinkers, 527
Problem patients, 519
  evaluation of, 519–520
  recognition of, 519
  specific disorders of, 520–521
  treatment of, 521–522
Probucol, cholesterol lowering effects of, 624
Procainamide, premature ventricular contractions and, 147, 149
Proctitis
  with gonococcal infection, 533
  sexually transmitted, 546
Proctosigmoidoscopy, 230
Progesterone, premenstrual syndrome and, 363–364
Progestins
  in osteoporosis prevention, 310
  recommended starting doses for in menopause, 377t
Progestogen-only contraceptive pills, 351
Prokinetic agents, for gastroesophageal reflux disease, 194
Propafenone
  for premature ventricular contractions, 149
  to prevent atrial fibrillation, 154
Propantheline bromide (Pro-Banthine)
  for diverticulosis, 211
  for irritable bowel syndrome, 208
Propionic acids, 297t
Propranolol
  for hypertension, 120
  for paroxysmal supraventricular tachycardia, 145
  for premature ventricular contractions, 150
Propylthiouracil (PTU), for hyperthyroidism, 419–420
Prostacyclin, for chronic arterial insufficiency, 180
Prostaglandin inhibitors
  for dysmenorrhea, 361–362
  side effects of, 361
Prostaglandins, in dysmenorrhea, 360
Prostate
  benign hyperplasia of, 249–251
  cancer of, 650–652
    prostate-specific antigen for detection of, 651
    screening for, 595, 650–652
  needle biopsy of, 652
  painful diseases of, 245–246
    treatment of, 246–248
  transurethral resection of, 251

Prostate-specific antigen (PSA), for detection of prostate cancer, 651
Prostatectomy, 251
Prostatitis
　acute, 245
　　treatment of, 246–247
　chronic
　　bacterial and nonbacterial, 245
　　treatment of, 247
　　pathogenesis of, 246
Prostatodynia, 246
　treatment of, 247–248
Prosthetic valves, 168
　endocarditis with, 166–168
　hemolysis with, 167
　longevity and breakdown of, 167
　patient monitoring with, 167
　thromboembolism with, 166
Proteinuria, 270–273
　angiotensin-converting enzyme inhibitors for, 272–273
　constant, 272
　detection of, 270
　diagnostic evaluation of, 270–271
　functional, 271
　with hematuria, 267
　isolated nonnephrotic, 271–272
　and nephrotic syndrome, 272
　orthostatic, 271–272
　pathophysiology of, 270
Prothrombin time, partial activated (aPTT), 451–452
Prothrombin time (PT), 451, 452
Pruritus ani, 228–229
Pseudodiverticulosis, esophageal, 189
Pseudoephedrine
　for nasal symptoms of cold, 61
　for rhinitis, 82, 82t
Pseudomonas infection, spreading, with otitis externa, 52
Pseudoseizures, 471
Psoriasis, of external ear, 51
Psychiatric disorders, 501–530
Psychogenic rheumatism, 337
Psychological counseling
　for chronic pain, 686
　for erectile failure, 388
Psychophysiologic insomnia, 513
Psychophysiologic reaction, 520
Psychotherapy
　for anxiety, 505
　for depression, 511
Psychotic decompensation, acute, 502
Psyllium seed preparations, cholesterol lowering effects of, 624
Pulmonary disease, edema with, 659
Pulmonary embolus, 656
Pulmonary nodules, solitary, 107–108
Pulmonary rehabilitation, 99
Pulmonary stenosis, peripheral, 160
Pulmonary tuberculosis, therapy for, 575–576
Pulmonic stenosis, infundibular, midsystolic murmur with, 159–160
Pulsatile tinnitus, 48–49

Puncture wounds, 675
Purine restriction, for renal stone disease, 262
Purpura simplex, 451
Pyelonephritis
　with indwelling catheters, 281
　treatment of in women, 244
Pyrantel pamoate
　for enterobiasis, 570
　for hookworm, 570
Pyrazoles, 299t
Pyrimethamine, for malaria, 634
Pyuria, with hematuria, 267

Q fever, 676
Quadriceps
　atrophy of, 327
　strengthening of, 330
Quazepam (Doral), for insomnia, 517
Quetelet index. *See* Body mass index (BMI)
Quinacrine, for giardiasis, 569
Quinamm, for nocturnal leg cramps, 338
Quinidine
　causing esophagitis, 196
　for intractable hiccups, 682
　for premature ventricular contractions, 149
　premature ventricular contractions with, 147
　to prevent atrial fibrillation, 154
Quinidine-like drugs
　for paroxysmal supraventricular tachycardia prevention, 145–146
　for premature ventricular contractions, 149
Quinine, for nocturnal leg cramps, 338
Quinolines, for pelvic inflammatory disease, 368
Quinolones, for cystitis, 244
Quinsy sore throat, 73–74

Rabies
　prophylaxis for, 679–680
　vaccination for, 613, 631
Radiation fibrosis, dysphagia with, 190
Radiation-induced esophageal injury, 196
Radioactive iodine therapy, 420
Radioallergosorbent tests (RASTs), 88
Radioisotope studies
　for angina pectoris, 129
　for polycythemia, 455
Range-of-motion exercises, 293
Ranitidine (Zantac), for gastroesophageal reflux disease, 193–194
Rapid plasma reagin (RPR), in HIV-infected patient, 552
Rectal bleeding, with hemorrhoids, 225–226
Rectal examination, digital. *See* Digital rectal examination
Red blood cells (RBCs)
　dysmorphic, 267
　in urine, 265–266
Red eye, 26–28. *See also* Conjunctivitis
Reflux esophagitis, 189–190
Refractive errors, 41–43
Refractory asthma, 88

Index 741

Rehabilitation
  after myocardial infarction, 139–142
  for osteoarthritis, 286
  with osteoporosis, 309
Relaxation techniques
  for anxiety, 505
  for chronic pain, 686
  for COPD, 98–99
  for headache, 464
Renal artery stenosis, 115
Renal biopsy, for hematuria, 268–269
Renal colic, acute, 262–264
  evaluation for, 262–263
  treatment of, 263
  urological intervention for, 264
Renal failure
  acute, 253–254
  anemia with, 447
  chronic, 252–256
  hypertension with, 115
  with NSAIDs, 301
  renal size in, 253
Renal stones, 258
  and acute renal colic, 262–263
  clinical manifestations of, 259
  evaluation for, 259–261
  follow-up of, 264
  with gout, 436
  increased solubility of constituents of, 262
  "metabolically active," 259
  pathogenesis of, 258–259
  predisposing factors in, 259–260
  reduced excretion of constituents of, 261–262
  treatment modalities for, 261–262
  treatment principles for, 261
  urologic approaches to, 264
Renal transplantation, 407
Reproductive system problems, 341–388
Reserpine, for hypertension, 122
Rest, for rheumatoid arthritis, 293
Restless legs syndrome, 514
Reticulocyte count, 443–444
Reticulocyte index, calculation of, 443
Reticulocytopenic anemia
  microcytic, 444–446
  normocytic, 447
Reticulocytosis
  anemia with, 447–448
  with iron therapy, 446
Retinal detachment, 43
Retinopathy
  diabetic, 406
  screening for, 595
Rewarming technique, in patients with hypothermia, 668–669, 670
Reye's syndrome, with influenza, 63
Rhabdomyolysis, 672
Rheumatic fever, prevention of, 70
Rheumatic mitral stenosis, 151
Rheumatism, psychogenic, 337
Rheumatoid arthritis, 287
  course of, 287
  disability with, 294–295
  drug therapy for, 287–293

  first-line drugs for, 288–289
  occupational therapy for, 294
  second-line drugs for, 289–292
  supportive care for, 293–295
  surgery for, 295
  third-line drugs for, 292–293
Rheumatoid vasculitis, 293
Rhinitis, 79
  allergic, 79–83
  differentiation of from sinusitis, 66–67
  medicamentosa, 84
  miscellaneous causes of, 84–85
  and nasal polyps, 85
  vasomotor, 83–84
Rifampin, for tuberculosis, 576–577
Rinne test, 45
RNA virus, 579
Roaring tinnitus, 48
Rocky Mountain spotted fever, 676
Romberg test, 1
Rotator cuff, 316
Rotator cuff syndrome, evaluation for, 317–318
Rubber band ligation, 227
Rubella
  immunization for in travelers, 630
  vaccination for, 600, 609

Salicylates, 299t, 302
  clinical pharmacology of, 302
  drug interactions of, 303
  for low back pain, 323
  for rheumatoid arthritis, 288, 290–291t
  for shoulder pain, 319
  side effects of, 302–303
Salivary gland tumors, 700
Salt restriction. *See* Sodium restriction diets
Saprophytic infections, of external ear, 50
Sarcoidosis
  associated with hypercalcemia, 432
  evaluation for, 433
Saturated fat, reduction of, 707
Saturated solution of potassium iodide (SSKI), 105
Sciatica, 321
Sclerotherapy, 176
Screening, 593
  for breast cancer, 646–649
  for cancer, 594–595
  for cardiovascular disease, 593–594
  for diabetes, 391
  for glaucoma, 39, 595
  hearing, 595–596
  for high blood cholesterol, 619–625
  for HIV infection, 596–597
  for prostate cancer, 650–652
  thyroid, 596
  for tuberculosis, 596
  for visual acuity, 595
Seasonal rhinitis, 79
Seborrhea
  of external ear, 51
  in HIV-infected patient, 558
Sedative-hypnotic drugs, for insomnia, 516t, 517

Sedatives
  avoidance of in COPD, 98
  for irritable bowel syndrome, 208
Sedentary life-style, and coronary heart disease risk, 617
Seizures
  activity limitations with, 479
  avoiding precipitants of, 479
  classification of, 469
  diagnostic evaluation for, 472–473
  discontinuing anticonvulsant medication with, 479–480
  distinguishing of from other conditions, 471
  drug therapy for, 474–478
  establishing diagnosis of, 469–471
  evaluation of, 469–473
  follow-up for, 473
  in HIV-infected patient, 557
  recurrent, 479
  versus syncope, 654t
  treatment of, 474–480
Selegilene (Eldepryl), for parkinsonism, 490
Senile purpura, 451
Senna (Senokot), side effects of, 223–224
Sensorineural hearing loss, 46
Sensory neuropathy, 407
Serologic tests
  for group A streptococcal pharyngitis, 71
  for hepatitis B, 581, 582t
  for syphilis in HIV-infected patient, 532
Serotonin-enhancing tertiary amines, 686
Serous otitis, 55
  treatment of, 55–56
Serum alpha-1-antitrypsin, 97–98
Sex therapists, 382–383
Sexual activity
  and chronic prostatitis, 247
  guilt about, 381–382
  after myocardial infarction, 140
  and risk of PID, 365
Sexual dysfunction
  drug-related, 381
  female, 380–383
  male, 384–388
Sexually Transmitted Disease Treatment Guidelines (1989), 538
Sexually transmitted diseases (STDs), 533.
  See also specific diseases
  common clinical syndromes of, 543–548
  common pathogens in, 533–543
  counseling for prevention of, 600
  prevention of transmission of, 547–548
  in travelers, 635
Shigella infections, sexually transmitted, 546–547
Shingles. *See* Herpes zoster
Shoulder joint
  anatomy of, 316
  physical examination of, 317
  structures of, 316f
Shoulder pain, 315–316
  evaluation for, 316–317
    with specific conditions, 317–318
  treatment of, 318–319
    with specific conditions, 319–320

Sigmoidoscopy
  for diarrhea, 219
  for occult GI bleeding, 231, 232
Single-positron emission computed tomography (SPECT), for dementia in elderly, 498
Sinuses, Water's view of, 67f
Sinusitis, 66
  causes of, 68
  diagnosis of, 66–68
  laboratory tests for, 68
  referral for, 69
  signs and symptoms of, 66–68
  transillumination for, 68
  treatment of, 68–69
Skin
  breakdown of around condom catheter, 282
  care of with chronic arterial insufficiency, 179
  hyperthyroidism effects on, 417
  hypothyroidism effects on, 422
  problems of
    with chronic venous insufficiency, 173–174
    in HIV-infected patient, 558
  ulceration of with chronic venous insufficiency, 174
Skinfold thickness measurement, 18
Skin-testing, for reactions to bee sting, 591–592
Sleep
  patterns of in insomnia, 515
  phenomena related to, 515
Sleep hygiene measures, 515–516
Sleep-wake schedule disorders, 514
Smoking
  and cardiovascular disease, 593
  cessation of, 640–641
    assessing obstacles to, 642
    counseling about, 597, 641–645
    financial savings from, 642
    follow-up for, 643–644, 645
    manuals and group programs for, 645
    motivation for, 642
    nationally available aids to, 644–645t
    role of physician in, 641
    setting date for, 643
  chronic arterial insufficiency and, 179
  and coronary heart disease risk, 616
  declining prevalence of, 640
  hoarseness with, 76
  myocardial infarction, risk of and, 141
  osteoporosis and, 308
  passive, 641
  and polycythemia, 454
Snellen chart testing, 41, 595
Social Security disability system, 639–640
Social services, for dementia in elderly, 499
Sodium balance, management of in chronic renal failure, 255
Sodium fluoride, for osteoporosis treatment, 310
Sodium restriction diets, 701–703
  for congestive heart failure, 135
  for hypertension, 116

Sodium retention
  with NSAIDs, 301
  orthostatic, 660
Soft tissue, minor injuries and infections of, 674–680
Solitary pulmonary nodule (SPN), 107
  causes of, 107
  diagnostic strategy for, 108
  diagnostic tests for, 107–108
Somatic delusion, 521
Somogyi phenomenon, 399
Sore throat, 70
  causes of, 70–74
  nonspecific presentations of, 72–73
  recurrent, 74–75
  severe syndromes of, 73–74
  symptomatic therapy for, 74
Spectinomycin
  for gonococcal infections, 535
  for PID, 368
Speech discrimination scores, 47
Speech reception threshold (SRT), 47
Sphenoid sinusitis, persistent, 69
Spider bites, 676
Spine
  osteoarthritis of, 283–284
    treatment of, 285
  stenosis of, 321
Spirometry, 97
Spironolactone, for premenstrual syndrome, 364
Sports
  disqualifying conditions for, 605
  physical examination for, 603–605
  recommendations for participation in, 606–607t
Sputum cultures, for acute lower respiratory tract infection, 105
Squamous cell carcinoma
  oral, 699
    single ulcers with, 697
    white lesions with, 698
Stage fright, 505
Stanozolol, for lipodermatosclerosis, 174
Staphylococcal folliculitis, 50
Staphylococcal infections, in HIV-infected patient, 558
Staphylococcus aureus
  causing hordeolum, 31
  corneal infection with, 28
Staphylococcus saprophyticus, in urinary tract infections in women, 241
Starr-Edwards prostheses, risk of embolization with, 166
Steroids. *See* Corticosteroids
Still's murmur, 158
Straight leg raising test, 321
Streptococcal infections, non-group A beta-hemolytic, 72–73
Streptococcal pharyngitis, group A
  antigen tests for, 71
  benefits of diagnosing and treating, 70
  clinical diagnosis of, 70–71
  laboratory diagnosis of, 71
  recommended clinical strategy for, 71–72
  treatment of, 72

Stress, steroid coverage for, 441
Stress incontinence, 275
Stress management
  for anxiety, 505
  for premenstrual syndrome, 364
Stretching exercises, for nocturnal leg cramps, 339
Stroke
  risk of with atrial fibrillation, 154
  risk of with mitral valve prolapse, 163
  risk of with TIAs, 481
Strongyloides infection, laboratory diagnosis of, 567–568
Strongyloidiasis, 570
  diagnosis of, 571
  therapy for, 571
Struvite stones, pathogenesis of, 259
Stye. *See* Hordeolum
Subconjunctival hemorrhage, 28
Sucralfate (Carafate), for peptic ulcer disease, 204
Suction lipectomy, 13
Sudden cardiac death
  exercise-related, 627
  with mitral valve prolapse, 164
  and premature ventricular contractions, 147
Suicide assessment, 508
Sulfacetamide (Sulamyd, Bleph-10), for blepharitis, 31
Sulfasalazine (Azulfidine), for rheumatoid arthritis, 292
Sulfinpyrazone, for gout, 306
Sulfisoxazole
  for chlamydial infections, 536
  for cystitis, 244
Sulfonylureas
  hypoglycemia with, 411
  for type II diabetes, 403, 405
Sulindac, 298t
  renal insufficiency with, 301
Superficial venous thrombosis (SVT), 182, 185
Supraglottitis, hoarseness with, 76
Supraventricular tachycardia, paroxysmal, 142–146
Surgery
  for benign prostatic hyperplasia, 251
  cataract, 34–36
  for chronic arterial insufficiency, 180–181
  for diverticulitis, 212
  for erectile failure, 388
  for gastroesophageal reflux disease, 194
  for hemorrhoids, 227
  for hyperthyroidism, 420
  for low back pain, 325
  for neck pain, 314
  for obesity, 12–13
  for osteoarthritis, 286
  for overflow incontinence, 276
  for parkinsonism, 492
  for peptic ulcer disease, 205
  prophylactic endarterectomy in patients undergoing, 486
  for prostatitis, 247
  for rheumatoid arthritis, 295

Surgery—*Continued*
  for transient ischemic attacks (TIAs) 484–485
  for varicose veins, 176
  for venous ulcers, 175
Swimmer's ear, vertigo with, 2
Sympatholytics
  and erectile dysfunction, 384
  for hypertension, 117t
Sympathomimetic decongestants, 81t
  for allergic rhinitis, 82–83
  topical
    overuse of, 84
    for sinusitis, 69
  for urticaria, 589
Sympathomimetic nasal drops, overuse of, 84
Syncope, 653
  approach to diagnosis of, 656
  causes of, 653–656
  differential diagnosis of, 471
  frequency of, 653
  versus seizures, 654t
Syphilis, 537
  clinical presentation of, 537
  diagnosis of, 537–538
  HIV and, 532, 538
  sexual contacts with, 538
  treatment of, 539t
  and follow-up, 538
Systolic blood pressure, 113
Systolic hypertension, isolated, 113
Systolic Hypertension in the Elderly (SHEP) study, 113, 616
Systolic murmurs, 158
  early, 158, 160
  innocent, 158
  later, 158, 160
  midsystolic in middle and old age, 158–159
  pansystolic, 160
  pathologic midsystolic, 159–160

Tachycardias, paroxysmal supraventricular, 142–146
Tamm-Horsfall protein, in urine, 270
Tamoxifen, for breast pain, 371
Temazepam (Restoril), for insomnia, 516t, 517
Temporomandibular joint (TMJ)
  headache with dysfunction of, 457
  tinnitus with arthritis of, 49
Tendinitis
  common syndromes of, 332–334
  definition of, 332
  evaluation for, 318
  knee, 330
  shoulder, 317
  treatment of, 320, 330
Tendon injury, common sites of, 332t
Tennis elbow, 333
Tenosynovitis, 332
Tension headache, 457
  abortive treatment of, 465
  prophylactic treatment for, 465–468
  symptomatic treatment for, 464
Tensor tympani spasm, 49

Terazosin, for hypertension, 122
Terfenadine (Seldane)
  for allergic rhinitis, 81t
  for asthma, 89
Terpin hydrate
  for COPD, 101
  for coughs, 61
Testosterone, for erectile failure, 387
Tetanus
  guidelines for booster immunization for in wounds, 677t
  prophylaxis for with wounds, 676
  toxoid, 608
  vaccination for, 600
    in travelers, 630
Tetracycline
  for chlamydial infections, 536
  derivatives of causing esophagitis, 196
  for diverticulitis, 211
  for PID, 368
Tetrahydroaminoacridine, for dementia in elderly, 498
Thalassemia, 448
Thalassemia major, abnormal uterine bleeding with, 357
Thallium scintigraphy, for angina pectoris, 129
Theophylline
  for asthma, 92
  for COPD, 100
Thermoregulatory mechanisms, impaired, 667–668, 672
Thiabendazole, for strongyloidiasis, 571
Thiazide diuretics
  causing hypercalcemia, 432–433
  for congestive heart failure, 136
  for hypertension, 118–119
  metabolic side effects of, 119
  for osteoporosis prevention, 311
  for renal stone disease, 261
Thioridazine (Mellaril), edema with, 601
Thiothixene (Navane), edema with, 601
Thoracic aortic aneurysms, 190
Thoracotomy
  for achalasia, 189
  for solitary pulmonary nodule diagnosis, 108
Throat cultures, for group A streptococcal pharyngitis, 71
Thromboangiitis obliterans, 181
Thrombocytopathy, Glanzmann's, 450
Thrombocytopenia, 450–451
Thrombocytopenic purpura, idiopathic (ITP), 449, 450
  abnormal uterine bleeding with, 357
Thromboembolism, with prosthetic valves, 166
Thrombolysis, enzymatic, 484
Thromboneurosis, 183–184
Thrombophlebitis
  diagnosis of, 182–183
  incidence of, 182
  management strategy for, 183–184
  predisposing conditions in, 185
  prevention of, 185

superficial, 185
treatment of, 184
and warfarin drug interactions, 185t
Thromboplastin time, activated partial (aPTT), 450, 451–452
Thrush, 74
Thyroid adenoma, 419
autonomously functioning, 427
treatment of, 421
Thyroidal hypothyroidism, 424
Thyroid-binding proteins, 413
Thyroid carcinoma, 425
medullary, 427
family history of, 426
risk factors for, 426
types of, 427
Thyroid function
abnormalities of in nonthyroidal illness, 415
evaluation of, 412–415
tests of, 412–414
drug effects on, 415
for weight loss, 17
Thyroid gland, 412–431
Thyroid hormone
for depression, 511
drugs to ameliorate effects of, 420
for obesity, 13
preparations of, 424–425
serum levels of in hyperthyroidism, 418
in treatment of hypothyroidism, 424–425
Thyroiditis
chronic autoimmune, 428–429
painless, 419
subacute, 419
thyroid enlargement in, 417
treatment of, 421
Thyroid nodules, 425
clinical findings of, 426
diagnostic strategies for, 426–427
diagnostic studies of, 426
hypofunctioning benign, 427
solitary, 425
specific types of, 427
Thyroid radioisotope scanning, 414, 426
Thyroid-stimulating hormone (TSH), serum levels of, 412
deficiency of, 424
elevated, 422–423
in hyperthyroidism, 418
measuring of, 413–414
Thyrotoxicosis
causing hypercalcemia symptoms, 433
evaluation for, 434
Thyrotropin. See Thyroid-stimulating hormone (TSH), serum levels of
Thyrotropin-releasing hormone (TRH), deficiency of, 424
Thyroxine (T_4)
for hypothyroidism, 424
serum free, 412–413
serum levels of, 412–413
low, 423
Thyroxine-binding prealbumin (TBPA), 413
Tick paralysis, 676

Ticks, 676
Timolol, for glaucoma, 38–39
Tinnitus, 48–49
Tocainide, for premature ventricular contractions, 149
Todd's paralysis, 471
Tonic-clonic seizures
drug therapy for, 476
generalized, 469, 470
Tonometry, 595
Topical medications, allergic reactions to, 30
Torulopsis glabrata, 341
Torus mandibularis, 699
Torus palatinus, 699
Total joint replacement, for osteoarthritis, 286
"Touch-me-not" syndrome, 337
Toxic substances, exposure to, 638
Traction
for low back pain, 323
for neck pain, 314
Transcutaneous electrical nerve stimulation (TENS), for chronic pain, 686
Transdermal patch, in nicotine replacement therapy, 642–643
Transient global amnesia, 471
Transient ischemic attacks (TIAs), 481
diagnosis of, 482–483
differentiation of, 471
evaluation in, 482–483
modification of risk factors for, 483
pathogenesis of, 482
prognosis for, 481
treatment of, 483–485
Transient motor paralysis, with herpes zoster, 561–562
Transillumination, of paranasal sinuses, 68
Transluminal balloon angioplasty, 180–181
Transmural infarctions, atrial fibrillation with, 151
Transrectal ultrasound, for detecting prostate cancer, 651–652
Transthoracic echocardiography, 482
Transurethral resection of prostate (TURP), 251
Transverse myelitis, 63
Trauma
corneal, 26
death due to in travelers, 635
mouth ulcers with, 696
neck pain with, 312
oral lesions with, 700
"unmentionable," and anxiety, 502
Trauma neurosis, 315
Traveler's diarrhea, 632–633
Travelers
disease in, 632–636
medical advice for, 630–636
medical kit for, 636
routine immunizations for, 630
vaccinations for, 631–632
Tremor, of parkinsonism, 489
Trench foot, 669
Trench mouth, 74
Treponema pallidum, 537–538

Treponema pallidum hemagglutination assay (TPHA-TP), 538
Triamcinolone cream, for eczematous dermatitis, 174
Triamcinolone hexacetonide (Aristospan), for rheumatoid arthritis, 293
Triazolam (Halcion), for insomnia, 516t, 517
Trichomonas vaginitis
  diagnosis of, 343
  prevalence of, 342
  symptoms of, 342
  treatment of, 343
Trichuriasis, 570
Tricuspid regurgitation, pansystolic murmur with, 160
Tricyclic antidepressants
  for chronic pain, 686
  for depression, 510
  premature ventricular contractions with, 147
Trifluoperazine (Stelazine), edema with, 601
Triglycerides serum levels, 621–622
  fasting, 621
  reduced, 708
Trihexyphenidyl (Artane), for parkinsonism, 491
Triiodothyronine, measuring serum concentrations of, 414
Trimethadione, during pregnancy, 480
Trimethoprim-sulfamethoxazole
  for cryptosporidiosis and isosporiasis, 571
  for cystitis, 243
  for epididymitis, 248
  for otitis media, 55
  for *Pneumocystis carinii* pneumonia, 553, 554
  for prostatitis, 246, 247
  for sinusitis, 68
Trophoblastic tumors, 419
Tropical illnesses, 634–635
TSH-secreting pituitary tumors, 419
TSH serum concentration
  in diagnosis of hyperthyroidism, 418
  in diagnosis of hypothyroidism, 423
Tuberculosis, 572
  incidence of, 572
  isoniazide preventive therapy for, 574–575
  screening for, 572–573
    and prophylaxis, 596
  standard therapy for, 575–578
  tuberculin skin test for, 573–574
Tuberculous adenitis, 665
Tuberculous salpingitis, 366
Tumors, hoarseness with, 76
Tuning fork test, 45
Tympanic membrane, examination of, 54
Tympanometry, 46, 84
  for fluttering tinnitus, 49
  for hearing loss evaluation, 47
  in otitis media diagnosis, 54
Tympanostomy tubes, 57
Type A behavior, and coronary heart disease risk, 617
Typhoid vaccination, 631
Tzanck smear
  for herpes zoster diagnosis, 561
  for HSV diagnosis, 541

Ulcers
  aphthous, 697
  genital, 540t, 545–546, 666
  ischemic, 179
  mouth, 696–698
  NSAID-associated, 300
  peptic, 200–206
  pharyngitis associated with, 74
Ultrasonography. *See also* Echocardiography
  abdominal, 234–235
  for breast lumps, 371
  for detecting gallstones, 234–235
  for detecting prostate cancer, 651–652
  for hematuria, 268
  for peripheral vascular disease, 178
  for PID, 367
  for thrombophlebitis diagnosis, 183
  for thyroid nodules, 426
  for TIAs, 482–483
Unna boots, 175
Upper respiratory infections (URIs), 59–64
  differentiation of from sinusitis, 66–67
  viral etiologies of, 59
Upper respiratory problems, 59–85
Urate, serum levels of, 435
Urate-lowering drugs, 306
Ureaplasma infections, 366
Urease-producing bacteria, with indwelling catheters, 281
Ureteroscopy, 264
Urethral sphincter insufficiency, 275
  treatment of, 277
Urethral trauma, with intermittent catheterization, 279
Urethritis, 533
  complications of, 545
  differential diagnosis of, 544
  with sexually transmitted disease, 543–545
  treatment and follow-up for, 544–545
Uric acid crystals, 304
Uric acid nephrolithiasis, 436
Uric acid nephropathy, acute, 436
Uric acid stones, 258–259
Uricosuric therapy, 306–307
Urinalysis
  in chronic renal failure, 253
  for hematuria, 267
  for hypertension workup, 116
  for renal stone evaluation, 262–263
  for urinary tract infections in men, 136
  for urinary tract infections in women, 242
Urinary catheterization
  external, 281–282
  indwelling, 280–281
  intermittent, 279
    complications of, 279
  problems with, 278–279
Urinary continence, neuroanatomy and physiology of, 274
Urinary excretion
  protein, 24-hour, in chronic renal failure, 253
  reduction of renal stone constituents in, 261–262
  of various solutes, 260t

Index 747

Urinary incontinence
  in elderly, 274–277
  evaluation for, 275–276
  pathophysiology of, 274–275
  treatment of, 276–277
  types of, 275
Urinary tract infections
  in men, 245
    epididymitis in, 248
    painful prostate disease in, 245–248
  recurrent, 241
  in women, 241
    evaluation of, 241–242
    laboratory tests for, 242–243
    management of, 243–244
    prevention of recurrences of, 244
Urinary tract problems, 241–282
Urine
  cultures of for urinary tract infections in women, 242–243
  cytology of for hematuria, 268
  red blood cells in, 265–266
Urine sediment, in chronic renal failure, 253
Urogenital atrophy, with menopause, 374
Urologic disorders, and erectile dysfunction, 385
Urosepsis, with indwelling catheters, 281
Ursodeoxycholic acid, 236–237
Urticaria, 587
  causes of, 587, 588t
  diagnostic approach to, 587–588
  treatment of, 589
Uterus
  abnormal bleeding of, 357–359
    in adolescents, 357–358
    in perimenopausal and postmenopausal women, 359
    in reproductive-aged women, 358–359
  estrogen effect on bleeding of, 376

Vaccinations. *See* Immunizations
Vaccine
  hypersensitivity to components of, 632
Vacuum constriction devices, for erectile failure, 388
Vagal maneuvers, for paroxysmal supraventricular tachycardia, 144
Vaginismus, 380
Vaginitis, 341
  abnormal bleeding with, 359
  atrophic, 344–345
  bacterial, 344
  candidal, 341–342
  incidence of, 241
  infectious, 345
  sexually transmitted, 546
  symptoms of, 341
  trichomonas, 342–343
Vaginosis, bacterial, 344
Valgus deformity, 327
Valproic acid (Depakene, Depakote)
  for absence seizures, 478
  for partial seizures, 477
  during pregnancy, 480
  for seizures, 475t, 478
Valves, prosthetic, 166–167

Valvular collagen abnormalities
  conditions associated with, 162
  with mitral valve prolapse, 162
Vapocoolant sprays, 337
Varicella zoster virus, 560
Varicose veins, 175
  clinical presentation of, 175
  diagnosis of, 175–176
  treatment of, 176
Varus deformity, 327
Vascular insufficiency, peripheral, 173–186
  and erectile dysfunction, 385
Vascular headache
  associated with menses, 462
  prophylactic treatment for, 465–468
Vasoconstrictors, for hay fever conjunctivitis, 30
Vasodilators
  for afterload reduction, 137, 138
  for chronic arterial insufficiency, 180
  and erectile dysfunction, 384
  for hypertension, 117t
  for TIAs, 484
Vasomotor rhinitis, 83
  symptoms of, 83–84
  treatment of, 84
Vasovagal syncope, 653–654
VDRL test, in HIV-infected patient, 552
  for syphilis, 537–538
Venereal warts, 547
Venography, 182–183
Venous digital subtraction angiography, 178
Venous disorders, chronic, 173–176
Venous thrombosis, 182–185
  superficial, 182, 185
Venous ulcers, 175
Ventricular response, control of, 154
Ventricular tachycardia, 147–148
  ECG of, 148
Ventriculoatrial shunts, endocarditis risk with, 169
Ventriculography, radionuclide
  for angina pectoris, 129
  for congestive heart failure, 135
Verapamil
  for angina pectoris, 131
  for atrial fibrillation, 153
  for hypertension, 121–122
  for nocturnal leg cramps, 338
  for paroxysmal supraventricular tachycardia, 144, 145
  for premature ventricular contractions, 149–150
Verapamil-like drugs, for premature ventricular contractions, 149–150
Vernal keratoconjunctivitis, 30
Vertebrobasilar ischemia, 2
Vertigo, 1–4
Vestibular neuritis, with vertigo, 3
Vestibular problems, 1–4
Vinblastine sulfate (Velban), for warts in HIV-infected patients, 558
Vincent's angina, 74
Very-low-density lipoprotein (VLDL)
  decreased production of, 623
  overproduction of, 708

Vinegar douches, 343, 345
Viral conjunctivitis, 29
Viral hepatitis. *See* Hepatitis, viral
Vision. *See* Visual impairment
Vision testing, 41
Visual disturbances, in HIV-infected patient, 557
Visual field testing, for glaucoma, 39
Visual impairment, 41–44
  causes of, 41
  measurement of, 41–42
  screening of, 595
  special problems of, 42–44
Vitamin A intoxication, causing hypercalcemia, 433
Vitamin B_{12} deficiency, 446
  treatment of, 447
Vitamin C, for cold prevention, 61
Vitamin D
  causing hypercalcemia, 432, 433
  deficiency of, 308
  for osteoporosis prevention, 310
  thiazide, 311
  tissue insensitivity to, 308
Vitamin E
  for breast pain, 371
  for nocturnal leg cramps, 338, 339
Vitamin K, in hepatitis management, 582
Vocal cord nodules, 77–78
Voiding reflexes, deconditioned, 275
Von Willebrand disease, 449–450
  abnormal uterine bleeding with, 357
Von Willebrand factor, 452
  activity of, 449
Vulvovaginal candidiasis, 546

Warfarin
  for atrial fibrillation, 154
  drug interactions of, 185*t*
  for thrombophlebitis, 184
  for patients with mechanical valves, 166
Wart-like oral lesions, 698
Warts
  in HIV-infected patient, 558
  venereal, 547
Weight
  ranges of for men and women, 9*t*
  relative (RW), 9
  tables for, age-specific, 9–10

Weight loss
  causes and mechanisms of, 15–16
  determining cause of, 16–17
  documentation of, 15
  in HIV-infected patient, 557–558
  laboratory studies for, 17
  in normal fluctuation, 15
  patient history of, 16–17
  physical examination for, 17
  psychological causes of, 16
  treatment for, 17–18
Westergren ESR, 367
Whiplash injury
  neck pain with, 312
  therapy for, 314–315
Wide-QRS complex tachycardia, 144
  treatment of, 148–149
Wolff-Parkinson-White (WPW) syndrome, 143
Women
  cholesterol level recommendations for, 622
  iron deficiency in, 445
  sexual dysfunction in, 380–383
  urinary tract infections in, 241–244
Worker's Compensation, 639
Work-related injury or illness, 637
  evaluation for, 637–638
  resources for information on, 639
Wounds
  tetanus booster immunization in, 677*t*
  tetanus prophylaxis for, 676
Wry neck, 312
Wyanoid HC, for hemorrhoids, 227

Xanthine oxidase inhibitors, for gout, 306–307
Xerosis, 558
Xylometazoline (Otrivin), 81*t*
  for allergic rhinitis, 83
  for nasal symptoms of cold, 60–61

Yeast infections, recurrent vaginal, 342. *See also* Vaginitis
Yellow fever vaccination, 631

Zidovudine (AZT)
  in HIV-infected patient, 552–553
  for HIV prophylaxis, 596
Zollinger-Ellison syndrome, refractory esophagitis with, 192

The Little, Brown Spiral® Manual Series,
The Little, Brown Handbook Series,
The Little, Brown Practical Approach Series
AVAILABLE AT YOUR BOOKSTORE

- **MANUAL OF ACUTE BACTERIAL INFECTIONS,** 2nd Edition – Gardner & Provine (#303895)
- **MANUAL OF ACUTE ORTHOPAEDIC THERAPEUTICS,** 4th Edition – Iversen & Swiotkowski (#434396)
- **MANUAL OF ACUTE RESPIRATORY CARE** – Zagelbaum & Pare (#984671)
- **MANUAL OF ALLERGY AND IMMUNOLOGY,** 3rd Edition – Lawlor, Fischer, & Adelman (#516813)
- **MANUAL OF ANESTHESIA,** 2nd Edition – Snow (#802220)
- **MANUAL OF CLINICAL EVALUATION** – Aronson & Delbanco (#052108)
- **MANUAL OF CLINICAL ONCOLOGY,** 2nd Edition – Casciato & Lowitz (#130672)
- **MANUAL OF CARDIAC ARRHYTHMIAS** – Vlay (#904767)
- **MANUAL OF CARDIOVASCULAR DIAGNOSIS AND THERAPY,** 3rd Edition – Alpert & Rippe (#035203)
- **MANUAL OF CLINICAL HEMATOLOGY,** 2nd Edition – Mazza (#552208)
- **MANUAL OF DERMATOLOGIC THERAPEUTICS,** 5th Edition – Arndt (#051756)
- **MANUAL OF ELECTROCARDIOGRAPHY,** 2nd Edition – Mudge (#589187)
- **MANUAL OF EMERGENCY AND OUTPATIENT TECHNIQUES** – Washington University Department of Surgery: Klippel & Anderson (#498688)
- **MANUAL OF EMERGENCY MEDICINE,** 2nd Edition – Jenkins & Loscalzo (#460559)
- **MANUAL OF ENDOCRINOLOGY AND METABOLISM,** 2nd Edition – Lavin (#516570)
- **MANUAL OF GASTROENTEROLOGY,** 2nd Edition – Eastwood & Avunduk (#199923)
- **MANUAL OF GYNECOLOGIC ONCOLOGY AND GYNECOLOGY** – Piver (#709360)
- **MANUAL OF INTENSIVE CARE MEDICINE,** 2nd Edition – Rippe (#747122)
- **INTRODUCTION TO CLINICAL MEDICINE: A STUDENT-TO-STUDENT MANUAL,** 3rd Edition – Macklis, Mendelsohn, & Mudge (#542431)
- **MANUAL OF MEDICAL CARE OF THE SURGICAL PATIENT,** 4th Edition – Coussons, McKee, & Williams (#774936)
- **MANUAL OF MEDICAL THERAPEUTICS,** 27th Edition – Washington University Department of Medicine: Woodley & Whelan (#924202)
- **MANUAL OF NEONATAL CARE,** 3rd Edition – Cloherty & Stark (#147621)
- **MANUAL OF NEPHROLOGY,** 3rd Edition – Schrier (#774863)
- **MANUAL OF NEUROLOGIC THERAPEUTICS,** 5th Edition – Samuels (#770043)
- **MANUAL OF NUTRITIONAL THERAPEUTICS,** 2nd Edition – Alpers, Clouse, & Stenson (#035122)
- **MANUAL OF OBSTETRICS,** 4th Edition – Niswander (#611735)
- **MANUAL OF OCULAR DIAGNOSIS AND THERAPY,** 3rd Edition – Pavan-Langston (#695475)
- **MANUAL OF OTOLARYNGOLOGY,** 2nd Edition – Strome, Fried, & Kelley (#819689)
- **MANUAL OF OUTPATIENT GYNECOLOGY,** 2nd Edition – Havens, Sullivan, & Tilton (#350982)
- **MANUAL OF PEDIATRIC THERAPEUTICS,** 5th Edition – The Children's Hospital Department of Medicine, Boston: Graef (#138754)
- **MANUAL OF PSYCHIATRIC EMERGENCIES,** 3rd Edition – Hyman & Tesar (#387282)
- **MANUAL OF PSYCHIATRIC THERAPEUTICS,** 2nd Edition – Shader (#782238)
- **MANUAL OF RHEUMATOLOGY AND OUTPATIENT ORTHOPEDIC DISORDERS,** 3rd Edition – Paget, Pellicci, & Beary (#688460)
- **MANUAL OF SURGICAL INFECTIONS** – Gorbach, Bartlett, & Nichols (#320706)
- **MANUAL OF SURGICAL THERAPEUTICS,** 8th Edition – Condon & Nyhus (#153672)
- **MANUAL OF UROLOGY** – Siroky & Krane (#792969)
- **PROBLEM-ORIENTED MEDICAL DIAGNOSIS,** 5th Edition – Friedman (#293873)
- **PROBLEM-ORIENTED PEDIATRIC DIAGNOSIS** – Barkin (#081027)
- **MANUAL OF CLINICAL PROBLEMS IN ADULT AMBULATORY CARE,** 2nd Edition – Dornbrand, Hoole, & Pickard (#190195)
- **MANUAL OF CLINICAL PROBLEMS IN CARDIOLOGY,** 4th Edition – Hillis, Lange, Wells, & Winniford (#364053)
- **MANUAL OF CLINICAL PROBLEMS IN DERMATOLOGY** – Olbricht, Bigby, & Arndt (#094250)
- **MANUAL OF DIAGNOSTIC IMAGING,** 2nd Edition – Straub (#818593)
- **MANUAL OF CLINICAL PROBLEMS IN GASTROENTEROLOGY,** 2nd Edition – Van Ness & Chobanian (#897264)
- **MANUAL OF CLINICAL PROBLEMS IN INFECTIOUS DISEASE,** 3rd Edition – Gantz, Gleckman, Brown, Esposito, & Berk (#303496)
- **MANUAL OF CLINICAL PROBLEMS IN INTERNAL MEDICINE,** 4th Edition – Spivak & Barnes (#807389)
- **MANUAL OF CLINICAL PROBLEMS IN NEPHROLOGY** – Rose & Black (#756377)
- **MANUAL OF CLINICAL PROBLEMS IN NEUROLOGY,** 2nd Edition – Mohr (#577480)
- **MANUAL OF CLINICAL PROBLEMS IN OBSTETRICS AND GYNECOLOGY,** 4th Edition – Rivlin & Martin (#747777)
- **MANUAL OF CLINICAL PROBLEMS IN ONCOLOGY,** 2nd Edition – Portlock & Goffinet (#714259)
- **MANUAL OF CLINICAL PROBLEMS IN OPHTHALMOLOGY** – Gittinger & Asdourian (#314714)
- **MANUAL OF CLINICAL PROBLEMS IN PEDIATRICS,** 4th Edition – Roberts (#750069)
- **MANUAL OF CLINICAL PROBLEMS IN PSYCHIATRY** – Hyman (#387223)
- **MANUAL OF CLINICAL PROBLEMS IN PULMONARY MEDICINE,** 3rd Edition – Bordow & Moser (#102725)
- **MANUAL OF CLINICAL PROBLEMS IN SURGERY** – Cutler, Dodson, Silva, & Vander Salm (#165751)
- **MANUAL OF CLINICAL PROBLEMS IN UROLOGY** – Resnick (#740543)

THE LITTLE, BROWN HANDBOOK SERIES

- CLINICAL ANESTHESIA PROCEDURES OF THE MASSACHUSETTS GENERAL HOSPITAL, 4th Edition – Davison, Eckhardt, & Perese (#177148)
- HANDBOOK OF ANTIBIOTICS, 2nd Edition – Reese & Betts (#737194)
- HANDBOOK OF CANCER CHEMOTHERAPY, 3rd Edition – Skeel (#795747)
- THE PRACTICE OF CARDIAC ANESTHESIA – Hensley & Martin (#357774)
- HANDBOOK OF CARDIAC DRUGS, 2nd Edition – Purdy, Boucek, & Boucek (#722464)
- HANDBOOK OF CARDIOVASCULAR AND INTERVENTIONAL RADIOLOGIC PROCEDURES – Kandarpa (#482552)
- HANDBOOK OF CLINICAL PHARMACOLOGY, 2nd Edition – Bochner, Carruthers, Kampmann, & Steiner (#100641)
- HANDBOOK OF COLPOSCOPY – Hatch (#350281)
- HANDBOOK OF CONTRACEPTION AND ABORTION – Burkman (#091677)
- HANDBOOK OF CORONARY CARE, 5th Edition – Alpert & Francis (#035262)
- HANDBOOK OF DIALYSIS, 2nd Edition – Daugirdas & Ing (#173835)
- HANDBOOK OF DRUG THERAPY IN RHEUMATIC DISEASE – Hardin & Longenecker (#346047)
- HANDBOOK OF DRUG THERAPY IN REPRODUCTIVE ENDOCRINOLOGY AND INFERTILITY – Rivlin (#747726)
- HANDBOOK OF DRUG THERAPY IN LIVER AND KIDNEY DISEASE – Schrier & Gambertoglio (#774855)
- HANDBOOK OF GASTROINTESTINAL DRUGS – Van Ness & Gurney (#897248)
- HANDBOOK OF HEMODYNAMIC MONITORING – Gore, Alpert, Benotti, Kotilainen, & Haffajee (#320854)
- HANDBOOK OF HEMOSTASIS AND THROMBOSIS – Ansell (#043311)
- HANDBOOK OF MEDICAL TOXICOLOGY – Viccellio (#902470)
- HANDBOOK OF OCULAR DRUG THERAPY AND OCULAR SIDE EFFECTS OF SYSTEMIC DRUGS – Pavan-Langston (#695459)
- HANDBOOK OF PATIENT CARE IN CARDIAC SURGERY, 5th Edition – Vlahakes, Lemmer, Behrendt, & Austen (#087793)
- HANDBOOK OF PEDIATRIC EMERGENCIES, 2nd Edition – Baldwin (#079189)
- HANDBOOK OF PEDIATRIC INFECTIOUS DISEASE – Edelson & Noel (#210749)
- HANDBOOK OF PEDIATRIC NEUROLOGY AND NEUROSURGERY – Gaskill & Marlin (#546399)
- HANDBOOK OF PEDIATRIC ONCOLOGY – Gottlieb (#321699)
- HANDBOOK OF PERINATAL INFECTIONS, 2nd Edition – Sever, Larsen, & Grossman (#781711)
- HANDBOOK OF PHARMACOLOGIC THERAPEUTICS – Bogner (#100889)
- HANDBOOK FOR PRESCRIBING MEDICATIONS DURING PREGNANCY, 2nd Edition – Berkowitz, Coustan, & Mochizuki (#091995)
- HANDBOOK OF PRESCRIBING MEDICATIONS FOR GERIATRIC PATIENTS – Ahronheim (#020427)
- HANDBOOK OF PSYCHIATRIC DRUG THERAPY, 2nd Edition – Arana & Hyman (#049387)
- HANDBOOK OF PULMONARY DRUG THERAPY – Spagnolo, Witorsch, & Nicklas (#804746)
- HANDBOOK OF REFRACTION, 4th Edition – Garcia (#798398)
- HANDBOOK OF VASCULAR SURGERY, 3rd Edition – Hallett, Brewster, & Darling (#340537)
- INTERPRETATION OF DIAGNOSTIC TESTS, 5th Edtion – Wallach (#920509)
- THE M.D. ANDERSON SURGICAL ONCOLOGY HANDBOOK – M.D. Anderson Cancer Center, Department of Surgery: Berger, Fuhrman, & Feig (#564311)
- NOMENCLATURE AND CRITERIA FOR DIAGNOSIS OF DISEASES OF THE HEART AND GREAT VESSELS, 9th Edition – The Criteria Committee of the New York Heart Association (#605387)
- POSTOPERATIVE CRITICAL CARE OF THE MASSACHUSETTS GENERAL HOSPITAL, 2nd Edition – Hoffman & Wasnick (#368385)
- THE JOHNS HOPKINS HANDBOOK OF IN VITRO FERTILIZATION AND ASSISTED REPRODUCTIVE TECHNOLOGIES – Damewood (#171948)

THE LITTLE, BROWN PRACTICAL APPROACH SERIES

- A PRACTICAL APPROACH TO BREAST DISEASE – O'Grady, Howell, Lindfors, & Rippon (#633771)
- A PRACTICAL APPROACH TO EMERGENCY MEDICINE, 2nd Edition – Stine & Chudnofsky (#816272)
- A PRACTICAL APPROACH TO INFECTIOUS DISEASES, 3rd Edition – Reese & Betts (#737178)
- A PRACTICAL APPROACH TO OCCUPATIONAL AND ENVIRONMENTAL MEDICINE, 2nd Edition – McCunney (#555347)

Visit your local bookstore or call **1 (800) 343-9204** for these and other Little, Brown Medical Publications.

For further information write to Little, Brown and Company, Medical Division, 200 West Street, Waltham, MA 02154

> "... probably the most comprehensive single medical textbook written on HIV disease."
> — from a review of the first edition in Annals of Internal Medicine

THE AIDS KNOWLEDGE BASE:
A Textbook on HIV Disease from the University of California, San Francisco and the San Francisco General Hospital, Second Edition

Edited by **P. T. Cohen, M.D., Ph.D., Merle A. Sande, M.D.,** and **Paul A. Volberding, M.D.**

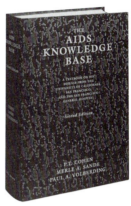

Published by the Massachusetts Medical Society in its first edition, the latest edition of this encyclopedic compendium is thoroughly revised and updated to give you:

- **Clinically tested and up-to-date strategies you can use to evaluate, manage, and treat HIV disease and associated problems**
- **A comprehensive guide to the current literature through extensive selected references**
- **A full, authoritative discussion of the ethical, legal, social, political, and fiscal implications of AIDS**

Authoritative...
This monumental work brings together 85 outstanding contributing authors who draw on more than a decade of unparalleled experience in treating HIV-related diseases at the University of California, San Francisco and the San Francisco General Hospital.

Complete...
From basic information to specific therapies, **THE AIDS KNOWLEDGE BASE, Second Edition,** is unsurpassed in its broad, current coverage of HIV disease. Extensive, current references at the end of each chapter point the way to detailed literature for deeper study of specific topics. **More than 200 charts, tables, and photos (including color) complete the text.**

THE AIDS KNOWLEDGE BASE, Second Edition, is an invaluable tool in combating HIV disease.

Scheduled for publication in Summer1994. Paperback, approx. 1,200 pages, illustrated, #770671, $125.00(T)

Available at your local medical bookstore or by calling toll-free 1(800)527-0145 (Mon. - Fri., 8:30-5:30 Eastern time) Call today for a Free 30–Day Trial!

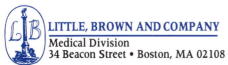

LITTLE, BROWN AND COMPANY
Medical Division
34 Beacon Street • Boston, MA 02108

All material copyright © 1994, Little, Brown and Company, Boston.
Prices subject to change without notice. (T) indicates tentative price.

Keep These Authoritative Guides by Your Side

Interpretation of Diagnostic Tests:
A Synopsis of Laboratory Medicine, Fifth Edition

By **Jacques Wallach, M.D.**

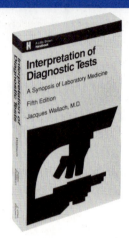

This popular handbook contains the most current information available on adult and pediatric laboratory tests. The book is conveniently divided into four sections, making it the ideal reference for on-the-spot consultation whenever you select or interpret laboratory tests.

The first section presents normal adult and pediatric values for common tests in both discussion and table formats. The second section covers specific lab exams with respect to the diseases or conditions in which test results are increased, normal, or decreased. Section Three lists 500 diseases by organ system, with abnormal and normal test findings. The final section shows you how test results may vary when a patient is taking a drug. For speedy consultation and current facts, **Interpretation of Diagnostic Tests, Fifth Edition,** is an indispensable companion.

1992. 960 pages, paperback, #920509, $36.50

HIV Infection:
A Clinical Manual, Second Edition

Edited by **Howard Libman, M.D.**, and **Robert A. Witzburg, M.D.**

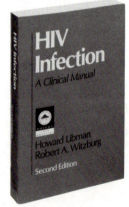

Written by internists for internists, this important manual is a practical guide to the full range of issues surrounding the diagnosis and treatment of the adult AIDS patient.

HIV Infection: A Clinical Manual offers a broad-based, multidisciplinary approach to the topic of HIV infected patients. Drs. Libman and Witzburg, in collaboration with 33 experts, present an overview of HIV infection, discuss epidemiology, explore clinical syndromes and clinical manifestations, and more. Numerous line drawings and photographs supplement the text, and useful tables and charts make information easily accessible.

1993. 576 pages, illustrated, paperback, #511625, $34.00

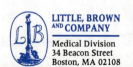

LITTLE, BROWN AND COMPANY
Medical Division
34 Beacon Street
Boston, MA 02108

Available at your local medical bookstore or by calling toll-free 1(800)527-0145 (Mon. - Fri., 8:30-5:30 Eastern time)